T0211682

Lecture Notes in Computer Science 11767

More information about this series at http://www.springer.com/series/7412

Dinggang Shen · Tianming Liu ·
Terry M. Peters · Lawrence H. Staib ·
Caroline Essert · Sean Zhou ·
Pew-Thian Yap · Ali Khan (Eds.)

Medical Image Computing and Computer Assisted Intervention – MICCAI 2019

22nd International Conference
Shenzhen, China, October 13–17, 2019
Proceedings, Part IV

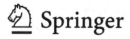 Springer

Editors
Dinggang Shen
University of North Carolina
at Chapel Hill
Chapel Hill, NC, USA

Terry M. Peters ⓘ
Western University
London, ON, Canada

Caroline Essert ⓘ
University of Strasbourg
Illkirch, France

Pew-Thian Yap
University of North Carolina
at Chapel Hill
Chapel Hill, NC, USA

Tianming Liu
University of Georgia
Athens, GA, USA

Lawrence H. Staib ⓘ
Yale University
New Haven, CT, USA

Sean Zhou
United Imaging Intelligence
Shanghai, China

Ali Khan
Western University
London, ON, Canada

ISSN 0302-9743   ISSN 1611-3349   (electronic)
Lecture Notes in Computer Science
ISBN 978-3-030-32250-2   ISBN 978-3-030-32251-9   (eBook)
https://doi.org/10.1007/978-3-030-32251-9

LNCS Sublibrary: SL6 – Image Processing, Computer Vision, Pattern Recognition, and Graphics

This Springer imprint is published by the registered company Springer Nature Switzerland AG
The registered company address is: Gewerbestrasse 11, 6330 Cham, Switzerland

Preface

We are pleased to present the proceedings for the 22nd International Conference on Medical Image Computing and Computer-Assisted Intervention (MICCAI), which was held at the InterContinental Hotel, Shenzhen, China, October 13–17, 2019. The conference also featured 34 workshops, 13 tutorials, and 22 challenges held on October 13 or 17. MICCAI 2019 had an approximately 63% increase in submissions and accepted papers compared with MICCAI 2018. These papers, which comprise six volumes of *Lecture Notes in Computer Science* (LNCS) proceedings, were selected after a thorough double-blind peer-review process. Following the example set by the previous program chairs of MICCAI 2018 and 2017, we employed Microsoft's Conference Managing Toolkit (CMT) for paper submissions and double-blind peer-reviews, and the Toronto Paper Matching System (TPMS) to assist with automatic paper assignment to area chairs and reviewers.

From 2625 original intentions to submit, 1809 full submissions were received and sent out to peer-review. Of these, 63% were considered as pure Medical Image Computing (MIC), 5% as pure Computer-Assisted Interventions (CAI), and 32% as both MIC and CAI. The MICCAI 2019 Program Committee (PC) comprised 69 area chairs, with 25 from the Americas, 21 from Europe, and 23 from Asia/Pacific/Middle East. Each area chair was assigned ~ 25 manuscripts, with up to 15 suggested potential reviewers using TPMS scoring and self-declared research areas. Subsequently, over 1200 invited reviewers were asked to bid for the papers for which they had been suggested. Final reviewer allocations via CMT took account of PC suggestions, reviewer bidding, and TPMS scores, finally allocating 5–6 papers per reviewer. Based on the double-blinded reviews, 306 papers (17%) were accepted immediately, and 920 papers (51%) were rejected, with the remainder being sent for rebuttal. These decisions were confirmed by the area chairs. During the rebuttal phase, two additional area chairs were assigned to each rebuttal paper using CMT and TPMS scores, who then independently scored them to accept or reject, based on the reviews, rebuttal, and manuscript, resulting in clear paper decisions using majority voting. This process resulted in the acceptance of further 234 papers for an overall acceptance rate of 30%. Regional PC teleconferences were held in late June to confirm the final results and collect PC feedback on the peer-review process.

For the MICCAI 2019 proceedings, 538 accepted papers have been organized in six volumes as follows:

Part I, LNCS Volume 11764: Optical Imaging; Endoscopy; Microscopy
Part II, LNCS Volume 11765: Image Segmentation; Image Registration; Cardiovascular Imaging; Growth, Development, Atrophy, and Progression
Part III, LNCS Volume 11766: Neuroimage Reconstruction and Synthesis; Neuroimage Segmentation; Diffusion-Weighted Magnetic Resonance Imaging; Functional Neuroimaging (fMRI); Miscellaneous Neuroimaging

Part IV, LNCS Volume 11767: Shape; Prediction; Detection and Localization; Machine Learning; Computer-Aided Diagnosis; Image Reconstruction and Synthesis
Part V, LNCS Volume 11768: Computer-Assisted Interventions; MIC Meets CAI
Part VI, LNCS Volume 11769: Computed Tomography; X-ray Imaging

We would like to thank everyone who contributed to the success of MICCAI 2019 and the quality of its proceedings, particularly the MICCAI Society for support, insightful comments, and providing funding for Kitty Wong to be the ongoing Conference System Manager. Given the increase in workload for this year's meeting, the Program Committee simply could not have functioned effectively without her, and she will provide ongoing oversight of the review process for future MICCAI conferences. Without the dedication and support of all of the organizers of the workshops, tutorials, and challenges, under the guidance of Kenji Suzuki, together with satellite event chairs Hongen Liao, Qian Wang, Luping Zhou, Hayit Greenspan, and Bram van Ginneken, none of these peripheral events would have been feasible.

Also, the Industry Forum (led by Xiaodong Tao and Yiqiang Zhan), the Industry Session (led by Sean Zhou), as well as the Doctoral Symposium (led by Junzhou Huang and Dajiang Zhu) brought new events to MICCAI 2019. The publication chairs, Li Wang and Gang Li, undertook the onerous task of assembling the camera-ready proceedings for publication by Springer.

Behind the scenes, MICCAI secretariat personnel, Janette Wallace and Johanne Langford, kept a close eye on logistics and budgets, while Doris Lam and her team from Momentous Asia, this year's Professional Conference Organization, along with the Local Organizing Committee chair, Dong Ni (together with Jing Qin, Qianjin Feng, Dong Liang, Xiaoying Tang), handled the website and local organization. The Student Travel Award Committee chaired by Huiguang He, Jun Shi, and Xi Jiang evaluated numerous applications, including awards for undergraduate students, which is new in the history of MICCAI. We also thank our sponsors for their financial support and presence on site. We are especially grateful to all members of the Program Committee for their diligent work in the reviewer assignments and final paper selection, as well as the reviewers for their support during the entire process. Finally, and most importantly, we thank all authors, co-authors, students/postdocs, and supervisors, for submitting and presenting their high-quality work that made MICCAI 2019 a greatly enjoyable, informative, and successful event. We are indebted to those reviewers and PC members who helped us resolve issues relating to last-minute missing reviews. Overall, we thank all of the authors and attendees for making MICCAI 2019 a spectacular success. We look forward to seeing you in Lima, Peru at MICCAI 2020!

October 2019

Dinggang Shen
Tianming Liu
Terry M. Peters
Lawrence H. Staib
Caroline Essert
Sean Zhou
Pew-Thian Yap
Ali Khan

Organization

General Chairs

Dinggang Shen   The University of North Carolina at Chapel Hill, USA
Tianming Liu   The University of Georgia, USA

Program Executive

Terry Peters   Robarts Research Institute, Western University, Canada
Lawrence H. Staib   Yale University, USA
Sean Zhou   United Imaging Intelligence (UII), China
Caroline Essert   University of Strasbourg, France
Pew-Thian Yap   The University of North Carolina at Chapel Hill, USA
Ali Khan   Robarts Research Institute, Western University, Canada

Submissions Manager

Kitty Wong   Robarts Research Institute, Western University, Canada

Workshops/Challenges/Tutorial Chairs

Kenji Suzuki   Illinois Institute of Technology, USA
Hayit Greenspan   Tel Aviv University, Israel
Bram van Ginneken   Radboud University Medical Center, The Netherlands
Qian Wang   Shanghai Jiao Tong University, China
Luping Zhou   The University of Sydney, Australia
Hongen Liao   Tsinghua University, China

MICCAI Society, Board of Directors

Leo Joskowicz (President)   The Hebrew University of Jerusalem, Israel
Stephen Aylward (Treasurer)   Kitware, Inc., NY, USA
Josien Pluim (Secretary)   Eindhoven University of Technology, The Netherlands
Wiro Niessen (Past President)   Erasmus Medical Centre, The Netherlands
Marleen de Bruijne   Erasmus Medical Centre, The Netherlands and University of Copenhagen, Denmark
Hervé Delinguette   Inria, Sophia Antipolis, France
Caroline Essert   University of Strasbourg, France
Alejandro Frangi   University of Leeds, UK
Lena Maier-Hein   German Cancer Research Center, Germany

Shuo Li	Western University, London, Canada
Tianming Liu	University of Georgia, USA
Anne Martel	University of Toronto, Canada
Daniel Racoceanu	Pontifical Catholic University of Peru, Peru
Julia Schnabel	King's College, London, UK
Guoyan Zheng	Institute for Surgical Technology & Biomechanics, Switzerland
Kevin Zhou	Chinese Academy of Sciences, China

Industry Forum

Xiaodong Tao	iFLYTEK Health, China
Yiqiang Zhan	United Imaging Intelligence (UII), China

Publication Committee

Gang Li	The University of North Carolina at Chapel Hill, USA
Li Wang	The University of North Carolina at Chapel Hill, USA

Finance Committee

Dong Ni	Shenzhen University, China
Janette Wallace	Robarts Research Institute, Western University, Canada
Stephen Aylward	Kitware, Inc., USA

Local Organization Chairs

Dong Ni	Shenzhen University, China
Jing Qin	The Hong Kong Polytechnic University, SAR China
Qianjin Feng	Southern Medical University, China
Dong Liang	Shenzhen Institutes of Advanced Technology, Chinese Academy of Sciences, China
Xiaoying Tang	Southern University of Science and Technology, China

Sponsors and Publicity Liaison

Kevin Zhou	Institute of Computing Technology, Chinese Academy of Sciences, China
Hongen Liao	Tsinghua University, China
Wenjian Qin	Shenzhen Institutes of Advanced Technology, Chinese Academy of Sciences, China

Keynote Lectures Chairs

Max Viergever   University Medical Center Utrecht, The Netherlands
Kensaku Mori   Nagoya University, Japan
Gözde Ünal   Istanbul Technical University, Turkey

Student Travel Award Committee

Huiguang He   Institute of Automation, Chinese Academy of Sciences,
                             China
Jun Shi   Shanghai University, China
Xi Jiang   University of Electronic Science and Technology
                             of China, China

Student Activities Liaison

Julia Schnabel   King's College London, UK
Caroline Essert   University of Strasbourg, France
Dimitris Metaxas   Rutgers University, USA
MICCAI Student Board Members

Area Chairs

Purang Abolmaesumi   The University of British Columbia, Canada
Shadi Albarqouni   The Technical University of Munich (TUM), Germany
Elsa Angelini   Imperial College London, UK
Suyash Awate   Indian Institute of Technology (IIT) Bombay, India
Ulas Bagci   University of Central Florida (UCF), USA
Kayhan Batmanghelich   University of Pittsburgh, USA
Christian Baumgartner   Swiss Federal Institute of Technology Zurich,
                             Switzerland
Ismail Ben Ayed   Ecole de Technologie Superieure (ETS), Canada
Weidong Cai   The University of Sydney, Australia
Xiaohuan Cao   United Imaging Intelligence (UII), China
Elvis Chen   Robarts Research Institute, Western University, Canada
Xinjian Chen   Soochow University, China
Jian Cheng   Beihang University, China
Jun Cheng   Cixi Institute of Biomedical Engineering, Chinese
                             Academy of Sciences, China
Veronika Cheplygina   Eindhoven University of Technology, The Netherlands
Elena De Momi   Politecnico di Milano, Italy
Ayman El-Baz   University of Louisville, USA
Aaron Fenster   Robarts Research Institute, Western University, USA
Moti Freiman   Philips Healthcare, The Netherlands
Yue Gao   Tsinghua University, China

Xiujuan Geng	Chinese University of Hong Kong, SAR China
Stamatia Giannarou	Imperial College London, UK
Orcun Goksel	Swiss Federal Institute of Technology Zurich, Switzerland
Xiao Han	AI Healthcare Center, Tencent Inc., China
Huiguang He	Institute of Automation, Chinese Academy of Sciences, China
Yi Hong	The University of Georgia, USA
Junzhou Huang	The University of Texas at Arlington, USA
Xiaolei Huang	The Pennsylvania State University, USA
Juan Eugenio Iglesias	University College London, UK
Pierre Jannin	The University of Rennes, France
Bernhard Kainz	Imperial College London, UK
Ali Kamen	Siemens Healthcare, USA
Jaeil Kim	Kyungpook National University, South Korea
Andrew King	King's College London, UK
Karim Lekadir	Universitat Pompeu Fabra, Spain
Cristian Linte	Rochester Institute of Technology, USA
Mingxia Liu	The University of North Carolina at Chapel Hill, USA
Klaus Maier-Hein	German Cancer Research Center, Germany
Anne Martel	Sunnybrook Research Institute, USA
Andrew Melbourne	University College London, UK
Anirban Mukhopadhyay	Technische Universität Darmstadt, Germany
Anqi Qiu	National University of Singapore, Singapore
Islem Rekik	Istanbul Technical University, Turkey
Hassan Rivaz	Concordia University, USA
Feng Shi	United Imaging Intelligence (UII), China
Amber Simpson	Memorial Sloan Kettering Cancer Center, USA
Marius Staring	Leiden University Medical Center, The Netherlands
Heung-Il Suk	Korea University, South Korea
Tanveer Syeda-Mahmood	University Medical Center Utrecht, The Netherlands
Xiaoying Tang	Southern University of Science and Technology, China
Pallavi Tiwari	Case Western Reserve University, USA
Emanuele Trucco	University of Dundee, UK
Martin Urschler	Graz University of Technology, Austria
Hien Van Nguyen	University of Houston, USA
Archana Venkataraman	Johns Hopkins University, USA
Christian Wachinger	Ludwig Maximilian University of Munich, Germany
Linwei Wang	Rochester Institute of Technology, USA
Yong Xia	Northwestern Polytechnical University, China
Yanwu Xu	Baidu Inc., China
Zhong Xue	United Imaging Intelligence (UII), China
Pingkun Yan	Rensselaer Polytechnic Institute, USA
Xin Yang	Huazhong University of Science and Technology, China
Yixuan Yuan	City University of Hong Kong, SAR China

Daoqiang Zhang	Nanjing University of Aeronautics and Astronautics, China
Miaomiao Zhang	Washington University in St. Louis, USA
Tuo Zhang	Northwestern Polytechnical University, China
Guoyan Zheng	Shanghai Jiao Tong University, China
S. Kevin Zhou	Institute of Computing Technology, Chinese Academy of Sciences, China
Dajiang Zhu	The University of Texas at Arlington, USA

Reviewers

Abdi, Amir
Abduljabbar, Khalid
Adeli, Ehsan
Aganj, Iman
Aggarwal, Priya
Agrawal, Praful
Ahmad, Ola
Ahmad, Sahar
Ahn, Euijoon
Akbar, Shazia
Akhondi-Asl, Alireza
Akram, Saad
Al-Kadi, Omar
Alansary, Amir
Alghamdi, Hanan
Ali, Sharib
Allan, Maximilian
Amiri, Mina
Anton, Esther
Anwar, Syed
Armin, Mohammad
Audigier, Chloe
Aviles-Rivero, Angelica
Awan, Ruqayya
Awate, Suyash
Aydogan, Dogu
Azizi, Shekoofeh
Bai, Junjie
Bai, Wenjia
Balbastre, Yaël
Balsiger, Fabian
Banerjee, Abhirup
Bano, Sophia

Barbu, Adrian
Bardosi, Zoltan
Bateson, Mathilde
Bathula, Deepti
Batmanghelich, Kayhan
Baumgartner, Christian
Baur, Christoph
Baxter, John
Bayramoglu, Neslihan
Becker, Benjamin
Behnami, Delaram
Beig, Niha
Belyaev, Mikhail
Benkarim, Oualid
Bentaieb, Aicha
Bernal, Jose
Beyeler, Michael
Bhatia, Parmeet
Bhole, Chetan
Bhushan, Chitresh
Bi, Lei
Bian, Cheng
Bilinski, Piotr
Bise, Ryoma
Bnouni, Nesrine
Bo, Wang
Bodenstedt, Sebastian
Bogunovic, Hrvoje
Bozorgtabar, Behzad
Bragman, Felix
Braman, Nathaniel
Bridge, Christopher
Broaddus, Coleman

Bron, Esther
Brooks, Rupert
Bruijne, Marleen
Bühler, Katja
Bui, Duc
Burlutskiy, Nikolay
Burwinkel, Hendrik
Bustin, Aurelien
Cabeen, Ryan
Cai, Hongmin
Cai, Jinzheng
Cai, Yunliang
Camino, Acner
Cao, Jiezhang
Cao, Qing
Cao, Tian
Carapella, Valentina
Cardenes, Ruben
Cardoso, M.
Carolus, Heike
Castro, Daniel
Cattin, Philippe
Chabanas, Matthieu
Chaddad, Ahmad
Chaitanya, Krishna
Chakraborty, Jayasree
Chakraborty, Rudrasis
Chang, Ken
Chang, Violeta
Charaborty, Tapabrata
Chatelain, Pierre
Chatterjee, Sudhanya
Chen, Alvin
Chen, Antong
Chen, Cameron
Chen, Chao
Chen, Chen
Chen, Elvis
Chen, Fang
Chen, Fei
Chen, Geng
Chen, Hanbo
Chen, Hao
Chen, Jia-Wei
Chen, Jialei
Chen, Jianxu

Chen, Jie
Chen, Jingyun
Chen, Lei
Chen, Liang
Chen, Min
Chen, Pingjun
Chen, Qingchao
Chen, Xiao
Chen, Xiaoran
Chen, Xin
Chen, Xuejin
Chen, Yang
Chen, Yuanyuan
Chen, Yuncong
Chen, Zhiqiang
Chen, Zhixiang
Cheng, Jun
Cheng, Li
Cheng, Yuan
Cheng, Yupeng
Cheriet, Farida
Chong, Minqi
Choo, Jaegul
Christiaens, Daan
Christodoulidis, Argyrios
Christodoulidis, Stergios
Chung, Ai
Çiçek, Özgün
Cid, Yashin
Clarkson, Matthew
Clough, James
Collins, Toby
Commowick, Olivier
Conze, Pierre-Henri
Cootes, Timothy
Correia, Teresa
Coulon, Olivier
Coupé, Pierrick
Courtecuisse, Hadrien
Craley, Jeffrey
Crimi, Alessandro
Cury, Claire
D'souza, Niharika
Dai, Hang
Dalca, Adrian
Das, Abhijit

Das, Dhritiman
Deeba, Farah
Dekhil, Omar
Demiray, Beatrice
Deniz, Cem
Depeursinge, Adrien
Desrosiers, Christian
Dewey, Blake
Dey, Raunak
Dhamala, Jwala
Ding, Meng
Distergoft, Alexander
Dobrenkii, Anton
Dolz, Jose
Dong, Liang
Dong, Mengjin
Dong, Nanqing
Dong, Xiao
Dong, Yanni
Dou, Qi
Du, Changde
Du, Lei
Du, Shaoyi
Duan, Dingna
Duan, Lixin
Dubost, Florian
Duchateau, Nicolas
Duncan, James
Duong, Luc
Dvornek, Nicha
Dzyubachyk, Oleh
Eaton-Rosen, Zach
Ebner, Michael
Ebrahimi, Mehran
Edwards, Philip
Egger, Bernhard
Eguizabal, Alma
Einarsson, Gudmundur
Ekin, Ahmet
Elazab, Ahmed
Elhabian, Shireen
Elmogy, Mohammed
Eltanboly, Ahmed
Erdt, Marius
Ernst, Floris
Esposito, Marco

Esteban, Oscar
Fan, Jingfan
Fan, Xin
Fan, Yong
Fan, Yonghui
Fang, Xi
Farag, Aly
Farzi, Mohsen
Fauser, Johannes
Fawaz, Hassan
Fedorov, Andrey
Fehri, Hamid
Feng, Chiyu
Feng, Jun
Feng, Xinyang
Feng, Yuan
Fenster, Aaron
Ferrante, Enzo
Feydy, Jean
Fischer, Lukas
Fischer, Peter
Fishbaugh, James
Fletcher, Tom
Flores, Kevin
Forestier, Germain
Forkert, Nils
Fotouhi, Javad
Fountoukidou, Tatiana
Franz, Alfred
Frau-Pascual, Aina
Freysinger, Wolfgang
Fripp, Jurgen
Fu, Huazhu
Funka-Lea, Gareth
Funke, Isabel
Funke, Jan
Fürnstahl, Philipp
Furukawa, Ryo
Gahm, Jin
Galassi, Francesca
Galdran, Adrian
Gan, Yu
Gao, Fei
Gao, Mingchen
Gao, Siyuan
Gao, Zhifan

Gardezi, Syed
Ge, Bao
Gerber, Samuel
Gerig, Guido
Gessert, Nils
Gevaert, Olivier
Gharabaghi, Sara
Ghesu, Florin
Ghimire, Sandesh
Gholipour, Ali
Ghosal, Sayan
Giraud, Rémi
Glocker, Ben
Goceri, Evgin
Goetz, Michael
Gomez, Alberto
Gong, Kuang
Gong, Mingming
Gonzalez, German
Gopal, Sharath
Gopinath, Karthik
Gordon, Shiri
Gori, Pietro
Gou, Shuiping
Granados, Alejandro
Grau, Vicente
Green, Michael
Gritsenko, Andrey
Grupp, Robert
Gu, Lin
Gu, Yun
Gu, Zaiwang
Gueziri, Houssem-Eddine
Guo, Hengtao
Guo, Jixiang
Guo, Xiaoqing
Guo, Yanrong
Guo, Yong
Gupta, Kratika
Gupta, Vikash
Gutman, Boris
Gyawali, Prashnna
Hacihaliloglu, Ilker
Hadjidemetriou, Stathis
Haldar, Justin
Hamarneh, Ghassan

Hamze, Noura
Han, Hu
Han, Jungong
Han, Xiaoguang
Han, Xu
Han, Zhi
Hancox, Jonny
Hanson, Erik
Hao, Xiaoke
Haq, Rabia
Harders, Matthias
Harrison, Adam
Haskins, Grant
Hatamizadeh, Ali
Hatt, Charles
Hauptmann, Andreas
Havaei, Mohammad
He, Tiancheng
He, Yufan
Heimann, Tobias
Heldmann, Stefan
Heller, Nicholas
Hernandez-Matas, Carlos
Hernandez, Monica
Hett, Kilian
Higger, Matt
Hinkle, Jacob
Ho, Tsung-Ying
Hoffmann, Nico
Holden, Matthew
Hong, Song
Hong, Sungmin
Hou, Benjamin
Hsu, Li-Ming
Hu, Dan
Hu, Kai
Hu, Xiaowei
Hu, Xintao
Hu, Yan
Hu, Yipeng
Huang, Heng
Huang, Huifang
Huang, Jiashuang
Huang, Kevin
Huang, Ruobing
Huang, Shih-Gu

Huang, Weilin
Huang, Xiaolei
Huang, Yawen
Huang, Yixing
Huang, Yufang
Huang, Zhongwei
Huaulmé, Arnaud
Huisman, Henkjan
Huo, Xing
Huo, Yuankai
Husch, Andreas
Hussein, Sarfaraz
Hutter, Jana
Hwang, Seong
Icke, Ilknur
Igwe, Kay
Ingalhalikar, Madhura
Irmakci, Ismail
Ivashchenko, Oleksandra
Izadyyazdanabadi, Mohammadhassan
Jafari, Mohammad
Jäger, Paul
Jamaludin, Amir
Janatka, Mirek
Jaouen, Vincent
Jarayathne, Uditha
Javadi, Golara
Javer, Avelino
Jensen, Todd
Ji, Zexuan
Jia, Haozhe
Jiang, Jue
Jiang, Steve
Jiang, Tingting
Jiang, Weixiong
Jiang, Xi
Jiao, Jianbo
Jiao, Jieqing
Jiao, Zhicheng
Jie, Biao
Jin, Dakai
Jin, Taisong
Jin, Yueming
John, Rogers
Joshi, Anand
Joshi, Shantanu

Jud, Christoph
Jung, Kyu-Hwan
Jungo, Alain
Kadkhodamohammadi, Abdolrahim
Kakileti, Siva
Kamnitsas, Konstantinos
Kang, Eunsong
Kao, Po-Yu
Kapoor, Ankur
Karani, Neerav
Karayumak, Suheyla
Kazi, Anees
Kerrien, Erwan
Kervadec, Hoel
Khalifa, Fahmi
Khalili, Nadieh
Khallaghi, Siavash
Khalvati, Farzad
Khan, Hassan
Khanal, Bishesh
Khansari, Maziyar
Khosravan, Naji
Kia, Seyed
Kikinis, Ron
Kim, Geena
Kim, Hosung
Kim, Hyo-Eun
Kim, Jae-Hun
Kim, Jinman
Kim, Jinyoung
Kim, Minjeong
Kim, Namkug
Kim, Seong
Kim, Young-Ho
Kitasaka, Takayuki
Klein, Stefan
Klinder, Tobias
Kolli, Kranthi
Kong, Bin
Kong, Xiang-Zhen
Konukoglu, Ender
Koo, Bongjin
Koohbanani, Navid
Kopriva, Ivica
Kose, Kivanc
Koutsoumpa, Christina

Mozaffari, Mohammad
Muetzel, Ryan
Müller, Henning
Muñoz-Barrutia, Arrate
Munsell, Brent
Nadeem, Saad
Nahlawi, Layan
Nandakumar, Naresh
Nardi, Giacomo
Neila, Pablo
Ni, Dong
Nichols, Thomas
Nickisch, Hannes
Nie, Dong
Nie, Jingxin
Nie, Weizhi
Niethammer, Marc
Nigam, Aditya
Ning, Lipeng
Niu, Shuaicheng
Niu, Sijie
Noble, Jack
Noblet, Vincent
Novo, Jorge
O'donnell, Thomas
Obeid, Mohammad
Oda, Hirohisa
Oda, Masahiro
Odry, Benjamin
Oeltze-Jafra, Steffen
Oksuz, Ilkay
Oliveira, Marcelo
Oliver, Arnau
Oñativia, Jon
Onofrey, John
Orasanu, Eliza
Orihuela-Espina, Felipe
Orlando, Jose
Osmanlioglu, Yusuf
Otalora, Sebastian
Pace, Danielle
Pagador, J.
Pai, Akshay
Pan, Yongsheng
Pang, Shumao
Papiez, Bartlomiej

Parajuli, Nripesh
Park, Hyunjin
Park, Jongchan
Park, Sanghyun
Park, Seung-Jong
Paschali, Magdalini
Paul, Angshuman
Payer, Christian
Pei, Yuru
Peng, Jialin
Peng, Tingying
Pennec, Xavier
Perdomo, Oscar
Pereira, Sérgio
Pérez-Carrasco, Jose-Antonio
Pesteie, Mehran
Peter, Loic
Peters, Jorg
Petitjean, Caroline
Pezold, Simon
Pfeiffer, Micha
Phellan, Renzo
Phophalia, Ashish
Pisharady, Pramod
Playout, Clement
Pluim, Josien
Pohl, Kilian
Portenier, Tiziano
Pouch, Alison
Prasanna, Prateek
Prevost, Raphael
Ps, Viswanath
Pujades, Sergi
Qi, Xin
Qian, Zhen
Qiang, Yan
Qiao, Lishan
Qiao, Yuchuan
Qin, Chen
Qin, Wenjian
Qirong, Bu
Qiu, Wu
Qu, Liangqiong
Raamana, Pradeep
Rabbani, Hossein
Rackerseder, Julia

Rad, Reza
Rafii-Tari, Hedyeh
Rajpoot, Kashif
Ramachandram, Dhanesh
Ran, Lingyan
Raniga, Parnesh
Rashwan, Hatem
Rathore, Saima
Ratnarajah, Nagulan
Raval, Mehul
Ravikumar, Nishant
Raviprakash, Harish
Raza, Shan
Reaungamornrat, Surreerat
Rekik, Islem
Remeseiro, Beatriz
Rempfler, Markus
Ren, Jian
Ren, Xuhua
Ren, Yudan
Reyes-Aldasoro, Constantino
Reyes, Mauricio
Riedel, Brandalyn
Rieke, Nicola
Risser, Laurent
Rittner, Leticia
Rivera, Diego
Ro, Yong
Robinson, Emma
Robinson, Robert
Rodas, Nicolas
Rodrigues, Rafael
Rohr, Karl
Roohani, Yusuf
Roszkowiak, Lukasz
Roth, Holger
Rouco, José
Roy, Abhijit
Ruijters, Danny
Rusu, Mirabela
Rutter, Erica
S., Sharath
Sabuncu, Mert
Sachse, Frank
Safta, Wiem
Saha, Monjoy

Saha, Pramit
Sahu, Manish
Samani, Abbas
Samek, Wojciech
Sánchez-Margallo, Francisco
Sánchez-Margallo, Juan
Sankaran, Sethuraman
Sanroma, Gerard
Sao, Anil
Sarhan, Mhd
Sarikaya, Duygu
Sarker, Md.
Sato, Imari
Saut, Olivier
Savardi, Mattia
Savitha, Ramasamy
Scarpa, Fabio
Scheinost, Dustin
Scherf, Nico
Schirmer, Markus
Schlaefer, Alexander
Schmid, Jerome
Schnabel, Julia
Schultz, Thomas
Schwartz, Ernst
Sdika, Michael
Sedai, Suman
Sekou, Taibou
Sekuboyina, Anjany
Selvan, Raghavendra
Semedo, Carla
Senouf, Ortal
Seoud, Lama
Sermesant, Maxime
Serrano, Carmen
Sethi, Amit
Shaban, Muhammad
Shaffie, Ahmed
Shah, Meet
Shalaby, Ahmed
Shamir, Reuben
Shan, Hongming
Shao, Yeqin
Sharma, Harshita
Shehata, Mohamed
Shen, Haocheng

Shen, Li
Shen, Mali
Shen, Yiru
Sheng, Ke
Shi, Bibo
Shi, Jun
Shi, Kuangyu
Shi, Xiaoshuang
Shi, Yonggang
Shi, Yonghong
Shigwan, Saurabh
Shin, Hoo-Chang
Shin, Jitae
Shontz, Suzanne
Signoroni, Alberto
Siless, Viviana
Silva, Carlos
Silva, Wilson
Simonovsky, Martin
Simson, Walter
Sinclair, Matthew
Singh, Vivek
Soans, Rajath
Sohel, Ferdous
Sokooti, Hessam
Soliman, Ahmed
Sommen, Fons
Sommer, Stefan
Song, Ming
Song, Yang
Sotiras, Aristeidis
Sparks, Rachel
Spiclin, Ziga
St-Jean, Samuel
Steinbach, Peter
Stern, Darko
Stimpel, Bernhard
Strait, Justin
Studholme, Colin
Styner, Martin
Su, Hai
Su, Yun-Hsuan
Subramanian, Vaishnavi
Subsol, Gérard
Sudre, Carole
Suk, Heung-Il

Sun, Jian
Sun, Li
Sun, Tao
Sung, Kyunghyun
Suter, Yannick
Tajbakhsh, Nima
Tan, Chaowei
Tan, Jiaxing
Tan, Wenjun
Tang, Min
Tang, Sheng
Tang, Thomas
Tang, Xiaoying
Tang, Youbao
Tang, Yuxing
Tang, Zhenyu
Tanner, Christine
Tanno, Ryutaro
Tao, Qian
Tarroni, Giacomo
Tasdizen, Tolga
Thung, Kim
Tian, Jiang
Tian, Yun
Toews, Matthew
Tong, Yubing
Topsakal, Oguzhan
Torosdagli, Neslisah
Toussaint, Nicolas
Troccaz, Jocelyne
Trzcinski, Tomasz
Tulder, Gijs
Tustison, Nick
Tuysuzoglu, Ahmet
Ukwatta, Eranga
Unberath, Mathias
Ungi, Tamas
Upadhyay, Uddeshya
Urschler, Martin
Uslu, Fatmatulzehra
Uyanik, Ilyas
Vaillant, Régis
Vakalopoulou, Maria
Valindria, Vanya
Varela, Marta
Varsavsky, Thomas

Vedula, S.
Vedula, Sanketh
Veeraraghavan, Harini
Vega, Roberto
Veni, Gopalkrishna
Verma, Ujjwal
Vetter, Thomas
Vialard, Francois-Xavier
Villard, Pierre-Frederic
Villarini, Barbara
Virga, Salvatore
Vishnevskiy, Valery
Viswanath, Satish
Vlontzos, Athanasios
Vogl, Wolf-Dieter
Voigt, Ingmar
Vos, Bob
Vrtovec, Tomaz
Wang, Bo
Wang, Changmiao
Wang, Chengjia
Wang, Chunliang
Wang, Dadong
Wang, Guotai
Wang, Haifeng
Wang, Haoqian
Wang, Hongkai
Wang, Hongzhi
Wang, Hua
Wang, Huan
Wang, Jiazhuo
Wang, Jingwen
Wang, Jun
Wang, Junyan
Wang, Kuanquan
Wang, Kun
Wang, Lei
Wang, Li
Wang, Liansheng
Wang, Manning
Wang, Mingliang
Wang, Nizhuan
Wang, Pei
Wang, Puyang
Wang, Ruixuan
Wang, Shanshan

Wang, Sheng
Wang, Shuai
Wang, Wenzhe
Wang, Xiangxue
Wang, Xiaosong
Wang, Xuchu
Wang, Yalin
Wang, Yan
Wang, Yaping
Wang, Yuanjun
Wang, Ze
Wang, Zhe
Wang, Zhinuo
Wang, Zhiwei
Wang, Zilei
Weber, Jonathan
Wee, Chong-Yaw
Weese, Jürgen
Wei, Benzheng
Wei, Dong
Wei, Donglai
Wei, Dongming
Weigert, Martin
Wein, Wolfgang
Wels, Michael
Wemmert, Cédric
Werner, Rene
Wesierski, Daniel
Williams, Bryan
Williams, Jacqueline
Williams, Travis
Williamson, Tom
Wilms, Matthias
Wiskin, James
Wittek, Adam
Wollmann, Thomas
Wolterink, Jelmer
Wong, Ken
Woo, Jonghye
Wu, Guoqing
Wu, Ji
Wu, Jian
Wu, Jiong
Wu, Pengxiang
Wu, Xi
Wu, Ye

Wu, Yicheng
Wuerfl, Tobias
Xi, Xiaoming
Xia, Jing
Xia, Wenfeng
Xiao, Deqiang
Xiao, Yiming
Xie, Hai
Xie, Hongtao
Xie, Jianyang
Xie, Long
Xie, Weidi
Xie, Yiting
Xie, Yuanpu
Xie, Yutong
Xing, Fuyong
Xiong, Tao
Xu, Chenchu
Xu, Jiaofeng
Xu, Jun
Xu, Kele
Xu, Rui
Xu, Ting
Xu, Yan
Xu, Yongchao
Xu, Zheng
Xu, Zhenlin
Xu, Zhoubing
Xu, Ziyue
Xue, Jie
Xue, Wufeng
Xue, Yuan
Yahya, Faridah
Yan, Chenggang
Yan, Ke
Yan, Weizheng
Yan, Yu
Yan, Yuguang
Yan, Zhennan
Yang, Guang
Yang, Guanyu
Yang, Hao-Yu
Yang, Jie
Yang, Lin
Yang, Shan
Yang, Xiao

Yang, Xiaohui
Yang, Xin
Yao, Dongren
Yao, Jianhua
Yao, Jiawen
Ye, Chuyang
Ye, Jong
Ye, Menglong
Ye, Xujiong
Yi, Jingru
Yi, Xin
Ying, Shihui
Yoo, Youngjin
Yousefi, Bardia
Yousefi, Sahar
Yu, Jinhua
Yu, Kai
Yu, Lequan
Yu, Renping
Yu, Weichuan
Yushkevich, Paul
Zanjani, Farhad
Zenati, Marco
Zeng, Dong
Zeng, Guodong
Zettinig, Oliver
Zhan, Liang
Zhang, Baochang
Zhang, Chuncheng
Zhang, Dongqing
Zhang, Fan
Zhang, Haichong
Zhang, Han
Zhang, Haopeng
Zhang, Heye
Zhang, Jianpeng
Zhang, Jiong
Zhang, Jun
Zhang, Le
Zhang, Lichi
Zhang, Mingli
Zhang, Pengyue
Zhang, Pin
Zhang, Qiang
Zhang, Rongzhao
Zhang, Shengping

Zhang, Shu
Zhang, Songze
Zhang, Tianyang
Zhang, Tong
Zhang, Wei
Zhang, Wen
Zhang, Wenlu
Zhang, Xiang
Zhang, Xin
Zhang, Yi
Zhang, Yifan
Zhang, Yizhe
Zhang, Yong
Zhang, Yongqin
Zhang, You
Zhang, Yu
Zhang, Yue
Zhang, Yueyi
Zhang, Yungeng
Zhang, Yunyan
Zhang, Yuyao
Zhang, Zizhao
Zhao, Haifeng
Zhao, Jun
Zhao, Qingyu
Zhao, Rongchang
Zhao, Shijie
Zhao, Shiwan
Zhao, Tengda
Zhao, Wei
Zhao, Yitian
Zhao, Yiyuan

Zhao, Yu
Zhao, Zijian
Zheng, Shenhai
Zheng, Yalin
Zheng, Yinqiang
Zhong, Zichun
Zhou, Bo
Zhou, Jianlong
Zhou, Luping
Zhou, Niyun
Zhou, S.
Zhou, Shoujun
Zhou, Tao
Zhou, Wenjin
Zhou, Yuyin
Zhou, Zhiguo
Zhu, Hancan
Zhu, Junjie
Zhu, Qikui
Zhu, Weifang
Zhu, Wentao
Zhu, Xiaofeng
Zhu, Xinliang
Zhu, Yingying
Zhu, Yuemin
Zhu, Zhuotun
Zhuang, Xiahai
Zia, Aneeq
Zimmer, Veronika
Zolgharni, Massoud
Zou, Ju
Zuluaga, Maria

Accepted MICCAI 2019 Papers

By Region of First Author

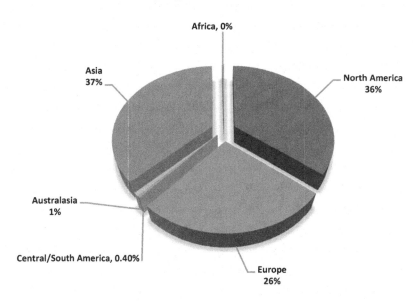

Africa, 0%

Asia
37%

North America
36%

Australasia
1%

Central/South America, 0.40%

Europe
26%

By Technical Keyword

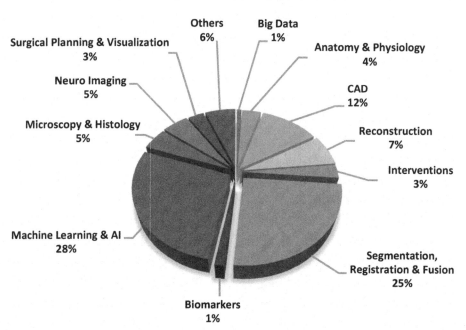

Others
6%

Big Data
1%

Surgical Planning & Visualization
3%

Anatomy & Physiology
4%

Neuro Imaging
5%

CAD
12%

Microscopy & Histology
5%

Reconstruction
7%

Interventions
3%

Machine Learning & AI
28%

Segmentation,
Registration & Fusion
25%

Biomarkers
1%

Awards Presented at MICCAI 2018, Granada, Spain

MICCAI Society Enduring Impact Award: The Enduring Impact Award is the highest award of the MICCAI Society. It is a career award for continued excellence in the MICCAI research field. The 2018 Enduring Impact Award was presented to Sandy Wells, Brigham and Women's Hospital/Harvard Medical School, USA.

MICCAI Society Fellowships: MICCAI Fellowships are bestowed annually on a small number of senior members of the society in recognition of substantial scientific contributions to the MICCAI research field and service to the MICCAI community. In 2018, fellowships were awarded to:

- Pierre Jannin (Université de Rennes, France)
- Anne Martel (University of Toronto, Canada)
- Julia Schnabel (King's College London, UK)

Medical Image Analysis Journal Award Sponsored by Elsevier: Jianyu Lin, for his paper entitled "Dual-modality Endoscopic Probe for Tissue Surface Shape Reconstruction and Hyperspectral Imaging Enabled by Deep Neural Networks," authored by Jianyu Lin, Neil T. Clancy, Ji Qi, Yang Hu, Taran Tatla, Danail Stoyanov, Lena Maier-Hein, and Daniel S. Elson.

Best Paper in *International Journal of Computer-Assisted Radiology and Surgery* (IJCARS) journal: Arash Pourtaherian for his paper entitled "Robust and Semantic Needle Detection in 3D Ultrasound Using Orthogonal-Plane Convolutional Neural Networks," authored by Arash Pourtaherian, Farhad Ghazvinian Zanjani, Svitlana Zinger, Nenad Mihajlovic, Gary C. Ng, Hendrikus H. M. Korsten, and Peter H. N. de With.

Young Scientist Publication Impact Award: MICCAI papers by a young scientist from the past 5 years were eligible for this award. It is made to a researcher whose work had an impact on the MICCAI field in terms of citations, secondary citations, subsequent publications, h-index. The 2018 Young Scientist Publication Impact Award was given to Holger R Roth: "A New 2.5D Representation for Lymph Node Detection Using Random Sets of Deep Convolutional Neural Network Observations" authored by Holger R. Roth, Le Lu, Ari Seff, Kevin M. Cherry, Joanne Hoffman, Shijun Wang, Jiamin Liu, Evrim Turkbey, and Ronald M. Summers.

MICCAI Young Scientist Awards: The Young Scientist Awards are stimulation prizes awarded for the best first authors of MICCAI contributions in distinct subject areas. The nominees had to be full-time students at a recognized university at, or within, two years prior to submission. The 2018 MICCAI Young Scientist Awards were given to:

- Erik J. Bekkers for the paper entitled: "Roto-Translation Covariant Convolutional Networks for Medical Image Analysis"
- Bastian Bier for the paper entitled: "X-ray-transform Invariant Anatomical Landmark Detection for Pelvic Trauma Surgery"

- Yuanhan Mo for his paper entitled: "The Deep Poincaré Map: A Novel Approach for Left Ventricle Segmentation"
- Tanya Nair for the paper entitled: "Exploring Uncertainty Measures in Deep Networks for Multiple Sclerosis Lesion Detection and Segmentation"
- Yue Zhang for the paper entitled: "Task-Driven Generative Modeling for Unsupervised Domain Adaptation: Application to X-ray Image Segmentation"

Contents – Part IV

Prediction

Detection and Localization

Machine Learning

Computer-Aided Diagnosis

Image Reconstruction and Synthesis

Shape (Including Neuroimage Shape)

A CNN-Based Framework for Statistical Assessment of Spinal Shape and Curvature in Whole-Body MRI Images of Large Populations

Philipp Ernst[(⊠)], Georg Hille, Christian Hansen, Klaus Tönnies, and Marko Rak

Faculty of Computer Science, University of Magdeburg, Magdeburg, Germany
philipp.ernst@ovgu.de

Abstract. The extraction of spines from medical records in a fast yet accurate way is a challenging task, especially for large data sets. Addressing this issue, we present a framework based on convolutional neural networks for the reconstruction of the spinal shape and curvature, making statistical assessments feasible on epidemiological scale. Our method uses a two-step strategy. First, anchor vertebrae and the spinal centerline in between them get extracted. Second, the centerlines are transformed into a common coordinate system to enable comparisons and statistical assessments across subjects. Our networks were trained on 103 subjects, where we achieved accuracies of 3.3 mm on average, taking at most 1 s per record, which eases the handling of even very large cohorts. Without any further training, we validated our model on study data of about 3400 subjects with only 10 cases of failure, which demonstrates the robustness of our method with respect to the natural variability in spinal shape and curvature. A thorough statistical analysis of the results underpins the importance of our work. Specifically, we show that the spinal curvature is significantly influenced by the body mass index of a subject. Moreover, we show that the same findings arise when Cobb angles are considered instead of direct curvature measures. To this end, we propose a generalization of classical Cobb angles that can be evaluated algorithmically and can also serve as a useful (visual) tool for physicians in everyday clinical practice.

1 Introduction

Recently, medical images have become an integral part of public health studies to get a broader insight into the data [12,13]. However, they are not suitable for direct analyses as the important information is not obtainable directly. For this reason, frameworks need to be established that extract information suitable for epidemiological purposes. Furthermore, non-experts in image processing should be able to apply the methodology. Our goal is to provide such a framework for

© Springer Nature Switzerland AG 2019
D. Shen et al. (Eds.): MICCAI 2019, LNCS 11767, pp. 3–11, 2019.
https://doi.org/10.1007/978-3-030-32251-9_1

quantification of spinal curvatures on large scale data sets. Following the idea behind visual analytics [8], the framework shall be suitable for the exploration of data sets with respect to certain factors to derive hypotheses on potential relations and to later validate these using statistical tests. We will show that our framework is well-suited to implement this workflow (exploration → hypothesis → testing). To this end, we will investigate the relation between the body mass index (BMI) and spinal curvature. Due to the heterogeneity that can be expected from public health studies, our framework is based on convolutional neural networks (CNNs), which achieve state-of-the-art results for many medical image processing tasks [5] with large natural variability between subjects.

Related Work. Many attempts have been made in the scope of spine analysis. Han et al. [2] use a Recurrent GAN for simultaneous semantic segmentation of spinal structures and classification of spinal diseases for 2D MR images. Hille et al. [3] present a hybrid level-set-based approach for robust and precise segmentation of vertebral bodies in 3D clinical routine MRI with minimal user interaction. Korez et al. [4] couple deformable models with CNNs for supervised segmentation of vertebral bodies from 3D MR spine images. Castro-Mateos et al. [1] introduce Statistical Interspace Models as an extension to Statistical Shape Models that take relative positions and orientations among objects into account and apply them to spine segmentation of CT images. Rak et al. [9] apply a combination of CNNs and graph cuts with star-convexity constraints to 3D patches of MR vertebra images to segment the whole spine. For further works please see the survey of Rak and Tönnies [10].

2   Method

Pretest Data Set. For the development of our framework, a pretest data set of the Study of Health in Pomerania (SHIP) [13] was used. It includes T_1-weighted whole spine MR images of 103 subjects that were acquired sagitally on a 1.5 T Siemens scanner with a field-of-view (FOV) of 50×50 cm and a voxel spacing of $1.1 \times 1.1 \times 4.4$ mm. We processed the images as follows: z-score normalization was applied to better generalize and the in-plane resolution was halved to $2.2 \times 2.2 \times 4.4$ mm to speed up training. Ground truth annotations for each subject were created by the authors. Specifically, the centers of all vertebrae from the topmost cervical vertebra (C1) to the first sacral vertebra (S1) were defined for each subject, whereby an isotropically resliced volume with a resolution of $1.1 \times 1.1 \times 1.1$ mm was used during creation to maximize ground truth precision.

Outline. The first step of our method extracts a centerline probability map (CPM) of the spine using a V-Net-like CNN (Fig. 1) [7]. It is not favorable to directly extract the individual vertebrae via regression since their number may vary between subjects, which is difficult to reflect at the output of a neural network. As an example, this natural variability occurs in 5 % of the Chinese population [14] and thus cannot be neglected in the context of public health studies. In parallel, a second CNN (Fig. 1 but with 2 output channels) extracts the positions of the anchor vertebrae (AVs), which in our case are C1 and S1. These AVs can be found reliably due to their specific appearance and shape, which will be shown in the experiments. Given the trained CNNs, the centerline is extracted by following the CPM in between the found AVs. Afterwards, the reconstructed centerline is transformed into a reference system. This high-level spine representation enables simple visual as well as statistical comparability, as will be shown later on.

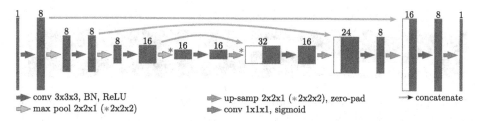

Fig. 1. Architecture of our CNN for extracting the centerline probability map. Blue boxes depict multi-channel feature maps. A white box corresponds to a copied feature map. The number above each box denotes the number of channels. (Color figure online)

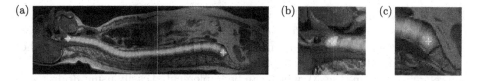

Fig. 2. (a) Predictions of our CNNs. Anchor vertebra CNN (red channel). Extracted anchor vertebra locations (crosses). Centerline probability map CNN (green channel). (b–c) Zoomed patches centered around the upper and lower vertebra, respectively. (Color figure online)

Anchor Vertebra Localization. For localization of the AVs, the CNN is trained to predict one probability map for each AV from the whole spine MRI. To create these maps, a white voxel is inserted into a zero-volume at the position of the respective AV and a Gaussian filter ($\sigma = 6\,\mathrm{mm}$) is applied to yield a smooth blob around the AV location. The size of the kernel was chosen to roughly reflect the size of an average vertebra. After prediction, the AV center locations can be extracted easily by searching for the global maximum per channel (Fig. 2, red channel, crosses). Preliminary tests showed that this fuzzy segmentation task results in more accurate and robust localizations compared to a coordinate regression task, which would have been the intuitive strategy.

Centerline Calculation. To create the CPM, we fit a cubic spline through the ground truth vertebra locations and rasterize the resulting curve into a volume that is initially filled with zeros. Afterwards, a Gaussian filter ($\sigma = 6\,\mathrm{mm}$) is applied to create a smooth ridge along the spine, which is then to be predicted via a dedicated CNN (Fig. 2 green channel). As for AV localization, this fuzzy segmentation task yields more accurate and robust predictions compared to direct coordinate regression. After prediction, the actual centerline is defined by locations of maximal probability for each axial slice between the AVs. A shortest path algorithm is reasonable, too, and also more robust in case of ambiguous CPM predictions, which was not the case for any of our data.

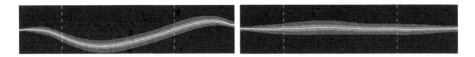

Fig. 3. Sagittal (left) and coronal projections (right) of the normalized centerlines of the about 3400 subjects of the SHIP study. The visualization encodes the distribution of shapes in boxplot-manner using different gray values. From white to black: median centerline, centerline range from 1st to 3rd quartile, centerline ranges for the 5th and 95th percentile. Dashed yellow lines separate the cervical, thoracic and lumbar area. (Color figure online)

Centerline Normalization. For further analyses, the extracted centerlines are transformed into a common reference system by applying a similarity transformation, i.e. translation, rotation and isotropic scaling, to each centerline. The transformation maps the extracted AV locations onto fixed targets in the common reference system (Fig. 3), which can be implemented easily using Rodrigues' rotation formula, yielding an angle- and ratio-preserving mapping by construction, which is suitable for later statistical analysis.

Cobb Angle Transformation. To compare our framework with earlier work, we utilize Cobb angles, which are typically measured between inflection points. Based on preliminary tests, we found that the localization of these points and the subsequent angle measurement is error-prone when directly applied inside a neural network. For this reason, we generalized the idea of Zukić et al. [15]: For each pair of positions along the centerline, the signed angle between the direction vectors along the centerline is calculated (Fig. 4(a)). We arrange the so-obtained values into a matrix representation (Fig. 4(b)), the so-called Cobb angle transformation (CAT). It contains the (signed) Cobb angles between any pair of points along the spine and can be seen as a generalization of classic Cobb angles which are calculated between inflection points only. Using the CAT, we can also reconstruct classic Cobb angles by finding the maximum (unsigned) angle in the matrix representation.

Data Augmentation. To cope with the rather small number of training samples available, a data augmentation was applied in each epoch, consisting of random flips along the sagittal or transverse axis as well as random pixel-wise translations along the coronal or transverse axis, avoiding errors introduced by interpolation. To constrain the translation during augmentation, we require that all vertebra locations remain inside the input domain even after augmentation.

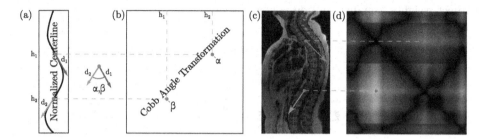

Fig. 4. (a) Normalized direction vectors d_1 and d_2 along the normalized centerline at positions h_1 and h_2. (b) Cobb angle transformation contains $\alpha = \angle(d_1, d_2)$ and $\beta = \angle(d_2, d_1)$ at positions (h_1, h_2) and (h_2, h_1) where $\angle(x, y)$ defines the signed angle between x and y. (c–d) Example for (a–b) using $\angle(a, b) = \operatorname{sgn}(a_x) \cdot \arccos(\langle a, b \rangle)$ depicting the part of the vertebral column with largest Cobb angle with respect to the sagittal plane. Cobb angles in the coronal plane are defined analogously.

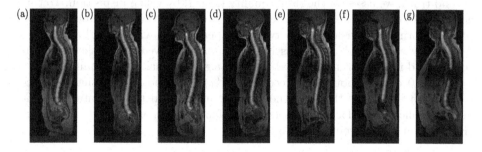

Fig. 5. Predictions on unseen data from the main SHIP study. Almost all results were classified as correct (a–d); few cases suffered from, for example, a weak prediction of the lower anchor vertebra (e), disappearing vertebrae due to acquisition artifacts (f) or bad illumination in the thoracic area (g).

Pretest Data Results. After training both CNNs using stochastic gradient descent (learning rate $= 0.01$, Nesterov momentum $= 0.7$) [11] on the fuzzy Dice loss [7] for 600 epochs (AV CNN) and 200 epochs (CPM CNN) on the training data (82 of 103 samples), our method achieves a mean absolute error of 3.3 mm between the predicted and the ground truth centerline on the validation data (21 of 103 samples), which is already well below the inter-slice spacing for our data and thus sufficient for our needs.

3   Experiments

Study Data Sets. After training both networks on the pretest data, the main SHIP data is evaluated without any further training. It consists of about 3400 records which also include interviews on the health status and laboratory data. The main SHIP data is stratified based on geographical regions, subject age and sex, which leads to near-uniform distributions across these attributes. Regarding subject weights, the distribution is nearly Gaussian.

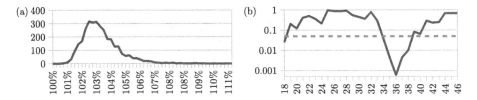

Fig. 6. (a) Histogram of lengths of normalized centerlines in the sagittal plane (100 % being a perfectly straight spine). (b) p-values of Mann-Whitney U tests on BMI thresholds, comparing the normalized centerline lengths above and below each BMI threshold for statistical differences; significance level $\alpha = 0.05$ (gray, dashed).

Study Data Results. Since the main SHIP data set does not include any ground truth, we assessed the result quality (Fig. 5) by visual inspection. To this end, the computed centerlines were used to create sagittal and coronal curved planar reformations yielding only two slices per subject with centerline overlay. A result was classified as success if the centerline stayed inside the vertebral column and its appearance seemed natural (e.g. no visual discontinuities).

Only 10 of the about 3400 records (0.3 %) could not be classified as success, which underpins the robustness of our method on unseen data and renders it applicable for large data sets. These failure cases are related to artifacts (Fig. 5(f)) or bad illumination (Fig. 5(g)).

Exploration and Hypotheses. To verify the suitability of our method for epidemiological analysis workflows, we used our centerline normalization to derive reasonable hypotheses about the data. Having a look at the distribution of spines with respect to attributes like subject size and weight, we came up with the hypothesis that subjects with a predisposition to obesity tend to have more bent spines than non-obese subjects. To verify this exemplary hypothesis, we set up according statistical tests, the results of which will now be discussed.

Statistical Testing. In our first experiment, we compare different body mass index (BMI) levels by spine curvature directly, exploiting our centerline normalization approach. In the common coordinate system, the centerline length directly corresponds to curvature. For statistical evaluation, the Mann-Whitney

U (MWU) test [6] was used which tests whether one random variable is statistically larger than the other one. Specifically, we test whether subjects with smaller BMIs have straighter spines. To this end, we split the set of subjects at each BMI level and perform MWU tests for each split. In Fig. 6 (right), the resulting p-values are depicted graphically. We observe significant results ($\alpha = 0.05$) for $34 \leq BMI \leq 38$. Looking at the actual centerline lengths, we observe that subjects of obesity class 1 or lower have significantly straighter spines ($\varnothing$ 102.5 % length) than those of obesity class 2 or higher ($\varnothing$ 103.2 % length). This finding looks intuitive at first glance, but due to the lack of large scale assessments, we have not found any consolidation in literature. This underpins the need for frameworks like ours.

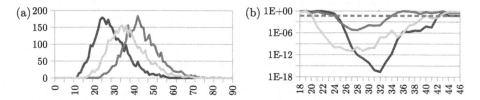

Fig. 7. (a) Histogram of maximum of the Cobb angle transformation in degrees. (b) p-values of Mann-Whitney U test on BMI thresholds, comparing the Cobb angles above and below each BMI threshold for statistical differences in the cervical (blue), thoracic (red) and lumbar (yellow) area; significance level $\alpha = 0.05$ (gray, dashed). (Color figure online)

We set up another experiment based on the CAT for further underpinning. Here, the Cobb angles were evaluated for the cervical, thoracic and lumbar area, using the very same procedure as described above. From the results (Fig. 7), we observe significant differences when splitting subjects at BMI levels $\{25 - 42\}, \{25 - 33\}, \{21 - 42\}$ for the three respective sections (Fig. 7(b)). Comparing the estimated Cobb angles after the subjects split, the cervical (less obese: 27° vs. more obese: 23°) and the thoracic area (less obese: 43° vs. more obese: 41°) are bent less and the lumbar area is bent more (less obese: 33° vs. more obese: 35°) for subjects with higher obesity levels.

4 Conclusion

Our goal was to enable analysis of large image data sets in the context of epidemiological public health studies. Specifically, we provide a CNN-based framework to extract the whole spinal centerline from MR images in a fast (at most 1 s for one whole-body MRI) yet accurate way (mean absolute error of 3.3 mm per centerline). To ease the comparison of the extracted centerlines, we introduced a normalization step, which maps all centerlines into a common reference system. The latter can be used to derive hypotheses about the data, which are then tested statistically. Furthermore, we generalized standard Cobb angles into the so-called

Cobb angle transformation, which proves a useful tool for detecting, classifying and quantifying spinal malformation at a glance in clinical daily routine. To underpin the importance of frameworks like ours, we derived hypotheses about the spine curvature on an epidemiological data set of about 3400 subjects. Using statistical tests, we found that the body mass index has a significant influence on the spinal curvature, i.e. subjects with at most obesity class 1 have straighter spines than more obese subjects. We also found that the spine in the cervical and thoracic section is bent less the higher the body mass index gets. Further tests, which were beyond the scope of this work, showed that even normal subjects have small but significant scoliotic tendencies (Cobb angles of $-7°$ to $9°$) and spines of females are bent more than those of males. Of course, with more attributes becoming available in the course of a public health study, more interesting questions will arise. For example, whether the curvature of the spine is influenced by diseases not related to the spine or by certain human habits.

Acknowledgments. We thank all parties and participants of the Study of Health in Pomerania. This work is funded by the EU and the federal state of Saxony-Anhalt, Germany (ZS/2016/08/80388 and ZS/2016/04/78123) as part of the initiative 'Sachsen-Anhalt WISSENSCHAFT Schwerpunkte'. This work was conducted within the context of the International Graduate School MEMoRIAL at Otto von Guericke University Magdeburg, Germany, kindly supported by the ESF under the program 'Sachsen-Anhalt WISSENSCHAFT Internationalisierung' (ZS/2016/08/80646). We thank the NVIDIA Corporation for donating the Titan Xp used for this research.

References

1. Castro-Mateos, I., Pozo, J.M., Pereañez, M., Lekadir, K., Lazary, A., Frangi, A.F.: Statistical interspace models (SIMS): application to robust 3D spine segmentation. IEEE Trans. Med. Imag. **34**(8), 1663–1675 (2015)
2. Han, Z., Wei, B., Mercado, A., et al.: Spine-GAN: semantic segmentation of multiple spinal structures. Med. Imag. Anal. **50**, 23–35 (2018)
3. Hille, G., Saalfeld, S., Serowy, S., Tönnies, K.: Vertebral body segmentation in wide range clinical routine spine MRI data. Comput. Methods Prog. Biomed. **155**, 93–99 (2018)
4. Korez, R., Likar, B., Pernuš, F., Vrtovec, T.: Model-based segmentation of vertebral bodies from MR images with 3D CNNs. In: Ourselin, S., Joskowicz, L., Sabuncu, M.R., Unal, G., Wells, W. (eds.) MICCAI 2016. LNCS, vol. 9901, pp. 433–441. Springer, Cham (2016). https://doi.org/10.1007/978-3-319-46723-8_50
5. Litjens, G.J.S., Kooi, T., Bejnordi, B.E., et al.: A survey on deep learning in medical image analysis. Med. Image Anal. **42**, 60–88 (2017)
6. Mann, H.B., Whitney, D.R.: On a test of whether one of two random variables is stochastically larger than the other. Ann. Math. Statist. **18**, 50–60 (1947)
7. Milletari, F., Navab, N., Ahmadi, S.: V-NET: fully convolutional neural networks for volumetric medical image segmentation. In: International Conference on 3D Vision (2016)
8. Pak, C.W., Thomas, J.: Visual analytics. IEEE Comput. Graph Appl. **24**(5), 20–21 (2004)

9. Rak, M., Steffen, J., Meyer, A., et al.: Combining convolutional neural networks and star convex cuts for fast whole spine vertebra segmentation in MRI. Comput. Methods Programs Biomed. **177**, 47–56 (2019)
10. Rak, M., Tönnies, K.D.: On computerized methods for spine analysis in MRI. Int. J. CARS **11**(8), 1445–1465 (2016)
11. Robbins, H., Monro, S.: A stochastic approximation method. Ann. Math. Stat. **22**, 400–407 (1951)
12. Tönnies, K.D., Gloger, O., Rak, M., et al.: Image analysis in epidemiological applications. it (2015)
13. Völzke, H.: Study of health in pomerania (ship). Bundesgesundheitsblatt - Gesundheitsforschung - Gesundheitsschutz (2012)
14. Yan, Y.Z., Li, Q.P., Wu, C.C., et al.: Rate of presence of 11 thoracic vertebrae and 6 lumbar vertebrae in asymptomatic Chinese adult volunteers. J. Orthop. Surg. Res. **13**, 124 (2018)
15. Zukić, D., Vlasák, A., Egger, J., et al.: Robust detection and segmentation for diagnosis of vertebral diseases using routine mr images. Comput Graph Forum (2014)

Exploiting Reliability-Guided Aggregation for the Assessment of Curvilinear Structure Tortuosity

Pan Su[1,2], Yitian Zhao[1(✉)], Tianhua Chen[3], Jianyang Xie[1], Yifan Zhao[1,4], Hong Qi[5], Yalin Zheng[1,6], and Jiang Liu[1,7]

[1] Cixi Institute of Biomedical Engineering, Ningbo Institute of Industrial Technology, Chinese Academy of Sciences, Ningbo, China
`yitian.zhao@nimte.ac.cn`
[2] School of Control and Computer Engineering, North China Electric Power University, Baoding, China
[3] School of Computing and Engineering, University of Huddersfield, Huddersfield, UK
[4] School of Aerospace, Transport and Manufacturing, Cranfield University, Cranfield, UK
[5] Department of Ophthalmology, Peking University Third Hospital, Beijing, China
[6] Department of Eye and Visual Science, University of Liverpool, Liverpool, UK
[7] Department of Computer Science and Engineering, Southern University of Science and Technology, Shenzhen, China

Abstract. The study on tortuosity of curvilinear structures in medical images has been significant in support of the examination and diagnosis for a number of diseases. To avoid the bias that may arise from using one particular tortuosity measurement, the simultaneous use of multiple measurements may offer a promising approach to produce a more robust overall assessment. As such, this paper proposes a data-driven approach for the automated grading of curvilinear structures' tortuosity, where multiple morphological measurements are aggregated on the basis of reliability to form a robust overall assessment. The proposed pipeline starts dealing with the imprecision and uncertainty inherently embedded in empirical tortuosity grades, whereby a fuzzy clustering method is applied on each available measurement. The reliability of each measurement is then assessed following a nearest neighbour guided approach before the final aggregation is made. Experimental results on two corneal nerve and one retinal vessel data sets demonstrate the superior performance of the proposed method over those where measurements are used independently or aggregated using conventional averaging operators.

Keywords: Tortuosity assessment · Curvilinear structure · Fuzzy clustering · Reliability guided aggregation

© Springer Nature Switzerland AG 2019
D. Shen et al. (Eds.): MICCAI 2019, LNCS 11767, pp. 12–20, 2019.
https://doi.org/10.1007/978-3-030-32251-9_2

1   Introduction

Tortuosity of curvilinear structures in ophthalmic images can be used as indicators to a number of diseases. For example, the tortuosity of corneal fibers shown in *in vivo* confocal microscopy images can be used to explain the nerve degeneration and subsequent regeneration [10], which is correlated with diabetic neuropathy, retinopathy of prematurity [9], and keratitis [11]. The assessment of curvilinear structures' tortuosity level could be utilised for early diseases prevention of further complications. In several studies, the tortuosity of curvilinear structures has been manually graded in the band of 3–5 levels [12] or ranked by ophthalmologists based on their clinical experiences. However, the imprecision and uncertainty inherently embedded in the subjective empirical assessment may lead to substantial inter-observer and intra-observer variability [2].

In the literature, the tortuosity grading may also be conducted using various measurements of curvilinear structures such as the angle [5], length [7], and curvature [8]. A fully automated pipeline on the basis of these measurements that takes raw images as inputs and outputs assessment results may be devised for tortuosity estimation. Typically, such automated methods employ segmentation algorithms to replace manual tracing of curvilinear structures. However, many of the existing tortuosity measurements are based on mathematical definitions, which are sensitive to pixel-level calculation. The jagged and inaccurate boundaries embedded in the automated segmentation, easily result in low performance of tortuosity estimates. On the other hand, hand-crafted tortuosity definitions only provide fixed models of subjective perception, which limits the generalisation ability of individual measurements across different tasks. The automated tortuosity assessment of curvilinear structures in ophthalmic images is therefore still a challenging problem.

As such, it is still prevalent to use different measurements of curvilinear structure to grade the tortuosity. To our best knowledge, there is no universal agreement as to which standard or measurement to apply. Recent studies suggest to simultaneously use multiple relevant measurements, in order to produce a robust overall assessment of tortuosity [2,14]. Indeed the use of multiple measurements may avoid the bias that may arise from using one particular tortuosity measurement. Inspired by this observation, This paper proposes a novel unsupervised pipeline for the automated grading of curvilinear structures' tortuosity, whereby multiple morphological measurements are aggregated on the basis of data-driven reliability to form a robust overall assessment. Experimental analysis on three data sets demonstrates the superior performance of the proposed method over those where measurements are used independently or aggregated using conventional averaging operators.

2   Method

2.1   Pipeline and Preprocessing of the Proposed Method

The proposed method is named Fuzzy Clustering and Measurement Reliability based Assessment of Tortuosity (FCMRAT). The working process starts by generating fuzzy clusters using fuzzy c-means algorithm [3] on each of the tortuosity measurements which are preselected (and predefined) by experts. The resultant fuzzy clusters (termed base clusters) can be associated with linguistic labels, which facilitate readability and validation against medical knowledge by clinicians. The reliability based aggregation operators are subsequently used to combine the base clusters that share the same linguistic label, resulting in the final fuzzy clusters of images. An illustrative flowchart of the proposed FCMRAT is shown in Fig. 1 with key operations detailed in the following subsections.

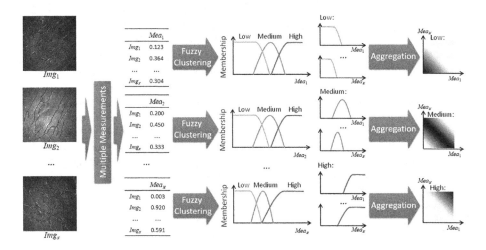

Fig. 1. Pipeline of FCMRAT. Firstly, the tortuosity of nerves in each image is evaluated by multiple measurements. Secondly, linguistic labelled fuzzy clusters are generated based on each measurement individually; Then, all the clusters are grouped by labels. Finally, an aggregation is applied on each group of fuzzy clusters with the same label.

Given a set of N images $\{Img_1, Img_2, \cdots, Img_N\}$ and M morphological measurements of tortuosity $mea_1, mea_2, \cdots, mea_M$, the curvilinear structures shown on $Img_i, i = 1, 2, \cdots, N$, can be traced and their tortuosity can be calculated by the M measurements. Typically, a measurement $mea_j, j = 1, 2, \cdots, M$, is deemed to be a mapping from the set of single curvilinear structures C to positive real-valued numbers $mea_j : C \rightarrow \mathbb{R}^+$, where large number indicates high tortuosity. An original image may contain a number of traced curvilinear structures. Therefore, an image-level tortuosity may be obtained by averaging all curvilinear structures traced in that image weighted by their length. Formally, given that H segments $c_h \in C, h = 1, 2, \cdots, H$ of curvilinear structures are traced in an image and the length of h-th structure is denoted as l_h, the image-level tortuosity can be defined as: $Mea_j(Img_i) = \sum_{h=1}^{H} l_h mea_j(c_h) / \sum_{h=1}^{H} l_h$ [2]. For images which contain only one single curvilinear structure c_1 (as in the RET-TORT [7]), $Mea_j(Img_i) = mea_j(c_1)$. Despite that the proposed FCMRAT is tested on segmentation results of curvilinear structures, both manually and automated segmentation can be embedded in the pipeline. However, it is worth noticing that in retina, certain diseases cause tortuosity alterations in portion of the eye, or just in capillaries. In such cases, the selection of curvilinear structures of interest is necessary in the preprocessing of images.

2.2 Generation of Fuzzy Clusters at Measurement Level

In case where there exists imprecision and vagueness that arise from the ophthalmologists' subjective empirical grading of tortuosity, fuzzy set theory is regarded as an effective means to dealing with vague concepts that are ubiquitous in natural languages and practical reasoning. It is a common practice to use fuzzification techniques to translate real-valued measurements into linguistic terms. In this paper, fuzzy clustering is employed for the fuzzification of each individual measurement. Suppose that $\{Img_1, Img_2, \cdots, Img_N\}$ are evaluated with regard to $Mea_1, Mea_2, \cdots, Mea_M$. For each measurement Mea_j, fuzzy c-means is utilised to form S base clusters $\widetilde{F}_1^j, \widetilde{F}_2^j, \cdots, \widetilde{F}_S^j$ on the set of images with respect to $\{Mea_j(Img_i)|i = 1, 2, \cdots, N\}$, with $\widetilde{F}_s^j(Img_i) \in [0, 1]$ representing the degree of Img_i belonging to an individual base cluster $\widetilde{F}_s^j, s = 1, 2, \cdots, S$, which satisfies $\sum_{s=1}^S \widetilde{F}_s^j(Img_i) = 1$ for all $j = 1, 2, \cdots, M$.

Linguistic terms are often used by clinicians in practice to describe the grading of curvilinear structure tortuosity in the ophthalmic images. A preference ordering relation is usually defined to describe the grading of tortuosity on a set of linguistic terms such as $Low \prec Medium \prec High$. In FCMRAT, labelling base clusters is not only helpful for ophthalmologists to investigate the relative tortuosity reflected in objective measurements, it also plays a significant role in organising base clusters into groups for subsequent aggregation process. Since the resulting clusters for a certain tortuosity measurement Mea_j on the set of images are totally ordered, the cluster centers $\widetilde{F}_1^j, \widetilde{F}_2^j, \cdots, \widetilde{F}_S^j$ can be employed to signify the overall relative tortuosity. Thus, given a set of S pre-defined linguistic terms $\mathbb{L} = \{L_1, L_2, \cdots, L_S\}$ which satisfy that $L_1 \prec L_2 \prec \cdots \prec L_S$, the fuzzy clusters $\widetilde{F}_1^j, \widetilde{F}_2^j, \cdots, \widetilde{F}_S^j$ can be readily sorted in ascending order with regard to their cluster centers and labelled with $L_1, L_2, \cdots, L_S$, respectively. From this, the notation $\widetilde{F}_{L_s}^j$ represents the base cluster generated by tortuosity measurement Mea_j and labelled with linguistic term $L_s, s = 1, 2, \cdots, S$.

2.3 Consensus of Base Clusters Guided by Reliability

Having gone through the fuzzification process as described in the preceding subsection, a total number of $M \times S$ fuzzy clusters are generated and labelled. They can be groupted into S sets of fuzzy sets $\mathbb{F}_{L_s}, s = 1, 2, \cdots, S$, where $\mathbb{F}_{L_s} = \{\widetilde{F}_{L_s}^j | j = 1, 2, \cdots, M\}$ consists of all the base clusters with label L_s. The base clusters in each group $\mathbb{F}_{L_s}$ is further aggregated to generate a final fuzzy cluster of images (denoted as $\widetilde{F}_{L_s}^*$) with their tortuosity graded into level L_s. The membership of an image Img_i to $\widetilde{F}_{L_s}^*$ can be computed by

$$\widetilde{F}^*_{L_s}(Img_i) = \frac{Agg(\widetilde{F}^1_{L_s}(Img_i),\widetilde{F}^2_{L_s}(Img_i),\cdots,\widetilde{F}^M_{L_s}(Img_i))}{\sum_{t=1}^{S} Agg(\widetilde{F}^1_{L_t}(Img_i),\widetilde{F}^2_{L_t}(Img_i),\cdots,\widetilde{F}^M_{L_t}(Img_i))} \quad \text{where } Agg : \mathbb{R}^M \to \mathbb{R}$$

is an aggregation operator.

As the effectiveness of certain measurements varies on different tasks, weighting all available tortuosity measurements equally may not reflect the deviations in the contribution made by individual measurements and therefore limit the quality of overall assessment. In addition, it is practically difficult and time-consuming for ophthalmologists to use empirical knowledge to agree on proper weights for different tortuosity measurements. In order to automate this complicated aggregation task, this paper employs the concept of K-Nearest-Neighbour guided Dependent Ordered Weighted Averaging (KNNDOWA) [4,15], in which an argument (such as a measurement in this case) whose value is similar to its neighbours is deemed reliable and can be highly weighted. In contrast, an argument that is largely different from its neighbours is discriminated as an unreliable member. Formally, the reliability of an argument a_j, $j = 1, 2, \cdots, M$, in KNNDOWA is defined as: $R^K_j = 1 - \frac{\sum_{k=1}^{K} d(a_j, n_k^{a_j})/K}{\max_{t,t' \in \{1,2,\cdots,M\}} d(a_t, a_{t'})}$.

where $n_k^{a_j} \in \{a_1, 2, \cdots, a_M\}/\{a_j\}$ is the value of k-th nearest neighbour ($k = 1, 2, \cdots, K$ and $K < M$) of the argument a_j, and the distance matric is $d(a_t, a_{t'}) = |a_t - a_{t'}|$ for $t, t' \in \{1, 2, \cdots, M\}$. Note that the distance metric is also used to perform neighbour-searching. Having obtained the reliability values of all arguments concerned, they are normalised to form the weighing vectors in KNNDOWA. Given the reliability value R^K_j of each argument $a_j, j = 1, 2, \cdots, M$, the corresponding aggregation operator Agg^K can be specified by $Agg^K(a_1, a_2, \cdots, a_M) = \sum_{j=1}^{M} R^K_j a_j / \sum_{j=1}^{M} R^K_j$.

In FCMRAT, KNNDOWA is adopted to aggregate the memberships of images with respect to base clusters in each labelled group. Computationally speaking, alternative aggregation operators can also be fitted into the FCMRAT pipeline. The advantages of selecting KNNDOWA out of alternatives are: 1) the weights used in the aggregation are purely data-driven, which are automatically learned from the memberships $\widetilde{F}^j_{L_s}(Img_i)$, and 2) the weight assigned to each argument $w(a_j) = R^K_j / \sum_{t=1}^{M} R^K_t, j = 1, 2, \cdots, M$, represents the reliability of a_j, which can be utilised as a meaningful indicator to ophthalmologists for further interpreting the effectiveness of the underlying tortuosity measurements.

2.4 Tortuosity Assessment Based on Aggregated Fuzzy Clusters

The final step of the proposed FCMRAT is to assess the tortuosity based on the aggregated fuzzy clusters. Consider an example where the set of pre-defined linguistic terms $\mathbb{L}$ is $\{Low, Medium, High\}$ with the preference ordering relation $Low \prec Medium \prec High$, the memberships of an image Img_i to the final fuzzy clusters is represented as a vector such as $(\widetilde{F}^*_{Low}(Img_i), \widetilde{F}^*_{Medium}(Img_i), \widetilde{F}^*_{High}(Img_i)) = (0.2, 0.5, 0.3)$, it is straightforward to defuzzify the assessment result by assigning Img_i to the linguistic label associated with the final fuzzy cluster that possesses the maximum membership degree among others. The final grade of Img_i is computed as $\arg\max_{L_s \in \mathbb{L}} \widetilde{F}^*_{L_s}(Img_i)$, i.e., the tortuosity of Img_i is graded to *Medium* in this example.

To utilise all available information, an alternative method is to assign a significance score to each of the linguistic terms and then, to sort the images with respect to the weighted sum of the scores and memberships to the final fuzzy clusters. In this paper, the significance score of L_s is set to s. Then, the ranking over a set of images can be obtained by sorting the images in a descending/ascending order, according to a ranking index: $\sum_{s=1}^{S} s\widetilde{F}^*_{L_s}(Img_i)$. In the previous example, the ranking index of Img_i is 2.1.

3 Experimental Analysis

The FCMRAT is tested on two public data sets: the NERVE TORTUOSITY (NT1) in which 30 images are graded into 3 levels [6] and the RET-TORT [7] in which the images of arteries (Art.) and veins (Vei.) are ranked and used independently. An in-house conrneal nerve data set (NT2) is also employed, in which 242 images are taken in the resolution of 384×384 pixels and are graded into 4 levels of tortuosity based on a protocol [12]. Five tortuosity measurements including the arc Length over Chord length ratio (LC), Total Curvature (TC), Total Squared Curvature (TSC), Inflection Count Metric (ICM) [1], and Absolute Direction Angle Change (DCI) [13] are employed for generating the base clusters of FCMRAT. An segmentation algorithm proposed in [17] is adopted on the NT1 and NT2 data sets to trace the curvilinear structures. Depending on whether the segmentation of curvilinear structures is implemented by automated algorithm or by manual annotation, a suffix -A or -M is used for annotation. The Spearman's coefficients between individual measurements and the ground truth of each data set are reported in Table 1, where the highest values are highlighted in boldface. The average and median values of the coefficients on each data set are provided as baselines.

Table 1. Spearman's coefficients of individual measurements

Dataset	Lc	Tc	Tsc	ICM	DCI	Average	Median
NT1-A	0.5990	0.7547	0.7924	0.4339	**0.8160**	0.6792	0.7547
NT1-M	**0.8254**	0.8018	0.7830	0.6226	0.7028	0.7471	0.7830
NT2-A	**0.6316**	0.6112	0.6013	0.3184	0.5210	0.5367	0.6013
Art.	0.8194	0.8945	**0.9017**	0.8269	0.7161	0.8317	0.8269
Vei.	0.6130	0.8143	**0.8346**	0.6397	0.7378	0.7279	0.7378

The Spearman's coefficients between ranks generated by the FCMRAT ranking index (the number of final clusters S is set to 5) and the ground truth are reported in Table 2. In addition to the KNNDOWA, four aggregation operators namely: Andness-OWA (an OWA operator with weighting vector $(0.300, 0.233,$

$0.167, 0.100, 0.033)$), Mean, Orness-OWA (an OWA operator with weighting vector $(0.033, 0.100, 0.167, 0.233, 0.300)$), and Dependent OWA [16] are also implemented under the FCMRAT pipeline for the consensus of base clusters to support systematic comparisons. Since there are five measurements to be aggregated, the number of nearest neighbours K in KNNDOWA is set to 2, which indicates the reliability of each measurement is estimated by half (2 out of 4) of its neighbours. The fuzzy c-means algorithm starts with random initialisation of memberships and each reported FCMRAT result is an average of 30 runs. The standard deviation of all the results are smaller than 0.0075. The performance for the NT1 and NT2 data set is also evaluated based on the weighted accuracy (wAcc) [2] through defuzzifying final fuzzy clusters. In order to generate the grade-based result, the number of final clusters (i.e., the number of base clusters for each measurements) S in this experiments is set to the number of grades in the ground truth (3 and 4 for NT1 and NT2, respectively).

Table 2. Results of FCMRAT with different aggregation operators

	Spearman's coefficient					wAcc		
	NT1-A	NT1-M	NT2-A	Art.	Vei.	NT1-A	NT1-M	NT2-A
FCMRAT+And	0.7309	0.8160	0.6156	**0.9132**	0.7972	0.8222	0.7333	0.5809
FCMRAT+Mean	0.7314	0.8242	0.6132	0.9119	0.7949	0.8222	0.7333	0.5831
FCMRAT+Or	0.7294	**0.8279**	0.6115	0.9052	0.7835	0.8222	0.7333	**0.5834**
FCMRAT+DOWA	0.7283	0.8174	0.6166	0.9119	0.8019	0.8222	0.7333	0.5828
FCMRAT+2NN	**0.7558**	0.8018	**0.6167**	0.9026	**0.8112**	0.8222	0.7333	0.5786

It can be seen from Table 1 that the most relevant single measurement, i.e., the one with highest Spearman's coefficient with the ground truth (in boldface) varies on different data sets, which supports the observation that there is no agreement as to which measurement to apply universally. As it is shown in Table 2, by applying the proposed FCMRAT pipeline, the aggregation based results are better than those obtained by averaging individual measurements across all the data sets. The FCMRAT based results are better than the median value of individual measurements for four out of five data sets. These observations show the effectiveness of the fuzzy clustering based aggregation of multiple measurements for tortuosity assessment. It is also worth noticing that the FCMRAT based aggregations can achieve results which are better than the best result achieved by individual measurements on the NT1-M and Art. data sets. This further demonstrates that the proposed aggregation of multiple measurements is effective in the tortuosity assessment for curvilinear structures. Furthermore, the weighted accuracies of all FCMRAT based aggregations on the NT1 data set are the same, which indicates the insensitivity and robustness of FCMRAT in the selection of aggregation operators. The performance of the proposed method on the in-house data set is lower than that on the public data sets, which is mainly attributed to the low performances achieved at the level of individual measurements, possibly resulting from the inaccurate segmentation of curvilinear structures and inconsistent grading in the ground truth.

Amongst all the tested aggregation operators, the KNNDOWA based FCM-RAT is the only one which achieves results better than the medians of individual measurements across all the tested data sets. In addition to the superior and stable performance of KNNDOWA in providing overall tortuosity assessment, the linguistic term labelled base clusters and the data-driven generated reliabilities during aggregation operation provide a supportive tool for ophthalmologists to interpret and fine-tune the assessment model. For each measurement Mea_j, its overall reliability can be evaluated by the mean of its weights in all the aggregations as $\sum_{i=1}^{N}\sum_{s=1}^{S} w(\widetilde{F}_{L_s}^{j}(Img_i))/(NS)$. Take the NT1-A data set as an example with the number of final clusters is set to 3, the overall reliability of the Lc, Tc, Tsc, ICM, and DCI is 0.1969, 0.2182, 0.2238, 0.1646, and 0.1965, respectively, with Tc and Tsc being considered more reliable than the other three measurements in the FCMRAT.

It is worth noticing that in practice, the 3-level (low, medium, high) or 4-level tortuosity grades may be more common in nerve fiber studies. In retinal studies, 5-level grading may be used. Theoretically, the clustering granularity can be defined as fine as possible by allowing a large number of clusters and associated linguistic labels. In practice, this is not encouraged, especially in cases where clearly divided stages for tortuosity grading may not exist, or for psychological reasons in order to linguistically interpret the labelled clusters to clinicians.

4 Conclusion and Future Work

This paper proposes a novel pipeline for the assessment of curvilinear structure tortuosity based on fuzzy clustering and reliability-guided aggregation of morphological measurements. The proposed work is verified on three real-world data sets with superior and stable results achieved over those at the level of individual tortuosity measurements, demonstrating the efficacy and effectiveness of the proposed method. Whist promising, the proposed pipeline could be naturally extended to cope with a broader range of medical imaging tasks such as investigation of unsupervised methods in automated tortuosity assessment systems.

Acknowledgement. This work was supported by Project funded by China Postdoctoral Science Foundation (2019M652156), National Science Foundation Program of China (61601029), Zhejiang Provincial Natural Science Foundation (LZ19F010001).

References

1. Abdalla, M., et al.: Quantifying retinal blood vessels' tortuosity - review. In: Science & Information Conference (2015)
2. Annunziata, R., et al.: A fully automated tortuosity quantification system with application to corneal nerve fibres in confocal microscopy images. Med. Image Anal. **32**, 216–232 (2016)

3. Bezdek, J.C., et al.: FCM: the fuzzy C-means clustering algorithm. Comput. Geosci. **10**(2), 191–203 (1984)
4. Boongoen, T., Shen, Q.: Nearest-neighbor guided evaluation of data reliability and its applications. IEEE Trans. Syst. Man Cybern. Part B Cybern. **40**(6), 1622–1633 (2010)
5. Bribiesca, E.: A measure of tortuosity based on chain coding. Pattern Recogn. **46**(3), 716–724 (2013)
6. Fabio, S., et al.: Automatic evaluation of corneal nerve tortuosity in images from in vivo confocal microscopy. Invest. Ophthalmol. Vis. Sci. **52**(9), 6404 (2011)
7. Grisan, E., et al.: A novel method for the automatic grading of retinal vessel tortuosity. IEEE Trans. Med. Imaging **27**, 310–319 (2008)
8. Hart, W.E., et al.: Measurement and classification of retinal vascular tortuosity. Int. J. Med. Inform. **53**(2–3), 239–252 (1999)
9. Heneghan, C., et al.: Characterization of changes in blood vessel width and tortuosity in retinopathy of prematurity using image analysis. Med. Image Anal. **6**(4), 407–429 (2002)
10. Kim, J., Markoulli, M.: Automatic analysis of corneal nerves imaged using in vivo confocal microscopy. Clin. Exp. Optom. **101**(2), 147–161 (2018)
11. Kurbanyan, K., et al.: Corneal nerve alterations in acute acanthamoeba and fungal keratitis: an in vivo confocal microscopy study. Eye **26**(1), 126 (2012)
12. Oliveira-Soto, L., Efron, N.: Morphology of corneal nerves using confocal microscopy. Cornea **20**(4), 374–384 (2001)
13. Patasius, M., et al.: Evaluation of tortuosity of eye blood vessels using the integral of square of derivative of curvature. In: IFMBE Proceedings of the 3rd European Medical and Biological Engineering Conference (EMBEC05), vol. 11 (2005)
14. Scarpa, F., Ruggeri, A.: Development of clinically based corneal nerves tortuosity indexes. In: Cardoso, M.J., Arbel, T., Melbourne, A., Bogunovic, H., Moeskops, P., Chen, X., Schwartz, E., Garvin, M., Robinson, E., Trucco, E., Ebner, M., Xu, Y., Makropoulos, A., Desjardin, A., Vercauteren, T. (eds.) FIFI/OMIA -2017. LNCS, vol. 10554, pp. 219–226. Springer, Cham (2017). https://doi.org/10.1007/978-3-319-67561-9_25
15. Su, P., et al.: Exploiting data reliability and fuzzy clustering for journal ranking. IEEE Trans. Fuzzy Syst. **25**(5), 1306–1319 (2017)
16. Xu, Z.: Dependent OWA operators. In: Torra, V., Narukawa, Y., Valls, A., Domingo-Ferrer, J. (eds.) MDAI 2006. LNCS (LNAI), vol. 3885, pp. 172–178. Springer, Heidelberg (2006). https://doi.org/10.1007/11681960_18
17. Zhao, Y., et al.: Automated vessel segmentation using infinite perimeter active contour model with hybrid region information with application to retinal images. IEEE Trans. Med. Imaging **34**(9), 1797–1807 (2015)

A Surface-Theoretic Approach
for Statistical Shape Modeling

Felix Ambellan$^{(\boxtimes)}$ (ID), Stefan Zachow (ID), and Christoph von Tycowicz (ID)

Visual Data Analysis, Zuse Institute Berlin, Berlin, Germany
{ambellan,zachow,vontycowicz}@zib.de

Abstract. We present a novel approach for nonlinear statistical shape modeling that is invariant under Euclidean motion and thus alignment-free. By analyzing metric distortion and curvature of shapes as elements of Lie groups in a consistent Riemannian setting, we construct a framework that reliably handles large deformations. Due to the explicit character of Lie group operations, our non-Euclidean method is very efficient allowing for fast and numerically robust processing. This facilitates Riemannian analysis of large shape populations accessible through longitudinal and multi-site imaging studies providing increased statistical power. We evaluate the performance of our model w.r.t. shape-based classification of pathological malformations of the human knee and show that it outperforms the standard Euclidean as well as a recent nonlinear approach especially in presence of sparse training data. To provide insight into the model's ability of capturing natural biological shape variability, we carry out an analysis of specificity and generalization ability.

Keywords: Statistical shape analysis · Principal Geodesic Analysis · Lie groups · Classification · Manifold valued statistics

1 Introduction

Statistical shape models (SSMs) have become an essential tool for medical image analysis with a wide range of applications such as segmentation of anatomical structures, computer-aided diagnosis, and therapy planning. SSMs describe the geometric variability in a population in terms of a mean shape and a hierarchy of major modes explaining the main trends of shape variation. Based on a notion of shape space, SSMs can be learned from a database of consistently parametrized instances from the object class under study. The resulting models provide a shape prior that can be used to constrain synthesis and analysis problems. Moreover, their parameter space provides a compact representation that is amenable to learning algorithms (e.g. classification or clustering), evaluation, and exploration.

Electronic supplementary material The online version of this chapter (https://doi.org/10.1007/978-3-030-32251-9_3) contains supplementary material, which is available to authorized users.

© Springer Nature Switzerland AG 2019
D. Shen et al. (Eds.): MICCAI 2019, LNCS 11767, pp. 21–29, 2019.
https://doi.org/10.1007/978-3-030-32251-9_3

Standard SSMs treat the space of shapes as a Euclidean vector space allowing for linear statistics to be applied (see e.g. [22] and the references therein). Linear methods, however, are often inadequate for capturing the high variability in biological shapes [12]. Nonlinear approaches have been developed based on geometric as well as physical concepts such as Hausdorff distance [8], elasticity [25,27,28], and viscous flows [6,17,20]. In general, these methods lack numerical robustness and fast response rates limiting their practical applicability especially in interactive applications. To address these challenges, one line of work models shapes by a collection of primitives [14,16,21] that naturally belong to Lie groups and effectively describe local changes in shape. Performing intrinsic calculus on the uncoupled primitives allows for fast computations while, at the same time, accounting for the nonlinearity in shape variation. However, solving the inverse problem, i.e. mapping from primitives back to surface meshes, is generally non-trivial. Recently, von Tycowicz et al. [26] presented a physically motivated approach based on differential coordinates for which the inverse problem is well-known and can be solved at linear cost. Despite their inherent nonlinear structure, the employed representations are not invariant under Euclidean motion and, thus, suffer from bias due to arbitrary choices. While the effect of rigid motions can be removed between pairs of shapes using alignment strategies, non-transitivity thereof prevents true group-wise alignment.

This work presents a novel shape representation based on discrete fundamental forms that is invariant under Euclidean motion. We endow this representation with a Lie group structure that admits bi-invariant metrics and therefore allows for consistent analysis using manifold-valued statistics based on the Riemannian framework. Furthermore, we derive a simple, efficient, robust, yet accurate (i.e. without resorting to model approximations) solver for the inverse problem that allows for interactive applications.

Although in computer graphics and vision communities, rotation invariant differential coordinates have also been successfully employed for geometry processing applications, e.g. [18,19,24], these approaches fall short of a fully intrinsic treatment (e.g. due to lack of bi-invariant group structure and linearization) and have not been adapted to the field of SSMs.

2   Rotation Invariant Surface Representation

In this section, we derive a discrete surface representation based on concepts from differential geometry of smooth surfaces.

Relation to Surface Theory. To every smooth surface there uniquely exist two smoothly pointwise varying and symmetric bilinear forms on the tangent plane, the so called *fundamental forms*. The *first* fundamental form I (a.k.a. metric tensor) is positive definite and allows for angle, length and area measurement. The *second* fundamental form II describes the curvature of the surface. A prominent result in classical mathematics, the *Fundamental Theorem of Surface Theory* due to Bonnet ($\approx$1860, e.g. [7] Sec. 4.3), states that if given two symmetric bilinear forms (one of them positive definite), s.t. for both certain integrability conditions hold (viz. the Gauß–Codazzi equations), then they (locally) determine uniquely, up to global rotation and translation, a surface embedded in three dimensional space with these two as its fundamental forms. Therefore, a discrete description of the fundamental forms is an excellent candidate for a rotation-invariant surface representation. In the following, we will denote our proposed shape model as the *fundamental coordinate model* (FCM).

Discretization. We consider shapes that belong to a particular population of anatomical structures, s.t. each digital shape S can be described as a left-acting deformation ϕ of a common reference shape $\bar{S}$ given as triangulated surface. Let deformation ϕ be affine on each triangle $\bar{T}_i$ of $\bar{S}$, then the deformation gradient $\nabla\phi$ is the 3×3 matrix of partial derivatives of ϕ and constant on each triangle $D_i := \nabla\phi|_{\bar{T}_i}$ (see e.g. [5] for detailed expressions). Assuming ϕ to be an orientation-preserving embedding of $\bar{S}$, we can decompose D_i uniquely into its rotational R_i and stretching U_i components by means of the polar decomposition $D_i = R_i U_i$. Note that U_i furnishes a complete description of the metric distortion of $\bar{T}_i$ and is defined in reference coordinates, hence invariant under rotation of S. Indeed, we can obtain a representation of the first fundamental form by restricting the stretches to the tangent plane. To this end, we define an arbitrary but fixed element-wise field $\{\bar{F}_i\}$ of orthonormal frames on $\bar{S}$, s.t. the last column of each frame is the normal of the respective element. Then, we represent the metric in terms of reduced stretch $\tilde{U}_i := [\bar{F}_i^T U_i \bar{F}_i]_{3,3} = \mathrm{I}|_{\bar{T}_i}^{1/2}$, where $[\cdot]_{3,3}$ denotes the submatrix with the third row and column removed.

As for the second fundamental form, we note that at a point $p \in S$ it is determined by the differential of the normal field N, viz. $\mathrm{II}_p(v, w) = \mathrm{I}_p(-dN_p(v), w)$ for tangent vectors v, w. For a triangulated surface, the differential dN is supported along the edges. In order to derive a representation thereof, we induce the frame field $\{F_i\}$ on S consistent to $\{\bar{F}_i\}$ using the rotational part of the deformation gradient, i.e. $F_i = R_i \bar{F}_i$. This allows us to define *transition rotations* $F_i C_{ij} = F_j$ for each inner edge (incident to triangles T_i, T_j) that fully describe the change in normal directions. Note that, while both the frames $\{F_i\}$ and the rotations $\{R_i\}$ are equivariant, the transition rotations $\{C_{ij}\}$ are invariant under global rotations of S and $\bar{S}$.

Group Structure. In order to perform intrinsic statistical analysis, we derive a distance that is compatible with the underlying representation space. In particular, we endow the space with a Lie group structure together with a bi-invariant Riemannian metric for which group and Riemannian notions of exponential and logarithm coincide. This allows us to exploit closed-form expressions to perform geodesic calculus yielding simple, efficient, and numerically robust algorithms. We recommend chapter two of [1] to readers interested in deeper insight about bi-invariant metrics on Lie groups. This regards especially their existence and the geometric consequences thereof.

Our shape representation consists of transition rotations $C_{ij} \in \mathrm{SO}(3)$ (one per inner edge) and tangential stretches $\tilde{U}_i \in \mathrm{Sym}^+(2)$ (one per triangle), where $\mathrm{SO}(3)$ is the Lie group of rotations in $\mathbb{R}^3$ and $\mathrm{Sym}^+(2)$ the space of symmetric and positive definite 2×2 matrices. Following the approach in [3], we equip $U, V \in$

$\mathrm{Sym}^+(2)$ with a multiplication $U \circ V := \exp(\log(U) + \log(V))$, s.t. $\mathrm{Sym}^+(2)$ turns into a commutative Lie group. It now allows for a bi-invariant metric induced by the Frobenius inner product yielding distance $d_{\mathrm{Sym}^+(2)}(U,V) = \|\log(V) - \log(U)\|_2$. $\mathrm{SO}(3)$ also admits a bi-invariant metric induced by the Frobenius inner product with distance $d_{\mathrm{SO}(3)}(Q,R) = \|\log(Q^T R)\|_2$, s.t. we define our representation space as the product group $G := \mathrm{SO}(3)^n \times \mathrm{Sym}^+(2)^m$ and m, n the number of triangles and inner edges. Finally, we define the distance of $S, T \in G$ as

$$d(S,T) = \frac{\omega^3}{\bar{A}_{\mathcal{E}}} \sum_{(i,j)\in\mathcal{E}} \bar{A}_{ij}\, d_{\mathrm{SO}(3)}\left(C_{ij}^S, C_{ij}^T\right) + \frac{\omega}{\bar{A}} \sum_{i=1}^{m} \bar{A}_i\, d_{\mathrm{Sym}^+(2)}\left(\tilde{U}_i^S, \tilde{U}_i^T\right),$$

where $\omega \in \mathbb{R}^+$ is a weighting factor, $\mathcal{E}$ is the set of inner edges, $\bar{A}_i$ is the area of triangle $\bar{T}_i$, $\bar{A}_{ij} = 1/3(\bar{A}_i + \bar{A}_j)$, $\bar{A}_{\mathcal{E}} = \sum_{(i,j)\in\mathcal{E}} \bar{A}_{ij}$, and $\bar{A} = \sum_{i=1}^{m} \bar{A}_i$. Here the area terms provide invariance under refinement of the mesh as well as simultaneous scaling of $\bar{S}, S, T$, whereas ω allows for commensuration of the curvature and metric contributions inspired by the Koiter thin shell model (e.g. [9] Sec. 4.1).

Model Construction. The derived representation carries a rich non-Euclidean structure calling for manifold-valued generalizations for first and second moment statistical analysis. To this end, we employ Principal Geodesic Analysis (PGA) [15]. Furthermore, to avoid systematic bias due to the choice of reference shape $\bar{S}$, we require it to agree with the mean of the training data as proposed in [23].

3   Efficient Numerics

In this section, we derive an efficient numerical solver for the inverse problem of mapping a point in representation space G to a corresponding shape $S = \phi(\bar{S})$. If the corresponding rotations $\{R_i\}$ were known, ϕ could be obtained as the minimizer of $\sum_{i=1}^{m} \bar{A}_i \|D_i - R_i U_i\|_2^2$ by solving the well-known Poisson equation (see e.g. [5,26]). However, in our representation the rotations are only given implicitly in terms of the transition rotations. In particular, an immediate computation shows that $R_j = R_i \bar{F}_i C_{ij} \bar{F}_j^T =: R_{i \to j}$ for an integrable field $\{C_{ij}\}$. Based on this condition, for each triangle T_i we can formulate a residual term $\varepsilon_i(\phi, \{R_i\}) = \sum_{j\in\mathcal{N}_i} 1/|\mathcal{N}_i| \|D_i - R_{j \to i} U_i\|_2^2$ in terms of the rotations of neighboring triangles (indexed by $\mathcal{N}_i$). Then, the objective for the inverse problem is given as $E(\phi) = \min_{\{R_i \in \mathrm{SO}(3)\}} E(\phi, \{R_i\})$, where $E(\phi, \{R_i\}) = \sum_{i=1}^{m} \bar{A}_i \varepsilon_i(\phi, \{R_i\})$. Although $E(\phi)$ is a nonlinear function calling for iterative optimization routines, it exhibits a special structure amenable to an efficient alternating minimization technique. Specifically, we employ a block coordinate descent strategy that alternates between a local and a global step:

Local Step: First, we minimize $E(\phi, \{R_i\})$ over the rotations $\{R_i\}$ keeping ϕ (hence D_i) fixed. Each summand in ε_i depends on a single rotation R_j, s.t. the problem decouples into individual low-dimensional optimizations that can be solved in closed-form and allow for massive parallelization.

Global Step: Second, we minimize $E(\phi, \{R_i\})$ over ϕ with rotations $\{R_i\}$ fixed leading to a quadratic optimization problem for which the optimally conditions are determined by a Poisson equation. As the system matrix is sparse and depends only on the reference shape, it can be factorized once during the preprocess allowing for very efficient global solves with close to linear cost.

Note that the objective is bounded from below and that both local and global steps feature unique solutions that are guaranteed to weakly decrease the objective making any numerical safeguards unnecessary. This contrasts with classical approaches that require precautions, such as line search strategies and modification schemes for singular or indefinite Hessians, to guarantee robustness.

Initialization. To provide the solver with a warm start, we compute an initial guess for the rotation field $\{R_i\}$. To this end, we employ the local integrability condition $R_j = R_{i \rightarrow j}$ to propagate an initial rotation matrix from an arbitrary seed along a precomputed spanning tree of the dual graph of $\bar{S}$. Note, that this strategy recovers the rotation field exactly for integrable $\{C_{ij}\}$. In case of non-integrable fields, one advantage of the Poisson-based reconstruction (global step) is that it distributes errors uniformly s.t. local inconsistencies are attenuated.

4 Experiments and Results

All experiments are performed employing a fixed commensuration weight $\omega = 10$ that empirically shows the best performance in our classification experiments (cf. suppl. material).

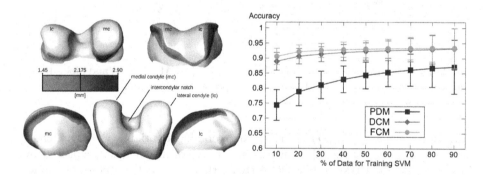

Fig. 1. Left: Mean shape of healthy distal femora overlaid with mean shape of the diseased femora wherever the distance is larger than 1.45 mm, colored accordingly. Right: OA classification experiment for the proposed FCM, PDM [10] and DCM [26].

Data. We employ three datasets: (i) Distal femora (see Fig. 1, left) from the Osteoarthritis Initiative (OAI) for 58 severely diseased and 58 healthy subjects that were also used for evaluation in [26] and are publicly available as segmentations [2], (ii) a male human body in two poses from the open-access FAUST [4] dataset (see Fig. 2, left) and (iii) synthetic pipe surfaces in a cylindrical and a helical configuration (see Fig. 2, right). For the former two, we used the surface meshes as provided by the authors (in particular the correspondences) and we refer to [4] and [26] for further details. A detailed list of the exact subjects that are included in (i) as well as their disease state can be found in the supplemental material.

Knee Osteoarthritis Classification. Osteoarthritis (OA) is a degenerative disease of the joints that is i.a. characterized by changes of the bone shape (see Fig. 1, left). Here, we investigate the proposed FCM's ability to classify knee OA for the OAI dataset of distal femora. To this end, we employ a support vector machine (SVM) with linear kernel on the 115-dimensional feature vectors comprising the coefficients w.r.t. the principal modes for each shape. The classifier is trained on a balanced set of feature vectors for different shares of data varying from 10% to 90% with testing on the respective complement. To address the randomness of our experimental design, we carried out the experiment 10000 times per partition. We compare to the popular *point distribution model* [10] (PDM) as well as to the differential coordinates model [26] (DCM), which recently achieved highly accurate classification results. Figure 1 (right) shows the results in terms of average accuracy and standard deviation. Note that solely the FCM achieves an accuracy of over 90% in case of sparse (10%) training data.

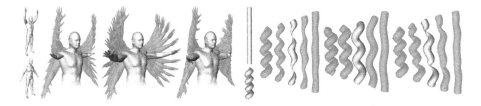

Fig. 2. Interpolating geodesic (mean highlighted) for the FAUST (left) and pipe surface (right) data within (f.l.t.r.) the PDM [10], the proposed FCM, and DCM [26], each.

Validity. Frequently, datasets feature a high nonlinear variability that are characterized by large rotational components, which are insufficiently captured by linear models like PDM. While DCM treats the rotational components explicitly, it requires them to be well-localized, s.t. the logarithm is unambiguous. This assumption may not be satisfied for data with large spread in shape space. Contrary, our model overcomes this limitation utilizing a relative encoding: Transition rotations will never exceed 180° in practical scenarios (cf. supplemental material for a quantitative evaluation). In Fig. 2 we illustrate the validity of our model for two extreme examples in comparison to PDM and DCM.

Computational Performance. We compare our framework in terms of performance to the state-of-the-art approaches: The *large deformation diffeomorphism metric mapping* (LDDMM) using the open-source Deformetrica [13] software, and the recent DCM. To this end, we compute the mean shape on 100 randomly sampled pairs from the OAI dataset. Overall, the LDDMM approach requires 172.8 s (±44.8 s) in average whereas the proposed FCM features an average run-time of only 2.3 s (±1.9 s), hence a two orders of magnitude speedup. In comparison to the highly efficient DCM—requiring 1.1 s (±0.3 s) in average—our model achieves runtimes within the same order of magnitude, despite the added nonlinearity in the inverse problem.

Specificity, Generalization Ability, Compactness. We perform a quantitative comparison with PDM and DCM using standard measures (detailed in [11]) w.r.t. a physically-based surface distance $\mathcal{W}$ [20] as proposed in [26]. *Specificity* (Fig. 3 middle) evaluates the validity of the model generated instances in terms of their distance to the training shapes. We estimate it using 1000 randomly generated instances according to the distribution estimated by the respective model. *Generalization ability* (Fig. 3 left) assesses how well a model represents unseen instances. It is calculated in a leave-one-out study. *Compactness* (Fig. 3 right) measures the relative amount of variability of the training set captured by every mode in an accumulated manner. The results show that the FCM is more specific than PDM and DCM. In terms of generalization ability, the FCM is superior to PDM, yet inferior to DCM. Finally, the FCM is less compact than PDM and DCM. Note that compactness is calculated for each model w.r.t its own metric, hence not directly comparable. In particular, we found that decreasing ω leads to increased compactness, albeit at the expense of classification accuracy (cf. suppl. material). Therefore, we conjecture that lower compactness allows for more expressiveness within the different modes of variation.

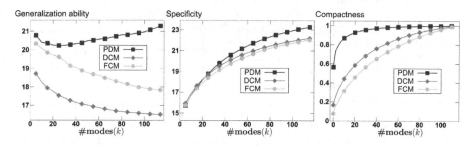

Fig. 3. Generalization ability (left), specificity (middle) and compactness (right) of the proposed FCM, PDM [10], and DCM [26].

5   Conclusion

In this work, we presented a novel nonlinear SSM based on a Euclidean motion invariant—hence alignment-free—shape representation with deep foundations in surface theory. The rich structure of the derived shape space assures valid shape instances even in presence of strong nonlinear variability. We perform manifold-valued statistics in a consistent Lie group setup allowing for closed-form evaluation of Riemannian operations. We show that this model yields highly discriminative shape descriptors that are superior to the state-of-the-art model [26] in experiments on OA classification. Furthermore, we devise an efficient and robust algorithm to solve the inverse problem that does not require any numerical safeguards. One possible and interesting way to proceed in the future is to replace the log-Euclidean metric with the affine-invariant one, which can be considered the natural metric on the symmetric positive definite matrices.

Acknowledgments. The authors are funded by the Deutsche Forschungsgemein-schaft (DFG, German Research Foundation) under Germany's Excellence Strategy – The Berlin Mathematics Research Center MATH+ (EXC-2046/1, project ID: 390685689). Furthermore we are grateful for the open-access datasets OAI[1] and FAUST [4] as well as for the open-source software Deformetrica [13].

References

1. Alexandrino, M.M., Bettiol, R.G.: Lie Groups and Geometric Aspects of Isometric Actions, vol. 8. Springer, Heidelberg (2015)
2. Ambellan, F., Tack, A., Ehlke, M., Zachow, S.: Automated segmentation of knee bone and cartilage combining statistical shape knowledge and convolutional neural networks. Med. Image Anal. **52**, 109–118 (2019)
3. Arsigny, V., Fillard, P., Pennec, X., Ayache, N.: Log-Euclidean metrics for fast and simple calculus on diffusion tensors. Magn. Reson. Med. **56**(2), 411–421 (2006)
4. Bogo, F., Romero, J., Loper, M., Black, M.J.: FAUST: dataset and evaluation for 3D mesh registration. In: CVPR. IEEE (2014)
5. Botsch, M., Sumner, R., Pauly, M., Gross, M.: Deformation transfer for detail-preserving surface editing. In: VMV, pp. 357–364 (2006)
6. Brandt, C., von Tycowicz, C., Hildebrandt, K.: Geometric flows of curves in shape space for processing motion of deformable objects. Comput. Graph. Forum **35**(2), (2016)
7. do Carmo, M.P.: Differential Geometry of Curves and Surfaces. Prentice-Hall, Englewood Cliffs (1976)
8. Charpiat, G., Faugeras, O., Keriven, R., Maurel, P.: Distance-based shape statistics. In: ICASSP, pp. V925–V928. IEEE (2006)
9. Ciarlet, P.G.: An introduction to differential geometry with applications to elasticity. J. Elast. **78**(1), 1–215 (2005)

---

[1] The Osteoarthritis Initiative is a public-private partnership comprised of five contracts (N01-AR-2-2258; N01-AR-2-2259; N01-AR-2-2260; N01-AR-2-2261; N01-AR-2-2262) funded by the National Institutes of Health, a branch of the Department of Health and Human Services, and conducted by the OAI Study Investigators. Private funding partners include Merck Research Laboratories; Novartis Pharmaceuticals Corporation, GlaxoSmithKline; and Pfizer, Inc. Private sector funding for the OAI is managed by the Foundation for the National Institutes of Health. This manuscript was prepared using an OAI public use data set and does not necessarily reflect the opinions or views of the OAI investigators, the NIH, or the private funding partners.

10. Cootes, T.F., Taylor, C.J., Cooper, D.H., Graham, J.: Active shape models-their training and application. Comput. Vis. Image Underst. **61**(1), 38–59 (1995)
11. Davies, R., Twining, C., Taylor, C.: Statistical Models of Shape: Optimisation and Evaluation. Springer, London (2008). https://doi.org/10.1007/978-1-84800-138-1
12. Davis, B.C., Fletcher, P.T., Bullitt, E., Joshi, S.: Population shape regression from random design data. Int. J. Comput. Vis. **90**(2), 255–266 (2010)
13. Durrleman, S., Prastawa, M., Charon, N., Korenberg, J.R., Joshi, S., Gerig, G., Trouvé, A.: Morphometry of anatomical shape complexes with dense deformations and sparse parameters. NeuroImage **101**, 35–49 (2014)
14. Fletcher, P.T., Lu, C., Joshi, S.: Statistics of shape via principal geodesic analysis on lie groups. In: CVPR, vol. 1, p. I-95. IEEE (2003)
15. Fletcher, P., Lu, C., Pizer, S., Joshi, S.: Principal geodesic analysis for the study of nonlinear statistics of shape. IEEE Trans. Med. Imaging **23**(8), 995–1005 (2004)
16. Freifeld, O., Black, M.J.: Lie bodies: a manifold representation of 3D human shape. In: Fitzgibbon, A., Lazebnik, S., Perona, P., Sato, Y., Schmid, C. (eds.) ECCV 2012. LNCS, vol. 7572, pp. 1–14. Springer, Heidelberg (2012). https://doi.org/10.1007/978-3-642-33718-5_1
17. Fuchs, M., Jüttler, B., Scherzer, O., Yang, H.: Shape metrics based on elastic deformations. J. Math. Imaging Vis. **35**(1), 86–102 (2009)
18. Gao, L., Lai, Y.K., Liang, D., Chen, S.Y., Xia, S.: Efficient and flexible deformation representation for data-driven surface modeling. ACM Trans. Graph. **35**(5), 158 (2016)
19. Hasler, N., Stoll, C., Sunkel, M., Rosenhahn, B., Seidel, H.P.: A statistical model of human pose and body shape. Comput. Graph. Forum **28**(2), 337–346 (2009)
20. Heeren, B., Zhang, C., Rumpf, M., Smith, W.: Principal geodesic analysis in the space of discrete shells. Comput. Graph. Forum **37**(5), 173–184 (2018)
21. Hefny, M.S., Okada, T., Hori, M., Sato, Y., Ellis, R.E.: A liver Atlas using the special euclidean group. In: Navab, N., Hornegger, J., Wells, W.M., Frangi, A.F. (eds.) MICCAI 2015. LNCS, vol. 9350, pp. 238–245. Springer, Cham (2015). https://doi.org/10.1007/978-3-319-24571-3_29
22. Heimann, T., Meinzer, H.P.: Statistical shape models for 3D medical image segmentation: a review. Med. Image Anal. **13**(4), 543–563 (2009)
23. Joshi, S., Davis, B., Jomier, M., Gerig, G.: Unbiased diffeomorphic Atlas construction for computational anatomy. NeuroImage **23**, S151–S160 (2004)
24. Kircher, S., Garland, M.: Free-form motion processing. ACM Trans. Graph. **27**(2), 12 (2008)
25. Rumpf, M., Wirth, B.: An elasticity-based covariance analysis of shapes. Int. J. Comput. Vis. **92**(3), 281–295 (2011)
26. von Tycowicz, C., Ambellan, F., Mukhopadhyay, A., Zachow, S.: An efficient Riemannian statistical shape model using differential coordinates. Med. Image Anal. **43**, 1–9 (2018)
27. von Tycowicz, C., Schulz, C., Seidel, H.P., Hildebrandt, K.: Real-time nonlinear shape interpolation. ACM Trans. Graph. **34**(3), 34:1–34:10 (2015)
28. Zhang, C., Heeren, B., Rumpf, M., Smith, W.A.: Shell PCA: statistical shapemodelling in shell space. In: ICCV, pp. 1671–1679. IEEE (2015)

One-Stage Shape Instantiation from a Single 2D Image to 3D Point Cloud

Xiao-Yun Zhou$^{(\boxtimes)}$, Zhao-Yang Wang, Peichao Li, Jian-Qing Zheng, and Guang-Zhong Yang

The Hamlyn Centre for Robotic Surgery, Imperial College London, London, UK
`xiaoyun.zhou14@imperial.ac.uk`

Abstract. Shape instantiation which predicts the 3D shape of a dynamic target from one or more 2D images is important for real-time intra-operative navigation. Previously, a general shape instantiation framework was proposed with manual image segmentation to generate a 2D Statistical Shape Model (SSM) and with Kernel Partial Least Square Regression (KPLSR) to learn the relationship between the 2D and 3D SSM for 3D shape prediction. In this paper, the two-stage shape instantiation is improved to be one-stage. PointOutNet with 19 convolutional layers and three fully-connected layers is used as the network structure and Chamfer distance is used as the loss function to predict the 3D target point cloud from a single 2D image. With the proposed one-stage shape instantiation algorithm, a spontaneous image-to-point cloud training and inference can be achieved. A dataset from 27 Right Ventricle (RV) subjects, indicating 609 experiments, were used to validate the proposed one-stage shape instantiation algorithm. An average point cloud-to-point cloud (PC-to-PC) error of 1.72 mm has been achieved, which is comparable to the PLSR-based (1.42 mm) and KPLSR-based (1.31 mm) two-stage shape instantiation algorithm.

Keywords: Shape instantiation · One-stage learning · PointOutNet · Chamfer distance loss

1 Introduction

Minimally-invasive and robot-assisted surgeries made significant advances in recent years. Compared to traditional open surgery, they decrease patient trauma and shorten the recovery time for patients. However, this development brings challenges to surgeons, as the operation environment is often not visually accessible. Clinicians need to perform very difficult interventions under poor, low-resolution and less-informative 2D navigation. Therefore, shape instantiation which instantiates the 3D shape of a dynamic target from limited 2D images is

X.-Y. Zhou and Z.-Y. Wang—Contribute equally to this paper. This work was supported by EPSRC project grant EP/L020688/1.

© Springer Nature Switzerland AG 2019
D. Shen et al. (Eds.): MICCAI 2019, LNCS 11767, pp. 30–38, 2019.
https://doi.org/10.1007/978-3-030-32251-9_4

important for mitigating this challenge. To achieve real-time navigation intra-operatively, there are two main requirements on shape instantiation algorithms: (1) the number of intra-operative 2D images should be kept minimal, otherwise it increases the input collection time and hence is harmful for real-time navigation; (2) fast inference speed during the application.

Shape instantiation is usually based on multiple 2D images, for example, six to seven prostate 2D images were needed in [2] for the reconstruction. In [8], to predict intra-operative 3D Abdominal Aortic Aneurysm (AAA) deformation caused by catheter insertion, 3D AAA shape was instantiated from two 2D fluoroscopic images with the as-rigid-as-possible method for navigation in Endovascular Aortic Repair (EVAR). Currently, many applications are focusing on using a single 2D intra-operative image as the input. The 3D shape of a fully-deployed, partially-deployed and fully-compressed stent graft was predicted from a single 2D intra-operative fluoroscopic image in [10–12] respectively for navigating Fenestrated Endovascular Aortic Repair (FEVAR). The 3D AAA skeleton was instantiated from a single intra-operative 2D fluoroscopic image with graph matching and skeleton deformation for FEVAR robotic path planning [9]. The 3D shape of a liver was instantiated from a single 2D image scanned at an optimal scan plane with Statistical Shape Model (SSM) and Partial Least Square Regression (PLSR) [5].

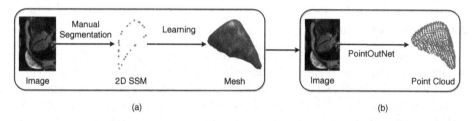

Fig. 1. Shape instantiation of (a) two-stage with manual image segmentation to generate 2D SSM and KPLSR-based learning for 3D mesh prediction; and (b) one-stage with PointOutNet to predict 3D point cloud from a single 2D image.

A general dynamic framework was proposed recently in [13] for 3D shape instantiation. First, it determined an optimal scan plane for a dynamic target by analyzing its pre-operative 3D SSM with Sparse Principal Component Analysis (SPCA). Second, Kernel Partial Least Square Regression (KPLSR) was used to learn the relationship between the pre-operative 2D and 3D SSM. Third, during the inference, with a new intra-operative 2D image at the same optimal scan plane as the input, the KPLSR-learned model was applied to predict the intra-operative 3D shape. However, in [13], the shape instantiation is two-stage with manual segmentation to generate 2D SSM first and then KPLSR-based learning for 3D mesh prediction, as shown in Fig. 1(a).

Recently, new neural network architectures were proposed to recover 3D shape from a single 2D image. In [1], based on the Long Short-Term Memory

(LSTM) framework, a 3D Recurrent Reconstruction Neural Network (3D-R2N2) was proposed to utilize one or more images from different viewpoints to recover a 3D volume. In [3], a point cloud prediction network called PointOutNet is proposed to generate un-ordered 3D point cloud from a single RGB image. In [6], a two-stage architecture called 3D-LMNet was proposed to improve 3D point cloud reconstruction: a 3D point cloud auto-encoder was used to learn the 3D point cloud latent space and then an image encoder was used to map the 2D image to the learned latent space. [4] proposed an approach recovering 3D hand mesh from a single image. Their architecture consists of image encoder, graph-convolution-based mesh auto-encoder and decoder.

In this paper, the previously designed shape instantiation is improved to be one-stage, as shown in Fig. 1(b). PointOutNet [3] with 19 convolutional layers, three fully-connected layers and Chamfer loss is used. The Right Ventricles (RVs) of 27 subjects, including both asymptomatic subjects and subjects with Hypertrophic Cardiomyopathy (HCM), were used to validate the one-stage shape instantiation with 609 experiments. The results show that the proposed one-stage shape instantiation algorithm can achieve comparable accuracy to previous two-stage ones based on PLSR or KPLSR learning, indicating potential end-to-end inference capability during practical applications.

2   Methodology

2.1   Framework Introduction

For a dynamic target, i.e. the RV, multiple 3D scans are acquired at different time frames in the dynamic cycle. A 3D mesh is reconstructed for the target at each time frame. For different time frames of a patient, these meshes are expressed into the same number of vertices and the same connectivity $\mathbf{Y}_{M \times numY \times 3}$ - 3D SSM with the method in [7], where M is the number of time frame, numY is the number of vertices, 3 represents the (x, y, z) coordinate of each vertex. Synchronized 2D images $\mathbf{I}_{M \times H \times W}$ at all time frames are acquired at the optimal scan plane, where H is the image height while W is the image width. PointOutNet is trained from $\mathbf{I}$ to $\mathbf{Y}$. In [13], the predicted $\hat{\mathbf{Y}}$ by KPLSR is with the same corresponding vertex order as the ground truth $\mathbf{Y}$. In this paper where PointOutNet is used, restricting the predicted point cloud with the same vertex order as the ground truth leads to an unsatisfactory result. Hence Chamfer distance is used as the loss function and the predicted $\hat{\mathbf{Y}}$ is a point cloud with different vertex order as $\mathbf{Y}$. During the inference, with a new intra-operative 2D input image $i_{H \times W}$, the intra-operative 3D RV point cloud will be predicted by the trained PointOutNet model as $\mathbf{y}_{numY \times 3}$.

2.2   PointOutNet

PointOutNet consists of an encoding part with convolutional layers to extract information from images and a prediction part with fully-connected layers to predict vertex coordinates. With an input of $\mathbf{F}^{in}_{N \times H \times W \times C^{in}}$, where N is the batch size, C^{in} is the input feature channel, multiple trainable convolutional kernels $\mathbf{T}_{C^{in} \times K \times K \times C^{out}}$ move along the input with a stride of S, resulting in an output feature map:

$$\mathbf{F}^{out}_{N \times H' \times W' \times C^{out}} = \mathbf{F}^{in}_{N \times H \times W \times C^{in}} \cdot \mathbf{T}_{C^{in} \times K \times K \times C^{out}} + \mathbf{B}_{C^{out}} \qquad (1)$$

where K is the kernel size, C^{out} is the output feature channel number, $H' = H//S$, $W' = W//S$, $//$ is floor division, $\mathbf{B}_{C^{out}}$ is the bias. In the encoding part, ReLU is used as the activation function. Convolutional layers with strides of 2 are used for feature map down-sampling. In order to avoid over-fitting, L2 regularization is applied after each convolutional layer. The channel number of the first convolutional layer is 16 and incrementally doubles after each down-sampling convolution. The output of the encoding part is received by the prediction part which consists of three fully-connected layers with ReLU activation functions and L2 regularizers. The output dimension of each fully-connected layer is 2048, 1024 and numY × 3 respectively. The final output layer uses a linear activation function. Details of the PointOutNet can be found in Fig. 2.

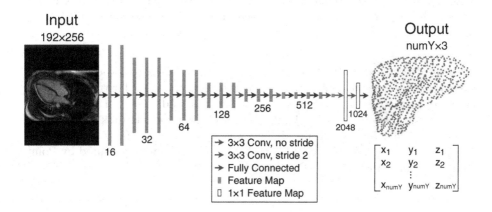

Fig. 2. Detailed network architecture of PointOutNet.

As point cloud is an unordered data format, Using the regular L1 or L2 loss to calculate the corresponding distance error between the predicted point cloud and the ground truth may cause regression difficulty. Hence Chamfer distance is used as the loss function. It calculates the distance between the predicted point cloud and the ground truth as:

$$Loss = \sum_{\hat{y} \in \hat{Y}} \min_{y \in Y} ||\hat{y} - y||^2_2 + \sum_{y \in Y} \min_{\hat{y} \in \hat{Y}} ||y - \hat{y}||^2_2 \qquad (2)$$

The advantage of this loss function is that it is easy to differentiate and robust against outliers [3].

2.3   Experimental Setup

Data Collection. 27 RV subjects including 9 Hypertrophic Cardiomyopathy (HCM) patients and 18 asymptomatic subjects were scanned by a 1.5 T Magnetic Resonance (MR) scanner (Sonata, Siemens, Erlangen, Germany) from the atrioventricular ring to the apex. The time frames are 19−25. The slice gap is 10 mm. The pixel spacing is 1.5–2 mm. Pre-operative 3D RV meshes were segmented manually from multiple short-axis 2D images for generating pre-operative 3D SSM. Synchronized 2D images were scanned at the four-chamber long axis scan plane which is the optimal scan plane based on [13]. Leave-one-out cross validation was performed as suggested by [13] where one time frame was used for the testing while all others were used for the training. In total, 609 experiments were performed.

Data Pre-processing. The 2D input images were of dimensions of 192×256. Their intensities were normalized to $[0, 1]$ according to the maximum intensity of each image. Batch size was set as one. Batches were fed into the network in a random order. The number of vertices for each patient varied from 800 to 2500, hence the feature channel number in the last layer of the PointOutNet needs to be adjusted individually for each patient. $\mathbf{Y}$ was centered at $(0, 0, 0)$ by subtracting its center coordinate.

Training Configuration. 1500 epochs were trained for each experiment. The learning rate was set as 0.003, and Adam optimizer was used for training. With a CPU of Intel Xeon (R) E5-1650 v4@3.60 GHz×12 and a GPU of Nvidia Titan XP, training one subject with 19–25 time frames or models took about seven hours. The time for testing one image was approximately 0.055 s. The error between the predicted point cloud and the ground truth was measured by Point Cloud-to-Point Cloud (PC-to-PC) error as:

$$Error = \sum_{\hat{\mathbf{y}} \in \hat{\mathbf{Y}}} min_{\mathbf{y} \in \mathbf{Y}} ||\hat{\mathbf{y}} - \mathbf{y}||_2^2 / \text{numY} \qquad (3)$$

3   Result

PC-to-PC errors for different time frames for 12 subjects are shown in Sect. 3.1. Four instantiated point clouds are shown in Sect. 3.2. The result compared with the two-stage shape instantiation by using PLSR and KPLSR learning are shown in Sect. 3.3.

3.1   PC-to-PC Error for Each Time Frame

The PC-to-PC errors for each time frame of 12 subjects selected randomly from the 27 subjects are shown in Fig. 3. We can see that errors are around 1–3 mm for

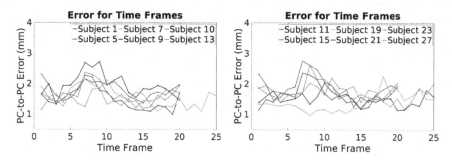

Fig. 3. The PC-to-PC error for each time frame for 12 subjects selected randomly from the 27 subjects.

all time frames. There are no excessively high peaks, which illustrates the stability of the proposed one-stage shape instantiation with PointOutNet. Slightly higher errors exist at the beginning and the end time frame (e.g. 1 and 25) and the middle time frame (e.g. 9), which is common as it was also observed in [13]. As these time frames are boundary time frames which are at either systole or diastole. By moving these time frames from the training data, the trained model can not see the boundaries. This happens only in this paper, as leave-one-out cross validation is used. In the real world application, this will be a minor issue, as the training data will cover all boundaries.

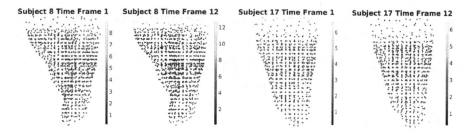

Fig. 4. Intuitive illustrations of the instantiation results of two randomly selected subjects at the systole and diastole time frame, color indicates the PC-to-PC error for each vertex in *mm*.

3.2   Instantiation Examples

The point clouds predicted by the PointOutNet at the systole and diastole time frames from two randomly selected subjects are shown in Fig. 4. Empirically, the predictions at the systole and diastole time frames are with slightly higher errors. We can see that most vertices in the middle part have an error of 2 mm while vertices at the top part - atrioventricular ring have higher errors. This is because the 2D MRI slices end at the atrioventricular ring, introducing plane area and sparse vertices at the top part in the 3D SSM mesh. This phenomenon increases the difficulty of vertices prediction at the top part and introduces a higher error.

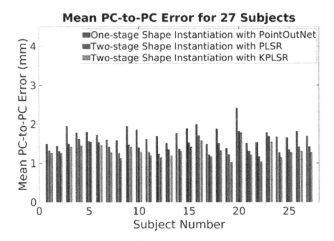

Fig. 5. The mean PC-to-PC error for 27 subjects with PLSR-based and KPLSR-based two-stage shape instantiation and PointOutNet-based one-stage shape instantiation.

3.3 Comparisons to Other Methods

The proposed one-stage shape instantiation with PointOutNet was compared to previous two-stage shape instantiation with PLSR and KPLSR. The mean PC-to-PC error for each subject is shown in Fig. 5. We can see that comparable accuracy was achieved by the proposed method. In general, the mean PC-to-PC error of the proposed method is around 1.5 mm.

4   Discussion

In the one-stage shape instantiation with PointOutNet, the predicted point cloud is not with a corresponding vertex order to the ground truth. This is due to the fact that the used loss function, Chamfer distance, takes the nearest distance of a predicted vertex to the ground truth into consideration rather than the distance of a predicted vertex to a single and corresponding vertex of the ground truth. Though the Chamfer distance loss loses the vertex correspondence information, it offers larger exploration space for the network to converge. Regular L1 and L2 loss function were tested with vertex correspondences, however, the network experienced convergence difficulty and generated poor predictions. Unlike [13] where the prediction is a point cloud with vertex correspondence and hence the 3D mesh can be achieved directly by applying the 3D SSM triangle connectivity, an additional 3D reconstruction algorithm is needed for a complete mesh instantiation in this paper.

Boundary effect where shape instantiation achieves worse performance at boundary time frames also exists in the one-stage shape instantiation with PointOutNet in this paper. In the real application, the training data will cover the boundary time frames and this effect will be alleviated. KPLSR-based two-stage shape instantiation has the kernel width as a sensitive hyper-parameter, which needs to be adjusted manually and carefully, whereas the proposed one-stage shape instantiation with PointOutNet is fully automatic. We think the main bottleneck for achieving higher instantiation accuracy is the loss function. We will explore this topic further in the future.

5 Conclusion

A one-stage shape instantiation algorithm with PointOutNet and Chamfer loss was proposed in this paper. A (2D image)-to-(3D point cloud) inference was achieved end-to-end with comparable accuracy and higher automation. To the best of the author's knowledge, this is the first work that applies deep learning into 3D shape instantiation in medical applications. It demonstrates the possibility of deep learning to achieve cross-modality tasks, which may indicate a wide application of deep learning in intra-operative and real-time navigation. For example, predicting 3D prosthesis pose or navigating medical robot's joint angle from 2D images directly.

References

1. Choy, C.B., Xu, D., Gwak, J.Y., Chen, K., Savarese, S.: 3D-R2N2: a unified approach for single and multi-view 3D object reconstruction. In: Leibe, B., Matas, J., Sebe, N., Welling, M. (eds.) ECCV 2016. LNCS, vol. 9912, pp. 628–644. Springer, Cham (2016). https://doi.org/10.1007/978-3-319-46484-8_38
2. Cool, D., Downey, D., Izawa, J., Chin, J., Fenster, A.: 3D prostate model formation from non-parallel 2D ultrasound biopsy images. Med. Image Anal. **10**(6), 875–887 (2006)
3. Fan, H., Su, H., Guibas, L.J.: A point set generation network for 3D object reconstruction from a single image. In: Proceedings of the IEEE Conference on Computer Vision and Pattern Recognition, pp. 605–613 (2017)
4. Kulon, D., Wang, H., Güler, R.A., Bronstein, M., Zafeiriou, S.: Single image 3D hand reconstruction with mesh convolutions. arXiv preprint arXiv:1905.01326 (2019)
5. Lee, S.-L., Chung, A., Lerotic, M., Hawkins, M.A., Tait, D., Yang, G.-Z.: Dynamic shape instantiation for intra-operative guidance. In: Jiang, T., Navab, N., Pluim, J.P.W., Viergever, M.A. (eds.) MICCAI 2010. LNCS, vol. 6361, pp. 69–76. Springer, Heidelberg (2010). https://doi.org/10.1007/978-3-642-15705-9_9
6. Mandikal, P., Murthy, N., Agarwal, M., Babu, R.V.: 3D-LMNet: latent embedding matching for accurate and diverse 3D point cloud reconstruction from a single image. arXiv preprint arXiv:1807.07796 (2018)
7. Manu: nonrigidicp (2016). https://uk.mathworks.com/matlabcentral/fileexchange/41396-nonrigidicp. Accessed 02 Apr 2019

8. Toth, D., Pfister, M., Maier, A., Kowarschik, M., Hornegger, J.: Adaption of 3D models to 2D X-Ray images during endovascular abdominal aneurysm repair. In: Navab, N., Hornegger, J., Wells, W.M., Frangi, A.F. (eds.) MICCAI 2015. LNCS, vol. 9349, pp. 339–346. Springer, Cham (2015). https://doi.org/10.1007/978-3-319-24553-9_42

9. Zheng, J.Q., Zhou, X.Y., Riga, C., Yang, G.Z.: 3D path planning from a single 2D fluoroscopic image for robot assisted fenestrated endovascular aortic repair. arXiv preprint arXiv:1809.05955 (2018)

10. Zheng, J.Q., Zhou, X.Y., Yang, G.Z.: Real-time 3D shape instantiation for partially-deployed stent segment from a single 2D fluoroscopic image in robot-assisted fenestrated endovascular aortic repair. arXiv preprint arXiv:1902.11089 (2019)

11. Zhou, X., Yang, G., Riga, C., Lee, S.: Stent graft shape instantiation for fenestrated endovascular aortic repair. In: The Hamlyn Symposium on Medical Robotics, pp. 78–79 (2016)

12. Zhou, X.Y., Lin, J., Riga, C., Yang, G.Z., Lee, S.L.: Real-time 3-D shape instantiation from single fluoroscopy projection for fenestrated stent graft deployment. IEEE Robot. Autom. Lett. **3**(2), 1314–1321 (2018)

13. Zhou, X.Y., Yang, G.Z., Lee, S.L.: A real-time and registration-free framework for dynamic shape instantiation. Med. Image Anal. **44**, 86–97 (2018)

Placental Flattening via Volumetric Parameterization

S. Mazdak Abulnaga[1]([✉]), Esra Abaci Turk[2], Mikhail Bessmeltsev[3],
P. Ellen Grant[2], Justin Solomon[1], and Polina Golland[1]

[1] Computer Science and Artificial Intelligence Lab, MIT, Cambridge, MA, USA
abulnaga@mit.edu
[2] Fetal-Neonatal Neuroimaging and Developmental Science Center, Boston
Children's Hospital, Harvard Medical School, Boston, MA, USA
[3] Department of Computer Science and Operations Research, Université de
Montréal, Montréal, QC, Canada

Abstract. We present a volumetric mesh-based algorithm for flattening the placenta to a canonical template to enable effective visualization of local anatomy and function. Monitoring placental function *in vivo* promises to support pregnancy assessment and to improve care outcomes. We aim to alleviate visualization and interpretation challenges presented by the shape of the placenta when it is attached to the curved uterine wall. To do so, we flatten the volumetric mesh that captures placental shape to resemble the well-studied *ex vivo* shape. We formulate our method as a map from the *in vivo* shape to a flattened template that minimizes the symmetric Dirichlet energy to control distortion throughout the volume. Local injectivity is enforced via constrained line search during gradient descent. We evaluate the proposed method on 28 placenta shapes extracted from MRI images in a clinical study of placental function. We achieve sub-voxel accuracy in mapping the boundary of the placenta to the template while successfully controlling distortion throughout the volume. We illustrate how the resulting mapping of the placenta enhances visualization of placental anatomy and function. Our implementation is freely available at https://github.com/mabulnaga/placenta-flattening.

Keywords: Placenta · Fetal MRI · Flattening · Injective maps ·
Volumetric mesh parameterization · Anatomy visualization

1 Introduction

The placenta is a critical organ that connects the fetus to the maternal blood system. Placental dysfunction increases the risk of pregnancy complications, with long-term effects on a child's health and development and the mother's health. It is therefore critical to monitor placental function and health *in vivo*. Ultrasound and MRI capture detailed information about the placental position, shape, and tissue properties [11]. Blood oxygen level dependent (BOLD) MRI has recently

© Springer Nature Switzerland AG 2019
D. Shen et al. (Eds.): MICCAI 2019, LNCS 11767, pp. 39–47, 2019.
https://doi.org/10.1007/978-3-030-32251-9_5

been demonstrated to assess oxygen transport within the placenta [5,11], providing initial evidence for clinical utility of MRI for functional assessment of the placenta. Compared with ultrasound, MRI provides direct measurements of placental function, which provides signals necessary to study function and assess pathology [5,11].

The *in vivo* shape of the placenta is determined by the curved surface of the uterine wall to which it is attached during pregnancy. This presents significant challenges for interpretation of the MRI scans. No common standard exists for visualizing the functional or anatomical images of the placenta whose *in vivo* shape and location of attachment to the uterine wall vary greatly across subjects. We present a novel algorithm for mapping the placental shape observed in an MRI scan to a flattened template that resembles the organ's well-studied *ex vivo* flattened shape, to alleviate visualization challenges during *in vivo* examination and to facilitate clinical research and development of placental health biomarkers. Our work offers the first step toward developing a common coordinate system to enable statistical analysis.

We build on state-of-the-art mesh parameterization methods to represent and estimate the deformation of the placenta onto a template. Mesh parameterization is a topic of active research in geometry processing for mapping surfaces to canonical domains such as planes or spheres while guaranteeing desirable properties of the mapping such as injectivity [8,10]. When applied to cortical mapping, this parameterization facilitates visualization and population studies [2,12,13]. The formulation may estimate the optimal map by minimizing a cost function that penalizes areal distortion [13], changes in geodesic distance [2], or more commonly a combination of different distortion measures [12]. In contrast to the inherently two-dimensional (2D) cortex however, the placenta is a fully three-dimensional (3D) organ. Image information along the depth direction from the maternal to the fetal side of the placenta is important for characterizing function. The parameterization must therefore map the entire volume.

In placenta imaging, a method for placental flattening has been recently demonstrated [6]. Their algorithm represents the placenta as a stack of parallel surfaces spanning the thickness of the organ. Each surface is flattened separately by mapping the boundary to a disk with each interior vertex moved to the average of its neighbors. This approach is limited in two ways. First, the lack of correspondence across surfaces throughout the volume results in through-plane artifacts, distorting important depth-wise information. Second, due to the variability in placental shape, constraining the mapping to a fixed boundary results in high distortion. In contrast, our method computes a continuous volumetric mapping with free boundary that ensures uniform consistency throughout the volume and enables explicit control of the resulting deformation.

To our knowledge, this is the first volumetric approach for mapping the placenta to a canonical domain. Our algorithm estimates the transformation of the volumetric mesh to a template as the solution of an optimization problem. This formulation readily accepts a broad family of templates and shape distortion functions. We choose to minimize the symmetric Dirichlet energy [9,10] to penalize local deformations of the volumetric mesh. We evaluate our method on images from a clinical MRI study, demonstrating effective mapping of the highly variable placental shape to the template with minimal distortion. We demonstrate improved visualization of anatomical structures and their surrounding context, illustrating the promise of our algorithm to support clinical use of MRI in placental imaging.

2   Methods

We represent the placental shape as a tetrahedral mesh that contains N vertices and K tetrahedra. In our experiments, we extract such meshes from segmented MRI scans as described later. We parameterize the mapping via mesh vertex locations in the template coordinate system and interpolate the deformation to the interior of each tetrahedron using a locally affine (piecewise-linear) model. The mapping is geometry-based so it is independent of imaging modality used.

2.1   Problem Formulation

Let $X \in \mathbb{R}^{3 \times N}$ be a matrix whose columns are the 3D coordinates of all mesh vertices in the template space with the M boundary vertices forming the first M columns. Let $X_k \in \mathbb{R}^{3 \times 4}$ be a matrix whose columns are the 3D coordinates of the four corner vertices of tetrahedron k $(k = 1, \ldots, K)$ in the template space. We formulate the mapping as an optimization problem over the mesh vertices that seeks to map to the template space while minimizing shape distortion. We formulate the general objective function as

$$\phi(X) = \underbrace{\sum_{m=1}^{M} A_m T\left(x_m\right)}_{\text{Template match}} + \lambda \underbrace{\sum_{k=1}^{K} V_k \mathcal{D}\left(X_k\right)}_{\text{Distortion}}, \tag{1}$$

where $\{x_m\}_{m=1}^{M}$ are the boundary vertex coordinates in the template system, $T\left(\cdot\right)$ is a measure of distance from the template shape, A_m is the normalized barycentric area of boundary vertex m in the original space, $\mathcal{D}\left(\cdot\right)$ measures local distortion, V_k is the normalized volume of tetrahedron k in the original space, and λ is a parameter that governs the trade-off between the template fit and the shape distortion. The distortion term regularizes the mapping.

We use a locally affine model to capture the deformation of tetrahedron Z_k in the original image space to X_k in the template space. The Jacobian matrix $J(X_k) = (X_k B)(Z_k B)^{-1}$ captures the linear transformation of the new vertex coordinates X_k while ignoring the shared translation component. The constant matrix $B \in \mathbb{R}^{4 \times 3}$ extracts three basis vectors defining the tetrahedron.

We measure local distortion using the symmetric Dirichlet energy density

$$\mathcal{D}(J) = \|J\|_F^2 + \|J^{-1}\|_F^2 = \sum_{i=1}^{3} \left(\sigma_i^2 + \sigma_i^{-2}\right), \tag{2}$$

where $\| \cdot \|_F$ is the Frobenius norm and $\{\sigma_1, \sigma_2, \sigma_3\}$ are the singular values of matrix J [8,10]. We chose the symmetric Dirichlet energy since it penalizes expansion and shrinking equally and favors a locally-injective mapping.

The image intensities are mapped to the template space using barycentric coordinates (BC). The BC represent a voxel in a tetrahedron as a convex combination of the tetrahedon's vertices. Since our mapping is injective and affine, the resulting voxel position is determined using its BC and the mapped vertices.

2.2   Template

After evaluating several volumetric templates (ellipsoid, sphere, cylinder; not shown), we find that the best results (i.e., clear anatomical structure and small local distortion) are achieved by encouraging constant height of the flattened placenta to mimic the post-delivery examination process, where the maternal side is placed on an examination table. The fetal side is flattened to the ease visualization. The function $T(\cdot)$ measures the distance to the appropriate plane:

$$T(x) = \begin{cases} (x^{(3)} - h)^2 & \text{if } x \in \mathcal{F}(\partial Z), \\ (x^{(3)} + h)^2 & \text{if } x \in \mathcal{M}(\partial Z), \\ 0 & \text{otherwise,} \end{cases} \tag{3}$$

where $x^{(3)}$ refers to the third coordinate of point x in the template coordinate system, ∂Z denotes the mesh boundary in the original image space, and $\mathcal{F}(\partial Z)$, $\mathcal{M}(\partial Z)$ denote the fetal and maternal sides of ∂Z. We identify the maternal and fetal sides via spectral clustering [7] as described below.

We employ a similarity metric based on the angle between unit normals of boundary vertices $(\hat{n})$. We construct an affinity matrix $W \in \mathbb{R}^{M \times M}$ whose (i, j) element $w_{i,j} = \exp\{\gamma (\hat{n}_i^\top \hat{n}_j)\}$ for any two boundary vertices i and j that are connected by a path of at most 3 edges (the 3-ring neighborhood), and $w_{i,j} = 0$ otherwise. The parameter γ penalizes the variation in the orientation of the normals. We cluster the boundary vertices by thresholding the values of the second smallest eigenvector of the Laplacian $L = I - D^{-\frac{1}{2}} W D^{-\frac{1}{2}}$, where D is a diagonal matrix with $d_{i,i} = \sum_j w_{i,j}$ and I is the identity matrix [7]. Since the maternal side is more curved, we assign the corresponding label to the cluster with the larger number of vertices on the convex hull of the mesh.

We use the term *rim* to denote the highly curved region that separates the fetal and maternal sides. We first assign to the rim all vertices on the boundary of the two clusters, i.e., those with neighbors in the other cluster. The rim is then dilated to a set width based on the approximated geodesic distance along the mesh boundary. The geodesic distance accounts for mesh irregularities and ensures a consistent rim width.

2.3   Optimization

We minimize cost function $\phi(\cdot)$ in (1) using gradient descent. We initialize the mapping using the identity transformation. The gradient of the template term is linear in the vertices, $\frac{\partial T(x)}{\partial x^{(3)}} = 2\left(x^{(3)} \pm h\right)$. We derive the gradient of the symmetric Dirichlet energy term defined in (2) using the chain rule for matrices:

$$\frac{d\,\|J(X_k)\|_F^2}{d\,X_k} = X_k\left[2B\left(Z_kB\right)^{-1}\left(Z_kB\right)^{-T}B^T\right],$$

$$\frac{d\,\|J(X_k)^{-1}\|_F^2}{d\,X_k} = -2X_kB\left(B^TX_k^TX_kB\right)^{-1}B^TZ_k^TZ_kB\left(B^TX_k^TX_kB\right)^{-1}B^T.$$

We employ line search to prevent tetrahedra from "flipping," i.e., from crossing the singularity point of zero volume, thereby enforcing local injectivity [10]. In every iteration, we determine the largest value η such that adjusting the current vertex locations X by $-\eta\nabla\phi(X)$ avoids singularities for all tetrahedra. The (signed) volume of tetrahedron k is computed as the determinant of matrix $(X_k - \eta\nabla\phi(X_k))B$ and is a cubic polynomial of η. The smallest, positive real root provides the upper limit for η in the line search [10].

2.4 Implementation Details

We generate tetrahedral meshes from segmentation labelmaps using iso2mesh [1]. Prior to mapping, we center the mesh and rotate it to align its principal axes with the template. We assume the algorithm convergences when the Frobenius norm of the gradient is lower than 1×10^{-4}. We implemented the algorithm in MATLAB using GPU functionality to parallelize computation, and ran our experiments on an NVIDIA Titan Xp (12 GB) GPU. The algorithm took an average of 4083 iterations and took less than 20 min to converge. Our implementation is freely available at https://github.com/mabulnaga/placenta-flattening.

3 Experiments

Data: We validate the approach on a set of 28 MRI scans from 2 studies. The first is a twin study on 7 pregnant women (gestational age (GA): 28–34 weeks). All twin pregnancies had one placenta shared by the 2 twins. The second is a singleton pregnancy study on 11 women (GA: 27–40 weeks). For 10 of 11 subjects, scans were acquired in the supine and left lateral positions, yielding 20 different segmentations. MRI BOLD scans were acquired on a 3 T Siemens Skyra scanner (GRE-EPI, 3 mm³, TR = 5.8–8 s, TE = 32–36 ms, FA = 90°). The placenta was manually segmented by a trained observer and input to the meshing software, which produced 6,500 tetrahedra and 2,800 surface triangles on average.

Parameters: We used a grid search to determine the values of the hyperparameters. We set shape distortion parameter $\lambda = 1$ as it was in the optimal trade-off range between the template match and distortion (Fig. 1a). We set the template half-height h to be half of the placenta thickness estimated from the histogram of the distance transform values inside the segmentation boundary. We set the spectral clustering parameter $\gamma = 20$ and used a boundary geodesic distance of 5 voxels as the width of the rim.

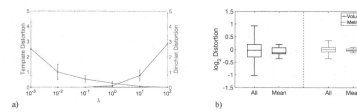

Fig. 1. (a) The final template matching term and distortion energy approaching optimality near $\lambda = 1$; (b) Distributions of distortion. We report (i) the statistics of volumetric and metric distortion across all tetrahedra (All), weighted by original tetrahedral volume, and (ii) of the mean distortion values across the 28 cases (Mean). The distributions are unimodal and well-contained at the extrema.

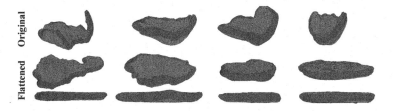

Fig. 2. Flattening results for four tetrahedral meshes: One twin (left) and three singleton pregnancies. Fetal sides are facing upwards and the rim is shown in red. The greatly differing shapes in the dataset are robustly mapped and the rim is a faithful representation of the curved area separating the fetal and maternal sides. (Color figure online)

Evaluation: We use the log-determinant of the Jacobian matrix $\log_2 \det (J(X_k))$ of tetrahedron k to quantify local volumetric distortion [4]. We quantify metric distortion using the ratio of edge lengths $\log_2 (x_{ij}/z_{ij})$. We visually assess the quality of the transformation by mapping the BOLD MRI to the template coordinate system.

We compare with the prior parameterization approach in [6] where 2D surfaces spanning the placenta were independently parameterized to a disk in $\mathbb{R}^2$. The surfaces were derived by cutting Euclidean level sets to minimize local curvature changes. To emulate this method, we derive such 2D surfaces by intersecting the flattened placenta volume with planes spaced one voxel apart. We harmonically parameterize each surface to a disk [3], each with a corresponding point mapped to the north point of the disk. We scale the areas and edge lengths in the parameterized space to have mean 0 areal and metric log-distortion.

3.1   Results

For all cases, our algorithm achieves sub-voxel accuracy of matching the template (median of 0.09 voxels, max. of 0.30 voxels). The resulting transformations achieve close to minimum values of the symmetric Dirichlet energy (median 3.87% higher, max. 9.04% higher than the smallest possible value), where the

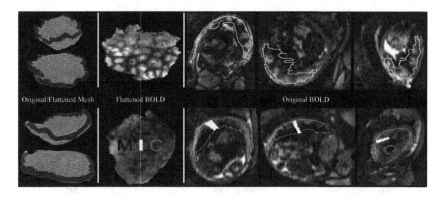

Fig. 3. Visual assessment of landmarks in two twin pregnancy subjects. Top: The cotyledons, characterized by a honeycomb structure of small hyperintense regions, are immediately apparent in the flattened view. The local anatomy surrounding the two cotyledons with marked centers is lost in the original images. Bottom: Mapping the fabricated landmark "MIC" to the original volume loses contextual information since the curved geometry distorts the letters and they are not easily seen together. Local anatomy is difficult to visualize in the original volume due to the curvature of the uterine wall that determines the *in vivo* shape of the placenta.

energy is minimized by the identity transformation. Figure 1b demonstrates the mapping achieves minimal local volumetric and metric distortions. We did not observe differences across twin and singleton pregnancies.

Figure 2 illustrates the mapping results for four placentae, highlighting the variability in shape encountered in the dataset. We are able to map difficult structures robustly such as the fold in the first placenta and bowl-shape in the last. The estimated rim also effectively separates the maternal and fetal regions.

Figure 3 demonstrates that the mapping enhances visualization of landmarks. The mapped BOLD intensity patterns clearly visualize local anatomy and function as is apparent in the honeycomb structure of the cotyledons, which are the circular structures that exchange oxygen and nutrients between the maternal blood and the fetal blood in the chorionic villi [5]. Cotyledons appear hyperintense in BOLD MRI. Similarly, contextual information is lost when visualizing a fabricated landmark (the letters "MIC") in the curved volume. Since the inherent geometry of the placenta is flat, the letters could represent biomarkers. The curved geometry of the *in vivo* placenta demonstrates immediate difficulty in visualizing the details that are clearly seen in the flattened view. Several views in the original image space are required to identify anatomical landmarks.

Figure 4 compares our method with the baseline 2D approach. Our method produces considerably lower distortion across all cases. Mapping to a fixed boundary results in higher distortion, and we observe image artifacts due to the lack of coupling across planes. These results confirm the need for a free boundary volumetric parameterization method. Finally, we note that the nested surfaces in the original space were derived from the volumetric parameterization to the flattened space. In practice, estimating these surfaces is challenging and requires a multi-step specialized pipeline as in [6].

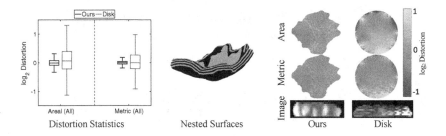

Fig. 4. Comparison with the baseline 2D parameterization approach. Left: Our method results in significantly lower distortion across all cases ($p < .001$). Right: Our free-boundary parameterization results in lower and more homogeneous spatial distributions of distortion as demonstrated on an interior surface. The baseline approach also creates through-plane imaging artifacts due to a lack of coupling across flattened planes.

4   Conclusion

We developed a volumetric mesh-based mapping of the placenta to a flattened template represented by two parallel planes, resembling the *ex vivo* flattened shape of the organ, thereby enabling visualization of local anatomy and function. An immediate next step is to assess the utility for clinical research by quantifying the improvement in identifying known key biomarkers and anatomical features. In future work, we will improve the template using anatomical data such as the umbilical cord insertion. We are collecting higher-resolution anatomical images to include landmarks that are not easily seen in the BOLD (functional) images. This work is the first step towards developing a common coordinate system to visualize, examine, and study the organ as well as to support statistical analysis across subjects and time. Such a framework promises to advance the state of the art in studies of the placenta and to provide MRI biomarkers of fetal health.

Acknowledgments. This work was supported in part by NIH NIBIB NAC P41EB015902, NIH NICHD U01HD087211, NSF IIS-1838071, Air Force FA9550-19-1-0319, Wistron, SIP, AWS, NSF Graduate Research Fellowship, and NSERC Post Graduate Scholarship.

References

1. Fang, Q., Boas, D.A.: Tetrahedral mesh generation from volumetric binary and grayscale images. In: 2009 IEEE ISBI, pp. 1142–1145 (2009)
2. Fischl, B., Sereno, M.I., Dale, A.M.: Cortical surface-based analysis: II: inflation, flattening, and a surface-based coordinate system. Neuroimage **9**, 195–207 (1999)

3. Joshi, P., Meyer, M., DeRose, T., Green, B., Sanocki, T.: Harmonic coordinates for character articulation. ACM Trans. Graph. **26**(3), 87–93 (2007)
4. Leow, A.D., et al.: Statistical properties of Jacobian maps and the realization of unbiased large-deformation nonlinear image registration. IEEE TMI **26**(6), 822–832 (2007)
5. Luo, J., et al.: In vivo quantification of placental insufficiency by BOLD MRI: a human study. Sci. Rep. **7**(1), 3713 (2017)
6. Miao, H., et al.: Placenta maps: in utero placental health assessment of the human fetus. IEEE TVCG **23**(6), 1612–1623 (2017)
7. Ng, A.Y., Jordan, M.I., Weiss, Y.: On spectral clustering: analysis and an algorithm. In: Advances in Neural Information Processing Systems, pp. 849–856 (2002)
8. Rabinovich, M., Poranne, R., Panozzo, D., Sorkine-Hornung, O.: Scalable locally injective mappings. ACM Trans. Graph. **36**(4) (2017)
9. Schreiner, J., Asirvatham, A., Praun, E., Hoppe, H.: Inter-surface mapping. ACM Trans. Graph. **23**(3), 870–877 (2004)
10. Smith, J., Schaefer, S.: Bijective parameterization with free boundaries. ACM Trans. Graph. **34**(4), 70:1–70:9 (2015)
11. Sørensen, A., Peters, D., Simonsen, C., Pedersen, M., Stausbøl-Grøn, B., Christiansen, O.B., et al.: Changes in human fetal oxygenation during maternal hyperoxia as estimated by BOLD MRI. Prenat. Diagn. **33**, 141–145 (2013)
12. Timsari, B., Leahy, R.M.: Optimization method for creating semi-isometric flat maps of the cerebral cortex. In: Proceedings of SPIE, Medical Imaging, pp. 698–709 (2000)
13. Tosun, D., Prince, J.L.: Hemispherical map for the human brain cortex. In: Proceeding of the SPIE, Medical Imaging, pp. 290–301 (2001)

Fast Polynomial Approximation to Heat Diffusion in Manifolds

Shih-Gu Huang[1(✉)], Ilwoo Lyu[2], Anqi Qiu[3], and Moo K. Chung[1]

[1] University of Wisconsin, Madison, WI, USA
shihgu@gmail.com, mkchung@wisc.edu
[2] Vanderbilt University, Nashville, TN, USA
[3] National University of Singapore, Singapore, Singapore

Abstract. Heat diffusion has been widely used in image processing for surface fairing, mesh regularization and surface data smoothing. We present a new fast and accurate numerical method to solve heat diffusion on curved surfaces. This is achieved by approximating the heat kernel using high degree orthogonal polynomials in the spectral domain. The proposed polynomial expansion method avoids solving for the eigenfunctions of the Laplace-Beltrami operator, which is computationally costly for large-scale surface meshes, and the numerical instability associated with the finite element method based diffusion solvers. We apply the proposed method to localize the sex differences in cortical brain sulcal and gyral curve patterns.

Keywords: Chebyshev polynomials · Diffusion wavelets · Heat diffusion · Laplace-Beltrami operator · Brain cortical surface · Sulcal graph patterns

1 Introduction

Heat diffusion has been widely used in image processing as a form of smoothing and noise reduction starting with Perona and Malik's groundbreaking study [15]. Over the years, the diffusion equation has been solved by various numerical techniques [1–4,17]. In [1,2], the isotropic heat equation was solved by the least squares estimation of the Laplace-Beltrami (LB) operator and the finite difference method (FDM). In [3,4], the heat diffusion was solved iteratively by the discrete estimate of the LB-operator using the finite element method (FEM) and the FDM. However, the FDM is known to suffer numerical instability if the sufficiently small step size is not chosen in the forward Euler scheme. In [3,16], diffusion was solved by expanding the heat kernel as a series expansion of the LB-eigenfunctions. Although the LB-eigenfunction approach avoids the numerical instability associated with the FEM based diffusion solvers [3,4], the computational complexity is very high for large-scale surface meshes.

Motivated by the diffusion wavelet transform [11,12,20] and convolutional neural networks (CNN) [5] on graphs, we propose a new fast and accurate numerical method to solve the heat diffusion on manifolds by expanding the heat kernel using orthogonal polynomials. Taking advantage of recurrence relations of

© Springer Nature Switzerland AG 2019
D. Shen et al. (Eds.): MICCAI 2019, LNCS 11767, pp. 48–56, 2019.
https://doi.org/10.1007/978-3-030-32251-9_6

orthogonal polynomials [14], the computational run time of solving diffusion is substantially reduced. We present three examples of the proposed methods based on the Chebyshev, Hermite and Laguerre polynomials. The proposed method is significantly faster than the LB-eigenfunction approach and FEM based diffusion solvers [3]. As an application, the proposed method is applied to a large number of magnetic resonance images (MRI) to localize the sex differences in the sulcal and gyral patterns of the human brain.

The main contributions of the paper are (1) a novel polynomial scheme to solve diffusion on manifolds, which is faster than the existing numerical schemes while achieving high numerical accuracy, and (2) an innovative way to analyze the sulcal and gyral patterns of the whole brain in a mass univariate fashion.

2 Methods

2.1 Heat Diffusion on Manifolds

Suppose functional data $f \in L^2(\mathcal{M})$, the space of square integrable functions on manifold $\mathcal{M}$ with inner product $\langle f, h \rangle = \int_\mathcal{M} f(p)h(p)d\mu(p)$, where $\mu(p)$ is the Lebesgue measure such that $\mu(\mathcal{M})$ is the total area or volume of $\mathcal{M}$. Let Δ denote the LB-operator on $\mathcal{M}$. The isotropic heat diffusion at diffusion time σ on $\mathcal{M}$ with initial condition f is given by

$$\frac{\partial g(p, \sigma)}{\partial \sigma} + \Delta g = 0, \quad g(p, \sigma = 0) = f(p). \tag{1}$$

It has been shown that the convolution of f with heat kernel K_σ is the unique solution of the heat diffusion equation [3]. Let ψ_j be the eigenfunctions of the LB-operator with eigenvalues λ_j, i.e., $\Delta \psi_j = \lambda_j \psi_j$, with $0 = \lambda_0 \leq \lambda_1 \leq \lambda_2 \leq \cdots$. The heat kernel can be expanded by the LB-eigenfunctions with exponential weight $e^{-\lambda \sigma}$ as $K_\sigma(p, q) = \sum_{j=0}^\infty e^{-\lambda_j \sigma} \psi_j(p)\psi_j(q)$ [3]. Then, with Fourier coefficients $f_j = \langle f, \psi_j \rangle$, the heat diffusion can be expressed as

$$g(p, \sigma) = K_\sigma * f(p) = \sum_{j=0}^\infty e^{-\lambda_j \sigma} f_j \psi_j(p). \tag{2}$$

2.2 Heat Diffusion Using Polynomial Expansion

Consider an orthogonal polynomial basis P_n such as Chebyshev, Hermite and Laguerre polynomials, which is often defined by the following second order recurrence [14],

$$P_{n+1}(\lambda) = (\alpha_n \lambda + \beta_n)P_n(\lambda) + \gamma_n P_{n-1}(\lambda), \quad n \geq 0, \tag{3}$$

with initial conditions $P_{-1}(\lambda) = 0$ and $P_0(\lambda) = 1$ in some interval $[a, b]$. We expand the exponential weight $e^{-\lambda \sigma}$ of the heat kernel as

$$e^{-\lambda \sigma} = \sum_{n=0}^\infty c_{\sigma,n} P_n(\lambda), \quad c_{\sigma,n} = \int_a^b e^{-\lambda \sigma} P_n(\lambda)d\mu(\lambda). \tag{4}$$

Table 1. The orthogonal conditions, expansion coefficients and recurrence relations of polynomials. I_n in Chebyshev are the modified Bessel functions of the first kind [14].

Method	Orthogonal conditions	Coefficients $c_{\sigma,n}$	Recurrence relations $\alpha_n, \ \beta_n, \ \gamma_n$
Chebyshev	$\int_{-1}^{1} \dfrac{T_n(\lambda)T_k(\lambda)}{\sqrt{1-\lambda^2}} d\lambda = \dfrac{(1+\delta_{n0})\pi}{2}\delta_{nk}$	$e^{-\frac{\lambda_{max}}{2}\sigma}(2-\delta_{n0})$ $\cdot (-1)^n I_n(\lambda_{max}\sigma/2)$	$\dfrac{2(2-\delta_{n0})}{\lambda_{max}}, \ \delta_{n0}-2, \ -1$
Hermite	$\int_{-\infty}^{\infty} H_n(\lambda)H_k(\lambda)e^{-\lambda^2} d\lambda = \sqrt{\pi}2^n n!\delta_{nk}$	$\dfrac{1}{n!}\left(\dfrac{-\sigma}{2}\right)^n e^{\frac{\sigma^2}{4}}$	$2, \ 0, \ -2n$
Laguerre	$\int_{0}^{\infty} L_n(\lambda)L_k(\lambda)e^{-\lambda} d\lambda = \delta_{nk}$	$\dfrac{\sigma^n}{(\sigma+1)^{n+1}}$	$\dfrac{-1}{n+1}, \ \dfrac{2n+1}{n+1}, \ \dfrac{-n}{n+1}$

Using (4), the heat kernel convolution (2) becomes

$$K_\sigma * f = \sum_{n=0}^{\infty} c_{\sigma,n} \sum_{j=0}^{\infty} P_n(\lambda_j)f_j\psi_j. \tag{5}$$

Since $P_n(\lambda)$ is a polynomial of degree n, we have $P_n(\lambda_j)\psi_j = P_n(\Delta)\psi_j$, and

$$K_\sigma * f = \sum_{n=0}^{\infty} c_{\sigma,n} P_n(\Delta) f. \tag{6}$$

The direct computation of $P_n(\Delta)f$ requires the computation of $\Delta f, \cdots, \Delta^n f$, which is costly. Instead, we compute $P_n(\Delta)f$ by the recurrence

$$P_{n+1}(\Delta)f = (\alpha_n\Delta + \beta_n)P_n(\Delta)f + \gamma_n P_{n-1}(\Delta)f, \quad n \geq 0, \tag{7}$$

with initial conditions $P_{-1}(\Delta)f = 0$ and $P_0(\Delta)f = f$. In the numerical implementation, we discretized the LB-operator using the cotan formulation [3,20].

Chebyshev, Hermite and Laguerre Polynomials. We present three examples based on the Chebyshev T_n, Hermite H_n and Laguerre L_n polynomials. The Chebyshev polynomials were used in the diffusion wavelet transform [11,20] and CNN on graphs [5]. Following [11], we shift and scale the Chebyshev polynomials to $\overline{T}_n(\lambda) = T_n\left(\frac{2\lambda}{\lambda_{max}} - 1\right)$ over interval $[0, \lambda_{max}]$, where λ_{max} is the maximum eigenvalue of LB-operator in the numerical implementation. We derived the closed-form expressions of the expansion coefficients $c_{\sigma,n}$ for $\overline{T}_n$, H_n and L_n using the orthogonal conditions (Table 1) [10,14]. The parameters $\alpha_n, \beta_n, \gamma_n$ in the recurrence relations (3) and (7) for $\overline{T}_n$, H_n and L_n are also given in Table 1.

Figure 1 is an illustration of the heat diffusion of the left hippocampus surface mesh coordinates ($\sigma = 1.5$, $m = 100$). The reconstruction error is measured by the mean squared error (MSE) (measured in voxel width squared) between the polynomial expansion method and the original surface mesh. Since the Chebyshev expansion method converges the fastest with the smallest error in various surface meshes, it will be used through the paper but other polynomial methods can be similarly applicable. The MATLAB code for generating Fig. 1 is given in http://www.stat.wisc.edu/~mchung/chebyshev.

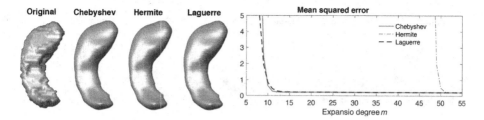

Fig. 1. Left: left hippocampus surface and heat diffusion with $\sigma = 1.5$ using the Chebyshev, Hermite and Laguerre polynomial expansion methods with degree $m = 100$. Right: MSE between the original surface mesh and the polynomial expansion methods for different m. The Chebyshev method converges the fastest in general.

Iterative Convolution. One can obtain diffusion related multiscale features at different time points by iteratively performing heat kernel smoothing. Instead of applying the polynomial expansion method separately for each σ, the computation can also be done quickly by the iterative heat kernel convolution [3]

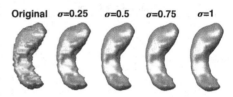

Fig. 2. Sequential application of Chebyshev expansion method with $\sigma = 0.25$ four times.

$$K_{\sigma_1 + \sigma_2 + \cdots + \sigma_m} * f = K_{\sigma_1} * K_{\sigma_2} \cdots * K_{\sigma_m} * f.$$

For example, if we compute $K_{0.25} * f$, then $K_{0.5} * f$ is simply computed as two repeated kernel convolution $K_{0.25} * (K_{0.25} * f)$, and diffusion with much larger diffusion time can be done similarly. Figure 2 displays heat diffusion with $\sigma = 0.25, 0.5, 0.75$ and 1 realized by iteratively applying the Chebyshev expansion method with $\sigma = 0.25$ sequentially four times.

2.3 Validation

We compared the Chebyshev expansion method against the FEM based diffusion solver [4] and the LB-eigenfunction approach [3] on the unit spheres with 2562, 10242, 40962 and 163842 mesh vertices. On the unit spheres, the ground truth of heat diffusion can be analytically constructed by the spherical harmonics (SPHARM) [18]. Consider the surface signal consisting of values 1, −1 and 0 (Fig. 3). The signal is represented using the SPHARM with degree 100, which is taken as the initial condition of heat diffusion. The SPHARM representation is taken as the ground truth since its diffusion can be analytically given. Figure 3 shows the result with $\sigma = 0.01$ on the unit sphere with 163842 vertices.

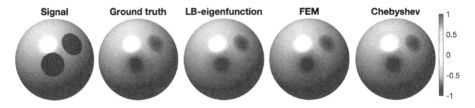

Fig. 3. Signal (initial condition) and ground truth of heat diffusion with $\sigma = 0.01$ are constructed by the SPHARM representation with degree 100. The LB-eigenfunction approach with 210 eigenfunctions, FEM based diffusion solver with 406 iterations, and Chebyshev expansion method with degree 45 have similar accuracy (MSE about 10^{-5}).

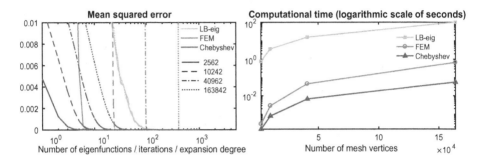

Fig. 4. Left: MSE of the LB-eigenfunction approach, FEM based diffusion solver and Chebyshev expansion method against the ground truth with different number of eigenfunctions, iterations and expansion degree respectively. Unit spheres with 2562, 10242, 40962 and 163842 mesh vertices and fixed $\sigma = 0.01$ were used. Right: computational run time against mesh size at similar accuracy (MSE about 10^{-5}).

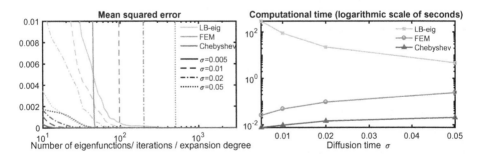

Fig. 5. Left: MSE of the LB-eigenfunction approach, FEM based diffusion solver and Chebyshev expansion method against the ground truth with different number of eigenfunctions, iterations and expansion degree respectively. Diffusion times $\sigma = 0.005, 0.01,$ 0.02 and 0.05 and 40962 mesh vertices were used. Right: computational run time versus σ at similar accuracy (MSE about 10^{-7}).

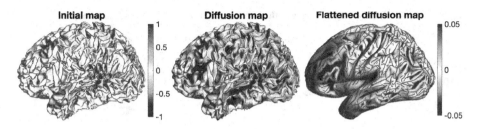

Fig. 6. Left: sulcal (blue) and gyral (red) curves are extracted and displayed on the white matter surface. Middle: heat diffusion using the Chebyshev expansion method with degree 1000 and diffusion time 0.001. Right: diffusion map was flattened to show the pattern of diffusion. (Color figure online)

Run Time over Mesh Sizes. For fixed σ, the FEM based diffusion solver and Chebyshev expansion method need more iterations and higher degree for larger meshes, while the LB-eigenfunction approach is nearly unaffected by the mesh sizes (Fig. 4-left). Since there is a trade-off between the accuracy and computational run time, we fixed the numerical accuracy with MSE at around 10^{-5} and compared the run time (Fig. 4-right).

Run Time over Diffusion Times. For fixed mesh resolution, the FEM based diffusion solver and Chebyshev expansion method need more iterations and higher degree for larger σ, while the LB-eigenfunction approach requires less number of eigenfunctions (Fig. 5-left). Figure 5-right displays the computational run time versus σ with similar MSE of about 10^{-7}.

From Figs. 4 and 5, in terms of reconstruction error, the LB-eigenfunction method is the slowest. The polynomial approximation method is up to twelve times faster than the FEM method.

3   Application

Preprocessing. We used the T1-weighted MRI dataset consisting of 268 females and 176 males collected as the subset of the Human Connectome Project [21]. The MRI data underwent image preprocessing including gradient distortion correction, skull-stripping, bias field correction, nonlinear image registration and white matter and pial surface mesh extractions in FreeSurfer [9]. The automatic sulcal curve extraction method [13] was used to detect concave regions (sulcal fundi) along which sulcal curves are traced. Sulcal points were determined by the line simplification method [7] that denoises the sulcal regions without significant loss of morphological details. A partially connected graph was constructed by the sulcal points, where edge weights are assigned based on geodesic distances. Finally, the sulcal curves were traced over the graph by the Dijkstra's algorithm [6]. Similarly, we extended the same method to the gyral curve extraction by finding convex regions (Fig. 6).

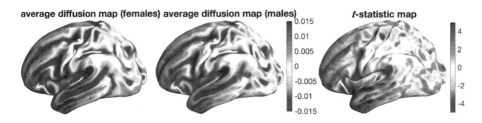

Fig. 7. Left and middle: average diffusion maps of 268 females and 176 males displayed on the average surface template. Right: t-statistic map shows localized sulcal and gyral pattern differences (female-male) thresholded at -4.96 and 4.96 (uncorrected p-value of 10^{-6}).

Diffusion Maps. The sulcal and gyral curves are represented as graphs embedded on the brain surface meshes. It is difficult to establish the precise mapping between curves across subjects. Thus, we applied the proposed method to smooth out sulcal and gyral curves. The gyral curves are assigned value 1, and sulcal curves are assigned value -1. All other parts of surface mesh vertices are assigned value 0 (Fig. 6). The difference in the initial temperature produces heat gradient. We used the Chebyshev expansion method with diffusion time $\sigma = 0.001$ and expansion degree $m = 1000$. On average, the construction of the discrete LB-operator took 5.8 s, and the Chebyshev expansion method took 3.2 s resulting in a total run time of 9 s per subject in a computer. The diffusion maps were subsequently used in localizing the regions of the brain that differentiates male and female differences.

Statistical Analysis. The average diffusion maps of females and males in Fig. 7 show major differences in the temporal lobe among other regions, which is responsible for processing sensory input into derived meanings for the appropriate retention of visual memory, language comprehension, and emotion association [19]. The two-sample t-statistic map (female-male) was constructed on the diffusion maps (max. t-stat. 7.02, min. t-stat. -6.5). The multiple comparisons are corrected using the false discovery rate at 0.05 via the Benjamini-Hochberg procedure [8]. t-statistic values larger than 2.75 and smaller than -2.75 are considered as significant (red and blue regions).

4 Conclusion

In this paper, we proposed a new fast and accurate numerical method to solve heat diffusion on curved surfaces by expanding the heat kernel in the spectral domain by orthogonal polynomials. The proposed polynomial expansion method speeds up the computation significantly compared to existing numerical schemes. The proposed method was applied in the sulcal and gyral curve pattern analysis.

The proposed polynomial method can be applied to multiscale shape analysis via the iterative kernel convolution. The method can be further extended to any arbitrary domain without much computational bottlenecks. Thus, the method can be easily applicable to large-scale images where the existing methods may not be applicable without additional computational resources, such as 3D volumetric meshes [22]. These are left as future studies.

Acknowledgements. This study was funded by NIH Grant R01 EB022856. We would like to thank Won Hwa Kim of University of Texas Arlington and Vikas Singh of University of Wisconsin-Madison for providing valuable discussions on the diffusion wavelets.

References

1. Andrade, A., et al.: Detection of fMRI activation using cortical surface mapping. Hum. Brain Mapp. **12**, 79–93 (2001)
2. Cachia, A., et al.: A primal sketch of the cortex mean curvature: a morphogenesis based approach to study the variability of the folding patterns. IEEE Trans. Med. Imaging **22**, 754–765 (2003)
3. Chung, M.K., Qiu, A., Seo, S., Vorperian, H.K.: Unified heat kernel regression for diffusion, kernel smoothing and wavelets on manifolds and its application to mandible growth modeling in CT images. Med. Image Anal. **22**, 63–76 (2015)
4. Chung, M.K., Worsley, K.J., Robbins, S., Evans, A.C.: Tensor-based brain surface modeling and analysis. In: IEEE Conference on Computer Vision and Pattern Recognition (CVPR), vol. I, pp. 467–473 (2003)
5. Defferrard, M., Bresson, X., Vandergheynst, P.: Convolutional neural networks on graphs with fast localized spectral filtering. In: Advances in Neural Information Processing Systems, pp. 3844–3852 (2016)
6. Dijkstra, E.W.: A note on two problems in connexion with graphs. Numer. Math. **1**, 269–271 (1959)
7. Douglas, D.H., Peucker, T.K.: Algorithms for the reduction of the number of points required to represent a digitized line or its caricature. Cartographica Int. J. Geograph. Inf. Geovisualization **10**, 112–122 (1973)
8. Genovese, C.R., Lazar, N.A., Nichols, T.: Thresholding of statistical maps in functional neuroimaging using the false discovery rate. NeuroImage **15**, 870–878 (2002)
9. Glasser, M.F., et al.: The minimal preprocessing pipelines for the Human Connectome Project. NeuroImage **80**, 105–124 (2013)
10. Gradshteyn, I.S., Ryzhik, I.M.: Table of Integrals, Series, and Products, 7th edn. Academic, San Diego (2007)
11. Hammond, D.K., Vandergheynst, P., Gribonval, R.: Wavelets on graphs via spectral graph theory. Appl. Comput. Harmonic Anal. **30**, 129–150 (2011)
12. Kim, W.H., Pachauri, D., Hatt, C., Chung, M.K., Johnson, S., Singh, V.: Wavelet based multi-scale shape features on arbitrary surfaces for cortical thickness discrimination. In: Advances in Neural Information Processing Systems, pp. 1241–1249 (2012)
13. Lyu, I., Kim, S., Woodward, N., Styner, M., Landman, B.: TRACE: a topological graph representation for automatic sulcal curve extraction. IEEE Trans. Med. Imaging **37**, 1653–1663 (2018)
14. Olver, F.W.J., Lozier, D.W., Boisvert, R.F., Clark, C.W.: NIST Handbook of Mathematical Functions. Cambridge University Press, Cambridge (2010)

15. Perona, P., Malik, J.: Scale-space and edge detection using anisotropic diffusion. IEEE Trans. Anal. Mach. Intell. **12**, 629–639 (1990)
16. Reuter, M.: Hierarchical shape segmentation and registration via topological features of Laplace-Beltrami eigenfunctions. Int. J. Comput. Vision **89**, 287–308 (2010)
17. Seo, S., Chung, M.K., Vorperian, H.K.: Heat Kernel smoothing using Laplace-Beltrami eigenfunctions. In: Jiang, T., Navab, N., Pluim, J.P.W., Viergever, M.A. (eds.) MICCAI 2010. LNCS, vol. 6363, pp. 505–512. Springer, Heidelberg (2010). https://doi.org/10.1007/978-3-642-15711-0_63
18. Shen, L., Chung, M.: Large-scale modeling of parametric surfaces using spherical harmonics. In: Third International Symposium on 3D Data Processing, Visualization and Transmission (3DPVT), pp. 294–301 (2006)
19. Smith, B., et al.: The OBO foundry: coordinated evolution of ontologies to support biomedical data integration. Nat. Biotechnol. **25**, 1251 (2007)
20. Tan, M., Qiu, A.: Spectral Laplace-Beltrami wavelets with applications in medical images. IEEE Trans. Med. Imaging **34**, 1005–1017 (2015)
21. Van Essen, D.C., et al.: The human connectome project: a data acquisition perspective. NeuroImage **62**, 2222–2231 (2012)
22. Wang, G., Zhang, X., Su, Q., Shi, J., Caselli, R.J., Wang, Y.: A novel cortical thickness estimation method based on volumetric Laplace-Beltrami operator and heat kernel. Med. Image Anal. **22**, 1–20 (2015)

Hierarchical Multi-geodesic Model for Longitudinal Analysis of Temporal Trajectories of Anatomical Shape and Covariates

Sungmin Hong[1]($\boxtimes$), James Fishbaugh[1], Jason J. Wolff[2], Martin A. Styner[3], Guido Gerig[1], and the IBIS Network

[1] Department of Computer Science and Engineering, Tandon School of Engineering, New York University, Brooklyn, NY, USA
sungmin.hong@nyu.edu
[2] Department of Educational Psychology, University of Minnesota, Minneapolis, MN, USA
[3] Departments of Computer Science and Psychiatry, University of North Carolina at Chapel Hill, Chapel Hill, NC, USA

Abstract. Longitudinal regression analysis for clinical imaging studies is essential to investigate unknown relationships between subject-wise changes over time and subject-specific characteristics, represented by covariates such as disease severity or a level of genetic risk. Image-derived data in medical image analysis, e.g. diffusion tensors or geometric shapes, are often represented on nonlinear Riemannian manifolds. Hierarchical geodesic models were suggested to characterize subject-specific changes of nonlinear data on Riemannian manifolds as extensions of a linear mixed effects model. We propose a new hierarchical multi-geodesic model to enable analysis of the relationship between subject-wise anatomical shape changes on a Riemannian manifold and multiple subject-specific characteristics. Each individual subject-wise shape change is represented by a univariate geodesic model. The effects of subject-specific covariates on the estimated subject-wise trajectories are then modeled by multivariate intercept and slope models which together form a multi-geodesic model. Validation was performed with a synthetic example on a S^2 manifold. The proposed method was applied to a longitudinal set of 72 corpus callosum shapes from 24 autism spectrum disorder subjects to study the relationship between anatomical shape changes and the autism severity score, resulting in statistics for the population but also for each subject. To our knowledge, this is the first longitudinal framework to model anatomical developments over time as functions of both continuous and categorical covariates on a nonlinear shape space.

Electronic supplementary material The online version of this chapter (https://doi.org/10.1007/978-3-030-32251-9_7) contains supplementary material, which is available to authorized users.

D. Shen et al. (Eds.): MICCAI 2019, LNCS 11767, pp. 57–65, 2019.
https://doi.org/10.1007/978-3-030-32251-9_7

1   Introduction

Recent advances in medical image analysis allow researchers to track an individual subject's development with multiple repeated observations [4]. Longitudinal regression analysis, which adequately accounts for intra-subject correlation, is essential to estimate unknown relationships between subject-specific temporal changes and characteristics of individuals via repeated observations [2].

Data derived from medical images, such as diffusion tensors, diffeomorphic deformations, or geometric shapes, are to be analyzed on their natural nonlinear spaces, e.g. Riemannian manifolds. For longitudinal analysis of nonlinear data on a Riemannian manifold, hierarchical geodesic models were suggested as extensions of a linear mixed effects model on Euclidean space [6,7,9]. These methods estimate the same model for both subject and population levels which is a direct reformulation of a linear mixed effects model on a Riemannian manifold. The previous methods face challenges from too few observations per subject to hierarchically solve a multivariate model at a subject level even though the number of subjects may be sufficient. Despite the importance of including subject-specific characteristics for longitudinal analysis, a hierarchical model that analyzes the relationship between subject-wise morphological changes over time and multiple covariates on a Riemannian manifold has not been shown before.

We propose a novel hierarchical multi-geodesic model for longitudinal analysis of subject-specific morphological changes of anatomical structures on a Riemannian manifold. Each subject-wise morphological change over time is modeled by a univariate geodesic model which only requires a minimum of two observations per subject. The effects of subject-specific characteristics, represented by subject-specific covariates, on subject-wise trajectories are modeled by a multi-geodesic model. The covariates are fixed for an individual subject but varying across a population. The multi-geodesic model consists of multivariate intercept and slope models which account for the effects of the subject-specific characteristics to subject-wise baselines and developments over time, respectively. It is worth noting that the proposed method is different from the direct extension of a linear mixed effects model because the relationship between subject-specific characteristics and the slopes of subject-wise temporal trajectories cannot be modeled by linearly adding the covariates as additional explanatory variables.

A synthetic example on a S^2 manifold with a comparison to the ground truth showed the feasibility of the proposed method. Experimental validation on 72 corpus callosum shapes represented on a nonlinear shape space from 24 autism spectrum disorder subjects with different autism severity scores demonstrate the capability of the proposed method for longitudinal analysis of the relationship between subject-specific morphological changes and multiple covariates.

2   Method

Background on Riemannian Geometry: A geodesic is a zero-acceleration curve on an n-dimensional Riemannian manifold M. It has the minimizing property that there is no curve shorter than a geodesic between any two points within a small neighborhood. An exponential map $Exp(p, v) = q$ is a mapping of $p \in M$ to $q \in M$ along a geodesic going out from p in the direction and magnitude of v. Its inverse, $Log(p, q) = v$, is defined onto a neighborhood $U(p)$ of p. The Riemannian distance between p and q is the length of a geodesic between the two, $d(p, q) = ||Log(p, q)||$. Parallel transport $\psi_{p \to q}(u)$ of a tangent vector $u \in T_p M$ along a differentiable curve $c(t) : I \to M$ from p to q is defined by a unique parallel vector field $V(t)$ along $c(t)$ where $I = [0, 1]$, $c(0) = p$, and $c(1) = q$. $V(t)$ satisfies $V(t_0) = u$ and $\frac{DV}{dt} = 0$, where $\frac{DV}{dt}$ is a covariant derivative of a vector field V. Parallel transport has the following angle and scale preserving properties: the angle of u along $c(t)$ does not change, $\frac{DV}{dt} = 0$, and the scale of u also does not change, $||u|| = ||V(t)||$, at any $t \in I$ [1]. $\psi_{p \to q}(u)$ is not unique and depends on a curve c that connects p and q. We will only use $\psi_{p \to q}$ along with the unique geodesic between p and q to guarantee the transport to be unique.

Subject-Wise Trajectory Estimation: Let $y_{ij} \in M$ be the jth observation of the ith subject associated with time $t_{ij} \in \mathbb{R}$, $i = 1, .., N_s$, $j = 1, ..., N_{obs}^i$. N_s and N_{obs}^i are the number of subjects and the number of observations of the ith subject, respectively. We estimate a subject-wise trajectory Y_i by the least squares geodesic regression model [3].

$$(\hat{a}_i, \hat{b}_i) = \underset{a_i, b_i}{\operatorname{argmin}} \sum_{j=1}^{N_{obs}^i} d^2(y_{ij}, Exp(a_i, b_i t_{ij})), \qquad Y_i = Exp(\hat{a}_i, \hat{b}_i t), \qquad (1)$$

where $a_i \in M$ and $b_i \in T_{a_i} M$ are an intercept and a slope tangent vector of the geodesic model Y_i for the ith subject's trajectory as shown in Fig. 1(a). It is worth noting that Eq. 1 only requires the minimum of two observations per subject to solve for two coefficients, an intercept a_i and a slope b_i.

Hierarchical Multi-geodesic Model: Let the ith subject be associated with two sets of subject-specific covariates for intercepts $\boldsymbol{\eta}^i = \{\eta_1^i, ..., \eta_{N_\eta}^i\}$ and slopes $\boldsymbol{\theta}^i = \{\theta_1^i, ..., \theta_{N_\theta}^i\}$, where N_η and N_θ are the numbers of the covariates.

We aim to model the effects of $\boldsymbol{\eta}$ and $\boldsymbol{\theta}$ on subject-wise trajectories. The proposed Hierarchical Multi-Geodesic model (HMG) consists of an intercept model $f(\boldsymbol{\eta})$ and a slope model $g(\boldsymbol{\theta})$,

$$Y = Exp(Exp(f(\boldsymbol{\eta}), g(\boldsymbol{\theta})t), \epsilon). \qquad (2)$$

Intercept Model: The intercept model $f(\boldsymbol{\eta})$ is formulated as a multivariate geodesic model with a base intercept $\beta_0 \in M$ and tangent vectors $\beta_k \in T_{\beta_0} M$ [5],

$$f(\boldsymbol{\eta}) = Exp(\beta_0, \beta_1 \eta_1 + ... + \beta_{N_\eta} \eta_{N_\eta}). \qquad (3)$$

β_k, $k = 1, ..., N_\eta$, are coefficients that represent the effects of subject-specific covariates η_k to the intercepts of subject-wise trajectories. For example, a hypothesis that a subject diagnosed with autism and a healthy subject might have different baseline corpus callosum shapes at 3-month after birth can be

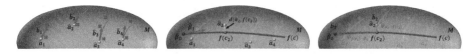

Fig. 1. Illustration of the proposed method. (a) Subject-wise geodesic trajectory estimation. (b) The example of an intercept model $f(c)$ with a single covariate c. (c) Stop-over parallel transport ϕ from $\hat{a}_2$ to $\hat{\beta}_0$.

modeled by the intercept model f. The coefficients β_k can be estimated by a least squares formulation of the multivariate geodesic model,

$$(\hat{\beta}_0, \hat{\beta}_1, ..., \hat{\beta}_{N_\eta}) = \underset{\beta_0,...,\beta_{N_\eta}}{\mathrm{argmin}} \sum_{i=1}^{N_s} d^2(f(\boldsymbol{\eta}^i), \hat{a}_i). \qquad (4)$$

We optimize Eq. 4 by a Euclideanized optimization scheme similar to [5] with an iterative update of an anchor point to the estimated intercept, instead of fixing it at the intrinsic mean of given data. The estimated intercept model is given as $\hat{f}(\boldsymbol{\eta}) = Exp(\hat{\beta}_0, \hat{\beta}_1\eta_1 + ... + \hat{\beta}_{N_\eta}\eta_{N_\eta})$ after optimization.

The least squares formulation Eq. 4 assumes that the distribution of subject-wise intercepts around $\hat{f}(\boldsymbol{\eta})$ is the generalized normal distribution [3],

$$\hat{a}_i = Exp(\hat{f}(\boldsymbol{\eta}^i), \epsilon_a), \qquad (5)$$

where $\epsilon_a \sim N(0, \sigma_a^2)$. ϵ_a can be directly interpreted as random effects of subject-wise intercepts that indicate longitudinal effects of repeated observations of individual subjects [2]. Figure 1(b) shows the illustration of the concept of the intercept model f with an example model with one continuous covariate c.

Tangent Vector Space of Slope Model: The effects of covariates on the slopes of subject-wise trajectories are modeled as a linear model $g_0(\boldsymbol{\theta})$ on a tangent vector space from a set of subject-wise slope tangent vectors $\hat{b}_i$,

$$g_0(\boldsymbol{\theta}) = \gamma_0 + \gamma_1\theta_1 + ... + \gamma_{N_\theta}\theta_{N_\theta}, \qquad (6)$$

where γ_k, $k = 0, ..., N_\theta$, are coefficient tangent vectors associated with θ_k. The model can explain a hypothesis on the relationship between covariates and the slopes. For example, a corpus callosum may develop differently from a baseline for a subject diagnosed with autism versus a healthy subject.

There are two problems that we need to consider to model subject-wise slopes. First, γ_k must be on a single tangent vector space to be linearly combined as in Eq. 6. For consistent modeling and comprehensible interpretation, we set γ_k to be on a tangent vector space of the base intercept of the intercept model, $T_{\hat{\beta}_0} M$, which makes $g_0(\boldsymbol{\theta}) \in T_{\hat{\beta}_0} M$. Second, $\hat{b}_i$ are not directly comparable to each other because they are on different tangent vector spaces $T_{\hat{a}_i} M$. Therefore, we need to properly transport $\hat{b}_i$ to $T_{\hat{\beta}_0} M$ to estimate γ_k.

Stop-Over Parallel Transport ϕ: Recall that subject-wise intercepts $\hat{a}_i$ are the combination of the fixed effects intercept model $\hat{f}(\eta^i)$ and the random effects ϵ_a on subject-wise intercepts as explained in Eq. 5. In other words, each $\hat{a}_i$ is randomly distributed in the normal distribution of the random effects centered at $\hat{f}(\eta^i)$ [8]. Therefore, we need to transport a tangent vector on $T_{\hat{a}_i}M$ to $T_{\hat{f}(\eta^i)}M$ first to account for the random effects and then from $T_{\hat{f}(\eta^i)}M$ to $T_{\hat{\beta}_0}M$ to account for the fixed effects as shown in Fig. 1(c) by a stop-over parallel transport ϕ,

$$\tilde{b}_i = \phi(\hat{b}_i) = \psi_{\hat{f}(\eta^i) \to \hat{\beta}_0}(\psi_{\hat{a}_i \to \hat{f}(\eta^i)}(\hat{b}_i)), \qquad (7)$$

where $\tilde{b}_i \in T_{\hat{\beta}_0}M$. ψ is a parallel transport along with a geodesic between two points with the angle and scale preserving properties that suit our need to consistently transport $\hat{b}_i$ at each stage of the stop-over transport. Figure A1 in the appendix shows the effect of the stop-over parallel transport with a synthetic experiment on a S^2 manifold. The direct parallel transportation to the intercept point may arbitrarily rotate tangent vectors when the stop-over transport preserves the directions of the tangent vectors consistently.

Slope Model Estimation: With $\tilde{b}_i$ transported to $T_{\hat{\beta}_0}M$ by ϕ, we estimate slope coefficients γ_k, $k = 0, ..., N_\theta$, in $g_0(\theta)$. It can be formulated as the least squares formulation of a standard multivariate linear regression problem [2],

$$(\hat{\gamma}_0, \hat{\gamma}_1, ..., \hat{\gamma}_{N_\theta}) = \underset{\gamma_0, \gamma_1, ..., \gamma_{N_\theta}}{\text{argmin}} \sum_{i=1}^{N_s} ||\gamma_0 + \gamma_1 \theta_1^i + ... + \gamma_{N_\theta} \theta_{N_\theta}^i - \tilde{b}_i||^2. \qquad (8)$$

Equation 8 is optimized by the closed-form solution of a multivariate linear regression problem with the assumption of no correlation in γ_k. The estimated slope model $\hat{g}_0(\theta) = \hat{\gamma}_0 + \hat{\gamma}_1 \theta_1 + ... + \hat{\gamma}_{N_\theta} \theta_{N_\theta}$ is transported to the respective tangent vector space of the intercept model $\hat{f}(\eta)$, $\hat{g}(\theta) = \psi_{\hat{\beta}_0 \to \hat{f}(\eta)}(\hat{g}_0(\theta))$.

The least squares formulation in Eq. 8 is related to the random effects of subject-wise slopes, similar to Eq. 5 for the intercept model. The complete estimated multi-geodesic model is then formulated as $y = Exp(\hat{f}(\eta), \hat{g}(\theta)t)$.

3 Experiments

Synthetic Example on S^2 Manifold: We tested our method with a synthetic example on a S^2 manifold. We used the exponential map, log map, and parallel transport of S^2 manifold as in [7]. 3527 points of 1000 subjects were generated by the following model with time $t \in (20, 70)$ and a continuous covariate $c \in (0, 5)$,

$$y = Exp(Exp(f(c), g(c)t)), \quad f(c) = Exp(\beta_0, \beta_1 c), \quad g(c) = \psi_{\beta_0 \to f(c)}(\gamma_0 + \gamma_1 c),$$

where we assigned $\beta_0 = [1, 0, 0]$, $\beta_1 = [0, 0, 0.4]$, $\gamma_0 = [0, 0.01, 0.02]$, and $\gamma_1 = [0, 0.002, -0.003]$ with random effects on intercepts $\epsilon_a \sim N(0, 0.05^2)$ and slopes $\epsilon_b \sim N(0, 0.001^2)$ and the data observation noise $\epsilon \sim N(0, 0.001^2)$.

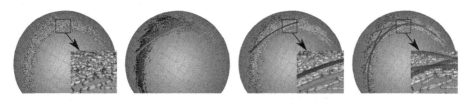

Fig. 2. Synthetic example on a S^2 manifold. (a) Generated data points colored by associated values of a covariate c (blue to green) with subject-wise trajectories (white lines). (b) Estimated single geodesic model (SG, magenta). Data points are colored by time (black to white). (c) Estimated hierarchical single geodesic model (HSG, brown). (d) Estimated hierarchical multi-geodesic model (HMG) and the ground truth (yellow) visualized with selected values of c. (Color figure online)

Figure 2(a) shows the synthetic data colored by c from blue to green. The estimated subject level geodesic models are plotted as translucent white curves. Figure 2(b) shows the estimated geodesic of a geodesic regression model (SG, magenta) with data points colored by t from black to white [3]. Figure 2(c) illustrates the results of a Hierarchical Single Geodesic model (HSG, brown) [5,7]. The results of the proposed Hierarchical Multi-Geodesic model (HMG) and the ground truth (yellow curves) are displayed in Fig. 2(d) with uniformly selected values of c with a unit interval from 0.5 to 4.5. The generalized R^2 with respect to individual data of SG, HSG, and the proposed HMG were 0.31, 0.29, and 0.96, respectively [3]. The R^2 with respect to subject-wise intercepts R_a^2 and slopes R_b^2 of the proposed HMG were 0.98 and 0.90. R_a^2 and R_b^2 of HSG are zero since the HSG is the average trajectory of the subject-wise trajectories [7]. Validation with respect to subject-wise trajectories is not available for non-longitudinal SG. Standard deviations of the random effects estimated by HMG of subject-wise intercepts and slopes are $\sigma_a = 0.09$ and $\sigma_b = 0.002$, respectively.

Longitudinal Corpus Callosum Shape Changes: Previous research demonstrated differences of corpus callosum (CC) size in autism [10], stating that it is thicker in infants later diagnosed with autism by multi-level linear analysis of derived features from shapes, such as mean thickness. Applying the proposed framework, quantitative exploration of longitudinal shape changes as a function of diagnostic scores becomes possible, resulting in population level and subject-specific models. We modeled HMG with sex s and Autistic Diagnostic Observation Schedule (ADOS) severity score AS, which combines symptoms related to a social interaction and a repetitive behavior with scores ranging from 4 to 10 for autism spectrum disorder (ASD) subjects. Larger AS indicate higher severity of autism. Seventy-two CC shapes from 24 ASD subjects (9 females and 15 males) from the ACE-IBIS study were used for the experiment [10]. Each subject was repeatedly scanned three times. Because the development of CC is known to be asymptotic to a logarithm [10], we reparametrized time t by taking the natural log to model the asymptotic shape changes over time.

Table 1. Quantitative comparisons of SG, HSG, and the proposed HMG. R^2 with respect to observations (R^2), subject-wise intercepts (R_a^2) and slopes (R_b^2), the standard deviations of subject-wise intercepts (σ_a) and slopes (σ_b), and the root mean squared boundary landmark distances (RMSE) are listed.

	Synthetic					CC-autism spectrum					
	R^2	R_a^2	R_b^2	σ_a	σ_b	R^2	R_a^2	R_b^2	σ_a	σ_b	RMSE (mm)
SG	0.31	N/A	N/A	N/A	N/A	0.23	N/A	N/A	N/A	N/A	0.287
HSG	0.29	0.0	0.0	0.58	$5.0e^{-3}$	0.23	0.0	0.0	$1.02e^{-2}$	$5.15e^{-3}$	0.287
HMG	**0.96**	**0.98**	**0.90**	**0.09**	**$2.0e^{-3}$**	**0.27**	**0.06**	**0.09**	**$9.55e^{-3}$**	**$4.68e^{-3}$**	**0.277**

$$y = Exp(Exp(f(s, AS), g(s, AS)\log(t))),$$
$$f(s, AS) = Exp(\beta_0, \beta_1 s + \beta_2 AS), \quad g(s, AS) = \psi_{\beta_0 \to f(s, AS)}(\gamma_0 + \gamma_1 s + \gamma_2 AS),$$

with sex s, 0 for male and 1 for female, age(month) $t = (6, 25)$, and $AS = (4, 10)$.

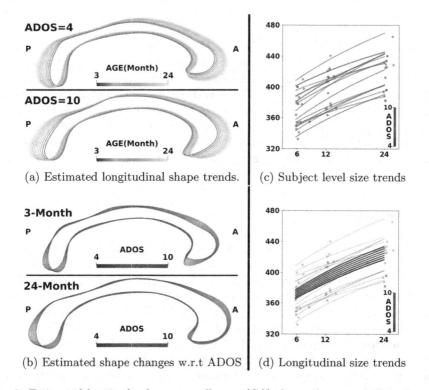

(a) Estimated longitudinal shape trends.

(b) Estimated shape changes w.r.t ADOS

(c) Subject level size trends

(d) Longitudinal size trends

Fig. 3. Estimated longitudinal corpus callosum (CC) shape changes of 15 male subjects (A: Anterior, P: Posterior). (a) Population level longitudinal shape trends of subjects with the lowest and the highest ADOS scores. (b) Shape changes with varying ADOS scores of baseline shapes at 3-month and end point shapes at 24-month. (c) The observed shape sizes with estimated subject-level trends. (d) Population level longitudinal size trends with varying ADOS scores.

CC shapes were represented on a product manifold $\mathbf{M} = \mathbb{R} \times \mathbb{C}P^{k-2}$ of a scale $\rho \in \mathbb{R}$, which represents a shape size, and a Kendall shape $\mathbf{z}$ with k points in 2D Kendall shape space $\mathbb{C}P^{k-2}$, where translation, rotation, and scale of shapes are removed. The squared distance between $p = (\rho_p, \mathbf{z}_p)$ and $q = (\rho_q, \mathbf{z}_q)$ on $\mathbf{M}$ is a weighted sum of the distances on the element spaces. The distance on $\mathbb{C}P^{k-2}$ is normalized by the ratio of variances of data distributions of scales ρ and Kendall shapes $\mathbf{z}$, $d^2(p, q) = ||Log(\rho_p, \rho_q)||^2 + \frac{\sigma_\rho^2}{\sigma_\mathbf{z}^2} ||Log(\mathbf{z}_p, \mathbf{z}_q)||^2$, where σ_ρ^2 and $\sigma_\mathbf{z}^2$ are the variances of the input data of scales ρ and shapes $\mathbf{z}$, respectively [8]. One hundred landmark points were sampled at corresponding locations from each shape boundary. We used the exponential map, log map, and parallel transport of $\mathbb{C}P^{k-2}$ as in [3]. The exponential and log maps of $\mathbb{R}$ are addition and subtraction, respectively. The parallel transport of $\mathbb{R}$ is an identity function.

Figure 3 displays the estimated longitudinal trends with fixed $s = 0$ of 15 male subjects. Figure 3(a) shows the estimated longitudinal shape trends of the lowest and the highest ADOS scores over time. The difference of the shape changes is more evident in Fig. 3(b) illustrating estimated baseline and end point shapes with varying ADOS scores at 3 and 24-month of age. One can observe the increased expansion of the anterior CC (the genu and rostral body) for subjects with higher ADOS scores which confirms previous clinical finding that subjects diagnosed with autism tend to have larger corpus callosum [10]. The population level longitudinal trends of shape sizes estimated from the subject-wise trends in Fig. 3(c) quantitatively show increasing trends of shape sizes with higher ADOS scores in Fig. 3(d). The overall R^2 values of SG, HSG, and HMG were 0.23, 0.23, and 0.27, respectively. The root mean squared error measured by average surface boundary landmark distances of SG, HSG, and HMG were 0.287, 0.287, and 0.277 (mm), respectively. Table 1 summarizes the quantitative evaluations. Mean and standard deviation of R^2 values of the subject-wise trends were 0.89 ± 0.04.

4   Discussion

The proposed hierarchical multi-geodesic model is a novel method for longitudinal analysis of subject-specific anatomical shape changes on a Riemannian manifold. It enables longitudinal analysis with multiple covariates directly on a nonlinear shape space which has not yet been possible for clinical studies. The application to subject-specific corpus callosum shape changes demonstrated promising results that confirmed clinical finding of the relationship between the anatomical development and diagnostic scores of individual subjects. We will focus on a hypothesis testing framework for the proposed model to further explore relationships between temporal change of anatomical structures and covariates.

Acknowledgements. Funding was provided by the IBIS (Infant Brain Imaging Study) Network, an NIH funded Autism Center of Excellence (2R01HDO55741) that consists of a consortium of 7 Universities in the U.S. and Canada. This research was also supported by NIH 1R01DA038215-01A1 (Cocaine effects), and R01EB021391 (SlicerSALT).

References

1. Carmo, M.P.D.: Riemannian Geometry. Birkhäuser, Basel (1992)
2. Fitzmaurice, G.M., Laird, N.M., Ware, J.H.: Applied Longitudinal Analysis, vol. 998. Wiley, Hoboken (2012)
3. Fletcher, P.T.: Geodesic regression and the theory of least squares on riemannian manifolds. Int. J. Comput. Vis. **105**(2), 171–185 (2013)
4. Gerig, G., Fishbaugh, J., Sadeghi, N.: Longitudinal modeling of appearance and shape and its potential for clinical use. Med. Image Anal. **33**, 114–121 (2016)
5. Kim, H.J., et al.: MGLM on riemannian manifolds with applications to statistical analysis of diffusion weighted images. In: CVPR. IEEE (2014)
6. Kim, H.J., Adluru, N., Suri, H., Vemuri, B.C., Johnson, S.C., Singh, V.: Riemannian nonlinear mixed effects models: analyzing longitudinal deformations in neuroimaging. In: CVPR. IEEE (2017)
7. Muralidharan, P., Fletcher, P.T.: Sasaki metrics for analysis of longitudinal data on manifolds. In: CVPR. IEEE (2012)
8. Pennec, X.: Intrinsic statistics on riemannian manifolds: basic tools for geometric measurements. J. Math. Imaging Vis. **25**(1), 127 (2006)
9. Singh, N., Hinkle, J., Joshi, S., Fletcher, P.T.: Hierarchical geodesic models in diffeomorphisms. Int. J. Comput. Vis. **117**(1), 70–92 (2016)
10. Wolff, J.J., et al.: Altered corpus callosum morphology associated with autism over the first 2 years of life. Brain **138**(7), 2046–2058 (2015)

Clustering of Longitudinal Shape Data Sets Using Mixture of Separate or Branching Trajectories

Vianney Debavelaere[1]([⊠]), Alexandre Bône[3], Stanley Durrleman[3], Stéphanie Allassonnière[2], and for the Alzheimer's Disease Neuroimaging Initiative

[1] CMAP, Ecole Polytechnique, Palaiseau, France
vianney.debavelaere@polytechnique.edu
[2] CRC, Université Paris Descartes, Paris, France
stephanie.allassonniere@parisdescartes.fr
[3] Inria, Aramis Team, ICM Institute, Paris, France
stanley.durrleman@inria.fr

Abstract. Several methods have been proposed recently to learn spatiotemporal models of shape progression from repeated observations of several subjects over time, i.e. a longitudinal data set. These methods summarize the population by a single common trajectory in a supervised manner. In this paper, we propose to extend such approaches to an unsupervised setting where a longitudinal data set is automatically clustered in different classes without labels. Our method learns for each cluster an average shape trajectory (or representative curve) and its variance in space and time. Representative trajectories are built as the combination of pieces of curves. This mixture model is flexible enough to handle independent trajectories for each cluster as well as fork and merge scenarios. The estimation of such non linear mixture models in high dimension is known to be difficult because of the trapping states effect that hampers the optimisation of cluster assignments during training. We address this issue by using a tempered version of the stochastic EM algorithm. Finally, we apply our algorithm on synthetic data to validate that a tempered scheme achieve better convergence. We show then how the method can be used to test different scenarios of hippocampus atrophy in ageing by using an heteregenous population of normal ageing individuals and mild cognitive impaired subjects.

Data used in preparation of this article were obtained from the Alzheimers Disease Neuroimaging Initiative (ADNI) database. As such, the investigators within the ADNI contributed to the design and implementation of ADNI and/or provided data but did not participate in analysis or writing of this report.

Electronic supplementary material The online version of this chapter (https:// doi.org/10.1007/978-3-030-32251-9_8) contains supplementary material, which is available to authorized users.

Keywords: Longitudinal data analysis · Mixture model · Branching population · Riemannian framework

1   Introduction

With the emergence of large longitudinal data sets (subjects observed repeatedly at different time points), construction of spatiotemporal atlases has become a central issue. From the repeated observations of individuals at different time points, such atlases aim at estimating a trajectory that will be representative of the population, as well as the spatiotemporal variability within this population. The representative trajectory is a long-term scenario of changes informed by sequences of short-term individual data. Being able to construct such an atlas has a large number of applications: understanding of a disease progression, highlighting of growth patterns, etc. Several statistical approaches have been proposed to address this problem. Descriptive [7] or generative [10,13] approaches have been derived for data taking the form of feature vectors. Generative longitudinal models have been proposed for shape data, usually using flows of deformations to construct shape trajectories [5,11,14]. All these methods however assumed that observations are drawn from an homogeneous population that may be summarized by a single representative trajectory.

In many situations, populations are likely to be heterogeneous but without prior knowledge on the sub-groups composing them, thus preventing the use of such supervised approaches. Developing unsupervised statistical learning methods is known to be challenging. The difficulty is further increased in the spatiotemporal setting since clustering may take various forms: sub-groups may follow independent trajectories, or they may follow trajectories that fork or merge at specific time-points. The former case is relevant to discover pathological sub-types having different disease course. The latter is interesting for a disease that is seen as a progressive deviation from a normal aging scenario.

In this paper, we address this issue by proposing a mixture model for longitudinal shape data. The scenario of each cluster results from the combination of successive pieces of trajectories. This framework enables to build complex broken line design. These pieces of trajectory may be different for different clusters, or certain parts may be shared among clusters to model forking or merging trajectories. The model offers therefore a very flexible framework for testing complex clustering scenarios.

In practice, we used the Large Deformation Diffeomorphic Metric Mapping (LDDMM) framework to build trajectories of shape changes, which may be seen as geodesics on a Riemannian manifold [12]. The construction of longitudinal atlases has been proposed in this framework, where the representative trajectory is a geodesic [5,13] or a piecewise geodesic [2] and the spatiotemporal variability is modeled using a tubular coordinate system around the common geodesic. Such methods are based on a generative mixed-effect model. We extend here this model to a mixture model, where each mixture component is described by a piecewise geodesic curve. Some part of this curve may be shared by several clusters. To estimate the different parameters, derivations of the Expectation-Maximization algorithm are known to be efficient [4]. However, estimating mixture components in such a high-dimension non-linear setting is known to be difficult. A central difficulty is the "trapping states" effect, where changing class assignment is always more costly than adjusting the parameters of the clusters, resulting in very few updates of class assignment during optimization. Pragmatic solutions have been proposed, for instance in [3] for cross sectional data but at high computational cost. Here we introduce tempered distributions into the stochastic approximation EM in order to avoid being trapped in the initial labelling.

We will finally quantitatively validate our model on simulated 2D data and then apply it on a data set of hippocampus shapes in the context of Alzheimer's disease to highlight different atrophy patterns between normal ageing individuals and subjects developing Alzheimer's disease.

2   Geometrical Model

In the following, we consider a longitudinal data set of n subjects, each being observed k_i times: $(y_{i,j})_{1 \leq i \leq n, 1 \leq j \leq k_i}$ at times $(t_{i,j})_{1 \leq i \leq n, 1 \leq j \leq k_i}$.

We recall the construction of geodesics in the Large Deformation Diffeomorphic Metric Mapping (LDDMM) framework [9]. Given an initial set of control points c_0 and momenta m_0 at a time t_0, we obtain a flow of diffeomorphisms $Exp_{c_0,t_0,t}(m_0)$ that deforms the ambient space continuously in time, and then any mesh embedded into this space. These flows define geodesics on the manifold $M = \{Exp_{c_0,t_0,1}(m_0) | m_0 \in \mathbb{R}^{n_{cp} \times d}\}$.

We want now to construct a piecewise geodesic representative trajectory γ_0 as a combination of K different geodesics following each other, generalizing the work done in [2] in dimension 1. Hence, we introduce a subdivision of $\mathbb{R}$: $(t_{R,1} < ... < t_{R,K-1} < t_{R,K} := +\infty)$ where $(t_{R,k})_{1 \leq k \leq K-1}$ are the rupture times i.e. times when the representative curve switches from one geodesic to the other. We also fix the value of the representative curve at the rupture times y_k for $k \geq 2$ to assure the continuity of the trajectory. More formally, given a set of control points $c_1 \in \mathbb{R}^{n_{cp} \times d}$, of rupture times $t_R \in \mathbb{R}^{K-1}$, an initial shape y_1 and K momenta $(m_0, m_1, ..., m_{K-1})$, we define the representative trajectory as:

$$
\begin{cases}
\gamma(t)(y_1) = Exp_{c_1,t_{R,1},t_{R,1}-t}(m_0) \cdot y_1 \mathbb{1}_{t \leq t_{R,1}} \\
\qquad\qquad + \sum_{k=1}^{K-1} Exp_{c_k,t_{R,k},t-t_{R,k}}(m_k) \cdot y_k \mathbb{1}_{t_{R,k} \leq t \leq t_{R,k+1}} \\
c_k = Exp_{c_{k-1},t_{R,k-1},t_{R,k}-t_{R,k-1}}(m_{k-1}) \cdot c_{k-1} \qquad \text{for } k \geq 2 \\
y_k = Exp_{c_{k-1},t_{R,k-1},t_{R,k}-t_{R,k-1}}(m_{k-1}) \cdot y_{k-1} \qquad \text{for } k \geq 2.
\end{cases}
\tag{1}
$$

It can be remarked that the first rupture time has a particular role as we must define a geodesic before it and another after.

Now that we can define a representative trajectory, we want to compute a transformation from this trajectory towards a subject taking into account both spatial and temporal differences. For each subject i, let $\xi_{i,0}, \ldots \xi_{i,K-1}$ be acceleration coefficients and $\tau_{i,0}, \ldots, \tau_{i,K-1}$ time shifts. We write for every subject i: $\psi_{i,0}(t) = t_{R,1} - e^{\xi_{i,0}}(t_{R,1} - t + \tau_{i,0})$ and, for each component $k \geq 1$, $\psi_{i,k}(t) = t_{R,k} + e^{\xi_{i,k}}(t - t_{R,k} - \tau_{i,k})$. Each subject has its own rupture times: $t_{R,i,k}$ such that $t_{R,k} = \psi_{i,k}(t_{R,i,k})$ i.e. $t_{R,i,k} = t_{R,k} + \tau_{i,k}$. To assure the continuity of the time reparametrization at each of those rupture times, we also fix all the time shifts but $\tau_{i,0}$, from now on noted τ_i, by continuity conditions. Finally, we set: $\psi_i(t) = \psi_{i,0}(t)\mathbb{1}_{t \leq t_{R,i,1}} + \sum_{k=1}^{K-1} \psi_{i,k}(t)\mathbb{1}_{t_{R,i,k} \leq t \leq t_{R,i,k+1}}$. The time shifts τ_i allow the subjects to be at different stage of evolution while the acceleration factors $\xi_{i,k}$ allow an inter-subject variability in the pace of evolution on each geodesic (quicker evolution if $\xi_{i,k} > 0$, slower if $\xi_{i,k} < 0$).

As proposed in [5], we also introduce for each subject a space-shift momenta w_i which accounts for geometric variability. We use the notion of parallel transport to define the spatial deformation at a time t. More precisely, we note P_γ the parallel transport which transports any vector $w \in \mathbb{R}^{n_{cp} \times d}$ along the trajectory γ. Then, to code the deformation field at a time t, we transport the momenta w along the curve $\gamma(t)$ and then compute the flow given by this new momenta. More precisely, we define: $\eta_t(w) = \mathrm{Exp}_{\gamma(t)(c_1),0,1}(P_{\gamma(t)}(w))$. Finally, the deformation of the representative curve γ by the space shift w is given by: $\gamma_w(t) = \eta_t(w) \circ \gamma(t) \circ y_1$. The space deformation process is summarized in Fig. 1.

We will model this space shift as a linear combination of n_s sources: we suppose that $w = A_{(m_0,\ldots,m_{K-1})^\perp} s$ with $A_{(m_0,\ldots,m_1)^\perp}$ a $n_{cp} \times n_s$ matrix called the modulation matrix and $s \in \mathbb{R}^{n_s}$ the sources. By projecting all the columns of $A_{(m_0,\ldots,m_{K-1})^\perp}$ on $(m_0,\ldots,m_{K-1})^\perp$ for the metric K_g, we impose orthogonality between the space shifts and the momenta vectors. It has been shown in [13] that this condition is necessary to assure the identifiability of the model by preventing a confusion between the space shifts and the acceleration factors. Finally, we deform the template $\gamma(t)(y_1)$ by setting: $\gamma_i(t) = \gamma_w(\psi_i(t))$.

This construction builds a piecewise geodesic model of progression. We now propose an extension for the analysis of heterogeneous populations. More precisely, we suppose it exists N different representative curves, each of the subjects i being in the cluster $cl(i)$ of the particular representative curve $\gamma^{cl(i)}$. This representative curve comes with its own set of rupture times $(t_{R,1}^{cl(i)} < \ldots < t_{R,K-1}^{cl(i)})$, initial shape $y_1^{cl(i)}$, control points $c_1^{cl(i)}$, momenta $(m_0^{cl(i)}, \ldots, m_{K-1}^{cl(i)})$ and modulation matrix $A_{(m_0^{cl(i)},\ldots,m_{K-1}^{cl(i)})^\perp}^{cl(i)}$.

This mixture framework enables to compare and test hypothesis on the clusters. For instance, all or part of the clusters can be shared on the first stage of evolution $(t < t_{R,1})$. This imposes all or part of the representative curves to have the same first component, i.e. $t_{R,1}^k$, y_1^k, c_1^k and m_0^k are equals for all or part of the clusters $k \in [\![1, N]\!]$. Similarly, we could impose the equality of some of the representative curves on other time segments, allowing us to handle populations forking or merging at the rupture times.

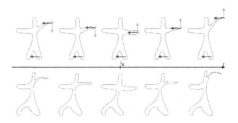

Fig. 1. Samples from a piecewise geodesic (top) and a parallel deformation (bottom). The red momenta codes the template evolution, lowering then raising an arm after the rupture time. The blue momenta is transported along the piecewise geodesic and defines the deformation frame. (Color figure online)

3 Statistical Model and Estimation

We now define the mixed effects statistical model: we note $z_{pop}^r = ((m_k^r)_{0 \leq k \leq K-1}, y_1^r, c_1^r, (t_{R,k}^r)_{0 \leq k \leq K-1}, A_{(m_0^r,\ldots,m_{K-1}^r)^\perp}^r)$ the population parameters of the cluster r and $z_i = ((\xi_{i,k})_{1 \leq k \leq K-1}, \tau_i, s_i)$ the deformation parameters of the subject i. Depending on the case, we place ourselves in the current [15] or varifold [6] framework, allowing us to compute distances between shapes without any point correspondence. We suppose that the subject i is obtained as a noised deformation of the representative curve $\gamma^{cl(i)}$: $\forall i \in [|1, n|], \forall j \in [|1, k_i|]$, $y_{i,j}|cl(i), z_{pop}^{cl(i)}, z_i \sim \mathcal{N}(\gamma_i(t_{i,j}), \sigma^2 Id)$, that the deformation parameters z_i verify: $z_i|cl(i) \sim \mathcal{N}(0, \Sigma^{cl(i)})$ where for all cluster r, Σ^r is a positive-definite matrix, that the cluster r is drawn with a probability p^r i.e. $cl(i) \sim \sum_{r=1}^N p^r \delta_r$ and that $z_{pop}^r \sim \mathcal{N}(\bar{z}_{pop}^r, v_{pop}^r)$ where v_{pop}^r are small fixed variances. Our model is thus defined with parameters $\theta = ((\Sigma^r, p^r, \bar{z}_{pop}^r)_{1 \leq r \leq N}, \sigma)$. For effectiveness in the high dimension low sample size setting, we work in the Bayesian framework and set as priors: $\Sigma^r \sim \mathcal{W}^{-1}(V, m_\Sigma)$, $\sigma \sim \mathcal{W}^{-1}(v, m_\sigma)$, $p \sim \mathcal{D}(\alpha)$ and $\bar{z}_{pop}^r \sim \mathcal{N}(\bar{\bar{z}}_{pop}^r, \bar{v}_{pop}^r)$ where $\mathcal{W}$ is the inverse Wishart distribution and $\mathcal{D}$ is the Dirichlet distribution. We can remark that the joint distribution is in the curved exponential family which guaranties the convergence of the Stochastic Approximation Expectation Maximization algorithm (SAEM) [4].

From now on, we write q the probability distribution. To estimate the parameters θ, we want to compute a maximum a posteriori estimator by using a stochastic version of the Expectation Maximization algorithm known as MCMC-SAEM [3]. It consists in the following steps: (i) simulation of (z, z_{pop}, cl) as an iterate of an ergodic Monte Carlo Markov Chain with stationary distribution $q(z_{pop}, z, cl|y, \theta)$, (ii) stochastic approximation of the sufficient statistics of the curved exponential model and (iii) maximization using the updated stochastic approximation.

However, using the algorithm as presented above yields to bad results in exploring the support of the conditional probability distribution. This issue is known as trapping states: once a label is given to an observation, the probability of changing to another is almost zero. This leads to no change of label after a

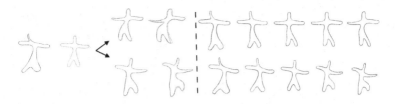

Fig. 2. In red, the exact simulated data, in black, the results given by our algorithm. On the left, the representative curves that split up at a certain rupture time. On the right side, two subjects given with their reconstructions. (Color figure online)

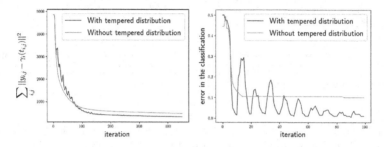

Fig. 3. Left: evolution of the varifold distances between the subjects and their reconstructions. Right: percentage of error in the classification along the first 100 iterations. With tempered distribution, the oscillating temperature coerces a lot of subjects to change classes. After 500 iterations, the error is 31.3% smaller.

few iterations. To solve this problem, we use a tempered version of the MCMC-SAEM. We choose to sample from $\frac{1}{C(T_k)}q(c|y,\theta)^{\frac{1}{T_k}}$ where T_k is a sequence of temperature converging towards 1 and $C(T_k)$ is the normalizing constant. The higher the temperature, the flatter the distribution and the more the clusters are likely to explore the entire set. We optimize the temperature sequence so that the Markov chain strides well the support with a dynamic similar to a simulated annealing [8]. By choosing a sequence of temperature converging towards 1, we do not affect the convergence of our algorithm, as showed in [1].

4   Results

We first test our algorithm on simulated data. We create 200 subjects by deforming a branching piecewise-geodesic representative curve with two components. More precisely, we draw three random momenta and apply them on a fixed shape to obtain the first common component and the two distinct ones forking at the rupture time. We then apply our algorithm to find the two clusters, the representative curves and the spatiotemporal deformations towards the data sequence of each subject. Results in Fig. 2 show that there is no noticeable differences between the true and estimated trajectories (left), nor between true and reconstructed observations (right). To quantify the reconstruction error, we compute

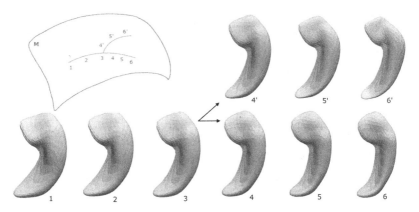

Fig. 4. Representative shape evolution at the ages 63.6y, 68.4y, 74.7y (i.e. rupture time), 77.9y, 81.5y and 85.1y. Bottom shapes: cluster with one dynamic. Top shapes: cluster with change of dynamic after rupture time.

the varifold norm of the errors for all subjects along the iterations on Fig. 3. In particular, all the errors in the estimation of the population and subjects parameters are under 5%. We also show the necessity of using tempered distributions by plotting the error of classification with and without temperature.

We want now to test hypothesis about the heterogeneity of the population. We run our algorithm supposing first that the two representative trajectories are different. We then run it again supposing that their first component is the same and that they fork at the rupture time. To select the model, we then compute the log-likelihood ratio test. As expected, the log-likelihood is smaller for the model without fork (difference of 24.6), confirming that the data are more likely to be drawn from a branching model than two unrelated components.

We now test our algorithm on 100 subjects obtained from the Alzheimer's Disease Neuroimaging Initiative database. 50 of those subjects are control patients (CN) and 50 are Mild Cognitive Impairment subjects eventually diagnosed with Alzheimer's disease (MCIc). Meshes of the right hippocampus is segmented from the rigidly registered MRI. We run our algorithm with a forking model as in the synthetic experiment. As there is no reason for the control subjects to have two different dynamics, we also ask one of the branch to follow the same geodesic after the rupture time. Our algorithm splits the patients in two clusters, one of them presenting a quicker and different pattern of atrophy (Figs. 4 and 5, left). In particular, 72% of the subjects are classified as expected: the CN in the cluster with one dynamic and a slower atrophy and the MCIc in the cluster with a quicker atrophy after the rupture time. Moreover, the individual rupture times are strongly correlated to the diagnostic age.

We run again the algorithm, looking for two clusters with separate trajectories, one of them with only one dynamic (see supplementary material and Fig. 5, center). This time, 70% of the subjects are classified as expected. We cannot compare the volume evolution of the different models as the time reparametriza-

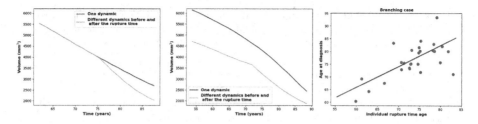

Fig. 5. Left: volume evolution for two branching clusters. Center: volume evolution for two clusters with separate trajectories. Right: comparison of the age at diagnosis with the individual rupture time for the MCIc patients, $R^2 = 0.91$

tion and so the time-line is different from one cluster to the other. We now want to select the model. The log-likelihood is bigger in this second case, which suggests that the MCI subjects are likely to deviate from a normal aging scenario at an earlier stage in life that is not observed in this data set.

5 Conclusion

We proposed a mixture model for longitudinal shape data sets where representative trajectories take the form of piecewise geodesic curves. Our model can be applied in a wide variety of situations to test whether sub-populations fork or merge at different time-points or follow unrelated trajectories on other time intervals. We showed on simulated examples that our tempered optimisation scheme is key to achieve convergence of such a mixed model combining discrete variables with continuous variables of high dimension. Its application on real data allowed us to investigate the relationship between normal and pathological ageing. Future work will focus on designing specific model selection criterion in this longitudinal setting.

Acknowledgements. This work has been partly funded by ERC grant No. 678304 and H2020EU grant No. 66699.

References

1. Allassonnière, S., Chevallier, J.: A New Class of EM Algorithms. Escaping Local. Minima and Handling Intractable Sampling (2019)
2. Allassonniere, S., Chevallier, J., Oudard, S.: Learning spatiotemporal piecewise-geodesic trajectories from longitudinal manifold-valued data. In: Advances in Neural Information Processing Systems, pp. 1152–1160 (2017)
3. Allassonnière, S., Kuhn, E.: Stochastic algorithm for Bayesian mixture effect template estimation. ESAIM: Probab. Stat. **14**, 382–408 (2010)
4. Allassonnière, S., Kuhn, E., Trouvé, A., et al.: Construction of Bayesian deformable models via a stochastic approximation algorithm: a convergence study. Bernoulli **16**(3), 641–678 (2010)

5. Bône, A., Colliot, O., Durrleman, S.: Learning distributions of shape trajectories from longitudinal datasets: a hierarchical model on a manifold of diffeomorphisms. In: Proceedings of the IEEE Conference on Computer Vision and Pattern Recognition, pp. 9271–9280 (2018)
6. Charon, N., Trouvé, A.: The varifold representation of nonoriented shapes for diffeomorphic registration. SIAM J. Imaging Sci. **6**(4), 2547–2580 (2013)
7. Donohue, M.C., et al.: Estimating long-term multivariate progression from short-term data. Alzheimer's Dement. **10**(5), S400–S410 (2014)
8. Duflo, M.: Algorithmes Stochastiques. Springer, Berlin (1996)
9. Durrleman, S., et al.: Morphometry of anatomical shape complexes with dense deformations and sparse parameters. NeuroImage **101**, 35–49 (2014)
10. Jedynak, B.M., et al.: A computational neurodegenerative disease progression score: method and results with the Alzheimer's disease neuroimaging initiative cohort. Neuroimage **63**(3), 1478–1486 (2012)
11. Lorenzi, M., Ayache, N., Pennec, X.: Schild's ladder for the parallel transport of deformations in time series of images. In: Székely, G., Hahn, H.K. (eds.) IPMI 2011. LNCS, vol. 6801, pp. 463–474. Springer, Heidelberg (2011). https://doi.org/10.1007/978-3-642-22092-0_38
12. Miller, M.I., Trouvé, A., Younes, L.: Geodesic shooting for computational anatomy. J. Math. Imaging Vis. **24**(2), 209–228 (2006)
13. Schiratti, J.B., Allassonnière, S., Colliot, O., Durrleman, S.: A Bayesian mixed-effects model to learn trajectories of changes from repeated manifold-valued observations. J. Mach. Learn. Res. **18**(1), 4840–4872 (2017)
14. Singh, N., Hinkle, J., Joshi, S., Fletcher, P.T.: Hierarchical geodesic models in diffeomorphisms. Int. J. Comput. Vis. **117**(1), 70–92 (2016)
15. Vaillant, M., Glaunès, J.: Surface matching via currents. In: Christensen, G.E., Sonka, M. (eds.) IPMI 2005. LNCS, vol. 3565, pp. 381–392. Springer, Heidelberg (2005). https://doi.org/10.1007/11505730_32

Group-Wise Graph Matching of Cortical Gyral Hinges

Tuo Zhang[1]($\boxtimes$), Xiao Li[1,2], Lin Zhao[1,2], Ying Huang[1], Zhibin He[1],
Lei Guo[1], and Tianming Liu[2]

[1] School of Automation, Northwestern Polytechnical University, Xi'an, China
tuozhang@nwpu.edu.cn
[2] Cortical Architecture Imaging and Discovery Lab,
Department of Computer Science and Bioimaging Research Center,
The University of Georgia, Athens, GA, USA

Abstract. Human brain image alignment has long been an intriguing research topic. The difficulty lies in the huge inter-individual variation. Also, it is not fully understood how structural similarity across subjects is related to functional correspondence. Recently, a gyral folding pattern, which is the conjunction of gyri from multiple directions and termed gyral hinge, was characterized. Gyral hinges have been demonstrated to have structural and functional importance and some of them were found to have cross-subject correspondences by manual labeling. However, there is no automatic method to estimate the cross-subject correspondences for whole-brain gyral hinges yet. To this end, we propose a novel group-wise graph matching framework, to which we feed structural connective matrices among gyral hinges from all subjects. The correspondence estimated by this framework is demonstrated by cross-subject consistency of both structural connective and functional profiles. Also, our results outperform the correspondences identified by pairwise graph matching and image-based registration methods.

Keywords: Gyral hinges · Structural connectivity · Cross-subject correspondence

1 Introduction

Identification of human brain structure correspondence enables cross-subject comparison and the studies of brain mechanisms [1]. In spite of the progresses made towards this goal, there is still much room to refine the solutions [1]. One of the obstacles is the cross-subject variation of brain structures, such as cortical folding [2–4]. Moreover, it is still not certain whether cortical folding pattern alignment across subjects could lead to structural connective wiring patterns and/or functional correspondences [2].

Recently, a unique cortical folding pattern was characterized in the literature [5, 7]. It is the conjunction of gyri from multiple directions and is termed gyral hinges (see their locations highlighted by green bubbles in Fig. 1(c)). Gyral hinges with more than three gyral spikes are rarely seen, and thus we focus on those with three gyral spikes, and use 3-hinges to denote them. In addition to the unique appearance, gyral hinges

© Springer Nature Switzerland AG 2019
D. Shen et al. (Eds.): MICCAI 2019, LNCS 11767, pp. 75–83, 2019.
https://doi.org/10.1007/978-3-030-32251-9_9

have the thickest cortex, the densest long-range fibers, and the most complex functional profiles, in contrast to other gyral counterparts and sulcal regions [5, 6]. The structural and functional importance of gyral hinges endorse them with critical roles as possible cortical hubs of cortex [5, 6]. Besides their importance, correspondence was found for six 3-hinges by manual labeling in [7] across subjects, showing possibility and promise in establishing the correspondence for whole-brain 3-hinges. However, given the huge variability in numbers and folding patterns of 3-hinges, a poor performance of alignment was obtained based on the conventional image registration methods [8]. Therefore, to better understand the regularity and variability of cerebral cortex, we propose a novel framework to group-wisely identify the correspondence for 3-hinges, by means of matching the structural connective diagram within the 3-hinges across subjects.

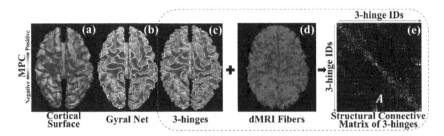

Fig. 1. Identification of 3-hinges (a–c) and construction of structural connective matrix within 3-hinges (dashed box). (a) Grayordinate white matter surfaces color-coded by maximum principal curvature (MPC). (b) White curves are the gyral net. (c) Bubbles highlight locations of 3-hinges. (d) DMRI-derived streamline fibers. (e) Structural connective matrix within 3-hinges system (Color figure online).

However, there are three challenges: (1) a solution is needed to match the whole 3-hinge systems including their structural connections; (2) subjects have different numbers of 3-hinges. The pairwise quadratic graph matching method [9] can tackle these two challenges but it is incapable for the third one: (3) a suboptimal choice of the template subject could result in a suboptimal matching when huge variation is found from a target subject. To solve these problems, we propose a group-wise scheme, where a group mean graph is produced to which all individual graphs are matched *via* the pairwise one in [9]. The group mean is updated as the weighted sum of all aligned individual graphs. Then the effectiveness of our method is demonstrated by the cross-subject consistency of structural connective diagrams as well as functional profiles on the aligned 3-hinges, and in these respects, our method outperforms image and surface-based registration method [4] and the pairwise graph matching method [9]. Our results provide novel insights to the relation between cortical folding patterns, the underlying structure connective diagram and brain function, and offer new clues to investigate brain alignment on different groups of brains, such as those of diseases and other primate species.

2 Materials and Methods

2.1 Datasets and Data Preprocessing

We use structural MRI and dMRI of 64 human brains from the Q1 release of WU-Minn Human Connectome Project (HCP) consortium [10] to develop the algorithms. The imaging parameters for structural MRI are: TR = 2400 ms, TE = 2.14 ms, flip angle = 8°, image matrix = 260 × 311 × 260 and resolution = 0.7 × 0.7 × 0.7 mm^3. The imaging parameters for dMRI are: TR = 5520 ms, TE = 89.5 ms, flip angle = 78°, FOV = 210 × 180, matrix = 168 × 144, resolution = 1.25 × 1.25 × 1.25 mm^3, echo spacing = 0.78 ms. A dMRI session includes 3 different gradient tables, each of which includes approximately 90 directions plus 6 $b = 0$ acquisitions. It consists of 3 shells of $b = 1000, 2000,$ and 3000 s/mm^2 interspersed with an approximately equal number of acquisitions on each shell. We use resting state fMRI, emotion and working memory task fMRI data to validate the results. The acquisition parameters are as follows: 90 × 104 matrix, 220 mm FOV, 72 slices, TR = 0.72 s, TE = 33.1 ms, flip angle = 52°, BW = 2290 Hz/Px, in-plane FOV = 208 × 180 mm, 2.0 mm isotropic voxels, 0.72 s temporal resolution. Time points for resting state are 1200 while they vary in different tasks, which are referred to [4].

Within each subject, the grayordinate white matter cortical surface (Fig. 1(a)) provided by HCP [4] is used as the standard space. Grayordinate surface was reconstructed from structural MRI data and has been registered to standard volume. Because of within-subject cross-modal registration, each surface vertex has a preprocessed functional MRI signal [4]. To align the dMRI data and the surface, we apply FSL-FLIRT and FNIRT to register the FA map to structural MRI. The warp field is inversely applied to the grayordinate surface obtained from the structural MRI to transpose the surface to dMRI space. The generalized Q-sampling imaging (GQI) method [11] in DSI Studio was adopted to estimate the voxel-wise axonal orientations on dMRI data. The deterministic streamline tracking algorithm in DSI Studio was used to reconstruct 4×10^4 fiber tracts for each subject with default parameters (max turning angle: 60°, streamline length: 30 mm–300 mm, step length: 1 mm, quantitative anisotropy threshold: 0.2).

2.2 Identification of 3-Hinges and Their Structural Connective Matrix

We identify 3-hinges *via* the automatic method in [8]. In general, a gyral net (curves in Fig. 1(b)) was obtained on the gyral regions, consisting of vertices with positive maximum principal curvatures (Fig. 1(a)). The intersection vertices of the three branches are defined as 3-hinges (bubbles in Fig. 1(c)). Within these 3-hinges, we construct a structural connective matrix (Fig. 1(d–e)) for each subject. We use the number of streamline fibers that simultaneously pass through the neighborhoods (a sphere with $r = 3$ mm) of a pair of 3-hinges as the connective strength [12]. No normalization is needed for the strength because the total fiber number on each subject is equal (4×10^4). It is noted that different subjects have different numbers of 3-hinges (267–369, 275.25 ± 34.64), such that the 3-hinge connective matrices are of different sizes.

2.3   Basics of Pairwise Graph Matching

Our aim is to estimate the correspondence of 3-hinges in Fig. 1(c) cross subjects by matching their structural connective matrices in Fig. 1(e). In this section, we introduce the basics of pairwise matching of two graphs and the quadratic re-weighted graph matching algorithm [9]. We use $\mathbf{G}^P = \left(\mathbf{V}^P, \mathbf{E}^P, \mathbf{A}^P \right)$ and $\mathbf{G}^Q = \left(\mathbf{V}^Q, \mathbf{E}^Q, \mathbf{A}^Q \right)$ to denote two graphs. $\mathbf{V}$ denotes nodes and $\mathbf{E}$ denotes edges. In our application, $a_{ij} \in \mathbf{A}$ is the structural connective strength for $e_{ij} \in \mathbf{E}$ between v_i and v_j defined in Sect. 2.2.

To quadratically match two graphs, we define an affinity matrix $\mathbf{W}$, where $\mathbf{W}_{ia;jb} = f\left(a_i^P, a_j^P, a_{ij}^P, a_a^Q, a_b^Q, a_{ab}^Q \right)$ describes the consistency of attributes between the node pairs of candidate correspondences (v_i^P, v_a^Q) and (v_j^P, v_b^Q). A non-diagonal element $\mathbf{W}_{ia;jb}$ measures the similarity between the pair of edges $e_{ij}^P \in \mathbf{E}^P$ and $e_{ab}^Q \in \mathbf{E}^Q$. A diagonal element $\mathbf{W}_{ia;ia}$ represents the nodal similarity which is not used in this work. The edge similarity is defined as $\exp(-\left| a_{ij}^P - a_{ab}^Q \right|^2 / \sigma^2)$, where σ is empirically set to 50 which is close to the mean value of $\left| a_{ij}^Q - a_{ab}^Q \right|$. Given an assignment matrix $\mathbf{X} \in \{0,1\}^{n^P \times n^Q}$, where $\mathbf{X}_{ia} = 1$ indicates that v_i^P corresponds to v_a^Q, the graph matching problem is formulated as a program that searches for the vector $\mathbf{x}^*$ ($\mathbf{x}$ is a column-wise vector converted from $\mathbf{X}$) that maximizes the quadratic score function in Eq. (1).

$$\mathbf{x}^* = \arg \max_{\mathbf{x}} \left(\mathbf{x}^T \mathbf{W} \mathbf{x} \right), \; s.t. \; \mathbf{x} \in \{0,1\}^{n^P n^Q}, \forall i \sum_{a=1}^{n^Q} \mathbf{x}_{ia} \leq 1, \forall a \sum_{i=1}^{n^P} \mathbf{x}_{ia} \leq 1 \quad (1)$$

where the two-way constrains $\forall i \sum_{a=1}^{n^Q} \mathbf{x}_{ia} \leq 1$ and $\forall a \sum_{i=1}^{n^P} \mathbf{x}_{ia} \leq 1$ enforce the one-to-one correspondence between $\mathbf{V}^P$ and $\mathbf{V}^Q$. Empty correspondence is allowed if two graphs are of different sizes, that is, a graph or subgraph matching between $\mathbf{G}^P$ and $\mathbf{G}^Q$.

	Algorithm 1. Reweighted random walk graph matching
1:	Given the affinity matrix $\mathbf{W}$, parameter α and β; initialize $\mathbf{x}$ as uniform
2:	Set $\mathbf{W}_{(ia,jb)} = 0$ for all conflicting match pairs
3:	Updated matrix $\mathbf{W} = \mathbf{W}/d_{max}$, where $d_{max} = \max_{ia} \sum_{jb} \mathbf{W}_{(ia,jb)}$
4:	**Begin A**: (Do A until $\mathbf{x}$ converges)
5:	$\bar{\mathbf{x}}^T = \mathbf{x}^T \mathbf{W}$
6:	$\bar{\mathbf{x}} = \exp(\beta \bar{\mathbf{x}} / \max \bar{\mathbf{x}})$
7:	**Begin B**: (Do B until $\bar{\bar{\mathbf{x}}}$ converges)
8:	Normalize across all rows: $\bar{\bar{\mathbf{x}}}_{ai} = \bar{\bar{\mathbf{x}}}_{ai} / \sum_{i=1}^{I} \bar{\bar{\mathbf{x}}}_{ai}$
9:	Normalize across all columns: $\bar{\bar{\mathbf{x}}}_{ai} = \bar{\bar{\mathbf{x}}}_{ai} / \sum_{a=1}^{A} \bar{\bar{\mathbf{x}}}_{ai}$
10:	**End B**
11:	$\bar{\mathbf{x}} = \bar{\mathbf{x}} / \sum \bar{\mathbf{x}}_{ai}$
12:	$\mathbf{x}^T = \alpha \bar{\mathbf{x}}^T + (1-\alpha) \bar{\bar{\mathbf{x}}}^T$
13:	$\mathbf{x} = \mathbf{x} / \sum \mathbf{x}_{ai}$
14:	**End A**

The re-weighted random walk algorithm [9] is used as a solution in this work: Finally, **x** is discretized by the Hungarian algorithm [14].

2.4   Group-Wise Graph Matching

Conceptually, the group-wise method is the major methodological contribution of this paper, which is detailed as follows. Suppose we have n subjects, and the 3-hinge structural connective matrices are represented by graphs $\{\mathbf{G}_n = (\mathbf{V}_n, \mathbf{E}_n, \mathbf{A}_n)\}$. In each iteration (Fig. 2), a group mean connective matrix **M** is obtained as the weighted sum of all individual matrices $\mathbf{A}_n$, and is used as the 'template' in the next iteration, to which each individual matrices $\mathbf{A}_n$ is matched. Specifically, in the tth iteration, Algorithm 1 is applied to each $(\mathbf{A}_n^t, \mathbf{M}^{t-1})$ pair to obtain a updated $\hat{\mathbf{A}}_n^t$ by the assignment vector $\mathbf{x}_n^t$ (black arrows in Fig. 2). Then, the similarity between $\hat{\mathbf{A}}_n^t$ and $\mathbf{M}^{t-1}$ is defined as the energy $s_n^t = \mathbf{x}_n^t{}^T \mathbf{W}_{\hat{\mathbf{A}}_n^t, \mathbf{M}^{t-1}} \mathbf{x}_n^t$, based on which the weight is defined as $w_n^t = s_n^t / \sum s_n^t$ and is used to update the group mean $\mathbf{M}^t$. To prevent a blur $\mathbf{M}^t$, we used $w_n^t = \exp(\varepsilon w_n^t)/\Sigma \exp(\varepsilon w_n^t)$ to make w_n^t with large value close 1. $\mathbf{M}^0$ is the sum of all the original $\mathbf{A}_n^0$s with equal weight. The algorithm stops when there is no difference between $\mathbf{M}$s of two successive iterations.

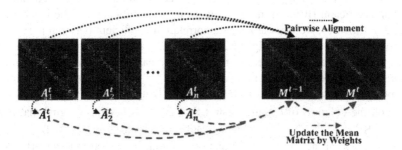

Fig. 2. The group-wise graph matching in the tth iteration. Black arrows represent pair-wise matching *via* Algorithm 1. Blue arrows represent update of $\mathbf{M}_n^t$ (Color figure online).

Another issue is the different sizes of $\mathbf{A}_n$s. We pre-define the node number k of the group mean **M** as that of the subject having the most nodes. For those that have fewer nodes, we add empty rows and columns to make the matrices up to the size of k.

The group-wise graph matching algorithm is summarized as follows:

Algorithm 2. Group-wise graph matching
1:        Given a group of adjacent matrices $\{\mathbf{A}_1, \mathbf{A}_2, \cdots, \mathbf{A}_n\}$, γ and δ
2:        Normalize the size: $\mathbf{A}_n = \begin{bmatrix} \mathbf{A}_n & \mathbf{0}_1 \\ \mathbf{0}_1^T & \mathbf{0}_2 \end{bmatrix}$, where the size of $\mathbf{A}_n$ is $k = \max(\{|\mathbf{A}_n|\})$
3:        Initialize weight vector w^0 as uniform and group mean $\mathbf{M}^0 = \sum \mathbf{A}_n * w_n^0$
4:        Initialize loop control parameters $t=0, r = 0$
5:        **Begin A**: (Do A until $r \leq \gamma$, or $t \geq \delta$)
6:        Update $\{\mathbf{A}_n^t\}$ by performing pairwise graph matching between $\mathbf{A}_n^t$ and $\mathbf{M}^{t-1}$ *via* feeding the affinity matrix $\mathbf{W}_n^t$ between them to *Algorithm 1* to yield $\mathbf{x}_n^t$
7:        Compute weights: $w_n^t = \mathbf{x}_n^{t\,T} \mathbf{W}_n^t \mathbf{x}_n^t$, and update weights: $w_n^t = w_n^t / \sum w_n^t$, $w_n^t = \exp(\varepsilon w_n^t) / \sum \exp(\varepsilon w_n^t)$ and $w_n^t = w_n^t / \sum w_n^t$
8:        Update group mean $\mathbf{M}^t = \sum \mathbf{A}_n^t * w_n^t$
9:        $r^t = \sum |\mathbf{M}^t - \mathbf{M}^{t-1}|$, $t=t+1$;
10:      **End A**

2.5   Anatomical, Structural and Functional Metrics for Result Evaluation

For anatomical metrics, we adopt Desikan-Killiany parcellation scheme [13]. Each subject has a label vector recording the brain sites of all aligned 3-hinges. The label vectors from different subjects are expected to be of the same. We used interclass correlation coefficient (ICC) to measure the group-wise similarity of the label vectors. For structural metrics, we use the Pearson correlation coefficient between a pair of the connective matrices from the aligned 3-hinges to measure the similarity. The mean coefficient averaged over all subject pairs is used to measure the group consistency. For functional metrics, we conduct a group-wise version of the sparse representation method in [6]. For each task, all m cortical fMRI signals (length of t) of the ith subject are arranged on the columns of a signal matrix $\mathbf{S}_i \in \mathbb{R}^{t \times m}$. A n-subject signal matrix $\mathbf{S} = [\mathbf{S}_1, \mathbf{S}_2, \cdots, \mathbf{S}_n] \in \mathbb{R}^{t \times (m \times n)}$ is then obtained and factorizes as $\mathbf{S} = \mathbf{D} \times \mathbf{A}$. $\mathbf{D} \in \mathbb{R}^{t \times k}$ is a group-wise temporal dictionary with k dictionary atoms ($k = 200$ in this work). $\mathbf{A}$ is a sparse coefficient weight matrix $\mathbf{A} = [\mathbf{A}_1, \mathbf{A}_2, \cdots, \mathbf{A}_n] \in \mathbb{R}^{k \times (m \times n)}$, where $\mathbf{A}_i \in \mathbb{R}^{k \times m}$ corresponds to the ith subject and is comparable across subjects. Because m^{th} column of $\mathbf{A}_i$ represents the weights of the k dictionary atoms that contribute to represent the fMRI signal of the mth vertex, we retrieve columns from $\mathbf{A}_i$ corresponding to 3-hinges as their functional profiles. We use the Euclidian distance between the functional profiles as the similarity between two matched 3-hinges. The mean distance averaged over all matched 3-hinges and all subject pairs is used to measure the group difference.

2.6   Other Matching Methods for Comparisons

We compare our algorithm to the one in Algorithm 1, in which the subject s with the most 3-hinges is the template and other subject was matched to it. The alignment provided by grayordinate surfaces themselves is compared with our method as well, which is achieved by a combination of image-based and surface-based registration methods [4]. The correspondences of 3-hinges are established by computing the Euclidean distance between all 3-hinges pairs between a subject and the template subject s. Finally, the Hungarian algorithm [14] is applied to the distance matrices to search for the 3-hinge correspondence with the closest distance while ensuring the one-to-one matching.

3   Results

We empirically used 30 and 10 for β and ε, respectively, because they do not strongly affect the matching. γ is 1×10^{-4} in our algorithm. The maximal iteration step δ is 100, which is far more than the algorithm need to converge. The algorithm is applied on all 64 subjects and it costs around 30 h on a typical desktop computer.

3.1   Correspondence of 3-Hinges and Validation by Anatomical Metrics

Figure 3(a) show the matched 3-hinges on 8 randomly selected subjects. The numbers show the consistency of their anatomical locations. For example, 3-hinges #82 and #271 are frequently found in the left and right post-central gyri, respective. In Fig. 3 (b)–(c), we show dMRI fiber bundles and functional profiles (on the columns) of the 154th 3-hinges. The consistency of both fiber bundle shape and functional profiles are observable. It is noted that only the 3-hinges that find correspondence on over 75% of

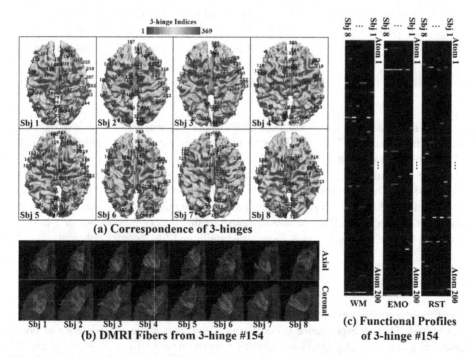

(a) Correspondence of 3-hinges

(b) DMRI Fibers from 3-hinge #154

(c) Functional Profiles of 3-hinge #154

Fig. 3. (a) 3-hinges with cross-subject correspondences (indicated by colors and numbers) on eight random subjects. Yellow arrows highlight some example 3-hinges (#82, #87, #154, #250 and #271). (b) Axial and coronal views of the fiber bundles of 3-hinge #154 (red arrows in (a)). (c) The functional profiles of 3-hinge #154 in resting state, emotional and working memory tasks (Color figure online).

all subjects are shown, because not all 3-hinges can find the correspondence on all subjects due to different 3-hinge numbers on subjects. This result suggests the co-existent regularity and variability of 3-hinges.

To quantify that corresponding 3-hinges are found at the same anatomical location, we segment the cortical surface to 72 gyral/sulcal based brain sites (the Desikan-Killiany parcellation scheme [13]). The ICC is computed for all 3-hinges to investigate if the corresponding 3-hinges have the same brain site label. Results from the pair-wise matching method and grayordinate system based matching method are also evaluated by this way. The r-value is 0.70 for our method, 0.62 for grayordinate method, and 0.51 for pairwise matching method, demonstrating the substantially better performance of our method with respect to anatomical consistency of corresponding 3-hinges.

3.2   Validation by Means of Structural Connective and Functional Metrics

Table 1. Comparison of the matching results from our method (Group), pairwise graph matching (Pair) and surface alignment in grayordinate system (Gray), in terms of functional difference and structural similarity. * indicates p-value < 0.001 in the t-tests conducted on Group-Pair and Group-Gray pairs. Abbreviations: RST: resting state; EMO: emotion; WM: working memory.

	Structural Connective Similarity (*avg.* $\pm$ *std.*)	Functional profile difference (*avg.* $\pm$ *std.*)		
		RST	EMO	WM
Group	0.40 $\pm$ 0.06*	0.08 $\pm$ 0.03*	0.06 $\pm$ 0.02*	0.06 $\pm$ 0.02*
Pair	0.24 $\pm$ 0.05*	0.21 $\pm$ 0.08*	0.15 $\pm$ 0.05*	0.16 $\pm$ 0.06*
Gray	0.32 $\pm$ 0.04*	0.21 $\pm$ 0.07*	0.16 $\pm$ 0.05*	0.16 $\pm$ 0.06*

We validate the 3-hinge correspondences with respect of structural connective patterns and functional profiles (Table 1). The structural connective patterns within the aligned 3-hinge system exhibit higher cross-subject consistency in our method, which significantly outperforms the pairwise method and grayordinate one (p-values < 0.001 for unpaired t-tests between our method and one of the other methods). The functional profile difference between corresponding 3-hinges is significantly lower in our method than other two methods. These results demonstrate that the correspondence of 3-hinges estimated by our method is much more structurally and functionally coherent.

4   Conclusions

We propose a novel group-wise framework to identify the cross-subject correspondence of 3-hinges. The correspondence is demonstrated by cross-subject consistency of both structural connective and functional profiles. Our results outperform those by pairwise graph matching and image-based registration methods and suggest that correspondences could be found for well-defined folding patterns, providing novel insights to the linkage between folding patterns and structure connectivity and brain function.

References

1. Derrfuss, J., Mar, R.A.: Lost in localization: the need for a universal coordinate database. Neuroimage **48**(1), 1–7 (2009)
2. Fischl, B., et al.: Cortical folding patterns and predicting cytoarchitecture. Cereb. Cortex **18**, 1973–1980 (2007)
3. Avants, B.B., Tustison, N.J., Song, G., Cook, P.A., Klein, A., Gee, J.C.: A reproducible evaluation of ANTs similarity metric performance in brain image registration. Neuroimage **54**(3), 2033–2044 (2011)
4. Glasser, M.F., et al.: WU-Minn HCP Consortium. the minimal preprocessing pipelines for the human connectome project. Neuroimage **80**, 105–124 (2013)
5. Ge, F., et al.: Denser growing fiber connections induce 3-hinge gyral folding. Cereb. Cortex **28**(3), 1064–1075 (2017)
6. Jiang, X., et al.: Sparse representation of HCP grayordinate data reveals novel functional architecture of cerebral cortex. Hum. Brain Mapp. **36**, 5301–5319 (2015)
7. Li, X., et al.: Commonly preserved and species-specific gyral folding patterns across primate brains. Brain Struct. Funct. **222**(5), 2127–2141 (2017)
8. Chen, H., et al.: Gyral net: a new representation of cortical folding organization. Med. Image Anal. **42**, 14–25 (2017)
9. Cho, M., Lee, J., Lee, K.M.: Reweighted random walks for graph matching. In: Daniilidis, K., Maragos, P., Paragios, N. (eds.) ECCV 2010. LNCS, vol. 6315, pp. 492–505. Springer, Heidelberg (2010). https://doi.org/10.1007/978-3-642-15555-0_36
10. https://www.humanconnectome.org/
11. Yeh, F.C., Wedeen, V.J., Tseng, W.Y.I.: Generalized q-sampling imaging. IEEE Trans. Med. Imaging **29**, 1626–1635 (2010)
12. Van Den Heuvel, M.P., Sporns, O.: Rich-club organization of the human connectome. J. Neurosci. Official J. Soc. Neurosci. **31**, 15775–15786 (2011)
13. Desikan, R.S., et al.: An automated labeling system for subdividing the human cerebral cortex on MRI scans into gyral based regions of interest. Neuroimage **31**(3), 968–980 (2006)
14. Munkres, J.: Algorithms for the Assignment and Transportation Problems. SIAM, Philadelphia (1957)

Multi-view Graph Matching of Cortical Landmarks

Ying Huang[1], Zhibin He[1], Lei Guo[1], Tianming Liu[2], and Tuo Zhang[1(✉)]

[1] School of Automation, Northwestern Polytechnical University, Xi'an, China
[2] Cortical Architecture Imaging and Discovery Lab, Department of Computer Science and Bioimaging Research Center, The University of Georgia, Athens, GA, USA

Abstract. Human brain image alignment based on cortical folding pattern has long been an intriguing yet challenging research topic. Recently, a new gyral folding pattern, termed gyral hinge, was proposed and characterized by the conjunction of gyri from multiple directions. The uniqueness and importance of gyral hinges lie in their structural and functional importance and potential cross-subject correspondence, making them possible to be used as cortical landmarks. However, such an anatomical correspondence based on these new cortical landmarks is not fully studied and not related to structural connective similarity and functional coherence. Thus, we investigate whether the single use of structural connective or functional interactive diagrams, or the joint use of them could improve the alignment of these gyral hinges. Based on the pairwise graph matching method, we propose a multi-view framework in which all gyral hinges within a subject are taken as a system and its structural and functional connective networks are used as inputs. The results demonstrate that the joint use of structural and functional profiles outperforms those based on either of them and outperform those based on image registration methods.

Keywords: Cortical landmarks · Cross-subject correspondence

1 Introduction

In the brain mapping field, there have been significant interests in establishing cross-subject cortical landmark correspondence in terms of structural/functional consistency [1–3]. However, due to the remarkable inter-individual variability of cortical folding patterns, it is still challenging to establish a common architecture of cortical landmarks that can comprehensively and simultaneously encode and characterize both structural and functional consistency across brains [4–6]. Recently, a group of novel cortical landmarks, termed gyral hinges, have been identified, which are widely spread across cortices and located at the crossings of multiple gyri [7]. Because most gyral hinges have three gyral spokes and those with more than three spokes are rarely seen, we use 3-hinge to denote them in this work. These 3-hinges possess the thickest cortices, the densest fiber connections and the most complicated functional network interactions [8–10], suggestive of their structural and functional uniqueness and importance. More

D. Shen et al. (Eds.): MICCAI 2019, LNCS 11767, pp. 84–92, 2019.
https://doi.org/10.1007/978-3-030-32251-9_10

importantly, cross-subject and cross-species correspondences for six such 3-hinges were found by manual labeling [10]. These 3-hinges exhibit similar structural connective patterns, suggestive of the possibility that 3-hinges could be used as cortical landmarks which simultaneously encode structural and functional cross-subject correspondence. In spite of these findings for 3-hinges, there still lacks an automatic method to establish the cross-subject correspondence for all of them and a comprehensive investigation of the relation between the correspondence and structural/functional characteristics at a connectome-scale is much needed.

To this end, we propose a multi-view graph matching method to estimate the cross-subject correspondences for these 3-hinge landmarks. The connectome-scale structural connective matrix and functional interaction matrix of all 3-hinges within a subject are simultaneously used as inputs to match those from other subjects in a group-wise manner. Our results demonstrate that the joint use of structural and functional connectome-scale features could improve the matching of these 3-hinges when compared to a single use of either of them or other image registration methods, in terms of simultaneous anatomical, structural and functional consistency. These results further suggest that cross-subject correspondences in terms of anatomical, structural and functional similarity could be found for well-defined cortical landmarks, such as 3-hinges in this work.

2   Materials and Methods

2.1   Datasets and Preprocessing

Ten subjects in the Q1 release of WU-Minn Human Connectome Project (HCP) consortium are used to develop the method [11]. Structural MRI imaging, diffusion MRI and fMRI parameters, as well as preprocessing steps, are referred to [11]. Within each subject, the grayordinate white matter cortical surface is used as the standard space across modalities. To estimate the voxel-wise axonal orientations and fibers, the generalized Q-sampling imaging (GQI) method and the deterministic streamline tracking algorithm in DSI Studio [12] are adopted with default parameters (max turning angle: $60°$, streamline length: 30 mm–300 mm, step length: 1 mm, quantitative anisotropy threshold: 0.2, fiber tract number: 4×10^4). Grayordinate surface is aligned to the dMRI space *via* FSL-flirt and FSL-fnirt applied to T1-weighted MRI and FA-map [12]. It is note that grayordinate surfaces have been resampled to be of the same vertex number across subjects. They are also registered to a common space to provide cross-subject vertex-wise correspondences. But the correspondences are not used in our method, but only used as the 3-hinge alignment results obtained based on registration methods in [13] and compared to our method.

2.2   Cortical Landmark Identification and Structural/Functional Connective Matrices Estimation

The 3-hinges are automatically identified *via* the published methods in [9]. In general, a gyral net (curves in Fig. 1(a)) is obtained on the gyral regions. The intersection vertices of the three branches are defined as 3-hinges (bubbles in Fig. 1(b)). For each subject, we construct a structural connective matrix (Fig. 1(c–d)) using these 3-hinges as nodes. The number of fibers that simultaneously pass through the neighborhoods (a sphere with $r = 3$ mm) of two 3-hinges is defined as the connective strength [14]. No normalization is needed for the strength as the total fiber number on each subject is equal (4×10^4). To construct a functional connective matrix, we conduct a group-wise version of the sparse representation method in [15] (Fig. 1(e)). FMRI signals (length of t) of all m cortical fMRI signals of all n subjects are arranged as a matrix $\mathbf{S} = [\mathbf{S}_1, \mathbf{S}_2, \cdots, \mathbf{S}_n] \in \mathbb{R}^{t \times (m \times n)}$. The matrix is factorized as $\mathbf{S} = \mathbf{D} \times \mathbf{A}$. $\mathbf{D} \in \mathbb{R}^{t \times k}$ is a group-wise temporal dictionary with k dictionary atoms ($k = 200$ in this work). $\mathbf{A}$ is a sparse coefficient weight matrix $\mathbf{A} = [\mathbf{A}_1, \mathbf{A}_2, \cdots, \mathbf{A}_n] \in \mathbb{R}^{k \times (m \times n)}$, where $\mathbf{A}_i \in \mathbb{R}^{k \times m}$ corresponds to the ith subject and is comparable across subjects. Because m^{th} column of $\mathbf{A}_i$ represents the weights of the k dictionary atoms that contribute to represent the fMRI signal of the mth vertex, we retrieve columns from $\mathbf{A}_i$ corresponding to 3-hinges (green columns in Fig. 1(e)) as their functional profiles. The Pearson correlation coefficients between two functional profiles across 3-hinges are computed and defined as the functional connective matrix (Fig. 1(f)). It is noted that subjects have different numbers of 3-hinges (267–369, 275.25 ± 34.64) and the 3-hinge connective matrices are of different sizes.

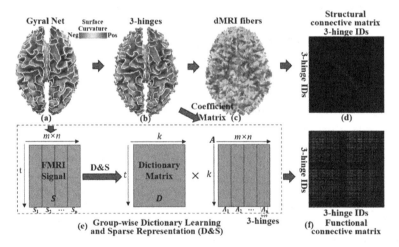

Fig. 1. Pipeline of structural and functional connective matrices estimation. (a) White curves are gyral crest lines which comprise the gyral net. The white matter cortical surface is color-coded by the surface curvatures. (b) Green bubbles highlight the locations of 3-hinges. (c) Streamline fibers from dMRI. (d) Structural connective matrix within 3-hinges. (e) Group-wise dictionary learning and sparse representation method on all subjects. (f) Functional connective matrix within 3-hinges. Matrices in (d) and (f) are binarized for the ease of presentation (Color figure online).

2.3   Two-View Graph Matching Methods

We firstly provide a summary of the basics of single-view graph matching method. $\mathbf{G}^P = (\mathbf{V}^P, \mathbf{E}^P, \mathbf{A}^P)$ and $\mathbf{G}^Q = (\mathbf{V}^Q, \mathbf{E}^Q, \mathbf{A}^Q)$ denote two subjects P and Q. $\mathbf{V}$ denotes nodes (3-hinges) and $\mathbf{E}$ denotes edges. $a_{ij} \in \mathbf{A}$ is the connective strength (fiber number or functional similarity) for $e_{ij} \in \mathbf{E}$ between v_i and v_j. To match two graphs, we define an affinity matrix $\mathbf{W}$, where $\mathbf{W}_{ia;jb} = f(a_i^P, a_j^P, a_{ij}^P, a_a^Q, a_b^Q, a_{ab}^Q)$ describes the consistency of attributes between the node pairs of candidate correspondences (v_i^P, v_a^Q) and (v_j^P, v_b^Q). A non-diagonal element $\mathbf{W}_{ia;jb}$ measures the similarity between the pair of edges $e_{ij}^P \in \mathbf{E}^P$ and $e_{ab}^Q \in \mathbf{E}^Q$. A diagonal element $\mathbf{W}_{ia;ia}$ represents the nodal similarity which is not used in this work. The edge similarity is defined as $\exp(-\left| a_{ij}^P - a_{ab}^Q \right|^2 / \sigma^2)$, where σ is set to be the mean value of $\left| a_{ij}^P - a_{ab}^Q \right|$. Given an assignment matrix $\mathbf{X} \in \{0,1\}^{n^P \times n^Q}$, where $\mathbf{X}_{ia} = 1$ indicates that v_i^P corresponds to v_a^Q, the graph matching problem is formulated as a program that searches for the vector $\mathbf{x}^*$ ($\mathbf{x}$ is a column-wise vector of $\mathbf{X}$) that maximizes the energy function in Eq. (1)

$$E(\mathbf{x}) = \mathbf{x}^T \mathbf{W} \mathbf{x} \; s.t. \; \mathbf{x} \in \{0,1\}^{n^P n^Q}, \forall i \sum_{a=1}^{n^Q} x_{ia} \leq 1, \forall a \sum_{i=1}^{n^P} x_{ia} \leq 1 \qquad (1)$$

where the constrains $\forall i \sum_{a=1}^{n^Q} x_{ia} \leq 1$ and $\forall a \sum_{i=1}^{n^P} x_{ia} \leq 1$ enforce the one-to-one matching between nodes. Empty matching is allowed if graphs are of different sizes.

We extend the graph matching method to a multi-view one. For clarity, we use two-views to introduce the method. Let subjects P and Q have two graphs (or two views): $\{\mathbf{G}_1^P, \mathbf{G}_2^P\}$ and $\{\mathbf{G}_1^Q, \mathbf{G}_2^Q\}$. The energy function can be written as the following one:

$$E(\mathbf{x}, \mathbf{y}) = \mathbf{x}^T \mathbf{W}_1 \mathbf{x} + \mathbf{y}^T \mathbf{W}_2 \mathbf{y} + \mathbf{x}^T \mathbf{W}_1 \mathbf{y} + \mathbf{y}^T \mathbf{W}_2 \mathbf{x} + \beta \mathbf{x}^T \mathbf{y} \; s.t. \; \mathbf{x}, \mathbf{y} \in$$
$$\{0,1\}^{n^P n^Q}, \forall i \sum_{a=1}^{n^Q} x_{ia} \leq 1, \forall a \sum_{i=1}^{n^P} x_{ia} \leq 1, \forall i \sum_{a=1}^{n^Q} y_{ia} \leq 1, \forall a \sum_{i=1}^{n^P} y_{ia} \leq 1 \qquad (2)$$

where $\mathbf{W}_1$ and $\mathbf{W}_2$ are the affinity matrices for two graphs, and $\mathbf{x}$ and $\mathbf{y}$ are the corresponding assignment vectors. Introduction of $\mathbf{x}^T \mathbf{y}$ is to minimize the disagreement between the assignments of two views. The Taylor series approximation is as follows:

$$E(\mathbf{x}, \mathbf{y}) \approx E(\mathbf{x}^{(0)}, \mathbf{y}^{(0)}) + \frac{\partial E}{\partial \mathbf{x}}\bigg|_{\mathbf{x}^{(0)}, \mathbf{y}^{(0)}} (\mathbf{x} - \mathbf{x}^{(0)}) + \frac{\partial E}{\partial \mathbf{y}}\bigg|_{\mathbf{x}^{(0)}, \mathbf{y}^{(0)}} (\mathbf{y} - \mathbf{y}^{(0)}) = a\mathbf{x} + b\mathbf{y} + c$$

$$(3)$$

where

$$\begin{cases} a = 2\mathbf{x}^{(0)T}\mathbf{W}_1 + \mathbf{y}^{(0)T}(\mathbf{W}_1 + \mathbf{W}_2 + \beta I) \\ b = 2\mathbf{y}^{(0)T}\mathbf{W}_2 + \mathbf{x}^{(0)T}(\mathbf{W}_1 + \mathbf{W}_2 + \beta I) \\ c = -\mathbf{x}^{(0)T}\mathbf{W}_1\mathbf{x}^{(0)} - \mathbf{y}^{(0)T}\mathbf{W}_2\mathbf{y}^{(0)} - \mathbf{y}^{(0)T}\mathbf{W}_1\mathbf{x}^{(0)} - \mathbf{x}^{(0)T}\mathbf{W}_2\mathbf{y}^{(0)} - \beta\mathbf{x}^{(0)T}\mathbf{y}^{(0)} \end{cases} \qquad (4)$$

and $\mathbf{I}$ is an identity matrix. Based on Eq. (3), $\mathbf{x}$ and $\mathbf{y}$ are updated in turns in each iteration. Details of the multi-viewgraph matching algorithm are in 'Algorithm 1' Table. The solution is proposed based on reweighted random walk graph matching [17].

The multi-view method above is applied to subjects in a group-wise manner. Given n subjects, the 3-hinge matrices of two views are represented by graphs $\{\mathbf{G}_v^n, v \in \{1, 2\}\}$. In each iteration, group mean connective matrices $\{\mathbf{M}_1, \mathbf{M}_2\}$ are obtained as the weighted sum of all individual matrices $\{\mathbf{A}_1^n, \mathbf{A}_2^n\}$, and are used as the 'templates' in the next iteration, to which matrices $\{\mathbf{A}_1^n, \mathbf{A}_2^n\}$ on each individual are matched. For example, in the tth iteration, Algorithm 1 is applied to $\{\mathbf{A}_1^n|_t, \mathbf{A}_2^n|_t\}$ and $\{\mathbf{M}_1|_{t-1}, \mathbf{M}_2|_{t-1}\}$ for each individual to obtain the updated $\{\hat{\mathbf{A}}_1^n|_t, \hat{\mathbf{A}}_2^n|_t\}$ by the assignment vectors $\{\mathbf{x}_n|_t, \mathbf{y}_n|_t\}$. Then, the similarity between $\hat{\mathbf{A}}_v^n|_t$ and $\mathbf{M}_v|_{t-1}$ is defined as the energy $s_v^n|_t = \mathbf{x}_n|_t^\mathsf{T} \mathbf{W}_{\hat{\mathbf{A}}_v^n|_t, \mathbf{M}_v|_{t-1}} \mathbf{x}_n|_t$, based on which the weight is defined as $w_v^n|_t = s_v^n|_t / \sum s_v^n|_t$ and is used to update the group mean $\mathbf{M}_v|_t$. In the 0th iteration, $\mathbf{M}_v$ is the sum of all the original $\mathbf{A}_v^n|_0$ s with equal weights. The algorithm stops when there is no difference between $\mathbf{M}_v$ s of two successive iterations.

2.4   Statistical Analyses

We segment the cortical surfaces to brain sites under the Automated Anatomical Labeling (AAL) parcellation scheme. Each subject has a label vector recording the brain site IDs of all 3-hinges. It is expected that the corresponding 3-hinges are located in the same brain site, and therefore the vectors from different subjects are expected to be the same. Interclass correlation coefficient (ICC) is used to measure the consistency of the label vectors over all subjects. To measure the inter-individual consistency of structural and functional connectomes within the aligned 3-hinges, we compute the Euclidean distance between structural/functional matrices from two subjects. The mean values averaged over all subject pairs are used as the consistency metric on the group. All these metrics are used on the aligned 3-hinges obtained by our method and single-view graph matching to compare the results. The 3-hinge correspondence provided by grayordinate is also compared, which is achieved by a combination of image and surface registration methods based on a variety of anatomical, structural and functional features [13]. To determine the correspondences of 3-hinges on grayordinates, we compute the Euclidean distance between all 3-hinges pairs between a subject and the template subject with the most 3-hinges. The Hungarian algorithm [16] is applied to the distance matrices to provide a one-to-one 3-hinge correspondence by searching for the closest distances.

Algorithm 1. Graph matching with two views

1 Given the affinity matrices $\mathbf{W_1}$ and $\mathbf{W_2}$, parameter α and β; initialize $\mathbf{x}$ and $\mathbf{y}$ as uniform

2 Set $\mathbf{W}_{k\,(ia,jb)} = 0, k \in \{1,2\}$ for all conflicting match pairs

3 Updated matrix $\mathbf{W}_k = \mathbf{W}_k / d_{k\,max}$, where $d_{k\,max} = \max_{ia} \sum_{jb} \mathbf{W}_{k\,(ia,jb)}, k \in \{1,2\}$

4 **Begin A**: (Do A until $\mathbf{x}$ and $\mathbf{y}$ converges)

5 $\quad \hat{\mathbf{x}}^T = 2\mathbf{x}^T\mathbf{W_1} + \mathbf{y}^T(\mathbf{W_1} + \mathbf{W_2} + \beta\mathbf{I}), \bar{\mathbf{y}}^T = 2\mathbf{y}^T\mathbf{W_2} + \mathbf{x}^T(\mathbf{W_1} + \mathbf{W_2} + \beta\mathbf{I})$

6 $\quad \hat{\mathbf{x}} = \exp(\beta\hat{\mathbf{x}}/max\,\hat{\mathbf{x}})$

7 $\quad$ **Begin B**: (Do B until $\hat{\mathbf{x}}$ converges)

8 $\quad\quad$ Normalize across all rows: $\hat{\mathbf{x}}_{ai} = \hat{\mathbf{x}}_{ai}/\sum_{i=1}^{I}\hat{\mathbf{x}}_{ai}$

9 $\quad\quad$ Normalize across all columns: $\hat{\mathbf{x}}_{ai} = \hat{\mathbf{x}}_{ai}/\sum_{a=1}^{A}\hat{\mathbf{x}}_{ai}$

10 $\quad$ **End B**

11 $\quad \hat{\mathbf{x}} = \hat{\mathbf{x}}/\sum\hat{\mathbf{x}}_{ai}$

12 $\quad \mathbf{x}^T = \alpha\hat{\mathbf{x}}^T + (1-\alpha)\hat{\mathbf{x}}^T$

13 $\quad \mathbf{x} = \mathbf{x}/\sum\mathbf{x}_{ai}$

14 $\quad \hat{\mathbf{y}} = exp(\beta\hat{\mathbf{y}}/max\,\hat{\mathbf{y}})$

15 $\quad$ **Begin C**: (Do B until $\hat{\mathbf{y}}$ converges)

16 $\quad\quad$ Normalize across all rows: $\hat{\mathbf{y}}_{ai} = \hat{\mathbf{y}}_{ai}/\sum_{i=1}^{I}\hat{\mathbf{y}}_{ai}$

17 $\quad\quad$ Normalize across all columns: $\hat{\mathbf{y}}_{ai} = \hat{\mathbf{y}}_{ai}/\sum_{a=1}^{A}\hat{\mathbf{y}}_{ai}$

18 $\quad$ **End C**

19 $\quad \hat{\mathbf{y}} = \hat{\mathbf{y}}/\sum\hat{\mathbf{y}}_{ai}$

20 $\quad \mathbf{y}^T = \alpha\hat{\mathbf{y}}^T + (1-\alpha)\hat{\mathbf{y}}^T$

21 $\quad \mathbf{y} = \mathbf{y}/\sum\mathbf{y}_{ai}$

22 **End A**

23 $\mathbf{x}$ is discretized by the Hungarian algorithm [16].

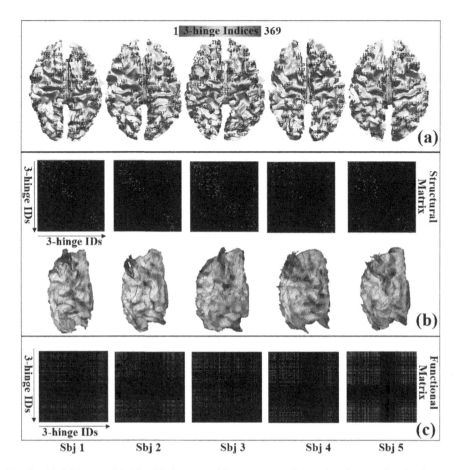

Fig. 2. (a) 3-hinges with identified cross-subject correspondence (numbers and color bar) on five randomly selected subjects as examples. Red, green and yellow arrows highlight three 3-hinges with correspondence. (b) Structural connective matrices of the aligned 3-hinge systems and DMRI fibers extracted from the 3-hinges highlighted by the red arrows in (a). (c) Functional connective matrices of the aligned 3-hinge systems (Color figure online).

3   Results

Figure 2(a) show the 3-hinge alignment results on 5 randomly selected subjects as examples. The cross-subject consistency of the 3-hinges highlighted by the numbers and color scales are observable by their locations. For example, 3-hinges #81, 287 and #260 are consistently found in the left and right post-central gyri, respectively. The structural and functional connective matrices (binarized for clarity) within the aligned 3-hinges are shown in Fig. 2(b) and (c), respectively. We also show the dMRI fiber bundles extracted from 3-hinge #260 as an example. The consistency of the global structural/functional connectome and local fiber bundle shape can be observed across subjects.

In addition to the visualization results, we also perform quantitative evaluations. To demonstrate the efficacy of our two-view graph matching method, we compare the alignment results with those obtained by single-view graph matching methods. Structural connective matrices (Str. column in Table 1) and functional connective matrices (Fun. column in Table 1) are used as the input to the single-view graph matching method, respectively. The grayordinate-based 3-hinge alignment is also compared to our method (Gray column in Table 1). We measure the similarity of both structural and functional connectome within the aligned 3-hinges *via* the metrics in Sect. 2.4.

Table 1. Comparison of inter-subject consistency in terms of structural (Struc.) and functional (Func.) connectomes between different methods. A smaller value indicates a higher consistency. * indicates p-value of t-test is < 0.05. The t-tests are between other methods and our two-view method. It is noted that the metrics are z-scores normalized across methods.

	Two-view ($\times 10^{-2}$)	Single-view		Gray ($\times 10^{-1}$)
		Str. ($\times 10^{-2}$)	Fun. ($\times 10^{-2}$)	
Struc.	-9.92 ± 0.99	$-9.37 \pm 1.00^*$	$-8.16 \pm 1.03^*$	$1.93 \pm 1.05^*$
Func.	-7.27 ± 1.01	$-1.42 \pm 1.02^*$	$-5.16 \pm 1.01^*$	$1.24 \pm 1.06^*$

The highest consistency in terms of both structural and functional 3-hinge connectomes is yield by our method, indicated by the lowest group-wise distance metrics in Table 1. It is noted that the metrics are z-scores normalized across all methods to make the results comparable without bias. The significance of the improvement of our results are demonstrated by the low p-values (<0.05) of t-tests between our method and one of the other methods in Table 1. Among the comparative result, it is interesting to see that our two-view method yield more consistent structural 3-hinge connectomes than single-view method based only on structural connective matrices. Similarly, our method yields more consistent functional connectomes than single-view method based only on functional connective matrices. This result demonstrates that the joint use of structural and functional connectome features could improve the alignment accuracy of cortical folding pattern when compared to the use of only one feature. Finally, we measure that whether corresponding 3-hinges are located at the same anatomical location (AAL atlas). The r-value of ICC measuring the group-wise consistency is 0.40 for our two-view method, which outperforms single-view methods based on structural matrices (0.29) and functional matrices (0.27) and grayordinate method (0.30).

4   Conclusion

We propose a novel multi-view framework to identify the correspondence of 3-hinge cortical landmarks across subjects. The effectiveness of this framework is demonstrated by cross-subject consistency of anatomical, structural connective and functional metrics, as well as the better performance over other methods. Our results provide new clues to the relationship between folding patterns and structure connectivity and brain function. In the future, we will apply this framework on larger scale multimodal datasets to further evaluate its robustness and accuracy, as well as other applications in neuroimage analysis domain such as brain image registration and alignment.

References

1. Zhu, D., Li, K., Guo, L.: DICCCOL: dense individualized and common connectivity-based cortical landmarks. Cereb. Cortex **23**(4), 786–800 (2013)
2. Sabuncu, M.R., Singer, B.D., Bryan, C., Bryan, R.E., Ramadge, P.J., Haxby, J.V.: Function-based intersubject alignment of human cortical anatomy. Cereb. Cortex **20**(1), 130–140 (2010)
3. Derrfuss, J., Mar, R.A.: Lost in localization: the need for a universal coordinate database. Neuroimage **48**(1), 1–7 (2009)
4. Zhang, S., Zhao, Y., Jiang, X., Shen, D., Liu, T.: Joint representation of consistent structural and functional profiles for identification of common cortical landmarks. Brain Imaging Behav. **12**(3), 728–742 (2018)
5. Avants, B.B., Tustison, N.J., Song, G., Cook, P.A., Klein, A., Gee, J.C.: A reproducible evaluation of ANTs similarity metric performance in brain image registration. Neuroimage **54**(3), 2033–2044 (2011)
6. Jiang, X., et al.: Sparse representation of HCP grayordinate data reveals novel functional architecture of cerebral cortex. Hum. Brain Mapp. **36**, 5301–5319 (2015)
7. Kaiming, L., et al.: Gyral folding pattern analysis via surface profiling. Neuroimage **52**(4), 1202–1214 (2010)
8. Ge, F., et al.: Denser growing fiber connections induce 3-hinge gyral folding. Cereb. Cortex **28**(3), 1–12 (2017)
9. Zhang, T., et al.: Exploring 3-hinge gyral folding patterns among HCP Q3 868 human subjects. Hum. Brain Mapp. **39**(10), 4134–4149 (2018)
10. Li, X., et al.: Commonly preserved and species-specific gyral folding patterns across primate brains. Brain Struct. Funct. **222**(5), 1–15 (2017)
11. https://www.humanconnectome.org/
12. http://dsi-studio.labsolver.org/
13. Glasser, M.F., et al.: WU-Minn HCP consortium. the minimal preprocessing pipelines for the human connectome project. Neuroimage **80**, 105–124 (2013)
14. Zhang, T., et al.: Characterization of U-shape streamline fibers: methods and applications. Med. Image Anal. **18**(5), 795–807 (2014)
15. Lv, J., et al.: Sparse representation of group-wise FMRI signals. Med. Image Comput. Comput. Assist. Interv. **2013**, 608–616 (2013)
16. Munkres, J.: Algorithms for the assignment and transportation problems. J. Soc. Ind. Appl. Math. **5**(1), 32–38 (1957)
17. Cho, M., Lee, J., Lee, K.M.: Reweighted random walks for graph matching. In: European Conference on Computer Vision 2010, pp. 492–505 (2010)

Patient-Specific Conditional Joint Models of Shape, Image Features and Clinical Indicators

Bernhard Egger[1(✉)], Markus D. Schirmer[1,2,3], Florian Dubost[2,4],
Marco J. Nardin[2], Natalia S. Rost[2], and Polina Golland[1]

[1] Computer Science and Artificial Intelligence Lab (CSAIL), MIT, Cambridge, USA
egger@mit.edu
[2] Massachusetts General Hospital (MGH), Harvard Medical School, Boston, USA
[3] German Centre for Neurodegenerative Diseases (DZNE), Bonn, Germany
[4] Erasmus MC - University Medical Center Rotterdam, Rotterdam, Netherlands

Abstract. We propose and demonstrate a joint model of anatomical shapes, image features and clinical indicators for statistical shape modeling and medical image analysis. The key idea is to employ a copula model to separate the joint dependency structure from the marginal distributions of variables of interest. This separation provides flexibility on the assumptions made during the modeling process. The proposed method can handle binary, discrete, ordinal and continuous variables. We demonstrate a simple and efficient way to include binary, discrete and ordinal variables into the modeling. We build Bayesian conditional models based on observed partial clinical indicators, features or shape based on Gaussian processes capturing the dependency structure. We apply the proposed method on a stroke dataset to jointly model the shape of the lateral ventricles, the spatial distribution of the white matter hyperintensity associated with periventricular white matter disease, and clinical indicators. The proposed method yields interpretable joint models for data exploration and patient-specific statistical shape models for medical image analysis.

Keywords: Statistical shape modeling · Copula · Gaussian processes · Attributes · Meta-data · White matter hyperintensities

1 Introduction

In medical imaging almost every image is at least weakly labeled with clinical indicators. A minimal set of such labels usually includes age, sex, demographics, and diagnostic or prognostic clinical values such as blood pressure, history of

Electronic supplementary material The online version of this chapter (https://doi.org/10.1007/978-3-030-32251-9_11) contains supplementary material, which is available to authorized users.

© Springer Nature Switzerland AG 2019
D. Shen et al. (Eds.): MICCAI 2019, LNCS 11767, pp. 93–101, 2019.
https://doi.org/10.1007/978-3-030-32251-9_11

smoking or outcome scores. The labels are of interest for clinical decisions or clinical research, however, they are rarely included in the analysis of shape or image features. We propose to construct joint statistical shape and attribute models to better understand and visualize the interplay between shape deformations and the variations of clinical indicators. The proposed model promises to reveal associations between anatomical shapes, image features, and clinical phenotypes, to help understand disease mechanisms and risk factors, and to improve predictions and patient stratification in clinical trials.

We demonstrate our approach in the context of a clinical cohort of ischemic stroke patients, where we investigate the relationships between the patterns of expansion of the lateral ventricles, the spatial patterns of white matter hyperintensity (WMH) indicative of the white matter disease, and patient data that include stroke outcome scores. Our model is built from segmentations of ventricles and white matter hyperintensities in T2-FLAIR magnetic resonance images.

We integrate copula [13] and Gaussian processes [11] to jointly analyze shape and other variables. Copula methods provide a decomposition of every continuous and multivariate distribution into its marginal distributions and a copula that captures the dependency structure [13]. The separate modeling of the marginal distributions and of the copula offers better flexibility than the classical statistical shape models. The marginal distributions can be modeled as Gaussian, or other parametric and non-parametric distributions. The choice of the model for each marginal distribution is separate from all others, e.g., a Gaussian distribution for the shape components and the empirical distributions for the clinical indicators. In this work, we use a Gaussian copula, which means we transform the data into a space where all marginal distributions are Gaussian. In this latent space, we then apply standard shape modeling techniques, such as the principal component analysis (PCA) or the Gaussian processes, to model the dependency structure between 3D coordinates of the shape and other indicators. The transformation to the latent space is invertible and our shape model remains generative. We can, therefore, construct the conditional distribution given clinical indicators using Gaussian process regression. Here we focus on the setting where some clinical indicators are given and we capture the conditional distribution of shapes, i.e., a patient-specific statistical shape model.

The main contributions of this paper are: (i) a novel approach for generating conditional shape models based on clinical indicators or image features; (ii) copula-based shape models that include binary, discrete, ordinal and continuous variables; (iii) novel associations between ventricle growth, WMH patterns and clinical indicators in the ischemic stroke patient cohort.

Related Work. Although many clinical indicators are collected and available with medical images, the idea of combining statistical shape models with clinical indicators is rarely explored. The work of Blanc *et al.* [2] includes patient attributes in femur modeling. The method assumes the data is Gaussian distributed and cannot handle binary, discrete, or ordinal variables. Pereanez *et al.* [10] proposed constraining shape models based on clinical indicators. They demonstrated that such constrained models are beneficial for model-based image segmentation. This approach is limited to a model prediction given a complete set of clinical indicators and handles ordinal variables as a set of binary attributes. Our method combines these ideas to employ the copula and uses the conditional distribution to capture the remaining variability given partial data. Han and Liu [7] proposed a variant of PCA called Copula Component Analysis that is inherently scale-invariant, more robust to outliers and handles arbitrary discrete ordinal marginal distributions. Hoff [8] presented the idea of an extended rank likelihood which can also account for non-continuous variables. In computer vision, Egger et al. [4,5] used copulas for shape and appearance modeling to account for the non-Gaussian appearance of human faces, however, they did not handle discrete or ordinal variables.

Conditional shape models without clinical indicators are well studied. A Bayesian approach was proposed by Albrecht et al. [1] to model the remaining variability of the femur given partial information. They showed that (probabilistic) PCA and Gaussian process regression with a statistical kernel are equivalent for such modeling. We build upon this model and include clinical indicators to construct patient-specific conditional shape models based on image features and/or clinical indicators. In our experiments, we visualize the conditional models and demonstrate superior performance in a reconstruction task when including all data in the statistical model.

2   Methods

We propose a joint model for anatomical shape, image features and clinical indicators based on the copula [13] and combine it with the idea of conditional shape models based on Gaussian processes [1]. To enable the use of not only continuous, but also binary, discrete and ordinal variables, we use a sampling strategy similar to [8].

We define an instance of our model to be a combination of 3D shape coordinates $x_k^{(1)}, x_k^{(2)}, x_k^{(3)}$ and image-based feature f_k associated with surface point k. All N surface points are in correspondence across training data, achieved via shape registration to an atlas in our experiments. In addition each instance includes K binary, discrete, ordinal or continuous variables $\{a_1 \ldots a_K\}$. Let $y = [x_1^{(1)}, x_1^{(2)}, x_1^{(3)}, \ldots, x_N^{(1)}, x_N^{(2)}, x_N^{(3)}, f_1, \ldots, f_N, a_1, \ldots, a_K]^T$ be the vector representation of the instance, $y \in \mathbb{R}^d$ with $d = 4N + K$. The training set of M shapes with image features and clinical indicators forms the data matrix $Y \in \mathbb{R}^{d \times M}$. Let random variable y_i represent component i of the instance and $W_i = p(y_i)$ represents its marginal distribution.

We use a Gaussian copula to capture the dependency pattern in combination with marginal distributions W_i [6,14]. According to Sklar's theorem [13] the copula C provides the dependency structure in the joint cumulative distribution function (CDF) F such that

$$F(y_1, \cdots, y_n) = C(W_1, \ldots, W_n) = \Phi_R(\Phi^{-1}(W_1), \ldots, \Phi^{-1}(W_n)) \qquad (1)$$

Where $\Phi^{-1}(\cdot)$ is the inverse standard normal CDF and $\Phi_R(\cdot)$ is the joint CDF of a zero-mean multivariate Gaussian distribution with covariance matrix R. The multivariate latent representation $\hat{y}_i = \Phi^{-1}(W_i), i = 1, \ldots, d$ distributed according to the standard normal distribution.

Marginal Distributions. To learn the model above from training data we first estimate the marginal distributions with parametric or nonparametric methods. For properties that cannot be naturally captured by a Gaussian distribution (e.g., image features, sex or outcome scores), we employ the empirical marginal distribution for all the components as proposed in [7]. If only limited data is available, various assumptions on the marginal distribution must be made, separately for each component. In statistical shape modeling, a Gaussian marginal distribution is usually assumed. To transform our data into the latent space, we first transform the empirical marginal distribution into a uniform distribution by replacing every entry of the data by the CDF of the empirical distribution. Second, we use the inverse CDF of a standard normal distribution to map to the latent space [4].

While the original copula framework is limited to continuous distributions, multiple solutions have been proposed to overcome this limitation. The first step, the transformation to a uniform distribution, relies on unique ranks (values of CDF). For binary, discrete and ordinal variables this sorting is not unique. In our experiments, we observed that the latent representation is stable when permuting elements with the same values for ranking, in the setting where we have many more variables than samples ($d \gg M$). To construct a consistent dependency structure we generate multiple (50) random rankings for non-unique values and average the resulting estimates of the model parameters. Once the data is transformed to its latent representation we estimate the covariance matrix R and represent it by its $M - 1$ eigenvectors (i.e. principal components).

Conditional Modeling. The Gaussian copula represents the dependency structure of our data y based on the latent representation $\hat{y}$. We use Gaussian processes to capture correlations in the latent space [11]. We define function $s_j : \Omega \to \mathbb{R}$ on a finite domain Ω such that $s_j(\hat{y}_i) \in \mathbb{R}$ refers to the ith element of the jth training example in our latent space, $i = 1, \ldots, d, j = 1, \ldots, M$. The Gaussian process is fully defined by the mean and covariance functions estimated from the training data:

$$\mu(\hat{y}) = \frac{1}{M} \sum_{j=1}^{M} s_j(\hat{y})$$

$$\Sigma(\hat{y}, \hat{y}') = \sum_{j=1}^{M} \left(s_j(\hat{y}) - \mu(\hat{y}) \right) \left(s_j(\hat{y}') - \mu(\hat{y}') \right)^T. \tag{2}$$

Given a subset z of the vector y as an observation, we construct component-wise its latent representation $\hat{z}$. The prediction of the missing parts reduces to a standard Gaussian process regression problem. We assume observations are corrupted by uncorrelated Gaussian noise $\epsilon = \mathcal{N}(0, \sigma^2)$ and obtain the prediction for the distribution of the complete vector $\hat{y}$ from the observed vector $\hat{z}$. The conditional distribution $p(\hat{y}|\hat{z})$ is again a Gaussian process with mean:

$$\mu_c(\hat{y}|\hat{z}) = \mu(\hat{y}) + \Sigma(\hat{y}, \hat{z})^T \left(\Sigma(\hat{z}, \hat{z}) + \sigma^2 \mathcal{I}\right)^{-1} (\hat{z} - \mu_{\hat{z}}) \tag{3}$$

and covariance

$$\Sigma_c(\hat{y}, \hat{y}'|\hat{z}) = \Sigma(\hat{y}, \hat{y}') - \Sigma(\hat{y}, \hat{z})^T \left(\Sigma(\hat{z}, \hat{z}) + \sigma^2 \mathcal{I}\right)^{-1} \Sigma(\hat{z}, \hat{y}') \tag{4}$$

where $\mathcal{I}$ is the identity matrix.

The parameter σ has an impact on the accuracy of the prediction and varies between different observations. The different modalities in our model have a different amount of uncertainty. For shape observations, σ is an estimate of the segmentation accuracy and the registration quality, for clinical indicators, it is a measurement of how accurate they are measured. We estimated the optimal parameters for observation uncertainty σ for each set of observations via cross-validation.

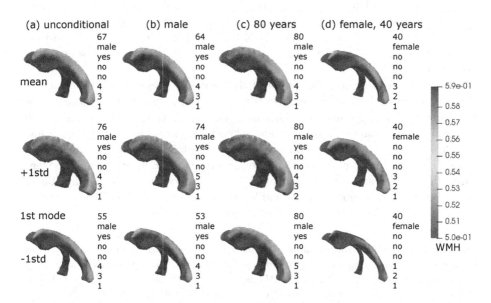

Fig. 1. Joint model of ventricle shape, WMH burden, and clinical indicators. Mean and variation along the first principal mode is shown. (a) the original model, (b), (c), (d) the model conditioned on sex = male, age = 80 years and (sex = female, age = 40 years) respectively. The color indicates the spatially varying amount of WMH burden. The variables per instance are ordered as age, sex, hypertension, hyperlipidemia, atrial fibrillation, smoking, NIHSS, and mRS.

3   Experiments

We produce a statistical model based on a dataset of T2-FLAIR magnetic resonance images from 793 acute ischemic stroke patients, without gross pathologies, such as mass effects, from the Genes Affecting Stroke Risk and Outcomes Study (GASROS), for which patients were enrolled at Massachusetts General Hospital between 2003 and 2011 [15]. Manual WMH segmentation was performed using MRIcro [12], and ventricles were automatically segmented (Dice: 0.89), using a 3D U-Net [3]. Subsequently, we isolated periventricular from subcortical WMH, based on connectivity of individual WMH lesions to the ventricles. After segmentation, we establish correspondence between every ventricle segmentation and the atlas ventricles by fitting a Gaussian process deformation model estimated via the iterative closest point algorithm [9]. The ventricles are represented as a surface triangle mesh with 1504 vertices. The WMH is modeled as a feature based on the vertices of the mesh. Every voxel labeled as periventricular WMH is assigned to the closest vertex point. This results in a WMH representation as a surface feature. In addition to the shape of the ventricles and the WMH burden feature, we include clinical indicators that represent age, sex, hypertension (binary), hyperlipidemia (binary), atrial fibrillation (binary), smoking (ordinal, 1–6) and NIHSS (stroke score, ordinal 0–42), mRS (outcome score, ordinal 0–6) and the overall WMH volume. With 1504 3D ventricle vertices, 1504 WMH burden features and 9 clinical indicators, the total dimensionality of a single data point is $d = 6025$.

Figure 1 presents the joint model of the ventricle shape, WMH burden features, and clinical indicators and also three conditional models for different clinical indicators, like age and sex. The conditional models have similar mean and variability as the unconditioned model when conditioned on features with low correlations to the remaining components Fig. 1b and show different means and less variability when conditioned on stronger correlated Fig. 1c or combined features Fig. 1d. The supplementary material contains a video of our graphical user interface for data exploration. It enables the user to fix clinical indicators and visualize the remaining variability in the conditional model.

Table 1. Clinical indicator prediction. Mean error and standard deviation are reported for the prediction of age, stroke outcome (mRS) and sex. The columns of the matrix correspond to the prediction based on the mean of the marginal distribution and conditioned on the ventricle shape, WMH burden, all other clinical indicators, indicators combined with WMH volume (ind + vol), and all available components except for the one being predicted. For sex, the percent of correct predictions is reported.

	Mean	Ventricles	WMH	Indicators	Ind + vol	Combined
Age	15.77 ± 9.49	11.27 ± 6.62	12.06 ± 7.58	13.21 ± 8.19	11.57 ± 7.04	**9.85 ± 5.76**
mRS	2.01 ± 1.50	1.88 ± 1.37	1.96 ± 1.45	**1.65 ± 1.20**	**1.65 ± 1.20**	**1.65 ± 1.19**
Sex	60.6%	62.7%	61.7%	65.3%	64.8%	**67.0%**

Table 2. Ventricle Shape and WMH burden prediction. The setting is the same as in Table 1 but we predict the shape of the ventricles and the WMH burden from the remaining values. Mean and standard deviation of distances between mesh vertices in mm is reported for the ventricle shape and WMH feature distance in voxels.

	Mean	Ventricles	WMH	Indicators	Ind + vol	Combined
Ventricles	1582.2 ± 34.5	–	132.9 ± 35.0	146.9 ± 45.1	144.8 ± 43.0	**132.3** ± 34.8
WMH	3980 ± 2830	2927 ± 2270	–	3073 ± 2419	1291 ± 897	**1254** ± 866

We evaluate the joint model in a reconstruction task of estimating the full vector from partial data in three different tasks: attribute prediction (Table 1), shape prediction, and WMH burden prediction (Table 2). For all tasks, we use the mean of the conditional distribution in the latent space to generate predictions. The values are obtained by randomly splitting the dataset into a training set of 600 patients and a validation set of the remaining 193 patients. The attribute prediction task (Table 1) aims to estimate clinical indicators, e.g., stroke outcome, given the shape and WMH burden. We observe that the ventricle shape and WMH burden are strong indicators for age whilst they contribute little to the stroke outcome score. For age and sex, using the combination of all modalities provides the best prediction. The shape and WMH prediction tasks (Table 2) reveal how the imaging data from a patient relates to the clinical indicators. The shape of the ventricles can be predicted from the WMH burden. The prediction in the other direction is more challenging, due to strong variability in WMH burden in the population. Clinical indicators including WMH volume combined with the ventricle shape produce the best prediction.

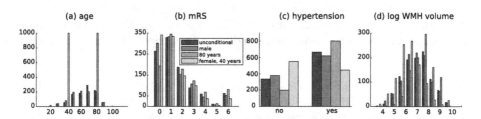

Fig. 2. Sample distributions of age, mRS (outcome score), hypertension and the log WMH volume for unconditional and conditional model conditioned on sex = male, age = 80 years and (sex = female, age = 40 years) respectively.

In the third experiment, we demonstrate the difference between the unconditional and conditional models. We produce the sample distributions by drawing 1,000 random samples from the corresponding model. Figure 2 reports those sample distributions before and after conditioning on the same three events as in Fig. 1. We observe that the conditioning on male has a weak effect whilst the conditioning on age or a combination of age and sex has a strong effect on the resulting marginal distributions.

We implemented the copula model based on the code provided in [4] in the Scalismo[1] framework for statistical shape modeling based on Gaussian processes. The computation of the conditional shape models based on the clinical indicators takes a few seconds for our dataset on a single core. Reducing the model via PCA will speed it up to real-time performance, enabling interactions with the model.

Limitations. The proposed model has two main limitations. First, we assume dense correspondence on the surface of the ventricles as well as correspondence across image features. This is especially limiting if some shape features have weak or no correspondence across the population. Second, the Gaussian model for the dependency structure we are using is limited to second-order dependency and does not reflect higher-order dependency. These two limitations and assumptions are very common in the statistical shape modeling, especially when working with small datasets.

4   Conclusion

We present a joint generative model of shape, image features, and clinical indicators. Conditional models for partially observed data can be straightforwardly derived. The copula can be implemented as a simple pre- and postprocessing step in existing pipelines relying on (probabilistic) PCA or Gaussian processes. In addition, conditional models can be constructed efficiently for interactive data exploration. Our work provides a highly effective approach to exploring high dimensional data, especially spatial correlations, for example between ventricle expansion and WMH burden patterns. Statistical shape models are commonly used as statistical priors for image analysis tasks, and the proposed conditional models can be interpreted as patient-specific statistical shape models for patient-specific medical image analysis. Our model includes binary, discrete, ordinal and continuous variables and hence can handle a vast variety of available clinical indicators.

Aknowledgments. This research was funded by SNSF P2BSP2_178643, NIH NIBIB NAC P41EB015902, NIH NINDS R01NS086905, Horizon2020 753896, De Drie Lichten 24/18, ZonMw 104003005, Wistron Corporation, AWS, SIP and NVIDIA.

References

1. Albrecht, T., Lüthi, M., Gerig, T., Vetter, T.: Posterior shape models. Med. Image Anal. **17**(8), 959–973 (2013)
2. Blanc, R., Seiler, C., Székely, G., Nolte, L., Reyes, M.: Statistical model based shape prediction from a combination of direct observations and various surrogates: application to orthopaedic research. Med. Image Anal. **16**(6), 1156–1166 (2012)

---

[1] Scalismo - A Scalable Image Analysis and Shape Modeling Software Framework https://github.com/unibas-gravis/scalismo.

3. Dubost, F., de Bruijne, M., Nardin, M., Dalca, A.V., Donahue, K.L., et al.: Automated image registration quality assessment utilizing deep-learning based ventricle extraction in clinical data. arXiv e-prints arXiv:1907.00695, July 2019

4. Egger, B., Kaufmann, D., Schönborn, S., Roth, V., Vetter, T.: Copula eigenfaces with attributes: semiparametric principal component analysis for a combined color, shape and attribute model. In: Braz, J., et al. (eds.) VISIGRAPP 2016. CCIS, vol. 693, pp. 95–112. Springer, Cham (2017). https://doi.org/10.1007/978-3-319-64870-5_5

5. Egger, B., Kaufmann, D., Schönborn, S., Roth, V., Vetter, T.: Copula eigenfaces - semiparametric principal component analysis for facial appearance modeling. In: Proceedings of the 11th Joint Conference on Computer Vision, Imaging and Computer Graphics Theory and Applications: Volume 1: GRAPP, pp. 50–58. SCITEPRESS-Science and Technology Publications, Lda (2016)

6. Genest, C., Ghoudi, K., Rivest, L.P.: A semiparametric estimation procedure of dependence parameters in multivariate families of distributions. Biometrika 82(3), 543–552 (1995)

7. Han, F., Liu, H.: Semiparametric principal component analysis. In: Advances in Neural Information Processing Systems, pp. 171–179 (2012)

8. Hoff, P.D.: Extending the rank likelihood for semiparametric copula estimation. Ann. Appl. Stat. 1, 265–283 (2007)

9. Lüthi, M., Gerig, T., Jud, C., Vetter, T.: Gaussian process morphable models. IEEE PAMI 40(8), 1860–1873 (2018)

10. Pereañez, M., Lekadir, K., Albà, X., Medrano-Gracia, P., Young, A.A., Frangi, A.: Patient metadata-constrained shape models for cardiac image segmentation. In: Camara, O., Mansi, T., Pop, M., Rhode, K., Sermesant, M., Young, A. (eds.) STACOM 2015. LNCS, vol. 9534, pp. 98–107. Springer, Cham (2016). https://doi.org/10.1007/978-3-319-28712-6_11

11. Rasmussen, C.E.: Gaussian processes in machine learning. In: Bousquet, O., von Luxburg, U., Rätsch, G. (eds.) ML-2003. LNCS (LNAI), vol. 3176, pp. 63–71. Springer, Heidelberg (2004). https://doi.org/10.1007/978-3-540-28650-9_4

12. Rost, N.S., Rahman, R.M., Biffi, A., et al.: White matter hyperintensity volume is increased in small vessel stroke subtypes. Neurology 75(19), 1670–1677 (2010)

13. Sklar, M.: Fonctions de répartition à n dimensions et leurs marges. Université Paris 8 (1959)

14. Tsukahara, H.: Semiparametric estimation in copula models. Can. J. Stat. 33(3), 357–375 (2005)

15. Zhang, C.R., et al.: Determinants of white matter hyperintensity burden differ at the extremes of ages of ischemic stroke onset. J. Stroke Cerebrovasc. Dis. 24(3), 649–654 (2015)

Surface-Based Spatial Pyramid Matching of Cortical Regions for Analysis of Cognitive Performance

Kristen M. Campbell[1]($\boxtimes$) (ID), Jeffrey S. Anderson[2](ID), and P. Thomas Fletcher[3]

[1] Scientific Computing and Imaging Institute, University of Utah, Salt Lake City, UT, USA
kris@sci.utah.edu
[2] Department of Radiology and Imaging Sciences, University of Utah, Salt Lake City, UT, USA
andersonjeffs@gmail.com
[3] University of Virginia, Charlottesville, VA, USA

Abstract. We propose a method to analyze the relationship between the shape of functional regions of the cortex and cognitive measures, such as reading ability and vocabulary knowledge. Functional regions on the cortical surface can vary not only in size and shape but also in topology and position relative to neighboring regions. Standard diffeomorphism-based shape analysis tools do not work well here because diffeomorphisms are unable to capture these topological differences, which include region splitting and merging across subjects. State-of-the-art cortical surface shape analyses compute derived regional properties (scalars), such as regional volume, cortical thickness, curvature, and gyrification index. However, these methods cannot compare the full extent of topological or shape differences in cortical regions. We propose icosahedral spatial pyramid matching (ISPM) of region borders computed on the surface of a sphere to capture this variation in regional topology, position, and shape. We then analyze how this variation corresponds to measures of cognitive performance. We compare our method to other approaches and find that it is indeed informative to consider aspects of shape beyond the standard approaches. Analysis is performed using a subset of 27 test/retest subjects from the Human Connectome Project in order to understand both the effectiveness and reproducibility of this method.

1 Introduction

Much work has been done to understand what parts of the brain are responsible for which functions. This localization of function is important for fundamental understanding of how the brain works and for neurosurgical tasks such as planning regions to target or avoid during the removal of tumors [2]. While localization of function is generally consistent across individuals, there is variability in the shape of functional regions.

© Springer Nature Switzerland AG 2019
D. Shen et al. (Eds.): MICCAI 2019, LNCS 11767, pp. 102–110, 2019.
https://doi.org/10.1007/978-3-030-32251-9_12

Glasser et al. showed in [3] that certain cortical regions can have multiple *topological* variants that are present in a significant percentage of the population. In particular, they highlight the 55b region, a lightly myelinated area of the premotor cortex that separates the frontal eye field (FEF) and premotor eye field (PEF). However, there is a consistent variant in which 55b is split into two disjoint pieces, with FEF in between the split sections. A second variant exists in which 55b can be shifted relative to FEF, so that FEF is now between 55b and PEF. See Fig. 1 for examples of the variety in 55b, FEF, and PEF configurations. Furthermore, it is possible that a region is missing in a subject. As an example, PEF is missing in the bottom-right subject in Fig. 1.

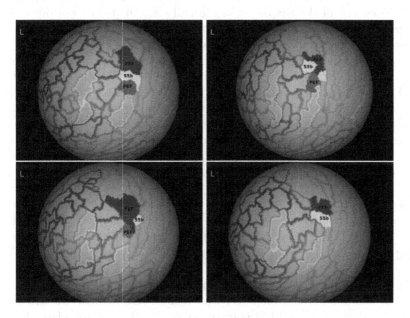

Fig. 1. Four examples of the variety of 55b, FEF, and PEF configurations. Each example is the cortical surface of a subject's left hemisphere projected onto a sphere.

The presence of these and other topological variations in a large subset of individuals leads to the question of whether these variants are related to any sort of change in cognitive or social ability, psychological well-being, or personality. To answer this question, we first need a statistical shape analysis method that can (1) compare shapes with differing topology and (2) handle the possibility of missing shapes, that is, the method allows the null set to be a valid shape.

Existing shape correspondence methods require shapes to be prealigned and need to find a one-to-one mapping for each point around the shape [10]. Diffeomorphic methods such as large deformation diffeomorphic metric mapping (LDDMM) [1] and spherical demons [12] assume that a diffeomorphism exists that can deform one shape into the other. Neither shape correspondence nor diffeomorphic methods can compare one region to a region split into two separate pieces.

Other shape analysis methods allow topologically different shapes, but do not allow missing shapes. Leventon et al. [6] represent shapes as level sets of the signed distance from the shape boundary. This method does not have a unique representation for a shape and cannot handle the null set. Another approach is the Gromov-Hausdorff metric [9], which provides a valid distance metric between shapes and allows multiple topologies, but does not allow for a shape to be the null set.

Another metric that we could use is the Jaccard distance that measures the difference between the size of union and the size of intersection of two sets. This metric allows one of the shapes to be the null set, but it does not differentiate between nonoverlapping sets that are near versus far away from each other. Both of these cases will have the same distance of 0.

We propose a new distance metric on shapes defined as regions on a sphere, called icosahedral spatial pyramid matching (ISPM). This metric is an extension of spatial pyramid matching (SPM) [5,13] defined for images. ISPM can measure distances between shapes that are not topologically equivalent and differences in configurations of shapes relative to each other. Our goal is to analyze relationships between the shapes of cortical regions and cognitive measures. However, standard correlation or regression approaches are not applicable, since our shapes do not live in a Euclidean vector space, but rather a non-trivial metric space defined through the ISPM metric. Instead, we use a statistic called distance correlation [11], which measures the dependency between two random values sampled from metric spaces.

2   Methods

ISPM computes spatial pyramid matching (SPM) on a mesh of a spherical surface using labeled borders of parcellated regions as features. We will review d-dimensional image space SPM here and then describe how we adapt the computation to an icosahedral mesh of a spherical surface. Once we can compute distances between shape complexes on a sphere, we show how to use distance correlation in order to find relationships between shape and cognitive performance measures.

2.1   Spatial Pyramid Matching

SPM [5] is a measure of similarity of features between two images, A and B, using the pyramid match kernel (PMK) from [4] while preserving spatial information on a rectangular d-dimensional image grid. SPM starts by separating each image into C channels, one channel per feature type, where each channel contains the spatial locations where that feature type is found in the image.

We then construct a pyramid of L resolution levels, where the finest resolution is level L, and the number of bins in a level, D, decreases by a factor of 2 in each direction at each level.

For each resolution level, l, in the pyramid, a spatial histogram is computed for each channel, c, that counts how many times that feature appears within the spatial extent covered by each bin. The amount a feature "matches" at a particular level of resolution can be measured by the intersection of the histograms $I(H^l_{A_c}, H^l_{B_c})$ for A_c and B_c. Histogram intersection is used here because it has the useful property of being positive-definite, as shown in [4]. The intersection of a channel histogram at a particular level is

$$I^l_c(H^l_{A_c}, H^l_{B_c}) = \sum_{i=1}^{D} \min(H^l_{A_c}(i), H^l_{B_c}(i)). \tag{1}$$

To avoid counting the same contribution at more than one level, we look at the number of new matches, N^l, at each level:

$$N^l_c(A_c, B_c) = I^l_c(H^l_{A_c}, H^l_{B_c}) - I^{l+1}_c(H^{l+1}_{A_c}, H^{l+1}_{B_c}), \tag{2}$$

$$N^L_c(A_c, B_c) = I^L_c(H^L_{A_c}, H^L_{B_c}). \tag{3}$$

The pyramid match kernel is the weighted combination of these new matches across all levels:

$$\kappa_c(A_c, B_c) = \sum_{l=0}^{L} \frac{1}{2^{L-l}} N^l_c(A_c, B_c). \tag{4}$$

The spatial pyramid matching is the normalized combination of these kernels across the different channels:

$$K_S(A, B) = \frac{\sum_{c=1}^{C} \kappa_c(A_c, B_c)}{\sqrt{\sum_{c=1}^{C} \kappa_c(A_c, A_c) * \sum_{c=1}^{C} \kappa_c(B_c, B_c)}}. \tag{5}$$

Because histogram intersection is used, and κ_c sums these intersections with a weight that is decreasing as the grid coarsens, the pyramid match kernel is positive-definite, as shown in [4]. The positive-definiteness continues to be maintained when summing across channels, and thus K_S is a Mercer kernel since κ_c is one. Since $K_S(A, A) = 1$ for all images, A, we convert this similarity kernel to a distance metric, $d_S(A, B)$, scaling by 0.5 to keep $0 \le d_S(A, B) \le 1$ as follows:

$$d_S(A, B) = \frac{1}{2}(K_S(A, A) + K_S(B, B) - 2K_S(A, B))$$

$$= 1 - K_S(A, B). \tag{6}$$

2.2 Icosahedral Spatial Pyramid Matching

We adapt SPM from a d-dimensional image grid to an icosahedral mesh approximation of a spherical surface so that we can compute the similarity of cortical surface features. One way to produce a regular mesh of a spherical surface is to start with an icosahedron, subdivide each triangle face into 4 smaller triangles, project the new vertices onto the sphere and repeat until the desired level of approximation of the sphere has been achieved.

We use this process in reverse to generate our sequence of pyramid levels. We start with triangles on the finest mesh, merging them with the 3 neighboring triangles that share a common edge into larger triangles. Whereas the SPM pyramid reduces the number of bin cells by a factor of 2^d at each level, ISPM reduces the number of bin faces by a factor of 4 at each level and the number of vertices by a factor of 2. We implemented this pyramid generation as a histogram resampling method added to the Connectome Workbench tool [8].

Once the pyramid is constructed, we proceed as for SPM, computing the histogram at each level by counting the number of features of a particular type that fall within a spatial bin and then summing across feature channels. We use the same weighting scheme as above to combine across pyramid levels. Since we are using a decreasing weighting scheme and summing positive-definite kernels, we preserve the Mercer kernel property, and ISPM is a distance metric.

We use the icosohedral mesh instead of a cuboid or uv mesh so that each bin in each spatial histogram has nearly equal area, and so that we have a simple way to generate the pyramid of histograms. If different features like structure tensors [13] are used instead of the region membership used here, then care must be taken to rotate the features appropriately as they are moved around on the surface of the sphere.

2.3   Distance Correlation

We want to look at whether there is a relationship between the shape of functional regions and cognitive measures, but we only have distances between shape complexes, not an individual measurement of shape. Therefore, we ask the question: *If two subjects have similar (or dissimilar) shapes of functional regions, do they also have similar (or dissimilar) cognitive measures?* We address this question by using the distance correlation, dCor [11], between two distance matrices, which tests the joint independence of two random variables of arbitrary dimension. The dCor is zero when the random variables are independent and otherwise ranges between 0 and 1. The dCor t test has a null hypothesis that the two variables are independent (i.e., dCor = 0). A small p-value of this test rejects this null hypothesis and indicates that the dCor is significantly different from 0, with dCor representing the amount of dependence.

Lyons [7] extended the theory of distance correlation to metric spaces and showed that it is necessary and sufficient for the metric space to be of the strong negative type to test independence. Because we were careful to ensure ISPM is a distance metric, we are able to use dCor to test independence. This property also holds for the Jaccard distance metric we evaluate in the results section.

To compare cognitive measures to the ISPM distances, we compute the pairwise distance between each subject's value of that cognitive measure. To analyze k cognitive measures concurrently, we can construct a k-vector of the measures and compute the pair-wise Euclidean distances between these vectors. One of the many attractive properties of the distance correlation is that it is scale-invariant.

Thus, we do not need to center or scale the variables prior to computing the distance correlation. Instead, *dcor.ttest* from the *energy* package in R performs a U-centering of each of the distance matrices and then provides a bias-corrected dCor and *p*-value. After bias correction, the dCor values are shifted, and may fall slightly below 0.

3   Results

To gain insight into whether the shape and topological variability of cortical regions is related to cognitive performance, we looked at the distance correlation between the ISPM of cortical regions and several cognitive measures. We also compared the ISPM distance metric performance to that of a more commonly used metric, the Jaccard index (JI). Finally, we looked at whether the ISPM metric is more informative than using measures like cortical thickness or surface area of cortical regions.

Because we were specifically interested in looking at topological variability of region configuration, we needed to start with a cortical region parcellation that allows for topological variation. The Glasser 2016 multi modal parcellation (MMP) finds high-quality subject-specific parcellations using an areal classifier that defines 180 regions per hemisphere based on features such as myelin maps, resting state fMRI, and cortical folding patterns. Regions are constrained to be in proximity to the group parcellation, but are not constrained to be topologically equivalent. The Glasser parcellations are publicly available for 27 subjects who are in the Test/ReTest subgroup of the Human Connectome Project (HCP) Young Adult dataset. Each subject was scanned twice and the subject scans were processed independently through the HCP pipelines. The cortical surfaces of each hemisphere were inflated onto a sphere where each vertex in channel, c, is labelled 1 if that vertex followed the border of a parcellation region c. We computed ISPM for each hemisphere and then summed them to get a total distance between subjects. We compared dCor and *p*-values for the Test and ReTest data sets to get a sense of the consistency of these results.

We chose four cognitive measures for analysis. The picture vocabulary test (PVT), reading test (Read), processing speed (Speed), and fluid cognition composite score (Fluid). PVT and Read were chosen to evaluate relationships between language-related areas and language ability, whereas Speed and Fluid where chosen since they are representative of more global relationships between all brain regions and cognitive ability. We used the age-adjusted version of cognitive measures whenever possible. All *p*-values shown were corrected for multiple comparisons with FDR.

We started by looking at the relationship between the ISPM of the cortical regions and each of these cognitive measures separately and then combined into a 4-vector (All). As shown in Table 1, we see that the distance correlation of 0.21 between ISPM and fluid cognition is consistently significant, but there is more variability in Test/ReTest in reading and processing speed.

We compared our results to a more standard metric for the comparison of segmentations, the Jaccard index, $d_J(A, B) = \frac{|A \cup B| - |A \cap B|}{|A \cup B|}$. Although JI is often used to compare segmentation results, this is the first time it has been used in shape analysis of cortical regions. We see in Table 1 that although JI did correlate significantly with fluid cognition, the distance correlation between JI and fluid cognition decreased to 0.15 for Test, 0.18 for ReTest. Other results were less significant or not significant compared to ISPM. As we expect, JI and ISPM were strongly related where the dCor of JI and ISPM was 0.905 with a p-value $< 2.2\mathrm{e}{-}16$.

We computed the surface area and mean cortical thickness of each of the 360 regions. We then compared the distances between each subject's 360-d thickness vector and the same cognitive measures as above. We repeated this comparison for the 360-d surface area vector. As you can see in Table 1, there were some significant correlations between surface area and fluid cognition and also correlations with the four combined measures for the ReTest dataset. The correlations were smaller and less consistent than the JI and ISPM results, with the exceptions of a significant correlation between surface area and Read in the ReTest data set, and a stronger correlation of the surface area vs all four com-

Table 1. Distance correlation between average cortical thickness (Thick), surface area (Area), Jaccard index (JI) or ISPM and cognitive measures.
* p-value < 0.05. ** p-value < 0.01. *** p-value < 0.001.

Test name	Test dCor	Test P-Value	ReTest dCor	ReTest P-Value
Thick vs PVT	−0.042	1	0.008	1
Thick vs Read	−0.003	1	0.058	0.573
Thick vs Speed	0.109	0.279	0.024	0.958
Thick vs Fluid	0.053	0.836	0.107	0.314
Thick vs All	0.043	0.836	0.066	0.573
Area vs PVT	−0.012	1	0.053	0.392
Area vs Read	0.001	1	0.135	**0.029***
Area vs Speed	0.048	0.732	0.088	0.161
Area vs Fluid	0.099	0.431	0.165	**0.00967****
Area vs All	0.060	0.732	0.162	**0.00967****
JI vs PVT	0.037	0.575	0.081	0.276
JI vs Read	0.099	0.106	0.070	0.294
JI vs Speed	0.102	0.106	0.022	0.787
JI vs Fluid	0.154	**0.0156***	0.179	**6.95e–3****
JI vs All	0.182	**5.61e–3****	0.134	**0.0436***
ISPM vs PVT	0.071	0.227	0.086	0.229
ISPM vs Read	0.128	**0.039***	0.042	0.509
ISPM vs Speed	0.117	**0.0494***	0.044	0.509
ISPM vs Fluid	0.212	**3.26e–4*****	0.211	**7.37e–4*****
ISPM vs All	0.239	**7.36e–5*****	0.144	**0.0267***

bined measures than JI and ISPM had for the ReTest dataset. The dCor of mean cortical thickness and ISPM was 0.275 with a p-value of 6.28e−4, while the dCor of surface area and ISPM was 0.445 with a p-value $< 2.2e−16$. These results demonstrate that considering aspects of shape beyond cortical thickness and surface area is informative. ISPM appears to be more discriminative than JI in this regard.

4   Conclusion

We propose a novel method of analyzing shapes on a spherical surface using two distance metrics, the Jaccard index and our icosahedral spatial pyramid matching metric. This measure is particularly useful to capture topological shape variants such as region splitting, region location changes relative to neighbors, and missing regions. Even though we only had 27 subjects, our distance correlation analysis finds statistically significant dependencies between the shape of functional cortical regions and fluid intelligence.

It would be interesting to perform a more extensive statistical analysis involving the Glasser MMP individual parcellations for all HCP subjects when this data become publicly available. Also, our ISPM method provides an interesting distance metric on shapes and complexes of shapes that can open up avenues for other types of statistical analysis involving shape metrics, e.g., Fréchet means.

Acknowledgements. Data were provided by the Human Connectome Project, WU-Minn Consortium (Principal Investigators: David Van Essen and Kamil Ugurbil; 1U54MH091657) funded by the 16 NIH Institutes and Centers that support the NIH Blueprint for Neuroscience Research; and by the McDonnell Center for Systems Neuroscience at Washington University.

References

1. Beg, M.F., Miller, M.I., Trouvé, A., Younes, L.: Computing large deformation metric mappings via geodesic flows of diffeomorphisms. Int. J. Comput. Vision **61**(2), 139–157 (2005)
2. Duffau, H.: A two-level model of interindividual anatomo-functional variability of the brain and its implications for neurosurgery. Cortex **86**, 303–313 (2017)
3. Glasser, M.F., et al.: A multi-modal parcellation of human cerebral cortex. Nature **536**(7615), 171–178 (2016)
4. Grauman, K., Darrell, T.: The pyramid match kernel: discriminative classification with sets of image features. In: Tenth IEEE International Conference on Computer Vision, ICCV 2005, vol. 2, pp. 1458–1465. IEEE (2005)
5. Lazebnik, S., Schmid, C., Ponce, J.: Beyond bags of features: spatial pyramid matching for recognizing natural scene categories. In: 2006 IEEE Computer Society Conference on Computer Vision and Pattern Recognition (CVPR 2006), vol. 2, pp. 2169–2178. IEEE (2006)
6. Leventon, M.E., Grimson, W.E.L., Faugeras, O.: Statistical shape influence in geodesic active contours. In: 5th IEEE EMBS International Summer School on Biomedical Imaging. IEEE (2002)

7. Lyons, R.: Distance covariance in metric spaces. Annal. Probab. **41**(5), 3284–3305 (2013)
8. Marcus, D., et al.: Informatics and data mining tools and strategies for the human connectome project. Front. Neuroinformatics **5**, 4 (2011)
9. Mémoli, F.: Gromov-Wasserstein distances and the metric approach to object matching. Found. Comput. Math. **11**(4), 417–487 (2011)
10. Oguz, I., et al.: Entropy-based particle correspondence for shape populations. Int. J. Comput. Assist. Radiol. Surg. **11**(7), 1221–1232 (2016)
11. Székely, G.J., Rizzo, M.L., Bakirov, N.K.: Measuring and testing dependence by correlation of distances. Annal. Stat. **35**(6), 2769–2794 (2007)
12. Yeo, B.T.T., Sabuncu, M., Vercauteren, T., Ayache, N., Fischl, B., Golland, P.: Spherical demons: fast surface registration. In: Metaxas, D., Axel, L., Fichtinger, G., Székely, G. (eds.) MICCAI 2008. LNCS, vol. 5241, pp. 745–753. Springer, Heidelberg (2008). https://doi.org/10.1007/978-3-540-85988-8_89
13. Zhu, P., Awate, S.P., Gerber, S., Whitaker, R.: Fast shape-based nearest-neighbor search for brain mris using hierarchical feature matching. In: Fichtinger, G., Martel, A., Peters, T. (eds.) MICCAI 2011. LNCS, vol. 6892, pp. 484–491. Springer, Heidelberg (2011). https://doi.org/10.1007/978-3-642-23629-7_59

Prediction

Diagnosis-Guided Multi-modal Feature Selection for Prognosis Prediction of Lung Squamous Cell Carcinoma

Wei Shao[1], Tongxin Wang[2], Zhi Huang[5], Jun Cheng[3], Zhi Han[1],
Daoqiang Zhang[4(✉)], and Kun Huang[1(✉)]

[1] School of Medicine, Indiana University, Indianapolis, IN 46202, USA
kunhuang@iu.edu
[2] Department of Computer Science, Indiana University Bloomington, Bloomington,
IN 47405, USA
[3] School of Biomedical Engineering, Shenzhen University, Shenzhen 518073, China
[4] College of Computer Science and Technology, Nanjing University of Aeronautics
and Astronautics, Nanjing 211106, China
dqzhang@nuaa.edu.cn
[5] School of Electrical and Computer Engineering, Purdue University, West Lafayette,
IN 47907, USA

Abstract. The existing studies have demonstrated that the integrative
analysis of histopathological images and genomic data can hold great
promise for survival analysis of cancers. However, direct combination of
multi-modal data may bring irrelevant or redundant features that will
harm the prognosis performance. Therefore, it has become a challenge to
select informative features from the derived heterogeneous data for survival analysis. Most existing feature selection methods only utilized the
collected multi-modal data and survival information to identify a subset of relevant features, which neglect to use the diagnosis information
to guide the feature selection process. In fact, the diagnosis information
(*e.g.,* TNM stage) indicates the extent of the disease severity that are
highly correlated with the patients' survival. Accordingly, we propose a
diagnosis-guided multi-modal feature selection method (DGM2FS) for
prognosis prediction. Specifically, we make use of the task relationship
learning framework to automatically discover the relations between the
diagnosis and prognosis tasks, through which we can identify important
survival-associated image and eigengenes features with the help of diagnosis information. In addition, we also consider the association between

This work was supported in part by the Indiana University Precision Health Initiative
to ZH and KH, the National Natural Science Foundation of China (61876082,
61861130366, 61703301) to DZ, and Shenzhen Peacock Plan (KQTD201605311205
1497) to JC.

Electronic supplementary material The online version of this chapter (https://
doi.org/10.1007/978-3-030-32251-9_13) contains supplementary material, which is
available to authorized users.

© Springer Nature Switzerland AG 2019
D. Shen et al. (Eds.): MICCAI 2019, LNCS 11767, pp. 113–121, 2019.
https://doi.org/10.1007/978-3-030-32251-9_13

the multi-modal data and use a regularization term to capture the correlation between the image and eigengene data. Experimental results on a lung squamous cell carcinoma dataset imply that incorporating diagnosis information can help identify meaningful survival-associated features, by which we can achieve better prognosis prediction performance than the conventional methods.

1   Introduction

One of the long-term goals of cancer research is to identify prognostic factors that affect patients' survival time, which in turn allows clinicians to make early decision on treatment [1]. So far, many biomarkers have been shown to be sensitive to the prognosis of cancers [2]. For example, quite a number of cancer prognosis models are based on the histopathological images, since they reveal the morphological attributes of cells that are closely associated with the progress of cancer disease. Moreover, it is known that mutations in genes can cause cancer by accelerating cell division rates. Accordingly, many researchers also use the genomic data such as gene expression signatures to drive cancer prognosis.

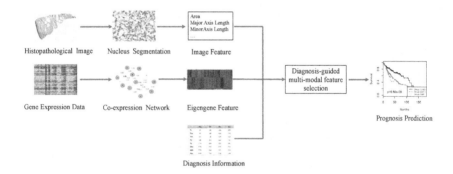

Fig. 1. The flowchart of the proposed method.

In many medical applications, it is common to acquire multiple biomarkers to predict the disease status more accurately. Recently, some researchers also integrated the histopathological imaging and gene-level data to predict the clinical outcome of cancer patients [3,4]. For instance, Yuan *et al.* [3] combined the pathological image data with copy number variation data to devise an integrated predictor of survival for breast cancer patients. Yao *et al.* [4] developed a novel correlational survival prediction framework for the integration of pathological images and genomic data on different cancer cohorts. All these results indicate that using multiple biomarkers can reveal hidden information that are overlooked by only using imaging or genomic data, and thus can better predict patients' clinical outcome.

Although integrating imaging and genomic features can achieve promising results, simply combining them may bring the problem of curse of dimensionalities. Thus, feature selection, which can be considered as the identification of key biomarkers, is commonly used to select useful features. Specifically, the studies in [2,3] firstly put the features from different modalities together and then applied the traditional single-modality feature selection method (*i.e.*, LASSO) to discover the key components that affect the patients' survival. Shao *et al.* [5] exploited and utilized the correlation across multi-modal data to select important imaging and genomic biomarkers related to cancer prognosis. However, these feature selection algorithms are only based on the collected multi-modal data and the survival information, which neglect to take the prior diagnosis information into consideration. As a matter of fact, the diagnosis information (*i.e.*, TNM stage) could also provide guidance to help predict the clinical outcome of patients. For example, the patients who are in stage III suffer from more aggressive cancers than those in stage I, and thus generally have higher survival risks.

Based on the above considerations, in this paper, we propose a diagnosis-guided multi-modal feature selection method (DGM2FS) to discover relevant imaging and genomic risk factors for survival analysis. Specifically, based on the task relationship learning approach, our method can automatically derive the correlation between the diagnosis and prognosis tasks to help identify survival-associated features. In addition, we also consider the association between multi-modal data by adding a regularization term that is capable of capturing the inter-correlation between the selected imaging and genomic components. The experimental results on a public available lung squamous cell carcinoma (LUSC) dataset demonstrate that the proposed method outperforms conventional methods in terms of prognosis prediction.

Table 1. Demographics and clinical characteristics of the LUSC dataset.

Characteristics	Summary	Characteristics	Summary
Patients:		Stage:	
Censored	258	Stage I	218
Non-censored	188	Stage II	151
Age (Y):	58.3 ± 13.1	Stage III	77
Follow-up (M):	47.4 ± 23.2		

2   Method

We summarize our framework in Fig. 1, which consists of the following 3 steps, *i.e.*, feature extraction, the proposed diagnosis-guided multi-modal feature selection method (DGM2FS), and prognostic prediction. We will firstly provide the description of the dataset used in this study.

Dataset: The Cancer Genome Atlas (TCGA) project has generated genomic and imaging data for thousands of tumour samples across more than 30 types of cancers. In this study, we test our method on the lung squamous cell carcinoma (LUSC) cohort derived from TCGA. Specifically, the LUSC dataset contains the H&E stained whole-slide images and gene expression data for 446 patients. For each patient, the corresponding survival information (*i.e.*, survival status, survival time) and the TNM stage information are all available. We show the details of the cohort information in Table 1, where censored patients mean that these patients did not suffer the outcome of death events during the follow-up period, while the non-censored category refers to the patients whose survival information are accurate from diagnosis to death.

Feature Extraction: For whole-slide images of each patient, $2-8$ regions of interest (ROI) of size 3K by 3K are extracted at first. Then, we apply an unsupervised method introduced in [6] to segment the nuclei from these extracted patches. Next, for each segmented nucleus, we extract seven cell-level features, including nuclei area (denoted as area), the major and minor axis length of cell nucleus, the ratio of major axis length to minor axis length (major, minor, and ratio), and mean, maximum, and minimum distances (distMean, distMax, and distMin) to its neighbouring nuclei. Finally, for each cell-level feature, a 10-bin histogram and five statistics (*i.e.*, mean, SD, skewness, kurtosis, and entropy) are used to aggregate the cell-level features into patient-level features, and thus a 105-dimensional imaging feature can be obtained for each patient. As to gene expression data, to overcome the large number of genes which poses a challenge to the statistical analysis, we use the co-expression network analysis algorithms [7] to cluster genes into co-expressed modules and summarize each module into an eigengene using singular value decomposition, and this process yields to 58-dimensional eigengene features.

Multi-modal Feature Selection for Prognosis Prediction: For the derived imaging and eigengene features, we firstly introduce the multi-modal feature selection (M2FS) algorithm for identifying survival-associated features without the guidance of diagnosis information. Specifically, let $X = [x_1, x_2, ..., x_N]^T = [X^H, X^G] \in R^{N \times (p+q)}$. Here, $X^H \in R^{N \times p}$ and $X^G \in R^{N \times q}$ correspond to the histopathological imaging data and eigengene data. N is the number of the patients, and p and q are the feature number of imaging data and eigengene data, respectively. We use a triplet (x_i, t_i, δ_i) to represent each observation in survival analysis, where $x_i \in R^{p+q}$ is the patient vector, t_i is the observed survival time, and δ_i is the censoring indicator. Here, $\delta_i = 1$ or $\delta_i = 0$ indicates a non-censored or a censored instance, respectively. Then, the objective function of M2FS is:

$$\min_{w_s} \sum_{i=1}^{N} l_S(x_i) + \alpha \left\| X^H w_S^H - X^G w_S^G \right\|_2^2 + \beta_S^H \left\| w_S^H \right\|_1 + \beta_S^G \left\| w_S^G \right\|_1 \quad (1)$$

$$s.t. \quad \left\| X^H w_S^H \right\|_2^2 \leq 1; \left\| X^G w_S^G \right\|_2^2 \leq 1;$$

In the M2FS model, $l_S(x_i) = c_i \|x_i w_S - t_i\|_2^2$ is a weighted regression term, where $w_s = [w_S^H, w_S^G] \in R^{p+q}$ and c_i is the weight of the survival regression loss for each patient defined as follows:

$$c_i = \begin{cases} 1 & if \ \delta = 1 \\ 0 & if \ \delta = 0 \ and \ x_i w_S - t_i > 0 \\ \sigma & if \ \delta = 0 \ and \ x_i w_S - t_i \leq 0 \end{cases} \qquad (2)$$

where $c_i = 1$ if x_i is a non-censored patient. By considering that the actual survival time for a censored instance should be larger than its observed time, we define c_i as 0 if $x_i w_S - t_i \geq 0$. Otherwise, we let c_i equal to a constant σ that is larger than 1 since the difference between actual survival time and the estimated survival time is indeed greater than $t_i - x_i w_S$. The second term in Eq. (1) is used to minimize the distance between the projections of imaging $i.e.$, $X^H w_S^H$ and genomic $i.e.$, $X^G w_S^G$ data, so that their inter-correlations can be captured. The third and fourth L1-norm terms are used to select a small number of image and eigengene features for the following prognosis prediction.

Diagnosis-Guided Multi-modal Feature Selection: In the above M2FS method, we only utilize the multi-modal data and the survival information for prognosis prediction, which overlooks the available diagnosis information ($i.e.$, TNM stage) is also correlated with patients' survival. To address this problem, we propose to incorporate the diagnosis information and use the task relationship learning term [8] to automatically discover the relationship between the diagnosis and prognosis tasks to boost the prognosis prediction performance. The task relationship learning term is defined as $tr(W M^{-1} W^T)$ with $M \geq 0$ and $tr(M) = 1$. Here, $W = [w_D, w_S] \in R^{(p+q) \times 2}$, where $w_D = [w_D^H, w_D^G]^T$ and $w_S = [w_S^H, w_S^G]^T$ correspond to the linear discriminant functions for the diagnosis and prognosis tasks on the multi-modal data, respectively. M^{-1} denotes the inverse of the matrix $M \in R^{2 \times 2}$, and M is defined as a task covariance matrix that will benefit learning on W by automatically inducing the correct relationship M between different tasks. The constraint term $M \geq 0$ is used to restrict M as positive semidefinite matrix, and $tr(M) = 1$ is used to penalize the complexity of M. By incorporating the above relationship induced term, the objective function of the proposed diagnosis-guided multi-modal feature selection ($i.e.$, DGM2FS) method can be formulated as:

$$\min_{W,M} \sum_{k \in \{S,D\}} \sum_{i=1}^{N} l_k(x_i) + \alpha \sum_{k \in \{S,D\}} \|X^H w_k^H - X^G w_k^G\|_2^2$$

$$+ \sum_{k \in \{S,D\}} \sum_{j \in \{H,G\}} \beta_k^j \|w_k^j\|_1 + \gamma tr(W M^{-1} W^T) \qquad (3)$$

$$s.t. \quad M \geq 0, tr(M) = 1$$

In comparison with the above M2FS model (shown in Eq. (1)), the first term of Eq. (3) further incorporates the empirical loss for the diagnosis task $i.e.$,

$l_D(x_i) = \|x_i w_D - y_i\|_2^2$, where y_i indicates the categorical TNM stage for patient i. The second term is used to capture the correlation between the imaging and eigengene data for both diagnosis and prognosis tasks. The third term enforces some elements of w_k^j to be zero, and thus can select important features for different tasks. In what follows, we will develop an efficient optimization algorithm to solve the objective function defined in Eq. (3).

Optimization: We adopt an alternating strategy to optimize W and M in the proposed DGM2FS model. Specifically, given a fixed M, we define $M^{-1} = [M_{DD}, M_{DS}; M_{DS}, M_{SS}] \in R^{2\times2}$. Then, the optimization problem for W is:

$$\min_W \left\|C(X^H w_S^H + X^G w_S^G - T)\right\|_2^2 + \left\|X^H w_D^H + X^G w_D^G - Y\right\|_2^2$$
$$+ \alpha \sum_{k\in\{S,D\}} \left\|X^H w_k^H - X^G w_k^G\right\|_2^2 + 2r M_{DS} \sum_{j\in\{H,G\}} (w_D^j)^T w_S^j \qquad (4)$$
$$+ \sum_{k\in\{S,D\}} \sum_{j\in\{H,G\}} (\beta_k^j \left\|w_k^j\right\|_1 + r M_{kk}(w_k^j)^T w_k^j)$$

Where, $T = [t_1, t_2, ..., t_N]^T \in R^N$ and $Y = [y_1, y_2, ..., y_N]^T \in R^N$ indicate the recorded survival time and TNM stage information for the patients in the training set. $C \in R^{N\times N}$ is a diagonal matrix, with the k-th element as c_i defined in Eq. (2). It is worth noting that, Eq. (4) is convex with respect to each $w_k^j(k \in \{S, D\}, j \in \{H, G\})$ in W, and thus can be solved alternatively to obtain the optimal W. After W is determined, we follow the method in [8] to get the closed-formed solution for $M = (W^T W)^{\frac{1}{2}}/tr((W^T W)^{\frac{1}{2}})$. Finally, we renew the weight of each instance *i.e.*, $c(i)$ according to Eq. (2). The above steps will repeat until W, M converge to fixed values.

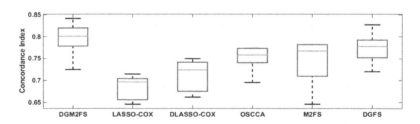

Fig. 2. Comparison of different feature selection methods on Concordance Index.

Prognostic Prediction: We build the Cox model [4] for prognosis prediction. Specifically, we firstly divide all patients into 5 folds, with 4 folds used for training and the remaining for testing, then the Cox proportional hazards model is built on the selected features in the training set, through which we calculate the Concordance Index (CI) [4] that measures the fraction of all pairs of patients whose survival risks are correctly ordered on the testing set to evaluate the performance of prognosis prediction. The CI value ranges from 0 to 1, where larger CI value means the better prediction performance and vice versa.

3   Experimental Results

Experimental Settings: The parameters $\alpha, \beta_k^j (k \in \{S, D\}, j \in \{H, G\})$ and r in the proposed DGM2FS are tuned from $\{0.5, 1, 1.5\}, \{0.1, 0.5, 1\}$ and $\{1, 1.5, 2\}$, respectively. The parameter σ in Eq. (2) is fixed as 1.5.

Results and Discussion: We compare DGM2FS with the following baseline methods by the measurement of CI. (1) LASSO-Cox [2]: use the LASSO method for variable selection in the Cox model. (2) DLasso-Cox: add the diagnosis information as a feature to the multi-modal data, then use the LASSO-Cox model for feature selection. (3) OSCCA [5]: a multi-modal feature selection method for survival analysis without the guidance of diagnosis knowledge. (4) M2FS: a variant of DGM2FS (shown in Eq. (1)), which neglects to take the diagnosis information into consideration. (5) DGFS: a variant of DGM2FS, which miss the second term in Eq. (3) that can capture the correlation between imaging and genomic data. The results are shown in Fig. 2. As can be seen from Fig. 2, DGM2FS and its variant DGFS achieve higher CI value than the competing methods. These results clearly demonstrate that the incorporation of the diagnosis information (*i.e.,* TNM stage) under task relationship learning framework can help improve the prognosis performance. In addition, we observe that the DGM2FS model could provide better prognostic prediction (0.795 ± 0.043) than the DGFS algorithm (0.769 ± 0.039), which also shows the advantage of taking the correlation among different modalities into account for feature selection.

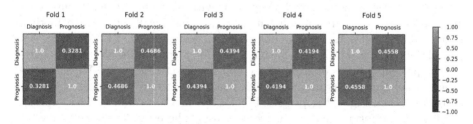

Fig. 3. The correlation coefficient matrix between the diagnosis and prognosis tasks for each fold of cross-validation learned by DGM2FS.

In addition, we visualize the learned correlation coefficient matrix (*i.e.,* calculated from M in Eq. (3)) between the diagnosis and prognosis tasks in Fig. 3. From Fig. 3, we observe that the diagnosis and prognosis tasks are *positively correlated* in each fold of cross-validation, which again verify that adding the diagnosis information could improve the performance of prognosis prediction.

Since it is of great importance to identify the biomarkers that affect prognosis
prediction. We focus on the biological significance of the selected imaging and
eigenegene features that are appeared at least four times in the 5-fold cross-
validation. Specifically, our method selects 6 image features including *major_-
bin6*, *distMean_bin2*, *distMin_kurtosis*, *distMin_bin3*, *distMean_entropy* and *dist-
Min_entropy*, where most of them are related to the distance among segmented
cells. The cells with smaller neighboring distance (*i.e., disMean_bin2 and dist-
Min_bin3*) usually correspond to the cancer cells or lymphocytes that cluster
together in the tissue images, which is generally considered to be the key factors
affecting the survival of lung cancer patients [9]. As to genomic features, three
eigenegenes *i.e., eigengene 10, eigengene 25, eigengene 29* are identified (details
are shown in Supplementary). The enrichment analysis on eigengene 10 shows
that its corresponding module contains 30 genes, and 14 of them are enriched
with the biological process of immune response, which is consistent with the
existing study [10] that the immune response plays an important role in the
development of lung cancer.

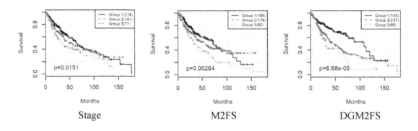

Fig. 4. Comparison of different feature selection methods for patient stratification.

Finally, we also compare the prognostic power of different approaches by
stratifying cancer patients into 3 subgroups with different predicted outcomes,
with the experimental results shown in Fig. 4. Specifically, the stage method
divides all the patients into 3 subgroups according to the TNM stage. For
DGM2FS or M2FS approach, k-means clustering algorithm is adopted to aggregate the patients into 3 subgroups based on the selected features. Then, we test
if these 3 subgroups has distinct survival outcome using log-rank test [2]. As
can be seen from Fig. 4, the proposed DGM2FS method could achieve superior
stratification performance than the competitors. These results further show the
promise of incorporating diagnosis information for patient stratification from
multi-modal data, which opens up the opportunity for building personalized
treatment plan in the stage of cancer development.

4   Conclusion

In this paper, we develop DGM2FS, an effective multi-modal feature selection
method that can identify survival associated biomarkers from both histopathological image and gene expression data. The main advantage of our approach

is its capability of utilizing the diagnosis information to guide the feature selection process, which can more accurately predict the clinical outcome for lung squamous cell carcinoma patients. DGM2FS is a general framework and can be easily transferred to other types of cancers or predict the response of a specific treatment, which opens up new opportunity in personalized treatment.

References

1. Liu, J., Lichtenberg, T.: An integrated tcga pan-cancer clinical data resource to drive high-quality survival outcome analytics. Cell **173**(2), 400–416 (2018)
2. Cheng, J., Huang, K.: Integrative analysis of histopathological images and genomic data predicts clear cell renal cell carcinoma prognosis. Cancer Res. **77**(21), 91–100 (2017)
3. Yuan, Y., Rueda, M.: Quantitative image analysis of cellular heterogeneity in breast tumors complements genomic profiling. Sci. Transl. Med. **4**(157), 143–157 (2012)
4. Yao, J., Huang, J.: Deep correlational learning for survival prediction from multi-modality data. In: International Conference on Medical Image Computing and Computer Assisted Intervention, pp. 406–414 (2017)
5. Shao, W., Cheng, J.: Ordinal multi-modal feature selection for survival analysis of early-stage renal cancer. In: International Conference on Medical Image Computing and Computer Assisted Intervention, pp. 648–656 (2018)
6. Phoulady, H., Dmitry, B.: Nucleus segmentation in histology images with hierarchical multilevel thresholding. In: International Conference on SPIE, pp. 1–8 (148)
7. Zhang, J., Lu, K.: Weighted frequent gene co-expression network mining to identify genes involved in genome stability. PLoS Comput. Biol. **8**(8), 1–14 (2012)
8. Zhang, Y.: A regularization approach to learning task relationships in multitask learning. ACM Trans. Knowl. Discov. Data **8**(3), 1–12 (2012)
9. Al-Shibli, K.I., Donnem, T., Al-Saad, S., Persson, M., Bremnes, R.M., Busund, L.T.: Prognostic effect of epithelial and stromal lymphocyte infiltration in non-small cell lung cancer. Clin. Cancer Res. **14**(16), 5220–5227 (2008)
10. Liu, Y.: Cancer and innate immune system interactions: translational potentials for cancer immunotherapy. J. Immunother. **35**(4), 299–299 (2012)

Graph Convolution Based Attention Model for Personalized Disease Prediction

Anees Kazi[1(✉)], Shayan Shekarforoush[1], S. Arvind Krishna[1],
Hendrik Burwinkel[1], Gerome Vivar[1,2], Benedict Wiestler[3], Karsten Kortüm[4],
Seyed-Ahmad Ahmadi[2], Shadi Albarqouni[1], and Nassir Navab[1,5]

[1] Computer Aided Medical Procedures (CAMP), Technical University of Munich,
Munich, Germany
anees.kazi@tum.de

[2] German Center for Vertigo and Balance Disorders, Ludwig Maximilians Universität
München, Munich, Germany

[3] Department of Neuroradiology, TU Munich University Hospital, Munich, Germany

[4] Augenklinik der Universität, Klinikum der Universität München, Munich, Germany

[5] Whiting School of Engineering, Johns Hopkins University, Baltimore, USA

Abstract. Clinicians implicitly incorporate the complementarity of multi-modal data for disease diagnosis. Often a varied order of importance for this heterogeneous data is considered for personalized decisions. Current learning-based methods have achieved better performance with uniform attention to individual information, but a very few have focused on patient-specific attention learning schemes for each modality. Towards this, we introduce a model which not only improves the disease prediction but also focuses on learning patient-specific order of importance for multi-modal data elements. In order to achieve this, we take advantage of LSTM-based attention mechanism and graph convolutional networks (GCNs) to design our model. GCNs learn multi-modal but class-specific features from the entire population of patients, whereas the attention mechanism optimally fuses these multi-modal features into a final decision, separately for each patient. In this paper, we apply the proposed approach for disease prediction task for Parkinson's and Alzheimer's using two public medical datasets.

1 Introduction

Recently, deep learning based methods for disease prediction have relied on training a classifier that learns class-specific structures. However, diversity in the condition leads to highly heterogeneous data. For instance, diagnosis and treatment may differ among patients with the same disease, based on demographic, clinical and imaging data. In case such as Alzheimer's disease drugs, especially APOE-targeting ones, may act differently in patients with different APOE genotypes but same disease condition. Moreover, other than the demographic and genetic factors, brain imaging and other biomarkers may also be used for patient-specific diagnosis. The importance of such personalized diagnosis of the disease has been

© Springer Nature Switzerland AG 2019
D. Shen et al. (Eds.): MICCAI 2019, LNCS 11767, pp. 122–130, 2019.
https://doi.org/10.1007/978-3-030-32251-9_14

shown in [1,2] respectively. A CAD system capable of learning such patient-specific decision is required to improve the clinical outcome.

Some of the recent studies [3,4] have demonstrated that personalized models can improve predictive performance compared to more general models. Such a pipeline for personalized disease prediction contains two stages: (1) measuring the similarity among patients, and (2) building a model for patient-specific disease condition using his/her specific risk factors. Such a framework is motivated by the clinical workflow, i.e., after reviewing or recollecting the diagnosed patients with similar diseases conditions, the experts then make a patient-specific decision.

To this end, Graph Convolutional networks (GCNs) have shown their power for extracting similarity among the patients for disease prediction [5,6]. GCNs use the relation between the patients often defined as a neighborhood graph built based on non-imaging data like gender, age, clinical scores, or any other meta-information. Each patient can be considered as a node on this graph with features from, e.g., imaging modalities. Eventually, GCNs provide a principled manner for learning optimal graph filters to minimize the objective. Several studies [6–9] have proposed GCN based models in parallel setting of GC layers to deal with multi-graph scenario fusing the information by pooling, concatenation, or averaging at the end. On the other hand, [10–12] have focused on node-level attention mechanism to learn the weights of the neighbors for training. All the methods discussed above show the superiority of graph convolutional networks over other traditional methods. Each one deals either with the multi-graph setting or node level attention mechanism. Our target in this paper is to consider both with an end to end pipeline for solving the disease classification task.

We propose a model that first clusters the patients based on certain similarities and then, learns patient specific traits for personalized diagnosis. More specifically, for each patient, our model learns multiple representations of features for each modality. The patient-specific attention mechanism is further incorporated using the LSTM based attention scheme to optimally fuse the multi-modal data to make a final decision, separately for each patient. Our methodological contributions are:

- incorporating GCNs with multi-graph setting to learn similarity among the patients at multiple levels.
- incorporating LSTM based attention mechanism to learn weights for each non-imaging factor for personalized disease prediction task.

Our method could be generalized to other multi-modal datasets for the disease prediction task. Here, we demonstrate its application on two publicly available multi-modal datasets for Alzheimer's and Parkinson's disease. We show the superiority of our model in terms of accuracy, f1 score, sensitivity, and PPV.

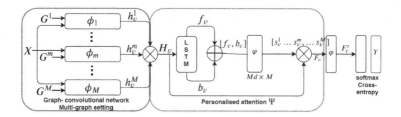

Fig. 1. The end to end pipeline of the proposed method. The red box indicates the GC layers extracting similarity among patients. The green box produces personalized attention scores later used for combining representations. In the end, logits and cross-entropy loss are calculated. (Color figure online)

2   Methodology

Let X denote the population of N patients. Each patient n_i has an imaging feature vector $x_i \in \mathbb{R}^D$ and a non-imaging feature vector $\eta_i \in \mathbb{R}^M$. Then, the imaging and non-imaging feature matrix for all the patients together is denoted by $X \in \mathbb{R}^{N \times D}$ and $\eta \in \mathbb{R}^{N \times M}$. The labels $Y \in \mathbb{R}^{N \times C}$ for C classes (one-hot encoded) are available only for the training set Y_{tr}. Therefore, given X, η and, Y_{tr} the task is to predict the classes for the test set Y_t. Next, to incorporate the similarity between the patients in the learning task, we leverage m non-imaging elements. We define affinity graph $G^m \in \mathbb{R}^{N \times N}$ corresponding to each element m in η. We obtain $G^1, ..., G^m, ..., G^M$ as different graphs from individual elements of non-imaging modality. Note that the procedure of graph construction is entirely described in later Sect. 2.1.

Given the graph information, we redefine the task of disease prediction for test set Y_t as,

$$\widehat{Y_t} = \Psi(\Phi_m(X, G^m, \Theta_1^m), \Theta_2). \tag{1}$$

where, $\widehat{Y}_t$ are the predicted labels for the test set, Φ_m is a function specific to η^m modality that learns feature representation for each patient as shown in Fig. 1, Ψ is the personalized attention function which weights the representations corresponding to each η^m. The set of learnable parameters of both the functions Φ_m and Ψ are represented by $[\Theta_1^1, ..., \Theta_1^m, ..., \Theta_1^M]$ and Θ_2 respectively.

As mentioned in the introduction section, the first step of this personalized prediction pipeline aims to capture the similarity among the patients. GCNs fit well with their remarkable ability to learn such similarities. Therefore, we design each of the Φ_m using graph convolutional (GC) layers. Each branch Φ_m consists of 2 GC layers. Further, the personalized attention mechanism Ψ is built using a bidirectional LSTM that learns the attention scores for representations obtained from each Φ_m. Due to its inherent property LSTM, learns final representation F_v for each patient by incorporating the inter-relation between each representation Φ_m for each patient individually. The entire end to end pipeline is shown in Fig. 1.

In the next subsection, we provide mathematical details of both the functions Φ_m and Ψ. Further, we show how they are connected to build the end to end model. Our model minimizes weighted cross entropy loss to learn the filters.

2.1 Definition of Φ_m

For Φ_m corresponding to the mth branch, we opt for Chebyshev polynomial approximated variant of spectral convolution g_ϕ defined on each graph G^m and feature vector x_v, where $x_v \in X$, for v^{th} node. Mathematically this spectral operation is defined as $h_v^m = g_\phi(L^m)x_v = \sum_{r=0}^{K-1} \phi_r T_r(L^m)x_v$, where $h_v^m \in \mathbb{R}^d$ is the output feature representation corresponding to η^m, $\phi_r \in \mathbb{R}^K$ is the vector of learnable Chebyshev coefficients, $T_r(L^m)$ is the Chebyshev polynomial of order k for L^m and $x \in \mathbb{R}^{N \times N}$ is the input features. The graph G^m defined on the entire population (including training and testing patients) plays role in spectral convolution to define the neighborhood for each patient in order to perform convolution. This information is incorporated in each of the normalized graph Laplacian L^m corresponding to G^m. Further mathematical details on GCNs can be found in [13]. Finally by concatenating the outputs of each branch, we obtain $H_v = [h_v^1, ..., h_v^m, ..., h_v^M]$ for each node. The representation h_v^m learnt from m^{th} branch of GC layers is specific to the mth element of non-imaging risk factor. H_v thus becomes personalized sequence of learnt multi-modal features for each patient.

We construct the required affinity graph $G = (V, E, W)$ where $|V| = $ N vertices, $E \in \mathbb{R}^{N \times N}$ is the binary edge connections matrix of the graph and $W \in \mathbb{R}^{N \times N}$ is the weight matrix. $Sim(x_i, x_j) \circ E_{i,j}^m = \begin{cases} 1 \ if \ \left| \eta_i^m - \eta_j^m \right| < \beta^m \\ 0 \quad otherwise \end{cases}$,

where $Sim(x_i, x_j) = exp(-\frac{[\rho(x_i, x_j)]^2}{2\sigma^2})$ with ρ being the 'correlation distance' and σ being the width of the kernel and β^m be the threshold for edge construction.

2.2 Personalized Attention Mechanism

In this section we provide details about the LSTM based attention scheme used for personalized attention. For $H_v = [h_v^1, ..., h_v^m, ..., h_v^M]$, we learn a scalar attention score s_v^m for each representation h_v^m such that $\sum_m s_v^m = 1$. Learning an attention for multiple representations for same patient makes our attention mechanism and the output personalized to the given patient. These attention scores $[s_v^1, ..., s_v^m, ..., s_v^M]$ represents the importance of the mth branch, for node v. Below we provide the step wise details of our node-level attention mechanism.

Step-1. The concatenated output H_v from GCN mimics a sequence and is fed to the LSTM attention cell with d units. Let f_v and b_v represent the forward and backward LSTM hidden activation for each node v, h_m is the feature representation of the mth branch, $r_{m \pm 1}$ is the hidden state of bi-directional LSTM and α is the tanh activation function.

Step-2. Generating node level attention scores for each graph is done by applying a linear mapping φ and a softmax to s_v as, $s_v = softmax(\varphi \{[f_v, b_v] \omega + b\})$

where, $s_v \in \mathbb{R}^M$, $[.,.]$ stands for concatenation. We apply φ as a dense layer without any non-linear activation, ω and b are the weights and biases of the dense layer.

Step-3. Fetching final representation for node v is done by taking the weighted sum of the representation as $F_v = \sum_m s_v^m \cdot h_v^m$, where $F_v \in \mathbb{R}^d$ is the personalized final representation obtained from weighted combination over all the graphs. F_v is given to a dense layer to output logits for each class F_v'. We minimize the weighted cross-entropy loss. The proposed node-level attention based method is described in Fig. 1.

3 Experiments and Results

We evaluate our proposed model using two publicly available datasets Parkinson's Progression Markers Initiative (PPMI) (www.ppmi-info.org/data) and TADPOLE [14]. PPMI dataset consists of 75 healthy and 249 diseased patients. Each patient in this dataset is provided with brain MRI volume and non-imaging risk factors such as Unified Parkinson's Disease Rating Scale (UPDRS) and Montreal Cognitive Assessment (MoCA) scores and demographics (age and gender). We pre-process the MRI volume by co-registering each 2D image to the SRI24 ATLAS, skull stripping using ROBEX, and finally normalizing each volume into the range [0, 1]. Later these volumes are fed to a 3D auto-encoder pretrained for anomaly detection. The details of the architecture and implementation are provided in [15]. We obtain the bottleneck feature vector with the dimensionality of 320 for each volume.

On the other hand, TADPOLE dataset consists of 564 patients divided into 160 for normal, 320 MCI and 84 AD patients, respectively. Each patient comes with a 354 dimensional feature vector extracted from brain MR and PET imaging, CSF, cognitive test, and non-imaging risk factors such as age, gender, APOE genotype, and average FDG PET imaging values. For both, the datasets we use non-imaging features to construct the affinity graph and imaging features are used as input feature matrix X. We choose the values of the thresholds β^m same as [6] for the fair comparison. For both the datasets the task at hand is to predict the disease for each patient. We divide our dataset in 90% train and 10% test for each dataset.

Our experiments are designed to show that (1) LSTM based attention mechanism is better than other representation fusing schemes, as shown in Table 2, and (2) proposed an end to end pipeline that works better than single/multi-graph global attention mechanism shown in Table 1. Baseline methods include concatenation, maxpool and average pooling techniques applied to H_v. Further, we compare the proposed method with five state of the art methods categorized into three as shown in Table 1. The methods in **(a)**, have multi-graph setting with global attention scheme [6] and personalized attention scheme [10]. Next, methods in **(b)** are both GCN based methods working with a single graph. We construct this single graph by averaging all the graph following the graph construction technique in [5]. Comparing the performance with these two methods show the superiority of multi-graph setting over the single-graph setting. Finally, it is compared with multi-layered perceptron (MLP) categorized as **(c)** to show its superiority over a conventional non-graph based method.

Interpretation: In general, all the attention based methods acquire higher performance compared to other methods with no attention, as shown in Table 1 (a) vs. (b) and (c) respectively. Since our personalized attention technique can weight different graphs for each patient separately, it achieves 4.32% and 1.07% improvement in accuracy for PPMI and TADPOLE, respectively. Further, as an ablation test of the proposed attention mechanism, we show its comparison with other feature fusing techniques. We obtain 1.01% and 0.89% improvement over other method (ref. Table 2). We perform Kolmogorov-Smirnov test (K-S test) shown by $*$ in all the tables, where $*$ represents that our results are statistically significant compared to the mentioned methods ($p < 0.05$). Minimum variance over the results of 10 folds shows the stability of our model toward new samples. We report F1 score, sensitivity, specificity, and PPV as both our datasets are highly imbalanced. For most of the reported metrics, the proposed method outperforms others.

Table 1. Performance comparison of proposed method to state of the art methods in term of five metrics for PPMI and TADPOLE dataset. Our results are statistically significant in the setting marked by Asterisk symbol.

PPMI

		Accuracy	F1score	Sensitivity	Specificity	PPV
	Proposed	**91.04 ± 04.68**	**76.12 ± 14.74**	79.28 ± 20.57	**91.93 ± 05.76**	**75.97 ± 13.18**
(a)	Kazi et al. [6]	86.72 ± 06.37*	53.25 ± 19.77*	52.85 ± 24.07*	88.30 ± 07.83	58.72 ± 19.80*
	Ma et al. [8]	45.06 ± 22.86*	39.57 ± 02.73*	**94.28 ± 09.98***	14.18 ± 17.36*	25.18 ± 02.47*
(b)	Kipf et al. [16]	28.39 ± 03.01*	33.49 ± 08.98*	43.03 ± 17.96*	66.71 ± 16.37*	28.82 ± 08.62*
	Parisot et al. [5]	86.72 ± 05.00	73.27 ± 10.66	79.64 ± 16.73*	89.11 ± 04.44	69.13 ± 09.95
(c)	MLP	50.30 ± 08.50*	27.53 ± 09.77*	42.14 ± 18.40*	52.16 ± 06.75*	20.63 ± 06.76*

TADPOLE

		Accuracy	F1score	Sensitivity	Specificity	PPV
	Proposed	**83.33 ± 03.89**	**72.55 ± 11.97**	76.87 ± 18.64	**86.64 ± 09.06**	72.06 ± 13.48
(a)	Kazi et al. [6]	82.26 ± 07.75	68.13 ± 14.89	72.50 ± 15.08*	83.11 ± 11.48	66.47 ± 20.59
	Ma et al. [8]	49.46 ± 06.79*	44.70 ± 05.58*	75.00 ± 15.30*	36.48 ± 16.16*	32.22 ± 04.47*
(b)	Kipf et al. [16]	50.88 ± 07.31*	51.88 ± 06.75*	76.38 ± 10.22*	52.84 ± 09.46*	39.45 ± 05.70*
	Parisot et al. [5]	72.69 ± 08.00*	61.95 ± 14.59*	68.75 ± 15.65*	78.18 ± 09.85*	57.11 ± 15.31*
(c)	MLP	79.60 ± 07.27	69.63 ± 09.82	80.00 ± 10.12*	79.89 ± 07.13	61.90 ± 10.30

4   Discussion and Conclusion

In this paper, we have presented a model for personalized disease prediction and shown its application to Alzheimer's and Parkinson's' using two publicly available datasets. Our model is built with graph convolutional layers which intake modality specific affinity graph and patient-specific features to performs

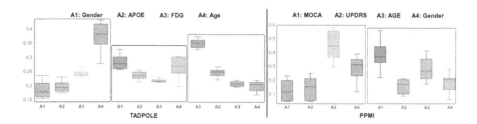

Fig. 2. Over all the figure shows the boxplot of the attention scores learnd for each patients for 10 folds for TADPOLE. The variance of each boxplot is computed for 10 folds. Each boxplot shows weights learnt for each class normal (left), MCI (center) and Alzheimer's (right) per patient for tadpole. For PPMI dataset Normal (left) and abnormal (right) for each patient respectively.

Table 2. Performance comparison of proposed method personalized attention method to the baseline methods for both the datasets to show that LSTM mechanism improves the over all classification of the model. Our results are statistically significant in the setting marked by Asterisk symbol.

PPMI

	Accuracy	F1score	Sensitivity	Specificity	PPV
Proposed	**91.04 ± 04.68**	76.12 ± 14.74	79.28 ± 20.57	**91.93 ± 05.76**	75.97 ± 13.18
Concat	90.53 ± 07.01	74.08 ± 08.44	**82.32 ± 15.87***	88.33 ± 04.06*	68.58 ± 07.45
MaxPool	86.40 ± 05.48	72.80 ±10.43	78.75 ± 14.61*	88.73 ± 06.25	69.39 ± 13.22
AvgPool	87.97 ± 04.62	74.75 ± 10.59	78.92 ± 16.27*	90.75 ± 04.27	72.65 ± 09.91

TADPOLE

	Accuracy	F1score	Sensitivity	Specificity	PPV
Proposed	**83.33 ± 03.89**	72.55 ± 11.97	76.87 ± 18.64	**86.64 ± 09.06**	72.06 ± 13.48
Concat	82.44 ± 08.95	**77.37 ± 08.55**	**92.36 ± 08.22***	80.96 ± 08.82	67.13 ± 10.11
MaxPool	68.41 ± 08.02*	56.58 ± 15.52*	55.62 ± 20.29	85.40* ± 06.54	60.40 ± 13.02
AvgPool	70.36 ± 06.36*	56.82 ± 10.72*	50.62 ± 11.94*	88.78 ± 09.97	70.65 ± 21.21

spectral convolution on features vectors. Further, our personalized LSTM based attention mechanism fuses these graph specific feature representations for each patient separately. These attentions given to each graph almost matches the clinical order of importance and is well suited for personalized disease prediction. As an ablation test on our attention mechanism, we have provided a comparison with the baseline methods (ref. Table 2) with various fusing approaches. We have compared our results with five different state of the art methods (ref. Table 1) and shown the superior performance of our model in terms of different metrics necessary to analyze the performance on much harder data setting such as class imbalance. The attention weights are shown in Fig. 2 obtained for all the patients for both the datasets. The variance of each boxplot represents the required heterogeneity in the weights for the given task. It depicts a particular pattern for each class for both the datasets. Our model is capable of learning a global pattern for each class. Further, the general order of importance followed by the clinicians for Alzheimer's is age, followed by gender, APOE, and FDG

[1,2]. Our method follows the same order except for gender. A similar observation is observed for the PPMI where our model is slightly incorrect in following the order of importance. This can be explained by the fact that the size of both of our datasets is 564 and 324 patients which represent only a subsample of the population.

Major points to be discussed are (1) scalability to larger number of affinity Graphs and (2) the problem of out of sample extension. The number of branches is equal to the number of non-imaging elements. However spectral convolution designed using Chebyshev parameterization are computationally inexpensive [13]. On the other hand, a spatial graph convolutional layers can be defined, which allows modifying the graph during training. Such a technique is suitable for out of sample extension and graph learning process where one graph can be learned from multi-graph setting together with better representation learning. In this paper, we focus on learning patient-specific attention for each graph using spectral convolutions to make it scalable and convergent enough to accommodate multiple graphs. Our method could be generalized to other multi-modal datasets. As a future work inductive version of the model can be explored to address the out of sample extension together with graph learning technique for the spectral domain can be explored.

Acknowledgement. The study was carried out with financial support of Freunde und Förderer der Augenklinik, München, Germany, Carl Zeiss Meditec AG, Germany and the German Federal Ministry of Education and Research (BMBF) in connection with the foundation of the German Center for Vertigo and Balance Disorders (DSGZ) (grant number 01 EO 0901).

References

1. Bu, L.-L., et al.: Toward precision medicine in parkinson's disease. Annal. Transl. Med. **4**(2), 26 (2016)
2. Peng, X., et al.: Towards personalized intervention for Alzheimer's disease. Genomics, Proteomics Bioinform. **14**(5), 289–297 (2016)
3. Ng, K., Sun, J., Hu, J., Wang, F.: Personalized predictive modeling and risk factor identification using patient similarity. Am. Med. Inform. Assoc. Summits Transl. Sci. Proc. **2015**, 132 (2015)
4. Suo, Q., et al.: Personalized disease prediction using a CNN-based similarity learning method. In: International Conference on Bioinformatics and Biomedicine 2017, pp. 811–816, IEEE (2017)
5. Parisot, S., et al.: Spectral graph convolutions for population-based disease prediction. In: Descoteaux, M., Maier-Hein, L., Franz, A., Jannin, P., Collins, D.L., Duchesne, S. (eds.) MICCAI 2017. LNCS, vol. 10435, pp. 177–185. Springer, Cham (2017). https://doi.org/10.1007/978-3-319-66179-7_21
6. Kazi, A., Shekarforoush, S., Kortuem, K., Albarqouni, S., Navab, N.: Self-attention equipped graph convolutions for disease prediction. arXiv preprint arXiv:1812.09954 (2018)
7. Zhang, X., He, L., Chen, K., Luo, Y., Zhou, J., Wang, F.: Multi-view graph convolutional network and its applications on neuroimage analysis for parkinson's disease. arXiv preprint arXiv:1805.08801 (2018)

8. Ma, T., Xiao, C., Zhou, J., Wang, F.: Drug similarity integration through attentive multi-view graph auto-encoders. In: International Joint Conferences on Artificial Intelligence (2018)

9. Ma, Y., Wang, S., Aggarwal, C.C., Yin, D., Tang, J.: Multi-dimensional graph convolutional networks. In: Social and Information Networks, pp. 657–665 (2018)

10. Veličković, P., Cucurull, P., Casanova, A., Romero, A., Lio, P., Bengio, Y.: Graph attention networks. In: International Conference on Learning Representations (2018)

11. Kazi, A., et al.: InceptionGCN: receptive field aware graph convolutional network for disease prediction. In: Chung, A.C.S., Gee, J.C., Yushkevich, P.A., Bao, S. (eds.) IPMI 2019. LNCS, vol. 11492, pp. 73–85. Springer, Cham (2019). https://doi.org/10.1007/978-3-030-20351-1_6

12. Fout, A., Byrd, J., Shariat, B., Ben-Hur, A.: Protein interface prediction using graph convolutional networks. In: Neural Information Processing Systems, pp. 6530–6539 (2017)

13. Defferrard, M., Bresson, X., Vandergheynst, P.: Convolutional neural networks on graphs with fast localized spectral filtering. In: Neural Information Processing Systems, pp. 3844–3852 (2016)

14. Marinescu, R.V., et al.: Tadpole challenge: prediction of longitudinal evolution in Alzheimer's disease. arXiv preprint arXiv:1805.03909 (2018)

15. Baur, C., Wiestler, B., Albarqouni, S., Navab, N.: Deep autoencoding models for unsupervised anomaly segmentation in brain MR images. In: Crimi, A., Bakas, S., Kuijf, H., Keyvan, F., Reyes, M., van Walsum, T. (eds.) BrainLes 2018. LNCS, vol. 11383, pp. 161–169. Springer, Cham (2019). https://doi.org/10.1007/978-3-030-11723-8_16

16. Kipf, T.N., Welling, M.: Semi-supervised classification with graph convolutional networks. In: International Conference on Learning Representations (2017)

Predicting Early Stages of Neurodegenerative Diseases via Multi-task Low-Rank Feature Learning

Haijun Lei[1], Yujia Zhao[1], and Baiying Lei[2(✉)]

[1] School of Computer Science and Software Engineering, Shenzhen University,
Shenzhen 518060, China
[2] National-Regional Key Technology Engineering Laboratory for Medical
Ultrasound, Guangdong Key Laboratory for Biomedical Measurements and
Ultrasound Imaging, School of Biomedical Engineering, Health Science Center,
Shenzhen University, Shenzhen 518060, China
leiby@szu.edu.cn

Abstract. Early stages of neurodegenerative diseases draw increasing recognition as obscure symptoms may appear before classical clinical diagnosis. For this reason, we propose a novel multi-task low-rank feature learning method, which takes advantages of the sparsity and low-rankness of neuroimaging data for Parkinson's Disease (PD) and Alzheimer's Disease (AD) multi-classification. First, the low-rank learning is proposed to unveil the underlying relationships between input data and output targets by preserving the most class-discriminative features. Multi-task learning is simultaneously performed to capture intrinsic feature relatedness. A sparse linear regression framework is designed to find the low-dimensional structure of high dimensional data. Experimental results on the Parkinson's progression markers initiative (PPMI) and Alzheimer's disease neuroimaging initiative (ADNI) datasets show that our proposed model not only enhances the performances of multi-classification tasks, but also outperforms the conventional algorithms.

Keywords: Parkinson's Disease · Alzheimer's Disease · Multi-task · Low-rank

1 Introduction

Parkinson's Disease (PD) and Alzheimer's Disease (AD) have gained increasing attention as the growing aging problem in the world. The chronic progression nature and imperceptible neuro-diminishment of neurodegenerative diseases make the treatment comparatively difficult [1]. There is suggestive evidence that olfaction changes, sleep behavior disorder, subtle cognitive changes, and depression can be presented at early PD stages, which indicates high potential of having PD. The occurrence of motor symptoms permits the clinical diagnosis of PD, about or above 50% of the dopaminergic neurons of the substantia nigra have degenerated [2]. The time span between the onset of neurodegeneration and manifestation of the typical motor symptoms is referred as prodromal phase of PD (PPD). On the other hand, SWEDD (scans without evidence

© Springer Nature Switzerland AG 2019
D. Shen et al. (Eds.): MICCAI 2019, LNCS 11767, pp. 131–139, 2019.
https://doi.org/10.1007/978-3-030-32251-9_15

for dopaminergic deficit) refers to the absence of an imaging abnormality in patients clinically presumed to have PD. Both PPD and SWEDD are different disorders of PD, whose patients require targeted treatment. Therefore, early PD diagnosis offers timely prevention treatment of the patients. Similarly for AD, identifying early stages patients (i.e., mild cognitive impairment (MCI)) provide better chance of getting treatment.

Using the rich information of different neuroimaging techniques (e.g., magnetic resonance imaging (MRI)), we can monitor the minor neural changes, which are not easy to perceive in normal clinical symptom-based diagnosis. Recently, many machine learning methods have been applied to utilize the neuroimages in the computer-aided diagnosis of neurodegenerative diseases [3]. Due to the challenges of high dimensionality and limited sample size, the overfitting problem could occur. Studies have demonstrated that feature selection is capable of overcoming this issue [4]. A L_1-regularizer (i.e., a sparse term) is introduced in the feature selection model when the sample size is significantly smaller than the feature dimension [5]. However, sparsity regularization is insufficient in multi-classification application since there are several progressive classification targets: normal control (NC), SWEDD, and PPD for PD, MCI, light MCI (lMCI), and stable MCI (sMCI) for AD.

In fact, the relationship between input data (i.e., MRI images) and output targets (i.e., prediction results) has more to be explored. Inspired by the fact that the brain is organized with modular structures [6], we intend to find the most representative features to train our multi-class classifiers by extracting the low-rank structure. On the other hand, gray matter (GM), white matter (WM), and cerebrospinal fluid (CSF) are the most significant biomarkers in the brain which are later used as features [2, 7]. The conventional feature extraction methods usually apply simple linear combination to use the three matters without considering their own contribution. Moreover, low-rank regression considers the relations among the response variables to conduct subspace learning under the assumption that the rank of the coefficient matrix in regression is no larger than each dimension [8]. In view of this, we model this problem as a multi-task learning framework that efficiently leverages the multi-modal data since the constructive neuroimaging data provides complement and sufficient information. Our model considers each modal for multi-classification as one task, which assumes that these tasks are related and can benefit each other for computer-aided diagnosis. The proposed multi-task sparse low-rank learning framework combines the sparsity and low-rank constraints together for each task. Then, we jointly perform three tasks to capture their intrinsic low-rank structure to achieve better classification performance.

2   Method

The proposed method intends to locate a subset of features that are most related to neurodegenerative disease. In our framework, we first extract neuroimaging features from MRI images, and then select informative features by the proposed multi-task sparse low-rank feature learning. Each task applies the same feature selection method in a jointly multi-task framework. The shared weight matrix obtains the selected features with reduced dimensions. The selected features are then fed into multi-classification algorithms (e.g., support vector machine (SVM) and random forest (RF))

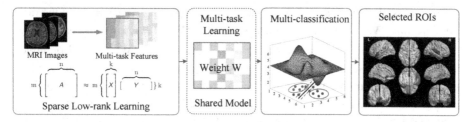

Fig. 1. General framework of our proposed method. The shared model is from the multi-task learning by considering each modal as a task.

to finally identify the clinical labels of testing data. Figure 1 shows the flowchart of our method.

2.1 Proposed Model

We denote matrices as boldface uppercase letters, vectors as boldface lowercase letters, and scalars as normal italic letters. For a matrix $\mathbf{X} = [x_{ij}]$, its i-th row and j-th column are denoted as $\mathbf{X}^i$ and $\mathbf{X}_j$, respectively. Also, we denote the Frobenius norm and the $l_{2,1}$-norm of a matrix $\mathbf{X}$ as $\|\mathbf{X}\|_F = \sqrt{\sum_i \|\mathbf{X}^i\|_2^2}$ and $\|\mathbf{X}\|_{2,1} = \sum_i \|\mathbf{X}^i\|_2 = \sum_i \sqrt{\sum_j x_{i,j}^2}$, respectively. The transpose operator, the trace operator, the rank, and the inverse of $\mathbf{X}$ are denoted as $\mathbf{X}^T$, $tr(\mathbf{X})$, $rank(\mathbf{X})$, and $\mathbf{X}^{-1}$, respectively.

Supposing that T tasks exist for the input and output data, we would have the input feature matrix $\mathbf{X}^{(t)} \in \mathbb{R}^{m \times n}$ for t-th task and the output label matrix $\mathbf{Y}^{(t)} \in \{0, 1\}^{m \times c}$ for t-th task, where m, n, and c denote the numbers of subjects, feature dimensions, and classes, respectively. In the linear regression model $\mathbf{Y} = \mathbf{XW}$, where $\mathbf{W}^{(t)} \in \mathbb{R}^{n \times c}$ is the weight coefficient matrix for each feature of t-th task, $\mathbf{W}$ is obtained by solving the following objective function with least square error

$$\min_{\mathbf{W}^{(t)}} \sum_1^t \left\| \mathbf{Y}^{(t)} - \mathbf{X}^{(t)} \mathbf{W}^{(t)} \right\|_F^2, \tag{1}$$

where Eq. (1) is a simple and straightforward linear regression model without constraint on any variable. However, it does not consider the properties of weight matrix, which results in inferior performance.

In our multi-classification tasks, we have multiple response variables. Equation (1) is equivalent to conduct the least square regression for each response variable separately. However, possible relationships among these variables have not been considered. On the other hand, we aim to find a weight matrix that represents the feature significance in the feature selection process. It is well-known that, the brain is divided into different parts known as regions of interest (ROIs) and neurodegenerative diseases are influenced by a block of brain regions that are responsible for certain human brain functions. For this reason, we assume that each group of features is related to others, which leads to a low-rank structure of the coefficient weight matrix because certain rows are dependent.

These possible factors are taken into account by imposing a constraint on the rank of $\mathbf{W}^{(t)}$ as $rank\left(\mathbf{W}^{(t)}\right) \leq \min(n, c)$. Suppose that $rank\left(\mathbf{W}^{(t)}\right) = r$, it implies each m row of $\mathbf{W}^{(t)}$ is actually a linear combination of r rows. Besides, $rank\left(\mathbf{W}^{(t)}\right) = r$ also implies $\mathbf{Y}^{(t)} = \mathbf{W}^{(t)}\mathbf{X}^{(t)} \leq r$, which indicates that each of c columns of $\mathbf{Y}^{(t)}$ is actually a linear combination of r columns. Such a low-rank constraint obviously considers the relations among response variables and different features. The low-rank constraint on $\mathbf{W}^{(t)}$ can be expressed as the product of two separate matrixes, one is the low-rank part and the other is the remaining part that makes $\mathbf{W}^{(t)}$ complete, which is denoted as

$$\mathbf{W}^{(t)} = \mathbf{P}^{(t)}\mathbf{Q}^{(t)\mathrm{T}}, \tag{2}$$

where $\mathbf{P}^{(t)} \in \mathbb{R}^{n \times r}$ is the low-rank structure and $\mathbf{Q}^{(t)} \in \mathbb{R}^{c \times r}$ is the orthogonal matrix. $\mathbf{Q}^{(t)}$ can be regard as the rotation operation to transfer low-rank structure into the original data space. In most machine learning applications, over-fitting is a common problem when the data matrix is unbalanced. Especially in the field of neuroimaging-aided diagnosis, the brain images are rare, and yet they provide extensive information, leading to high dimensionality. However, some of these features may not be useful in prediction. To this end, we employ the $l_{2,1}$-norm also known as $l_{2,1}$ sparse regularizers to perform feature selection on the low-rank framework. We can formulate the objective function using sparse representation as

$$\min_{\mathbf{P}^{(t)}\mathbf{Q}^{(t)}}\left\|\mathbf{Y}^{(t)} - \mathbf{X}^{(t)}\mathbf{P}^{(t)}\mathbf{Q}^{(t)T}\right\|_F^2 + \alpha\left\|\mathbf{P}^{(t)}\right\|_{2,1}, \tag{3}$$

where α is the tuning parameter. The $l_{2,1}$-norm regularizer on $\mathbf{P}^{(t)}$ penalizes the coefficients of $\mathbf{P}^{(t)}$ for joint selection or un-selection of the features in predicting the clinical labels. The sparse low-rank feature learning framework selects informative features by considering the relations between the neuroimaging features and the response variables via $l_{2,1}$-norm regularizer and utilizing the relations among features via low-rank constraints. For each task, model is built on the assumption that features are closely related with group of features while the relevance between these groups may be sparse. Multiple tasks share the same low-rank and sparse weight coefficients and orthogonal constraints $\mathbf{Q}^{(t)}$. Thus, we can establish the final objective function in the multi-task learning as

$$\min_{\mathbf{P},\mathbf{Q}}\sum_1^t\left\|\mathbf{Y}^{(t)} - \mathbf{X}^{(t)}\mathbf{P}^{(t)}\mathbf{Q}^{(t)T}\right\|_F^2 + \alpha\|\mathbf{P}\|_{2,1}, \tag{4}$$

where α is the tuning parameter. After optimizing Eq. (4), we have different zero row vectors in $\mathbf{P}$. Therefore, the irrelevant features whose regression coefficient vectors are zero in the rows can be discarded. The reduced features are then concatenated and eventually use them to train classifiers for further prediction.

2.2   Optimization

Specifically, we iteratively conduct the following two steps with fixed values until convergence: (a) update $\mathbf{Q}$ with fixed $\mathbf{P}$. (b) update $\mathbf{P}$ with fixed $\mathbf{Q}$. When fixing $\mathbf{P}$, solving $\mathbf{Q}$ becomes an orthogonal Procrustes problem. The optimal solution of $\mathbf{Q}$ is $\mathbf{Q} = \mathbf{SD}^\mathrm{T}$, where $\mathbf{S}$ and $\mathbf{D}$ are obtained from the singular value decomposition of $\mathbf{Q} = \mathbf{Y}^\mathrm{T}\mathbf{X} = \mathbf{SVD}^\mathrm{T}$.

When fixing $\mathbf{Q}$, the objective function is equivalent to

$$\min_{\mathbf{P}} \sum_1^t \left\| \mathbf{Y}^{(t)}\mathbf{Q}^{(t)} - \mathbf{X}^{(t)}\mathbf{P}^{(t)T} \right\|_F^2 + \alpha tr\left(\mathbf{P}^T\mathbf{H}\mathbf{P}\right). \tag{5}$$

where $\mathbf{H} \in \mathbb{R}^{n \times n}$ are the diagonal matrices with $h_{i,j} = \frac{1}{2\|\mathbf{P}^j\|_2^2}$. By setting Eq. (5) to zero, we can obtain $\mathbf{P} = \left(\mathbf{X}^\mathrm{T}\mathbf{X} + \alpha\mathbf{H}\right)^{-1}\mathbf{X}^\mathrm{T}\mathbf{Y}\mathbf{Q}$. Accordingly, $\mathbf{P}$ and $\mathbf{Q}$ are solved by iteratively updating values until convergence.

3   Experiments

3.1   Experimental Setting

The data used in this experiment are MRI images from the PPMI and ADNI datasets [9, 10]. All the original images are preprocessed by the anterior commissure-posterior commissure correction and skull-stripping for later operation. Then, we segment the images into GM, WM, and CSF using Statistical Parametric Mapping (SPM) toolbox [11]. Following the automated anatomical labeling atlas which divides the brain into 116 regions, GM/WM/CSF tissue volume in the ROI region are computed by integrating the tissue segmentation result of this subject. In this work, we collected 347 PD subjects (127 NC, 130 PD, 56 SWEDD and 34 PPD) and 407 AD subjects (107 NC, 98 AD, 86 lMCI, and 116 sMCI).

Our method is evaluated by classifying different stages of PD and AD subjects. Multiple classifiers are applied for efficiency comparison with logistic regression (LR), SVM, and RF. Besides, we also compare capped-norm SVM classifier (cSVM), which can deal with both light and heavy outliers to boost classification performance. The main parameters used are α in Eq. (4). The initial value of α is set in the range $[2^{-5}, 2^{-4}, ...,2^5]$. The fine-tuned parameter value is specified by a 5-fold cross-validation strategy. The results are evaluated using different metrics, accuracy (ACC), sensitivity (SEN), specificity (SPE), precision (PRE) and area under the receiver operating characteristic curve (AUC). For fair evaluation, the classification performance of the proposed method is evaluated via a 10-fold cross-validation strategy.

3.2   Classification Performance

To further validate the effectiveness of our method, we compare with other similar methods as sparse learning (SL), low-rank learning (LRL), sparse low-rank learning (SLRL). The experiments are divided into 4 parts. NC vs. PD vs. SWEDD (PD3), NC vs. PD vs. SWEDD vs. PPD (PD4), NC vs. AD vs. MCI (AD3), and NC vs. AD vs. lMCI vs. sMCI (AD4). The classification performance results are summarized in Tables 1 and 2, respectively (bold faces represent the best performance). It is clear the

Table 1. Classification performances of competing methods with different classifiers for PD.

Method	Classifier	PD3					PD4				
		ACC	PRE	SEN	SPE	AUC	ACC	PRE	SEN	SPE	AUC
SL	LR	67.84	65.32	73.17	84.11	86.23	53.29	47.84	63.74	64.11	71.57
	RF	65.27	65.40	73.45	85.23	84.65	54.05	55.27	63.64	75.24	73.48
	SVM	73.55	69.30	80.05	94.05	88.23	56.32	54.55	70.04	74.69	78.23
	cSVM	73.81	68.30	81.55	97.45	89.45	57.46	55.81	71.43	65.65	73.72
LRL	LR	72.10	66.18	75.24	85.38	87.54	53.65	52.10	65.26	73.83	77.54
	RF	72.46	68.35	78.20	87.79	89.07	56.39	63.46	68.20	77.38	76.65
	SVM	73.09	69.34	79.80	86.38	91.75	55.40	53.74	67.43	78.50	75.64
	cSVM	76.43	69.89	78.46	87.44	90.34	56.77	57.82	67.03	77.86	72.58
SLRL	LR	74.59	69.33	79.56	89.32	91.76	60.69	55.72	65.47	74.24	75.33
	RF	75.32	70.20	79.63	91.05	92.36	62.86	58.67	68.98	78.56	74.63
	SVM	76.54	70.46	82.54	91.88	90.33	64.57	57.63	70.50	79.43	77.50
	cSVM	76.40	70.83	82.33	91.20	92.72	63.22	63.65	72.74	80.12	77.39
MSLRL	LR	73.50	69.88	83.22	90.10	93.55	65.44	59.63	73.59	80.54	78.54
	RF	75.76	70.57	85.78	93.39	93.32	66.43	59.76	72.57	80.35	78.92
	SVM	79.25	71.29	88.65	95.34	94.23	67.43	**67.60**	74.58	**84.59**	80.14
	cSVM	**80.43**	**74.23**	**89.21**	**96.40**	**96.12**	**67.56**	66.55	**74.43**	83.46	**80.53**

Table 2. Classification performances of competing methods with different classifiers for AD.

Method	Classifier	AD3					AD4				
		ACC	PRE	SEN	SPE	AUC	ACC	PRE	SEN	SPE	AUC
SL	LR	64.56	70.75	73.55	64.56	80.33	53.25	47.84	43.17	71.23	66.23
	RF	63.67	73.60	73.63	65.96	80.69	53.14	45.27	43.45	72.75	64.56
	SVM	72.45	80.05	86.04	63.86	81.35	60.03	54.55	50.05	72.43	65.03
	cSVM	72.3	81.55	76.63	61.51	86.03	61.54	55.81	51.57	73.97	64.82
LRL	LR	65.45	75.75	76.55	62.26	86.92	55.82	42.10	45.24	76.34	67.14
	RF	67.31	78.80	74.70	65.14	83.56	53.70	43.46	48.20	75.16	69.44
	SVM	66.55	73.55	74.37	63.56	86.53	53.55	48.72	43.55	77.05	68.59
	cSVM	69.74	74.82	75.88	68.96	84.32	53.82	49.76	43.62	78.30	69.18
SLRL	LR	86.61	80.95	79.63	69.34	87.54	60.42	46.43	55.45	78.28	68.23
	RF	81.55	77.87	81.55	67.84	85.37	61.55	53.53	58.61	79.46	69.25
	SVM	81.11	84.11	78.25	65.68	83.43	64.11	55.58	57.56	82.11	72.77
	cSVM	83.23	86.23	80.95	74.55	89.55	63.22	54.24	55.25	83.23	73.54
MSLRL	LR	84.30	88.30	81.55	75.81	91.18	56.34	55.05	**58.63**	84.30	74.85
	RF	82.05	91.05	75.34	72.10	94.25	64.05	52.50	55.65	83.05	73.67
	SVM	84.79	**91.45**	**85.24**	76.85	93.94	64.73	54.29	56.14	83.38	74.54
	cSVM	**85.30**	87.79	85.11	**77.03**	**95.07**	**65.42**	**55.76**	54.22	**84.79**	**76.45**

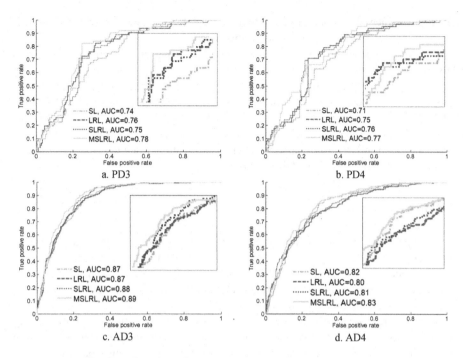

Fig. 2. ROC plots of the comparing methods with the cSVM.

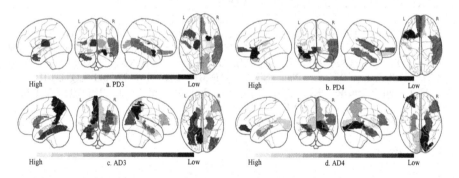

Fig. 3. Top 10 selected ROIs most-related with PD and AD. Each color indicates one ROI. High indicates higher relevance with the disease classification. (Color figure online)

proposed method achieves higher accuracy than other similar feature selection methods. SLRL turns out to be more effective than LRL and SL since sparsity and low-rank structure are jointly considered. Furthermore, our method outperforms SLRL with each classifier, which proves that multitask learning successfully explores the intrinsic relations within features. However, the best performance with different classification varies as AD3 is better than PD3 while AD4 is worse than PD4. This result indicates higher distinctiveness in AD3 and PD4. Receiver operating characteristic curves (ROC) for algorithm comparison are shown in Fig. 2. Our method obtains the best

ROC performance in all competing methods in the selected classifier, which shows the advantage and potential for early disease diagnosis.

We further exploit potential disease-related ROIs, we choose the top 10 related ROIs using our feature selection method, shown in Fig. 3. In each of the ROI plot, from left to right, sagittal left hemisphere, coronal, sagittal right hemisphere, and axial views are shown, respectively. Each figure contains the top 10 most disease-related ROIs with different degree of red color. Obviously, affecting areas are not the same for PD and AD. As for the specific classification task, as 3-classification or 4-classification, significance also differs. Some areas need special attention when considering multiple prodromal stages like lMCI, sMCI and PPD.

4 Conclusion

In this paper, we introduced a multi-task sparse low-rank learning framework for neurodegenerative diseases diagnosis between multiple progression stages. Specifically, for each task, we added the sparsity and low-rank regularization to the weight coefficients, which unveils the underlying relationships within data. By exploring the intrinsic relationships among multiple tasks, this framework selects the most representative features by jointly considering the dimension reduction of neuroimaging feature vectors and the relevant dependency properties of disease-related brain region features. Using neuroimaging data from PPMI and ADNI neuroimaging dataset, extensive experiments demonstrated that our method has the best multi-class classification results among all the traditional methods.

Acknowledgments. This work was supported partly by National Natural Science Foundation of China (Nos. 61871274, 61801305 and 81571758), National Natural Science Foundation of Guangdong Province (No. 2017A030313377), Guangdong Pearl River Talents Plan (2016 ZT06S220), Shenzhen Peacock Plan (Nos. KQTD2016053112051497 and KQTD20150330 16104926), and Shenzhen Key Basic Research Project (Nos. JCYJ20180507184647636, JCYJ20170818142347251 and JCYJ20170818094109846).

References

1. Lei, H., et al.: Joint detection and clinical score prediction in Parkinson's disease via multi-modal sparse learning. Expert Syst. Appl. **80**(1), 284–296 (2017)
2. Emrani, S., McGuirk, A., Wei, X.: Prognosis and diagnosis of parkinson's disease using multi-task learning. In: ACM SIGKDD International Conference on Knowledge Discovery and Data Mining, pp. 1457–1466 (2017)
3. Bhatkoti, P., Paul, M.: Early diagnosis of Alzheimer's disease: a multi-class deep learning framework with modified k-sparse autoencoder classification. In: International Conference on Image and Vision Computing New Zealand, pp. 1–5 (2017)
4. Lei, B., Yang, P., Wang, T., Chen, S., Ni, D.: Relational-regularized discriminative sparse learning for Alzheimer's disease diagnosis. IEEE Trans. Cybern. **47**(4), 1102–1113 (2017)

5. Zhu, Y., Zhang, X., Hu, R., Wen, G.: Robust features selection via structure learning and multiple subspace learning. In: IEEE International Conference on Big Knowledge, pp. 326–331 (2017)
6. Zhu, X., Suk, H.-I., Shen, D.: Low-rank dimensionality reduction for multi-modality neurodegenerative disease identification. World Wide Web **22**(2), 907–925 (2019)
7. Chaudhuri, K.R., Healy, D.G., Schapira, A.H.V.: Non-motor symptoms of Parkinson's disease: diagnosis and management. Lancet Neurol. **5**(3), 235–245 (2006)
8. Fang, X., et al.: Approximate low-rank projection learning for feature extraction. IEEE Trans. Neural Netw. Learn. Syst. **29**(11), 5228–5241 (2018)
9. Marek, K., et al.: The parkinson progression marker initiative (PPMI). Prog. Neurobiol. **95**(4), 629–635 (2011)
10. Mueller, S.G., et al.: The Alzheimer's disease neuroimaging initiative. Neuroimaging Clin. North Am. **15**(4), 869 (2005)
11. Penny, W.D., Friston, K.J., Ashburner, J.T., Kiebel, S.J., Nichols, T.E.: Statistical Parametric Mapping: The Analysis of Functional Brain Images. Elsevier (2011)

Improved Prediction of Cognitive Outcomes via Globally Aligned Imaging Biomarker Enrichments over Progressions

Lyujian Lu[1], Saad Elbeleidy[1], Lauren Baker[1], Hua Wang[1]($\boxtimes$) (iD),
Heng Huang[2,3] (iD), Li Shen[4] (iD), and for the ADNI

[1] Department of Computer Science, Colorado School of Mines, Golden, CO, USA
{lyujianlu,selbeleidy,laurenzoebaker}@mymail.mines.edu,
huawangcs@gmail.com
[2] Department of Electrical and Computer Engineering, University of Pittsburgh,
Pittsburgh, PA, USA
[3] JD Finance America Corporation, Mountain View, CA, USA
heng.huang@pitt.edu
[4] Department of Biostatistics, Epidemiology and Informatics, University
of Pennsylvania, Philadelphia, PA, USA
Li.Shen@pennmedicine.upenn.edu

Abstract. Incomplete or inconsistent temporal neuroimaging records of patients over time pose a major challenge to accurately predict clinical scores for diagnosing Alzheimer's Disease (AD). In this paper, we present an unsupervised method to learn enriched imaging biomarker representations that can simultaneously capture the information conveyed by all the baseline neuroimaging measures and the progressive variations of the available follow-up measurements of every participant. Our experiments on the Alzheimer's Disease Neuroimaging Initiative (ADNI) dataset show improved performance in predicting cognitive outcomes thereby demonstrating the effectiveness of our proposed method.

Keywords: Alzheimer's Disease · Longitudinal representations · Representation enrichment · Imaging biomarker

1 Introduction

Alzheimer's Disease (AD) is a chronic neurodegenerative disease that severely impacts patients' thinking, memory, and behavior. AD is listed as the sixth

---

ADNI—Data used in preparation of this article were obtained from the Alzheimer's Disease Neuroimaging Initiative (ADNI) database (ad-ni.loni.usc.edu). As such, the investigators within the ADNI contributed to the design and implementation of ADNI and/or provided data but did not participate in analysis or writing of this report. A complete listing of ADNI investigators can be found at: https://adni.loni.usc.edu/wp-content/uploads/howtoapply/ADNIAcknowledgementList.pdf.

D. Shen et al. (Eds.): MICCAI 2019, LNCS 11767, pp. 140–148, 2019.
https://doi.org/10.1007/978-3-030-32251-9_16

leading cause of death in the United States of America, threatening 5.7 million American and 44 millions individuals worldwide [1]. Over the past decade, neuroimaging measures have been widely studied to predict disease status and/or cognitive performance [14]. However, there are some critical limitations in many predictive models, *i.e.*, they routinely perform learning at each time points *separately*, ignoring the longitudinal variations among temporal brain phenotypes. First, since AD is a progressive neurodegenerative disorder, multiple consecutive neuroimaging records are usually required to monitor the disease progressions. It would be beneficial to explore the temporal relations among the longitudinal records of the biomarkers. Second, the records of neuroimaging biomarkers are often missing at some time points for some participants over the entire courses of the AD progressions, because it is difficult to conduct medical scans consistently across a large group of participants. To be more specific, higher mortality risk and cognitive impairment hinder older adults from staying in studies requiring multiple visits and thus result in incomplete data.

To overcome the first limitation of longitudinal data, many studies [3,9,17,18] explore the temporal data structures of brain phenotypes over time. However, these models often formulate the temporal neuroimaging records as a tensor, which inevitably complicates the prediction problems. To handle the second limitation of data inconsistency, most longitudinal studies of AD only utilize the samples with complete temporal records for model analysis and ignore the samples with fewer time points. But discarding of observed samples may potentially neglects substantially valuable information in the data. To solve this problem, data imputation methods [4,10] have been used to generate missing records over AD progressions, after which temporal regression studies can then be conducted. However, missing data imputation methods can introduce undesirable artifacts, which in turn can worsen the predictive power of the longitudinal models.

To deal with the longitudinal prediction problem with incomplete temporal inputs, we propose a novel method to learn an enriched biomarker representation to integrate the baseline records of the neuroimaging biomarkers of the entire cohort and the dynamic measures across all following time points of the individuals. First, it learns a global projection from the baseline records of the biomarkers from all the participants to preserve the global structure of a given neuroimaging dataset. Then, for each participant we learn a local projection from available follow-up neuroimaging records in the later couple of years to maintain the local data structure for the participant. Finally, a soft constraint is used to build consistency between the global and local projections. A schematic illustration of this formulation is shown in Fig. 1. Armed with the learned projection, we can transform the records with inconsistent sizes in a neuroimaging dataset into fixed-length vectors. With these fixed-length biomarker representations, we can make use of conventional regression methods to predict clinical scores.

2   Problem Formalization and the Solution Algorithm

In the task of representation learning for predicting cognitive outcomes, our goal is to learn a fixed-length biomarker representation vector for a participant from

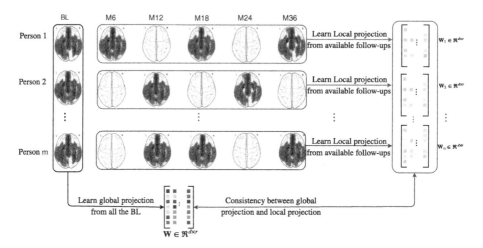

Fig. 1. Illustration of the proposed framework to learn the global and local projections. The blank plots denote the absence of scans for the participants of an AD dataset.

her or his baseline neuroimaging measures and all available follow-up measures. For the observed neuroimaging measures of a participant, we denote this information as: $\mathcal{X}_i = \{\mathbf{x}_i, \mathbf{X}_i\}$, where $i = 1, 2, \cdots, m$ is the index of a participant in a neuroimaging dataset. In every $\mathcal{X}_i$, $\mathbf{x}_i \in \Re^d$ is the baseline neuroimaging measure of the i-th participant where d denotes the dimensions of the neuroimaging feature set, and $\mathbf{X}_i = \left[\mathbf{x}_1^i, \ldots, \mathbf{x}_{n_i}^i \right] \in \Re^{d \times n_i}$ collects all available follow-up biomarker records of the i-th participant after the baseline where n_i denotes the number of available follow-up neuroimaging records of the same participant. Here we note that n_i varies over the dataset, because many participants of a cohort may have some missing records at certain time points.

Because the neuroimaging measures usually reside in a high-dimensional space, they can be redundant and noisy. Thus, we learn the compact representations of these measures via a global projection to only keep the most useful information of an input dataset. To achieve this goal, Principal Component Analysis (PCA) is the right tool, because it learns from the input data a linear projection to preserve as much information as possible in a low-dimensional projected subspace. Mathematically, PCA minimizes the reconstruction error via the projection $\mathbf{W} \in \Re^{d \times r}$ (usually $r \ll d$) that minimizes the following objective:

$$\mathcal{J}_{\text{Global}}(\mathbf{W}) = \sum_{i=1}^{m} \left\| \mathbf{x}_i - \mathbf{W} \mathbf{W}^T \mathbf{x}_i \right\|_2^2, \quad s.t. \ \mathbf{W}^T \mathbf{W} = \mathbf{I}. \tag{1}$$

Usually the neuroimaging measures of each participant do not experience drastic changes in a short time, thus we still want to preserve the local consistency in the projected space for each participant. To uncover the local consistency among the neuroimaging records of each participant, we keep the local pairwise patterns of measures in the projected subspace. To achieve this, locality preserving projections (LPP) is the right tool to leverage. Given a pairwise similarity matrix $\mathbf{S}_i \in \Re^{n_i \times n_i}$ of the i-th participant of the neuroimaging dataset, LPP preserves the local relationships and maximizes the smoothness of the manifold of the data in the embedding space by minimizing the following objective:

$$\mathcal{J}_{\text{Local}}(\mathbf{W}_i) = \sum_{\mathbf{x}_j^i, \mathbf{x}_k^i \in \mathbf{X}_i} s_{jk}^i \left\| \mathbf{W}_i^T \mathbf{x}_j^i - \mathbf{W}_i^T \mathbf{x}_k^i \right\|_2^2, \quad s.t. \ \mathbf{W}_i^T \mathbf{W}_i = \mathbf{I}, \quad (2)$$

where s_{jk}^i is the pairwise relationship coefficient between the available records of the i-th participant at j-th and k-th time points.

To integrate the global and local consistencies of the neuroimaging measures at the same time, following the same idea in our previous works [6,7,15,16] we can develop a combined objective using the above two objectives to minimize:

$$\mathcal{J}_{\ell_2^2}(\mathcal{W}) = \sum_{i=1}^m \left\| \mathbf{x}_i - \mathbf{W}\mathbf{W}^T \mathbf{x}_i \right\|_2^2 + \alpha \sum_{i=1}^m \sum_{\mathbf{x}_j^i, \mathbf{x}_k^i \in \mathbf{X}_i} s_{jk}^i \left\| \mathbf{W}_i^T \mathbf{x}_j^i - \mathbf{W}_i^T \mathbf{x}_k^i \right\|_2^2$$

$$+ \beta \sum_{i=1}^m \left\| \mathbf{W} - \mathbf{W}_i \right\|_2^2, \quad s.t. \ \mathbf{W}^T \mathbf{W} = \mathbf{I}, \ \mathbf{W}_i^T \mathbf{W}_i = \mathbf{I}, \quad (3)$$

where we denote $\mathcal{W} = \{\mathbf{W}, \mathbf{W}_1, \cdots, \mathbf{W}_m\}$. Through the third term of Eq. (3), the projections $\mathbf{W}_i$ learned from each participant are aligned with the projection $\mathbf{W}$ learned globally from the baseline measures of the entire dataset, such that the information conveyed by the global projection $\mathbf{W}$ learned from all the participants as a whole can be transferred to each individual participant.

Taking into account that the squared ℓ_2-norm is notorious for being very sensitive to the outliers in a dataset which usually results in the failure of traditional regression models, to improve the robustness of the learned enriched representations by our new method, we substitute the squared ℓ_2-norm terms in Eq. (3) by their *not-squared* counterparts as follows:

$$\mathcal{J}_{\ell_2}(\mathcal{W}) = \sum_{i=1}^m \left\| \mathbf{x}_i - \mathbf{W}\mathbf{W}^T \mathbf{x}_i \right\|_2 + \alpha \sum_{i=1}^m \sum_{\mathbf{x}_j^i, \mathbf{x}_k^i \in \mathbf{X}_i} s_{jk}^i \left\| \mathbf{W}_i^T \mathbf{x}_j^i - \mathbf{W}_i^T \mathbf{x}_k^i \right\|_2$$

$$+ \beta \sum_{i=1}^m \left\| \mathbf{W} - \mathbf{W}_i \right\|_2^2, \quad s.t. \ \mathbf{W}^T \mathbf{W} = \mathbf{I}, \ \mathbf{W}_i^T \mathbf{W}_i = \mathbf{I}. \quad (4)$$

Upon solving the optimization problem in Eq. (4), we learn a fixed-length representation for each participant by computing $\{\mathbf{y}_i = \mathbf{W}_i^T \mathbf{x}_i\}_{i=1}^m$, which can be readily fed into traditional machine learning models.

Although the motivations of the formulation of our new method in Eq. (4) is clear and justifiable, it is a non-smooth objective, which is difficult to efficiently solve in general. Using the optimization framework presented in our earlier work [8] that solves non-smooth objectives using not-squared ℓ_2-norm terms, we can solve Eq. (4) by an iterative procedure [8, Algorithm 1] in which the key step is to minimize the following objective:

$$\mathcal{J}_{\ell_2}^{R}(\mathcal{W}) = \mathrm{tr}\left(\mathbf{X} - \mathbf{W}\mathbf{W}^T\mathbf{X}\right)\mathbf{\Gamma}\left(\mathbf{X} - \mathbf{W}\mathbf{W}^T\mathbf{X}\right)^T + \alpha\sum_{i=1}^{m}\mathrm{tr}\left(\mathbf{W}_i^T\mathbf{X}_i\mathbf{L}_i\mathbf{X}_i^T\mathbf{W}_i\right)$$

$$+ \beta\sum_{i=1}^{m}\|\mathbf{W} - \mathbf{W}_i\|_2^2, \quad s.t. \quad \mathbf{W}^T\mathbf{W} = \mathbf{I}, \ \mathbf{W}_i^T\mathbf{W}_i = \mathbf{I}, \tag{5}$$

where $\mathbf{X} = [\mathbf{x}_1, \mathbf{x}_2, \cdots, \mathbf{x}_m] \in \Re^{d\times m}$ summarizes all the baseline measurements, and $\mathbf{\Gamma} \in \Re^{m\times m}$ is a diagonal matrix whose i-th element is $\gamma^i = \frac{1}{2\sqrt{\|\mathbf{x}_i - \mathbf{W}\mathbf{W}^T\mathbf{x}_i\|_2^2 + \delta}}$. Defining $\theta_{jk}^i = \frac{1}{2\sqrt{\|\mathbf{W}_i^T\mathbf{x}_j^i - \mathbf{W}_i^T\mathbf{x}_k^i\|_2^2 + \delta}}$ and $\tilde{\mathbf{S}}_i \in \Re^{n_i\times n_i}$ whose element value is $\tilde{s}_{jk}^i = \theta_{jk}^i s_{jk}^i$, in Eq. (5) we compute $\mathbf{L}^i = \mathbf{D}^i - \tilde{\mathbf{S}}^i$ where $\mathbf{D}^i$ is a diagonal matrix whose diagonal entries are the column (or row) sums of $\tilde{\mathbf{S}}_i$, i.e., $d_{jj} = \sum_j \tilde{s}_{jk}$.

The objective in Eq. (5) can be solved by the Alternating Direction Method of Multipliers (ADMM) [2] that minimizes the following equivalent objective:

$$\mathcal{J}_{\ell_2}^{ADMM}(\mathcal{W}, \mathcal{P}) = \mathrm{tr}\left(\mathbf{X} - \mathbf{W}\mathbf{W}^T\mathbf{X}\right)\mathbf{\Gamma}\left(\mathbf{X} - \mathbf{W}\mathbf{W}^T\mathbf{X}\right)^T$$

$$+ \alpha\sum_{i=1}^{m}\mathrm{tr}\left(\mathbf{W}_i^T\mathbf{X}_i\mathbf{L}_i\mathbf{X}_i^T\mathbf{W}_i\right) + \beta\sum_{i=1}^{m}\|\mathbf{P} - \mathbf{P}_i\|_F^2 + \frac{\mu}{2}\left\|\mathbf{W} - \mathbf{P} + \frac{1}{\mu}\mathbf{\Lambda}\right\|_2^2$$

$$+ \sum_{i=1}^{m}\frac{\mu}{2}\left\|\mathbf{W}_i - \mathbf{P}_i + \frac{1}{\mu}\mathbf{\Lambda}_i\right\|_2^2, \quad s.t. \quad \mathbf{P}^T\mathbf{P} = \mathbf{I}, \ \mathbf{P}_i^T\mathbf{P}_i = \mathbf{I}, \tag{6}$$

where $\mathcal{P} = \{\mathbf{P}, \mathbf{P}_1, \mathbf{P}_2, \cdots, \mathbf{P}_m\}$, $\mathbf{\Lambda} \in \Re^{d\times r}$ is the Lagrangian multiplier for the constraint of $\mathbf{W} = \mathbf{P}$, and $\mathbf{\Lambda}_i \in \Re^{d\times r}$ is the Lagrangian multiplier for the constraint of $\mathbf{W}_i = \mathbf{P}_i$. Algorithm (1) summaries the solution to Eq. (6).

3   Experiments

Data used in our experiments were obtained from the ADNI database (adni.loni.usc.edu). We downloaded 1.5T MRI scans and the demographic information for 821 ADNI-1 participants. We performed voxel-based morphometry (VBM) on the MRI data by following [12] and extracted mean modulated gray matter (GM) measures for 90 target regions of interest (ROI). These measures were adjusted for the baseline intracranial volume (ICV) using regression weights derived from the Healthy Control (HC) participants at the baseline. We also downloaded the longitudinal scores of the participants in the cognitive assessment of Mini-Mental State Examination (MMSE). The time points examined in this study for both imaging biomarkers and cognitive assessments include baseline (BL), Month 6 (M6), Month 12 (M12), Month 18 (M18) Month 24 (M24) and Month 36 (M36). All the participants' data used in our enriched biomarker representation study are required to have a BL MRI measurement, BL cognitive score and at least two available measures from M6/M12/M18/M24/36. A total

---

Algorithm 1: Solve the optimization problem in Eq. (6).

Initialization: $\mathbf{W}$, $\mathbf{W}_i$, $\mathbf{P}$, $\mathbf{P}_i$, $\boldsymbol{\Lambda}$, $\boldsymbol{\Lambda}_i$, $1 < \rho < 2$, $\mu, \alpha, \beta > 0$;

while *not converge* **do**

> **1.** Update $\mathbf{W}_i$ by $\mathbf{W}_i = \left(2\alpha \mathbf{X}_i \mathbf{L}_i \mathbf{X}_i^T + \mu \mathbf{I}\right)^{-1} (\mu \mathbf{P}_i - \boldsymbol{\Lambda}_i)$;
>
> **2.** Update $\mathbf{P}_i$ by $\mathbf{P}_i = \mathbf{U}_i \mathbf{V}_i^T$, where $\mathbf{N}_i = 2\beta \mathbf{P} + \mu \mathbf{W}_i + \boldsymbol{\Lambda}_i$ and svd $(\mathbf{N}_i) = \mathbf{U}_i \boldsymbol{\Sigma}_i \mathbf{V}_i^T$;
>
> **3.** Update $\mathbf{W}$ by $\mathbf{W} = \left(\mu \mathbf{I} - 2\mathbf{X}\boldsymbol{\Gamma}\mathbf{X}^T\right)^{-1} (\mu \mathbf{P} - \boldsymbol{\Lambda})$;
>
> **4.** Update $\mathbf{P}$ by $\mathbf{P} = \mathbf{U}\mathbf{V}^T$, where $\mathbf{N} = 2\beta \sum_{i=1}^{m} \mathbf{P}_i + \mu \mathbf{W} + \boldsymbol{\Lambda}$ and svd $(\mathbf{N}) = \mathbf{U}\boldsymbol{\Sigma}\mathbf{V}^T$;
>
> **5.** Update $\boldsymbol{\Lambda}_i$ by $\boldsymbol{\Lambda}_i = \boldsymbol{\Lambda}_i + \mu (\mathbf{W}_i - \mathbf{P}_i)$;
>
> **6.** Update $\boldsymbol{\Lambda}$ by $\boldsymbol{\Lambda} = \boldsymbol{\Lambda} + \mu (\mathbf{W} - \mathbf{P})$;
>
> **7.** Update μ by $\mu = \rho\mu$;

Output: $\mathbf{W}$, $\mathbf{W}_i$.

---

of 544 sample subjects are selected to perform in our study, among which we have 92 AD samples, and 205 Mild Cognitive Impairment (MCI) samples and 247 HC samples.

Experiment Settings. To validate the usefulness of our proposed method, we compare the performance to predict cognitive outcomes using two types of the neuroimaging inputs—the learned enriched representation and BL biomarker measurement. In our experiments, several methods proven to generalize well, such as ridge regression (RR), Lasso, support vector regression (SVR), and convolutional neural networks (CNN), are leveraged. For RR, Lasso and SVR models, we conduct a standard 5-fold cross-validation to fine tune the parameters and compute the root mean square error (RMSE) between the predicted values and ground truth values of the cognitive scores on the testing data. For the SVR model, the linear kernel is leveraged, for which the box constraint parameters are fine tuned by a grid search in standard 5-fold cross-validation as well. For the CNN regression model, we randomly select 70% of the neuroimaging measurements as the training set, 20% of the neuroimaging measurements as the validation set and the remaining 10% of the neuroimaging measurements as the testing set. The evaluation metrics are reported based on the results on the testing dataset. We construct a two-layer convolution architecture for the cognitive outcomes prediction and the dropout technique [13] is also leveraged to reduce overfitting in CNN models and prevent complex co-adaptations on training data. For the model parameters, α, β are fine tuned by searching the grid of $\{10^{-5}, \ldots, 10^{-1}, 1, 10, \cdots, 10^5\}$.

Experiment Results. From Table 1, we can see that the proposed enriched neuroimaging representation is consistently better than baseline representations when we use the four different methods, LR, RR Lasso, SVR and CNN. It can be attributed to the following reasons. First, the original baseline neuroimaging biomarker representation only contains the cognitive information of a participant at one single time point, which does not benefit from the correlation across different cognitive measures over the time. Instead, our proposed enriched neuroimaging biomarker representation could capture not only the baseline cognitive measurement, but also the temporal information conveyed by the longitudinal biomarkers over AD progressions. Our enriched neuroimaging representation could integrate the neuroimaging measurement at the fixed time point and the dynamic temporal changes. As AD is a progressively degenerative disease, incorporation of future information about subjects benefits the prediction model. Second, the original baseline neuroimaging measurements exhibits high dimensionality, which could be redundant and noisy. Thus the traditional methods easily suffer from "the curse of dimensionality". Via the projection, we map the baseline cognitive measurement into a low dimensional space thereby mitigating the issue of high dimensionality.

Table 1. RMSE values (smaller is better) when predicting MMSE score using the VBM biomarkers.

	RR	Lasso	SVR	CNN
Baseline	0.4398	0.3845	0.5035	0.1572
Enriched (our method)	0.3192	0.3509	0.3898	0.1546

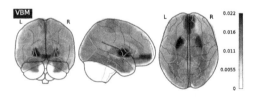

Fig. 2. Frequency map of regions of interest of brain.

Apart from the cognitive outcomes prediction task, another primary goal of our regression analysis is to identify a subset of imaging biomarkers which are highly correlated to AD progressions. Therefore, we examine the imaging biomarkers of each participant identified by the proposed methods encoded by the cognitive scores. A brief summary of all the patients' projections can be conducted to determine the most important biomarkers across patients. We select the 10 most frequently appearing regions of interest from each patient's projection coefficients to reconstruct a global frequency map, shown in Fig. 2. The bilateral hippocampus, amygdala, fusiform, putamen regions are found to be in the top selected biomarkers by our model, which are in nice accordance with the known clinical knowledge [5,11].

4   Conclusion

Missing data is a critical challenge in longitudinal AD studies. In this paper, we proposed a formulation to learn a consistent-length representation for all the participants in the ADNI dataset. The enriched fixed length biomarker representation could capture the global consistency from baseline measurements and local pairwise pattern from available follow-up measurements of each participant at the same time. Our results show that the learned enriched representation beat the performance of the baseline measurement in predicting the clinical scores. Furthermore, the identified biomarkers are highly suggestive and strongly agree with existing research findings, which warrants the correctness of our approach.

Acknowledgements. L. Lu, S. Elbeleidy, L. Baker and H. Wang were partially supported by the National Science Foundation (NSF) under the grants of IIS 1652943 and IIS 1849359; H. Huang was partially supported by the National Institutes of Health (NIH) under the grant of NIH R01 AG049371 and by the NSF under the grants of NSF IIS 1836938, DBI 1836866, IIS 1845666, IIS 1852606, IIS 1838627, IIS 1837956; L. Shen was partially supported by the NIH under the grant of NIH R01 EB022574 and by the NSF under the grant of NSF IIS 1837964.

References

1. Association, A., et al.: 2018 Alzheimer's disease facts and figures. Alzheimer's Dement. **14**(3), 367–429 (2018)
2. Boyd, S., Parikh, N., Chu, E., Peleato, B., Eckstein, J., et al.: Distributed optimization and statistical learning via the alternating direction method of multipliers. Found. Trends® Mach. Learn. **3**(1), 1–122 (2011)
3. Brand, L., et al.: Joint high-order multi-task feature learning to predict the progression of Alzheimer's disease. In: The Twenty-First International Conference on Medical Image Computing and Computer Assisted Intervention (MICCAI 2018), pp. 555–562 (2018)
4. Campos, S., Pizarro, L., Valle, C., Gray, K.R., Rueckert, D., Allende, H.: Evaluating imputation techniques for missing data in ADNI: a patient classification study. Progress in Pattern Recognition, Image Analysis, Computer Vision, and Applications. LNCS, vol. 9423, pp. 3–10. Springer, Cham (2015). https://doi.org/10.1007/978-3-319-25751-8_1
5. De Jong, L.: Strongly reduced volumes of putamen and thalamus in Alzheimer's disease: an MRI study. Brain **131**(12), 3277–3285 (2008)
6. Liu, K., Wang, H., Han, F., Zhang, H.: Visual place recognition via robust ℓ_2-norm distance based holism and landmark integration. In: The thirty-Third AAAI Conference on Artificial Intelligence (AAAI 2019) (2019)
7. Liu, K., Wang, H., Nie, F., Zhang, H.: Learning multi-instance enriched image representations via non-greedy ratio maximization of the ℓ_1-norm distances. In: Proceedings of the IEEE Conference on Computer Vision and Pattern Recognition 2018 (CVPR 2018), pp. 7727–7735 (2018)
8. Liu, Y., Guo, Y., Wang, H., Nie, F., Huang, H.: Semi-supervised classifications via elastic and robust embedding. In: The thirty-First AAAI Conference on Artificial Intelligence (AAAI 2017) (2017)

9. Lu, L., Wang, H., Yao, X., Risacher, S., Saykin, A., Shen, L.: Predicting progressions of cognitive outcomes via high-order multi-modal multi-task feature learning. In: IEEE ISBI 2018, pp. 545–548. IEEE (2018)

10. Minhas, S., Khanum, A., Riaz, F., Alvi, A., Khan, S.A.: Early Alzheimer's disease prediction in machine learning setup: empirical analysis with missing value computation. In: Jackowski, K., Burduk, R., Walkowiak, K., Woźniak, M., Yin, H. (eds.) IDEAL 2015. LNCS, vol. 9375, pp. 424–432. Springer, Cham (2015). https://doi.org/10.1007/978-3-319-24834-9_49

11. Poulin, S.P., Dautoff, R., Morris, J.C., Barrett, L.F., Dickerson, B.C., Initiative, A.D.N., et al.: Amygdala atrophy is prominent in early Alzheimer's disease and relates to symptom severity. Psychiatry Res. Neuroimaging $194(1)$, 7–13 (2011)

12. Risacher, S.L., et al.: Longitudinal MRI atrophy biomarkers: relationship to conversion in the ADNI cohort. Neurobiol. Aging $31(8)$, 1401–1418 (2010)

13. Srivastava, N., Hinton, G., Krizhevsky, A., Sutskever, I., Salakhutdinov, R.: Dropout: a simple way to prevent neural networks from overfitting. J. Mach. Learn. Res. 15, 1929–1958 (2014)

14. Stonnington, C.M., et al.: Predicting clinical scores from magnetic resonance scans in Alzheimer's disease. Neuroimage $51(4)$, 1405–1413 (2010)

15. Wang, H., Huang, H., Ding, C.: Discriminant laplacian embedding. In: The twenty-Fourth AAAI Conference on Artificial Intelligence (AAAI 2010) (2010)

16. Wang, H., Nie, F., Huang, H.: Globally and locally consistent unsupervised projection. In: The twenty-Eighth AAAI Conference on Artificial Intelligence (AAAI 2014), pp. 1328–1333 (2014)

17. Wang, H., et al.: High-order multi-task feature learning to identify longitudinal phenotypic markers for Alzheimer's disease progression prediction. In: NIPS, pp. 1277–1285 (2012)

18. Wang, X., et al.: Longitudinal genotype-phenotype association study via temporal structure auto-learning predictive model. In: Sahinalp, S.C. (ed.) RECOMB 2017. LNCS, vol. 10229, pp. 287–302. Springer, Cham (2017). https://doi.org/10.1007/978-3-319-56970-3_18

Deep Granular Feature-Label Distribution Learning for Neuroimaging-Based Infant Age Prediction

Dan Hu, Han Zhang, Zhengwang Wu, Weili Lin, Gang Li[(✉)],
Dinggang Shen[(✉)] and for UNC/UMN Baby Connectome Project
Consortium

Department of Radiology and BRIC, University of North Carolina at Chapel Hill,
Chapel Hill, NC 27599, USA
{gang_li, dgshen}@med.unc.edu

Abstract. Neuroimaging-based infant age prediction is important for brain development analysis but often suffers insufficient data. To address this challenge, we introduce label distribution learning (LDL), a popular machine learning paradigm focusing on the small sample problem, for infant age prediction. As directly applying LDL yields dramatically increased number of day-to-day age labels and also extremely scarce data describing each label, we propose a new strategy, called granular label distribution (GLD). Particularly, by assembling the adjacent labels to granules and designing granular distributions, GLD makes each brain MRI contribute to not only its own age but also its neighboring ages at a *granule* scale, which effectively keeps the information augmentation superiority of LDL and reduces the number of labels. Furthermore, to extremely augment the information supplied by the small data, we propose a novel method named *granular feature distribution* (GFD). GFD leverages the variability of the brain images at the same age, thus significantly increases the learning effectiveness. Moreover, deep neural network is exploited to approximate the GLD. These strategies constitute a new model: deep granular feature-label distribution learning (DGFLDL). By taking 8 types of cortical morphometric features from structural MRI as predictors, the proposed DGFLDL is validated on infant age prediction using 384 brain MRI scans from 35 to 848 days after birth. Our proposed method, approaching the mean absolute error as 36.1 days, significantly outperforms the baseline methods. Besides, the permutation importance analysis of features based on our method reveals important biomarkers of infant brain development.

Keywords: Infant age prediction · Cortical features · Label distribution learning

1 Introduction

Neuroimaging-based infant age prediction is important for tracking early brain development [1], identifying potential neurodevelopmental disorders [2], and discerning environmental influences on the brains [3]. Although there are many studies on

© Springer Nature Switzerland AG 2019
D. Shen et al. (Eds.): MICCAI 2019, LNCS 11767, pp. 149–157, 2019.
https://doi.org/10.1007/978-3-030-32251-9_17

brain imaging-based age prediction [1, 4], little work has been dedicated to infants, who are in a crucial period with neurodevelopmental disorders possibly emerging [5]. To this end, this paper focuses on predicting infant age from birth to 2 years of age using brain MR images, as well as identifying some development-related biomarkers. Conventionally, neuroimaging-based age prediction is considered as a regression problem and many machine learning algorithms have been adopted, e.g., support vector regression [6], convolutional neural network, Gaussian process regression [1], and multiple linear regression with elastic-net penalty [7]. On the other hand, age prediction can be taken as a classification problem as well by setting each age as a class label [8]. However, all these methods suffer from insufficient training data issue. Label distribution learning (LDL), as an effective strategy of learning from insufficient data, has become a popular learning paradigm in the past few years [8, 10, 11]. Taking advantage of the similarity of the features at close ages, LDL realizes the information augmentation by utilizing the images at the neighboring ages while learning a particular age. This merit attracts us introducing LDL to handle the data insufficiency issue in infant age prediction. However, there are still two major challenges while applying LDL method to the infant neuroimaging data: (1) high computational burden caused by a large number of "age labels", since there are nearly 800 different age labels in a day-to-day infant age prediction problem; (2) ineffective learning due to scarce training samples for each age label (384 MR images distributed on over 800 labels).

To overcome these challenges, we propose a deep granular feature-label distribution learning (DGFLDL) method for infant age prediction. First, we exploit the concept of granule, the collection of values that are arranged together due to their adjacency, to assemble the labels with high similarity, and propose a new strategy called granular label distribution (GLD). With GLD, the number of labels is sharply reduced to the number of granules by designing the distribution on granules rather than each single label. Then, by utilizing the inter-subject and noise-caused variability of the brain images at the same age, a novel concept granular feature distributions (GFD) is defined to replace the original single feature vector. The introduction of GFD further augments the information in the small data and effectively increases the robustness of the age prediction model. Furthermore, a deep neural network is employed to fit the granular label distribution by taking its advantage on nonlinear function approximation. Finally, some biomarkers for infant brain development are identified by permutation importance analysis based on our proposed model.

2   Method

2.1   Granular Label Distribution and Granular Feature Distribution

Conventional label distribution learning (LDL) assigns distribution for each label to measure the relative importance of different labels in describing an image. This causes great computational burden when the total number of labels is large (and day-to-day age prediction is such a problem). Since a brain MRI contributes to the neighboring labels analogously, it is unnecessary to define the contribution of the image on each label individually. Instead, we assemble the adjacent labels to a *granule* and define the contribution of the image to such a granule rather than many seemly independent labels, which is a good choice to solve the challenge of a large number of labels. Thus, by transforming the label set to granule set and assigning distributions on the granules, the label distribution is replaced by granular label distribution (as shown in Fig. 1(a)). Based on this strategy, the large number of labels involved in age learning is substantially reduced to a relatively small number of granules. As such, each granule has more corresponding data samples than a single label has, thus improves the effectiveness of learning as well.

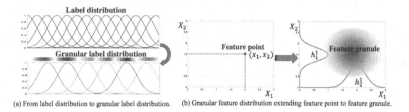

(a) From label distribution to granular label distribution.   (b) Granular feature distribution extending feature point to feature granule.

Fig. 1. Illustration of the granular label distribution and granular feature distribution.

The design of the granular label distribution is important for the whole model. Suppose *all the granules are disjoint intervals*, the distance from a granule to an age label is defined as the absolute difference between the midpoint of the granule and the age. Then, for a brain image x with the age a, the granular label distribution of x should be designed by satisfying the following requirement: the probability that a belongs to the granule decreases with the increase of the distance between a and the granule. A collection of adjacent Gaussian distributions centered at the midpoints of the granules is one of the possible choices satisfying the above requirement.

Except for granular label distribution, the information lying in the data could be further augmented by considering inter-subject and noise-caused variability existing in the brain image features. That is, a certain age can be associated with *not only* its own brain image *but also* many neighboring images with certain probabilities. To this end, we propose a new concept of granular feature distribution (GFD), which assigns distributions to the features on a granular scale. As shown in Fig. 1(b), the information lying in the point $x = (x_1, x_2)$ is augmented to a feature granule based on GFD. Starting from label learning (LL), the data transformation processes in LDL, granular label distribution learning (GLDL), and granular feature-label distribution learning (GFLDL) are illustrated in Fig. 2. Finally, our new model, *deep granular label feature distribution learning* (DGFLDL), is established by exploiting a deep neural network to approximate the granular label distribution and performing the infant age prediction based on the transformed data obtained from granular label distribution and granular feature distribution.

2.2   Problem Formulation

Let $X = \prod_{m=1}^{M} X_m$ denote a brain image feature space and $Y = \{y_1, y_2, \cdots, y_N\}$ denote a set of possible ages. The granular label space is defined as $Y^* = \{g_j = (\mu_j, \sigma_j),$

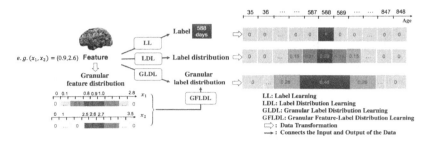

Fig. 2. An illustration of the data transformation in LL, LDL, GLDL, and GFLDL.

$j = 1, \cdots, c_Y\}$, $\mu_j \in Y$, $\sigma_j \in R$, $c_Y \ll N$. Each (μ_j, σ_j) represents a Gaussian distribution granule with mean μ_j and standard deviation σ_j. The granular feature space is defined as $X^* = \prod_{m=1}^{M} X_m^*$, where $X_m^* = \{h_m^i = (\varphi_m^i, \psi_m^i), i = 1, \cdots, c_X^m\}$, $\varphi_m^i \in X_m$, $\psi_m^i \in R$. Based on X^* and Y^*, the original training data $D = \{(x, a) | x \in X, a \in Y\}$ is transformed into a new data $D^* = \{(x^*, a^*) | x^* \in \prod_{m=1}^{M} [0, 1]^{c_X^m}, a^* \in [0, 1]^{c_Y}\}$, where $x^* = (P_{11}(x_1), \cdots, P_{1c_X^m}(x_1), \cdots, P_{M1}(x_M), \cdots, P_{Mc_X^M}(x_M))$, $\sum_{i=1}^{c_X^m} P_{mi}(x_m) = 1$, $a^* = (d_{g_1 x}, \cdots, d_{g_j x}, \cdots, d_{g_{c_Y} x})$, and $\sum_{j=1}^{c_Y} d_{g_j x} = 1$. $P_{mi}(x_m)$ is the probability that x_m belongs to the granule h_i^m, and $d_{g_j x}$ is the probability that a belongs to the granule g_j.

$$P_{mi}(x_m) = \frac{1}{\psi_m^i \sqrt{2\pi Z}} \exp\left(-\frac{(x_m - \varphi_m^i)^2}{2(\psi_m^i)^2}\right), Z = \frac{1}{\psi_m^i \sqrt{2\pi}} \sum_{i=1}^{c_X^m} \exp\left(-\frac{(x_m - \varphi_m^i)^2}{2(\psi_m^i)^2}\right) \quad (1)$$

$$d_{g_j x} = \frac{1}{\sigma_j \sqrt{2\pi V}} \exp\left(-\frac{(y - \mu_j)^2}{2\sigma_j^2}\right), V = \frac{1}{\sigma_j \sqrt{2\pi}} \sum_{j=1}^{c_Y} \exp\left(-\frac{(y - \mu_j)^2}{2\sigma_j^2}\right) \quad (2)$$

Then, the problem of granular feature-label distribution learning for infant age prediction can be formulated. Given a training set $S = \{(x_1, a_1), (x_2, a_2), \cdots, (x_K, a_K)\}$, where $x_k \in X$, $k = 1, \cdots, K$, represents the cortical feature vector of a brain MRI and $a_k \in Y$ is the chronological age of x_k. Based on granular feature space X^* and granular label space Y^*, S is transformed to $S^* = \{(x_1^*, a_1^*), (x_2^*, a_2^*), \cdots, (x_K^*, a_K^*)\}$. After learning a conditional probability mass function (p.m.f.) $P(g|x^*)$ from S^*, for $g \in Y^*$, the age could be estimated as

$$\hat{a} = E(g|x^*) = \sum_{j=1}^{c_Y} \frac{\mu_j P(g|x^*)}{\sum_{j=1}^{c_Y} P(g|x^*)} \quad (3)$$

Thus, DGFLDL aims to learn the parametric model $\hat{a} = f(x; \theta, W)$, where $\theta = (\mu, \sigma, \varphi, \psi)$ is the parameter vector in distributions defined by Eqs. 1 and 2, which corresponds to granular feature and label distributions; W is the parameter vector of a deep neural network (DNN), $P(g|x^*; W)$, which generates a mapping similar to S^*.

2.3   DGFLDL Model

Framework of DGFLDL is depicted in Fig. 3 and also detailed as follows.

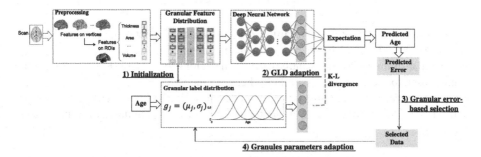

Fig. 3. The framework of our proposed DGFLDL method.

(1) Initialization: μ and φ are first initialized by the equal-distance partition of $\{X_m | m = 1, \cdots, M\}$ and Y, respectively. For each feature, ψ is designed as the standard deviation of its values on the training set. σ is designed as the same value (set as 20 in our experiment) for all granules of the label. To simplify the learning, only σ will be learned, while keeping μ, φ, and ψ fixed. Suppose $(\mu, \sigma_0, \varphi, \psi)$ are the predefined initial values, each training image x is transformed to its feature distribution x^* and associated with an initial label distribution a_0^*.

(2) GLD adaption: In the tth iteration, the target is to find W_t that can generate the granular label distribution most similar to a_{t-1}^*. As Kullback-Leibler (K-L) divergence is used to measure the dissimilarity between distributions, the best W_t is learned by solving the following minimization problem:

$$W_t = \operatorname{argmin}_W \sum\nolimits_{j=1}^{c_Y} P\big(g_j | x^*; W\big) \ln \frac{P\big(g_j | x^*; W\big)}{d_{g_j, x}^{t-1}} \tag{4}$$

(3) Granular error-based sample selection: After the GLD adaption, the conditional p.m.f. $P(g | x^*; W_t)$ is obtained. Thus, the age of each training image x can be estimated as the expectation of $P(g | x^*; W_t)$, i.e.,

$$\hat{a} = E(g | x^*) = \sum\nolimits_{j=1}^{c_Y} \frac{\mu_j P(g | x^*)}{\sum_{j=1}^{c_Y} P(g | x^*)} \tag{5}$$

A granular based mean absolute error strategy is designed to select images from the training set to fit the granule parameter vector σ. For each granule $g_j = (\mu_j, \sigma_j)$, the granule induced interval $\left[\alpha_j^-, \alpha_j^+\right]$ is obtained by the upper percentile of the corresponding Gaussian distribution, where $P\big(y \geq \alpha_j^-\big) = 1 - \beta, P\big(y \geq \alpha_j^+\big) = \beta$, β is a threshold and set as 0.05 in our experiment. In total, the selected images are

$$B = \cup_{j=1}^{c_Y} \left\{ (\boldsymbol{x}, a) \| a - \hat{a} | \leq \mathrm{MAE}_j, a \in \left[\alpha_j^-, \alpha_j^+ \right] \right\} \tag{6}$$

$$\mathrm{MAE}_j = \mathrm{mean} \left(|a - \hat{a}|, a \in \left[\alpha_j^-, \alpha_j^+ \right] \right) \tag{7}$$

(4) Granules parameters adaption: Based on the selected image set B, σ is learned to be the best parameter vector that can generate the granular label distribution most similar to the predicted granular label distributions in B. Here, K-L divergence is again chosen to measure the dissimilarity between the two distributions. Together with K-L divergence, the prediction loss is included to estimate the effectiveness of σ as well. These two losses are weighted-combined with a regularization parameter $0 \leq \lambda \leq 1$.

$$\sigma_t = \mathrm{argmin}_\sigma \left(\lambda \mathcal{L}_{Exp} + (1 - \lambda) \mathcal{L}_{KL} \right) \tag{8}$$

$$
\begin{aligned}
\mathcal{L}_{Exp} &= \sum_{x_b \in B} (a_b - \sum_{i=1}^{C} \frac{\mu_j d_{g_i, x_b}}{\sum_i d_{g_i, x_b}})^2, \\
\mathcal{L}_{KL} &= \sum_{x_b \in B} \sum_{j=1}^{c_Y} P(g_i | x_b; W_t) ln \frac{P(g_i | x_b; W_t)}{d_{g_j, x_b}}
\end{aligned}
\tag{9}
$$

Substituting Eq. 9 into Eq. 8 yields a nonlinear programming problem, which can be effectively solved by the sequential least squares programming method. W in the DNN and the parameters of feature-label distributions are optimized alternatively until the training error stop decreasing or the specified maximum number of epochs reaches.

Furthermore, the most contributive features in the age prediction model could be taken as the important infant brain development biomarkers, since they have high discriminative capability for age estimation. Based on the well-trained DGFLDL model, permutation importance was calculated for measuring the contribution of each feature for age prediction.

3   Experiments

We verified the effectiveness of our proposed DGFLDL method on the brain MRI based infant age prediction by using a high-quality dataset obtained from the UNC/UMN Baby Connectome Project [12]. In experiments, we used 185 subjects (97 females) with 384 longitudinal MRI scans acquired at different ages ranging from 35 to 848 days. All infant MR images were preprocessed by a well-established infant-specific computational pipeline [13]. Briefly, the pipeline includes intensity inhomogeneity correction, skull stripping, cerebellum removal, tissue segmentation, separation of left/right hemispheres, cortical topology correction, and inner and outer surface reconstruction. Since using the morphological features of each vertex for prediction is redundant and computationally expensive, a region-based analysis is used. Each individual cortical surface of each hemisphere was parcellated into 180 cortical regions of interest (ROIs) [9] by aligning onto the public 4D Infant Cortical Surface Atlas (https://www.nitrc.org/projects/infantsurfatlas/) [14]. With the ROIs on each surface of each hemisphere, 6 types of morphological features (i.e., sulcal depth measured with Euclidean distance (SDE), myelin content, local gyrification index (LGI), average convexity, mean curvature, and cortical thickness) were obtained by averaging the corresponding values of all vertices inside each ROI; and 2 types of features (i.e., surface area and cortical volume) were obtained by summing the corresponding values of all vertices inside each ROI. Therefore, for each scan, 2880 imaging features (8 feature types × 180 ROIs × 2 hemispheres) were acquired.

Four state-of-the-art regression methods for age prediction and 2 label distribution related methods are chosen as the baseline methods, which include support vector regression (SVR), Gaussian process regression (GPR), random forest (RF), deep neural network (DNN) applying to the original data, deep label distribution learning applying to the data with ordinary label distribution (DLDL), and deep granular label distribution applying to the data with our granular label distribution (DGLDL). These age prediction algorithms were assessed by 10 times of 10-fold cross validation with 3 criteria, i.e., the mean absolute error (MAE), the mean relative absolute error (MRAE), and the correlation value r between the predicted ages and the chronological ages. For r, the 95% confidence interval was computed by the 2.5 and 97.5 percentiles of the correlation values obtained from 1,000 bootstrap samples. During the cross-validation, for the longitudinal scans from the same subject, we guaranteed that the scans in the training data were scanned earlier than the scans in the testing data. The DNN employed in our DGLDL and DGFLDL model consists of 10 fully-connected layers with ReLU as the activation function of the first 9 layers and softmax as the activation function of the last layer.

The prediction results were presented in Table 1. Scatter plots of the predicted ages and the chronological ages are shown in Fig. 4, where r is the average of r_L and r_R. Our DGFLDL model outperformed the other 6 models and reduced the mean absolute error to 36.1 days. The correlation coefficient of the predicted ages and the chronological ages reached 0.963. These comparison results demonstrate that replacing label distribution learning (LDL) with the proposed granular label distribution method (GLDL) improved the prediction accuracy. In addition, when the granular feature distribution was adopted, the performance was further significantly improved.

Table 1. The comparison of the DGFLDL with SVR, GPR, RF, DNN, DLDL, and DGLDL. r_L and r_R are the left and right endpoints of the 95% confidence interval of r.

	MAE (days)	MRAE (%)	r_L	r_R
SVR	60.3 ± 3.5	23.6 ± 2.3	0.902 ± 0.005	0.928 ± 0.004
GPR	55.9 ± 2.8	18.5 ± 1.7	0.925 ± 0.007	0.949 ± 0.005
RF	65.3 ± 3.6	26.1 ± 2.1	0.872 ± 0.006	0.921 ± 0.004
DNN	66.1 ± 2.5	19.2 ± 1.5	0.889 ± 0.004	0.933 ± 0.002
DLDL	41.5 ± 2.7	12.2 ± 1.4	0.934 ± 0.004	0.966 ± 0.003
DGLDL (ours)	39.2 ± 2.6	11.9 ± 0.9	0.943 ± 0.005	0.971 ± 0.003
DGFLDL (ours)	$\mathbf{36.1 \pm 2.3}$	$\mathbf{11.1 \pm 0.5}$	$\mathbf{0.951 \pm 0.003}$	$\mathbf{0.976 \pm 0.002}$

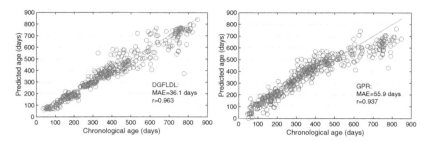

Fig. 4. Scatter plots of the chronological ages and predicted ages obtained by DGFLDL (our method) and GPR (one of the competing methods with the best performance).

The permutation importance of each feature type (or ROI) was obtained by summing the permutation importance of its corresponding 360 ROIs (or 8 features), respectively, as shown in Fig. 5. We found that cortical thickness, surface area, and cortical volume are the most important feature types in the prediction. This possibly results from the most dramatic development of these features in the first 2 years after birth. Furthermore, we revealed the top 5 important ROIs in age prediction, which includes the bilateral medial prefrontal cortex, left frontal opercular cortex, left posterior opercular cortex, and the left primary visual cortex.

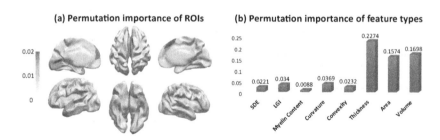

Fig. 5. The permutation importance of 360 ROIs and 8 feature types.

4   Conclusion

In this paper, we proposed deep granular feature-label distribution learning to address the insufficient data challenge of neuroimaging-based infant age prediction. Granular label distribution was introduced, which *not only* solved the problem of dramatically increased number of labels *but also* improved the learning efficiency. We further proposed granular feature-label distribution to realize *dual information augmentation* of the data, which utilizes the inter-subject and noise-caused variability of the brain images and has been validated as an effective method with high prediction accuracy. Moreover, the importance analysis of features based on our proposed model revealed the importance of cortical thickness in infant age prediction. Some brain regions were also identified as important infant brain development biomarkers. Our proposed

DFGLDL serves as a model for prediction with insufficient data and a potentially powerful method for studying normal and abnormal infant brain development.

Acknowledgments. This work was partially supported by NIH grants (MH107815, MH116225, and MH117943). This work also utilizes approaches developed by an NIH grant (1U01MH110274) and the efforts of the UNC/UMN Baby Connectome Project Consortium.

References

1. Cole, J.H., Franke, K.: Predicting age using neuroimaging: innovative brain ageing biomarkers. Trends Neurosci. **40**(12), 681–690 (2017)
2. Nenadic, I., Dietzek, M., Langbein, K., et al.: BrainAGE score indicates accelerated brain aging in schizophrenia, but not bipolar disorder. Psychiatry Res. Neuroimaging **266**, 86–89 (2017)
3. Jason, S., Christian, H.: Differences between chronological and brain age are related to education and self- reported physical activity. Neurobiol. Aging **40**, 138–144 (2016)
4. Toews, M., Wells, W.M., Zollei, L.: A feature-based developmental model of the infant brain in structural MRI. In: MICCAI 2012, vol. 15, no. 2, pp. 204–211(2012)
5. Gilmore, J.H., Kang, C., Evans, D.D., et al.: Prenatal and neonatal brain structure and white matter maturation in children at high risk for schizophrenia. Am. J. Psychiatry **167**, 1083–1091 (2010)
6. Liem, F., Varoquaux, G., Kynast, J., et al.: Predicting brain-age from multimodal imaging data captures cognitive impairment. Neuroimage **148**, 179–188 (2017)
7. Lewis, J.D., Evans, A.C., Tohka, J., Brain Development Cooperative Group: T1 white/gray contrast as a predictor of chronological age, and an index of cognitive performance. Neuroimage **173**, 341–350 (2018)
8. Antipov, G., Baccouche, M., Berrani, S.A., Dugelay, J.L.: Effective training of convolutional neural networks for face-based gender and age prediction. Pattern Recogn. **72**, 15–26 (2017)
9. Glasser, M., Coalson, T.S., Robinson, E.C., et al.: A multi-modal parcellation of human cerebral cortex. Nature **536**, 171–178 (2016)
10. Geng, X.: Label distribution learning. IEEE Trans. Knowl. Data Eng. **28**(7), 1734–1748 (2016)
11. Gao, B.B., Xing, C., Xie, C.W., Wu, J., Geng, X.: Deep label distribution learning with label ambiguity. IEEE Trans. Image Process. **26**(6), 2825–2838 (2017)
12. Brittany, R.H., Martin, A.S., Wei, G., et al.: The UNC/UMN baby connectome project (BCP): an overview of the study design and protocol development. Neuroimage **185**, 891–905 (2019)
13. Li, G., Wang, L., Yap, P.T., et al.: Computational neuroanatomy of baby brains: a review. Neuroimage **185**, 906–925 (2019)
14. Li, G., Wang, L., Shi, F., et al.: Construction of 4D high-definition cortical surface atlases of infants: Methods and applications. Med. Image Anal. **25**(1), 22–36 (2015)

End-to-End Dementia Status Prediction from Brain MRI Using Multi-task Weakly-Supervised Attention Network

Chunfeng Lian, Mingxia Liu[(✉)], Li Wang, and Dinggang Shen[(✉)]

Department of Radiology and BRIC, University of North Carolina at Chapel Hill,
Chapel Hill, NC 27599, USA
{mxliu,dgshen}@med.unc.edu

Abstract. Computer-aided prediction of dementia status (e.g., clinical scores of cognitive tests) from brain MRI is of great clinical value, as it can help assess pathological stage and predict disease progression. Existing learning-based approaches typically preselect dementia-sensitive regions from the whole-brain MRI for feature extraction and prediction model construction, which might be sub-optimal due to potential heterogeneities between different steps. Also, based on anatomical prior knowledge (e.g., brain atlas) and time-consuming nonlinear registration, these preselected brain regions are usually the same across all subjects, ignoring their *individual specificities* in dementia progression. In this paper, we propose a multi-task weakly-supervised attention network (MWAN) to jointly predict multiple clinical scores from the baseline MRI data, by explicitly considering individual specificities of different subjects. Leveraging a fully-trainable dementia attention block, our MWAN method can automatically identify subject-specific discriminative locations from the whole-brain MRI for end-to-end feature learning and multi-task regression. We evaluated our MWAN method by cross-validation on two public datasets (i.e., ADNI-1 and ADNI-2). Experimental results demonstrate that the proposed method performs well in both the tasks of clinical score prediction and weakly-supervised discriminative localization in brain MR images.

1 Introduction

As the most common cause of dementia, Alzheimer's disease (AD) is characterized by progressive and irreversible loss of intellectual skills [3]. In clinical practice, the dementia status can be comprehensively assessed by different cognitive tests, e.g., mini-mental state examination (MMSE), clinical dementia rating sum of boxes (CDRSB), and Alzheimer's disease assessment scale cognitive subscale (ADAS-Cog). Clinical scores of these cognitive tests have been proven to be reliably correlated with disease progression [7]. Therefore, automatically predicting these clinical scores is of great clinical value, which helps evaluate the stage of dementia pathology and forecast the disease progression.

© Springer Nature Switzerland AG 2019
D. Shen et al. (Eds.): MICCAI 2019, LNCS 11767, pp. 158–167, 2019.
https://doi.org/10.1007/978-3-030-32251-9_18

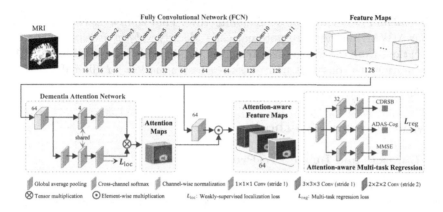

Fig. 1. Illustration of our multi-task weakly supervised attention network (MWAN).

Structural magnetic resonance imaging (MRI) is widely used in computer-aided diagnosis (CAD) of AD and mild cognitive impairment (MCI), due to its sensitivity to brain atrophy caused by dementia [2]. While diverse CAD methods have been proposed to identify categorical labels (e.g., AD/MCI) [4,8], there is relatively fewer studies on clinical score prediction, considering that regressing continuous variables is practically more challenging [6,9]. Several machine learning and deep learning techniques have been applied for clinical score prediction using brain MR images. Machine learning methods usually predefine dementia-sensitive locations (e.g., according to anatomical prior knowledge [13]) from the whole-brain MRI, and then extract hand-crafted features to construct regression models. Deep learning methods, e.g., with convolutional neural networks (CNNs) [5], typically combine feature extraction and model construction, potentially yielding better results due to task-oriented feature learning. However, most of the existing learning-based models require *preselecting dementia-sensitive locations* in MRI, since it is very challenging to directly capture subtle structural changes from the whole-brain image. This precondition may hamper the performance and efficiency of computer-aided clinical score prediction, mainly because 1) the isolated selection of dementia-sensitive brain locations might not be well coordinated with the latter stages of feature learning and model construction, and 2) this procedure usually relies on time-consuming non-linear registration in both training and test phases. Also, existing methods usually restrict all studied subjects to share exactly the same dementia-sensitive locations in brain MRIs, *ignoring individual variations* of different subjects in disease progression.

In this paper, we propose a multi-task weakly-supervised attention network (MWAN) to jointly predict multiple clinical scores from the baseline whole-brain MRI. Figure 1 shows a schematic diagram of our MWAN model, which consists of (1) a backbone fully convolutional network (FCN), (2) a trainable dementia attention block, and (3) an attention-aware multi-task regression block. Different from existing CAD methods for dementia diagnosis, our MWAN is an *end-to-end* and *fully-trainable* deep architecture. That is, in a task-oriented manner, our MWAN method can automatically identify *subject-specific* discriminative locations from the whole-brain image, and seamlessly learn high-level feature representations to construct multi-task regression models for clinical score prediction.

2   Materials and Method

2.1   Datasets and Image Pre-Processing

Two public datasets (i.e., ADNI-1 and ADNI-2 with 1,396 subjects in total) downloaded from Alzheimer's Disease Neuroimaging Initiative[1] were studied in this paper. For the independent test, subjects that appear in both ADNI-1 and ADNI-2 were removed from ADNI-2. The baseline ADNI-1 dataset consists of 1.5T T1-weighted MR images acquired from 797 subjects, including 226 normal control (NC), 225 stable MCI (sMCI), 165 progressive MCI (pMCI), and 181 AD subjects. The baseline ADNI-2 dataset contains 3T T1-weighted MR images acquired from 599 subjects, including 185 NC, 234 sMCI, 37 pMCI, and 143 AD subjects. The definition of pMCI/sMCI is based on whether MCI would convert to AD within 36 months after baseline evaluation. Each subject has baseline clinical scores for three cognitive tests, i.e., CDRSB, ADAS-Cog, and MMSE.

All brain MR images were processed following a standard pipeline, including anterior commissure (AC)-posterior commissure (PC) correction, intensity correction, skull stripping, and cerebellum removing. An affine registration was performed to linearly align all MRI data onto a template to remove global linear difference, and also to resample all imaging data to have the same spatial resolution (i.e., $1 \times 1 \times 1$ mm^3). Finally, all linearly-aligned brain MR images were cropped to have the identical size of $144 \times 184 \times 152$.

2.2   Multi-task Weakly-Supervised Attention Network

Backbone: As shown in Fig. 1, we employ a fully convolutional network (FCN) as the backbone to generate relatively high-dimensional feature maps that model global information of the whole-brain MRI. The backbone FCN in our current implementation contains eight $3 \times 3 \times 3$ convolutional (Conv) layers and three $2 \times 2 \times 2$ Conv layers, all with zero padding, followed by batch normalization (BN) and rectified linear unit (ReLU) activation. The numbers of channels for Conv1 to Conv11 are 16, 16, 16, 32, 32, 32, 64, 64, 64, 128, and 128, respectively. The stride for the $3 \times 3 \times 3$ kernels is set as 1, while the stride for the $2 \times 2 \times 2$ kernels is set as 2 to downsample feature maps and increase receptive fields. As a plug-in unit, this basic backbone in our MWAN model can be easily replaced by any other FCN architectures (e.g., by including residual or dense blocks).

---

[1]   http://adni.loni.usc.edu.

Weakly-Supervised Dementia Attention: It is worth noting that different cognitive tests actually evaluate the dementia status from complementarily different views. In addition, the respective clinical scores are intrinsically correlated with four categorical labels of dementia (i.e., NC, sMCI, pMCI, or AD), considering that they point to semantically similar targets [9]. Therefore, leveraging the image-wise categorical labels as weakly-supervised guidance, a *trainable* attention block is designed in our MWAN to automatically identify discriminative brain locations that are strongly relevant to *subject-specific* dementia status.

To this end, as the input to our dementia attention block, feature maps generated by the backbone FCN are first squeezed across channels by using an $1 \times 1 \times 1$ Conv layer. Denote the corresponding output as $\mathbf{F} = [\mathbf{F}_1, \ldots, \mathbf{F}_M]$, where $\mathbf{F}_m \in \mathbb{R}^{W \times H \times L}$ $(m = 1, \ldots, M)$ is the feature map (size: $W \times H \times L$) at the m-th channel and $M = 64$ is the number of channels. We then apply a global average pooling (GAP) layer on $\mathbf{F}$ to produce a holistic feature representation $\mathbf{f} \in \mathbb{R}^M$ capturing the semantic information of the whole-brain MRI. The feature representation $\mathbf{f}$ is further mapped by another $1 \times 1 \times 1$ Conv layer, followed by softmax normalization, onto the categorical label space (i.e., with $C = 4$ units). Inspired by [10,12], but operating distinctively in another fully-trainable way, we capitalize on the categorical label information to detect dementia-sensitive MRI locations. Specifically, in parallel with the mapping of $\mathbf{f}$, we also apply an $1 \times 1 \times 1$ Conv layer (with C channels) on $\mathbf{F}$, where the convolutional operations on $\mathbf{F}$ and $\mathbf{f}$ share the same set of learnable weights $\mathbf{w} = [\mathbf{w}_1, \ldots \mathbf{w}_C]$, with $\mathbf{w}_c \in \mathbb{R}^M$ $(c = 1, \ldots, C)$. Since the estimated score $\mathbf{s}_c = \text{ReLU}(\mathbf{w}_c^T \mathbf{f})$ explicitly indicates the individual score for the c-th categorical label, we can expect that

$$\mathbf{A}_c = \text{ReLU} \left(\sum\nolimits_{m=1}^{M} \mathbf{w}_{c,m} \mathbf{F}_m \right), \tag{1}$$

which describes the spatially-varying contributions of different regions in quantifying the score for the c-th categorical label ($\mathbf{A}_c \in \mathbb{R}^{W \times H \times L}$). After element-wisely normalizing $\mathbf{A} = [\mathbf{A}_1, \ldots, \mathbf{A}_C]$ for each channel, we finally aggregate the attention maps for different categorical labels as

$$\bar{\mathbf{A}} = \sum\nolimits_{c=1}^{C} \mathbf{s}_c \mathbf{A}_c. \tag{2}$$

Considering that such an attention block is jointly trained with other parts in our proposed MWAN model, the resulting $\bar{\mathbf{A}}$ can highlight discriminative brain regions that are strongly relevant to subject-specific dementia status.

Attention-Aware Multi-task Regression: With the subject-specific spatial attention map in (2), we further design a multi-task regression block to jointly predict multiple clinical scores (i.e., CDRSB, ADAS-Cog, and MMSE). To this end, feature maps generated by the backbone FCN are squeezed across channels via an $1 \times 1 \times 1$ Conv layer with $M = 64$ channels, which are then element-wisely weighted by $\bar{\mathbf{A}}$ across channels to enhance the influence of features extracted from discriminative brain locations (i.e., with large weights in $\bar{\mathbf{A}}$). A GAP operation is then performed on the spatially-weighted feature maps to yield an attention-aware holistic feature representation describing the semantic information of the whole-brain MRI. Finally, for each clinical score (or regression task), two successive fully-connected (FC) layers, with 32 and 1 unit(s), respectively, are applied on the attention-aware feature representation to predict its value. Notably, as a flexible module, the classification task (e.g., differentiation between NC, sMCI, pMCI, and AD) could also be potentially included here to provide auxiliary guidance for clinical score regression.

End-to-End Localization and Prediction: Let $\{(\mathbf{X}_n, \mathbf{y}_n, \mathbf{z}_n)\}_{n=1}^N$ be a training set containing N samples, where $\mathbf{X}_n$ is the n-th subject, $\mathbf{y}_n \in \{1, \ldots, C\}$ is the categorical label, and $\mathbf{z}_n = [\mathbf{z}_n^1, \ldots, \mathbf{z}_n^T]$ denotes T types of clinical scores. Our MWAN model performs end-to-end discriminative localization and clinical score prediction from the whole-brain MRI. It jointly optimizes the learnable parameters for the backbone FCN, the dementia attention block, and the attention-aware multi-task regression block, denoted as $\mathbf{W}^{\mathrm{fcn}}$, $\mathbf{W}^{\mathrm{loc}}$, and $\mathbf{W}^{\mathrm{reg}}$, respectively. As shown in Fig. 1, the loss functions $\mathfrak{L}$ to this end is the combination of the loss for weakly-supervised discriminative localization (i.e., $\mathfrak{L}_{loc}$) and the loss for multi-task regression (i.e., $\mathfrak{L}_{reg}$). Specifically, $\mathfrak{L}_{loc}$ is defined as

$$\mathfrak{L}_{loc} = -\frac{1}{N} \sum\nolimits_{n=1}^{N} \sum\nolimits_{c=1}^{C} \mathbf{1}\left(\mathbf{y}_n = c\right) \log\left(\mathbf{s}_c\left(\mathbf{X}_n | \mathbf{W}^{\mathrm{fcn}}, \mathbf{W}^{\mathrm{loc}}\right)\right), \quad (3)$$

where $\mathbf{1}(\cdot)$ is a binary indicator, and $\mathbf{s}_c\left(\mathbf{X}_n | \mathbf{W}^{\mathrm{fcn}}, \mathbf{W}^{\mathrm{loc}}\right)$ indicates the score for classifying $\mathbf{X}_n$ as the c-th category in terms of network parameters $\mathbf{W}^{\mathrm{fcn}}$ and $\mathbf{W}^{\mathrm{loc}}$. Besides, $\mathfrak{L}_{reg}$ is defined as

$$\mathfrak{L}_{reg} = \frac{1}{N} \sum\nolimits_{n=1}^{N} \left\| \mathbf{z}_n - \hat{\mathbf{z}}\left(\mathbf{X}_n | \mathbf{W}^{\mathrm{fcn}}, \mathbf{W}^{\mathrm{loc}}, \mathbf{W}^{\mathrm{reg}}\right) \right\|_2, \quad (4)$$

where $\hat{\mathbf{z}}\left(\mathbf{X}_n | \mathbf{W}^{\mathrm{fcn}}, \mathbf{W}^{\mathrm{loc}}, \mathbf{W}^{\mathrm{reg}}\right)$ denotes the predicted T clinical scores for $\mathbf{X}_n$ in terms of network parameters $\mathbf{W}^{\mathrm{fcn}}$, $\mathbf{W}^{\mathrm{loc}}$, and $\mathbf{W}^{\mathrm{reg}}$. We finally define $\mathfrak{L} = \alpha \mathfrak{L}_{loc} + \mathfrak{L}_{reg}$, where α (empirically set as 0.01 in this work) is a parameter to balance the contributions of the two terms. Based on (3) and (4), it is worth noting that, both the localization and regression losses will be back-propagated to optimize the backbone FCN, while the regression loss will also be merged into the dementia attention block to assist its training.

Implementation: Our MWAN model was implemented using Python based on Keras, trained with the Adam optimizer (mini-batch size: 2; dropout for Conv layers: 0.5). The input was the linearly-aligned MRI (size: $144 \times 184 \times 152$), and our network was constructed for end-to-end prediction of $T = 3$ clinical scores (i.e., CDRSB, ADAS-Cog, and MMSE). At the training stage, four ($C = 4$) categorical labels (i.e., NC, sMCI, pMCI, and AD) are used for weakly-supervised dementia attention detection. The training set was augmented online by randomly re-scaling brain MRIs in a tiny range and flipping them in the axial plane.

3 Experiments

Experimental Setup: We performed dataset-wise 2-fold cross-validation in the experiments. That is, we first trained a regression model on ADNI-1 and evaluated it on ADNI-2, and then trained another model on ADNI-2 and evaluated it on ADNI-1. As for the validation set at each iteration, we randomly selected 15% subjects from ADNI-1 and 10% subjects from ADNI-2, since ADNI-1 has more subjects than ADNI-2. The performance of score prediction was quantified by the correlation coefficient (CC) and the root mean square error (RMSE).

Table 1. Prediction results on *ADNI-2* obtained by models trained on ADNI-1.

Method	CDRSB		ADAS-Cog		MMSE	
	CC	RMSE	CC	RMSE	CC	RMSE
VBM	0.278	2.010	0.290	7.406	0.289	2.889
ROI	0.380	1.893	0.360	7.358	0.325	2.899
LBM	0.431	1.772	0.527	6.245	0.331	2.754
DM^{2}L	0.533	1.666	0.565	6.200	0.567	2.373
MTN	0.447	1.685	0.539	6.308	0.458	2.595
MWAN-S	0.616	1.589	0.631	5.874	0.603	2.263
MWAN (Ours)	**0.621**	**1.503**	**0.648**	**5.701**	**0.613**	**2.244**

We compared our MWAN method with 3 conventional methods using hand-crafted features, including (1) voxel-based morphometry (**VBM**) [1], (2) ROI-based pattern analysis (**ROI**), and (3) anatomical landmark-based morphometry (**LBM**) [11], as well as a deep learning method, i.e., (4) deep multi-task multi-channel learning (**DM^{2}L**) [5]. In VBM method, all brain MRIs were non-linearly aligned onto the anatomical automatic labeling (AAL) template, and then the voxel-wise gray matter (GM) tissue density was quantified as features. A feature selection operation using t-test was then performed to select informative features to train support vector regressors (SVRs) for clinical score prediction. In ROI method, the AAL template with 90 ROIs was non-linearly aligned onto each brain MRI. Then, the normalized GM volumes in the 90 ROIs were quantified as features to train SVRs for clinical score prediction. In LBM method, 50 anatomical landmarks [11] were used to locate 50 patches (size: $24 \times 24 \times 24$) from each brain MRI. Then, morphological features were extracted from these patches to train SVRs for clinical score prediction. In DM^{2}L method, the same set of patches used in LBM was used to construct a multi-task multi-branch CNN, where the identification of categorical labels was included as an auxiliary task to assist the prediction of clinical scores. Each patch was processed by a specific sub-network to learn patch-wise features, and then all patch-wise features were merged to learn higher-level feature for joint regression and classification.

To evaluate the contributions of two major components of our method (i.e., dementia attention and joint clinical score prediction), we compare MWAN with its two variants, called **MTN** and **MWAN-S**, respectively. In MTN, we removed the dementia block and trained the backbone FCN for joint clinical score prediction. In MWAN-S, we trained the weakly-supervised attention network to predict clinical scores independently. Note that three competing methods (i.e., VBM, ROI, and LBM) also construct individual SVRs to predict three types of clinical scores. To evaluate the effectiveness of the trainable dementia attention block in MWAN, we compared it with the offline method based on class activation map (**CAM**) [12]. Specifically, we built the CAM upon the backbone FCN to perform weakly-supervised discriminative localization after network training.

Prediction Results: The experimental results obtained by seven methods trained on ADNI-1 and tested on ADNI-2 (or trained on ADNI-2 and tested on ADNI-1) are summarized in Table 1 (or Table 2). From these tables, we at least have the following four observations. *First*, deep learning methods (i.e., DM^2L, MTN, MWAN-S, and MWAN) yield better results than conventional learning methods (i.e., VBM, ROI, and LBM) on both datasets, suggesting the effectiveness of task-oriented feature learning for regression model construction. *Second*, our MWAN and the state-of-the-art DM^2L methods perform better than MTL (i.e., a variant of MWAN without automated dementia attention). This implies that, without preselecting (in DM^2L) or automatically detecting (in our MWAN) discriminative brain regions, it is practically challenging to develop deep learning models with the whole-brain MRI for dementia diagnosis, considering that the early stage of dementia may only cause subtle structural changes. *Third*, MWAN consistently outperforms DM^2L on both datasets, which implies that performing task-oriented discriminative localization in an end-to-end framework is desired in the task of clinical score prediction. *Fourth*, MWAN is superior to its variant MWAN-S, which suggest that jointly predicting multiple clinical scores could provide complementary information to further improve the performance.

Table 2. Prediction results on *ADNI-1* obtained by models trained on ADNI-2.

Method	CDRSB		ADAS-Cog		MMSE	
	CC	RMSE	CC	RMSE	CC	RMSE
VBM	0.197	1.851	0.146	6.382	0.208	2.685
ROI	0.190	2.024	0.205	6.507	0.211	2.710
LBM	0.417	1.922	0.512	5.835	0.435	2.664
DM^2L	0.468	1.628	0.580	**5.426**	0.502	2.428
MTN	0.463	1.680	0.526	5.944	0.424	2.594
MWAN-S	0.512	1.639	0.556	5.593	0.488	2.503
MWAN (Ours)	**0.564**	**1.569**	**0.611**	5.525	**0.532**	**2.414**

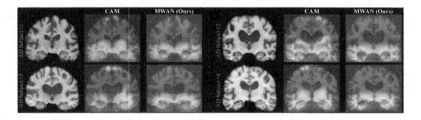

Fig. 2. Attention maps predicted by CAM [12] (with the backbone FCN) and our MWAN method, respectively, for four different AD subjects from ADNI-2.

Localization Results: In Fig. 2, we show the attention maps predicted by the offline CAM and our end-to-end MWAN models for 4 AD subjects from ADNI-2, with models trained on ADNI-1. From Fig. 2, we can see that the attention maps generated by our MWAN method are relatively more precise than those generated by CAM. For example, MWAN clearly highlights the regions of *hippocampus* and *amygdala*, and the discriminative capacity of these brain regions for dementia diagnosis has been validated in previous studies. In contrast, the attention maps generated by CAM contain more noise. These results imply that learning the dementia attention block in an end-to-end framework can more precisely localize discriminative brain regions for clinical score prediction.

In Fig. 3, we show four subjects with different categorical labels (i.e., NC, sMCI, pMCI, and AD) and their corresponding attention maps generated by our MWAN method. From Fig. 3, we can see that the attention map for the NC subject nearly highlights all spatial locations with heat values (i.e., red color), which implies that there is no clear difference between these locations in identifying NC subjects (i.e., no abnormalities). Along the progression from NC to AD, we can observe that the heat values (i.e., red color) in the attention maps are gradually decreased (i.e., changed to blue) at most brain locations, while they are eventually accumulated at the hippocampal regions. These results suggest that the attention maps generated by our MWAN method could also

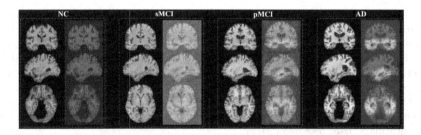

Fig. 3. Attention maps produced by our MWAN for MRIs with four different categorical labels (i.e., NC, sMCI, pMCI, and AD) shown in three views, respectively. (Color figure online)

provide additional information regarding the disease progression, by uncovering the potentially gradual atrophic process of the human brain due to dementia.

4   Conclusion

In this paper, we have proposed a multi-task weakly-supervised attention network to automatically identify dementia-sensitive brain locations from the whole-brain MR images for end-to-end prediction of multiple clinical scores. Experimental results on two public datasets have demonstrated the effectiveness of our method in both automated discriminative localization and clinical score prediction. As the future work, we will extend our current model to jointly predict longitudinal clinical scores for dementia prognosis. In addition, considering that our current dementia attention block works on downsampled FCN feature maps, further improving it for discriminative localization at higher resolution could also be an interesting and promising direction.

Acknowledgements. This work was supported in part by NIH grants (EB008374, AG041721, AG042599, and EB022880).

References

1. Baron, J., et al.: In vivo mapping of gray matter loss with voxel-based morphometry in mild Alzheimer's disease. NeuroImage **14**(2), 298–309 (2001)
2. Frisoni, G.B., et al.: The clinical use of structural MRI in Alzheimer disease. Nat. Rev. Neurol. **6**(2), 67 (2010)
3. Jagust, W.: Vulnerable neural systems and the borderland of brain aging and neurodegeneration. Neuron **77**(2), 219–234 (2013)
4. Lian, C., et al.: Hierarchical fully convolutional network for joint atrophy localization and Alzheimer's disease diagnosis using structural MRI. IEEE Trans. Pattern Anal. Mach. Intell. (2019, in press). https://doi.org/10.1109/TPAMI.2018.2889096
5. Liu, M., et al.: Joint classification and regression via deep multi-taskmulti-channel learning for Alzheimer's disease diagnosis. IEEE Trans. Biomed. Eng. **66**, 1195–1206 (2018)
6. Liu, M., et al.: Weakly supervised deep learning for brain disease prognosis using MRI and incomplete clinical scores. IEEE Trans. Cybern. (2019, in press). https://doi.org/10.1109/TCYB.2019.2904186
7. O'Bryant, S.E., et al.: Staging dementia using clinical dementia rating scale sum of boxes scores: a Texas Alzheimer's research consortium study. Arch. Neurol. **65**(8), 1091–1095 (2008)
8. Rathore, S., et al.: A review on neuroimaging-based classification studies and associated feature extraction methods for Alzheimer's disease and its prodromal stages. NeuroImage **155**, 530–548 (2017)
9. Sabuncu, M.R., et al.: Clinical prediction from structural brain MRI scans: a large-scale empirical study. Neuroinformatics **13**(1), 31–46 (2015)
10. Yang, J., et al.: Weakly supervised coupled networks for visual sentiment analysis. In: CVPR, pp. 7584–7592 (2018)

11. Zhang, J., et al.: Detecting anatomical landmarks for fast Alzheimer's disease diagnosis. IEEE Trans. Med. Imaging **35**(12), 2524–2533 (2016)
12. Zhou, B., et al.: Learning deep features for discriminative localization. In: CVPR, pp. 2921–2929. IEEE (2016)
13. Zhou, J., et al.: Modeling disease progression via multi-task learning. NeuroImage **78**, 233–248 (2013)

Unified Modeling of Imputation, Forecasting, and Prediction for AD Progression

Wonsik Jung[1], Ahmad Wisnu Mulyadi[1], and Heung-Il Suk[1,2(✉)]

[1] Department of Brain and Cognitive Engineering, Korea University,
Seoul, Republic of Korea
{ssikjeong1,wisnumulyadi,hisuk}@korea.ac.kr
[2] Department of Artificial Intelligence, Korea University,
Seoul, Republic of Korea

Abstract. In this paper, we propose a novel deep recurrent neural network as an Alzheimer's Disease (AD) progression model, capable of jointly conducting tasks of missing values imputation, phenotypic measurements forecast, and clinical state prediction of a subject based on his/her longitudinal imaging biomarkers. Unlike the existing methods that mostly ignore missing values or impute them by means of an independent statistical model before training a disease progression model, we devise a unified recurrent network architecture for jointly performing missing values imputation, biomarker values forecast, and clinical state prediction from the longitudinal data. For these tasks to be handled in a unified framework, we also define an objective function that can be efficiently optimized by means of stochastic gradient descent in an end-to-end manner. We validated the effectiveness of our proposed method by comparing with the comparative methods over the TADPOLE challenge cohort.

Keywords: Disease Progression Modeling · Alzheimer's Disease · Deep learning · Recurrent neural networks · Missing value imputation · Longitudinal data · Mild Cognitive Impairment

1 Introduction

Alzheimer's Disease (AD) is a progressive neurodegenerative disease with no pharmaceutical treatments available yet [10]. However, since some treatments, when applied at the early stage of the AD spectrum, are possibly effective to delay its symptomatic developments, *e.g.*, memory loss, it has been of great importance to monitor the progression over time. Researchers and clinicians use different types of potential biomarkers including volumetric information measurable in Magnetic Resonance Image (MRI) for monitoring.

With recent advances in machine learning, especially deep learning, data-driven Disease Progression Modeling (DPM) has emerged as one of the major tools for AD prognosis in the field. The main tasks in AD progression modeling

© Springer Nature Switzerland AG 2019
D. Shen et al. (Eds.): MICCAI 2019, LNCS 11767, pp. 168–176, 2019.
https://doi.org/10.1007/978-3-030-32251-9_19

are to predict the changes of measurable imaging biomarkers and to make a prognosis for the stages, *i.e.*, Cognitively Normal (CN), Mild Cognitive Impairment (MCI), and dementia. From a methodological development point of view, it is very challenging to learn a robust DPM for AD from the longitudinal imaging measurements due to many missing values in data and arbitrary missing data patterns. With regard to handling missing values in machine learning, the previous methods used a masking trick such that the missing values are either ignored during training or imputed the missing values by means of statistics [1,5,7].

For example, Jarret *et al.* devised a Convolutional Neural Network (CNN), where the longitudinal data were processed by temporal convolutions with a mask matrix of indicating missingness, to capture heterogeneous feature representations among observed covariates [7]. Moore *et al.* summarized the time series historical vectors and then predicted the progression of AD with a random forest classifier over the 'complete' observations by exploiting the relationship between pairs of data at different time points [11]. Ghazi *et al.* formulated the task of predicting AD progression in a sequence-to-sequence framework and used a Recurrent Neural Network (RNN) with Long-Short Term Memory (LSTM) cells. In training their LSTM-RNN, they simply imputed zeros to all missing values [5]. That is, by imputing with zeros, their method simply tried to ignore the respective values in learning model parameters and forecasting biomarker values. As for the AD prognosis, a separate classifier with Linear Discriminant Analysis (LDA) was trained based on the predicted imaging biomarker values.

To our best knowledge, many of the previous studies on DPM tried to build their models by either ignoring missing values or imputing those by means of statistical techniques. Further, when involving an imputation step in their framework, the predictive model was independent to an imputation model. In this work, we hypothesize that (1) it is helpful to use imputed values in training deep models rather than ignoring them; (2) it is beneficial for imputation to exploit the temporal and multivariate relations among variables jointly; (3) it is optimal to build a single model that can impute missing values and also conduct the target tasks of forecasting future values of biomarkers and predicting a clinical state. To this end, we propose a novel deep recurrent network that jointly handles the above-mentioned hypotheses in a unified framework. Further, all the network parameters are trained in an end-to-end manner with a well-designed objective function. As we based our model on Ghazi *et al.*'s work that considered both progressive prediction and identification from longitudinal data, in our experiment, we validated the effectiveness of our proposed method by comparing with their work over the TADPOLE challenge cohort.

2   Dataset and Preprocessing

The Alzheimer's Disease Prediction Of Longitudinal Evolution (TADPOLE)[1] is the Alzheimer's Disease Neuroimaging Initiative (ADNI) cohort as longitudinal dataset containing 1,500 biomarkers from 1,737 patients with 12,741 visits at

---

[1] https://tadpole.grand-challenge.org/Data/.

Table 1. Demographic of the TADPOLE dataset. Note that the number of subjects was measured at the baseline time point.

Clinical stage	# of subjects	# of visits		Age	
		Male	Female	Male	Female
Cognitively Normal	633	1,356	1,389	76.67 ± 6.44	75.85 ± 6.28
Mild Cognitive Impairment	869	2,454	1,604	75.59 ± 7.47	73.87 ± 8.09
Alzheimer's Disease	235	1,208	900	77.22 ± 7.11	75.45 ± 7.92
All	1,737	12,741		76.00 ± 7.38	

22 different time points in total [5,10]. From the total visits, we obtained the disease-stage labeled samples with 21.52% as CN, 31.85% as MCI, and 16.55% as AD. Table 1 summarized the demographic information [10].

Although TADPOLE basically offers numerous useful biomarkers to forecast the AD stages [10], in this paper, we utilize the MR features including volumes of ventricles, hippocampus, fusiform gyrus, middle temporal gyrus, entorhinal cortex, and whole brain as employed in [5,8]. Regarding the clinical status, we categorized into three groups as CN (CN, SMC (Significant Memory Concern), and normal), MCI (early and late MCI), and AD (AD and dementia) similar to the previous work. As for the subjects converting from MCI to AD, the status was labeled as AD. As our main objective in this work is to predict the yearly progression, we considered 11 regular visits out of 22 total visits. Subjects with no visit on the baseline or having less than 3 visits were filtered out, resulting in 773 subjects in total. Normalization was conducted by using their respective Intra-Cranial Volume (ICV) because of the inter-subject variability in brain size and volume [4,5]. Additionally, we adopted feature-wise linear normalization based on their min-max values to be in the range of $[-1, 1]$.

3   Proposed Method

Given a training set of $\left\{ \mathbf{X}^{(n)}, \mathbf{Y}^{(n)} \right\}_{n=1}^{N}$, where $\mathbf{X}^{(n)} = \left[\mathbf{x}_1^{(n)}, \ldots, \mathbf{x}_t^{(n)}, \ldots, \mathbf{x}_T^{(n)} \right]$ is a T-length sequence of observable variables $\mathbf{x}_t^{(n)} \in \mathbb{R}^D$ of a subject n, $\mathbf{Y}^{(n)} = \left[\mathbf{y}_1^{(n)}, \ldots, \mathbf{y}_t^{(n)}, \ldots, \mathbf{y}_T^{(n)} \right]$ is the corresponding clinical label $\mathbf{y}_t^{(n)} \in \{0,1\}^K$ sequence, with D, K, and N denotes the number of features, classes, and subjects, respectively. We aim to tackle two tasks of predicting the future MR features and identifying a clinical status jointly in an RNN with LSTM by efficiently estimating and imputing missing values. The overall network architecture at one time point is illustrated in Fig. 1.

Hereafter, we omit the superscript (n) for uncluttered. As there are missing values in either MR features $\mathbf{x}_t$ or clinical labels $\mathbf{y}_t$, we define two auxiliary variables $\mathbf{M_x} \in \{0,1\}^{D \times T}$ and $\mathbf{m_y} \in \{0,1\}^T$ to indicate missingness of the respective variables as follows:

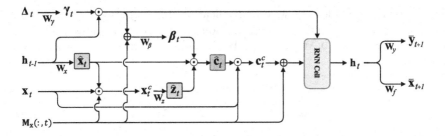

Fig. 1. Operations to impute missing values of the current input, forecast the biomarker values and to predict the clinical state at the next time point.

$$M_\mathbf{x}(d,t) = \begin{cases} 1 & \text{if } x_t^d \text{ is observed} \\ 0 & \text{otherwise} \end{cases}, \quad m_\mathbf{y}(t) = \begin{cases} 1 & \text{if } \mathbf{y}_t \text{ is observed} \\ 0 & \text{otherwise.} \end{cases}$$

We further utilize time delay information indicating the last observed variables in time. The larger the time delay is, the less amount of information should be utilized. We define this time delay variable $\mathbf{\Delta} \in \mathbb{R}^{D \times T}$ as follows:

$$\Delta(d,t) = \begin{cases} \mathbf{s}(t) - \mathbf{s}(t-1) + \Delta(d, t-1) & \text{if } t > 1, M_\mathbf{x}(d, t-1) = 0, \\ \mathbf{s}(t) - \mathbf{s}(t-1) & \text{if } t > 1, M_\mathbf{x}(d, t-1) = 1, \\ 0 & \text{if } t = 1 \end{cases}$$

where $\mathbf{s} \in \mathbb{R}^T$ records the time of visits.

3.1   Missing Value Imputation

We describe our method of imputing missing values by jointly utilizing temporal and multivariate relations by adopting Cao *et al.*'s work [2]. Provided a sequence of observations up to time $t - 1$, the hidden units represent compressed information, based on which we predict the MR features of the next time step. Given the hidden state $\mathbf{h}_{t-1}$ from a recurrent network at time step t, we first estimate MR features $\hat{\mathbf{x}}_t$ by utilizing only the temporally compressed information for all the previous time points, *i.e.*, temporal relations:

$$\hat{\mathbf{x}}_t = \mathbf{W}_x \mathbf{h}_{t-1} + \mathbf{b}_x. \tag{1}$$

Then, we get a complement vector $\mathbf{x}_t^c$ by replacing the missing values on the MR features observed at time t with the estimated values:

$$\mathbf{x}_t^c = \mathbf{M}_\mathbf{x}(:, t) \odot \mathbf{x}_t + (\mathbf{1} - \mathbf{M}_\mathbf{x}(:, t)) \odot \hat{\mathbf{x}}_t \tag{2}$$

where $\odot$ denotes an element-wise multiplication. In temporal relation, we basically further use the time delay information in $\mathbf{\Delta}(:, t)$ by defining a decay factor $\boldsymbol{\gamma}_t = \exp\{-\max(0, \mathbf{W}_\gamma \mathbf{\Delta}(:, t) + \mathbf{b}_\gamma)\}$. Then we introduce two auxiliary variables

$$\hat{\mathbf{z}}_t = \mathbf{W}_z \mathbf{x}_t^c + \mathbf{b}_z \tag{3}$$

$$\boldsymbol{\beta}_t = \mathbf{W}_\beta [\boldsymbol{\gamma}_t \oplus \mathbf{M}_\mathbf{x}(:, t)] + \mathbf{b}_\beta \tag{4}$$

where $\hat{\mathbf{z}}_t$ denotes the latent representation of the observed and estimated values in $\mathbf{x}_t^c$, $\boldsymbol{\beta}_t$ carries integrated information of the temporal decaying factors and the missing patterns at the current time step, and $\oplus$ is a concatenation operator. These two auxiliary variables are further exploited to better estimate the missing values via an interpolation between $\hat{\mathbf{x}}_t$ and $\hat{\mathbf{z}}_t$ with $\boldsymbol{\beta}_t$ as coefficients as follows:

$$\hat{\mathbf{c}}_t = \boldsymbol{\beta}_t \odot \hat{\mathbf{z}}_t + (1 - \boldsymbol{\beta}_t) \odot \hat{\mathbf{x}}_t \tag{5}$$

which combines the one vector estimated via temporal relations and the other vector computed by multiple variable relations. Lastly, we obtain a 'complete' observation by replacing the missing values with the estimated ones

$$\mathbf{c}_t^c = \mathbf{M}_\mathbf{x}(:, t) \odot \mathbf{x}_t + (1 - \mathbf{M}_\mathbf{x}(:, t)) \odot \hat{\mathbf{c}}_t. \tag{6}$$

3.2 Recurrent Computation

After imputing missing values as in Eq. (6), we get the complete vector $\mathbf{c}_t^c$ to be fed into RNN cells along with the corresponding mask vector $\mathbf{M}_\mathbf{x}(:, t)$ in the form of $[\mathbf{c}_t^c \oplus \mathbf{M}_\mathbf{x}(:, t)]$ and update the hidden state at the current time point as follows:

$$\mathbf{h}_t = \tanh(\mathbf{W}_h [\mathbf{h}_{t-1} \odot \boldsymbol{\gamma}_t] + \mathbf{U}_h [\mathbf{c}_t^c \oplus \mathbf{M}_\mathbf{x}(:, t)] + \mathbf{b}_h) \tag{7}$$

where $[\mathbf{h}_{t-1} \odot \boldsymbol{\gamma}_t]$ reflects the temporal decaying of the previous hidden state being aware of the time delay for different variables. As for the RNN cells, basically different forms of vanilla RNN, LSTM, or Gated Recurrent Unit (GRU) cells can be applied but in this work, we use LSTM cells. While we use the typical operations for various gates in an LSTM, as we consider the tasks of forecasting biomarker values and predicting the clinical state of a subject jointly, we devise the output operations as follows:

$$\bar{\mathbf{y}}_{t+1} = \mathrm{softmax}(\mathbf{W}_y \mathbf{h}_t + \mathbf{b}_y) \tag{8}$$

$$\bar{\mathbf{x}}_{t+1} = \mathbf{W}_f \mathbf{h}_t + \mathbf{b}_f. \tag{9}$$

3.3 Loss Function

In order to learn the network parameters[2], we define an imputation loss, a forecasting loss, and a prognosis loss. First, for the imputation loss, we measure the

---

[2] $\{\mathbf{W}_x, \mathbf{b}_x, \mathbf{W}_\gamma, \mathbf{b}_\gamma, \mathbf{W}_z \mathbf{b}_z, \mathbf{W}_\beta, \mathbf{b}_\beta, \mathbf{W}_h, \mathbf{U}_h, \mathbf{b}_h, \mathbf{W}_y, \mathbf{b}_y, \mathbf{W}_f, \mathbf{b}_f\}$.

similarity of the estimated vectors in different perspectives of Eqs. (1), (3) and (5) with the original vector

$$\mathcal{L}_{\text{imputation}} = \sum_{t=1}^{T} \mathcal{L}_{\text{reg}}(\mathbf{x}_t, \hat{\mathbf{x}}_t) + \mathcal{L}_{\text{reg}}(\mathbf{x}_t, \hat{\mathbf{z}}_t) + \mathcal{L}_{\text{reg}}(\mathbf{x}_t, \hat{\mathbf{c}}_t) \qquad (10)$$

where $\mathcal{L}_{\text{reg}}(\cdot, \cdot)$ is defined as Mean Absolute Error (MAE). Second, the loss for forecasting future features is defined by comparing with the observed values marked with a masking vector as follows:

$$\mathcal{L}_{\text{forecast}} = \sum_{t=1}^{T} \mathcal{L}_{\text{reg}}(\mathbf{x}_{t+1} \odot \mathbf{M_x}(:, t+1) , \ \bar{\mathbf{x}}_{t+1} \odot \mathbf{M_x}(:, t+1)). \qquad (11)$$

Lastly, regarding the task of clinical state prognosis, we use a cross-entropy loss but if and only if the target label is available

$$\mathcal{L}_{\text{prognosis}} = -\sum_{t=1}^{T} m_{\mathbf{y}}(t) \left[\sum_{k=1}^{K} y_t(k) \log(\bar{y}_t(k)) \right]. \qquad (12)$$

By integrating these three losses with hyperparameters of $\alpha, \lambda,$ and ξ, we define our full loss as follows:

$$\mathcal{L}_{\text{total}} = \alpha \mathcal{L}_{\text{imputation}} + \lambda \mathcal{L}_{\text{forecast}} + \xi \mathcal{L}_{\text{prognosis}} \qquad (13)$$

and train all the parameters jointly via stochastic gradient descent in an end-to-end manner.

4   Experimental Settings and Results

4.1   Experimental Settings

For performance evaluation, we used a stratified five-fold cross-validation, where one fold for validating, another one for testing and the remaining folds for training. We evaluated the performance in terms of MAE for regression and multi-class AUC (mAUC) [6] for classification tasks, respectively. Before we calculate the MAE, we normalized the range of both original and estimated features using the minimum and maximum values of original features. As for classification, we considered two scenarios: (i) training an independent LDA classifier (Single-Task) and (ii) jointly training a classifier in our framework (Multi-Task). In order to confirm the robustness of our proposed model, we considered three comparative methods, namely, Ghazi *et al.*'s model [5], mean (M+L) [3], and forward imputation combined with an RNN-LSTM (F+L) [9]. As for a network architecture, we used a single layer LSTM with 64 hidden units. We trained the model using Adam optimizer with a learning rate of 10^{-3}, a mini-batch size of 64, and an epoch of 2000. In addition, to avoid overfitting and to make the training curve converge considerably, we applied an l_2-regularization by setting

Table 2. Model performance in terms of MAE on regression task. Note that the original values were multiplied by 10^3 to get these reported values, and the best performance is in **bold**. (M/F: Mean/Forward imputation, L: vanilla LSTM)

Features	Competing methods			Ours	
	Ghazi *et al.* [5]	M+L [3]	F+L [9]	Single-Task	Multi-Task
Ventricles	2.266 ± 0.209	6.110 ± 1.199	5.505 ± 0.914	**1.227 ± 0.155**	1.381 ± 0.201
Hippocampus	0.229 ± 0.014	1.290 ± 0.087	1.309 ± 0.069	**0.141 ± 0.010**	0.148 ± 0.011
Entorhinal	0.195 ± 0.022	1.056 ± 0.045	1.108 ± 0.072	**0.187 ± 0.027**	0.194 ± 0.030
Fusiform	0.440 ± 0.044	2.435 ± 0.104	2.517 ± 0.315	**0.387 ± 0.049**	0.416 ± 0.049
MidTemp	0.490 ± 0.062	2.529 ± 0.152	2.646 ± 0.289	**0.424 ± 0.059**	0.449 ± 0.065
Whole Brain	12.788 ± 3.152	13.081 ± 3.636	10.186 ± 2.971	**9.415 ± 1.735**	9.857 ± 1.882

Table 3. Clinical state classification performance (AUC/mAUC). Note that the best performance for the entire method in **bold**. (M/F: Mean/Forward imputation, L: vanilla LSTM)

Tasks	Competing methods			Ours	
	Ghazi *et al.* [5]	M+L [3]	F+L [9]	Single-Task	Multi-Task
CN vs. MCI	0.669 ± 0.064	0.567 ± 0.040	0.531 ± 0.035	**0.672 ± 0.060**	–
CN vs. AD	0.899 ± 0.051	0.730 ± 0.033	0.724 ± 0.090	**0.902 ± 0.052**	–
MCI vs. AD	0.776 ± 0.046	0.680 ± 0.071	0.712 ± 0.059	**0.785 ± 0.055**	–
CN vs. MCI vs. AD	0.740 ± 0.011	0.644 ± 0.031	0.638 ± 0.043	**0.744 ± 0.021**	0.721 ± 0.034

the corresponding hyperparameter to 10^{-4}. To solve the convergence problem, we applied the weight of the loss function using α of 0.3, λ of 0.3, and ξ of 1.0. For network optimization, we choose parameters that yield the highest mAUC based on the validation set. We implement all of the LSTM-based models with PyTorch, a commonly used package for deep learning. All models are trained with GPU GTX 1080 TI.

4.2   Experimental Results

Regression. To forecast the future features estimated from imputation methods, we evaluate the difference between the estimated features and the ground truth features of the next time step using MAE. As shown in Table 2, we compared our model performance of regression with other competing methods. For all the features, our proposed method significantly outperformed all the competing methods in a single task. Also, we observed that the multi-task MAE score is worse than that of single task with a small margin in all feature types, but still better than other competing methods.

Classification. The other objective of the framework is to assess its classification performance of the clinical state. We set up the multi-class classification using a one-vs-one manner with CN vs. MCI, CN vs. AD, and MCI vs. AD. Furthermore, we classified three classes altogether, CN vs. MCI vs. AD.

We reported the classification results in Table 3. In the case of a single task, our proposed method is higher than the others in most cases. The imputation method that considered both temporal and correlated features at each time step indeed affected a positive role to classification. However, in multi-task for multi-class classification (CN vs. MCI vs. AD), Ghazi et al. [5] shows slightly better performance.

5   Conclusion

In this paper, we proposed a unified framework that jointly tackled the missing values imputation, phenotypic measurements forecast and clinical state prediction for AD progression. The temporal and multivariate relations of observations were effectively exploited to impute missing values. Also, the overall network structures were trained in an end-to-end manner. We evaluated two scenarios, which were single-task and multi-task, using the TADPOLE challenge cohort and observed that the proposed framework resulted in better performance in terms of forecasting the future biomarker values and predicting the AD progression stages than other competing methods in a single task.

Acknowledgement. This work was supported by Institute for Information & communications Technology Planning & Evaluation (IITP) grant funded by the Korea government (MSIT) (No. 2017-0-01779, A machine learning and statistical inference framework for explainable artificial intelligence). According to ADNI's data use agreement (https://ida.loni.usc.edu/collaboration/access/appLicense.jsp).

References

1. Albright, J.: Forecasting the Progression of Alzheimer's Disease using Neural Networks and a Novel Pre-Processing Algorithm. arXiv preprint arXiv:1903.07510 (2019)
2. Cao, W., Wang, D., Li, J., Zhou, H., Li, L., Li, Y.: BRITS: bidirectional recurrent imputation for time series. Adv. Neural Inf. Process. Syst. **31**, 6775–6785 (2018)
3. Che, Z., Purushotham, S., Cho, K., Sontag, D., Liu, Y.: Recurrent neural networks for multivariate time series with missing values. Sci. Rep. **8**, 6085 (2018)
4. Davis, W.: A new method for measuring cranial cavity volume and its ppplication to the assessment of cerebral atrophy at autopsy. Neuropathol. Appl. Neurobiol. **3**(5), 341–358 (1977)
5. Ghazi, M.M., et al.: Training recurrent neural networks robust to incomplete data: application to Alzheimer's disease progression modeling. Med. Image Anal. **53**, 39–46 (2019)
6. Hand, D.J., Till, R.J.: A simple generalisation of the area under the ROC curve for multiple class classification problems. Mach. Learn. **45**(2), 171–186 (2001)
7. Jarrett, D., Yoon, J., van der Schaar, M.: MATCH-Net: dynamic prediction in survival analysis using convolutional neural networks. In: Machine Learning for Health (ML4H) Workshop, Neural Information Processing Systems, vol. 31 (2018)
8. Li, K., Chan, W., Doody, R.S., Quinn, J., Luo, S.: Prediction of conversion to Alzheimer's disease with longitudinal measures and time-to-event data. J. Alzheimer's Dis. **58**(2), 361–371 (2017)

9. Lipton, Z.C., Kale, D.C., Wetzel, R.: Modeling missing data in clinical time series with RNNs. In: Proceedings of Machine Learning for Healthcare, vol. 56 (2016)
10. Marinescu, R.V., et al.: TADPOLE Challenge: Prediction of Longitudinal Evolution in Alzheimer's Disease. arXiv preprint arXiv:1805.03909 (2018)
11. Moore, P.J., Lyons, T.J., Gallacher, J.: Random forest prediction of Alzheimer's disease using pairwise selection from time series data. PLoS ONE **14**(2), e0211558 (2019)

LSTM Network for Prediction of Hemorrhagic Transformation in Acute Stroke

Yannan Yu[1], Bhargav Parsi[2], William Speier[3], Corey Arnold[3], Min Lou[4], and Fabien Scalzo[2(✉)]

[1] Department of Radiology, Stanford University, Stanford, CA 94305, USA
[2] Department of Neurology, UCLA, Los Angeles, CA 90095, USA
fab@cs.ucla.edu
[3] Department of Radiology, UCLA, Los Angeles, CA 90095, USA
[4] Second Affiliated Hospital, Zhejiang University, Hangzhou, Zhejiang, China

Abstract. Hemorrhagic transformation (HT) is one of the most devastating complications of reperfusion therapy in acute ischemic stroke. Prediction of an upcoming HT remains beyond current techniques in routine clinical practice. If made available, such information would benefit the management of acute ischemic stroke patients and help to tailor therapeutic strategies. This study aims at providing a machine learning framework for predicting occurrence and extent of HT from source perfusion-weighted magnetic resonance imaging (PWI) combined with diffusion weighted imaging (DWI). The model relies on a LSTM network based on PWI combined with DWI imaging features into a fully connected neural network. A retrospective comparative analysis performed on 155 acute stroke patients demonstrate the efficacy of the LSTM model (AUC-ROC: 89.4%) against state-of-the-art machine learning models. Predicted likelihood of HT at the voxel level was evaluated against HT annotations of stroke neurologists obtained from follow-up gradient recalled echo (GRE) imaging.

1 Introduction

Acute ischemic stroke (AIS) has a lifetime risk of 25% worldwide. It is often associated with significant disability, including motor and cognitive deterioration. Recent advances in treatment of acute stroke have demonstrated that reperfusion therapy, which dissolves or mechanically retrieves the clot, can significantly improve the outcome of the patients [14]. However, reperfusion therapy is also associated with complications; the most critical of which being intracerebral bleeding, also referred to as hemorrhagic transformation (HT). The risks of HT are particularly challenging to be assessed prior to reperfusion therapy. As HT may occur in eloquent brain areas, the consequences of HT have been shown to be associated with deteriorating symptoms, delayed neurological improvement, and poor outcome. The development of a computational model that could predict the occurrence and spatial extent of an upcoming HT before the reperfusion

© Springer Nature Switzerland AG 2019
D. Shen et al. (Eds.): MICCAI 2019, LNCS 11767, pp. 177–185, 2019.
https://doi.org/10.1007/978-3-030-32251-9_20

therapy would be very useful to refine eligibility criteria for reperfusion therapy. In this study, we introduce and evaluate a computational model based on a Long Short-Term Memory (LSTM) network that uses source perfusion-weighted magnetic resonance imaging (PWI) (i.e. after reconstruction from k-space but before feature extraction).

PWI imaging of the brain is obtained via a series of T2*-weighted MRI after the venous injection of a contrast bolus and is represented as a 4D dataset characterizing blood flow through the vasculature and tissue. In the context of stroke, it is common to process the contrast concentration time curve obtained for each voxel and extract specific features related to physiological changes of the tissue, such as cerebral blood volume (CBV) and time-to-maximum of the residue function (Tmax) [3]. In addition, pre-established permeability metrics can also be computed [11], including contrast slope, final contrast, and maximum concentration, reflecting brain-blood-barrier permeability. Some of these perfusion parameters, such as low CBV, prolonged Tmax, increased permeability, and lesion size on diffusion-weighted imaging (DWI), are known predictors of parenchymal hemorrhage. Yet, most of studies have limited their predictions to the simple occurrence of HT [15]. The severity, cerebral territory involved, and eloquence have not been addressed. Recent works have demonstrated that the use of source/native PWI has demonstrated an advantage over pre-defined maps in the context of tissue fate prediction in acute stroke [1,7] and time from stroke onset [8]. In these frameworks, the relevant features of the PWI are learned by a machine learning algorithm rather than being pre-defined. The main rationale is that the source PWI may contain additional information that is not captured by pre-defined features and that could improve the prediction of the target variable.

The key contribution of this work is a predictive model of HT that explicitly models the temporal features of the PWI signal using an LSTM network. LSTMs have outperformed standard machine learning models on a wide variety of applications related to temporal signals. Inspired by these findings, our framework goes beyond the prediction of occurrence of HT and aims at estimating the spatial extent of the injury by identifying the voxels that will undergo HT. Such predictions could bring valuable insights to stroke neurologists about the affected territory and the chances of good outcome. We provide a comparative analysis with standard models, including linear regression, kernel spectral regression, SVM, and random forests.

2   Methods

MRI data was collected from patients identified with AIS within six hours of symptom onset and admitted at a Chinese University Hospital from 06/2009 to 10/2016. Inclusion criteria were as follows: (1) acute ischemic lesions confirmed on DWI; (2) baseline perfusion MRI and DWI performed before reperfusion therapy; and (3) Enhanced 3D gradient recalled echo (GRE) T2*-weighted angiography performed 24 h after reperfusion therapy. Patients with significant motion artifacts were excluded. The ethics committee of the Hospital approved the study protocol.

All patients underwent MRI on 3.0 T systems equipped with 8-channel head coils. The routine MRI protocol including PWI, DWI, and GRE was performed in AIS patients at baseline and 24 h after reperfusion therapy. Although the acquisition parameters slightly varied during the seven-year period, the median parameters of PWI were as follows: field of view (FOV) = 240 mm, repetitive time (TR) = 1800 ms, echo time (TE) = 30 ms, acquisition matrix = 128 × 128, repetitive scanning times = 60, gadolinium dose = 15 ml, contrast speed = 4–5 ml/s, average duration = 1 min 48 s. The parameters of DWI b1000 and b0 were: FOV = 240 mm, TR = 4000 ms, TE = 80 ms, slice sickness = 5 mm, acquisition matrix = 160 × 160. The parameters of GRE: TE = 4.5 ms (first echo), matrix size = 256 × 256, flip angle = 20°, slice thickness = 2.0 mm.

Baseline PWI, DWI, and 24 h follow-up GRE images were co-registered automatically using SPM12. The arterial input function (AIF) was automatically detected using Olea Sphere and computed from the average of the time-intensity curve from several voxel locations. Because of the difference in acquisition settings across subjects, AIF and PWI values were interpolated temporally using bilinear interpolation to 60 time points with a 1.8s time interval. Presence of HT at 24 h on GRE images was assessed by a stroke neurologist and delineated on each patient using Osirix software.

2.1 Predictive Model

The predictive model of HT makes use of an LSTM architecture which captures the temporal information stored in the PWI signal. The model aims at predicting the occurrence of HT at the voxel level. The target output $y_i \in Y$ of the classifier is a binary variable indicating the presence of bleeding at follow-up in the pixel i. As a standard pre-processing, the concentration of the contrast agent $C_i(t)$ at time t in a voxel i is obtained from the pre-intervention PWI signal I by:

$$C_i(t) = -TE^{-1} \log\left(\frac{I_i(t)}{I_i(0)}\right) \tag{1}$$

where TE is the echo time, and I_0, I_t are the image intensity measured before bolus arrival and time t, respectively. The contrast concentration time curve C over a 3 × 3 local patch is used as the input data to an LSTM model and is therefore composed of 9 features over 60 time points. The LSTM is described by 60 output values that are connected to the output y_i using a fully connected neural network.

Long Short-Term Memory Network. LSTM [9] is a variation of the recurrent neural network (RNN) which allows information to persist inside the network via a loopy architecture. LSTMs are particularly well suited to represent time series and are used in our framework to model the relationship between a PWI image patch captured over time and the occurrence of HT post-intervention. An LSTM cell is defined by a state that changes according to three types of gates:

- Input Gates $i_t \in \mathcal{R}^N$ update the state of the cell and decide which values should be updated.
- Forget Gates $f_t \in \mathcal{R}^N$ are used to select relevant information with respect to a previous state.
- Output Gates $o_t \in \mathcal{R}^N$ determine the final cell state and the output value.

Given an input sequence $x = \{x_1, x_2, \ldots, x_T\}$ of length T with corresponding memory cell unit $C_t \in \mathcal{R}^N$ and hidden unit $h_t \in \mathcal{R}^N$ at time t, the parameters of the model are updated sequentially, as follows:

$$f_t = \sigma(W_f.[h_{t-1}, x_t] + b_f) \tag{2}$$
$$i_t = \sigma(W_i.[h_{t-1}, x_t] + b_i) \tag{3}$$
$$o_t = \sigma(W_o[h_{t-1}, x_t] + b_o) \tag{4}$$
$$\tilde{C}_t = \tanh(W_c.[h_{t-1}, x_t] + b_C) \tag{5}$$
$$C_t = f_t * C_{t-1} + i_t * \tilde{C}_t \tag{6}$$
$$h_t = o_t * \tanh C_t \tag{7}$$

The function $\sigma(x) = (1 + e^{-x})^{-1}$ used to compute f_t, i_t, o_t is a sigmoid whose values lie within the range $[0, 1]$. In addition to input, forget, and output gates previously described, the LSTM makes use of a memory cell unit C_t obtained from the sum of the previous memory cell unit C_{t-1} modulated by f_t, and a function of the current input x_t and previous hidden state h_{t-1} modulated by the input gate i_t. The output gate o_t is then used to determine what parts should be considered and then multiplied with the tanh of the memory cell state C_t to produce the hidden unit h_t. By learning how much of the memory cell state C_t should be transferred to the hidden state h_t based on the input x_t and previous state, this structure allows the LSTM to capture complex temporal dynamics.

Operating Modes. In addition to building an LSTM model from the contrast concentration C_i, we allow the framework to utilize additional inputs, including: the contrast concentration of the AIF $C_{aif} \in \mathcal{R}^T$, and the value of the DWI at b0 and b1000 $X_{dwi} \in \mathcal{R}^S$. A fully connected layer is used to combine the output of the LSTM and additional inputs. The binary output is obtained with a Softmax operator. We distinguish between several modes of operation depending on which input is used:

Mode 1: LSTM PWI. The 3×3 PWI patches for each time-point are used as input to the LSTM model, corresponding to 9 features over 60 time-points. The LSTM is defined by 60 output values.

Mode 2: LSTM PWI+AIF. Because the AIF is represented as a vector of 60 time-points, the input data now corresponds to 10 features by 60 time-points.

Mode 3: LSTM PWI+DWI. The outputs of the LSTM are combined with two 3×3 patches obtained from DWI b0 and b1000 to form a 78 input vector to the fully connected layer.

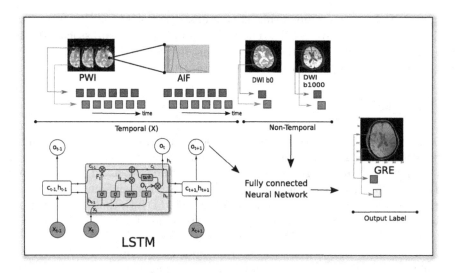

Fig. 1. Illustration of our LSTM-NeuralNet Framework. Local patches extracted on perfusion-weighted MRI (PWI) are combined together with the arterial input function (AIF) to train a LSTM model (bottom left, diagram modified from [13]). The output of the LSTM model is combined with local DWI image patches through a fully connected neural network that maps the features to the presence of HT as observed on gradient recalled echo (GRE) at followup.

Mode 4: LSTM PWI+DWI+AIF. The most comprehensive mode of operation combines the LSTM output (60) with the DWI b0 and b1000 patches, leading to 78 features combined in the fully connected layer (Fig. 1).

2.2   Experiments

We evaluate the framework using a 10-fold cross-validation performed at the voxel level. The accuracy of the model trained under 4 different modes is compared to Linear Regression, SR-KDA [2], SVM [4], and Random Forests. The LSTM training setup was defined with 60 cells of LSTM, 20 epochs, and trained with Adam optimizer [10] using binary cross-entropy as loss function. The outputs of the LSTM cells are converted to a binary output by using a fully connected neural network with a softmax optimization. The final output represents the probabilities of the HT class or the Non-HT class. The training of our machine learning model took place on 50,000 input samples equally distributed between HT and Non-HT voxels from various subjects as it has previously been shown that balanced classes provides a more representative estimation of the performance. The sampling method used in these experiments is similar to the one described in previous work [16]. As part of the cross-validation, we ensure that the data from a given patient were not included both in the training set and the test set. The accuracy is calculated on the basis of the area under the curve of the receiver operating characteristic curve (AUC-ROC) and the precision-recall curve (AUC-PR). The 95% confidence interval associated with each result is obtained using the Bootstrapping method [5]. Optimization of the hyperparameters was performed using a nested cross-validation.

3   Results

A total of 155 AIS patients satisfied the inclusion criteria and were included in this study, among whom 41 patients were diagnosed with HT. The results of each machine learning algorithm evaluated in this study are listed in Table 1 and illustrated in Fig. 2. For all models, the best performing configuration was the one that combines all inputs available (PWI, AIF and DWI), thus demonstrating the complementary information contained in these input variables. The LSTM model with PWI, DWI and AIF as inputs reached an AUC-ROC = $89.4 \pm 4\%$, AUC-PR = $87.4 \pm 6\%$. In addition, we also reported the predictive accuracy of manually defined ROI on Ktrans parametric map that was obtained in another study [12] (64%). It should be noted, however, that it is not directly comparable as the study was performed on another patient population and a different cross validation setup.

Table 1. Accuracy of the models in predicting voxel-wise HT occurrence.

Model	Input (s)	AUC-ROC	AUC-PR
LSTM	PWI	$83.1 \pm 2.9\%$	$82.3 \pm 5.8\%$
LSTM-NeuralNet	PWI+AIF	$79.6 \pm 2.6\%$	$71.9 \pm 5.8\%$
LSTM-NeuralNet	PWI+DWI	$88.3 \pm 3.6\%$	$86.4 \pm 6.4\%$
LSTM-NeuralNet	PWI+AIF+DWI	$\mathbf{89.4 \pm 4.3\%}$	$\mathbf{87.4 \pm 5.9\%}$
Linear regression	PWI+AIF+DWI	$58.5 \pm 7.5\%$	$44.4 \pm 9.8\%$
Random forests	PWI+AIF+DWI	$79.8 \pm 3.1\%$	$67.1 \pm 6.0\%$
SR-KDA [2]	PWI+AIF+DWI	$83.7 \pm 2.6\%$	$70.4 \pm 5.8\%$
SVM [4]	PWI+AIF+DWI	$82.1 \pm 2.9\%$	$69.9 \pm 5.8\%$
ROI-based [12]	K^{trans}	$64.1 \pm 6.0\%$	NA

4   Discussion

The aim of this paper is to introduce a predictive model for HT in acute ischemic stroke. The multi-input LSTM model achieved an AUC-ROC accuracy of 89% which is very promising considering the challenging nature of the problem. A significant finding of this paper is that the use of an LSTM improves the results over standard models.

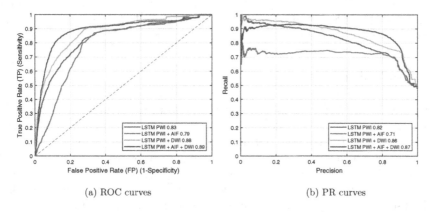

(a) ROC curves   (b) PR curves

Fig. 2. Illustration of the accuracy in terms of ROC and PR curves for various predictive models of HT based on LSTM-NeuralNet architecture.

The development of hemorrhagic transformation in AIS is a complex pathophysiological process, which is influenced by multiple factors such as reperfusion, age, serum glucose level, stroke severity, and blood-brain barrier (BBB) damage. Perfusion-weighted imaging is rich in information about brain tissue and blood flow. It is particularly useful in detecting BBB permeability disruptions that are linked to ongoing or future HT. PWI remains largely under-utilized in the context of AIS due to the non-standard way of detecting these BBB impairments. The relationship and causal influence of PWI imaging markers remains poorly understood. In this context, the fact that machine learning models can predict HT from imaging alone is particularly encouraging and could be considered as part of new therapeutic strategies.

We can improve our present model by giving it additional features which may or may not be related to MRI features. Similar to the multi-input LSTM model, we can have these features fed to a different layer and the output of that layer can be concatenated with the output of the LSTM.

While the prediction of future occurrence of HT has been successful on a multi-center study [15], it is not clear that the presence of a small hemorrhage would prevent the patient from being treated with endovascular clot-retrieval therapy. In this paper, we are predicting the risk of HT at the voxel level, which can be used to infer volumetric and eloquence measures that would be more helpful in the clinical setting to rule out clot-retrieval therapy.

A limitation of this study is to include data with various degrees of revascularization which is typically assessed using the Thrombolysis in Cerebral Infarction (TICI) score [6]. The TICI score, which varies from 0 (no reperfusion) to 3 (complete reperfusion), is useful to quantify the degree of success in restoring blood flow after clot-retrieval intervention. A multi-center evaluation of the model on a more representative set of cases would be beneficial. A specific predictive model could be trained for various degrees of revascularization. During diagnosis, predicted maps of likelihood of HT development could help clinicians to visualize the risks/benefits of the intervention and the dependency to the degree of revascularization.

5 Conclusion

This paper introduces a computational framework for the prediction of HT in acute ischemic stroke. The contribution of the model is two-fold; first it utilizes the source/native PWI signal and maps it to the development of HT using an LSTM model which captures the temporal signature of tissue voxels at risk of HT, second it does not only produce a prediction about overall presence of HT in the follow-up images but rather provides predictions at the voxel level that can be used to predict the severity of the HT and therefore better characterize the risks associated with an endovascular intervention.

Acknowledgements. This work was partially supported by a NIH award R01 NS100806. The GPU used for this research was donated by the NVIDIA Corporation.

References

1. Bertels, J., Robben, D., Vandermeulen, D., Suetens, P.: Contra-lateral information CNN for core lesion segmentation based on native CTP in acute stroke. In: Crimi, A., Bakas, S., Kuijf, H., Keyvan, F., Reyes, M., van Walsum, T. (eds.) BrainLes 2018. LNCS, vol. 11383, pp. 263–270. Springer, Cham (2019). https://doi.org/10.1007/978-3-030-11723-8_26
2. Cai, D., He, X., Han, J.: Spectral regression for efficient regularized subspace learning. In: ICCV (2007). https://doi.org/10.1109/ICCV.2007.4408855
3. Calamante, F., Christensen, S., Desmond, P.M., Ostergaard, L., Davis, S.M., Connelly, A.: The physiological significance of the time-to-maximum (Tmax) parameter in perfusion MRI. Stroke **41**(6), 1169–1174 (2010)
4. Chang, C.C., Lin, C.J.: LIBSVM: a library for support vector machines (2001). http://www.csie.ntu.edu.tw/~cjlin/libsvm
5. DiCiccio, T.J., Efron, B.: Bootstrap confidence intervals. Stat. Sci. **11**, 189–212 (1996)
6. Higashida, R.T., et al.: Trial design and reporting standards for intra-arterial cerebral thrombolysis for acute ischemic stroke. Stroke **34**(8), e109–137 (2003)
7. Ho, K.C., Scalzo, F., Sarma, K.V., Speier, W., El-Saden, S., Arnold, C.: Predicting ischemic stroke tissue fate using a deep convolutional neural network on source magnetic resonance perfusion images. J. Med. Imaging (Bellingham) **6**(2), 026001 (2019)
8. Ho, K.C., Speier, W., Zhang, H., Scalzo, F., El-Saden, S., Arnold, C.W.: A machine learning approach for classifying ischemic stroke onset time from imaging. IEEE Trans. Med. Imaging **38**(7), 1666–1676 (2019)
9. Hochreiter, S., Schmidhuber, J.: Long short-term memory. Neural Comput. **9**, 1735–80 (1997)
10. Kingma, D.P., Ba, J.: Adam: a method for stochastic optimization. arXiv preprint arXiv:1412.6980 (2014)

11. Leigh, R., et al.: Pretreatment blood-brain barrier damage and post-treatment intracranial hemorrhage in patients receiving intravenous tissue-type plasminogen activator. Stroke **45**(7), 2030–2035 (2014)
12. Li, Y., et al.: Focal low and global high permeability predict the possibility, risk, and location of hemorrhagic transformation following intra-arterial thrombolysis therapy in acute stroke. AJNR Am. J. Neuroradiol. **38**(9), 1730–1736 (2017)
13. Olah, C.: Understanding LSTM networks (2015). https://colah.github.io/posts/2015-08-Understanding-LSTMs/
14. Powers, W., et al.: 2015 AHA/American stroke association focused update of the 2013 guidelines for the early management of patients with acute ischemic stroke regarding endovascular treatment. Stroke **46**(10), 3020–3035 (2015)
15. Scalzo, F., et al.: Multi-center prediction of hemorrhagic transformation in acute ischemic stroke using permeability imaging features. Magn. Reson. Imaging **31**(6), 961–969 (2013)
16. Scalzo, F., Hao, Q., Alger, J.R., Hu, X., Liebeskind, D.S.: Regional prediction of tissue fate in acute ischemic stroke. Ann. Biomed. Eng. **40**(10), 2177–2187 (2012)

Inter-modality Dependence Induced Data Recovery for MCI Conversion Prediction

Tao Zhou[1], Kim-Han Thung[2], Yu Zhang[3], Huazhu Fu[1], Jianbing Shen[1(✉)], Dinggang Shen[2(✉)], and Ling Shao[1]

[1] Inception Institute of Artificial Intelligence, Abu Dhabi, UAE
jianbing.shen@inceptioniai.org
[2] Department of Radiology and BRIC, University of North Carolina, Chapel Hill, USA
dgshen@med.unc.edu
[3] Department of Psychiatry and Behavioral Sciences, Stanford University, Stanford, CA 94305, USA

Abstract. Learning complementary information from multi-modality data often improves diagnostic performance of brain disorders. However, it is challenging to obtain this complementary information when the data are incomplete. Existing methods, such as low-rank matrix completion (which imputes the missing data) and multi-task learning (which restructures the problem into the joint learning of multiple tasks, with each task associated with a subset of complete data), simply concatenate features from different modalities without considering their underlying correlations. Furthermore, most methods conduct multi-modality fusion and prediction model learning in separated steps, which may render to a sub-optimal solution. To address these issues, we propose a novel diagnostic model that integrates missing data recovery, latent space learning and prediction model learning into a unified framework. Specifically, we first recover the missing modality by maximizing the dependency among different modalities. Then, we further exploit the modality correlation by projecting different modalities into a common latent space. Besides, we employ an ℓ_1-norm to our loss function to mitigate the influence of sample outliers. Finally, we map the learned latent representation into the label space. All these tasks are learned iteratively in a unified framework, where the label information (from the training samples) can also inherently guide the missing modality recovery. Experimental results on the Alzheimer's Disease Neuroimaging Initiative (ADNI) dataset show the effectiveness of our method.

1 Introduction

Alzheimer's Disease (AD), one of the most common neurodegenerative diseases that impairs a patient's memory and other cognitive functions, is widely found in people over 65 years old. As AD is currently incurable, it is important to devise a Computer-Aided Diagnosis (CAD) method to detect AD at its prodromal stage, *i.e.*, Mild Cognitive Impairment (MCI), so that early intervention

© Springer Nature Switzerland AG 2019
D. Shen et al. (Eds.): MICCAI 2019, LNCS 11767, pp. 186–195, 2019.
https://doi.org/10.1007/978-3-030-32251-9_21

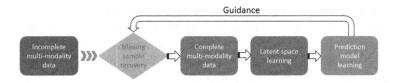

Fig. 1. Overview of the proposed MCI conversion prediction model, which integrates missing sample recovery, latent space learning, and prediction model learning into a unified framework.

can be carried out. To this end, recent studies have reported that structural Magnetic Resonance Imaging (MRI) [15,20] and fluorodeoxyglucose Positron Emission Tomography (PET) [19] measurements are among the best biomarkers for AD progression and MCI conversion prediction [5]. Since neuroimaging data (e.g., MRI and PET) are very high-dimensional, existing CAD approaches often use Region-Of-Interest (ROI) based features instead of the original voxel based features for analysis [8,12], and achieve promising results. Additionally, recent studies have also shown that fusing multi-modality data can provide complementary information to improve the diagnostic performance [12,18].

One of the main challenges in multi-modality fusion is the existence of missing modalities, which occurs for various reasons, such as poor data quality and patient dropouts. Several approaches have been developed to handle this incomplete multi-modality data issue. For example, some studies simply exclude subjects with missing modalities [8] from their analysis. However, this results in discarding a large amount of useful information as well and leads to a smaller subset of data for analysis. Another approach is to impute the missing data using techniques such as k-nearest neighbour (KNN) [13], expectation maximization (EM), and low-rank matrix completion (LRMC) [10]. However, these imputation techniques only work well if a small portion of data is missing, and their overall performances degrades if a large portion of data is missing. A third approach avoids the drawbacks of data imputation by dividing the dataset into several subsets of complete multi-modality data and jointly learning the prediction models for all data subsets [16]. Although many methods have been proposed and have significantly advanced CAD studies using incomplete multi-modality data, there still exist several drawbacks. *First*, the existing methods directly concatenate features from multi-modalities without considering their underlying correlations. *Second*, most existing imputation methods in the literature are based on a two-step strategy, where the missing data is first imputed, and then a classification model is learned. As the data imputation (or recovery) in the first step might not be optimal for the classification model in the second step, the final prediction model could be sub-optimal.

Accordingly, we propose to exploit the inter-modality dependence to learn a novel MCI conversion prediction model with incomplete multi-modalities. As shown in Fig. 1, our model can seamlessly integrate missing modality recovery, latent representation learning and prediction model learning into a unified framework. Specifically, we first recover the missing modalities by maximizing the inter-modality dependence using all the multi-modality data. Then, we project the multi-modality data into a common latent space to further exploit their correlation and alleviate the heterogeneity among different modalities. Additionally, we use an ℓ_1-norm to measure the projection error to mitigate the influences of sample outliers. Then, we map the learned representation from the latent space into the label space for prediction model learning. It is worth noting that we integrate all the above learning tasks into a unified framework, thus enabling all components to work together to learn a reliable diagnostic model using multi-modality data that could be incomplete. Experimental results on the Alzheimer's Disease Neuroimaging Initiative (ADNI) dataset have verified the effectiveness of our proposed method.

2   Dataset and Preprocessing

We use incomplete multi-modality data (*i.e.*, MRI and PET) from the ADNI dataset in this study. Note that only subjects that are labeled as MCI at baseline are used. Among all the MCI subjects, those that progressed to AD within 24 months are retrospectively defined as progressive MCI (pMCI) subjects, while the remaining are defined as stable MCI (sMCI) subjects. Thus, we have 124 pMCI and 118 sMCI subjects. Further, we extract features based on ROIs from MR and PET images. Specifically, we follow a standard pipeline [18] to process each MR images, and conduct template registration to 93 pre-defined ROIs. Finally, for each subject, we extract the volumes of gray matter tissue inside the 93 ROIs as features. For PET images, we align each one onto its corresponding MR image via a rigid registration, and then compute the mean intensity of each ROI in the PET image as features. Thus, we have 93 ROI-based features for both MRI and PET data.

3   The Proposed Method

Preliminary. We use Hilbert-Schmidt Independence Criterion (HSIC) [1] to measure the dependency between two random variables (see[1] for notations). HSIC is able to measure the intrinsic relationship between two variables by considering their correlation in kernel spaces. Let $\mathbf{x} \in \mathcal{X}$ and $\mathbf{y} \in \mathcal{Y}$ denote two different variables, which are mapped to kernel spaces $\mathcal{F}$ and $\mathcal{G}$ via $\phi(\cdot)$. Then an empirical definition of HSIC is given as follows.

Definition 1. Considering a set of n independent observations drawn from p_{xy}, *i.e.*, $\mathbf{Z} = \{(\mathbf{x}_1, \mathbf{y}_1), \ldots, (\mathbf{x}_N, \mathbf{y}_N)\} \subseteq \mathcal{X} \times \mathcal{Y}$, then $\text{HSIC}(\mathbf{Z}, \mathcal{F}, \mathcal{G})$ is defined as

$$\text{HSIC}(\mathbf{Z}, \mathcal{F}, \mathcal{G}) = (n-1)^{-2} tr(\mathbf{K}_1 \mathbf{H} \mathbf{K}_2 \mathbf{H}), \tag{1}$$

---

[1] Bold capital letters denotes matrices (*e.g.*, $\mathbf{X}$), bold small letters denote vectors (*e.g.*, $\mathbf{x}$), and non-bold letters denote scalar variables (*e.g.*, d_1). $\| \cdot \|_F$, $\| \cdot \|_1$, and $\| \cdot \|_{2,1}$ denote the F, ℓ_1, and $\ell_{2,1}$ norms, respectively. Besides, $\mathbf{X}^\top$ denotes the transpose operator of a matrix $\mathbf{X}$.

where $\mathbf{K}_1$ and $\mathbf{K}_2$ denote Gram matrices with their (i, j)-th elements given as $k_1(\mathbf{x}_i, \mathbf{x}_j) = \langle \phi(\mathbf{x}_i), \phi(\mathbf{x}_j) \rangle$ and $k_2(\mathbf{y}_i, \mathbf{y}_j) = \langle \phi(\mathbf{y}_i), \phi(\mathbf{y}_j) \rangle$, respectively. Besides, $\mathbf{H}$ is a centering matrix with its (i, j)-th element given as $h_{ij} := \delta_{ij} - 1/n$, which centralizes the two Gram matrices so that they have zero mean.

3.1   Methodology

Consider a two-modality neuroimaging dataset $\mathbf{X} = [\mathbf{X}_1, \mathbf{X}_2]$ with $\mathbf{X}_1 \in \mathbb{R}^{n \times d_1}$ and $\mathbf{X}_2 \in \mathbb{R}^{n \times d_2}$, where n is the number of samples in $\mathbf{X}$, and d_1 and d_2 denote the feature dimensions of $\mathbf{X}_1$ and $\mathbf{X}_2$, respectively. Due to missing data issue, some samples have only certain modalities available. Thus, we denote $\mathbf{X}_1 = [\mathbf{X}_1^{n_c}; \mathbf{X}_1^{n_1}; \mathbf{X}_1^{n_2}]$ and $\mathbf{X}_2 = [\mathbf{X}_2^{n_c}; \mathbf{X}_2^{n_1}; \mathbf{X}_2^{n_2}]$, where n_c samples have both modalities complete, n_1 samples have only the first modality data, and n_2 samples have only the second modality data. Obviously, $\mathbf{X}_1^{n_2}$ and $\mathbf{X}_2^{n_1}$ are unknown and need to be estimated. Assuming the existence of an inherent correlation between $\mathbf{X}_1$ and $\mathbf{X}_2$ (i.e., data from two different but related modalities), we estimate the missing modality from the incomplete samples by maximizing the dependency between the two modalities [2] as follows,

$$\max_{\mathbf{X}_1^{n_2}, \mathbf{X}_2^{n_1}} tr(\mathbf{H}\mathbf{K}_1\mathbf{H}\mathbf{K}_2), \tag{2}$$

where $\mathbf{K}_1 = \mathbf{X}_1\mathbf{X}_1^\top$ and $\mathbf{K}_2 = \mathbf{X}_2\mathbf{X}_2^\top$. Following [2], we first impute the missing data using the averaged values from the k-nearest samples (k is set to be 10 in our study), and update the imputed values using Eq. (2). After recovering the missing data, the general formulation for a prediction model is as follows:

$$\mathcal{L}(\mathbf{X}_1, \mathbf{X}_2; \mathbf{Y}) + \lambda \Psi(\mathbf{W}), \tag{3}$$

where $\mathcal{L}$ is the loss function of the prediction model, $\Psi(\cdot)$ is a regularizer on $\mathbf{W}$, and $\mathbf{Y} \in \mathbb{R}^{c \times n}$ is the label matrix with c number of classes. Generally, a least square loss function is used to measure the prediction error, i.e., $\mathcal{L}(\cdot) = \|\mathbf{W}^\top \mathbf{X}^\top - \mathbf{Y}\|_F^2$, where $\mathbf{X}$ denotes the concatenated multi-modality data, i.e., $\mathbf{X} = [\mathbf{X}_1, \mathbf{X}_2] \in \mathbb{R}^{n \times (d_1 + d_2)}$. Though simple and easy to implement, there are two main issues with this loss function: (1) not only does simple concatenation increase the feature dimension, which may lead to a dimensionality issue, but the complementarity among different modalities is also not fully exploited; (2) this formulation does not consider the influences of noise and outliers. To overcome these issues, we propose to first project the multi-modality data into a latent space before learning the prediction model, as follows,

$$\mathcal{L}_1(\mathbf{X}_1, \mathbf{X}_2; \mathbf{B}) + \mathcal{L}_2(\mathbf{B}; \mathbf{Y}) + \lambda \Psi(\mathbf{W}_1, \mathbf{W}_2, \mathbf{P}), \tag{4}$$

where $\mathbf{B} \in \mathbb{R}^{h \times n}$ is the common latent representation, and $\mathbf{W}_v \in \mathbb{R}^{d_v \times h}$ is the coefficient matrix that projects the original features of the v-th modality into $\mathbf{B}$, where h is the dimension of the latent space. The third term in Eq. (4) regularizes all the coefficient matrices to achieve a better solution for them. Specifically, we employ the $\ell_{2,1}$-norm regularizer to penalize $\mathbf{W}_v$, so that only certain rows in $\mathbf{W}_v$ are non-zero [14,20]. This is equivalent to assigning relatively large weights to informative features, while assigning zero or small weights to uninformative or less informative features. In addition, we employ an ℓ_1-norm for the loss function of the first term in Eq. (4) to alleviate the influence of sample outliers during the latent space learning. Finally, $\mathbf{P}$ is the coefficient matrix that maps the learned latent representation into the label space (*i.e.*, $\mathbf{Y}$). To avoid a trivial solution for $\mathbf{P}$, we employ an orthogonal constraint on $\mathbf{P}$, *i.e.*, $\mathbf{P}\mathbf{P}^\top = \mathbf{I}$.

By integrating the data imputation, latent space learning, and prediction model learning into a unified framework, the formulation of our proposed method is given as

$$
\min_{\substack{\mathbf{X}_1^{n_2},\mathbf{X}_2^{n_1},\mathbf{B},\mathbf{P}, \\ \{\mathbf{W}_v\}|_{v=1,2}}} \underbrace{-tr\left(\mathbf{H}\mathbf{X}_1\mathbf{X}_1^\top\mathbf{H}\mathbf{X}_2\mathbf{X}_2^\top\right)}_{\text{data imputation}} + \lambda \underbrace{\sum_{v=1}^2 \|\mathbf{W}_v^\top\mathbf{X}_v^\top - \mathbf{B}\|_1}_{\text{latent space learning}} + \gamma \underbrace{\sum_{v=1}^2 \|\mathbf{W}_v\|_{2,1}}_{\text{regularization}}
$$
$$
+ \underbrace{\beta\|\mathcal{P}_O(\mathbf{P}\mathbf{B} - \mathbf{Y})\|_F^2}_{\text{prediction model}}, \quad s.t. \ \mathbf{P}\mathbf{P}^\top = \mathbf{I}, \tag{5}
$$

where λ, β, and γ are the regularization parameters. $\mathcal{P}_O$ denotes a filter function, which forces the label prediction loss to only account for the labeled subjects (*i.e.*, training data). Specifically, $\mathcal{P}_O(\mathbf{P}\mathbf{B} - \mathbf{Y}) = (\mathbf{P}\mathbf{B} - \mathbf{Y})\mathbf{O}$, where $\mathbf{O}$ is a diagonal matrix with its diagonal elements denoting the indicator variables, *i.e.*, $\mathbf{O}_{ii} = 1$ if the i-th subject is labeled, and 0 otherwise. Accordingly, $\mathbf{Y} = [\mathbf{Y}_l, \mathbf{Y}_u]$, where $\mathbf{Y}_l$ and $\mathbf{Y}_u$ denote the matrices of labeled (*i.e.*, training) and unlabeled (*i.e.*, testing) data, respectively. Thus, we exploit the underlying data structure of the whole dataset (including the unlabeled samples) to better learn the prediction model.

Optimization. We use the ALM [4] algorithm to solve Eq. (5) efficiently and effectively. To this end, we first introduce an auxiliary variable $\mathbf{E}_v$ to make the problem separable. Then, the augmented Lagrangian function for Eq. (5) is given as

$$
\min_{\substack{\mathbf{X}_1^{n_2},\mathbf{X}_2^{n_1},\mathbf{B},\mathbf{P}, \\ \{\mathbf{W}_v,\mathbf{E}_v,\mathcal{Q}_v\}|_{v=1,2}}} - tr(\mathbf{H}\mathbf{X}_1\mathbf{X}_1^\top\mathbf{H}\mathbf{X}_2\mathbf{X}_2^\top) + \lambda \sum_{v=1}^2 \|\mathbf{E}_v\|_1 + \gamma \sum_{v=1}^2 \|\mathbf{W}_v\|_{2,1}
$$
$$
+ \beta\|(\mathbf{P}\mathbf{B} - \mathbf{Y})\mathbf{O}\|_F^2 + \sum_{v=1}^2 \Phi(\mathcal{Q}_v, \mathbf{E}_v - \mathbf{W}_v^\top\mathbf{X}_v^\top + \mathbf{B}), \ s.t. \ \mathbf{P}\mathbf{P}^\top = \mathbf{I}, \tag{6}
$$

where $\Phi(\mathcal{Q}, \mathbf{Q}) = \frac{\mu}{2}\|\mathbf{Q}\|_F^2 + \langle\mathcal{Q}, \mathbf{Q}\rangle$ with $\langle\cdot,\cdot\rangle$ denoting the matrix inner product, μ is a positive penalty scalar, and $\mathcal{Q}_v$ ($v = 1, 2$) are the Lagrangian multipliers. Using ALM, we iteratively optimize each variable in $\{\mathbf{X}_1^{n_2}, \mathbf{X}_2^{n_1}, \mathbf{W}_v, \mathbf{E}_v, \mathbf{B}, \mathbf{P}, \mathcal{Q}_v\}$, while fixing the others. Specifically, we obtain the closed-form solutions for $\mathbf{X}_1^{n_2}$ and $\mathbf{X}_2^{n_1}$ by taking the derivatives of the objective function in Eq. (6) with respect to these two variables and setting them to zero. To solve $\mathbf{W}_v$, we first compute the derivative of the term $\|\mathbf{W}_v\|_{2,1}$ *w.r.t.* $\mathbf{W}_v$, *i.e.*, $\frac{\partial\|\mathbf{W}_v\|_{2,1}}{\partial\mathbf{W}_v} = \Lambda\mathbf{W}_v$, where $\Lambda \in \mathbb{R}^{d_v \times d_v}$ is a diagonal matrix with $\Lambda_{jj} = \frac{1}{2\|\mathbf{W}_{v,j:}\|_2}$, and $\mathbf{W}_{v,j:}$ denotes the

j-th row of $\mathbf{W}_v$. Then, taking the derivative of Eq. (6) *w.r.t.* $\mathbf{W}_v$ and setting it to zero, we iteratively update $\mathbf{W}_v$ and Λ until convergence. We can use a shrinkage thresholding operator to solve $\mathbf{E}_v$. Further, we solve $\mathbf{B}$ by setting the derivative of the objective function in Eq. (6) *w.r.t.* $\mathbf{B}$ to zero. Besides, we adopt the method in [17] to obtain the optimal solution for $\mathbf{P}$. Finally, we update the multipliers $\mathcal{Q}_v$ using $\mathcal{Q}_v \leftarrow \mathcal{Q}_v + \mu(\mathbf{E}_v - \mathbf{W}_v^\top \mathbf{X}_v^\top + \mathbf{B})$. We iteratively update $\mathbf{X}_1^{n_2} \rightarrow \mathbf{X}_2^{n_1} \rightarrow \mathbf{W}_v \rightarrow \mathbf{E}_v \rightarrow \mathbf{B} \rightarrow \mathbf{P} \rightarrow \mathcal{Q}_v$ until it satisfies the convergence conditions (*i.e.*, $\|\mathbf{E}_v - \mathbf{W}_v^\top \mathbf{X}_v^\top + \mathbf{B}\|_\infty < \varepsilon$, ε is set to 10^{-4}).

4   Experiments

4.1   Experimental Settings

We evaluate the effectiveness of our proposed model by conducting experiments to predict MCI conversion, *i.e.*, to differentiate pMCI from sMCI subjects. In the ADNI dataset, all subjects have complete MRI data, while only half of the subjects have PET data. Thus, to evaluate our method for different combinations of missing modalities, we perform two groups of experiments in this study. In the first group, we use the whole dataset (including the complete MRI and incomplete PET data) to test our model, where it only recovers missing PET data. In the second group, we randomly remove $r\%$ ($r = 5, 10, 15, 20$ in this study) of subjects from the MRI data, and use our model to simultaneously recover the missing MRI and PET data. We adopt five metrics for performance evaluation, including accuracy (ACC), sensitivity (SEN), specificity (SPE), positive predictive value (PPV), and F-score.

Our comparison methods include a "Baseline" method, which only uses the complete MRI data to train a linear SVM classifier, a k-Nearest Neighbor (KNN) based imputation method [13], a multi-task learning method (*i.e.*, least-squared loss based incomplete Multi-Source Feature (iMSF) [16]), and a Low-Rank Matrix Completion method (LRMC) [10]. We also include two state-of-the-art methods in handling incomplete multi-view data, *i.e.*, Incomplete Multi-View Weak-label Learning (iMVWL) [9] and Doubly Aligned Incomplete Multi-view Clustering (MADIC) [3]. Furthermore, to verify the effectiveness of our proposed data imputation model, we include a degraded version of our model, which imputes the missing data via a KNN method without iteratively updating (denoted as "Ours-ablation"). In all experiments, a 10-fold cross-validation strategy is used for performance evaluation. This process is repeated 10 times and the mean results are reported. To optimize the parameters for different methods, we further perform an inner cross-validation using the training set for each fold of the experiment. For our method, we use the following range of values during the hyper-parameter search: $\lambda, \beta, \gamma \in \{10^{-4}, 10^{-3}, \ldots, 10^4\}$, and $h \in \{10, 20, \ldots, 60\}$. Note that iMSF, LRMC and our method can directly obtain the prediction results, while other methods feed the features into an SVM for classification. Here, the search space for the hyperparameter C of the SVM is $\{0.0001, 0.001, \ldots, 100\}$.

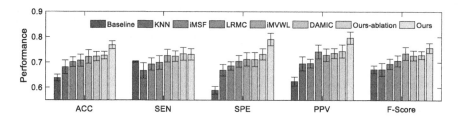

Fig. 2. Comparisons between the proposed method and the comparison methods for MCI conversion prediction. Note that we use complete MRI data and incomplete PET data.

4.2   Comparison of MCI Conversion Prediction

Figure 2 shows the comparison results for the first group of experiments. From Fig. 2, we can observe the following: (1) The proposed method consistently outperforms the comparison methods with regards to all five evaluation metrics for the pMCI vs. sMCI classification task. This verifies the effectiveness of our proposed framework for joint missing modality recovery and prediction model learning, which is likely due to the fact that it simultaneously conducts data imputation, feature learning, and prediction model learning, in a unified framework. These learning tasks are typically mutually beneficial, where the learning of one can improve the others. (2) All comparison methods that use multi-modality data (*i.e.*, MRI and PET) perform better than the Baseline method, which only uses MRI data. This indicates that multi-modality fusion, even when some samples are incomplete, can effectively improve the diagnostic performance. (3) Our full method outperforms the degraded model (*i.e.*, "Ours-ablation"), indicating the effectiveness of our HSIC based iterative imputation startegy. Further, Fig. 3 shows the classification results for the second group of experiments, *i.e.*, the ACC achieved by different methods using different missing rates of MRI data. It can be seen that, though the overall performance degrades when numbers of missing samples increase, our method consistently outperforms all the comparison methods under different missing rates for MRI data.

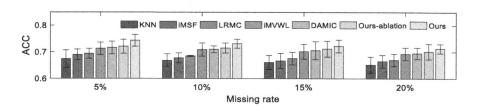

Fig. 3. Classification results (*i.e.*, ACC) achieved by different methods using different missing rates (*i.e.*, $r\%$) for MRI data. Note that, we use incomplete MRI and PET data.

4.3   Comparison with State-of-the-Art Methods

In Table 1, we briefly summarize several state-of-the-
art results reported in the
literature for MCI con-
version prediction using
ADNI data. Note that a
direct comparison between
these methods is impossi-
ble since different subjects
were used (see Table 1).

Table 1. A brief description of the state-of-the-art studies using ADNI data for MCI conversion prediction.

Algorithm	Modality	Subject	ACC
Ritter *et al.* [7]	MRI+PET	151sMCI + 86pMCI	0.730
Shi *et al.* [8]	MRI+PET	56sMCI + 43pMCI	0.743
Liu *et al.* [5]	MRI+PET+CSF	226sMCI + 169pMCI	0.733
Thung *et al.* [11]	MRI+PET	65sMCI + 53pMCI	0.737
Ours	MRI+PET	118sMCI + 124pMCI	0.768

However, though rough comparison, we can still observe that the proposed
method achieves the best ACC values and outperforms these state-of-the-art
methods. Besides, the two methods [5,11] also use the incomplete multi-modality
data, thus the results further demonstrate the effectiveness of our method in
recovering missing modalities using a self-supervised strategy.

4.4   Identifying Most Related Brain Regions

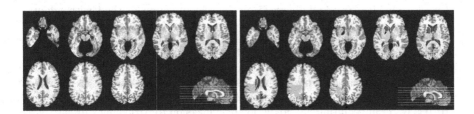

Fig. 4. Top ten selected regions from MRI (Left) and PET (Right) data.

We have also identified potential brain regions as biomarkers for MCI conversion
prediction based on the selected frequency of the ROIs. We ranked the ROIs
based on their weight values (*i.e.*, $\|\mathbf{W}_v\|_2^2$). The top selected regions from MRI
and PET data are shown in Fig. 4. Specifically, for MRI data, the top selected
ROIs are hippocampal formation right/left, uncus right/left, perirhinal cortex
left, amygdala right/left, and middle temporal gyrus right; whereas, for PET
data, the top selected ROIs are globus palladus left, precuneus right, precuneus
left, parietal lobe WM left, inferior temporal gyrus right, and angular gyrus left.
These regions are consistent with the findings from previous studies [6,19] and
can be used as potential biomarkers for MCI conversion prediction in clinical
practice.

5   Conclusion

In this paper, we propose a novel MCI conversion prediction model (using incomplete multi-modality data) that includes inter-modality dependence data imputation, feature selection, latent space learning, and prediction learning, in a unified framework. Our model imputes the missing modalities using a semi-supervised strategy, where the inter-modality dependence and the labels of the training data inherently guide the missing modalities recovery. Experimental results on the ADNI dataset demonstrate the efficacy of our model for the MCI conversion prediction task with incomplete multi-modalities.

References

1. Gretton, A., Bousquet, O., Smola, A., Schölkopf, B.: Measuring statistical dependence with Hilbert-Schmidt norms. In: Jain, S., Simon, H.U., Tomita, E. (eds.) ALT 2005. LNCS (LNAI), vol. 3734, pp. 63–77. Springer, Heidelberg (2005). https://doi.org/10.1007/11564089_7
2. Guo, J., Zhu, W.: Partial multi-view outlier detection based on collective learning. In: Thirty-Second AAAI Conference on Artificial Intelligence (2018)
3. Hu, M., Chen, S.: Doubly aligned incomplete multi-view clustering. In: IJCAI (2018)
4. Lin, Z., Liu, R., Su, Z.: Linearized alternating direction method with adaptive penalty for low-rank representation. In: NIPS, pp. 612–620 (2011)
5. Liu, M., Gao, Y., Yap, P.T., Shen, D.: Multi-hypergraph learning for incomplete multimodality data. IEEE J. Biomed. Health Inf. **22**(4), 1197–1208 (2018)
6. Misra, C., et al.: Baseline and longitudinal patterns of brain atrophy in MCI patients, and their use in prediction of short-term conversion to AD: results from ADNI. NeuroImage **44**(4), 1415–1422 (2009)
7. Ritter, K., et al.: Multimodal prediction of conversion to Alzheimer's disease based on incomplete biomarkers. Alzheimer's Dement. Diagn. Assess. Dis. Monit. **1**(2), 206–215 (2015)
8. Shi, J., et al.: Multimodal neuroimaging feature learning with multimodal stacked deep polynomial networks for diagnosis of Alzheimer's disease. IEEE JBHI **22**(1), 173–183 (2018)
9. Tan, Q., et al.: Incomplete multi-view weak-label learning. In: IJCAI, pp. 2703–2709 (2018)
10. Thung, K.-H., Adeli, E., Yap, P.-T., Shen, D.: Stability-weighted matrix completion of incomplete multi-modal data for disease diagnosis. In: Ourselin, S., Joskowicz, L., Sabuncu, M.R., Unal, G., Wells, W. (eds.) MICCAI 2016. LNCS, vol. 9901, pp. 88–96. Springer, Cham (2016). https://doi.org/10.1007/978-3-319-46723-8_11
11. Thung, K.H., et al.: Conversion and time-to-conversion predictions of mild cognitive impairment using low-rank affinity pursuit denoising and matrix completion. Med. Image Anal. **45**, 68–82 (2018)
12. Tong, T., Gray, K., Gao, Q., Chen, L., Rueckert, D.: Multi-modal classification of Alzheimer's disease using nonlinear graph fusion. Pattern Recogn. **63**, 171–181 (2017)
13. Troyanskaya, O., Cantor, M., et al.: Missing value estimation methods for DNA microarrays. Bioinformatics **17**(6), 520–525 (2001)

14. Wang, J., Wang, Q., Zhang, H., Chen, J., Wang, S., Shen, D.: Sparse multiview task-centralized ensemble learning for asd diagnosis based on age-and sex-related functional connectivity patterns. IEEE Trans. Cybern. **49**(8), 3141–3154 (2018)
15. Wang, Z., Liu, C., Cheng, D., Wang, L., Yang, X., Cheng, K.T.: Automated detection of clinically significant prostate cancer in mp-MRI images based on an end-to-end deep neural network. IEEE Trans. Med. Imaging **37**(5), 1127–1139 (2018)
16. Xiang, S., Yuan, L., Fan, W., Wang, Y., Thompson, P.M., Ye, J.: Bi-level multi-source learning for heterogeneous block-wise missing data. NeuroImage **102**, 192–206 (2014)
17. Zhang, C., Hu, Q., et al.: Latent multi-view subspace clustering. In: IEEE CVPR, pp. 4279–4287 (2017)
18. Zhou, T., Liu, M., Thung, K.H., Shen, D.: Latent representation learning for Alzheimers disease diagnosis with incomplete multi-modality neuroimaging and genetic data. IEEE Trans. Med. Imaging (2019)
19. Zhou, T., Thung, K.H., Zhu, X., Shen, D.: Effective feature learning and fusion of multimodality data using stage wise deep neural network for dementia diagnosis. Hum. Brain Mapp. **40**(3), 1001–1016 (2019)
20. Zhou, T., Thung, K.H., Liu, M., Shen, D.: Brain-wide genome-wide association study for Alzheimer's disease via joint projection learning and sparse regression model. IEEE Trans. Biomed. Eng. **66**(1), 165–175 (2018)

Preprocessing, Prediction and Significance: Framework and Application to Brain Imaging

Martin Nørgaard[1,2], Brice Ozenne[1,4], Claus Svarer[1,2],
Vibe G. Frokjaer[1], Martin Schain[1], Stephen C. Strother[5],
and Melanie Ganz[1,3(✉)]

[1] Neurobiology Research Unit, Rigshospitalet, Copenhagen, Denmark
mganz@nru.dk
[2] Faculty of Health and Medical Sciences, University of Copenhagen,
Copenhagen, Denmark
[3] Department of Computer Science, University of Copenhagen,
Copenhagen, Denmark
[4] Department of Biostatistics, University of Copenhagen, Copenhagen, Denmark
[5] Rotman Research Institute, Baycrest, University of Toronto, Toronto, Canada

Abstract. Brain imaging studies have set the stage for measuring brain function in psychiatric disorders, such as depression, with the goal of developing effective treatment strategies. However, data arising from such studies are often hampered by noise confounds such as motion-related artifacts, affecting both the spatial and temporal correlation structure of the data. Failure to adequately control for these types of noise can have significant impact on subsequent statistical analyses. In this paper, we demonstrate a framework for extending the non-parametric testing of statistical significance in predictive modeling by including a plausible set of preprocessing strategies to measure the predictive power. Our approach adopts permutation tests to estimate how likely we are to obtain a given predictive performance in an independent sample, depending on the preprocessing strategy used to generate the data. We demonstrate and apply the framework on examples of longitudinal Positron Emission Tomography (PET) data following a pharmacological intervention.

1 Introduction

Modern neuroimaging studies are complicated and comprised of many steps including subject selection, data acquisition, preprocessing and some form of statistical analysis. In the past decade, there has been a growing concern about the validity and reproducibility of produced findings in such studies, and this has largely been attributed to low statistical power, software errors and flexible data analysis strategies [1,10].

Data sharing initiatives such as OpenNeuro (openneuro.org) are now enabling researchers to open up the subject selection and data acquisition factors of a

© Springer Nature Switzerland AG 2019
D. Shen et al. (Eds.): MICCAI 2019, LNCS 11767, pp. 196–204, 2019.
https://doi.org/10.1007/978-3-030-32251-9_22

study by sharing raw image data publicly. Statistical analysis tools are also widely available in the major neuroimaging software packages (e.g. SPM, FSL, AFNI and FreeSurfer) or on GitHub, and the outputs of statistical analyses can be shared (e.g. on Neurovault). Furthermore, the analysis and statistical methods have been under intense scrutiny in the last years and concerns about errors in software packages as well as in the appropriate application of statistical methods have been heatedly discussed [2,4].

Conversely, the influence of preprocessing on the outcome of the data analysis has besides a few initiatives in fMRI [2,3] been an overlooked factor. Many laboratories have set up preprocessing pipelines that are used for all their studies and large research collaborations such as the Human Brain Project (HBP) have implemented a single preprocessing pipeline[1] that is used daily to extract features from subjects enrolled in neuroscience research studies. Hence, while researchers are focusing intensely on new statistical model development, the interaction of different types of preprocessing steps with the following statistical analysis is largely ignored [3].

One solution to limit the "researcher degrees of freedom" that has been proposed is the pre-registration of complete analysis pipelines e.g. with the Open Science Framework or AsPredicted [10]. The argument for pre-registration is that researchers should not be constrained to a single analysis method, but rather pre-define which approach they will use. Additionally, there might not even exist a single best workflow for all studies of a given type, even though there is evidence that different workflows might be optimal for different studies or even for different individuals [3]. However, at the same time it seems to be implausible that out of thousands of possible workflows only the chosen pre-registered one would be able to show a true biological effect. It is much more likely that a range of different processing pipelines would have yielded the same conclusion of a given study. In the case of a strong effect, one might even hope that most processing pipelines - so no matter how the data has been preprocessed - would be able to detect the effect. Hence, it is also of interest to analyze not only the variance arising from the preprocessing [2,3], but to take the step further and analyze the variance that different preprocessing pipelines add to the statistical analysis of a study and its conclusions. On the one hand, this approach can highlight spurious findings due to a specific preprocessing pipeline, since most preprocessing pipelines would not be able to produce the same result. On the other, it can also give strong evidence for an effect if most preprocessing pipelines arrive at the same or very similar result.

In this work, we present a comprehensive framework to test the influence of preprocessing choices on the subsequent statistical analysis. We demonstrate how the choice of preprocessing can affect our belief in the available sample data, $\mathbf{x}$, with class labels y, to generalize to the true underlying joint distribution $p(\mathbf{x}, y)$. Our approach adopts a range of preprocessing choices as a generative model for $\mathbf{x}$, and evaluates the predictive performance for the conditional distribution $p(y|\mathbf{x})$ using permutations [6] and the maximum statistic [8]. By permuting and

---

[1] See https://github.com/HBPMedical/mri-preprocessing-pipeline.

evaluating across preprocessing choices, the framework provides a measure of how likely we are to obtain the observed prediction by chance, only because the preprocessing strategy interacted with the predictive model to identify a pattern that happened to correlate with the class labels. We first detail the framework and then give an example of its application based on a published study involving the serotonin transporter and PET imaging [5].

2   Non-parametric Framework for Joining Multiple Preprocessing Strategies with Prediction

The framework that we are proposing can roughly be broken into three major components: (**A**) definition of a subset of equally plausible preprocessing strategies, (**B1**) definition of the set of predictive models and the performance metric, (**B2**) cross validation to select the optimal predictive model and estimate the prediction, and (**C**) estimation of the statistical significance of the prediction accuracy (Fig. 1).

2.1   Defining a Subset of Preprocessing Strategies

In all fields of neuroimaging, before any statistical model is applied to a given data set $\{(\mathbf{x}_n, y_n)\}_{n=1}^{N}$, with N observations, the data is commonly preprocessed using a set of steps such as motion correction, co-registration and partial volume correction (Fig. 1A). The data set $\mathbf{x}_n \in \mathbf{R}^p$ are observations with p features and $y_n \in \{-1, 1\}$ are the corresponding class labels. The entire sequence of preprocessing steps is often referred to as a pipeline, designed to remove artifacts and noise from the data. Designing the optimal sequence of preprocessing steps is a challenging problem, mainly due to the high dimensionality of the data and due to the complex spatio-temporal noise structure. Therefore, several preprocessing algorithms have been proposed and refined over the years, with limited consensus in the community on the optimal strategy. The preprocessed data can for pipeline j be defined as $\{(\mathbf{x}_{n,j}, y_n)\}_{n=1}^{N}$.

2.2   Model Selection and Cross-Validation

Once the data has been preprocessed it is ready for statistical analysis. Next, we need to (1) select a predictive model and tune the model parameters to the data, and (2) assess the chosen predictive model by estimating its ability to predict on unseen data. For both (1) and (2), one common approach is to use cross-validation and evaluate the model in an independent test set (Fig. 1B). For this purpose, the data has to be randomly divided into a training data set and validation set. The training data may be further split into an inner cross-validation loop (nested cross-validation) [11]. Finally, the entire cross-validation has to be repeated M times to obtain an unbiased mean predictive accuracy. This approach aligns with community guidelines on model selection and cross-validation [11].

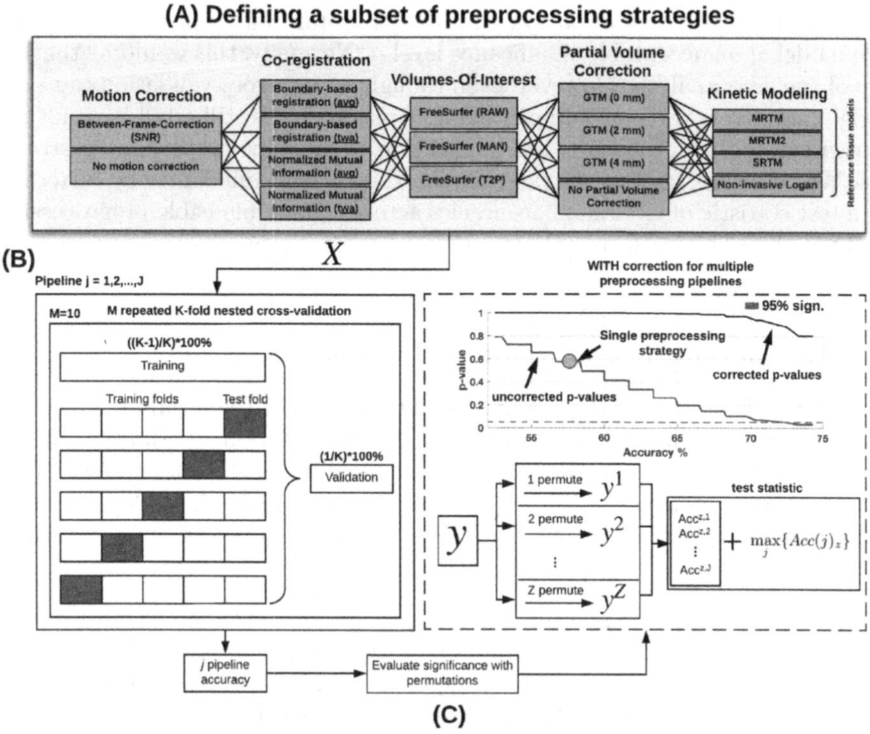

(A) Defining a subset of preprocessing strategies

Fig. 1. (**A**) Definition of a subset of preprocessing strategies $j = 1, ..., J$: This includes preprocessing steps such as motion correction, co-registration, delineation of volumes of interest, partial volume correction, and kinetic modeling. (**B**) Model selection and cross-validation: For each pipeline j, select a classification model (e.g. Linear Discriminant), and a K-fold nested cross-validation scheme with M repetitions. (**C**) Evaluate the significance with permutations: Randomly permute the class labels $y \in \{-1, 1\}$, and re-run (B) for each pipeline j to obtain a classification accuracy for the $z = 1, .., Z$ permutation. For each permutation z select the maximum accuracy across all preprocessing pipelines J and for Z permutations generate a null-distribution of maximum accuracies. Use the null-distribution of the max-accuracies to obtain the p-value for each pipeline at a significance level α. NOTE: uncorrected p-values refer to original accuracies according to their permuted null-distribution at a significance level α.

2.3 Permutation Test for a Single Pipeline

Once a model has been selected and evaluated to provide a predictive accuracy, the gold standard is to estimate the statistical significance of the observed accuracy using permutations (Fig. 1C). The significance of each model and pipeline is estimated by randomly permuting the class labels Z times (i.e., sampling a permutation z from a uniform distribution π^z over the set, $\mathbf{\Pi}_N$, of all permutations of indices $1, ..., N$) and re-running the above M times repeated K-fold cross-validation procedure, and after Z replications generate an empirical null-distribution. This distribution may be used to obtain an empirical p-value for each model at an acceptable significance level α. Normally, this would be the last step of the data analysis. However, even though nested cross-validation can tune model parameters while avoiding circularity bias, there is still a hidden multiple comparison problem following the application of different preprocessing strategies. We therefore propose an extension to the current guidelines, by introducing a test statistic of maximum accuracies across equally plausible preprocessing pipelines. This approach should have a strong control over experiment-wise type I error.

2.4   Permutation Test for Multiple Pipelines

Rather than computing the permutation distribution of the accuracy for a single preprocessing pipeline j, we compute the permutation distribution of the maximum accuracy across all preprocessing pipelines. Let $\mathbf{\Pi}_N$ be a set of all permutations of indices $1, ..., N$, where N is the number of independent observations in the data set. The permutation test procedure that consists of Z iterations is defined as follows:

- Repeat Z times (with index $z = 1, ..., Z$)
    - sample a permutation π^z from a uniform distribution over $\mathbf{\Pi}_N$
    - compute the accuracy for each pipeline j for this permutation of labels
    - save the maximum accuracy across all pipelines J

$$t^z_{max} = \max_j \{Acc(\mathbf{x}_{1,j}, y_{\pi^z_1}, ..., \mathbf{x}_{N,j}, y_{\pi^z_N})\}$$

- Construct an empirical cumulative distribution of maximum accuracies

$$\hat{P}_{max}(T \leq t) = \frac{1}{Z} \sum_{1=z}^{Z} \Theta(t - t^z_{max})$$

where Θ is a Heaviside step function ($\Theta(x) = 1$, if $x \geq 0$; 0 otherwise).
- Compute the accuracy for the true labels (non-permuted) for each pipeline j, $t_{0,j} = Acc(\mathbf{x}_{1,j}, y_1, ..., \mathbf{x}_{N,j}, y_N)$, and its corresponding p-value p^j_0 under the empirical distribution $\hat{P}_{max}$.

In our case, the null hypothesis assumes that the two classes have identical distributions, $\forall \mathbf{x} : p(\mathbf{x}|y = 1) = p(\mathbf{x}|y = -1)$, hence we deal with class balanced data. We reject the null hypothesis at level α if the accuracy for the true labeling of the data is in the α times 100% of the permuted distribution of the maximum accuracy. We can reject the null hypothesis for any preprocessing pipeline with an accuracy exceeding this threshold.

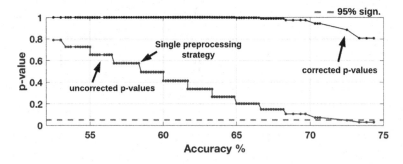

Fig. 2. Accuracy as a function of p-value for 384 preprocessing strategies. The blue dots indicate the p-value for each pipeline according to its permuted null distribution (uncorrected) and the black dots indicate the p-value according to the maximum permuted null distribution (corrected). The red dotted line is the 95% significance level.

2.5   Use of the Maximum Statistic in Neuroimaging

Correction of p-values using the maximum statistic has been used before in statistical studies of neuroimaging data [7,8]. Furthermore, several studies have examined the effects of multiple preprocessing options in combination with prediction [2,3]. The latter studies mainly focused on increasing predictive accuracy by examining multiple preprocessing strategies, but did not evaluate the prediction relative to random. Our work extends the non-parametric testing of statistical significance in predictive modeling by including a plausible set of preprocessing strategies to measure the predictive power.

3   Experiments

We illustrate the use of the framework in an experiment with data from a longitudinal PET study with a baseline and a re-scan, following a pharmacological intervention [5]. This data is publicly available through the CIMBI database (www.cimbi.dk). The data, $\mathbf{x}$, consists of 60 observations (30 baseline and 30 intervention scans) each with levels of serotonin transporter binding (BP$_{\mathrm{ND}}$) in 34 cortical brain regions covering the entire neocortex. The corresponding class labels are $y_n \in \{baseline, intervention\}$. For quantification of BP$_{\mathrm{ND}}$, we preprocessed the data using a fixed sequence of five preprocessing steps, each with varying parameter choices: (1) motion correction (with/without), (2) co-registration (four choices), (3) delineation of volumes-of-interest (three choices), (4) partial volume correction (four choices), and (5) kinetic modeling for quantification of BP$_{\mathrm{ND}}$ (MRTM, SRTM, Non-invasive Logan and MRTM2). This results in $2 \times 3 \times 4^3 = 384$ combinations of preprocessing (Fig. 1A). Details are described in [9]. In the experiment, we used a Linear Discriminant classifier to predict the classes (baseline and intervention). The number of M repeated cross-validation iterations was 10, the number of K cross-validation folds was 5, and the number of permutation iterations Z was 1,000. To obtain true independence between

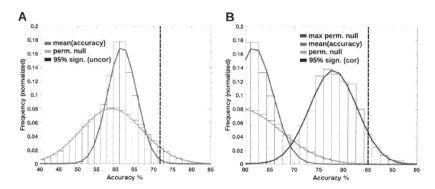

Fig. 3. (**A**) Average classification accuracies across preprocessing pipelines obtained using nested cross-validation with 10 repeats (red). The permuted null distribution of classification accuracies (1000 permutations) across preprocessing pipelines is visualized by the green distribution. The vertical dotted line is the 95% significance level of the permuted null distribution of classification accuracies across pipelines (**B**) The blue distribution is the permuted null distribution (1000 permutations) of maximum classification accuracies across preprocessing pipelines. The vertical dotted line is the 95% significance level for the permuted null distribution of maximum accuracies. (Color figure online)

the data and the labels, observations for each subject (i.e. baseline and intervention) were always stratified in the cross-validation. To summarize, the goal is to predict whether an observation in **x** is either a baseline or an intervention scan.

We start by studying the behaviour of accuracies and p-values, when varying the preprocessing strategy, reported in Fig. 2. Every point in Fig. 2 represents a preprocessing strategy with an accuracy and a p-value, either uncorrected (blue) or corrected (black). By changing the preprocessing strategy, this substantially improves the accuracy, with values ranging from 52% to 75%. There also exists a subset of preprocessing strategies that are significantly different ($p < 0.05$) from their permuted null distribution. The black line in Fig. 2 shows the p-values relative to the maximum permuted null distribution. The p-values decrease with increasing accuracy, but a much higher accuracy is needed compared to the blue line to obtain a significant p-value.

Figure 3 shows the distribution of accuracies for the estimated mean accuracies with the true labels (red), for the randomly permuted (green), and the maximum permuted (blue). Most preprocessing strategies fall within the permuted null distribution, but a subset of the preprocessing strategies are able to obtain statistical significance at $p < 0.05$ (i.e. less than 5% chance of observing better than 75% accuracy if the data and labels are truly independent). But to reject the null hypothesis under the empirical distribution of the maximum classification accuracies across pipelines, one would need an expected classification accuracy of 85% to obtain statistical significance at $\alpha = 0.05$ (Fig. 3).

4   Discussion and Conclusion

In this work, we extend the non-parametric testing of statistical significance in predictive modeling by including a plausible set of preprocessing strategies to measure the predictive power. We demonstrate its application in a longitudinal PET study. In this case, there are a few choices of preprocessing that lead to a significant prediction while the majority of preprocessing choices lead to a non-significant prediction (uncorrected). When correcting using knowledge about all the applied pipelines, no significant predictions survive (corrected using the maximum statistic).

While the statistical analysis of each individual preprocessing pipeline is carried out in an optimal fashion due to the use of M times repeated K-fold nested cross-validation, some of the preprocessing pipelines can still result in a significant prediction by chance. The reason for this can be that the preprocessing pipeline introduces spurious relations between the features and the labels, consequently overestimating the generalizability of the learning method. Our approach enables the examination of predictions across multiple preprocessing choices, providing a measure of the variance of the predictions across pipelines. Based on this we advise that care must be taken in a statistical analysis to avoid attributing an effect to a treatment/condition that was due to a single pipeline and/or predictive model.

The framework that we are proposing is not without limitations. First, while the goal of preprocessing is to factor out correlated features from the feature one is interested in, this is not necessarily a guarantee. For example, if one preprocessing strategy fails at factoring out correlated features and produces a "significant finding", and a different pipeline correctly removes correlated features and produces a "non-significant finding", this cannot be detected. This is one of the major drawbacks of data-driven selection of preprocessing strategies, and one risks drawing wrong conclusions if blindly selecting the preprocessing in a data-driven manner. In addition, as we are assuming independence between the preprocessing choices, one could worry that the effect we are observing, is simply due to the effect of assigning too much probability mass to strategies that no one would ever use. However, if we assume that all the included strategies are equally likely to be used, the proposed framework provides the researcher with a strong belief in the prediction under a set of plausible preprocessing strategies. This belief is both useful for the researcher carrying out the study, but also for colleagues reviewing the work for publication, as the impact of minor variations in acquisition/preprocessing is challenging to evaluate. The framework is also very flexible, and may be expanded to include a larger subset of preprocessing pipelines, a larger subset of features, but also a larger subset of statistical models (SVM, ANOVA, t-test etc.) with varying model complexities. However, it is noteworthy that the inclusion of more pipelines will also broaden the permuted null distribution further due to increased noise, so an increase in the number of pipelines will punish the ability to obtain statistical significance for any pipeline. The main point we hope to convey is that in future studies, researchers should not only pre-register their preprocessing or analysis as proposed by [10], but should also provide the variance of their results across a set of plausible preprocessing pipelines by using our framework. Because data acquisition is the most costly part of any experiment, spending resources on computing power by employing a framework as we propose is negligible in comparison. For future work, we still need to find a way of assigning appropriate non-uniform probability mass to strategies with different levels of relevance, otherwise we risk that the variance of the null distribution of maximum accuracies will be grossly overestimated. However, this is beyond the scope of this paper, and is left for future work.

References

1. Button, K.S., et al.: Power failure: why small sample size undermines the reliability of neuroscience. Nat. Rev. Neurosci. **14**(5), 365 (2013)
2. Carp, J.: On the plurality of (methodological) worlds: estimating the analytic flexibility of fMRI experiments. Front. Neurosci. **6**, 149 (2012)
3. Churchill, N.W., et al.: An automated, adaptive framework for optimizing preprocessing pipelines in task-based functional MRI. PLoS ONE **10**(7), e0131520 (2015)
4. Eklund, A., et al.: Cluster failure: why fMRI inferences for spatial extent have inflated false-positive rates. PNAS **113**(28), 7900–7905 (2016)
5. Frokjaer, V.G., et al.: Role of serotonin transporter changes in depressive responses to sex-steroid hormone manipulation: a positron emission tomography study. Biol. Psychiatry **78**(8), 534–543 (2015)
6. Golland, P., Fischl, B.: Permutation tests for classification: towards statistical significance in image-based studies. In: Taylor, C., Noble, J.A. (eds.) IPMI 2003. LNCS, vol. 2732, pp. 330–341. Springer, Heidelberg (2003). https://doi.org/10.1007/978-3-540-45087-0_28
7. Holmes, A.P., et al.: Nonparametric analysis of statistic images from functional mapping experiments. JCBFM **16**(1), 7–22 (1996)
8. Nichols, T.E., Holmes, A.P.: Nonparametric permutation tests for functional neuroimaging: a primer with examples. Hum. Brain Mapp. **15**(1), 1–25 (2002)
9. Nørgaard, M., et al.: Optimization of preprocessing strategies in Positron Emission Tomography (PET) neuroimaging: a [11C] DASB study. NeuroImage **199**, 466–479 (2019)
10. Poldrack, R.A., et al.: Scanning the horizon: towards transparent and reproducible neuroimaging research. Nat. Rev. Neurosci. **18**(2), 115 (2017)
11. Varoquaux, G., et al.: Assessing and tuning brain decoders: cross-validation, caveats, and guidelines. NeuroImage **145**, 166–179 (2017)

Early Prediction of Alzheimer's Disease Progression Using Variational Autoencoders

Sumana Basu[1,2]($\boxtimes$), Konrad Wagstyl[3], Azar Zandifar[1], Louis Collins[1], Adriana Romero[1], and Doina Precup[1,2]

[1] School of Computer Science, McGill University, Montreal, Canada
{sumana.basu,azar.zandifar}@mail.mcgill.ca, louis.collins@mcgill.ca, adriana.romsor@gmail.com, dprecup@cs.mcgill.ca
[2] Mila, Montreal, Canada
[3] Department of Psychiatry, University of Cambridge, Cambridge, UK
kw350@cam.ac.uk

Abstract. Prediction of Alzheimer's disease before the onset of symptoms is an important clinical challenge, as it offers the potential for earlier intervention to interrupt disease progression before the development of dementia symptoms, as well as spur new prevention and treatment avenues. In this work, we propose a model that learns how to predict Alzheimer's disease *ahead of time* from *structural Magnetic Resonance Imaging* (sMRI) data. The contributions of this work are two-fold: (i) We use the latent variables learned by our model to visualize areas of the brain, which contribute to confident decisions. Our model appears to be focusing on specific areas of the neocortex, cerebellum, and brainstem, which are known to be clinically relevant. (ii) There are various ways in which disease might evolve from a patient's current physiological state. We can leverage the latent variables in our model to capture the uncertainty over possible future patient outcomes. It can help identify and closely monitor people who are at a higher risk of disease, despite the current lack of clinical indications.

Keywords: Alzheimer's disease · Disease evolution prediction · Uncertainty · 3-dimensional relevance map

1 Introduction

Alzheimer's disease (AD) is a progressive, neurodegenerative disease that causes irreversible damage to the brain tissue. It impairs the ability to form and retrieve memories, and eventually disrupts the natural flow of life, by affecting the ability to carry out even daily activities. The disease is diagnosed from a history of cognitive decline and clinical cognitive testing (e.g., Mini-Mental State Examination [8]). MMSE indicates an impairment in cognitive abilities rather than the structural changes in the brain that cause it. However, cognitive changes can be

© Springer Nature Switzerland AG 2019
D. Shen et al. (Eds.): MICCAI 2019, LNCS 11767, pp. 205–213, 2019.
https://doi.org/10.1007/978-3-030-32251-9_23

relatively non-specific, and there is increasing evidence that neuropathological changes begin decades before the manifestation of the symptoms [13].

On post mortem histology, Alzheimer's pathology is characterized by neu-rofibrillary tangles and amyloid plaques, with associated neuronal loss and atro-phy [22]. There is a broad pattern of progression from early entorhinal changes with subsequent hippocampal and later neocortical atrophy [3]. However, it is impossible to acquire a longitudinal histological characterization of patients. Therefore, while histology remains the gold standard for confirming AD, the development of in vivo diagnostic and staging methods is essential for under-standing disease etiology and improving medical management. Using Magnetic Resonance Imaging (MRI), it is possible to capture in vivo morphological brain changes in AD, without the radiation risks associated with Positron Emission Tomography (PET). Visually, on MRI, AD is associated with cortical atrophy, ventricular enlargement, and hippocampal shrinkage. Using computational tech-niques, it has become possible to detect more subtle and informative quantitative changes such as hippocampal volume loss and cortical thinning [7]. While com-putational techniques enable detection and quantification of changes too subtle for conventional visual analysis, they are generally driven by subjectively chosen imaging features, such as cortical thickness. In this work, we aim to predict a sub-ject's *future* Alzheimer's disease progression from their *structural MRI* (sMRI). Specifically, we aim to build a model able to predict an individual's disease-state (Healthy/AD) *6 months after the MRI scan was acquired*. Because the disease exhibits large variability across the population, we use a deep generative model, the variational auto-encoder (VAE) [14], because it produces latent variables which are probabilistic and can be sampled. We leverage these variables in two different ways: (i) to visualize the areas of the brain which are the focus of attention in the model for particular patients (ii) to quantify the distribution of possible disease evolution paths for a given patient, and to produce an empirical risk measure which can inform early interventions. Results on the Alzheimer's Disease Neuroimaging Initiative (ADNI) dataset [19] suggest that the sMRI con-tains useful information for predicting patient transition to AD ahead of time, generating data-driven areas of importance for different stages of disease pro-gression and highlighting the potential of distribution-based models to identify currently healthy cases which may require additional monitoring.

2   Related Work

ADNI [19] is a multimodal longitudinal dataset launched in 2003. Alexiou et al. [2] used Bayesian models to assess the association of different biomarkers such as hippocampal volume loss, Tau protein aggregation etc. with disease progression. Ortiz et al. [20] applied Sparse Inverse Covariance Estimation [10] methods to understand the functional and structural relationships of different brain regions in the context of AD. Wolz et al. [27] fused features such as hippocampal volume, tensor-based morphometry and cortical thickness to train a classifier based on Support Vector Machine and Linear Discriminant Analysis. Other works, includ-ing [16,17,25], extracted neural network-based features from multiple modalities

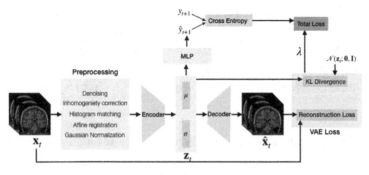

Fig. 1. Flow diagram for training.

such as sMRI and PET to predict future conversion to AD from healthy and mildly impaired cognitive state. However, the requirement of multiple diagnostic tests imposes a financial burden on the patient. Several works [11,12,21] used Convolutional Neural Networks (CNN) to classify patients into healthy and AD at the current time point (not predicting future evolution). Such methods can exhibit high accuracy but do not produce actual identifiable biomarkers. Finally, significant effort has also been devoted to showing that sMRI contains important information for the early prediction of AD [1].

3   Proposed Method

We denote an MRI taken at time step t by $\mathbf{x_t} \in \mathcal{R}^{D \times H \times W}$, where D is depth, H is height and W is width of the 3 dimensional (3D) scan. Our goal is to predict the disease label $y_{t+1} \in \{0, 1\}$ for the next scan (taken at time step $t+1$). We propose to model y_{t+1} by means of a generative classifier because discriminative models fail to capture the fact that progression depends on various factors and hence, a patient might evolve in various ways from their current physiological state. In contrast, generative classifiers model the distribution over possible disease progressions, providing a measure of *risk* for each patient. We define risk as the empirical probability of a healthy person getting diagnosed with either Mild Cognitive Impairment (MCI) or AD at the next time point $t + 1$. In particular, we propose to use Variational Autoencoder (VAE) [14] as the backbone for our model. VAEs learn a posterior distribution, from which we can sample multiple times.

Figure 1 depicts the proposed model, which consists of a 3D convolutional variational encoder q_ϕ that approximates the true posterior $p_\theta(\mathbf{z}_t|\mathbf{x}_t)$ as $q_\phi(\mathbf{z}_t|\mathbf{x}_t)$, a 3D convolutional decoder p_θ that calculates the reconstruction loss, and a Multi-Layer Perceptron (MLP) d_φ that predicts the likelihood of the next disease label $d_\varphi(y_{t+1}|\mathbf{z}_t)$. As in [14], we assume the prior over latent space $p_\theta(\mathbf{z}_t)$ to be isotropic multivariate Gaussian $\mathcal{N}(\mathbf{z}_t; \mathbf{0}, \mathbf{I})$ and the posterior to be a multivariate Gaussian with diagonal covariance $\mathcal{N}(\mathbf{z}_t; \mu, \sigma^2\mathbf{I})$. The objective of the

Table 1. Performance on the test set.

Model	Parameters	Accuracy	F1-score	Cross-entropy
CNN	97.34M	77.35%	0.71	0.48
CNN-AE	98.43M	81.93%	0.78	0.46
VAE	74.9M	$74.40 \pm 0.01\%$	0.66	0.73

MLP is to minimize the cross-entropy loss $\mathcal{L}_{CE}$. We train an end-to-end model by minimizing:

$$\mathcal{L}(\phi, \theta, \varphi; \mathbf{x}_t, \mathbf{y}_{t+1}) = \mathcal{L}_{CE} + \frac{\lambda}{2} \sum_{j=1}^{J} \left(1 + \log \sigma_j^2 - \mu_j^2 - \mu_j^2 - \sigma_j^2 \right) + ||\mathbf{x}_t - \hat{\mathbf{x}}_t||_2^2 \quad (1)$$

where J is the latent dimension and $\hat{\mathbf{x}}$ the reconstructed image. During inference, we calculate $p(\hat{y}|\mathbf{x}; \phi, \varphi)$ to predict the probability of the disease progression.

4   Experimental Setup

4.1   Data Processing

We used 1.5 T1-weighted sMRI from the ADNI dataset [19], which are of size $233 \times 197 \times 189$ and are mapped to two classes based on diagnosis at timestep $t + 1$: Healthy/Diseased (Diseased class includes both MCI and AD patients)[1]. We grouped the MCI and AD classes from the original data in order to have more cases in the disease category, and in order to avoid arbitrary, noisy labels.

All images went through a preprocessing pipeline, consisting of denoising [5], inhomogeneity correction using N3 [24], intensity normalization using histogram matching between the image and the average template, and an affine registration to ICBM152 template space with $1 \times 1 \times 1$ mm^3 resolution [4]. In this study, a population-specific template from the ADNI-1 database has been used [9]. Eventually, image intensities were normalized within each image and among the whole database. Final images are of $233 \times 197 \times 189$ voxels. We considered 4046 MRIs from 1092 patients, for whom at least 2 MRIs were available throughout the course of the study and split the data into 8:1:1 ratio at the patient level[2]. Training, validation and test set consists of 3257, 396 and 393 MRIs from 873, 109 and 110 patients, respectively. In the test set, 145 out of 393 are diseased.

4.2   Implementation Details

As a discriminative baseline, we trained a 3D CNN with binary cross-entropy loss. The model uses the same architecture as the encoder and classifier head of

---

[1] Each MRI is associated with the label of the next MRI of the same patient.

[2] All the MRIs corresponding to a patient in the training set lie in the training set only.

our VAE model. As a second baseline, we regularized the CNN with the reconstruction loss. This model has an associated decoder, with the same architecture as the decoder network of the VAE. We call this model CNN-AE.

All the models are trained with Adam optimizer, with $\beta_1 = 0.9, \beta_2 = 0.999, \epsilon = e^{-08}$ and a learning rate of 0.0001, which was reduced by a factor of 10 after 15, 25 and 35 epochs. Dropout of 0.2 was added to all CNN layers along with ReLU activation. The reconstruction hyper-parameter was set to 2.5 for CNN-AE. All the optimization and architecture hyper-parameters were chosen using cross-validation. The encoder consists of four 3D CNN layers and the decoder consists of four transposed CNN layers, all with filters of size $3 \times 3 \times 3$. Each layer in the encoder and decoder is followed by 3D max pooling and batch-normalization operations. The dimension of the latent space is 1024. Finally, the MLP is composed of two fully connected layers with 4096 dimensions followed by a classification layer.

5   Results and Discussion

5.1   Quantitative Results

Performance Analysis. Classification performance on the test set is reported in Table 1 and Fig. 3. As shown in the table, CNN-AE provides the best accuracy and F1-score. The high cross-entropy loss in the VAE is due to the fact that maximizing the likelihood of the target labels is not its sole objective, and the model loss is dominated by the Kullback-Leibler (KL) divergence. Similarly, cross-entropy is low for the discriminative classifiers, but high for VAE classifier. Figure 2 depicts the t-Distributed Stochastic Neighbor Embedding (t-SNE) [18] plots of the representations extracted from the final fully connected layers of the models. From the Figure, CNN and CNN-AE learns distinctly separated clusters of embeddings. This leads to mis-classification of the boundary cases. VAE on the other hand learns a Gaussian distribution and hence acts as a soft classifier for the overlapping cases. The Receiver operating characteristic (ROC) curves for all models, depicted in Fig. 3 show that the Area Under the Curve (AUC) of the VAE and CNN are comparable, even though the CNN has a better F1-score.

Risk Analysis. For each MRI in the test set, we draw 100 samples from the latent space of the trained VAE and predict the corresponding future disease status. As depicted in Table 2, the model suggests 59.27% patients are not at risk, but rest of the patients are at varying degree of risk. We repeat the same experiment for discriminative baselines by sampling from the softmax output distribution. As shown in the table, CNN and CNN-AE consider most of the patients in the test set are at risk, predicting only 2.79% and 9.16% of the cases at no risk. To validate the claims of the models, we extracted the patient data which had labels for timestep $t + 2$, which turned out for only 40% of the full test set. In this subset, we did not find any example of disease progression from healthy to diseased state, suggesting the prediction of the VAE is closer

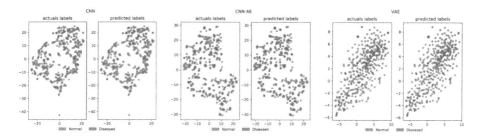

Fig. 2. Pre-activation t-SNE embedding of thee final layer of the classifier on test set. 2 principal components are visualized.

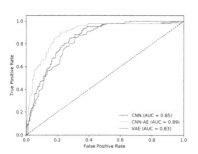

Fig. 3. Test set ROC curve.

Table 2. Percentage risk of currently healthy patients, based on 100 sample prediction on each MRI in the test set.

Risk band	VAE	CNN	CNN-AE
0	59.27%	2.79%	9.16%
1–19	16.13%	32.82%	29.51%
20–39	5.24%	11.19%	9.16%
40–59	2.42%	21.12%	15.52%
60–79	2.82%	22.90%	23.16%
80–100	14.11%	9.16%	13.49%

to the test data statistics. The patients indicated as being at risk by the VAE can be followed more closely, since they are fewer than for the CNN, and early intervention may prevent future problems.

5.2 Qualitative Results

Visualization of the features on which the model focuses is important for interpretability and can also aid clinicians discover new biomarkers of the disease. Akin to [28], we visualized the 3D relevance map of the final encoder layer conditioned on the input MRI. For the relevance maps visualized in Fig. 4, the model makes decisions with more than 90% confidence. Visually, the model appears to be focusing on specific areas of the neocortex, cerebellum and brainstem. Based on cognitive labels alone, the network learned that patterns of structural change, most likely relating to cerebral atrophy, are predictive of future AD diagnosis. These findings are consistent with neuroimaging and post mortem analyses of that have demonstrated a link between cognitive symptom burden and pathology in the brainstem [23], cerebellum [26], and neocortex, particularly in the temporo-parietal cortex [7]. Interestingly, the hippocampus and entorhinal cortex, which are associated with neuropathological change in Alzheimer's [3], did not emerge as areas with high relevance. These discrepancies may in part be due to the predictive nature of the task. Most neuroimaging studies have looked

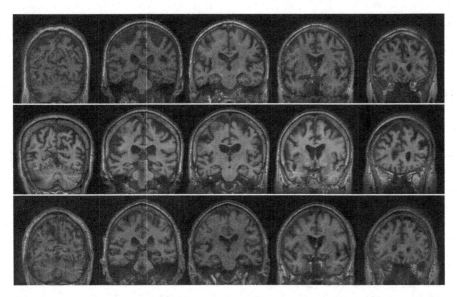

Fig. 4. Relevance maps for 3 subjects. Row 1: HL at baseline, HL at follow-up, row 2: HL at baseline, AD at follow-up, row 3: AD at baseline, AD at follow-up. Consistent areas of relevance include cerebellum (column 1), neocortex (columns 2–4) and brain stem (column 2).

at measures that correlate with current cognitive symptoms. In contrast, our network is trained to predict future cognitive state. Thus, the areas highlighted by these maps are learned as static biomarkers of a dynamic disease process.

One limitation of these maps is that they are regionally specific, but give no indication of what features the network is identifying in these areas. Future work is necessary to explore in more detail how the cerebral anatomy is changing. Nevertheless, data-driven maps are useful to corroborate existing targeted neuroanatomical markers in AD and to highlight areas for further research.

6   Conclusion

Based on our results, VAEs are a promising alternative to predict early the potential AD progression. The relevance maps from our trained models showed that the model pays attention correctly to areas of the brain affected by AD. The results also show the potential of our approach to detect healthy patients which may require close follow-up. Future directions include learning a predictive model based on past image acquisitions, reminiscent of recent work on video generation [6] or segmentation of ambiguous medical images [15]. Training similar models on skull stripped images to classify MCI and AD and further validation of this model on other, larger datasets would also be very useful.

Acknowledgement. This work was generously funded by Healthy Brains for Healthy Lives (HBHL) through CFREF grant. We would also like to thank Koustuv Sinha for useful discussions, comments and reviews of the manuscript.

References

1. Adaszewski, S., et al.: How early can we predict Alzheimer's disease using computational anatomy? Neurobiol. Aging **34**(12), 2815–2826 (2013)
2. Alexiou, A., et al.: A Bayesian model for the prediction and early diagnosis of Alzheimer's disease. Front. Aging Neurosci. **9**, 77 (2017)
3. Braak, H., Braak, E.: Staging of Alzheimer's disease-related neurofibrillary changes. Neurobiol. Aging **16**(3), 271–278 (1995)
4. Collins, D.L., et al.: Automatic 3D intersubject registration of mr volumetric data in standardized talairach space. J. Comput. Assist. Tomogr. **18**(2), 192–205 (1994)
5. Coupé, P., et al.: An optimized blockwise nonlocal means denoising filter for 3-D magnetic resonance images. IEEE Trans. Med. Imaging **27**(4), 425–441 (2008)
6. Denton, E., Fergus, R.: Stochastic video generation with a learned prior. In: ICML, vol. 80, pp. 1174–1183 (2018)
7. Dickerson, B.C., et al.: The cortical signature of Alzheimer's disease: regionally specific cortical thinning relates to symptom severity in very mild to mild AD dementia and is detectable in asymptomatic Amyloid-Positive individuals. Cereb. Cortex **19**(3), 497–510 (2009)
8. Folstein, M.F., et al.: Mini-mental state. A practical method for grading the cognitive state of patients for the clinician. J. Psychiatric Res. **12**(3), 189–98 (1975)
9. Fonov, V., et al.: Unbiased average age-appropriate atlases for pediatric studies. Neuroimage **54**(1), 313–327 (2011)
10. Friedman, J., et al.: Sparse inverse covariance estimation with the graphical lasso. Biostatistics **9**, 432–441 (2007)
11. Gupta, A., et al.: Natural image bases to represent neuroimaging data. In: ICML, pp. III-987–III-994 (2013)
12. Hosseini-Asl, E., et al.: Alzheimer's disease diagnostics by a deeply supervised adaptable 3D convolutional network. Front. Biosci. (Landmark Ed) **23**, 584–596 (2018)
13. Jack Jr., C.R., et al.: NIA-AA research framework: toward a biological definition of Alzheimer's disease. Alzheimers. Dement. **14**(4), 535–562 (2018)
14. Kingma, D.P., Welling, M.: Auto-encoding variational bayes. In: ICLR (2013)
15. Kohl, S.A.A., et al.: A probabilistic u-net for segmentation of ambiguous images. In: NeurIPS, June 2018
16. Lee, G., et al.: Predicting Alzheimer's disease progression using multi-modal deep learning approach. Sci. Rep. **9**, 1952 (2019)
17. Liu, S., et al.: Early diagnosis of Alzheimer's disease with deep learning. In: ISBI, pp. 1015–1018 (2014)
18. van der Maaten, L., Hinton, G.: Visualizing data using t-SNE. J. Mach. Learn. Res. **9**, 2579–2605 (2008)
19. Mueller, S.G., et al.: Alzheimer's disease neuroimaging initiative. Neuroimaging Clin. North Am. **15**(4), 869–877 (2005)
20. Ortiz, A., et al.: Exploratory graphical models of functional and structural connectivity patterns for Alzheimer's disease diagnosis. Front. Comput. Neurosci. **9**, 132 (2015)

21. Payan, A., Montana, G.: Predicting Alzheimer's disease: a neuroimaging study with 3D convolutional neural networks. In: ICPRAM, vol. 2 (2015)
22. Perl, D.P.: Neuropathology of Alzheimer's disease. Mt Sinai J. Med. **77**(1), 32–42 (2010)
23. Simic, G., et al.: Does Alzheimer's disease begin in the brainstem? Neuropathol. Appl. Neurobiol. **35**(6), 532–554 (2009)
24. Sled, J.G., et al.: A nonparametric method for automatic correction of intensity nonuniformity in MRI data. IEEE Trans. Med. Imaging **17**(1), 87–97 (1998)
25. Suk, H.-I., Shen, D.: Deep learning-based feature representation for AD/MCI classification. In: Mori, K., Sakuma, I., Sato, Y., Barillot, C., Navab, N. (eds.) MICCAI 2013. LNCS, vol. 8150, pp. 583–590. Springer, Heidelberg (2013). https://doi.org/10.1007/978-3-642-40763-5_72
26. Wegiel, J., et al.: Cerebellar atrophy in Alzheimer's disease-clinicopathological correlations. Brain Res. **818**(1), 41–50 (1999)
27. Wolz, R., et al.: Multi-method analysis of MRI images in early diagnostics of Alzheimer's disease. PLoS ONE **6**(10), e25446 (2011)
28. Zhou, B., et al.: Learning deep features for discriminative localization. In: CVPR, pp. 2921–2929, June 2016

Integrating Heterogeneous Brain Networks for Predicting Brain Disease Conditions

Yanfu Zhang[1], Liang Zhan[1], Weidong Cai[2], Paul Thompson[3],
and Heng Huang[1,4(✉)]

[1] Department of Electrical and Computer Engineering, University of Pittsburgh,
Pittsburgh, USA
heng.huang@pitt.edu
[2] School of Computer Science, University of Sydney, Sydney, Australia
[3] Imaging Genetics Center, Institute for Neuroimaging and Informatics,
University of Southern California, Los Angeles, USA
[4] JD Finance America Corporation, Mountain View, CA, USA

Abstract. Human brain networks convey important insights in understanding the mechanism of many mental disorders. However, it is difficult to determine a universal optimal among various tractography methods for general diagnosis tasks. To address this issue, tentative studies, aiming at the identification of some mental disorders, make an effective concession by exploiting multi-modal brain networks. In this paper, we propose to predict the clinical measures as a more comprehensive and stable assessment of brain abnormalities. We develop a graph convolutional network (GCN) framework to integrate heterogeneous brain networks. Particularly, an adaptive pooling scheme is designed, catering to the modal structural diversity and sharing the advantages of *locality, loyalty* and *likely* as in standard convolutional networks. The experimental results demonstrate that our method achieves state-of-the-art prediction results, and validates the advantages of the utilization of multi-modal brain networks in that, more modals are always at least as good as the best modal, if not better.

1 Introduction

Large-scale connection in the brains convey important insights in understanding the underlying yet unknown mechanism of many mental disorders [3,7,16]. With whole brain tractography, brain's anatomical networks represented as major fiber bundles can be reconstructed from diffusion-weighted MRI (DWI). There are various brain networks, generated from different tractography algorithms based on either voxel-wise diffusion model or cross-voxel fiber tracking, each finding the place in revealing targeted brain abnormalities, such as autism spectrum disorder [12], Parkinson's disease [4], and even in genetics. Nevertheless, for distinctive diagnosis tasks it is elusive to decide a universally optimal method and

© Springer Nature Switzerland AG 2019
D. Shen et al. (Eds.): MICCAI 2019, LNCS 11767, pp. 214–222, 2019.
https://doi.org/10.1007/978-3-030-32251-9_24

accompanied processing, e.g. dimension reduction [19], as that these tractography algorithms differ in the selection and accuracy of fiber extraction, robustness, and particularly the relevance between the extracted fiber bundles and the tasks. Essentially, tentative studies have demonstrated that multi-modal brain networks can provide complementary viewpoint toward the classification tasks, in leveraging the scattered information from acquisitions with diverse tractography algorithms. For example, it is showed that multi-view graph convolutional network [20] has state-of-the-art performance in classifying Parkinson's disease (PD) status.

To take one step further, we propose to predict the clinical measures, instead of directly classifying the disease status. The behind motivation lies in that, many mental disorders are degenerative, which can be inferred from the gradual progress of brain connectivity patterns, and that clinical measures, compared to simply classification, better capture the progress. Through integrating multi-modal brain networks in our prediction, a comprehensive assessment is constructed, and the potential deterioration from sub-optimal of single tractography is alleviated. To address the prediction problem, we resort to a cascade model, composed of a heterogeneous graph convolutional network (GCN) for brain network embeddings and a multi-layer perceptron (MLP) for regression. Our contributions are two-folded: first, we propose a heterogeneous GCN to predict the clinical scores from multi-modal brain networks, which benefits from the natural graph structures of diverse brain networks; second, an adaptive pooling scheme, driven by both graph structure and network patterns, is proposed, which is beneficial from gathering local information, yielding a faithful graph with smaller size, and enjoying efficiency in both computation and training. We name the proposed method as "heterogeneous" in that the graph convolution and pooling are customized for varied modal. The proposed method is verified on the data from the Parkinson Progression Marker Initiative (PPMI) [13], a cohort study aiming at identifying and validating PD progression markers. The experimental results show that our method outperforms related baselines significantly. It is also demonstrated that by integrating multi-modal brain networks, the proposed method achieves higher accuracy, and yields more stable prediction.

The rest of this paper is organized as follow. Sect. 2 provides the preliminary and describes the detail of the proposed method. Sect. 3 shows the experiments and the results. Sect. 4 concludes the paper.

2   Methodology

2.1   Preliminary

A graph can be represented as $\{V, E, W\}$, with $V = \{v_1, v_2, \cdots, v_n\}$ the set of n vertices, $E \subseteq V \times V$ the set of m edges, and $W \in \mathcal{R}^{n \times n}$ the weighted adjacency matrix of the graph. In this paper, vertices are Region Of Interest (ROIs). Graph Laplacian is an operation in spectral graph analysis, typically defined as $L_c = D - W$ in combinatorial form and $L_n = I_n - D^{-1/2}WD^{-1/2}$

in normalized form, with $D \in \mathcal{R}^{n \times n}$ the diagonal matrix and I_n an identity matrix. Graph convolutional network (GCN) [5] is designed as an extension of convolutional neural network (CNN), to analysis the signals on nodes, with a given graph structure. One strategy is to conduct graph convolution in frequency domain using the eigenvalue decomposition of graph Laplacian, $L = U^T \Lambda U$, and $U = [u_0, u_1, \cdots, u_{n-1}]$ specifies a Fourier basis. The graph Fourier transform [15] is then defined as $\hat{x} = U^T x$, with $x \in \mathcal{R}^n$ the signal, and the inverse transform $x = U\hat{x}$. The spectral representation of node signals, $\hat{x}$, allows the fundamental filtering operation for graphs. For computational accessibility, polynomial parametrization for localized filters [5] is proposed through learning the coefficients Θ_K of a K-order Chebyshev polynomial. The filter is defined as $g_\theta(\Lambda) = \sum_{k=0}^{K-1} \theta_k T_k(\Lambda)$, and the graph convolution is defined as $y = U g_\theta(\Lambda) U^T x$, with y the filtered signal, θ_k the trainable parameters and $T_k(\Lambda)$ the polynomials. Parallel to CNN, pooling operation in graph settings is accomplished by the graph coarsening [6] procedure. By truncating the Chebyshev polynomial to only first order, a faster version of GCN can be reformulated [11] similar to multi-layer perceptron, with each layer defined as $y = \sigma(\tilde{D}^{-1/2} \tilde{A} \tilde{D}^{-1/2} x \Theta)$, with $\tilde{A} = A + I_n$, $\tilde{D}$ accordingly defined as D, Θ the trainable parameters, and $\sigma(\cdot)$ an activation function.

In graph classification, a major concern is to represent graphs with embeddings. Previous approaches [18] include averaging all the node embeddings in a final layer, computing "virtual node" connected to all nodes, operating over sets using deep node aggregation, concatenating all embeddings, and training hierarchical structure. A majority of these methods apply a deterministic graph clustering subroutine, while some end-to-end [18,21] methods require additional structure to compute the pooling structure.

At last we want to include a short discussion on the relation of graph convolution and traditional methods. Essentially GCN is a flexible and mixed model of classical methods: it is rooted in graph spectral theory, in the manner the node signals are analyzed; meanwhile, the convolution is closely related and can be re-formulated as random-walk [8] or Weisfeiler-Lehman Method [17].

2.2   Predicting PD Clinical Scores via Heterogeneous GCN

The proposed method has two stages, as illustrated in Fig. 1. In the first stage, the per-modal embeddings for brain networks are generated via heterogeneous GCN; in the second, the concatenated embeddings are regressed to the clinical scores via MLP. Parallel to convolutional neural networks, the proposed GCN is formed by stacking graph convolutional layer and pooling layer sequentially. The fast graph convolutional [11] is applied, using corresponding rows of brain network matrix as node features. We also propose a novel efficient adaptive pooling scheme to learn data-driven pooling windows, which in turns can construct reduced while structural-preserving graphs and aggregate pooled features.

Although graph convolution is a quite established technique, pooling on graphs is challenging in many senses. A major difficulty is the structural irregularity of graph data, compared to naive application scenarios such as images. For

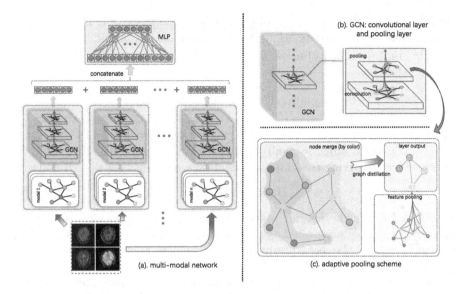

Fig. 1. The proposed heterogeneous GCN for PD clinical scores prediction. (a) illustrates the entire structure, in which multi-modal brain networks are generated from MRIs, and sequentially processed by GCN and MLP; (b) depicts the stacked convolutional layer and pooling layer; (c) provides a detailed description of the pooling procedure, including node merge, graph distillation and feature pooling.

CNNs, typically pooling layer defines the operation on a window sliding along images with strides, which shrinks the input size and augments the receptive field of convolution. However, the window and the minified graph are ambiguous due to the diverse topology. Another issue dedicated to our task is that the heterogeneity of brain networks calls for modal-specific designs. Last but not least, practical models should avoid potential computational inefficiency caused by complicated node operation. We prefer graph pooling sharing several appealing properties as CNN:

- **Locality**: The pooling windows aggregate local information from neighbor or related nodes.
- **Loyalty**: The reduced graph characterizes the structure of primary graph and data.
- **Likely**: The computation is efficient. Additionally, the data-driven pooling scheme should be end-to-end trainable, subject to deep learning principle.

To address these challenges, we imitate the process of CNN pooling, and decompose the graph pooling into two steps, node merge and graph distillation [18]. In the first step, nodes are clustered and features are computed accordingly; in the second, graph is reduced for follow-up graph convolution. Formally, the l-th pooling layer is defined as,

$$H_p^l = P^l H^l, \tag{1}$$

here $H^l \in \mathcal{R}^{n^{l-1} \times k^l}$ is the output of graph convolutional layer l, $P^l \in \mathcal{R}^{n^l \times n^{l-1}}$ is a trainable pooling matrix, $H_p^l \in \mathcal{R}^{n^l \times k^l}$ is the output of pooling layer, and n^l and k^l are the number of nodes and feature length, respectively. The reduced graph is defined as,

$$A^l = \arg\min_{A} \|A^{l-1} - P^l A P^{l^T}\|_F + f(A, x), \qquad (2)$$

here A^l is the graph matrix from layer l, and $f(A, x)$ are defined to coincide in the naive regression objective, and $\|\cdot\|_F$ is Frobenius norm. The first term can be derived by preserving the graph convolution consistency for pooled nodes,

$$U_P H_p^l \approx U P^l H^l, \qquad (3)$$

here U_P and U are the Fourier basis of after and before pooling, respectively. Naturally, it can be interpreted as the eccentricity of the reduced graph to the graph at hand, and the second term considers the data fidelity. In principle, this pooling structure is defined using P^l and A^l, learned from both graph and data.

Now we delve into the details and discuss how the aforementioned concerns are resolved through some further consideration. We decompose the pooling matrix,

$$P^l = A_p^l A^{l-1}, \qquad (4)$$

here $A_p^l \in \mathcal{R}^{n^l \times n^{l-1}}$ is a sparse assigning matrix, and each row of A_p^l represents a cluster in the reduced graph. Each cluster aggregates the vicinity of assigned nodes; meanwhile, the co-occurrence of assigned (perhaps distant) nodes represent a high-level relation beyond neighboring. Therefore, *locality* is attained by sparsity regularization related to A_p^l. *Loyalty* is also maintained via compelling A^l to satisfy (2). Combining the above arguments boils down to the objective,

$$\mathcal{L} = \|x - \hat{x}\|_F + \lambda_1 \sum_l \|A^{l-1} - P^l A^l P^{l^T}\|_F + \lambda_2 \sum_l \|A_P^l\|_1, \qquad (5)$$

here the first term is the tedious regression loss, λ_1 and λ_2 are tunable parameters. This formulation only exerts slight computation burden to naive graph convolutional layer in the inference stage; the training is also an end-to-end routine on an integral structure and avoids some potential redundancy [18]. Jointly, these indicate the *likely* of the adaptive scheme in both training and computation. Finally, each modality is dealt with using individual GCN, with modal-specified graph and pooling setup, which leads to an intuitive explanation for the effectiveness of the proposed method, that *heterogeneity* is contained in the first stage, modal-fusion in the second.

3   Experiments

3.1   Data Description

We analyzed the data from PPMI (http://www.ppmi-info.org), which includes 145 healthy controls (HC) (mean $age = 66.70 \pm 10.95$, 96 males) and 474 subjects with PD (mean age = 67.33±9.33, 318 males). No significant differences was identified in age between HC and PD ($P = 0.5$). We utilized the diffusion-weighted MRI-derived structure connectome to predict several PD clinical scores, including the Montreal Cognitive Assessment (MoCA) Test, the Tremor Dominant (TD) scores and the Postural Instability and Gait Difficulty (PIGD) scores, REM Sleep Behavior Disorder (RBD) scores, the Geriatric Depression Scale (GDS), and the University of Pennsylvania Smell Identification Test (UPSIT).

For each subject's T1-weighted MRI, we applied ROBEX, a robust automated brain extraction program trained on manually "skull-stripped" MRI data [9], to remove the extra-cerebral tissue. These skull-stripped volumes were carefully examined and manually edited if needed. Anatomical scans were then underwent the standard FreeSurfer (V6.0, http://surfer.nmr.mgh.harvard.edu/) parcellation, based on which 84 cortical and subcortical ROIs are defined.

For each subject's diffusion-weighted MRI, firstly *bet* and *eddy_correct* functions in FSL (http://www.fmrib.ox.ac.uk/fsl) were applied to remove the non-brain tissue and correct for the possible distortions, and then the gradient table was adjusted correspondingly for each subject. In order to avoid the distortions at tissue-fluid interfaces, echo-planar induced susceptibility artifacts were corrected by elastically aligning skull-stripped b0 images to each subject's T1 MRI using Advanced Normalization Tools (ANTs, http://stnava.github.io/ANTs/) with SyN algorithm. The resulted 3D deformation was then applied to the remaining diffusion-weighted volumes to generate the full preprocessed diffusion-weighted MRI data. Finally, based on the 84 ROIs derived from the T1 data, we reconstructed three brain structural graphs using three whole brain probabilistic tractography algorithms, including Orientation Distribution Function-based Hough voting [1] and PICo [14] as well as ball-and-sticks-based Probtrackx [2]. (please refer to [19] for more details). Each brain network was normalized by dividing the maximum values in the matrix to reduce the potential computation biases from the differences in scale and range from different tractography algorithms.

3.2 Experiment Settings

Throughout the experiments, ROIs are defined as vertices, the corresponding rows in each human brain networks are defined as features, and the graph is defined as the average of all brain networks. We compare the proposed method with several related methods: multivariate Ridge Regression (RR), Least Absolute Shrinkage and Selection Operator (LASSO), combined l_1 and l_2 norm (ElasticNet), Neural Networks (NN), and Convolutional Neural Network (CNN). For RR, LASSO and ElasticNet, we search the coefficient of the regularization term ranging from 0.001 to 100 and report the best results. For neural network, we use a two layer structure with 100 hidden units and Relu activation function. For the proposed method, we use two layer GCN for each modality. The feature length for each layer is [16, 32] respectively, and the graph size after pooling is [32, 8]. An one-layer perceptron is used for regression. Both λ_1 and λ_2 are set to 0.001 in the objective. We use Adam optimizer [10] with a learning rate 0.001,

Table 1. The comparison of the proposed method with baselines. For both metrics, smaller values indicate better results. The values are displayed as mean (μ) ± standard deviation (σ) from five tests. Bold font indicates the best performance.

Method	RMSE	MAE
RR	0.2382 ± 0.0069	0.1699 ± 0.0038
LASSO	0.2293 ± 0.0041	0.1613 ± 0.0033
ElasticNet	0.1969 ± 0.0011	0.1546 ± 0.0015
NN	0.1965 ± 0.0102	0.1544 ± 0.0057
CNN	0.1965 ± 0.0081	0.1545 ± 0.0049
Our method	$\mathbf{0.1922 \pm 0.0128}$	$\mathbf{0.1455 \pm 0.0064}$

and a batch size of 128. All clinical measures are normalized to $[0, 1]$ by different tests. We reported the root mean square error (RMSE) and mean absolute value (MAE) on 5-fold cross validation as the evaluation metrics.

3.3   Results

We first present the comparison of the performance of the proposed method with multiple baselines, and the results are summarized in Table 1. On both metrics, we observe that the proposed method outperforms baselines consistently. For linear methods, sparse methods achieve better prediction accuracy compared to non-sparse methods, RR. Non-linear models, including NN, CNN, and the proposed model, also improve the prediction performances against linear models in general. The baseline deep methods, NN and CNN, have similar results. Particularly, the proposed method outperforms NN with much less parameters and has better performance with similar parameter size compared to CNN.

In Table 2 we also include the prediction performance of different combination of generated graphs. Obviously, the network using single modal brain network yields much worse prediction, compared to multi-modal networks. The results also imply some interesting observations: particular subsets of involved modals may attain decent results, though the optimal combination require brutal search; the prediction yielded by the network integrating all modals, generally, is the best or at least comparable with the best. To this end it is fair to claim that multi-modality helps the prediction of PD clinical measures, and that more modals are always preferred. Besides, the brain graphs generated by *Hough* show worth-noting prediction ability, which indicates potential direction for future study.

Table 2. Predictions with different combination of modals. Values follow the instruction in Table 1. Bold font indicates the best performance.

Modality	RMSE	MAE
Hough+Probtrackx+PICo	0.1922 ± 0.0128	$\mathbf{0.1455 \pm 0.0064}$
Hough+Probtrackx	$\mathbf{0.1909 \pm 0.0111}$	0.1458 ± 0.0060
Probtrackx+PICo	0.1948 ± 0.0123	0.1472 ± 0.0067
Hough+PICo	0.1927 ± 0.0126	0.1458 ± 0.0061
Hough	0.1941 ± 0.0124	0.1470 ± 0.0071
Probtrackx	0.1958 ± 0.0135	0.1488 ± 0.0070
PICo	0.1970 ± 0.0127	0.1501 ± 0.0068

4 Conclusion

In this paper, we propose a graph convolutional network to predict the PD clinical measures, using multi-modal brain networks. Particularly, we propose an adaptive pooling scheme driven by both graph structure and brain data, which is efficient in computing and end-to-end training. The experiment results demonstrate that the proposed method attains state-of-the-art results compared to related baselines, and integrating multi-modal brain network is highly effective in the prediction task.

Acknowledgements. This study was partially funded by NSF IIS 1836938, DBI 1836866, IIS 1845666, IIS 1852606, IIS 1838627, IIS 1837956, and NIH R21 AG056782, R01 AG049371, U54 EB020403, P41 EB015922, R56 AG058854.

References

1. Aganj, I., et al.: A hough transform global probabilistic approach to multiple-subject diffusion MRI tractography. Med. Image Anal. **15**(4), 414–425 (2011)
2. Behrens, T.E., et al.: Probabilistic diffusion tractography with multiple fibre orientations: what can we gain? Neuroimage **34**(1), 144–155 (2007)
3. Bullmore, E., et al.: Complex brain networks: graph theoretical analysis of structural and functional systems. Nat. Rev. Neurosci. **10**(3), 186 (2009)
4. Caspell-Garcia, C., et al.: Multiple modality biomarker prediction of cognitive impairment in prospectively followed de novo Parkinson disease. PLoS ONE **12**(5), e0175674 (2017)
5. Defferrard, M., et al.: Convolutional neural networks on graphs with fast localized spectral filtering. In: NeurIPS, pp. 3844–3852 (2016)
6. Dhillon, I.S., et al.: Weighted graph cuts without eigenvectors a multilevel approach. IEEE TPAMI **29**(11), 1944–1957 (2007)
7. Fornito, A., et al.: Graph analysis of the human connectome: promise, progress, and pitfalls. Neuroimage **80**, 426–444 (2013)
8. Hamilton, W., et al.: Inductive representation learning on large graphs. In: Advances in Neural Information Processing Systems, pp. 1024–1034 (2017)

9. Iglesias, J.E., et al.: Robust brain extraction across datasets and comparison with publicly available methods. IEEE Trans. Med. Imaging **30**(9), 1617–1634 (2011)

10. Kingma, D.P., et al.: Adam: a method for stochastic optimization. arXiv preprint arXiv:1412.6980 (2014)

11. Kipf, T.N., et al.: Semi-supervised classification with graph convolutional networks. arXiv preprint arXiv:1609.02907 (2016)

12. Ktena, S.I., et al.: Distance metric learning using graph convolutional networks: application to functional brain networks. In: Descoteaux, M., Maier-Hein, L., Franz, A., Jannin, P., Collins, D.L., Duchesne, S. (eds.) MICCAI 2017. LNCS, vol. 10433, pp. 469–477. Springer, Cham (2017). https://doi.org/10.1007/978-3-319-66182-7_54

13. Marek, K., et al.: The parkinson progression marker initiative (PPMI). Prog. Neurobiol. **95**(4), 629–635 (2011)

14. Parker, G.J., et al.: A framework for a streamline-based probabilistic index of connectivity (PICO) using a structural interpretation of MRI diffusion measurements. J. Magn. Reson. Imaging Off. J. Int. Soc. Magn. Reson. Med. **18**(2), 242–254 (2003)

15. Shuman, D.I., et al.: The emerging field of signal processing on graphs: extending high-dimensional data analysis to networks and other irregular domains. IEEE Signal Process. Mag. **30**(3), 83–98 (2013)

16. Sporns, O., et al.: The human connectome: a structural description of the human brain. PLoS Comput. Biol. **1**(4), e42 (2005)

17. Xu, K., et al.: How powerful are graph neural networks? arXiv preprint arXiv:1810.00826 (2018)

18. Ying, Z., et al.: Hierarchical graph representation learning with differentiable pooling. In: Advances in Neural Information Processing Systems, pp. 4805–4815 (2018)

19. Zhan, L., et al.: Comparison of nine tractography algorithms for detecting abnormal structural brain networks in Alzheimer's disease. Front. Aging Neurosci. **7**, 48 (2015)

20. Zhang, X., et al.: Multi-view graph convolutional network and its applications on neuroimage analysis for Parkinson's disease. arXiv preprint arXiv:1805.08801 (2018)

21. Zhang, Y., Huang, H.: New graph-blind convolutional network for brain connectome data analysis. In: Chung, A.C.S., Gee, J.C., Yushkevich, P.A., Bao, S. (eds.) IPMI 2019. LNCS, vol. 11492, pp. 669–681. Springer, Cham (2019). https://doi.org/10.1007/978-3-030-20351-1_52

Detection and Localization

Uncertainty-Informed Detection of Epileptogenic Brain Malformations Using Bayesian Neural Networks

Ravnoor S. Gill$^{(\boxtimes)}$, Benoit Caldairou, Neda Bernasconi,
and Andrea Bernasconi

Neuroimaging of Epilepsy Laboratory, McConnell Brain Imaging Center,
Montreal Neurological Institute (MNI), Montreal, QC, Canada
ravnoor.gill@mail.mcgill.ca

Abstract. Focal cortical dysplasia (FCD) is a prevalent surgically-amenable epileptogenic malformation of cortical development. On MRI, FCD typically presents with cortical thickening, hyperintensity, and blurring of the gray-white matter interface. These changes may be visible to the naked eye, or subtle and be easily overlooked. Despite advances in MRI analytics, current machine learning algorithms fail to detect FCD in up to 50% of cases. Moreover, the deterministic nature of current algorithms does not allow conducting risk assessments of such predictions, an essential step in clinical decision-making. Here, we propose an algorithm formulated on Bayesian convolutional neural networks (CNN) providing information on prediction uncertainty, while leveraging this information to improve classification performance. Our classifier was trained on a patch-based augmented dataset derived from 56 patients with histologically-validated FCD to distinguish the lesion from healthy tissue. The algorithm was trained and cross-validated on multimodal 3T MRI data. Compared to a non-Bayesian learner with the same network architecture and complexity, the uncertainty-informed Bayesian CNN classifiers showed significant improvement in sensitivity (89% *vs* 82%; p < 0.05) while specificity was high for both classifiers. We demonstrate empirically the effectiveness of our uncertainty-informed CNN algorithm, making it ideal for large-scale clinical diagnostics of FCD.

Keywords: Magnetic resonance imaging · Clinical diagnostics · Epilepsy · Deep learning · Uncertainty · Dropout Monte Carlo · Classification

1 Introduction

Focal cortical dysplasia (FCD), a malformation of cortical development, is a frequent cause of drug-resistant epilepsy. This surgically-amenable lesion is characterized on histology by altered cortical laminar structure and cytological anomalies together with gliosis and demyelination, which may extend into the underlying white matter [1].

Electronic supplementary material The online version of this chapter (https://doi.org/10.1007/978-3-030-32251-9_25) contains supplementary material, which is available to authorized users.

© Springer Nature Switzerland AG 2019
D. Shen et al. (Eds.): MICCAI 2019, LNCS 11767, pp. 225–233, 2019.
https://doi.org/10.1007/978-3-030-32251-9_25

Complete lesion resection is associated with good post-surgical outcome [2]. On MRI, FCD typically presents with cortical thickening, hyperintensity and blurring of the gray-white matter interface. These changes may be visible to the naked eye on T1- and T2-weighted MRI, or subtle and easily overlooked (often referred to as "MRI-negative" FCD) [3].

Over the last decade, a number of automated FCD detection algorithms have been developed [4]. Recent methods rely on surface-based approaches [5–7], which allow to effectively model sulco-gyral morphology. Nevertheless, current algorithms fail to detect subtle FCD [3]. Also, arduous pre-processing and specialized expertise preclude their broader integration into clinical workflows. Importantly, they have not quantified the degree of uncertainty in predictions, a desirable information particularly when training datasets are small.

Convolutional neural networks (CNN) extract hierarchically increasing complex features from the data [8] without the need for user-defined feature engineering; they have achieved state-of-the-art performances in medical imaging (see Litjens el al. [9] for review). A standard approach to assess the reliability of CNN predictions is to rely on the probabilities obtained from the Softmax layer. However, such raw confidence scores may be miscalibrated [10]. Also, CNN predictions are typically deterministic. In contrast, traditional Bayesian machine learning assigns the degree of uncertainty (or confidence) to predictions through a probability density function. In clinical domains, uncertainty information has insofar been used to evaluate the robustness of predictions in multiple sclerosis [11] and diabetic retinopathy [12].

Dropout variational inference approximates Bayesian inference in models with large number of learnable parameters, for which exact Bayesian inference is computationally intractable [13]. This training strategy includes dropout after every convolutional layer; subsequently, a Monte Carlo dropout procedure, applied during testing, samples the posterior distribution to provide predictions [14]. The model's epistemic uncertainty is then derived from the mean and variance of the distribution of predictions. Here, we exploited the complementary diagnostic power of T1- and T2-weighted contrasts paired with an uncertainty-informed Bayesian CNN. Compared to a non-Bayesian CNN classifier with the same network architecture and complexity, the uncertainty-informed Bayesian classifier showed significant improvement in sensitivity, while maintaining high specificity.

2   Methods

2.1   MRI Acquisition

Multimodal MRI was acquired on a 3T Siemens scanner using a 32-channel head coil, including: 3D T1-weighted MPRAGE (T1w; TR = 2300 ms, TE = 2.98 ms, flip angle = 9°, FOV = 256 mm^2, voxel size = 1 × 1 × 1 mm^3), and T2-weighted 3D fluid-attenuated inversion recovery (FLAIR; TR = 5000 ms, TE = 389 ms, flip angle = 120°, FOV = 230 mm^2, 0.9 × 0.9 × 0.9 mm^3).

2.2 Image Pre-Processing

T1w and FLAIR images underwent intensity non-uniformity correction [15] and normalization. T1w images were then linearly registered (affine, 9 degrees of freedom) to the MNI152 symmetric template ($1 \times 1 \times 1$ mm^3) [16]. FLAIR images were linearly mapped to T1w images in MNI space. Skull-stripping excluded non-brain tissue.

2.3 Patch-Based Data Augmentation

MRI Sampling Procedure. To prevent biasing the classifier towards healthy voxels, we constructed a patch-based dataset by randomly under-sampling healthy voxels such that the feature set was composed of equal number of examples from both classes. To this end, we sub-sampled multi-contrast 3D patches from the co-registered 3D T1w and FLAIR images, with each input image modality representing a channel. The data was normalized within each input modality with zero mean and unit variance. For each normalized training image, we computed 3D patches ($16 \times 16 \times 16$) centered on the voxel of interest. The set of all multimodal patches served as training dataset.

Sampling Heuristics. We sampled hyperintense voxels based on FLAIR contrast by thresholding the subject-level z-normalized images and discarding the bottom 10 percentile intensities. This thresholding yielded a crude gray matter mask partially extending into the hyperintense white matter. This approach is biologically plausible since FCD lesions are primarily located in the gray matter [17]; moreover, their gray matter and white matter components are consistently hyperintense on FLAIR [18].

2.4 Network Architecture and Design

A typical convolutional neural network (CNN) consists of three stages: convolutions, nonlinearity, and pooling. We used a two-phase cascaded CNN training architecture [19] in which weights of two identical CNNs are optimized independently, a procedure yielding efficient training when the distribution of labels is unbalanced [5, 7]. CNN$_1$ was trained to maximize putative lesional voxels, while CNN$_2$ reduced the number of misclassified voxels (*i.e.*, removing false positives while maintaining optimal sensitivity). Each fully convolutional network was composed of three stacks of convolution (filter size: $3 \times 3 \times 3$) and max-pooling layers with 48, 96 and 2 filters, respectively. The rectified linear activation (ReLU) non-linearity function was applied to the first two of the three convolutional layers. Softmax non-linearity was used after the final convolution to normalize the result of the kernel convolutions into a binominal distribution over healthy and lesional labels. See Figure S1 (in supplementary material) for detailed network parameters.

2.5 Classification Paradigm

Training Algorithm. We used a validation set (75/25 training data split) to optimize the CNN weights. The training set is used to adjust the weights of the neural network, while the validation set measures the performance of the trained CNN after each epoch and continues until the validation error plateaus. The model is randomly initialized, and network parameters are learned iteratively via the adaptive learning rate method (AdaDelta) by minimizing the binary cross-entropy loss. Batch-normalization (BN) and Dropout were implemented to prevent overfitting.

Uncertainty Estimation. We computed the posterior distribution p(w|X, y), where {X, y} is the training dataset and {w} is the learned weights of the CNN. In practice, while the solution of this posterior is analytically intractable, variational inference (VI) methods approximate it with a parameterized distribution $q(w)$, while θ summarizes network parameters over a space of functions, and x* represents a new input point (see Eq. 1).

$$p(\theta|X,y,x^*) \approx \int p(\theta|x^*,w)p(w|X,y)dw \approx \int p(\theta|X^*,w)q(w)dw \qquad (1)$$

$$\mathcal{L}_{VI} := \int p(y|X,w)q(w)dw - KL(q(w)\|p(w)) \qquad (2)$$

The first term in Eq. (2) maximizes the likelihood of the training data {X, y}, whereas the second term approximates the true distribution $p(w)$ by $q(w)$. Gal and Ghahramani [13] empirically associates Eq. (2) with dropout training to approximate the intractable integral with Monte Carlo sampling. This results in the conventional Softmax loss for dropout networks, for which units are dropped by drawing from a Bernoulli prior with probability drop for setting a unit to zero. The Kullback-Leibler (KL) term in Eq. (2) was shown to correspond to a L2-regularization term in dropout networks.

Inference Algorithm. The proposed pipeline (Fig. 1) was trained and cross-validated using a 5-fold scheme on a cohort of 56 consecutive patients with histologically-confirmed FCD lesions. This trained model cascade served probabilistic predictions on held-out fold data. For each test subject, input images were first partitioned into patches with voxel sampling limited to the FLAIR mask (intra-subject Z-score > 0.1). The balanced patch dataset served as input to CNN_1. To discard improbable lesion candidates, we applied the following thresholding criteria. For the non-Bayesian classifier, we used a single forward pass at >0.1. For the Bayesian classifier, we used separately the mean ($\mu_{bayesian}$) and variance ($\sigma_{bayesian}$; i.e. uncertainty) of 20 stochastic forward passes thresholded at >0.1 and >0.05, respectively. For each of the three thresholding schemes, the resulting candidate voxels served as the input mask to sample patches for CNN_2. For the non-Bayesian classifier, the remaining voxels (threshold > 0.1) provided the final probabilistic lesion mask. For each Bayesian experiment, we computed the mean and uncertainty of the predictions resulting from 50 forward passes and thresholded the mean at >0.7. These thresholds are empirically determined by limiting the average cluster-level false positive rate to below 5 per patient. Finally, a simple post-processing routine involving successive morphological erosion, dilation, and extraction of connected components (>75 voxels) removed flat blobs and noise. The final segmentation masks were compared to manual expert annotations of the lesions.

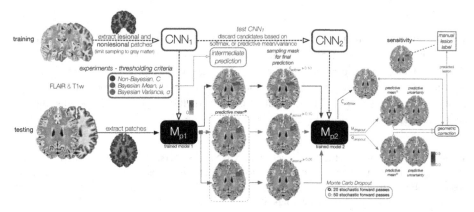

Fig. 1. Training and testing scheme using the two-stage CNN cascade (CNN$_1$ and CNN$_2$) that incorporates uncertainty information using dropout Monte Carlo.

3   Experiment and Results

3.1   Subjects

We studied a cohort of FCD lesions histologically-confirmed after surgery at a tertiary epilepsy center (n = 56). The pre-surgical workup included assessment of seizure history, video-EEG telemetry, and clinical neuroimaging. Since routine MRI was initially reported as unremarkable in 45 patients (80%), the location of the seizure focus was established using intracranially-implanted electrodes; in all, retrospective inspection revealed a subtle FCD in the seizure onset region.

Training and Cross-Validation Cohort. The dataset comprised 56 patients (28 females, 45 adults; mean ± SD age = 26 ± 10 years).

Independent Testing Cohorts. The control group consisted of 38 healthy individuals (age = 30 ± 7 years) and 63 disease controls with temporal lobe epilepsy (TLE) and histologically-verified hippocampal sclerosis (age = 31 ± 8), matched for age and sex to training cohort.

3.2   Performance Evaluation

Evaluation of Classification. Two experts manually segmented independently 56 lesions on co-registered T1w and FLAIR images. Inter-rater Dice agreement index was 0.93 ± 0.10. The union of the two ground truth labels served to train the classifier. The classifier was trained using 5-fold cross validation repeated 5 times. Sensitivity was the proportion of patients in whom a detected cluster co-localized with the lesion label. Specificity was determined with respect to controls (*i.e.*, proportion of controls in whom no FCD lesion cluster was falsely identified), and disease controls with TLE. We also report the number of clusters detected in patients remote from the lesion label (*i.e.*, false positives; FP).

3.3   Results

The 5-fold cross-validation of the Bayesian CNN classifiers resulted in a sensitivity of 89%, with an average of 50/56 lesions detected, compared to 82% using the non-Bayesian CNN, at an identical cluster-wise FP rate. Non-parametric permutation tests (one-tailed, 10,000 iterations) assessing the pair-wise predictive accuracy based on area under the curves (AUCs) showed that sensitivity of the Bayesian CNNs was significantly higher than the non-Bayesian CNN (see Table 1).

Table 1. Performance metrics for the three CNN classifiers. Sensitivity is derived after averaging across 5 trials and thresholding to aggregate voxel as clusters. The rate of false positives (FP) clusters is averaged across patients with FCD. The Dice index represents FCD lesion coverage compared to manual labeling.

CNN classifier	Sensitivity	FP	Dice	AUC permutation tests
Non-Bayesian (C1)	82% (46/56)	4 ± 5	0.49	–
Bayesian (C2; mean-based threshold)	89% (50/56)	5 ± 4	0.47	C2 > C1 (p < 0.05)
Bayesian (C3; uncertainty-based threshold)	89% (50/56)	5 ± 5	0.47	C3 > C1 (p < 0.05)

Voxel-wise receiver operating characteristics (ROC) curves are shown in Fig. 2A. Higher AUC scores signify better classification performance. Uncertainty values positively correlated with predictive probabilities at the individual level for both the mean-based thresholding (healthy controls: Pearson's $r = 0.81 \pm 0.03$, $p < 0.05$; TLE disease controls: Pearson's r: 0.77 ± 0.04, $p < 0.05$) and uncertainty-based thresholding (healthy controls: 0.78 ± 0.04, $p < 0.05$; TLE: 0.81 ± 0.03, $p < 0.05$). Specificity was 84% in healthy controls (no findings in 32/38; 1 ± 0 FPs) using Bayesian CNNs and the non-Bayesian CNN. Specificity was 87% (no findings in 55/63; 1 ± 0 FPs) in TLE controls using Bayesian CNNs, and slightly higher at 92% (no findings in 58/63; 1 ± 0 FPs) using the non-Bayesian CNN.

4   Discussion

We present the first deep learning-based method to segment FCD that leverages uncertainty for clinical decision-making with the highest sensitivity to date. Notably, epistemic uncertainty is important for safety-critical applications and instances with small datasets [14].

Our framework exploits uncertainty both during the intermediate testing and the final prediction. The calibration of posterior probabilities during the intermediate step is apparent in Fig. 2B (group evaluation) and Figure S2 (individual evaluation) showing that Bayesian CNN is more effective in separating tissue classes than the non-Bayesian CNN, a result attributable to fitting multiple hyperplanes in the former rather than just

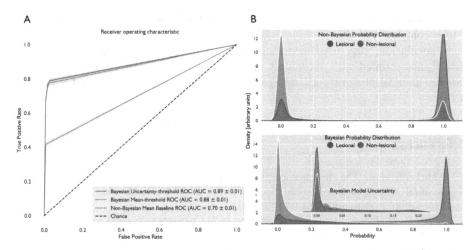

Fig. 2. A. Receiver operating characteristic (ROC) curves of the three CNN classifiers. The opaque error line represents the ±1 standard deviation of the area under the curve (AUC) around the mean AUC (solid colored line). The dotted line represents the AUC for a random classifier. B. The posterior predictive distributional profiles for FCD lesions and non-lesional tissue of the non-Bayesian CNN (top panel) and Bayesian CNN (bottom panel – only mean based thresholding depicted). The Bayesian model uncertainty is shown (inset) in the bottom panel.

one. This also explains why the Bayesian classifier detected lesions that were missed by the non-Bayesian learner (as exemplified by P2 in Fig. S2).

While being superior to the non-Bayesian classifier, both Bayesians CNNs yielded equal performance at the patient level. Notably, the number of FPs in healthy and disease controls were minimal, and highly correlated with their degree of uncertainty. Moreover, the overall high performance across cohorts strongly suggests that the CNN learns and optimizes parameters specific to FCD pathology, a fact validated by histological confirmation in all cases.

FCD lesions manifest on a biological spectrum ranging from subtle to severe. Subtle FCD resembles the healthy cortex and may thus present with high uncertainty, while the predictive mean may be high or low. Within the automated framework, the choice of parameters is based on the whole dataset since it is not possible to anticipate where a new, test FCD may lie along the spectrum. While we have shown that the automated approach is effective, a human-in-the-loop is more appropriate for the final clinical decision. Therefore, on account of the variability stemming from overlap in distributions of lesional and non-lesional tissue (as is evident from Fig. 2B and Figure S2), the uncertainty map would be best suited for an individualized analysis where the clinician rules out false positives in conjunction with converging evidence from other independent exams. Thus, uncertainty estimates can be used to refer uncertain predictions to experts for further evaluation This is especially important when considering that 80% of the FCD lesions detected by the CNN were missed by conventional radiological inspection. Finally, these estimates have the added benefit of being readily computed without the need to re-train the existing models or increasing model or time complexity.

In conclusion, easy implementation, minimal pre-processing, significant performance gains coupled with uncertainty information about predictions make our CNN classifier an ideal platform for large-scale clinical use, particularly in "MRI-negative" FCD.

References

1. Blümcke, I., et al.: The clinicopathologic spectrum of focal cortical dysplasias: a consensus classification proposed by an ad hoc Task Force of the ILAE Diagnostic Methods Commission. Epilepsia **52**, 158–174 (2011)
2. Fauser, S., et al.: Long-term seizure outcome in 211 patients with focal cortical dysplasia. Epilepsia. **56**, 66–76 (2015)
3. Bernasconi, A., Bernasconi, N., Bernhardt, B.C., Schrader, D.: Advances in MRI for "cryptogenic" epilepsies. Nat. Rev. Neurol. **7**, 99–108 (2011)
4. Kini, L.G., Gee, J.C., Litt, B.: Computational analysis in epilepsy neuroimaging: a survey of features and methods. NeuroImage Clin. **11**, 515–529 (2016)
5. Hong, S.-J., Kim, H., Schrader, D., Bernasconi, N., Bernhardt, B.C., Bernasconi, A.: Automated detection of cortical dysplasia type II in MRI-negative epilepsy. Neurology. **83**, 48–55 (2014)
6. Adler, S., et al.: Novel surface features for automated detection of focal cortical dysplasias in paediatric epilepsy. NeuroImage Clin. **14**, 18–27 (2017)
7. Gill, R.S., et al.: Automated detection of epileptogenic cortical malformations using multimodal MRI. In: Cardoso, M.J., et al. (eds.) DLMIA/ML-CDS 2017. LNCS, vol. 10553, pp. 349–356. Springer, Cham (2017). https://doi.org/10.1007/978-3-319-67558-9_40
8. LeCun, Y., Bengio, Y., Hinton, G.: Deep learning. Nature **521**, 436–444 (2015)
9. Litjens, G., et al.: A survey on deep learning in medical image analysis. Med. Image Anal. **42**, 60–88 (2017)
10. Guo, C., Pleiss, G., Sun, Y., Weinberger, K.Q.: On Calibration of Modern Neural Networks. http://arxiv.org/abs/1706.04599v2 (2017)
11. Nair, T., Precup, D., Arnold, D.L., Arbel, T.: Exploring Uncertainty Measures in Deep Networks for Multiple Sclerosis Lesion Detection and Segmentation. http://arxiv.org/abs/1808.01200v2 (2018)
12. Leibig, C., Allken, V., Ayhan, M.S., Berens, P., Wahl, S.: Leveraging uncertainty information from deep neural networks for disease detection. Sci. Rep. **7**, 17816 (2017)
13. Gal, Y., Ghahramani, Z.: Bayesian Convolutional Neural Networks with Bernoulli Approximate Variational Inference. http://arxiv.org/abs/1506.02158v6 (2015)
14. Kendall, A., Gal, Y.: What Uncertainties Do We Need in Bayesian Deep Learning for Computer Vision? http://arxiv.org/abs/1703.04977v2 (2017)
15. Sled, J.G., Zijdenbos, A.P., Evans, A.C.: A nonparametric method for automatic correction of intensity nonuniformity in MRI data. IEEE Trans. Med. Imaging **17**, 87–97 (1998)
16. Fonov, V.S., Evans, A.C., McKinstry, R.C., Almli, C.R., Collins, D.L.: Unbiased nonlinear average age-appropriate brain templates from birth to adulthood. Neuroimage **47**, S102 (2009)
17. Sisodiya, S.M., Fauser, S., Cross, J.H., Thom, M.: Focal cortical dysplasia type II: biological features and clinical perspectives. Lancet Neurol. **8**, 830–843 (2009)

18. Hong, S.-J., et al.: Multimodal MRI profiling of focal cortical dysplasia type II. Neurology **88**, 734–742 (2017)
19. Gill, R.S., et al.: Deep convolutional networks for automated detection of epileptogenic brain malformations. In: Frangi, A.F., Schnabel, J.A., Davatzikos, C., Alberola-López, C., Fichtinger, G. (eds.) MICCAI 2018. LNCS, vol. 11072, pp. 490–497. Springer, Cham (2018). https://doi.org/10.1007/978-3-030-00931-1_56

Automated Lesion Detection
by Regressing Intensity-Based Distance
with a Neural Network

Kimberlin M. H. van Wijnen[1(✉)], Florian Dubost[1], Pinar Yilmaz[2],
M. Arfan Ikram[2,3], Wiro J. Niessen[1,4], Hieab Adams[2], Meike W. Vernooij[2],
and Marleen de Bruijne[1,5]

[1] Biomedical Imaging Group Rotterdam, Department of Radiology and Nuclear
Medicine, Erasmus MC, Rotterdam, The Netherlands
{k.vanwijnen,f.dubost,marleen.debruijne}@erasmusmc.nl
[2] Departments of Radiology and Nuclear Medicine and of Epidemiology,
Erasmus MC, Rotterdam, The Netherlands
[3] Department of Neurology, Erasmus MC, Rotterdam, The Netherlands
[4] Imaging Physics, Faculty of Applied Sciences, TU Delft, Delft, The Netherlands
[5] Department of Computer Science, University of Copenhagen,
Copenhagen, Denmark

Abstract. Localization of focal vascular lesions on brain MRI is an
important component of research on the etiology of neurological disorders. However, manual annotation of lesions can be challenging, time-
consuming and subject to observer bias. Automated detection methods
often need voxel-wise annotations for training. We propose a novel approach for automated lesion detection that can be trained on scans only
annotated with a dot per lesion instead of a full segmentation. From
the dot annotations and their corresponding intensity images we compute various distance maps (DMs), indicating the distance to a lesion
based on spatial distance, intensity distance, or both. We train a fully
convolutional neural network (FCN) to predict these DMs for unseen
intensity images. The local optima in the predicted DMs are expected to
correspond to lesion locations. We show the potential of this approach to
detect enlarged perivascular spaces in white matter on a large brain MRI
dataset with an independent test set of 1000 scans. Our method matches
the intra-rater performance of the expert rater that was computed on
an independent set. We compare the different types of distance maps,
showing that incorporating intensity information in the distance maps
used to train an FCN greatly improves performance.

Keywords: Lesion detection · Geodesic distance · Fully convolutional
neural network · Dot annotations · Perivascular spaces

K.M.H. van Wijnen and F. Dubost—Both authors contributed equally to this work.

© Springer Nature Switzerland AG 2019
D. Shen et al. (Eds.): MICCAI 2019, LNCS 11767, pp. 234–242, 2019.
https://doi.org/10.1007/978-3-030-32251-9_26

1 Introduction

Obtaining the location of focal vascular lesions on brain scans, such as white matter hyperintensities, lacunes, enlarged perivascular spaces or microbleeds is extremely useful for studying the association of these lesions with neurological disorders. However the manual annotation of these lesions can be challenging, time-consuming and subject to observer bias due to the difficulty of distinguishing a specific type of lesion from other similarly appearing structures. An automated method for detecting lesions could improve reliability, generalization and speed of lesion detection, which could greatly advance neuropathology research.

Various promising automated methods have been proposed to detect lesions. Deep learning methods often provide the best accuracy, but depend on expensive manual annotations for training like voxel-wise segmentations [5,11] or bounding boxes [8] marking the lesions. This hinders applicability of these techniques in practice.

Annotating by placing a single dot per lesion instead is considerably more time-efficient, allowing to collect larger annotated datasets for training and evaluation. In this paper we therefore propose a novel method for lesion detection that requires only dot annotations. Dot annotations have been effectively used to train convolutional neural networks (CNNs) for other applications, such as cell detection in histology images [18], lacune detection in placental ultrasound [15] and landmark detection in retinal images [14]. An approach that has shown great promise is regression of a distance map (DM) that is computed from these dot annotations [14,15,18]. Contrary to many other deep learning detection methods that use a two-stage approach [8], this approach directly outputs predicted detections and is optimized in an end-to-end fashion.

We use a similar approach for detecting lesions based on dot annotations. Previous distance regression approaches for detection [14,18] have used Euclidean distance. This is especially suited for the detection of circular objects such as cells. Brain lesions on the other hand often have a morphology that is complex and discriminative [4].

In this paper we investigate the effect of including intensity information in DMs for lesion detection. Intensity distance incorporates local image context enabling the DM to capture complicated morphologies. Voxels surrounding dot annotations which have similar intensity values (inside the lesions) will have a lower value in the DM than dissimilar voxels (outside the lesions). This could encourage the CNN to learn the characteristic morphology of the lesions and propose more accurate detections than when trained on a Euclidean distance map (EDM) that does not make this distinction. We compare Euclidean distance, intensity distance, and geodesic distance that combines both Euclidean and intensity distances. For geodesic distance the image is seen as a curved surface defined by the spatial coordinates and one intensity coordinate, where the shortest path on the surface is the geodesic distance [17].

In this paper we show that including image intensity information in the DM improves optimization of a CNN for detecting lesions in brain MRI. We compute DMs from the dot annotations and their corresponding intensity images.

Subsequently we train a fully convolutional neural network (FCN) to predict these DMs for unseen intensity images. The local minimal distances in the predicted DMs correspond to the proposed detection candidates.

We show the potential of regressing intensity-based DMs for the detection of enlarged perivascular spaces (PVS). PVS burden has been associated with cerebral small vessel disease [6]. As PVS follow the course of the vessel they surround, they appear as elongated structures on 3D brain MRI scans. Several methods have been proposed to detect PVS. The majority of the proposed algorithms is however evaluated on a relatively small sets (less than 30 images) due to the need for voxel-wise annotations for testing (and training) [4,13]. We train and validate on a set of 1202 MRI scans and test on a separate set of 1000 images. As the centrum semiovale (CSO) is seen as the most difficult brain region for PVS detection and most clinically relevant, we focused on this brain region [3].

2   Method

We train an FCN to regress a DM for a given intensity image. Our approach requires MRI scans with dot annotations for training. The local optima in the predicted DMs are expected to correspond to lesion locations. We compare geodesic distance maps (GDMs), EDMs and intensity distance maps (IDMs).

2.1   Distance Transform

To compute DMs we use a distance transform, that requires a definition of the foreground – in our case the set of dot annotations Φ – and a gray-scale image $G(x)$ in the case of intensity and geodesic distances, with x the position in the image. The distance map $DM(x)$ is defined by

$$DM(x) = min(\Lambda(\gamma), \gamma \in \Psi(x, \Phi)) \tag{1}$$

with $\Psi(x, \Phi)$ the set of possible paths γ between a position x in the image and the set of dot annotations Φ. The length $\Lambda(\gamma)$ of the path γ is

$$\Lambda(\gamma) = \sum_{i=1}^{n-1} d(x_i, x_{i+1}) \tag{2}$$

with n the number of voxels in the path γ between a position x and a dot annotation $x_{dot} \in \Phi$ and d the distance measure. The geodesic distance d_G in a 2D gray-scale image between voxel x_i and the next voxel in the path x_{i+1}, with intensities $G(x_i)$ and $G(x_{i+1})$ respectively, is defined by [17] as

$$d_G(x_i, x_{i+1}) = \sqrt{d_I(x_i, x_{i+1})^2 + d_E(x_i, x_{i+1})^2} \tag{3}$$

with the intensity distance $d_I(x_i, x_{i+1}) = G(x_i) - G(x_{i+1})$ and the Euclidean distance $d_E(x_i, x_{i+1})$ which is 1 for $x_{i+1} \in N_4(x_i)$ (voxels connected horizontally and vertically) and $\sqrt{2}$ for $x_{i+1} \in N_8(x_i) \setminus N_4(x_i)$ (voxels connected diagonally). EDMs are consequently computed by setting $d_I = 0$ in Eq. 3, while IDMs are computed by setting $d_E = 0$. We approximate these DMs using the optimization algorithm *iterative raster scan* described in [17]. This approach is for computing DMs in 2D, though it can easily be extended to 3D.[1]

The resulting $DM(x)$ is normalized by dividing by the maximum distance in the $DM(x)$ and inverted as this is convenient for implementation. Furthermore, we add a parameter p to influence how steeply the distance decays. The final map $M_p(x)$ is calculated using

$$M_p(x) = \left(1 - \frac{DM(x)}{max\big(DM(x)\big)}\right)^p \tag{4}$$

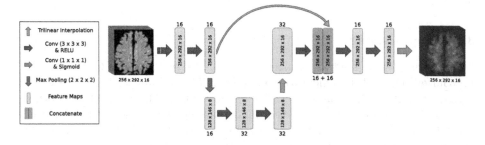

Fig. 1. Network architecture, on the left the input preprocessed brain scan is shown and the output predicted distance map is shown on the right

2.2 Fully Convolutional Neural Network

We use an architecture similar to a shallow U-Net for our FCN shown in Fig. 1, which was shown to work well for regressing the number of perivascular spaces in the basal ganglia [9, 16]. For optimization we use mean square error loss $MSE = \frac{1}{N} \sum_x \left(\widehat{M}_p(x) - M_p(x)\right)^2$, with $\widehat{M}(x)$ the predicted map and N the number of voxels in $M_p(x)$.

Non-maximum suppression is applied to the predicted distance map to detect local optima. We use a 5×5 maximum filter with a connectivity of 8. By thresholding the local optima the proposed detections are acquired.

---

[1] Our code for computing 2D as well as 3D distance maps is available at https://github.com/kimvwijnen/geodesic_distance_transform.

3   Experiments

3.1   Data

Our data set consists of 2202 T2-weighted MRI scans from the Rotterdam Scan Study. All scans were from different individuals and were acquired on a 1.5 T MRI scanner. The images have a size of $512 \times 512 \times 192$ with a voxel resolution of $0.49 \times 0.49 \times 0.8$ mm^3. Further details on the image acquisition of this data are discussed by Ikram et al. [12].

The number of PVS in the axial slice 1 cm above the lateral ventricles is highly correlated with the total number of PVS in the CSO [2]. The rater selected this specific slice and annotated it with dots indicating PVS between 1–3 mm in diameter in line with the guidelines described by Adams et al. [1]. The intra-rater performance was evaluated on a separate set of 40 MRI scans (see Table 1 and Fig. 3).

3.2   Preprocessing

Images are preprocessed as proposed by [10]. We segment the CSO with the FreeSurfer multi-atlas segmentation algorithm [7] producing a binary mask that we smooth with a Gaussian kernel. The image are multiplied with the smoothed mask and cropped to a fixed size containing only the slices close to the annotated slice. The resulting images are normalized to the range [0, 1] by dividing by the maximum intensity in the image.

Annotated dots were not always inside the PVS. To solve this problem, we shift the dots to the highest intensity value within the same connected component and within 3 voxels distance. The shifted dots were only used to compute the distance maps for the training and validation set. For evaluation of the detection performance, the original annotated dots were used.

3.3   Experimental Setup

Random sampling was used to split the 2202 scans into a set of 1202 for development of the method (1000 for training and 202 for validation) and a separate set of 1000 for testing. As only one slice per scan was annotated, DMs were computed in 2D and the loss was only evaluated for this slice. Non-maximum suppression and evaluation of detection performance was also only done on the slice that was annotated.

Weights for the convolutional layers were initialized by random sampling from a truncated normal distribution with zero mean and unit variance. For optimization we use Adadelta and a batch of one due to memory limitations. We use on-the-fly augmentation for the training set. For every image a random rotation around the depth direction with a maximum of 20° in both directions is applied combined with random flipping in horizontal and in vertical direction. Methods were implemented in Python and Keras with Tensorflow as backend.

3.4   Detection Performance

The candidate detections of each method are compared to the expert annotations using the hungarian algorithm to find a one-to-one mapping between these sets. Only detections within a 6 voxel radius of the annotations were counted as true positive. We use 6 voxels as this is the maximum PVS diameter (corresponds to 3 mm [1]).

The detection performance is mainly evaluated with the Free-Response Operating Characteristic (FROC) curve and its area under the curve (FAUC) until 10 FP_{avg}, which is approximately twice the FP_{avg} of the rater. The FAUC is calculated as the percentage of the highest possible area. We used bootstrapping to quantify the uncertainty, resulting in a mean FAUC and confidence interval based on 1000 sampled sets. Bootstrapping was performed by random sampling with replacement from the test set.

3.5   Evaluation Approach

We ran experiments varying the decay parameter p (see Fig. 2). For higher values of p the FCN did not train, we expect because of label imbalance. Based on the FAUC on the validation set we set p to 5 for geodesic distance, to 6 for intensity distance and 9 for euclidean distance. During training, the model parameters were chosen as the ones minimizing the FAUC computed on the validation set. Only the best model per distance type ($GDM_5(x)$, $EDM_9(x)$, $IDM_6(x)$) was tested on the test set of 1000 scans.

The operating point on the FROC was chosen per model as the threshold with a sensitivity on the validation set closest to the average intra-rater sensitivity. For $GDM_5(x)$ the threshold was chosen at 0.525, for $EDM_9(x)$ at 0.500 and for $IDM_6(x)$) at 0.495. This threshold was used as the detection threshold during evaluation on the test set.

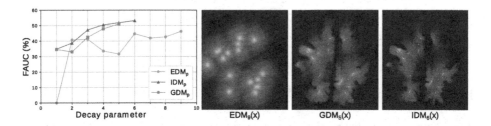

Fig. 2. Influence of decay parameter p on detection performance on the validation set and the chosen distance maps

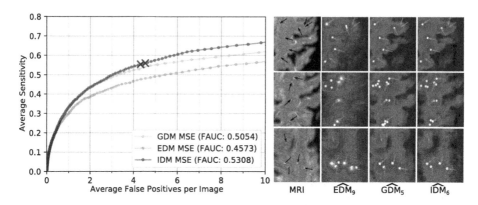

Fig. 3. FROC curves and crops of the output of the FCNs and their proposed detections (intra-rater performance indicated with red crosses, annotations with red arrows and predictions with blue stars) (Color figure online)

3.6 Results

Figure 3 shows the FROC curves computed on the test set and examples of the output of the FCNs. Table 1 shows the corresponding FAUCs, the sensitivity and FP_{avg} of the methods on the test set at the chosen thresholds (based on the validation set) and the average intra-rater performance.

Table 1. PVS detection performance on the test set for the detection methods and the average intra-rater performance on a smaller independent set

	FAUC	FP_{avg}	Sensitivity
$EDM_9(x)$	45.761 ($\pm$ 0.052)	7.49	53.63
$GDM_5(x)$	50.575 ($\pm$ 0.050)	5.10	55.26
$IDM_6(x)$	53.078 ($\pm$ 0.051)	4.35	55.35
Average intra-rater	-	4.43	55.66

4 Discussion and Conclusion

Our experiments indicate that incorporating image intensity information in a distance map used to train an FCN substantially improves performance of PVS detection. Results show that using GDMs and IDMs both result in a similar detection performance, with IDMs sometimes reaching higher performance than GDMs. This indicates that intensity difference is the most discriminative information, and that Euclidean distance could even be ignored. Using higher values of the decay parameter also increases the PVS detection performance, and stabilizes the optimization.

The FCN trained using IDMs reaches a sensitivity and FP_{avg} similar to the intra-rater performance computed on a smaller independent set (Fig. 3).

We expect our method could perform well for detecting other types of focal vascular lesions in the brain. Using intensity information in the computation of DMs could help the detection lesions that either have a complex morphology, or can have substantial variation in their size, such as microbleeds, white matter hyperintensities or lacunes. Additionally, in this work we evaluate the intensity-based distance maps only for their performance in detecting PVS. However, we observe that the PVS detections in the output maps of the FCNs trained on intensity-based distance maps (Fig. 3) seem to approximate the PVS shape quite well. We therefore expect our approach might also work well for segmentation.

Acknowledgments. This research is part of the research project Deep Learning for Medical Image Analysis (DLMedIA) with project number P15-26, funded by the Dutch Technology Foundation STW (part of the Netherlands Organisation for Scientific Research (NWO), which is partly funded by the Ministry of Economic Affairs), and with co-financing by Quantib. This research was also funded by the Netherlands Organisation for Health Research and Development (ZonMw), Project 104003005. Part of this work was carried out on the Dutch national e-infrastructure with the support of SURF Cooperative and on a Quadro P6000 donated by the NVIDIA Corporation.

References

1. Adams, H.H.H., et al.: Rating method for dilated Virchow-Robin spaces on magnetic resonance imaging. Stroke **44**, 1732–1735 (2013)
2. Adams, H.H., et al.: A priori collaboration in population imaging: the uniform neuro-imaging of Virchow-Robin spaces enlargement consortium. Alzheimer's Dement. Diagn. Assess. Dis. Monit. **1**(4), 513–520 (2015)
3. Ballerini, L., et al.: Perivascular spaces segmentation in brain MRI using optimal 3D filtering. Sci. Rep. **8**(1), 2132 (2018)
4. Boespflug, E.L., Schwartz, D.L., Lahna, D., Pollock, J., Iliff, J.J., Kaye, J.A., et al.: MR imagingbased multimodal autoidentification of perivascular spaces (mMAPS): automated morphologic segmentation of enlarged perivascular spaces at clinical field strength. Radiology **286**(2), 632–642 (2018)
5. Brosch, T., Tang, L.Y.W., Yoo, Y., Li, D.K.B., Traboulsee, A., Tam, R.: Deep 3D convolutional encoder networks with shortcuts for multiscale feature integration applied to multiple sclerosis lesion segmentation. IEEE T-MI **35**(5), 1229–1239 (2016)
6. Charidimou, A., et al.: Enlarged perivascular spaces as a marker of underlying arteriopathy in intracerebral haemorrhage: a multicentre MRI cohort study. J. Neurol. Neurosurg. Psychiatry **84**(6), 624–629 (2013)
7. Desikan, R.S., Ségonne, F., Fischl, B., Quinn, B.T., Dickerson, B.C., Blacker, D., et al.: An automated labeling system for subdividing the human cerebral cortex on MRI scans into gyral based regions of interest. NeuroImage **31**(3), 968–980 (2006)
8. Dou, Q., Chen, H., Yu, L., Zhao, L., Qin, J., Wang, D., et al.: Automatic detection of cerebral microbleeds from MR images via 3D convolutional neural networks. TMI **35**(5), 1182–1195 (2016)

9. Dubost, F., et al.: GP-Unet: lesion detection from weak labels with a 3D regression network. In: Descoteaux, M., Maier-Hein, L., Franz, A., Jannin, P., Collins, D.L., Duchesne, S. (eds.) MICCAI 2017. LNCS, vol. 10435, pp. 214–221. Springer, Cham (2017). https://doi.org/10.1007/978-3-319-66179-7_25

10. Dubost, F., et al.: Enlarged perivascular spaces in brain MRI: automated quantification in four regions. NeuroImage **185**, 534–544 (2019)

11. Ghafoorian, M., et al.: Deep multi-scale location-aware 3D convolutional neural networks for automated detection of lacunes of presumed vascular origin. NeuroImage: Clin. **14**, 391–399 (2017)

12. Ikram, M.A., et al.: The rotterdam scan study: design update 2016 and main findings. Eur. J. Epidemiol. **30**(12), 1299–1315 (2015)

13. Lian, C., et al.: Multi-channel multi-scale fully convolutional network for 3D perivascular spaces segmentation in 7T MR images. Med. Image Anal. **46**, 106–117 (2018)

14. Meyer, M.I., Galdran, A., Mendonça, A.M., Campilho, A.: A pixel-wise distance regression approach for joint retinal optical disc and fovea detection. In: Frangi, A.F., Schnabel, J.A., Davatzikos, C., Alberola-López, C., Fichtinger, G. (eds.) MICCAI 2018. LNCS, vol. 11071, pp. 39–47. Springer, Cham (2018). https://doi.org/10.1007/978-3-030-00934-2_5

15. Qi, H., Collins, S., Noble, J.A.: Automatic lacunae localization in placental ultrasound images via layer aggregation. In: Frangi, A.F., Schnabel, J.A., Davatzikos, C., Alberola-López, C., Fichtinger, G. (eds.) MICCAI 2018. LNCS, vol. 11071, pp. 921–929. Springer, Cham (2018). https://doi.org/10.1007/978-3-030-00934-2_102

16. Ronneberger, O., Fischer, P., Brox, T.: U-Net: convolutional networks for biomedical image segmentation. In: Navab, N., Hornegger, J., Wells, W.M., Frangi, A.F. (eds.) MICCAI 2015. LNCS, vol. 9351, pp. 234–241. Springer, Cham (2015). https://doi.org/10.1007/978-3-319-24574-4_28

17. Toivanen, P.J.: New geodosic distance transforms for gray-scale images. Pattern Recogn. Lett. **17**(5), 437–450 (1996)

18. Xie, Y., Xing, F., Shi, X., Kong, X., Su, H., Yang, L.: Efficient and robust cell detection: a structured regression approach. Med. Image Anal. **44**, 245–254 (2018)

Intracranial Aneurysm Detection from 3D Vascular Mesh Models with Ensemble Deep Learning

Mingsong Zhou[1], Xingce Wang[1(✉)], Zhongke Wu[1], Jose M. Pozo[2], and Alejandro F. Frangi[2]

[1] Information Science and Technology College, Beijing Normal University, Beijing, China
wangxingce@bnu.edu.cn
[2] Centre for Computational Imaging and Simulation Technologies in Biomedicine (CISTIB), School of Computing and School of Medicine, University of Leeds, Leeds, UK

Abstract. Intracranial aneurysm rupture can cause a serious stroke, which is related to the decline of daily life ability of the elderly. Although deep learning is now the most successful solution for organ detection, it requires myriads of training data, consistent of the image format, and a balanced sample distribution. This work presents an innovative representation of intracranial aneurysm detection as a shape analysis problem rather than a computer vision problem. We detected intracranial aneurysms in 3D cerebrovascular mesh models after segmentation of the brain vessels from the medical images, which can overcome the barriers of data format and data distribution, serving both clinical and screening purposes. Additionally, we propose a transferable multi-model ensemble (MMEN) architecture to detect intracranial aneurysms from cerebrovascular mesh models with limited data. To obtain a well-defined convolution operator, we use a global seamless parameterization converting a 3D cerebrovascular mesh model to a planar flat-torus. In the architecture, we transfer the planar flat-torus presentation abilities of three GoogleNet Inception V3 models, which were pre-trained on the ImageNet database, to characterize the intracranial aneurysms with local and global geometric features such as Gaussian curvature (GC), shape diameter function (SDF) and wave kernel signature (WKS), respectively. We jointly utilize all three models to detect aneurysms with adaptive weights learning based on back propagation. The experimental results on the 121 models show that our proposed method can achieve detection accuracy of 95.1% with 94.7% F1-score and 94.8% sensitivity, which is as good as the state-of-art work but is applicable to inhomogeneous image modalities and smaller datasets.

X. Wang and Z. Wu—Equally contributed to this work.

Electronic supplementary material The online version of this chapter (https://doi.org/10.1007/978-3-030-32251-9_27) contains supplementary material, which is available to authorized users.

D. Shen et al. (Eds.): MICCAI 2019, LNCS 11767, pp. 243–252, 2019.
https://doi.org/10.1007/978-3-030-32251-9_27

1 Introduction

Severe stroke is most often caused by the rupture of intracranial aneurysms (IAs) [9]. Early detection and quantification of IAs is essential for the prevention and treatment of aneurysm rupture and cerebral infarction. However, the detection, or identification of intracranial aneurysms is challenging due to the complexity and variability of their shapes. The location, shape boundary and size of IAs in a population are different. Previous algorithms detected IAs using the traditional machine learning method combined hand-crafted features with an enhancement filter, such as blobness and vesselness filters, applied on medical images [7]. More recently, deep learning, particularly the deep convolutional neural network (DCNN), has become the most successful technique in IAs detection and provides a unified framework for joint feature extraction and detection. Jerman [4] first utilized 7-layer 2D CNN to detect IAs with an intra-vascular distance map. Nakao [10] utilized 6-layer 2D CNN on 9-direction MIP images of each cube VOI. Ueda [16] applied ResNet-18 on four types of parameters from TOF-MRA, which extended IAs detection to multi-parameter images. Sichtermann [12] utilized "DeepMedic" with a network of 2 pathways and 11-layers to solve both 3T and 1.5T 3D TOF-MRA together. Jin [5] detected IAs with 2D-DSA sequences combining U-net and BiConvLSTM. In previous works based on hand-crafted feature selection, curvature, Hessian matrix, writhe number, skeleton information, and spherical harmonics function were used to describe the boundary of the sphere-like aneurysm shape, while illumination and texture were scarcely used, which shows that IAs detection is a graphical problem rather than a vision problem. A major difference between traditional and deep learning methods is that traditional methods rely more on domain knowledge such as sphere-like shape, whereas deep learning relies on access to massive datasets. Ideally, the advantages of both methods should be combined.

There are two limits in all previous works. First, there coexist different selection criteria for different image modalities. For example, CTA and 3DRA containing IAs are often used in clinic, while MRI without IAs is often used in targeted screening of the population. This difference causes an imbalance of the sample distribution in each medical image modality. Second, due to economic and ethical reasons, acquiring of a sufficiently large number of images as training data for directly applying deep learning is prohibitive. In this paper, we construct comparable 3D cerebrovascular models from the 3D image modalities, with which we can address different medical images and partially solve the data imbalance problem. We propose a transferable multi-model ensemble network (MMEN) for IAs detection from cerebrovascular models. We then apply deep learning to the 3D mesh model with a well-defined convolution operator on a global seamless parameterization to transfer the 3D cerebrovascular model to a planar flat-torus [6]. Three types of seamless counter-clóckwise covers fine-tune pre-trained GoogleNet Inception V3 models (V3 models) [14], palliating the need for large data sets, with which we aimed to characterize the overall appearance of IAs in 3D mesh models. These V3 models are used jointly to detect IAs with an adaptive weighting scheme learned during the error back propagation, which enables the cerebrovascular mesh model to be trained in an *end-to-end* manner. The proposed method allows us to bridge the gap of different data formats, break the barrier of the imbalance of sample distribution and obtain enough training data. Compared to those of the state-of-the art methods, our results show that the proposed algorithm provides substantial performance improvement.

2 Methods

Problem Formulation. Each 3D cerebrovascular structure can be modelled as a series of connected tubular-like 3D branches model. Our aim is to detect whether the IAs are in the 3D cerebrovascular model. The training data consist of a set of triplets $\{(S_i, \mathbf{x}_i, \hat{z}_i)\}_{i \in I}$ with 2D cerebrovascular watertight manifold models embedded in a three-dimensional space, $S_i \subset \mathbb{R}^3$, d-dimensional vector valued functions over the surface, $\mathbf{x}_i \in f(S_i, \mathbb{R}^d)$, and ground truth labelling functions $\hat{z}_i \in g(S_i, L)$, where $L = \{0, 1\}$ is the label set. Our goal is to find a non-linear mapping function as $F : f(S_i, \mathbb{R}^d) \to g(S_i, L)$ to produce a vector of confidences $F(\mathbf{x}_i) \in L$ per model S_i that correctly predicts its ground-truth label $\hat{z}_i$.

System Architecture. The proposed MMEN algorithm is summarized in Fig. 1. The algorithm has four steps: (1) Constructing the conformal mapping from the input cerebrovascular mesh model S to the sphere-like surface S' and conformal mapping from S' to the planar flat-torus τ with seamless counterclockwise covers of S' (2) Building a MMEN architecture for 3D mesh models based on classification (3) Training the MMEN with the input dataset $\{S_i\}$ described with d-dimensional features until convergence, and (4) Detecting IAs in each model based on the labels of the aneurysms.

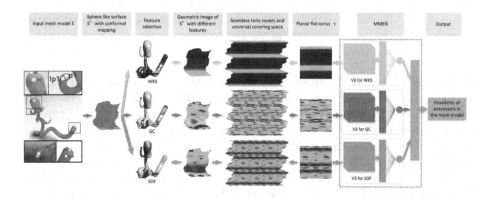

Fig. 1. Framework of our proposed MMEN algorithm.

Although the CNN is a powerful tool, existing architectures cannot directly run over S_i. We propose a transfer function to a planar flat-torus, denoted as τ, and train a CNN over τ with traditional 2D convolution operator on τ discretized in a grid. The key component is mapping S to τ, which is a non-trivial problem for the different topology between S and τ.

Seamless Parameterization and Convolution Operator. We define a sphere-like surface S' as an intermediate surface to create a desired seamless map between S and image τ. For given quarter-points $P = \{p_1, p_2, p_3, p_4\}$, we can obtain a unique transfer operation along the path $p_1 \to p_2 \to p_3 \to p_4$ to obtain the torus-like surface S'. Then we construct the universal covering space through stitching the surface S' with the method in [1], duplicating the planar mesh until we cover the representative square tile of the planar flat-torus with the orbifold as $\{\pi, \pi, \pi, \pi\}$. We use the cotan weights with negative values clamped to 10^{-2} to ensure positivity and hence bijective mapping. The quarter-points P can be computed efficiently of the approximated-conformal map by solving a sparse system of linear equation. We use ϕ_P as the transfer function between the sphere-like surface S' and the flat-torus τ, its push-forward to the flat image is defined as $\text{push}_P(x) = x \circ \varphi \circ \phi_P^{-1}$, where φ is the projection map from S' to S. We evaluate x at that point and assign the corresponding d-dimensional feature vector to it.

The convolution operator on the surface S requires the translation to be invariant. First, the definition of the map $S \to S'$ guarantees that a translation on S' is a local Euclidean translation on S. Second, according to the Poincaré-Hopf Theorem [8], for closed orientable surfaces, only torus-like surfaces, whose Euler characteristic is zero, have non-vanishing vector fields. Given two closed surfaces: S' (sphere-like) and τ (planar flat-torus) with a conformal homeomorphism $\phi : S' \to \tau$, a convolution operator $*_{(\tau)}$ on τ defines a corresponding convolution operator on S', by $f *_{(S')} g = ((f \circ \phi^{-1}) *_{(\tau)} (g \circ \phi^{-1})) \circ \phi$. As the convolution on the planar flat-torus τ is invariant to Euclidean translations σ, the convolution on S' is invariant to its translation $\phi^{-1} \circ \sigma \circ \phi$. Since the ϕ^{-1}, σ and ϕ are all conformal maps, these translations are also conformal maps. Therefore, no previous alignment on the cerebrovascular model is needed in this work.

Data and Material Generation. The used database gathers the 3D model reconstruction resulting from medical images of different modalities, in which the location and presence of aneurysms were evaluated by up to four experienced neuro-radiologists. The positive dataset (with aneurysms) of 56 patients was drawn from a large multicenter database created within the EU-funded project @neurIST [17] based on the 3DRA image. The negative dataset (without aneurysms), derived from the public dataset distributed by the MIDAS Data Server at Kitware Inc. [2], contains 50 MRAs of the cerebral vascular from healthy volunteers. Because MRA images include a larger portion of the cerebral vasculature than 3DRA images do, we selected only segments with branches similar to those present in the 3DRA mesh models, such as the anterior cerebral artery (ACA) or the internal carotid artery (ICA) bifurcation. No other information was considered during the selection process.

To train the network, we first need to push the training data to images defined over the planar flat-torus τ with seamless counter-clockwise covers. Given the training data $\{(S_i, x_i, \hat{z}_i)\}_{i \in I}$, for each i we sample ρ quarter-points $P = \{p_1, p_2, p_3, p_4\} \subset S_i$. The skeleton of the vascular model is computed by [15], and each skeleton endpoint is related to the corresponding vertices of the mesh model. The longest road in the skeleton is identified, and its two endpoints are labelled as lp_1 and lp_4. The endpoint with the largest number of binding vertices (likely representing a big aneurysm), excluding lp_1 and lp_4, is labelled as lp_2. A fourth point lp_3 is identified as the endpoint with the shortest skeleton length to lp_1 or lp_4. If the skeleton has only three branches, we set lp_3 equal to lp_2. Then, each point p_i is randomly selected (without repetition) from the binding points of lp_i. This choice of quarter-points follows the rationale of well-covering the surface to allow each point to be represented with a reasonable scale factor in at least one map. Hence, we sampled a small number ($\rho = 10$) of uniformly spread points P on the surface. We cut the square flat-image τ. To avoid data similarity, we set the random cut in their universal covering space with sphere-like surface S' computed with different points P for their close positions. The number of training samples can be increased by data augmentation, which can play an important role in deep learning with small data sets. We used 6x data augmentation in our experiments with mirroring, rotation and flipping operations.

Feature Selection. Conformal mapping can only convert a 3D mesh model S to a flat image τ with the smallest twist. Different types of features must describe the shape of the models. Our map provides a relatively small space of possible parameterizations, which make learning easier. For the local features, we choose the shape diameter function (SDF) and Gaussian curvature (GC) of each point in the model. For the global features, we use the spectral decomposition of the Laplace-Beltrami operator on the manifold to create spectral shape descriptors: wave kernel signature (WKS). The multi-model neural network is used to aggregate all these three feature maps.

Multi-model Ensemble Neural Network on the Planar Flat-Torus τ. We present a multi-model ensemble architecture with cerebral mesh models to three-dimensional features on τ. The V3 model pre-trained on the ImageNet dataset is adopted with one fully connected (FC) layer (GV3F) as the fundamental classifier for each feature image on τ. Three copies of this V3 model are fine-tuned using the input of three-dimensional features on τ in Fig. 1. The output neurons in the last fully connected layer of the classifiers are connected with one fully connected layer (MMEN) to give the final decision. This architecture is a non-linear function that takes three-dimensional functions over the image τ to L valued functions over the image which can be defined as $F(, \mathbf{w}) : \mathbb{R}^{m \times n \times 3} \to \mathbb{R}^{m \times n} \times L$.

A two-step training is used. For each classifier j, the loss function is defined as the binary cross entropy $E_j(w) = -\sum_i [\hat{z}_i \log(p(x_i^j)) + (1 - \hat{z}_i) \log(1 - p(x_i^j))$, where $p(x_i^j)$ denotes the result predicted by j-th V3 model. We use the stochastic gradient decent method with a batch size of 128 and learning rate of 0.01. The initial weights are stochastically selected with a truncated normal

Gaussian distribution in $[-1, 1]$. We stop training when the total loss is less than 0.2 for 500 iterations. When all the features are stably trained on τ, we begin the multi-model ensemble architecture training. The ultimate prediction result of the ensemble model is calculated as $P_i = \sum_{j=1}^{b} w_j p(x_i^j)$, where P_i is the likelihood of the input model S_i belonging to category $L \in \{0, 1\}$ and $b = 3$. The binary cross entropy loss function is used again in this ensemble model, and the change of weight is $\Delta w_j = -\eta \sum_i (\frac{\hat{z}_i}{P_i} - (\frac{1-\hat{z}_i}{1-P_i}))$, for learning rate $\eta = 0.01$. Stochastic gradient decent with a batch size 64 is adopted due to our small number of training data. A 5-fold cross validation is used, with which the whole dataset is split into five equal subsets, combining training set (80%) and a testing set (20%). To avoid over-fitting, the training set is further split into a proper training set (95%) and a validation set (5%). The training is terminated even before reaching the maximum iteration number of 1000.

3   Experiments

We conduct our research platform based on TensorFlow using an NVIDIA 960 M GPU on an Ubuntu 16.10 Linux OS 64-bit operating system. The proposed MMEN architecture has been applied to the dataset 5 times independently, with 5-fold cross validation. The mean and standard deviation of the obtained false positive ratio, specificity, accuracy and sensitivity in the full dataset are presented in Table 1 and are compared with the performance of 6 state-of-the-art methods with different datasets. Our results are superior in some metrics, depending on the compared study, although a more global and direct comparison is hindered by the differences in the datasets and evaluation criteria. Our algorithm obtains similar or superior results to both the hand-crafted feature-based traditional methods and the other deep leaning methods [4,5,10,12,16], which require more homogeneous data formats. Our results indicate that (1) The conformal parameterization method provides a valid mesh representation. (2) The

Table 1. Comparison of the performance of out proposed method to that of 6 state-of-the-art aneurysm detection methods on different datasets. *I: input data format; N: number of cases; F: false positive ratio; S: Specificity; A: Accuracy; SE: Sensitivity;*

Algorithms	I	N	F	S (%)	A (%)	SE (%)
Sichtermann *et al.* 19 [12]	3D TOF-MRA (1.5T,3T)	85	8.14	Poor	–	87
Ueda *et al.* 19 [16]	3D TOF-MRA (1.5T,3T)	748	10	–	–	91
Jin *et al.* 19 [5]	2D-DSA	493	3.77	–	–	89.3
Nakao *et al.* 18 [10]	3D TOF-MRA (3T)	450	2.9	–	–	94.2
Jerman *et al.* 17 [4]	3D-DSA	15	2.4	–	95	100
MIKI *et al.* 16 [7]	3D MRI(3T)	2701	–	–	–	82
Proposed (Mean ± standard deviation)	3DRA+3D TOF MRI(1.5T)	**121**	**0.8 ± 0.6**	**95.4 ± 6.2**	**95.1 ± 4.0**	**94.8 ± 6.7**

pre-trained and fine-tuned V3 model can effectively transfer the image representation ability learned on the ImageNet dataset to characterize the parameterization method model. (3) An adaptive ensemble of these images has superior ability in identifying aneurysms in cerebrovascular mesh models.

4   Discussion

Different Parameterization Methods. The parameterization of the mesh model S plays an important role in applying a deep model to the 3D mesh model problem. On one hand, the conformal mapping from S to τ provides the parameterization involving the least twist. On the other hand, the computational complexity of our method is small. We re-performed the experiments using conformal parameterization and sphere parameterization. The obtained performances are listed in Table 2. AP is the index of the area changing in the parameterization. If the surface area ratio between the aneurysm part and the branch part is similar to the original, the area twist would be small, just as our method. These two parameterization methods are conducted with the same quarter-point $P = \{p1, p2, p3, p4\}$ in each positive model.

Table 2. Comparison of the performance between our conformal parametrization and the sphere parameterization [11] on 3D mesh models with aneurysms. *SP: sphere parameterization; M number of missing aneurysms in parameterization images of each cerebrovascular model; AP: surface area ratio between the aneurysms part and the branch part. R: running time for the parameterization. Mean ± standard deviation.*

Parameterization	M	AP (%)	R(s)
Orginal mesh model S	–	2.36 ± 0.48	–
SP [11]	3.90 ± 2.69	0.14 ± 0.14	104.072
Proposed	0	**1.77 ± 0.58**	**12.6**

Ensemble Learning. To demonstrate the improvement in performance provided by the feature combination by the adaptive ensemble, we compared the performance with five features-WKS, GC, SDF, mean curvature (MC) and global point signature (GPS) on the same data set of intracranial aneurysms (Table 3). We can obtain the highest accuracy and F1-score with SDF geometric feature map and the highest sensitivity with WKS. For the GPS, the F1-score and sensitivity are both the lowest. Therefore, we choose the WKS, GC and SDF as the final features. Although each V3 model achieves a relatively good performance, the adaptive ensemble of them achieves a better performance.

Other Pre-trained DCNN Models. In addition to GoogLeNet, ResNet-50 [3], and VGGNet [13] are two of the most successful DCNN models. Using each of those three models to characterize from each of the three perspectives, we have

Table 3. Performance comparison of each component V3 model, considering only one feature, and the proposed MMEN model combining WKS,GC and SDF. *F1: F1-score*

Models (V3)	A (%)	SE (%)	S (%)	P (%)	F1
WKS	82.6	**91.2**	75.4	76.9	82.9
GC	86.8	87.7	**86.2**	85.8	86.0
SDF	**88.4**	91.1	**86.2**	**86.0**	**88.0**
MC	85.1	83.9	86.2	84.9	84.1
GPS	63.6	67.7	60.0	59.1	62.8
Proposed	**95.1**	**94.8**	**95.4**	**95.1**	**92.4**

27 configurations. To evaluate the performance of using other DCNN models, we tested all these configurations and gave the F1-score, accuracy and sensitivity of the configurations. Table 3 shows the best six configurations with F1-score. The other results are shown in the supplied materials for space limits. It shows that V3 model is very powerful, using three V3 models results in the highest F1-score and sensitivity with quite the same training time complexity as the shortest one. Nevertheless, the results also suggest that ResNet50 is also a good choices as well and using it to replace GoogLeNet may produce very similar good F1-score and sensitivities in some configurations. VGGNet must be trained with more time to converge with low accuracy and F1-score. For fairness of the comparision, we set the optimization method and hyper-parameters of all these DCNN model to be the same (Table 4).

Table 4. Performance of top-6 models from 27 ensemble models. *V3: GoogLeNet Inception V3;RN5:ResNet-50; VN:VGGNet*

DNN-WKS	DNN-GC	DNN-SDF	F1 (%)	A (%)	SE (%)	T (s)
V3	V3	V3	**94.7**	**95.1**	**94.9**	92.4
V3	RN5	V3	93.8	94.3	93.0	89.2
RN5	V3	V3	93.1	93.4	93.0	89.0
RN5	RN5	V3	92.1	92.6	91.2	**85.1**
V3	V3	RN5	91.4	91.7	94.7	86.5
VN	V3	RN5	91.0	90.9	92.9	258.6

Other Things: Computational Complexity and Failed Results. In our experiments, it took about 92.4 s to train the proposed model and less than 0.5 s for aneurysms detection in each mesh model. This result suggest that the proposed algorithm is very efficient for offline training and online testing. In the positive data set, model 2, 10 and 50 with failed detection have an average diameter smaller than 4 mm with irregular shape boundary, which is also very difficult for the radiologist to decide. More details on further aspects are described in the supplementary material.

5   Conclusion

We propose the MMEN algorithm to detect intracranial aneurysms in cerebrovascular mesh model from 3DRA data and MRA data. We seamlessly parameterize the input mesh model to the planar flat-torus with universal covering space. We use three pre-trained and fine-tuned GoogleNet Reception V3 models to characterize the cerebrovascular mesh model with three geometrical features (WKS, GC and SDF), and combine these models using an adaptive weighting scheme learned during the back-propagation process. The results show that our algorithm produces more accurate results, having good potential as a novel IA detection framework.

Acknowledgement. The authors want to thank the anonymous reviewers for their constructive comments. This research was partially supported by the National Key Cooperation between the BRICS of China (No. 2017YFE0100500), National Key R&D Program of China (No. 2017YFB1002604, No. 2017YFB1402105) and Beijing Natural Science Foundation of China (No. 4172033). AFF is supported by the Royal Academy of Engineering Chair in Emerging Technologies Scheme (CiET1819\19), and the OCEAN project (EP/M006328/1) and the MedIAN Network (EP/N026993/1) both funded by the Engineering and Physical Sciences Research Council (EPSRC).

References

1. Aigerman, N., Lipman, Y.: Orbifold tutte embeddings. TOG **34**(6), 1–12 (2015)
2. Aylward, S.R., Bullitt, E.: Initialization, noise, singularities, and scale in height ridge traversal for tubular object centerline extraction. TMI **21**(2), 61–75 (2002)
3. He, K., Zhang, X., Ren, S., et al.: Deep residual learning for image recognition. In: CVPR, pp. 770–778 (2016)
4. Jerman, T., Pernus, F., Likar, B., et al.: Aneurysm detection in 3D cerebral angiograms based on intra-vascular distance mapping and convolutional neural networks. In: ISBI, pp. 612–615 (2017)
5. Jin, H., Yin, Y., Hu, M., et al.: Fully automated unruptured intracranial aneurysm detection and segmentation from digital subtraction angiography series using an end-to-end spatiotemporal deep neural network. In: SPIE Medical Imaging 2019, pp. 1–8 (2019)
6. Maron, H., Galun, M., Aigerman, N., et al.: Convolutional neural networks on surfaces via seamless toric covers. TOG **36**(4), 71–1 (2017)
7. Miki, S., Hayashi, N., Masutani, Y., et al.: Computer-assisted detection of cerebral aneurysms in MR angiography in a routine image-reading environment: effects on diagnosis by radiologists. AJNR **37**(6), 1038–1043 (2016)
8. Milnor, J.W., Weaver, D.W.: Topology from the Differentiable Viewpoint. Princeton University Press, Princeton (1997)
9. Mozaffarian, D., Benjamin, E.J., Go, A.S., et al.: Executive summary: heart disease and stroke statistics-2016 update: a report from the american heart association. Circulation **133**(4), 447–454 (2016)

10. Nakao, T., Hanaoka, S., Nomura, Y., et al.: Deep neural network-based computer-assisted detection of cerebral aneurysms in MR angiography. JMRI **47**(4), 948–953 (2018)
11. Praun, E., Hoppe, H.: Spherical parametrization and remeshing. TOG **22**(3), 340–349 (2003)
12. Sichtermann, T., Faron, A., Sijben, R., et al.: Deep learning-based detection of intracranial aneurysms in 3D TOF-MRA. AJNR **40**(1), 25–32 (2019)
13. Simonyan, K., Zisserman, A.: Very deep convolutional networks for large-scale image recognition. arXiv:1409.1556 (2014)
14. Szegedy, C., Liu, W., Jia, Y., et al.: Going deeper with convolutions. In: CVPR, pp. 1–9 (2015)
15. Tagliasacchi, A., Alhashim, I., Olson, M., et al.: Mean curvature skeletons. CGF **31**(5), 1735–1744 (2012)
16. Ueda, D., Yamamoto, A., Nishimori, M.: Deep learning for MR angiography: automated detection of cerebral aneurysms. Radiology **290**, 187–194 (2019)
17. Villa-Uriol, M.C., Berti, G., Hose, D.R., et al.: @ neurist complex information processing toolchain for the integrated management of cerebral aneurysms. Interface Focus **1**(3), 308–319 (2011)

Automated Noninvasive Seizure Detection and Localization Using Switching Markov Models and Convolutional Neural Networks

Jeff Craley[1(✉)] , Emily Johnson[2] , Christophe Jouny[2] ,
and Archana Venkataraman[1]

[1] Department of Electrical and Computer Engineering, Johns Hopkins University,
Baltimore, USA
jcraley2@jhu.edu
[2] Department of Neurology, Johns Hopkins Medical Institute, Baltimore, USA

Abstract. We introduce a novel switching Markov model for combined epileptic seizure detection and localization from scalp electroencephalography (EEG). Using a hierarchy of Markov chains to fuse multichannel information, our model detects seizure onset, localizes the seizure focus, and tracks seizure activity as it spreads across the cortex. This model-based seizure tracking and localization is complemented by a nonparametric EEG likelihood using convolutional neural networks. We learn our model with an expectation-maximization algorithm that uses loopy belief propagation for approximate inference. We validate our model using leave one patient out cross validation on EEG acquired from two hospitals. Detection is evaluated on the publicly available Children's Hospital Boston dataset. We validate both the detection and localization performance on a focal epilepsy dataset collected at Johns Hopkins Hospital. To the best of our knowledge, our model is the first to perform automated localization from scalp EEG across a heterogeneous patient cohort.

1 Introduction

Epilepsy is one of the most common neurological disorders, and 20–40% of patients are medically refractory and do not respond anti-epileptic drugs [3]. When refractory epilepsy is *focal*, i.e. originating from a single seizure onset zone [7], surgical resection of this area may be the only treatment available. Scalp EEG is the first modality used to localize the seizure onset zone. While scalp EEG is non-invasive and easy to acquire, it is plagued by artifacts, such as muscle and eye movements, which may completely obscure the seizure characteristics. In addition, visual inspection of EEG recordings is time consuming and requires extensive training due to the inherent difficulty in identifying seizure activity.

Automated seizure localization methods fall into three general categories: spike detection, source localization, and signal decomposition. Spike detectors

© Springer Nature Switzerland AG 2019
D. Shen et al. (Eds.): MICCAI 2019, LNCS 11767, pp. 253–261, 2019.
https://doi.org/10.1007/978-3-030-32251-9_28

identify epileptiform activity between seizures. Channels containing this activity are noted as potential onset areas. However, the accuracy of these algorithms is hard to evaluate, as inter-rater agreement between clinicians for interictal epileptiform activity is low [10]. Source localization methods solve an inverse problem to identify the location within the brain the seizure activity originates from. However, these methods require manual identification of the seizure interval beforehand. Additionally, inverse methods require more expensive imaging, such as MRI, for accurate coregistration [8]. Decomposition methods, such as canonical decomposition, are used to localize the seizure in the sensor space but also require annotated onsets [9]. These methods are difficult to use in practice and do not provide much information beyond clinical review.

The work of [1,2] proposes an interesting alternative for seizure detection based on a coupled hidden Markov model (CHMM). The coupling between EEG channels acts as a spatio-temporal regularizer for the estimated seizure activity. While the CHMM achieves better detection accuracy, its ability to localize seizure activity requires heuristic evaluation of the output posterior probabilities.

We propose a novel Regime-Switching Markov Model for Propagation and Localization (R-SMMPL) and demonstrate it on both seizure detection and onset zone localization. Our model decouples detection, propagation, and localization into three interacting sets of variables. A switching variable controls the dynamic regime of the system, acting as a seizure onset and offset detector. In response to changes in this switching variable, we use a modified CHMM [1] to track the spread of seizure activity when seizures are detected. Our formulation includes a set of hierarchically linked location variables which allows us to tie onset location distributions between multiple recordings. We equip the R-SMMPL with nonparametric likelihoods using convolutional neural networks (CNNs) as in [2].

Unlike prior work, the R-SMMPL allows us to pool information across multiple seizure recordings into an onset zone hypothesis for each patient. Furthermore, it can easily incorporate expert information about the seizure onset times and locations. We validate our model on Johns Hopkins Hospital (JHH) dataset containing exclusively focal seizures and the Children's Hospital Boston (CHB) dataset of unspecified seizure types. To our knowledge, the R-SMMPL is the first unified framework for both seizure detection and localization from scalp EEG.

2   R-SMMPL Formulation

Figure 1 shows our graphical model (left) and variable descriptions (right). The plate notation in Fig. 1 describes how multiple seizure recordings are aggregated for a single patient. Bold variables represent collections across time and, if applicable, EEG channel. Figure 3 illustrates the temporal evolution of a seizure as represented by the inner plate of Fig. 1. Seizure propagation pathways are defined by the graph S, shown by the channel nodes and blue lines in Fig. 3. Notice that we have coupled neighboring and contralateral channels, as these are the most common propagation patterns observed in EEG seizure recordings.

Let N be the total number of patients, J^n be the number of recordings belonging to patient n, and let superscript nj denote recording j in patient n. M is the

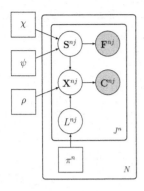

Symbol	Description
$S^{nj}[t]$	Switching chain for regime-switching
$X_i^{nj}[t]$	Seizure state of EEG channel i
L^{nj}	Seizure onset location
$C_i^{nj}[t]$	EEG observation in channel i
$F^{nj}[t]$	Full EEG observation for all channels
$\mathcal{S}$	Seizure propagation graph
π^n	Onset distribution for patient n
χ	Seizure onset probability
ψ	Seizure offset probability
ρ	Seizure propagation constant

Fig. 1. Left: R-SMMPL plate model. Squares denote parameters while circles indicate random variables. Observed variables are shaded gray. **Right:** Variable descriptions. $\mathbf{S}^{nj} \triangleq \{S^{nj}[t]\}_{t=0}^{T}$, $\mathbf{X}^{nj} \triangleq \{X_i^{nj}[t]\}_{t=0,i=1}^{T,M}$, and similarly for $\mathbf{F}^{nj}$ and $\mathbf{C}^{nj}$, respectively.

number of EEG channels (typically 18–20) and T is the recording duration. The switching chain $S^{nj}[t]$ tracks the overall state of the system as a seizure occurs and progresses. The chains $X_i^{nj}[t]$ track the spread of seizure activity through EEG channel i. Each recording has an onset location $L^{nj} \in \{1, 2, \ldots, M\}$. Emission variables $F^{nj}[t]$ and $C_i^{nj}[t]$ are observed from the switching chain S^{nj} and the individual CHMM chains $X_i^{nj}[t]$, respectively. The joint distribution is:

$$P(\mathbf{L}, \mathbf{S}, \mathbf{X}, \mathbf{F}, \mathbf{C}) = \prod_{n=1}^{N} \prod_{j=1}^{J^n} P\left(L^{nj}\right) \prod_{t=1}^{T} P\left(S^{nj}[t] \mid S^{nj}[t-1]\right) P\left(F^{nj}[t] \mid S^{nj}[t]\right)$$

$$\prod_{i=1}^{M} P\left(X_i^{nj}[t] \mid X_i^{nj}[t-1], L^{nj}, S^{nj}[t], X_{nes(i)}^{nj}[t-1]\right) P\left(C_i^{nj}[t] \mid X_i^{nj}[t]\right)$$

Localization: For each patient, a multinomial location parameter π^n represents the probability that a seizure from patient n will exhibit onset in a particular EEG channel. For each recording, the onset location L^{nj} is drawn from π^n.

Regime-Switching and Propagation: The variables $S^{nj}[t]$ progress through five states: pre-seizure baseline, seizure onset, seizure spreading, seizure offset, and post-seizure baseline. The variables $X_i^{nj}[t]$ are binary and denote either normal ($X_i^{nj}[t] = 0$) or seizure ($X_i^{nj}[t] = 1$) in channel i at time t. Each recording begins in pre-seizure baseline with all channels exhibiting normal EEG activity.

Seizure onset and spread are shown on the right side of Fig. 3. At each time step, there is probability χ of a seizure occurring, represented by the switching chain $S^{nj}[t]$ transitioning into the onset state. At onset, chain $X_{L^{nj}}^{nj}[t]$

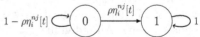

Fig. 2. Transition diagram for $X_i^{nj}[t]$ when $S^{nj}[t]$ is in the spreading state.

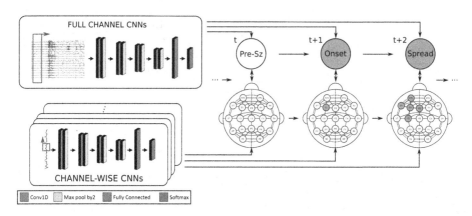

Fig. 3. Model schematic. The left side depicts the CNNs used for likelihood scoring prior to inference. The orientations of the kernels and convolutions are shown in red. At right the system is shown at seizure onset. Channel nodes and blue connections define the propagation graph $\mathcal{S}$. The seizure switching chain is shown above, where seizure activity is shown in red while normal activity is white. During spreading, seizure propagates through $\mathbf{X}^{nj}$ (below) along the blue propagation pathways. (Color figure online)

enters the seizure state, representing abnormal activity at the seizure onset zone. The switching chain $S^{nj}[t]$ then immediately transitions to the spreading state.

During spreading, seizure activity is allowed to spread through the seizure propagation graph $\mathcal{S}$ defined in Fig. 3. This spreading is governed by the probabilities in the transition diagram in Fig. 2. The probability that $X_i^{nj}[t]$ enters the seizure state (1) from the non-seizure state (0) at time t is proportionate to the number of possible ways a seizure can spread to channel i in $\mathcal{S}$. Let $\eta_i^{nj}[t] \triangleq \sum_{j \in ne\mathcal{S}} X_j^{nj}[t]$ be the number of neighbors in $\mathcal{S}$ that are in the seizure state at time t. The probability $X_i^{nj}[t]$ enters the seizure state at time $t+1$ is $\rho \eta_i^{nj}[t]$, where ρ is the parameter that governs how quickly the seizure spreads.

During the seizure, the probability of seizure offset at any time is ψ. When the switching chain $S^{nj}[t]$ enters an offset state, all EEG channels $X_i^{nj}[t]$ return to normal activity. This offset is immediately followed by a post-seizure baseline state for the remainder of the recording where no seizure activity is observed.

CNN Likelihood: Implemented in PyTorch, each CNN contains four convolution and pool layers as shown in Fig. 3. Convolution layers use eight kernels of five samples with two sample zero padding and LeakyReLU activation. Max pooling with a kernel size of two was used to halve the size of the representation at each layer. Softmax classification was performed on the concatenated result of the final pooling. All individual CNNs for $P(C_i^{nj}[t] \mid X_i^{nj}[t])$ were trained for 60 epochs; those for all channels $P(F^{nj}[t] \mid S^{nj}[t])$ were trained for 100 epochs using Adam, batches of 32 samples, a learning rate of 0.5, and cross entropy loss.

Algorithm 1. Approximate inference using loopy belief propagation.

1: **function** APPROXIMATE INFERENCE($\mathbf{F}^{nj}, \mathbf{C}^{nj}, \chi, \psi, \rho, \pi^n$)
2:     Pass the location variable, L^{nj}, to the $\mathbf{X}^{nj}$ chains
3:     **for** Two Iterations **do**
4:         Forward-backward algorithm on $\mathbf{S}^{nj}$ chain to update $\gamma_S^{nj}[t]$
5:         Pass detection messages from $\mathbf{S}^{nj}$ chain down to $\mathbf{X}^{nj}$ chains
6:         Approximate forward-backward on $\mathbf{X}^{nj}$ to update $\gamma_{X_i}^{nj}[t]$, $\xi_i^{nj}[t]$, and $\phi_i^{nj}[t]$.
7:         Pass the $\mathbf{X}^{nj}$ messages upward to the $\mathbf{S}^{nj}$ chain
8:     **end for**
9:     Pass the $\mathbf{X}^{nj}$ messages to L^{nj} to perform localization and update τ^{nj}
10:     **return** $\gamma_S^{nj}[t]$, $\gamma_{X_i}^{nj}[t]$, $\xi_i^{nj}[t]$, $\phi_i^{nj}[t]$, and τ^{nj}
11: **end function**

By construction, the CNN outputs the posterior probability $P(X_i^{nj}[t] \mid C_i^{nj}[t])$ and $P(S^{nj}[t] \mid F^{nj}[t])$. Therefore, to obtain the likelihood factor, the discriminative CNN outputs are rescaled using Bayes rule, e.g. $P(C_i^{nj}[t] \mid X_i^{nj}[t]) \approx \frac{P(X_i^{nj}[t]|C_i[t])P(C_i^{nj}[t])}{\hat{P}(X_i^{nj}[t])} \propto \frac{P(X_i^{nj}[t]|C_i^{nj}[t])}{\hat{P}(X_i^{nj}[t])}$. We only require the likelihood up to a constant factor for inference and thus drop the $P(C_i[t])$ term. $P(X_i^{nj}[t])$ is approximated by the empirical distribution of seizure in the dataset, i.e. $\hat{P}(X_i^{nj} = 1) = \frac{\# \text{ seizure windows}}{\# \text{ windows}}$, $\hat{P}(X_i^{nj} = 0) = 1 - \hat{P}(X_i^{nj} = 1)$ as in [2].

3 Inference and Learning

The hierarchical and coupled nature of our R-SMMPL renders exact inference intractable. Therefore, we rely on loopy belief propagation [6] for approximate inference. Loopy belief propagation is a general class of algorithms where local marginal beliefs are passed as messages between neighboring random variables. These messages between represent the current local beliefs. By multiplying and summing these messages we can find posterior marginal beliefs of random variables in our model. The marginals needed for learning our model are defined below. Our message passing schedule is detailed in Algorithm 1. While loopy belief propagation provides no convergence guarantees, we observe this procedure to yield robust marginals, with little change after further message passing.

We use an expectation-maximization (EM) type algorithm for fitting the R-SMMPL to data. Our model contains three unknown transition parameters: the seizure onset probability χ, the offset probability ψ, and the spreading rate ρ. In addition we learn the onset distribution π^n for each patient. The updates are derived by setting the first derivative of the expected log-likelihood of the joint distribution with respect to the parameter of interest to zero.

The parameters χ and ψ are updated by dividing the total number of onset and offset transitions by the expected number of timesteps spent in the pre-seizure and seizure spreading state, respectively. Let the singleton posterior marginals of $S^{nj}[t]$ be defined as $\gamma_S^{nj}[t](k) \triangleq P(S^{nj}[t] = k \mid \mathbf{F}^{nj}, \mathbf{C}^{nj})$ where

$k = 0$ represents pre-seizure baseline and $k = 2$ is the spreading state.

$$\chi = \frac{\sum_{n=1}^{N} J^n}{\sum_{n=1}^{N} \sum_{j=1}^{J^n} \sum_{t=0}^{T} \gamma_S^{nj}[t](0)}, \qquad \psi = \frac{\sum_{n=1}^{N} J^n}{\sum_{n=1}^{N} \sum_{j=1}^{J^n} \sum_{t=0}^{T} \gamma_S^{nj}[t](2)}$$

The spreading parameter ρ is updated by calculating the ratio of times channels enter a seizure state versus times channels remain in non-seizure states, weighted by the number of neighboring channels exhibiting seizure activity. Here we require the singleton and pairwise marginals $\gamma_{X_i}^{nj}[t](k) \triangleq P(X_i^{nj}[t] = k \mid \mathbf{F}^{nj}, \mathbf{C}^{nj})$ and $\xi_{X_i}^{nj}[t](k, l) \triangleq P(X_i^{nj}[t] = l, X_i^{nj}[t - 1] = k \mid \mathbf{F}^{nj}, \mathbf{C}^{nj})$. In addition, let the expected number of neighbors in the seizure state be $\phi_i^{nj}[t] = E\left[\eta_i^{nj}[t] \mid \mathbf{F}^{nj}, \mathbf{C}^{nj}\right]$.

$$\rho = \frac{\sum_{n=1}^{N} \sum_{j=1}^{J^n} \sum_{i=1}^{M} \sum_{t=1}^{T} \xi_{X_i}^{nj}[t](0, 1)}{\sum_{n=1}^{N} \sum_{j=1}^{J^n} \sum_{i=1}^{M} \sum_{t=0}^{T} \phi_i^{nj}[t] \gamma_{X_i}^{nj}[t](0)}$$

Let $\tau^{nj}[t](i) \triangleq P(L^{nj} = i \mid \mathbf{F}^{nj}, \mathbf{C}^{nj})$ be the posterior belief of onset in channel i. For patient n, we update π^n via $\pi^n(i) \propto \sum_{j=1}^{J^n} \tau^{nj}(i)$. This update pools the expected beliefs regarding onset location across all of a patient's recordings.

4   Experimental Results

CHB Dataset: Our first dataset consists of publicly available seizure recordings acquired at Children's Hospital Boston (CHB) [4]. We selected 185 seizures from 24 patients for our experiment. Clinical annotations for CHB include onset and offset times. The type of seizure, general or focal, and potential onset localization are not provided. Recordings in this dataset were made at 256 Hz in a longitudinal montage using the standard 10/20 electrode placement system [5].

JHH Dataset: Our second dataset consists of focal seizure recordings from the epilepsy monitoring unit of Johns Hopkins Hospital. Expert clinical annotations from this hospital include rough onset and offset times as well as consensus of rough onset zone localizations, allowing us to evaluate both detection and localization. The dataset includes 88 seizure recordings from 15 patients. Recordings were sampled at 200 Hz using 10/20 electrode placement.

Preprocessing: We extracted seizure recordings with up to 10 min of baseline before and after the seizure annotations. Channels were normalized to mean zero and variance one. High- and low-pass filters were applied at 1.6 Hz and 50 Hz to remove DC offsets and noise. A notch filter at 60 Hz was applied to remove any possible power line contamination. One second windows with 250 ms overlap were extracted from all EEG channels. Test and train sets were separated using leave one patient out cross validation. Unlike studies which train patient-specific detectors, our evaluation focuses on generalizability to unseen patients.

Baseline Comparisons: We compare detection accuracies to the discriminative CNNs trained on the individual EEG channels (I-CNN) and those trained on all channels (S-CNN). These baselines let us assess the effect of the propagation model in fusing information across time and channels. We also compare to the CHMM model in [1] using the same I-CNN for likelihood scoring. The CHMM was shown to outperform standard machine learning classifiers in [1].

Seizure Detection: Table 1 reports the detection performance of our R-SMMPL and baseline methods. We evaluate each algorithm's performance in terms of true positive rate (TPR), true negative rate (TNR), area under the curve (AUC), precision (P), and F1 score on a frame-wise basis. Performance was evaluated based on how well the methods detected the entire seizure interval. This evaluation is more stringent than prior work, which flags a single correct detection.

The R-SMMPL outperforms all baselines in TPR, P, and F1 scores. We observe that higher TPR comes at the cost of more false positives, reflected by lower TNR. Both the R-SMMPL and CHMM outperform the CNN baselines, illustrating the positive effect of data fusion through the use of spatio-temporal models. The main difference is that the CHMM provides localization information only via heuristic analysis, whereas the R-SMMPL provides it automatically.

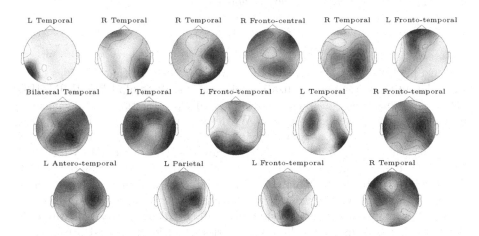

Fig. 4. Localization results from the JHH dataset. Posterior distributions over onset locations for each patient are shown with clinician provided onset diagnoses above.

Localization Results: We evaluate the localizing ability of our model when provided with a rough seizure onset time. We stipulate that the switching variable should remain in pre-seizure baseline until the clinician annotated onset. The R-SMMPL is free to switch on any time after this point.

Figure 4 shows the estimated location distribution π^n for each patient, along with the clinically diagnosed onset location. In this figure, red regions represent areas our model assigns high probability for the onset location. In the top

Table 1. Detection results for both datasets

Trial	JHH dataset					CHB dataset				
	TPR	TNR	AUC	P	F1	TPR	TNR	AUC	P	F1
R-SMMPL	**0.62**	0.84	<u>0.84</u>	**0.65**	**0.53**	**0.67**	0.94	**0.86**	**0.58**	**0.58**
CHMM	0.46	**0.96**	**0.86**	**0.65**	0.51	0.59	**0.96**	0.85	0.57	0.54
S-CNN	0.34	0.92	0.76	0.41	0.32	0.48	0.95	0.84	0.48	0.44
I-CNN	0.28	0.92	0.77	0.33	0.27	0.30	0.95	0.82	0.34	0.29

row we show cases where our algorithm reported a primary mode in agreement with clinical consensus of the seizure onset zone. The second row shows cases in which the secondary modes agrees with the clinical annotations. By pooling seizure localization information across all of each patient's recordings, our model identifies likely seizure onset zones in agreement with clinical consensus in 11 of 15 patients. The R-SMMPL misidentifies the seizure onset location in just four patients. In summary, not only does the R-SMMPL *automatically* detect and track the seizure, but also leverages multiple seizure presentations to create an onset zone hypothesis for each patient. These results demonstrate the promise of R-SMMPL for clinical evaluation of epilepsy.

5 Conclusion

We have presented R-SMMPL, the first unified framework that provides clinically relevant detection and localization information from scalp EEG. R-SMMPL combines a probabilistic graphical model of seizure propagation with deep learning for data driven likelihood scoring. We derive an inference and learning procedure for the model and demonstrate its detection and localization abilities on wholly unseen patients, mirroring clinical conditions. Our methodology for automatic seizure onset zone localization by tracking seizure propagation is the first of its kind. In the future, we plan to integrate clinically informative seizure semiology into the prior distribution for the seizure onset. We also plan to reweight onset posteriors when pooling individual recordings to automatically distinguish between noisy recordings and those with better onset location evidence.

Acknowledgment. This work was supported by a JHMI Synergy Award (Venkataraman/Johnson) and NSF CAREER 1845430 (Venkataraman).

References

1. Craley, J., Johnson, E., Venkataraman, A.: A novel method for epileptic seizure detection using coupled hidden markov models. In: Frangi, A.F., Schnabel, J.A., Davatzikos, C., Alberola-López, C., Fichtinger, G. (eds.) MICCAI 2018. LNCS, vol. 11072, pp. 482–489. Springer, Cham (2018). https://doi.org/10.1007/978-3-030-00931-1_55

2. Craley, J., Johnson, E., Venkataraman, A.: Integrating convolutional neural networks and probabilistic graphical modeling for epileptic seizure detection in multichannel EEG. In: Chung, A.C.S., Gee, J.C., Yushkevich, P.A., Bao, S. (eds.) IPMI 2019. LNCS, vol. 11492, pp. 291–303. Springer, Cham (2019). https://doi.org/10.1007/978-3-030-20351-1_22
3. French, J.A.: Refractory epilepsy: clinical overview. Epilepsia **48**, 3–7 (2007)
4. Goldberger, A.L., et al.: Physiobank, physiotoolkit, and physionet: components of a new research resource for complex physiologic signals. Circulation **101**(23), e215–e220 (2000)
5. Jurcak, V., et al.: 10/20, 10/10, and 10/5 systems revisited: their validity as relative head-surface-based positioning systems. Neuroimage **34**(4), 1600–1611 (2007)
6. Kschischang, F.R., et al.: Factor graphs and the sum-product algorithm. IEEE Trans. Inf. Theory **47**(2), 498–519 (2001)
7. Lüders, H.O., et al.: The epileptogenic zone: general principles. Epileptic Disord. **8**(2), 1–9 (2006)
8. Plummer, C., Harvey, A.S., Cook, M.: EEG source localization in focal epilepsy: where are we now? Epilepsia **49**(2), 201–218 (2008)
9. Vos, D., et al.: Canonical decomposition of ictal scalp eeg reliably detects the seizure onset zone. NeuroImage **37**(3), 844–854 (2007)
10. Wilson, S.B., Emerson, R.: Spike detection: a review and comparison of algorithms. Clin. Neurophysiol. **113**(12), 1873–1881 (2002)

Multiple Landmark Detection Using Multi-agent Reinforcement Learning

Athanasios Vlontzos$^{(\boxtimes)}$, Amir Alansary, Konstantinos Kamnitsas,
Daniel Rueckert, and Bernhard Kainz

BioMedIA, Computing Department, Imperial College London, London, UK
athanasios.vlontzos14@imperial.ac.uk

Abstract. The detection of anatomical landmarks is a vital step for medical image analysis and applications for diagnosis, interpretation and guidance. Manual annotation of landmarks is a tedious process that requires domain-specific expertise and introduces inter-observer variability. This paper proposes a new detection approach for multiple landmarks based on multi-agent reinforcement learning. Our hypothesis is that the position of all anatomical landmarks is interdependent and non-random within the human anatomy, thus finding one landmark can help to deduce the location of others. Using a Deep Q-Network (DQN) architecture we construct an environment and agent with implicit inter-communication such that we can accommodate K agents acting and learning simultaneously, while they attempt to detect K different landmarks. During training the agents collaborate by sharing their accumulated knowledge for a collective gain. We compare our approach with state-of-the-art architectures and achieve significantly better accuracy by reducing the detection error by 50%, while requiring fewer computational resources and time to train compared to the naïve approach of training K agents separately. Code and visualizations available: https://github.com/thanosvlo/MARL-for-Anatomical-Landmark-Detection

1 Introduction

The exact localization of anatomical landmarks in medical images is a crucial requirement for many clinical applications such as image registration and segmentation as well as computer-aided diagnosis and interventions. For example, for the planning of cardiac interventions it is necessary to identify standardized planes of the heart, *e.g.* short-axis and 2/4-chamber views [1]. It also plays a crucial role for prenatal fetal screening, where it is used to estimate biometric measurements like fetal growth rate to identify pathological development [17]. Moreover, the mid-sagittal plane, commonly used for brain image registration and assessing anomalies, is identified based on landmarks such as the Anterior

---

Electronic supplementary material The online version of this chapter (https://doi.org/10.1007/978-3-030-32251-9_29) contains supplementary material, which is available to authorized users.

D. Shen et al. (Eds.): MICCAI 2019, LNCS 11767, pp. 262–270, 2019.
https://doi.org/10.1007/978-3-030-32251-9_29

Commissure (AC) and Posterior Commissure (PC) [2]. Manual annotation of landmarks is often a time consuming and tedious task that requires significant expertise about the anatomy and suffers from inter- and intra-observer errors. Automatic methods on the other hand can be challenging to design because of the large variability in the appearance and shape of different organs, varying image qualities and artefacts. Thus, there is a need for methods that can learn how to locate landmarks with highest accuracy and robustness; one promising approach is based on the use Reinforcement Learning (RL) algorithms [2,8].

Contributions: This work presents a novel Multi-Agent Reinforcement Learning (MARL) approach for detecting multiple landmarks efficiently and simultaneously by sharing the agents' experience. The main contributions can be summarized as: *(i)* We introduce a novel formulation for the problem of multiple landmark detection in a MARL framework; *(ii)* A novel collaborative deep Q-network (DQN) is proposed for training using implicit communication between the agents; *(iii)* Extensive evaluations on different datasets and comparisons with recently published methods are provided (decision forests, Convolutional Neural Networks (CNNs), and single-agent RL).

Related Work. In the literature, automatic landmark detection approaches have adopted machine learning algorithms to learn combined appearance and image-based models, for example using regression forests [16] and statistical shape priors [6]. Zheng et al. [19] proposed using two CNNs for landmark detection; the first network learns the search path by extracting candidate locations, and the second learns to recognize landmarks by classifying candidate image patches. Li et al. [13] presented a patch-based iterative CNN to detect individual or multiple landmarks simultaneously. Ghesu et al. [8] introduced a single deep RL agent to navigate in a 3D image towards a target landmark. The artificial agent learns to search and detect landmarks efficiently in an RL scenario. This search can be performed using fixed or multi-scale step strategies [7]. Recently, Alansary et al. [2] proposed the use of different Deep Q-Network (DQN) architectures for landmark detection with novel hierarchical action steps. The agent learns an optimal policy to navigate using sequential action steps in a 3D image (environment) from any starting point towards the target landmark. In [2] the reported experiments have shown that such an approach can achieve state-of-the-art results for the detection of multiple landmarks from different datasets and imaging modalities. However, this approach was designed to learn a single agent for each landmark separately. In [2] it has also been shown that performance of different strategies and architectures strongly depends on the anatomical location of the target landmark. Thus we hypothesize that sharing information while attempting simultaneous detection reduces the aforementioned dependency.

Background: Reinforcement Learning (RL) allows artificial agents to learn complex tasks by interacting with an environment E using a set of actions A. The agent learns to take an action a at every step (in a state s) towards the target solution guided by a reward signal r during training. The main goal is to maximize the expected rewards in order to find the optimal policy π^*. In Q-Learning, a state-action value function $Q(s, a)$ is used to approximate the value of taking an action in a given state. The Q-function is defined as the expected value of the accumulated discounted future rewards, which can be approximated iteratively as: $Q_{t+1}(s, a) = E[r + \gamma \max_a(Q_t(s', a'))]$. Here $\gamma \in [0, 1]$ is a discount factor that is used to incorporate the notion of uncertainty in future events. Mnih et al. [15] proposed an approximation of the Q-function using a CNN by optimizing the network cost $L(\theta) = E\left[\left(r + \gamma \max_{a'} Q_{target}(s', a'; \theta^-) - Q_{net}(s, a; \theta)\right)^2\right]$. Q_{target} is a temporary fixed version of Q_{net}, which gets updated every N_{target} steps, used in order to avoid destabilization caused by rapid policy changes.

In single-agent RL scenarios, individual models learn solely from states that result from the actions of an agent. Complementary to this, MARL models learn from states that result from multiple agents dynamically interacting with their shared environment. In MARL models, there are K agents interacting with environment E. Each learns to take an action a_t^k during a state s_t^k using a reward signal r_t^k. Thus, the environment is subjected to the actions of all agents, as shown in Fig. 1. Hence, the environment becomes non-stationary as action a_i in state s_k will not always lead to the same future, since the future state is also a function of the other agents. This causes a violation of the Markov assumptions needed for the formulation of a RL scenario as a Markov Decision Process (MDP). To address this issue, [5,18] proposed to establish communication between the agents, thus taking all agents actions into account.

Any agent communication signifies the exchange of information or knowledge about the underlying Markov state of the environment. Communication between agents can be achieved explicitly via a communication protocol like in [4], where a limited bandwidth channel is learned by the agents, or implicitly by sharing knowledge in the parameter space or by combining value functions [10]. MARL scenarios can be classified as collaborative or competitive depending on the relation of the communication between agents. In this paper, we define the collaborative scenario as agents that attempt to minimize a common loss function. Competition between agents signifies a scenario in which agents try to minimize their own loss function through increasing the loss function of other agents.

2   Proposed Method

In this work, we formulate the problem of multiple anatomical landmark detection as a multi-agent reinforcement learning scenario. Building upon the work of [2,8] we extend the formulation of landmark detection as a Markov Decision Process (MDP), where artificial agents learn optimal policies towards their target landmarks, which defines a concurrent Partially Observable Markov Decision Process (co-POMDP) [9]. We consider our framework concurrent as the agents train together but each learns its own individual policy, mapping its private observations to a personal action [10]. We hypothesize that this is necessary as the localization of different landmarks requires learning partly heterogeneous policies. This would not be possible with the application of a centralized learning system.

Our RL framework is defined by the *States* of the environment, the *Actions* of the agent, their *Reward Function* and the *Terminal State*. We consider the environment to be a 3D scan of the human anatomy and define a state as a Region of Interest (ROI) centred around the location of the agent. This makes our formulation a POMDP as the agents can only see a subset of the environment [11]. We define the frame history to be comprised of four ROIs. In this setup each agent can move along the x, y, z axis creating thus a set of six actions. The agents evaluate their chosen actions based on the maximization of the rewards received from the environment. The reward function is defined as the relative improvement in Euclidean distance between their location at time t and the target landmark location. In our multi-agent framework, each agent calculates its individual reward as their policies are disjoint.

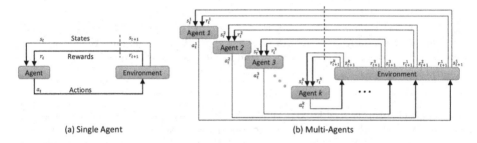

(a) Single Agent   (b) Multi-Agents

Fig. 1. (a) A single agent and (b) multi agents interact within an RL environment.

During training, we consider the search to have converged when the agent reaches a region within 1 mm of the target landmark. Episodic play is introduced in both training and testing. In training, the episode is defined as the time the agents need to find the landmarks or until they have completed a predefined maximum number of steps. In case one agent finds its landmark before all others, we freeze the training and disable network updates derived from this agent while allowing the other agents to continue exploring the environment. During testing, we terminate the episode when the agent starts to oscillate around a position or exceeds a defined maximum number of frames seen in the episode similar to [2].

Collaborative Agents. Previous approaches to the problem of landmark detection by [2,7,8] considered a single agent looking for a single landmark. This means that further landmarks needs to be trained with separate instances of the agent making a large scale application unfeasible. Our hypothesis is that the position of all anatomical landmarks is interdependent and non-random within the human anatomy, thus finding one landmark can help to deduce the location of other landmarks. This knowledge is not exploited when using isolated agents. Thus, in order to reduce the computational load in locating multiple landmarks and increase accuracy through anatomical interdependence, we propose a collaborative multi agent landmark detection framework (Collab-DQN). The following description will assume just two agents for simplicity of presentation. However, our approach scales up to K agents. For our experiments we show evaluations using two, three and five agents trained together.

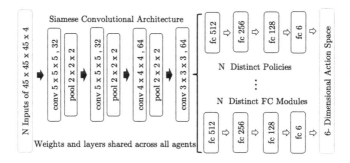

Fig. 2. Proposed Collaborative DQN for the case of two agents; The `convolutional` layers and corresponding weights are shared across all agents making them part of a Siamese architecture, while the policy making fully connected layers are separate for each agent

A DQN is composed of three `convolutional` layers interleaved with `maxpool` layers followed by three `fully connected` layers. Inspired by Siamese architectures [3], in our Collab-DQN we build K DQN networks with the difference that weights are shared across the `convolutional` layers. The `fully connected` layers remain independent since these will make the ultimate action decisions constituting the policy for each agent. In this way, the information needed to navigate through the environment are encoded into the shared layers while landmark specific information remain in the fully connected ones. In Fig. 2, we graphically represent the proposed architecture for two agents. Sharing the weights across the `convolutional` layers helps the network to learn more generalized features that can fit both inputs while adding an implicit regularization to the parameters avoiding overfitting. The shared weights enable indirect knowledge transfer in the parameter space between the agents, thus, we can consider this model as a special case of collaborative learning [10].

3   Experimentation

Dataset: We evaluate our proposed framework and model on three tasks: (i) brain MRI landmark detection with 728 training and 104 testing volumes [12]; (ii) cardiac MRI landmark detection with 364 training and 91 testing volumes [14] and (iii) landmark detection in fetal brain ultrasound with 51 training and 21 testing volumes. Each modality includes 7–14 anatomical ground truth landmark locations annotated by expert clinicians [2].

Training: During training an initial random location is chosen from the inner 80% of the volume, in order to avoid sampling outside a meaningful area. The initial ROI is $45 \times 45 \times 45$ pixels around the randomly chosen point. The agents follow an ϵ-greedy exploration strategy, where every few steps they choose a random action from a uniform distribution while during the remaining steps they act greedily. Episodic learning with the addition of freezing action updates for the agents that have reached their terminal state until the end of the episode is used, as detailed in Sect. 2.

Table 1. Results in millimeters for the various architectures on landmarks across brain MRI and fetal brain US. Our proposed Collab DQN performs better in all cases except the CSP where we match the performance of the single agent.

Method	AC	PC	RC	LC	CSP
Supervised CNN	–	–	–	–	5.47 ± 4.23
DQN	2.46 ± 1.44	2.05 ± 1.14	3.37 ± 1.54	3.25 ± 1.59	$\mathbf{3.66 \pm 2.11}$
Collab DQN	$\mathbf{0.93 \pm 0.18}$	$\mathbf{1.05 \pm 0.25}$	$\mathbf{2.52 \pm 2.25}$	$\mathbf{2.41 \pm 1.52}$	3.78 ± 5.55

Testing: For each agent, we fixed 19 different starting points in order to have a fair comparison among the different approaches. These points were used for all testing volumes for each modality at 25%, 50% and 75% of the volume's size. For each volume the Euclidean distance between the end location and the target location was averaged for each agent for each of the 19 runs. The mean distance in mm was considered to be the performance of the agent in the specific volume.

Multiple tests have been performed using our proposed architecture. Comparisons are made against the performance on multi-scale RL landmark detection [7], fully supervised deep Convolutional Neural Networks (CNN) [13] as well as a single agent DQN landmark detection algorithm [2]. In case of cardiac landmarks we compare with [16] that utilizes decision forests. Different DQN variations like the Double DQN or Duelling DQNs are not evaluated since their performance provides little to no improvement for the task of anatomical landmark detection as exhibited in [2].

Even though our method can scale up to K agents given enough computational power we limited our comparison to the Anterior Commissure (AC) and the Posterior Commissure (PC) of the brain; the Apex (AP) and Mitral Valve Centre (MV) of the heart; the Right Cerebellum (RC), Left Cerebellum (LC) and Cavum Septum Pellucidum (CSP) for the fetal brain. These are common, diagnostically valuable landmarks used in the clinical practice and by previous automatic landmark detection algorithms. For completeness and to facilitate future comparisons, we provide our performance comparison also for the training of three and five agents simultaneously. In Table 1, we show the performance of the brain MRI and fetal brain US landmarks using the different approaches. In Table 2 we exhibit the results for three and five agents trained simultaneously and the results for cardiac MRI landmarks.

Discussion: As shown in Tables 1 and 2 our proposed method significantly outperforms the current state-of-the-art in landmark detection. p-values from a paried student-t test for all experiments were in the range 0.01 to 0.0001. We perform an ablation study by training instances of a single agent with double the iterations and double the batch size. The study has been conducted on the Cardiac MRI landmarks that have exhibited the biggest localization difficulties because of larger anatomical variations across subjects than observed in brain data. Our results confirm that the agents share basic information across them, which helps all of them perform their tasks more efficiently. These results support our hypothesis that the regularization effect from the gradients collected from the increased experience and knowledge of the multi-agent system is advantageous. Furthermore, we created a single agent with doubled memory but due to the random initialization of experience memory, the agent failed to learn. In addition, as shown in Table 2(a), the inclusion of more agents leads to similar or improved results across all landmarks. It is interesting to note that even though we perform better in all landmarks, our approach can only match the performance of a single agent DQN for the CSP landmark. We theorize that this is due to the different anatomical nature of the RC, LC landmarks compared to the CSP landmark, thus the joint detection does not present an advantage. We chose to utilize the DQN in this paper rather than existing policy gradient methods like A3C as the DQN is represented by a single deep CNN that interacts with a single environment. A3C use many instances of the agent that interact asynchronously and in parallel. Multiple A3C agents with multiple incarnations of such environments are computationally expensive. In future work, we will investigate the application of other methods for multiple-landmarks detection using either collaborative or competitive agents.

Computational Performance: Training multiple agents together does not only provide benefits in performance of landmark localization, it also reduces the time and memory requirements of training. Sharing the weights between the convolutional layers helps to reduce the trainable parameters by 5% in case of

Table 2. (a) Multiple agent performance, training and testing were conducted in the Brain MRI; Landmarks 3, 4, 5 represent respectively the outer aspect, the inferior tip and the inner aspect of the splenium of corpus callosum; (b) multi-agent performance on cardiac MRI dataset;

Landmark	3 Agents	5 Agents
AC	0.94 ± 0.17	0.98 ± 0.25
PC	0.96 ± 0.20	0.90 ± 0.18
Landmark 3	1.45 ± 0.51	1.39 ± 0.45
Landmark 4	N/A	1.42 ± 0.90
Landmark 5	N/A	1.72 ± 0.61

(a)

Method	AP	MV
Inter-Obs. Error	5.79 ± 3.28	5.30 ± 2.98
Decision Forest	6.74 ± 4.12	6.32 ± 3.95
DQN	4.47 ± 2.64	5.73 ± 4.16
DQN Batch $\times 2$	4.30 ± 12.07	5.01 ± 4.49
DQN Iterations $\times 2$	4.78 ± 13.87	5.70 ± 18.11
Collab DQN	$\mathbf{3.96 \pm 5.07}$	$\mathbf{4.87 \pm 0.26}$

(b)

two agents and by 6% in case of three agents when compared with the parameters of two and three separate networks respectively. Furthermore, the addition of a single agent to our architecture reduces the required number of parameters by 6% compared to a single standalone agent. Due to the regularization effect that multiple agents have on their training and the implicit knowledge transfer, the training time our approach needs on average 25.000–50.000 less time steps to converge compared with a single DQN and each training epoch needs approximately 30 min less than the training of 2 epochs in a separate single DQN (NVIDIA Titan-X, 12 GB). Inference is on par with a single agent at $\sim$20fps.

4 Conclusion

In this paper we formulated the problem of multiple anatomical landmark detection as a multi-agent reinforcement learning scenario, we also introduced Collab-DQN, a Collaborative DQN for landmark detection in brain and cardiac MRI volumes and 3D US. We train K agents together looking for K landmarks. The agents share their convolutional layer weights. In this fashion we exploit the knowledge transferred by each agent to teach the other agents. We achieve significantly better performance than the next best method of [2] decreasing the error by more than 1 mm while taking less time to train and less memory than training K agents serially. We believe that a Bayesian exploration approach is a natural next step, which will be addressed in future work.

Acknowledgements. Wellcome Trust IEH Award [102431], EPSRC EP/ S013687/ 1, NVIDIA for their GPU donations. Brain MRI: adni.loni.usc.edu, US data: access only with informed consent, subject to approval and formal Data Sharing Agreement. Caridac data: digital-heart.org.

References

1. Alansary, A., et al.: Automatic view planning with multi-scale deep reinforcement learning agents. In: Frangi, A.F., Schnabel, J.A., Davatzikos, C., Alberola-López, C., Fichtinger, G. (eds.) MICCAI 2018. LNCS, vol. 11070, pp. 277–285. Springer, Cham (2018). https://doi.org/10.1007/978-3-030-00928-1_32
2. Alansary, A., et al.: Evaluating reinforcement learning agents for anatomical landmark detection. Med. Image Anal. **53**, 156–164 (2019)
3. Bromley, J., Guyon, I., LeCun, Y., Säckinger, E., Shah, R.: Signature verification using a "siamese" time delay neural network, pp. 737–744 (1993)
4. Foerster, J., Assael, I.A., de Freitas, N., Whiteson, S.: Learning to communicate with deep multi-agent reinforcement learning. In: NIPS, vol. 29, pp. 2137–2145 (2016)
5. Foerster, J., Chen, R.Y., Al-Shedivat, M., Whiteson, S., Abbeel, P., Mordatch, I.: Learning with opponent-learning awareness. In: Proceedings of 17th International Conference on Autonomous Agents and MultiAgent Systems AAMAS 2018, pp. 122–130 (2018)

6. Gauriau, R., Cuingnet, R., Lesage, D., Bloch, I.: Multi-organ localization with cascaded global-to-local regression and shape prior. Med. Image Anal. **23**(1), 70–83 (2015)
7. Ghesu, F., Georgescu, B., Zheng, Y., Grbic, S., Maier, A., Hornegger, J., Comaniciu, D.: Multi-scale deep reinforcement learning for real-time 3D-landmark detection in CT scans. IEEE PAMI **41**(1), 176–189 (2019)
8. Ghesu, F.C., Georgescu, B., Mansi, T., Neumann, D., Hornegger, J., Comaniciu, D.: An artificial agent for anatomical landmark detection in medical images. In: Ourselin, S., Joskowicz, L., Sabuncu, M.R., Unal, G., Wells, W. (eds.) MICCAI 2016. LNCS, vol. 9902, pp. 229–237. Springer, Cham (2016). https://doi.org/10.1007/978-3-319-46726-9_27
9. Girard, J., Emami, R.: Concurrent Markov decision processes for robot team learning. EAAI **39**, 223–234 (2015)
10. Gupta, J.K., Egorov, M., Kochenderfer, M.: Cooperative multi-agent control using deep reinforcement learning. In: Sukthankar, G., Rodriguez-Aguilar, J.A. (eds.) AAMAS 2017. LNCS (LNAI), vol. 10642, pp. 66–83. Springer, Cham (2017). https://doi.org/10.1007/978-3-319-71682-4_5
11. Jaakkola, T., Singh, S.P., Jordan, M.I.: Reinforcement learning algorithm for partially observable Markov decision problems. In: NIPS (1995)
12. Jack Jr., C.R., et al.: The Alzheimer's disease neuroimaging initiative (ADNI): MRI methods. J. Magn. Reson. Imaging **27**(4), 685–691 (2008)
13. Li, Y., et al.: Fast multiple landmark localisation using a patch-based iterative network. In: Frangi, A.F., Schnabel, J.A., Davatzikos, C., Alberola-López, C., Fichtinger, G. (eds.) MICCAI 2018. LNCS, vol. 11070, pp. 563–571. Springer, Cham (2018). https://doi.org/10.1007/978-3-030-00928-1_64
14. de Marvao, A., Dawes, T.J., Shi, W., Minas, C., Keenan, N.G., Diamond, T., Durighel, G., Montana, G., Rueckert, D., Cook, S.A., et al.: Population-based studies of myocardial hypertrophy: high resolution cardiovascular magnetic resonance atlases improve statistical power. J. Cardiovasc. Magn. Reson. **16**(1), 16 (2014)
15. Mnih, V., et al.: Human-level control through deep reinforcement learning. Nature **518**, 529 (2015)
16. Oktay, O., et al.: Stratified decision forests for accurate anatomical landmark localization in cardiac images. IEEE Trans. Med. Imaging **36**(1), 332–342 (2017)
17. Rahmatullah, B., Papageorghiou, A.T., Noble, J.A.: Image analysis using machine learning: anatomical landmarks detection in fetal ultrasound images. In: 2012 IEEE 36th Annual Computer Software and Applications Conference, pp. 354–355, July 2012
18. Rashid, T., Samvelyan, M., de Witt, C.S., Farquhar, G., Foerster, J.N., Whiteson, S.: QMIX: monotonic value function factorisation for deep multi-agent reinforcement learning. CoRR abs/1803.11485 (2018)
19. Zheng, Y., Liu, D., Georgescu, B., Nguyen, H., Comaniciu, D.: 3D deep learning for efficient and robust landmark detection in volumetric data. In: Navab, N., Hornegger, J., Wells, W.M., Frangi, A.F. (eds.) MICCAI 2015. LNCS, vol. 9349, pp. 565–572. Springer, Cham (2015). https://doi.org/10.1007/978-3-319-24553-9_69

Spatiotemporal Breast Mass Detection Network (MD-Net) in 4D DCE-MRI Images

Lixi Deng[1,2], Sheng Tang[1(✉)], Huazhu Fu[3], Bin Wang[1,2], and Yongdong Zhang[1]

[1] Key Lab of Intelligent Information Processing, Institute of Computing Technology, Chinese Academy of Sciences, Beijing, China
ts@ict.ac.cn
[2] University of the Chinese Academy of Sciences, Beijing, China
[3] Inception Institute of Artificial Intelligence, Abu Dhabi, UAE

Abstract. Automatic mass detection in breast dynamic contrast-enhanced magnetic resonance imaging (DCE-MRI) helps to reduce the workload of radiologists and improves diagnostic accuracy. However, most of the existing methods rely on hand-crafted features followed by rule-based or shallow machine learning based detection methods. Due to the limited expressive power of hand-crafted features, the diagnostic performances of existing methods are usually unsatisfactory. In this work, we aim to leverage recent deep learning techniques for breast lesion detection and propose the Spatiotemporal Breast Mass Detection Networks (MD-Nets) to detect the masses in the 4D DCE-MRI images automatically. Simulating the clinical diagnosis process, we initially generate image-based candidates from all individual images and then construct a spatiotemporal 4D data to classify mass by using the convolutional long short-term memory network (ConvLSTM) to incorporate kinetic and spatial characteristics. Moreover, we collect a DCE-MRI dataset containing 21,294 annotated images from 172 studies. In experiments, we achieve an AUC of 0.9163 with a sensitivity of 0.8655 and a specificity of 0.8452, which verifies the effectiveness of our method.

1 Introduction

Breast cancer is the most common invasive cancer in women and the second primary cause of cancer death in women [3]. Fortunately, the prognoses of breast cancer achieve good results, and the cure rate reaches more than 90% [11]. Dynamic contrast-enhanced magnetic resonance imaging (DCE-MRI), which dynamically acquires images after injecting the contrast agent that depicts physiological features of tissues, provides a valuable tool to observe the mass in

This work was supported by the National Key Research and Development Program of China (2017YFB1002202), and the National Natural Science Foundation of China (61871004, 61572472, 61525206).

early diagnosis. However, a study of 4D DCE-MRI data (3D over time) usually contains more than 700 images, leading the mass detection in DCE-MRI images become a challenging and time-consuming task. Therefore, automatic mass detection significantly reduces the diagnosis time and helps radiologists release themselves from the tedious works.

The existing methods of automatic mass detection can be summarized into two categories: (1) the hand-crafted feature methods; (2) the deep learning methods. **Hand-crafted features** have been extensively studied in medical image analysis. Gubern-Mrida et al. [6] localized breast cancer in DCE-MRI images by combining blob and voxel features. Ertas et al. [5] used volumetric principal component maps in 3D data to detect the lesion in breast MRI data. Mean-shift clustering and graph-cuts were applied by McClymont et al. [9] to segment the suspicious tissues in breast MRI. However, these methods were validated in a relatively small dataset with limited generalization. **Deep learning methods** were also applied to mass detection in DCE-MRI images, while they had been introduced into breast mass detection in other types of images, such as in ultrasound images [2]. Amit et al. [1] detected the mass in breast DCE-MRI images by using a hybrid framework which used CNN to reduce the false positives resulting from the previous saliency-based candidate detection. Maicas et al. [8] adopted an extended deep Q-network (DQN) with the attention mechanism to detect breast lesions, which reduced running time complexity while keeping the high detection accuracy. However, these approaches have certain limitations. The method proposed by Amit et al. [1] relays on the saliency-based method, which generates a large number of non-mass regions, leading a high false positive rate. The DQN method extended by Maical et al. [8] is unsatisfied for 4D DCE-MRI data. Even applying deep learning methods, the representations of kinetic features in these works are acquired through manually designed methods. Moreover, the datasets used in these works are labeled at slice-level, which confuses the morphological and kinetic features in the annotation data.

To address the above issues, we first collect a new DCE-MRI dataset with 21,294 annotated images from 172 studies. Then we propose a spatiotemporal breast mass detection Network (MD-Net) to detect the masses by taking full advantages of kinetic and spatial features. Our MD-Net generates image-based candidates to recall most of the lesion regions in the breast. With these candidates, a 4D input data is constructed by combining the corresponding representations from the nearby slices across all temporal phases to utilize the spatiotemporal information. Then, a convolutional long short term memory (ConvLSTM) [12] is used to learn the temporal variation characteristics from the constructed 4D data. The sequence-to-one classification model eliminates the erroneous image-based candidates and produces satisfying slice-based detection results. The main contributions of our work are threefold: (1) We introduce deep learning to obtain the discriminative representation to detect breast mass in 4D DCE-MRI images. (2) We build a large dataset of breast DCE-MRI images with bounding boxes annotations in each image rather than each slice. (3) We propose an MD-Net to automatically identify the mass in the breast DCE-MRI images by combining morphological, kinetic and spatial features.

2   Breast 4D DCE-MRI Dataset

While 4D DCE-MRI data is a few 3D MRI images over phases (time), in this paper, we use 'slice' to refer a set of images obtained from different phases of one slice of the breast. The annotations of existing datasets [1,8] are roughly delineated only on each slice, treating images on one slice as equal, which ignores the morphological features shown in images at different phases. To address this issue, we construct a new breast DCE-MRI image dataset with label on each image in which radiologists can observe a mass. We collect 126,112 images extracted from 172 studies. Each study has an average of 733 images which distribute between 104 to 112 slices and 5 to 8 phases. Slice refers to the spatial axis, and phase refers to different imaging times.

Three sophisticated radiologists were recruited to label the images, and one of them reviewed the labeled annotations. Ignoring the clinical diagnosis information and pathological information, the three radiologists label all images only by examining the images and the kinetic curve provided by labeling software. The labeling procedure is divided into two steps, diagnosis of mass and labeling. If the radiologist confirms the location of the mass in the breast, he is asked to mark the bounding box of the mass only in the images where the mass can be directly observed, rather than in all images of the slice. According to this principle, our image annotation can accurately capture morphological features, while the mass may only be observed in the specified phase, as shown in Fig. 1. All images are labeled with bounding boxes which consists of two coordinates: top left corner $(x1, y1)$ and bottom right corner $(x2, y2)$. Finally, we have 21,294 annotated images which spread in 4564 slices. Each image has 2.05 bounding boxes in average.

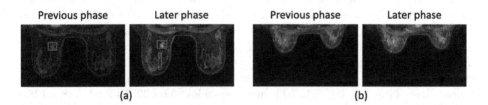

Fig. 1. Two subjects with previous and later phases. (a) More masses appear in later phases. (b) The mass only can be observed from previous phases.

3   Methodology

Figure 2 shows the framework of MD-Net, which consists of two stages: image-based candidate generation and slice-based mass detection. In our MD-Net, the

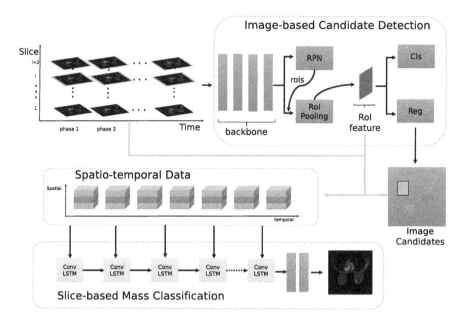

Fig. 2. The framework of our proposed MD-Net.

candidate regions in 2D images are generated based on the morphological features. Then constructing the 4D features to combine kinetic and spatial information, a sequential deep learning model is used to detect the slice-based results.

3.1 Image-Based Candidate Generation

In our MD-Net, Faster R-CNN [10] is employed to generate mass-like candidates in breast DCE-MRI, as Faster R-CNN has been demonstrated to be effective in the object detection task. It is worth to mention that any other object detectors can be also utilized in our framework. We generate the mass-like candidates in all phases, in order to make effective use of morphological features and recall most candidate regions. In our method, We choose ResNet 101 [7] as the backbone network of Faster R-CNN. In addition, we define size of bounding box with five aspect ratios {1:3, 1:2, 1:1, 2:1, 3:1} and four scales {32 × 32, 64 × 64, 128 × 128, 256 × 256} to cover masses of different shapes. Note that the aspect ratios with 1:3 and 3:1 are defined because of the existence of the catheter-related lesions which are critical in the diagnosis of breast cancer.

3.2 Slice-Based Mass Detection

After image-based candidate generation, we apply a sequence model to achieve slice-based results that correspond to clinical diagnosis. Analyzing the kinetic features helps to reduce the false positives that look suspiciously like masses in an individual image, hence it is crucial to perform mass detection in DCE-MRI images. As the kinetic feature is displayed in a sequence of images rather than in one single image, we need to process the sequential data to capture the information. Besides, the sequence length of DCE-MRI is not uniform because different devices have different configurations, resulting in the variable-length data which is difficult to handle. In our dataset, the length ranges from 5 to 8. Furthermore, incorporating morphological features and spatial features can help to detect the mass. Therefore, we construct a 4D data and adopt ConvLSTM [12], which not only has the timing modeling capability but also portrays local features to classify the candidates at slice-level.

Spatiotemporal Data Construction. We construct a spatiotemporal 4D data from the detected candidate regions in three steps:

- Generating slice-wise candidate regions. For each image, a set of candidate bounding boxes are generated with confidence scores. Resultantly, each slice has several sets of candidates. We filter the candidates with low confidence by setting a threshold. In order to balance between the recall and precision of masses detection, the threshold is set as 0.05. In addition, non-maximum suppression (NMS) is also adopted to refine the generated candidate regions. With NMS, candidates generated in similar positions in images from different phases will be filtered. The threshold of NMS is set as 0.7 and validated to be effective on the validation set.
- Assigning labels to the filtered candidates. The label is assigned according to the intersection-over-union (IoU) overlap between the detected candidate regions and the labeled ground-truth. As following the default settings in Faster-RCNN [10], the candidate regions with IoU lager than 0.7 are selected as the positive samples. In contrast, if the IoU is smaller than 0.3, it will be considered as a negative sample.
- Constructing 4D input data for the slice-wise candidates for the training of ConvLSTM. Instead of cropping patches from the original images in a trivial way, we obtain the features of backbone network of Faster R-CNN corresponding to each candidate bounding boxes to retain the learned morphological traits. For each slice-based candidate, we use RoI-pooling to crop several $1024 \times 7 \times 7$ D features in the fourth block feature maps from each of the images in the slice and form a sequence data. Moreover, to incorporate the spatial information, we crop the features in the contiguous slices based on the candidate. Specifically, for the candidates in i^{th} slice, we additional crop the features from $(i-2)^{th}$ and $(i+2)^{th}$ slices. Finally, all three features are concatenated in the channel-wise with generating a Time $\times 3072 \times 7 \times 7$ D feature as the input of sequence model.

Temporal-Spatial Classification Model. With the spatiotemporal data, we build up a sequence-to-one model to identify the mass. Keeping the ability of recording and transferring the information of sequential data, ConvLSTM is utilized to establish the three gates with adopting convolution operations to all input, cell state and hidden state. The ConvLSTM could capture the spatiotemporal feature from our data. We set the dimension of the hidden layer to $128 \times 7 \times 7$ D. Then, two fully connected layers follow the hidden states of the last time with 6272×1024 and 1024×2 D. We use L2 loss function to optimize our model. Finally, ConvLSTM yields a final inference by processing the input candidate in one slice, and identify the mass.

4   Experiment

4.1   Experiment Setting

For evaluation, we split the collect DCE-MRI dataset into the training set, validation set and test set in patient-wise to avoid the dependencies between them. 104 studies are prepared for training with 12,932 labeled images. 34 studies are selected as the validation set, and 34 studies are prepared for the test, containing 20,872 images which consist of 4,635 labeled images and 16,237 images of normal tissues. We train the detection model with training data which only contains label image. The validation data is used for training the sequence model. We construct training data of ConvLSTM by feeding the validation data into detection model as mentioned before. At last, we test our pipeline on the test set.

In training, we flip the images horizontally as the data augmentation approach and rescale all training images to 1000×1000 for detecting the small lesions more effectively in the breast. The backbone network ResNet 101 [7] of Faster R-CNN is pre-trained on ImageNet [4]. We optimize the model using stochastic gradient descent (SGD). Learning rate is set to 0.001 at the beginning and decays to 0.0001 after 8 epochs of training. For the ConvLSTM, we use Adam optimizer with learning rate of 0.001. The convolutional layer in ConvLSTM is initialized from a Gaussian distribution with a zero mean and standard deviation of 0.01.

To measure the performance of our framework, we employ sensitivity (Sen) and specificity (Spe) to evaluate our mass detection results. The Sen is defined as $\frac{TP}{nPos}$ instead of $\frac{TP}{TP+FN}$, where TP and FN denote the number of true positives and false negative respectively, and the $nPos$ is the number of mass in annotation at slice-level, for the TP + FN can only cover a part of the mass depends on the recall of detection. The Spe is defined as $\frac{TN}{TN+FP}$ as usual. Besides, we report the area under the ROC curve (AUC) and False-positives per slice (FPS).

4.2   Comparison Methods and Results

For comparing with our pipeline, we construct several other methods: (1) The baseline method which extends all the image-based results as slice-based results directly, with only applying NMS with a threshold of 0.7 on them. The extension procedure is as same as the slice candidates generation aforementioned. It demonstrates the performance of the candidates generation model. (2) The rule-based method which eliminates the image-based candidates by manual rule. More specifically, we increase the scores of candidates which have been detected in more than 4 images in one slice by Faster R-CNN and decrease those of others. We choose 4 as the hyperparameter by conducting experiments on the validation dataset. We multiply the scores of candidates with 1.2 and 0.8 for increasing and decreasing the probabilities respectively. (3) Sequence model with temporal data which only crop the feature from the corresponding slice rather than three slices. The results are reported in Table 1.

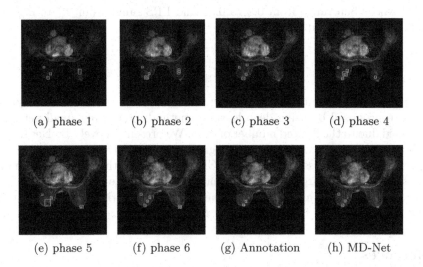

| (a) phase 1 | (b) phase 2 | (c) phase 3 | (d) phase 4 |
| (e) phase 5 | (f) phase 6 | (g) Annotation | (h) MD-Net |

Fig. 3. (a)–(f) The candidates in the single images at different phases for one slice. In different phases, the candidates are diverse. (g) The ground truth on this slice. (h) The output of the MD-Net that eliminates a number of false positives.

Table 1. Slice-based Results on DCE-MRI dataset

	AUC	Sensitivity	Specificity	False-positives
Baseline	0.8846	0.8643	0.7714	1.14/slice
Rule based	0.9021	0.8547	0.8231	0.84/slice
Temporal model	0.9127	**0.8684**	0.8367	0.77/slice
MD-Net	**0.9163**	0.8655	**0.8452**	**0.73**/slice

The baseline model directly considering all candidates as the final results lead to a large number of false positives. Thus, it achieves a Sen of 0.8652 with a Sep of 0.7714. While the rule-based method improves AUC from 0.8846 to 0.9021, the Sen drops from 0.8672 to 0.8547. Sequence model with temporal data shows better results than the rule-based method. Both Sen and Sep have been improved to verify the effectiveness of the kinetic features. Even without spatial information, the sequence model performs better than the rule-based method. Our temporal-spatial model outperforms other methods with the highest AUC of 0.9163, demonstrating that the proposed combination of morphological, kinetic and spatial features is effective for mass detection in DCE-MRI images. Figure 3 further shows the candidates, annotation and output of MD-Net of a sample, which demonstrates the effect of our method. Lacking a common benchmark, the reported results in other works show large variability [1]. Nevertheless, compared to [1,8] whose Sen range from 0.8 to 0.85 and FPS range from 0.7 to 3.2, our method achieves a comparable result.

5   Conclusion

Although there are some algorithms for lesion detection in DCE-MRI images have been proposed by using deep learning methods [1,8], only small networks are applied due to the limited number of data. We present a novel MD-Net framework for incorporating kinetic, morphological and spatial features to achieve better performance on mass detection of DCE-MRI. Due to the lacking of a public dataset, we collect a large number of images and annotate them independently in each image to train and test our framework. The experimental results verify the effectiveness of our framework.

References

1. Amit, G., et al.: Hybrid mass detection in breast MRI combining unsupervised saliency analysis and deep learning. In: Descoteaux, M., Maier-Hein, L., Franz, A., Jannin, P., Collins, D.L., Duchesne, S. (eds.) MICCAI 2017. LNCS, vol. 10435, pp. 594–602. Springer, Cham (2017). https://doi.org/10.1007/978-3-319-66179-7_68
2. Cao, Z., et al.: Breast tumor detection in ultrasound images using deep learning. In: Wu, G., Munsell, B.C., Zhan, Y., Bai, W., Sanroma, G., Coupé, P. (eds.) Patch-MI 2017. LNCS, vol. 10530, pp. 121–128. Springer, Cham (2017). https://doi.org/10.1007/978-3-319-67434-6_14
3. Chen, W., et al.: Cancer statistics in china, 2015. CA: Cancer J. Clin. **66**(2), 115–132 (2016)
4. Deng, J., Dong, W., Socher, R., Li, L.J., Li, K., Fei-Fei, L.: Imagenet: a large-scale hierarchical image database. In: CVPR, pp. 248–255. IEEE (2009)
5. Ertas, G., Doran, S., Leach, M.O.: Computerized detection of breast lesions in multi-centre and multi-instrument dce-mr data using 3D principal component maps and template matching. Phys. Med. Biol. **56**(24), 7795 (2011)
6. Gubern-Mérida, A., et al.: Automated localization of breast cancer in DCE-MRI. Med. Image Anal. **20**(1), 265–274 (2015)
7. He, K., Zhang, X., Ren, S., Sun, J.: Deep residual learning for image recognition. In: CVPR, pp. 770–778 (2016)

8. Maicas, G., Carneiro, G., Bradley, A.P., Nascimento, J.C., Reid, I.: Deep reinforcement learning for active breast lesion detection from DCE-MRI. In: Descoteaux, M., Maier-Hein, L., Franz, A., Jannin, P., Collins, D.L., Duchesne, S. (eds.) MICCAI 2017. LNCS, vol. 10435, pp. 665–673. Springer, Cham (2017). https://doi.org/10.1007/978-3-319-66179-7_76

9. McClymont, D., Mehnert, A., Trakic, A., Kennedy, D., Crozier, S.: Fully automatic lesion segmentation in breast MRI using mean-shift and graph-cuts on a region adjacency graph. J. Magn. Reson. Imaging 39(4), 795–804 (2014)

10. Ren, S., He, K., Girshick, R., Sun, J.: Faster R-CNN: towards real-time object detection with region proposal networks. In: Advances in Neural Information Processing Systems, pp. 91–99 (2015)

11. Siegel, R.L., Miller, K.D., Jemal, A.: Cancer statistics, 2016. CA: Cancer J. Clin. 66(1), 7–30 (2016)

12. Xingjian, S., Chen, Z., Wang, H., Yeung, D.Y., Wong, W.K., Woo, W.C.: Convolutional LSTM network: a machine learning approach for precipitation nowcasting. In: Advances in Neural Information Processing Systems, pp. 802–810 (2015)

Automated Pulmonary Embolism Detection from CTPA Images Using an End-to-End Convolutional Neural Network

Yi Lin[1], Jianchao Su[1], Xiang Wang[2], Xiang Li[2], Jingen Liu[3], Kwang-Ting Cheng[4], and Xin Yang[1(✉)]

[1] Huazhong University of Science and Technology, Wuhan, China
xinyang2014@hust.edu.cn
[2] The Central Hospital of Wuhan, Wuhan, China
[3] JD AI Research, Mountain View, USA
[4] Hong Kong University of Science and Technology, Hong Kong, Hong Kong

Abstract. Automated methods for detecting pulmonary embolisms (PEs) on CT pulmonary angiography (CTPA) images are of high demand. Existing methods typically employ separate steps for PE candidate detection and false positive removal, without considering the ability of the other step. As a result, most existing methods usually suffer from a high false positive rate in order to achieve an acceptable sensitivity. This study presents an end-to-end trainable convolutional neural network (CNN) where the two steps are optimized jointly. The proposed CNN consists of three concatenated subnets: (1) a novel 3D candidate proposal network for detecting cubes containing suspected PEs, (2) a 3D spatial transformation subnet for generating fixed-sized vessel-aligned image representation for candidates, and (3) a 2D classification network which takes the three cross-sections of the transformed cubes as input and eliminates false positives. We have evaluated our approach using the 20 CTPA test dataset from the PE challenge, achieving a sensitivity of 78.9%, 80.7% and 80.7% at 2 false positives per volume at 0 mm, 2 mm and 5 mm localization error, which is superior to the state-of-the-art methods. We have further evaluated our system on our own dataset consisting of 129 CTPA data with a total of 269 emboli. Our system achieves a sensitivity of 63.2%, 78.9% and 86.8% at 2 false positives per volume at 0 mm, 2 mm and 5 mm localization error.

Keywords: Convolutional neural network · Pulmonary embolism detection · End-to-end

This work was supported by the National Natural Science Foundation of China (61502188), the Hubei Provincial Natural Science Foundation (ZRMS2017000375), the Wuhan Science and Technology Bureau under Award (2017010201010111), the Fundamental Research Funds for the Central Universities (2019kfyRCPY118) and the Program for HUST Acadamic Frontier Youth Team.

D. Shen et al. (Eds.): MICCAI 2019, LNCS 11767, pp. 280–288, 2019.
https://doi.org/10.1007/978-3-030-32251-9_31

1   Introduction

Pulmonary Embolism (PE) is a thrombus that obstructs central, lobar, segmental, or subsegmental pulmonary arteries when it travels from the heart to the lungs. The morality rate of untreated PE is around 30%; however, early detection and treatment of PE could effectively decrease the morality rate to as low as 2% [11]. Computed tomography pulmonary angiography (CTPA), in which PE appears as a filling defect (i.e. a dark region surrounded by the bright vessel lumen), is the primary means for diagnosing PE in today's clinical practice. However, manually interpreting a CTPA volume demands a radiologist to carefully trace each pulmonary artery across 300–500 slices for any suspected PEs, which is time consuming and could suffer from a large inter-/intra-observer variety due to the different radiologists' experience, attention span and eye fatigue.

Automated detection of PE is of high demand for improving the accuracy and efficiency of PE detection and diagnosis. Existing methods typically consists of two separate steps: (1) generating a set of PE candidates based on voxel-level features; and (2) extracting region-level features of PE candidates and eliminating false positives (FPs) based on a classifier. For example, in [9] Masutani et al. extracted handcrafted features based on CT values, local contrast and the second derivatives of voxels for candidate detection. The volume, effective length and mean local contrast of grouped voxels were then extracted from the detected candidates for false positive removal. In [3], Bouma et al. used similar voxel-level features as [9] for candidate proposal and developed new region-level features based on the isophote curvature and circularity of the bright lumen for FP removal. However, due to the limited representation ability of these handcrafted features, conventional methods often suffer from a high number of false positives in order to achieve an acceptable sensitivity. Nima et al. [11] investigated the feasibility of CNN features for eliminating false positives in the task of PE detection. A novel vessel-aligned multi-planar image representation based on CNN was developed in [11] and demonstrated to be highly effective, efficient and robust for distinguishing true PEs from false positives. In this study, we also adopt such vessel-aligned image representation for its good robustness and distinctiveness. While different from [11] which utilized handcrafted feature based method [6] for detecting candidate PEs and a separate CNN for FP removal, this work for the first time integrates all steps including PE candidate proposal, the generation of vessel-aligned image representation and FP removal into an end-to-end trainable CNN for a jointly optimized PE detector.

As shown in Fig. 1, our PE detection network is a cascade of three subnets: candidate proposal subnet, spatial transformation network, and false positive removal network. The first subnet performs PE candidate proposal via a 3D fully convolutional network (FCN) to extract 3D feature hierarchies, followed by two 3D convolutional layers to generate candidate cubes containing PEs. The second subnet aims to transform the candidate cubes so as to align the suspected embolus with the orientation of the affected vessel segment. We implement the goal using two parametric-free layers, i.e. a spatial transformation layer and a 3D region-of-interest (ROI) pooling layer, which are derivable and can facilitate error

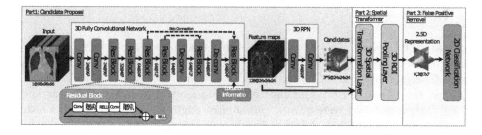

Fig. 1. Framework of our end-to-end PE detection network.

back-propagation in end-to-end training. The third subnet is a 2D classification CNN which takes three cross-sections of the transformed candidate cube as input and outputs its probability of being a PE. Our method is very efficient since convolutional features are shared among the proposal, spatial transformation and classification pipelines. We have evaluated our approach using the entire 20 CTPA test dataset from the PE challenge, achieving a sensitivity of 78.9%, 80.7% and 80.7% at 2 false positives per volume at 0 mm, 2 mm and 5 mm localization error. This performance is superior to the winning system in the literature, which achieves a sensitivity of 60.5%, 66.4% and 75.8% at the same level of false positives. We have further evaluated our system on our own dataset consisting of 129 CTPA data. Our system achieves a sensitivity of 63.2%, 78.9% and 86.8% at 2 false positives per volume at 0 mm, 2 mm and 5 mm localization error.

To summarize, the main contributions of our paper are:

- an end-to-end PE detection network with combined candidate proposal, spatial transformation for vessel-aligned image representation, and classification stages that detects arbitrary size embolisms;
- a derivable and parametric-free implementation of vessel-aligned representation using a 3D spatial transformation subnet;
- extensive evaluations on two diverse datasets consists of totally 149 patients data that demonstrate the general applicability and superior performance of our model to the state-of-the-art methods.

2   Method

Figure 1 illustrates the framework of our PE detection network which consists of three subnets: a 3D candidate proposal subnet, a derivable 3D spatial transformation subnet, and a false positive removal subnet.

2.1   Candidate Proposal Subnet

3D FCN for Feature Extraction. Our proposal subnet extracts features using a 3D FCN that employs an autoencoder network architecture with skip connections. Specifically, the encoder starts with two 3D convolution layers, followed by a max-pooling layer. Then, four residual blocks [4] are applied to encode hierarchical feature maps. In the decoder, the feature maps are up-sampled by two de-convolution layers and two residual blocks. Skip connections are utilized to connect the last two residual blocks in the encoder and the corresponding two residual blocks in the decoder. The size of a 3D pulmonary CTPA volume is typically very large, e.g. $512 \times 512 \times 400$. Directly inputting the entire 3D volume into the network could involve extremely high memory cost. To meet the constraint of GPU memory, we divide the entire volume into overlapping cubes size of $96 \times 96 \times 96$ and input each cube into the network, rather than the entire 3D volume. We also combine location information with the FCN feature maps as we believe location is an important indicator for identifying PEs which usually reside at some unique locations, i.e. bifurcations of the main pulmonary artery or lobar branches [2]. To this end, we form a feature map with the same size as FCN feature maps. Each voxel of the location feature map is a 3-dimensional vector indicating the x, y and z coordinates in the entire 3D volume. We concatenate this 3-channel feature map with the FCN feature map.

3D Region Proposal. The size of PEs could vary significantly depending on its locations in pulmonary arteries. Inspired by Faster R-CNN [10], we incorporate anchor cubes into a region proposal subnet to facilitate accurate detection of variable size proposals. Specifically, the anchor cues are pre-defined multi-scale 3D windows centered at every voxel location of the feature map. Each voxel location specifies $N = 3$ anchor cubes, each at a different fixed scale s (i.e. $s = 10\,mm$, $30\,mm$ and $60\,mm$ respectively) to ensure that the proposal prediction is scale invariant. For each anchor cube of a scale s, we design five detectors to regress five values $(\Delta x_s, \Delta y_s, \Delta z_s, \Delta d_s, p_s)$ which are offsets in locations $(\Delta x_s, \Delta y_s, \Delta z_s)$ and size (Δd_s) of the proposal cube with respect to the anchor cubes, as well as the probability (p) of the proposal containing a PE. To this end, we first apply a 3D convolution layer with 64 kernels size of $1 \times 1 \times 1$ to the feature map, then we apply another 3D convolution layer with $5N$ kernels size of $1 \times 1 \times 1$ to output a feature map, each voxel of which is a $5N$-dimensional vector indicating $(\Delta x_s, \Delta y_s, \Delta z_s, \Delta d_s, p_s)$, $s \in \{1, ..., N\}$.

Training. To train the candidate proposal subnet, we assign a binary class label to each anchor. If an anchor overlaps with some ground-truth with Intersection-over-Union (IoU) greater than 0.5, we label it as positive. If the anchor has an IoU overlap smaller than 0.02 with all ground-truth, we label it as negative. Anchors that are neither positive nor negative are excluded for training. The objective function of the candidate proposal subnet is defined as:

$$L(\{p_i\}, \{t_i\}) = \frac{1}{N_{cls}} \sum_i L_{cls}(p_i, p_i^*) + \lambda \frac{1}{N_{reg}} \sum_i p_i^* L_{reg}(t_i, t_i^*) \qquad (1)$$

which consists of two losses: the classification loss L_{cls} is the binary cross entropy loss, and the regression loss L_{reg} is the smooth L_1 loss. This two terms are normalized by N_{cls} and N_{reg}, and weighted by λ. Note that L_{reg} only applies to the positive anchor. In Eq. 1, i denotes the ith anchor in a mini-batch, p_i

and p_i^* denote the predicted probability of being PE and the ground-truth label ($p^* = \{0, 1\}$). t_i and t_i^* denote the predicted position and ground-truth position associated with a positive anchor, which consists of 4 parameters:

$$\Delta x = (x - x_a)/d_a, \ \Delta y = (y - y_a)/d_a,$$
$$\Delta z = (z - z_a)/d_a, \ \Delta d = log(d/d_a) \tag{2}$$

where (x, y, z, d) are predicted or ground-truth cube's center coordinates and its side length, and (x_a, y_a, z_a, d_a) are for anchor cube.

We use online hard sample mining to balance hard and easy samples in the training phase. In each mini-batch we randomly select M negative samples, sort them in a descending order based on their classification score. The top k samples are chosen as hard samples and contribute to the calculation of the loss function, the rest are abandoned by setting its loss to 0.

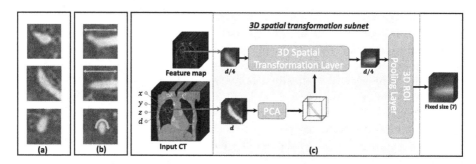

Fig. 2. (a)–(b) cross-section views of a proposal cube before and after being processed by the 3D spatial transformation subnet. The yellow arrows denote v_1, v_2 and v_3 the affected vessel. (c) Vessel-aligned fixed-sized proposal cube generation. (Color figure online)

2.2 3D Spatial Transformation Subnet

The proposal network could generate many false positives in order to achieve a satisfactory sensitivity. To exclude false positives, an intuitive solution is to apply an addition classification CNN which takes the proposal cubes as input and distinguish between true PE cubes and false positives. The problem, however, is that the appearance variations of all possible PEs is very large in practice. Training a classifier using a limited number of PE samples could yield severe overfitting and in turn exhibit poor performance for unseen testing cases. To alleviate this problem, Nima et al. [11] proposed a vessel-aligned image representation, which aligns each candidate proposal to the orientation of the affected vessel to reduce the appearance variations of PEs in the three cross-section slices. Inspired by their method, in this work we develop a 3D spatial transformation subnet which generates vessel-aligned fixed-sized cubes from arbitrary-sized candidate proposals (see Fig. 2). The vessel-aligned 2.5D representation (as shown in Fig. 2(b)) of the candidate is then derived by extracting the axial, sagittal and coronal slices from the vessel-aligned cube.

To implement our 3D spatial transformation subnet, we crop two proposal cubes (i.e. C_{ori} and C_{feat}) from both the original CTPA volume and the corresponding feature maps with stride of four, respectively. We compute the vessel orientation from C_{ori} by first segmenting vessels via simple intensity thresholding. Then we apply principle component analysis (PCA) to the segmented vessels to obtain three eigen vectors (v_1, v_2, v_3) and their corresponding eigen value ($\lambda_1 \geq \lambda_2 \geq \lambda_3$). The first eigen vector v_1 represents the direction in which the artery elongates, while v_2 and v_3 represent two orthogonal directions in the plane vertical to v_1. We align C_{feat} to vessel's orientation via the 3D affine transformation [5], according to Eq. 3:

$$
\begin{bmatrix} x^s \\ y^s \\ z^s \end{bmatrix} = A_\theta \begin{bmatrix} x^t \\ y^t \\ z^t \\ 1 \end{bmatrix} = \begin{bmatrix} s_x e_1^T v_1 & s_y e_1^T v_2 & s_z e_1^T v_3 & t_x \\ s_x e_2^T v_1 & s_y e_2^T v_2 & s_z e_2^T v_3 & t_y \\ s_x e_3^T v_1 & s_y e_3^T v_2 & s_z e_3^T v_3 & t_z \end{bmatrix} \begin{bmatrix} x^t \\ y^t \\ z^t \\ 1 \end{bmatrix} \tag{3}
$$

where (x^t, y^t, z^t) and (x^s, y^s, z^s) are the normalized target coordinates of the regular grid in the transformed cube and the normalized source coordinates in the feature map. A_θ is the affine transformation matrix, where t_x, t_y, t_z represent the offsets of the candidate center to the CT center, s_x, s_y, s_z represent the scaling ratio between the candidate's size and the CT's size, e_1, e_2, e_3 forms a unit matrix. We input vessel-aligned feature maps C_{feat} to a 3D ROI pooling layer to extract fixed-sized feature maps (i.e. $7 \times 7 \times 7$) for FP removal. Figure 2(c) illustrates the pipeline of 3D spatial transformation subnet.

2.3   False Positive Removal Subnet

We extract three cross sections to form a 2.5D representation and feed it to a simple classification subnet consisting of two fully connected layers for FP removal. In training, a sample is labeled as positive if its central point is within an embolus. Otherwise, it is considered as negative. To avoid any bias to negative samples, we randomly select 128 training samples in an iteration, where the radio of positive to negative samples is up to 1:3. If there are insufficient positive samples in an iteration, we pad negative ones in the mini-batch.

3   Experiments

3.1   Datasets

We evaluated our method using two datasets: (1) the test set of the PE challenge [1] consisting of 20 patients CTPA scans, and (2) the PE129 dataset consisting 129 CTPA scans with a total of 269 embolisms. 99 scans of the PE129 are collected in a local hospital and 30 of them are from [8].

3.2   Implementation Details

We pre-process the CTPA data before inputting it to our network. First, we segment the lung region to exclude the background tissues based on [7]. Then, we re-sample the data to achieve an isotropic resolution (1 mm × 1mm × 1 mm). After that, we adjust the contrast by clipping the data into [−1200, 600] HU and linearly transforming it into [−1, 1].

To train the candidate proposal subnet, we augment the dataset by randomly flipping, rotating (0–180°) and scaling (0.75X–1.25X) each original sample. The 3D FCN was pretrained on a large public dataset LUNA16 for nodule detection. We train the candidate proposal subnet in 100 epochs using SGD optimization with the learning rate 0.001, momentum 0.9, weight decay 10^{-4}.

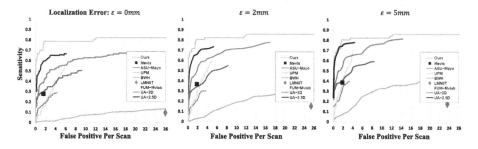

Fig. 3. Comparison with the state-of-the-art methods on the PE challenge dataset. We plot the FROC curve per scan at 0 mm, 2 mm and 5 mm localization error.

3.3   Comparison with Other Methods

We compared our PE detection network with the methods [1] on the PE challenge test set. As the ground truth labels are not available on the website, we asked a radiologist with over 10 years' reading experience to manually delineate PEs in each test scan. The manual annotations were further validated by a 2nd observer. We will also release our manual annotations for a fair comparison in the future studies. The evaluation metrics is FROC curve per CTPA scan. A detection is counted as positive if it locates within a certain range (i.e. 0 mm, 2 mm and 5 mm) to an embolus manual mask. Figure 3 shows that our method achieves a sensitivity of 78.9%, 80.7% and 80.7% at 2FPs/scan when the localization error is 0 mm, 2 mm and 5 mm, outperforming the winning system UA-2.5D which achieves 60.8%, 66.4% and 75.8% at 2FPs/scan at 0 mm, 2 mm and 5 mm localization error.

3.4   Ablation Studies

We further examine the impact of each subnets on the final performance on the PE challenge test set and our PE129 dataset. For simplicity, we denote the candidate proposal subnet, spatial transformation subnet and FP removal subnet

Table 1. Impact of the three subnets in our PE detection candidate network. Numbers indicate sensitivities at 2 FPs/scan at 0 mm localization error.

Method	PE challenge	PE129
S_1	71.9%	42.1%
$S_1 + S_3$	73.7%	44.7%
$S_1 + S_2 + S_3$	**78.9%**	**63.2%**

as S_1, S_2 and S_3 respectively. Quantitative results in terms of sensitivity at 2 FPs/scan at 0 mm localization error are reported in Table 1. On the PE challenge test set, our proposal subnet achieves a sensitivity of 71.9% at 2FPs. Directly removing FPs using the proposal cubes could improve the sensitivity by 1.8%. Integrating the vessel-aligned representation using S_2 could further improving the sensitivity by 5.2%. For PE129 dataset, the proposal subnet achieves 42.1% sensitivity at 2FPs, and the false positive removal subnet and spatial transformation subnet could improve the sensitivity by 2.6%, 21.1%, respectivity. Greater improvements achieved by S_2 on our PE129 dataset than PE challenge might be due to many small emboli with various rotations in our dataset. Aligning them with the vessel orientation can effectively reduce the variations.

4 Conclusion

This work presents an end-to-end PE detection network which achieves superior performance to the state-of-the-art methods. The main advantages of our network are three folds. First, it takes full advantage of 3D contextual information of a 3D CTPA volume via 3D FCN feature extraction. The FCN features are shared among three 3 subnets. Second, it utilizes an affine transformation layer with a ROI pooling layer to realize the vessel-aligned fixed-sized representation for arbitrary size PE candidates. The two layers can effectively reduce the appearance variations and meanwhile are completely derivable to enable end-to-end training. Third, it facilitates joint optimization of all steps for PE detection.

References

1. CAD-PE challenge. http://www.cad-pe.org/
2. Araoz, P.A., et al.: Pulmonary embolism: prognostic CT findings. Radiology **242**(3), 889–897 (2007)
3. Bouma, H., et al.: Automatic detection of pulmonary embolism in CTA images. IEEE Trans. Med. Imaging **28**(8), 1223–1230 (2009)
4. He, K., et al.: Deep residual learning for image recognition. In: Proceedings of the IEEE Conference on Computer Vision and Pattern Recognition, pp. 770–778 (2016)
5. Jaderberg, M., et al.: Spatial transformer networks. In: Advances in Neural Information Processing Systems, pp. 2017–2025 (2015)

6. Liang, J., Bi, J.: Computer aided detection of pulmonary embolism with toboggan-ing and mutiple instance classification in CT pulmonary angiography. In: Karsse-meijer, N., Lelieveldt, B. (eds.) IPMI 2007. LNCS, vol. 4584, pp. 630–641. Springer, Heidelberg (2007). https://doi.org/10.1007/978-3-540-73273-0_52

7. Liao, F., et al.: Evaluate the malignancy of pulmonary nodules using the 3-D deep leaky noisy-or network. In: IEEE Transactions on Neural Networks and Learning Systems (2019)

8. Masoudi, M., et al.: A new dataset of computed-tomography angiography images for computer-aided detection of pulmonary embolism. Sci. Data **5**, 1–9 (2018)

9. Masutani, Y., et al.: Computerized detection of pulmonary embolism in spiral CT angiography based on volumetric image analysis. IEEE Trans. Med. Imaging **21**(12), 1517–1523 (2002)

10. Ren, S., et al.: Faster r-cnn: Towards real-time object detection with region pro-posal networks. arXiv preprint arXiv:1506.01497 (2015)

11. Tajbakhsh, N., Gotway, M.B., Liang, J.: Computer-aided pulmonary embolism detection using a novel vessel-aligned multi-planar image representation and con-volutional neural networks. In: Navab, N., Hornegger, J., Wells, W.M., Frangi, A.F. (eds.) MICCAI 2015. LNCS, vol. 9350, pp. 62–69. Springer, Cham (2015). https://doi.org/10.1007/978-3-319-24571-3_8

Unsupervised Anomaly Localization
Using Variational Auto-Encoders

David Zimmerer$^{(\boxtimes)}$, Fabian Isensee, Jens Petersen, Simon Kohl,
and Klaus Maier-Hein

German Cancer Research Center (DKFZ), Heidelberg, Germany
`d.zimmerer@dkfz.de`

Abstract. An assumption-free automatic check of medical images for potentially overseen anomalies would be a valuable assistance for a radiologist. Deep learning and especially Variational Auto-Encoders (VAEs) have shown great potential in the unsupervised learning of data distributions. In principle, this allows for such a check and even the localization of parts in the image that are most suspicious. Currently, however, the reconstruction-based localization by design requires adjusting the model architecture to the specific problem looked at during evaluation. This contradicts the principle of building assumption-free models. We propose complementing the localization part with a term derived from the Kullback-Leibler (KL)-divergence. For validation, we perform a series of experiments on FashionMNIST as well as on a medical task including >1000 healthy and >250 brain tumor patients. Results show that the proposed formalism outperforms the state of the art VAE-based localization of anomalies across many hyperparameter settings and also shows a competitive max performance.

Keywords: Anomaly localization · Anomaly detection

1 Introduction

Unsupervised anomaly detection is a key technique that could allow us to overcome the data bottleneck that is ever so present especially in the medical domain. Unsupervised models can directly learn the data distribution from a large cohort of unannotated subjects and then be used to detect out of distribution samples and thus ultimately identify diseased or suspicious cases. By decoupling abnormality detection from reference annotations, these approaches are completely independent of human input and can therefore be applied to any medical condition or image modality. First approaches on unsupervised anomaly detection were built on explicit assumptions, often preventing generalizability to other tasks. Juan-Abarrachin et al. [10] manually designed a set of image features for brain tumor detection. By mapping the original image into carefully

Electronic supplementary material The online version of this chapter (https:// doi.org/10.1007/978-3-030-32251-9_32) contains supplementary material, which is available to authorized users.

D. Shen et al. (Eds.): MICCAI 2019, LNCS 11767, pp. 289–297, 2019.
https://doi.org/10.1007/978-3-030-32251-9_32

chosen feature representations, they were able to separate tumorous from healthy tissue by clustering of the voxels in feature space and combining this with an atlas-based approach. Erihov et al. [8] instead relied on the natural symmetry of the brain (as well as some other organs) to identify regions that behave abnormally. Only the era of deep-learning has allowed to address the problem in a more principled fashion, with the aim of learning normal data distributions in order to detect abnormal samples. Ideally, anomaly detection should not build upon case-specific assumptions in the form of medical domain knowledge or specific annotated validation sets to optimize for, which should be interpreted as an unwanted form of supervision implicitly added by design of the method. Variational Auto-Encoders (VAEs) and their extensions are, alongside flow-based and auto-regressive models, a current de-facto standard for density estimation and particularly anomaly/out-of-distribution sample detection tasks [1,3,12,14]. Here, the evidence lower bound (ELBO), by definition a combination of the reconstruction error with the Kullback-Leibler (KL)-divergence, commonly serves as a proxy for the sample likelihood [3,12]. Recent work has even demonstrated the ability of VAEs to localize and segment the parts in the image that are most suspicious, which is of particular importance in medical applications. Pawlowski et al. [16] compare different auto-encoders for CT based pixel-wise segmentation and Baur et al. [4] propose a VAE with an adversarial loss on the reconstructions to improve performance. Chen et al. [5,6] use a VAE with an additional adversarial latent loss. The localization part in these studies is currently solely based on the reconstruction error, thus outlining regions as suspicious if they cannot be adequately reconstructed by the model. You et al. [22] include the KL-term for reconstructions closer to the data manifold. In this work, we demonstrate that reconstruction-based anomaly detection is sub-optimal. One obvious deficiency is that the capability of a VAE to reconstruct anomalies is by design tightly coupled to the expressiveness (size and configuration) of the latent space. This, at the same time, also explains why reconstruction-based techniques are still able to achieve high performance scores on unsupervised tasks: their deficiencies can be compensated for to a certain extent by tuning the model architecture towards being optimally suited for a specific tasks (see also [6,9,16]), as is common practice when hyperparameters are optimized on annotated validation sets. Task specific hyperparameter optimization, however, contradicts the principle of assumption-free anomaly detection. To investigate this we analyze the robustness of the reconstruction-based anomaly detection on a sample-wise and pixel-wise level and compare it to the ELBO and the KL-divergence. Inspired by the results, we propose to integrate the KL-divergence of a VAE into a pixel-wise anomaly detection as well. This is in analogy to sample-wise anomaly detection, where the ELBO is also based on both the reconstruction error and the KL-divergence. The proposed approach outperforms reconstruction-based localization in a broad variety of different model configurations, demonstrating the robustness with respect to hyperparameters. When allowing task-specific fine-tuning, the model as well outperforms previously reported deep-learning based results.

2 Methods

2.1 Variational Autoencoders for Anomaly Detection

VAEs can approximate data distributions by optimizing a lower bound $\mathcal{L}$, often termed evidence lower bound (ELBO) [7,11,18]. It is defined as

$$\log p(x) \geq \mathcal{L} = -D_{KL}(q(z|x)\|p(z)) + \mathbb{E}_{q(z|x)}[\log p(x|z)], \tag{1}$$

where $q(z|x)$ and $p(x|z)$ are diagonal normal distributions parameterized by neural networks f_μ, f_σ, and g_μ and constant c:

$$
\begin{aligned}
q(z|x) &= \mathcal{N}(z; f_{\mu,\theta_1}(x), f_{\sigma,\theta_2}(x)^2), \\
p(x|z) &= \mathcal{N}(x; g_{\mu,\gamma}(z), \mathbb{I} * c),
\end{aligned}
\tag{2}
$$

However VAEs have design choices and data dependent parameters which can influence the performance, such as the network architecture, the number of latent variables, the standard deviation c of $p(x|z)$ and the data dimension. Given sufficiently powerful neural networks f_μ, f_σ, and g_μ and a large enough latent space, VAEs with Gaussian encoders and decoders can (and under some conditions will [7]) approximate the true data distribution. Thus, after optimization, $\mathcal{L}$ is often used as a proxy for the likelihood of a data sample and consequently as an anomaly score.

2.2 Pixel-Wise Anomaly Detection

For medical applications a pixel-wise localization, similar to a segmentation, is often more desirable than a sample-wise score. Related methods typically generate a segmentation map by thresholding the pixel-wise reconstruction error [4–6,16,19]. However, in contrast to anomaly detection in the common sample-wise setting, this discards the KL-term and potentially ignores useful information, since a low $\mathcal{L}$ and consequently high anomaly score can be caused by the reconstruction-term ($\mathbb{E}_{q(z|x)}[\log p(x|z)]$) and/or the KL-term ($D_{KL}(q(z|x)\|p(z))$). To alleviate this problem we aim to include, in addition to the pixel-wise reconstruction error ("**Rec-Error**"), the KL-term for a pixel-wise anomaly scoring. Our experiments include different strategies of achieving this as well as strategies for each term separately:

- "**ELBO-grad**": Building on the assumption that $\mathcal{L}$ allows for a good enough approximation of the true data distribution, we propose to use the derivative of $\mathcal{L}$ with respect to the input, yielding a pixel-wise vector pointing towards a data sample with a lower $\mathcal{L}$:

$$ELBO\text{-}Grad_{score}(x_i) = |[\frac{\partial \mathcal{L}}{\partial x}]_i|. \tag{3}$$

Given that $\mathcal{L}$ is locally convex, the magnitude of the pixel gradient should correspond to a pixel-wise anomaly score [2].

- **"KL-grad"**: To get a pixel-wise score for only the KL-term of $\mathcal{L}$, we differentiate the KL-term with respect to the input.
- **"Rec-Grad"**: To get a pixel-wise score for only the reconstruction-term of $\mathcal{L}$, we differentiate the reconstruction-term of $\mathcal{L}$ with respect to the input.
- **"Combi"**: Instead of differentiating the reconstruction-term of $\mathcal{L}$, we can directly use the reconstruction error and combine it with "KL-grad". This should be less prone to noise artifacts. For this model, we combine the derivative of the KL-term with the reconstruction error by multiplication, since the terms differ by several orders of magnitude.

2.3   Generalization and Robustness Across Different Parameters

We compare the discriminative performance of the ELBO $\mathcal{L}$, the KL-term, and the reconstruction-term separately to inspect the information they contain about the data distribution and consequentially the abnormality. We further analyze the robustness and generalizability across different parameter settings and different (medical and non-medical) datasets.

First, we use the FashionMNIST dataset [21], where we train and validate the model on 54000 images using 9 out of the 10 provided classes and then evaluate the performance by attempting to discriminate between the classes seen during training and the 10th unseen class. In analogy to [15], we used a model with a 3-layer fully connected encoder and decoder with 400 hidden units and ReLU non-linearities. To analyze the robustness we vary the number of latent variables, the standard deviation c of $p(x|z)$ (resulting in a down or up-weighing of the reconstruction loss), the image-size/scaling and class left out during training. By default we use 20 latent variables, $c = 1$, a scaling factor of 1 and class 0 is left out during training.

Second, we train and validate on the patient data from the HCP dataset [20] ($N = 1000$ patients) and test on the BraTS2017 dataset [13] ($N = 250$ patients). While the HCP patients are all young healthy subjects, the patients in the BraTS dataset all have brain tumours. Finding tumours in this setting is a particularly hard problem because additionally to the challenging nature of the task itself there is a considerable domain shift between the datasets. The BraTS dataset includes tumor annotations which we can use for model evaluation. We treat slices without annotations as healthy whereas slices with at least 20 annotated tumor voxels are considered diseased. Our model consists of a 5-Layer fully-convolutional encoder and decoder with feature-map size of 16-32-64-256. We use strided convolutions (stride 2) as downsampling and transposed convolutions as upsampling operations, each followed by a LeakyReLU non-linearity (inspired by DCGAN [17]). To analyze the robustness and generalizability of the different methods, we vary the number of latent variables (default 256), the standard deviation c of $p(x|z)$ (default 1) and the image-size (default 64×64 pixels).

The models are trained with Adam and an initial learning rate of 0.0001. Whenever the validation loss $\mathcal{L}_{val}$ reaches a plateau, the learning rate is decreased by multiplying it with 0.1. The training is stopped once the validation loss does not decrease for more than 3 epochs. For each model we perform 5 runs

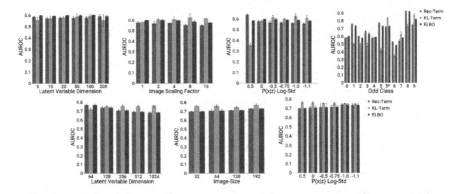

Fig. 1. Sample-wise anomaly detection AUROC for reconstruction-term (Rec), the KL-term, and the ELBO $\mathcal{L}$ for the FashionMNIST dataset (first row) and the BraTS2017 dataset (second row) over different VAE design choices. 5* shows a fine-tuned performance with odd-class 5 ($\log c = 1.4$).

and report the mean as well as the max/min performance. The code to replicate the results is available at https://github.com/MIC-DKFZ/vae-anomaly-experiments.

3 Results

3.1 Sample-Wise Performance

The sample-wise results across different parameter settings can be seen in Fig. 1. It is apparent that in most cases the reconstruction-term shows lower discriminative power than either the KL-term or the ELBO. Consequently, important information is lost when focusing only on the reconstruction error. Furthermore, cases where it has better performance, the model is severely constrained, for example by having a small latent variable dimension (which was shown in [7] to hinder VAEs from approximating the data distribution and to lead to poor reconstruction). Thus the robustness of the KL-term can perhaps be intuitively explained by [7], which states that for VAEs the ELBO best approximates the data distribution having "perfect reconstructions using the fewest number of clean, low-noise latent dimensions". So far, no hyperparameters were specifically tuned to specifically improve one of the losses. However we want to demonstrate that by using an annotated validation set to tune the parameters, the performance of the reconstruction error as well as the KL-term individually can give competitive performance. This is done by choosing the odd class with the largest gap between the rec-loss and the kl-loss (class 5) and using a single hyperparameter adjustment (setting $\log c = 1.4$). By doing so, we were able to achieve an area under the receiver operator curve (AUROC) of 0.82 for the KL-loss, which now significantly outperformed the reconstruction loss. However, when no annotated dataset is available our results indicate that in general including

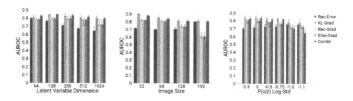

Fig. 2. Pixel-wise AUROC over different VAE design choices on the BraTS2017 dataset. We compare the reconstruction loss, the KL-term gradient, the reconstruction-term gradient, the ELBO $\mathcal{L}$ gradient and our *combi* method.

the KL-loss for anomaly scoring not just for a sample-wise level, but also on a pixel-wise level could increase performance, as analyze next.

3.2   Pixel-Wise Performance

The pixel-wise performance on the BraTS2017 dataset across different hyper-paramater settings is summarized in Fig. 2. Here the model was trained on the healthy HCP subjects and then applied to BraTS2017 for anomaly detection. We used the same model and data setting as before, but in this case evaluate the performance to detect pixel-wise whole tumor annotations. We compare the methods presented in Sec. 2.2: The pixel-wise reconstruction-error (*Rec-Error*), the backpropagated $\mathcal{L}$ (*Elbo-Grad*), its backpropagated KL-term (*KL-Grad*) and reconstruction-term (*Rec-Grad*) separately as well as the *combi* model. Similar to the previous cases, it is obvious that in most cases the reconstruction error alone is outperformed by other methods. Furthermore, for most choices the *KL-Grad* and the *combi* model perform best, indicating a more robust performance at least for this particular dataset (similar observations can be made for the ISLES2015 dataset, as shown in the Suppl.).

3.3   Hyperparameter Tuning

The top performing methods in the experiments shown above already exhibit high AUROC > 0.9. In particular, the often ignored KL-term shows robust performance across a variety of tested settings. The *combi* approach exhibits a similar robustness. We were interested in investigating the top performance of the KL-term approach in a scenario where an annotated validation set can be employed for hyperparameter tuning, just as it is often done in the literature when presenting reconstruction-based approaches. Results are shown in Table 1 and Fig. 3. Dice scores are calculated by thresholding the anomaly values at a value that was determined using $\frac{1}{5}$ of the test dataset. The reported dice scores were then taken from the other $\frac{4}{5}$th of the dataset.

Table 1. Dice of unsupervised whole tumor detection on the BraTS Dataset (the number in brackets specifies the year of the BraTS dataset that was used). While our approach is outperformed by non-deep learning approaches that were specifically designed with domain knowledge of the dataset in mind, it is competitive with other deep-learning based anomaly detection approaches.

Deep-learning		Ours		Non deep-learning		
α-GAN [6] (15)	VAE-Rec [6] (15)	Default (17)	Fine-tuned (17)	GHMRF [10] (13)	X-Saliency [8] (HGG 14)	GMM [6] (15)
0.37	0.42	0.36	0.44	0.72	0.75	0.22

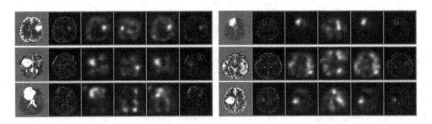

Fig. 3. Anomaly detection of the fine-tuned model on six test set samples. For each example, the reconstruction-error, the backpropagated KL-term, the backpropagated reconstruction-term, the backpropagated $\mathcal{L}$ and the *combi* is plotted from left to right.

4 Discussion and Conclusion

In this work we compared different approaches of detecting anomalies with VAEs over many different hyperparameter settings. However, a hyperparameters are regularly chosen by task specific optimization on an annotated validation set, which contradicts the principle of unsupervised anomaly detection. We showed that for a pixel-wise anomaly detection the reconstruction error does not always have the best performance and can regularly be improved by combining it with the backpropagated KL-term. This is in analogy to common VAE-based anomaly detection methods that consider the ELBO $\mathcal{L}$, which constitutes definition the combination of the KL-term with the reconstruction-term, as a proxy score. The proposed approaches shows promising performance across a broad range of hyperparameters and thus effectively reduce the need for manually tuning towards a validation set and thus keep the unsupervised property intact. If an annotated validation set is available, however, our approach can still be fine tuned to achieve the same competitive performance as other methods. On a first glance, our method is outperformed by non-deep learning methods on the BraTS dataset. This however neglects the fact that these models incorporate specific domain knowledge via their algorithmic design. While this results in a strong performance, it renders them unsuitable for application to a different organs or modalities. Our proposed approach does not make such assumptions, is robust with respect to the exact choice of hyperparameters and could therefore effectively be transferred to new problems or datasets without requiring any modification.

We believe that our proposed method constitutes a step in improving anomaly detection for medical imaging applications. In the future anomaly detection algorithms have the potential of making use of the increasing amounts of available raw data, offering the perspective of effective radiological support tools that are not affected by the annotation data bottleneck.

References

1. Abati, D., Cucchiara, R., et al.: AND: autoregressive novelty detectors (2018)
2. Alain, G., Bengio, Y.: What regularized auto-encoders learn from the data-generating distribution. JMLR **15**, 3563–3593 (2014)
3. An, J., Cho, S.: Variational autoencoder based anomaly detection using reconstruction probability (2015)
4. Baur, C., Navab, N., et al.: Deep autoencoding models for unsupervised anomaly segmentation in brain MR images. CoRR (2018)
5. Chen, X., Konukoglu, E.: Unsupervised detection of lesions in brain MRI using constrained adversarial auto-encoders. CoRR (2018)
6. Chen, X., Konukoglu, E., et al.: Deep generative models in the real-world: an open challenge from medical imaging. CoRR (2018)
7. Dai, B., Wipf, D.: Diagnosing and enhancing VAE models. In: ICLR (2019)
8. Erihov, M., Alpert, S., Kisilev, P., Hashoul, S.: A cross saliency approach to asymmetry-based tumor detection. In: Navab, N., Hornegger, J., Wells, W.M., Frangi, A.F. (eds.) MICCAI 2015. LNCS, vol. 9351, pp. 636–643. Springer, Cham (2015). https://doi.org/10.1007/978-3-319-24574-4_76
9. Goldstein, M., Uchida, S.: A Comparative evaluation of unsupervised anomaly detection algorithms for multivariate data. PLoS ONE **11**(4), e0152173 (2016)
10. Juan-Albarracín, J., García-Gómez, J.M., et al.: Automated glioblastoma segmentation based on a multiparametric structured unsupervised classification. PLoS ONE **10**(5), e0125143 (2015)
11. Kingma, D.P., Welling, M.: Auto-encoding variational Bayes. CoRR (2013)
12. Kiran, B., Parakkal, R., et al.: An overview of deep learning based methods for unsupervised and semi-supervised anomaly detection in videos. J. Imaging **4**(2), 36 (2018)
13. Menze, B.H., Van Leemput, K., et al.: The multimodal brain tumor image segmentation benchmark (BRATS). IEEE Trans. Med. Imaging **34**, 1993–2024 (2015)
14. Nalisnick, E., Lakshminarayanan, B., et al.: Do deep generative models know what they don't know? In: ICLR (2019)
15. Paszke, A., Lerer, A., et al.: Automatic differentiation in PyTorch (2017)
16. Pawlowski, N., Glocker, B., et al.: Unsupervised lesion detection in brain CT using Bayesian convolutional autoencoders (2018)
17. Radford, A., Chintala, S., et al.: Unsupervised representation learning with deep convolutional generative adversarial networks (2015)
18. Rezende, D.J., Wierstra, D., et al.: Stochastic backpropagation and approximate inference in deep generative models. In: ICML (2014). JMLR.org
19. Schlegl, T., Seeböck, P., Waldstein, S.M., Schmidt-Erfurth, U., Langs, G.: Unsupervised anomaly detection with generative adversarial networks to guide marker discovery. In: Niethammer, M., et al. (eds.) IPMI 2017. LNCS, vol. 10265, pp. 146–157. Springer, Cham (2017). https://doi.org/10.1007/978-3-319-59050-9_12

20. Van Essen, D.C., WU-Minn HCP Consortium, et al.: The human connectome project: a data acquisition perspective. Neuroimage **62**(4), 2222–2231 (2012)
21. Xiao, H., Rasul, K., Vollgraf, R.: Fashion-MNIST: a novel image dataset for benchmarking machine learning algorithms (2017)
22. You, S., Konukoglu, E., et al.: Unsupervised lesion detection via image restoration with a normative prior. In: International Conference on Medical Imaging with Deep Learning - Full Paper Track (2019)

HR-CAM: Precise Localization of Pathology Using Multi-level Learning in CNNs

Sumeet Shinde[1], Tanay Chougule[1], Jitender Saini[2],
and Madhura Ingalhalikar[1(✉)]

[1] Symbiosis Center for Medical Image Analysis,
Symbiosis International University, Pune 412115, India
head@scmia.edu.in
[2] National Institute of Mental Health and Neurosciences,
Bengaluru 560029, India

Abstract. We propose a CNN based technique that aggregates feature maps from its multiple layers that can localize abnormalities with greater details as well as predict pathology under consideration. Existing class activation mapping (CAM) techniques extract feature maps from either the final layer or a single intermediate layer to create the discriminative maps and then interpolate to upsample to the original image resolution. In this case, the subject specific localization is coarse and is unable to capture subtle abnormalities. To mitigate this, our method builds a novel CNN based discriminative localization model that we call high resolution CAM (HR-CAM), which accounts for layers from each resolution, therefore facilitating a comprehensive map that can delineate the pathology for each subject by combining low-level, intermediate as well as high-level features from the CNN. Moreover, our model directly provides the discriminative map in the resolution of the original image facilitating finer delineation of abnormalities. We demonstrate the working of our model on a simulated abnormalities data where we illustrate how the model captures finer details in the final discriminative maps as compared to current techniques. We then apply this technique: (1) to classify ependymomas from grade IV glioblastoma on T1-weighted contrast enhanced (T1-CE) MRI and (2) to predict Parkinson's disease from neuromelanin sensitive MRI. In all these cases we demonstrate that our model not only predicts pathologies with high accuracies, but also creates clinically interpretable subject specific high resolution discriminative localizations. Overall, the technique can be generalized to any CNN and carries high relevance in a clinical setting.

Keywords: Class Activation Map (CAM) · Convolutional Neural Networks (CNN) · High resolution · Ependymoma · Gliobastoma · Parkinson's disease

1 Introduction

Convolutional neural networks (CNNs) have become one of the most powerful tools for analyzing medical images and have demonstrated exceptional performance in image classification tasks [1] as well as in structure segmentation [2] often becoming the new

---

S. Shinde and T. Chougule—Equally contributed.

© Springer Nature Switzerland AG 2019
D. Shen et al. (Eds.): MICCAI 2019, LNCS 11767, pp. 298–306, 2019
https://doi.org/10.1007/978-3-030-32251-9_33

state of art in several use cases. The ability of CNNs in extracting the discriminative pixel based features, automatically, is attractive as it often accounts for better classification performance, particularly on large datasets, when compared to a similar task on empirically drawn features. This superior performance, however, comes with certain tradeoffs as the predictions are not intuitive and explanation of objects/regions that contribute towards the classification is crucial, especially for problems in medical imaging where gaining clarity is particularly imperative as the classification output has to be supported with clinical interpretation.

To this date, multiple techniques have been proposed to visualize the discriminative regions that allow us to gain insights into the functioning of the CNNs. Earlier, techniques were based on mapping activations back to the input space via deconvolutions to highlight the most discriminative regions [3]. However, the applicability of this deconv-net was limited owing to its complexity. Existing techniques are mainly based on class activation mapping (CAM) that have the capability to localize the regions either by extracting information from the final layer [4] using global average pooling (GAP) or any layer of choice using gradient information (Grad-CAM) [5]. These techniques are more applicable, and further have been adapted for medical imaging 2D and 3D applications [6, 7], for extracting multiple object instances [8] and for refining the classification output by revisiting the discriminative regions [9].

The challenge with CAMs is that they provide insights usually only from a single layer of the CNN. Moreover, the extracted CAM is a low resolution map especially when extracted from intermediate to final layers of CNN as the input is max-pooled multiple times. This facilitates a coarse output which fails to capture subtle details that discriminate the classes under consideration. Particularly, this is crucial in medical imaging, where the pathology under consideration may demonstrate highly heterogeneous and diffuse patterns of abnormalities that may not be characterized by current CAM techniques. It is therefore important to extract these subtle discriminative image based markers as these can support prognosis, diagnosis, risk prediction and treatment efficacy.

In this paper we address the aforementioned issues. We create high resolution class activation maps (HR-CAMs) to visualize and highlight the discriminative regions in pathologies with high precision. We achieve this by capturing feature maps from multiple layers (pre-max-pooling layers) and aggregating these for a single layer classifier that also facilitates improved classification accuracies. We first validate our novel technique on simulated abnormalities dataset where we demonstrate its superior working even on noisy data and then apply it to (1) predict Parkinson's disease from neuromelanin contrast MRI (brain-stem region) (2) classify ependymomas from glioblastomas on T1-CE MRI. The multi-layer aggregation provides better interpretability with higher accuracy while the HR maps facilitate precise localization. The method gives state-of-art performance when compared to current techniques, and is generalizable to any CNN model.

2 Method

In this work, we demonstrate that by employing a novel CNN based architecture, we can automate and generalize its ability in identifying the exact regions of an image that are important in the classification by generating HR-CAMs. Figure 1 gives the overview of our HR-CAM architecture.

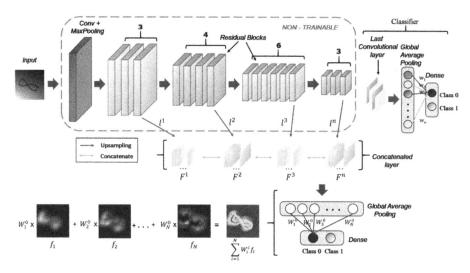

Fig. 1. Schematic diagram of the proposed model. The input images are first trained using CNN layers with a classifier at the end. The feature maps of each layer before max-pooling are sampled and concatenated and given as input to a global average pooling layer that is trained to optimize the weights (W_1, W_2,..., W_N) while keeping the previous layers frozen. These weights are used to create the HR-CAMs.

2.1 HR-CAM

Specifically, if we choose k number of convolutional layers $L = \{l^1, l^2, \ldots, l^k\}$, the feature maps $F^i = \{f_1^i, f_2^i, \ldots, f_m^i\}$ corresponding to the convolutional layers l^i are first upsampled using a bilinear interpolation to match the original input image dimensions. The number of feature maps corresponding to the kth layer is given by m_k. The feature maps are then stacked together to form a concatenated layer with total N feature maps where N is given by Eq. 1.

$$N = \sum_{i=1}^{k} m_k \tag{1}$$

These N feature maps are then average pooled globally thereby representing every feature map in the concatenated layer by a single value. The vector obtained after average pooling is given as input to a single fully-connected layer that is trained to minimize the categorical cross entropy loss function (Eq. 2), where y_n is target output probability, $\hat{y}_n$ is predicted output probability, S is number of samples and $J(w)$ is categorical cross-entropy loss and is achieved by using the Adam optimizer. The optimization is performed by freezing the convolutional layers.

$$J(w) = \frac{-1}{S} \sum_{n=1}^{S} [y_n \log \hat{y}_n + (1 - y_n) \log(1 - \hat{y}_n)] \tag{2}$$

This assigns new weights to all the feature maps according to their importance for classification and supports weighted aggregation. Finally, to obtain the discriminative activations, we forward propagate the input image and acquire the weights (W_1, W_2 ..., $W_{N)}$ at the output layer for the respective class, as given in Zhou et al. [4]. To create the class activation map, the weights W_i^c for the respective class are then multiplied with the feature maps f_i and then added together, as shown in Fig. 1. The resulting class activation map A can therefore demonstrate the most discerning regions in the image in high resolution.

$$A = \sum_{i=1}^{N} W_i^c f_i \tag{3}$$

Although Fig. 1 uses Resnet50 architecture [10] with global average pooling (GAP) and fully connected layers for binary classification, the proposed technique is generalizable to any CNN based classifier.

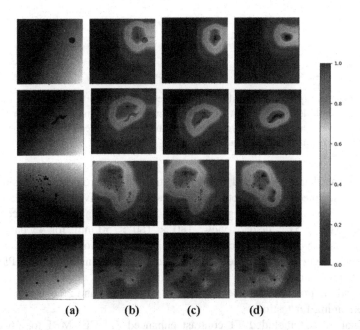

(a)   (b)   (c)   (d)

Fig. 2. Simulated dataset results. (a) demonstrates the simulated abnormities, (b) CAMs produced using Zhou et al.'s method (c) results from GradCAM (d) results from HR-CAM (proposed technique). The maps produced from our method are high resolution as can be clearly seen (especially in top 2 rows). Moreover, in case of diffuse abnormalities, our method can capture it more finely (bottom 2 rows).

3   Experiments and Results

3.1   Datasets

Our dataset consisted of two classes of simulated images. Class 1 included 1000 images of normative data without abnormalities but with added random noise and Class 2 consisted of 1000 images with simulated pathology with added random noise. We created abnormalities that were localized as well as abnormalities that were diffuse in nature as shown in Fig. 2. The data was divided into train and test groups with 1500 images for training and 500 for testing.

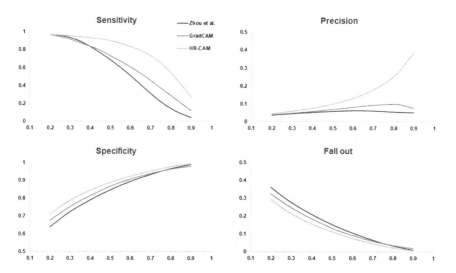

Fig. 3. Comparative quantitative analysis of the three CAM methods. The x-axis in all 3 plots denotes the threshold level for the CAMs. We demonstrate that at any threshold our HR-CAMs are more sensitive, specific with a very low fall out and high precision when the simulated abnormalities were considered as ground truth.

The second dataset included high resolution 3D neuromelanin sensitive MRI (NMS-MRI) scanned using spectral pre-saturation with inversion recovery (SPIR) sequence and was acquired using TR/TE: 26/2.2 ms, flip angle: 20°; reconstructed matrix size: 512 × 512; field of view: 180 × 180 × 50 mm, for 45 patients with Parkinson's disease (PD) and 35 controls. The NMS-MRI provides a good contrast in the substantia nigra pars compacta (SNc) and is useful in identifying PD as PD manifests depigmentation of the SNc [11]. The CNN was employed on the boxed region around the brainstem on the axial slices, with 30 PD and 25 controls in training and the remaining for testing.

Our final dataset included T1 contrast enhanced (T1-CE) MRI for 26 cases of ependymomas and 26 cases of grade IV glioblastoma. Majority ependymoma's tend to mimic grade IV glioblastomas and therefore it is crucial to be identified at a radiological level. We used a large boxed region around the lesion in the axial slices as an input to the CNNs with 3811 images for training with augmentation and 1004 images for testing.

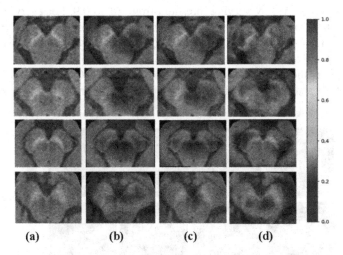

Fig. 4. Qualitative Comparison of Class Activation Maps obtained on the neuromelanin contrast images to predict PD. (a) Section of brainstem used in classification where the bright region is the SNc. (b) Results from Zhou.et al.'s CAMs (c) Results from GradCAM (d) Results from our proposed technique (HR-CAMs). Our methods can delineate the abnormal areas (SNc in this case) better than both the comparative techniques that produce a diffuse map.

3.2   Experiment Details

The CNN architecture was derived from ResNet50 design that consisted of 16 residual blocks each of which contains 3 convolutional layers and an identity connection. A max-pooling layer, that downsamples the image, was applied before the first block and after 3, 4, 6 and 3 residual blocks as shown in Fig. 1. The final layers included a GAP layer followed by fully connected layers and a 'softmax' classifier. Throughout the CNN architecture, we employed rectified linear unit (ReLU) activations and a learning rate of 0.0001. The cross entropy loss was minimized as shown in Eq. 2. To reduce the susceptibility to over-fitting, as a standard practice, data augmentation was performed which increases the dataset by several folds. We performed image translations, rotations, minor shifting as well as horizontal and vertical flipping. To increase the total dataset, we applied a random combination of these transformations on each image.

To compare our results with existing techniques we employed GAP based CAMs by Zhou et al. [4] that uses the final layer feature maps and Grad-CAMs where we used the layer before the final layer on the same ResNet50 model. Our models were trained on Nvidia Quadro P6000 with 24 GB of graphics RAM. The code was implemented in Python 3.6 and the deep-learning Framework used was Keras with a TensorFlow backend.

A discriminative ground truth area is necessary for quantifying the localization ability of CAMs. Therefore, we compared the three techniques- Zhou-CAMs, Grad-CAM, and HR-CAM (ours), with simulated abnormalities as the ground truth. All the class activation maps were intensity normalized (0 to 1.0) and compared with the ground truth masks (A_T) by varying threshold from 0.1 to 0.9. For every threshold, a binary image (A_C) was obtained and the foreground pixels were considered as positive labels (P_c) and the rest as negative labels (N_c). These were then matched with the ground-truth positive (P_T) and negative (N_T) labels where P_T is given by the abnormality and N_T is the noisy background. We compared the CAM localization performance based on sensitivity, specificity, precision and fall-out.

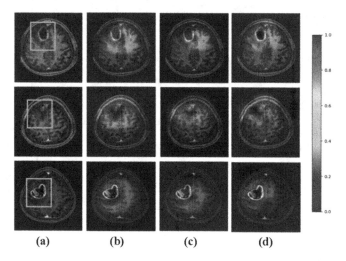

(a)   (b)   (c)   (d)

Fig. 5. Figure showing results for tumor classification (a) original image (boxed region is used for training/testing) (b) Results from Zhou et al.'s CAMs (c) Results from GradCAM (using one layer before the final layer) (d) HR-CAMs (proposed technique). It can be clearly seen by optimizing the weights and summing the feature maps from multiple layers, we obtain more accuracy in locating the abnormality.

Table 1. Quantitative comparison of CAMs on simulated data.

Mean values	Zhou et al.	GradCAM	HR-CAM (proposed)
Sensitivity	0.556	0.620	**0.774**
Specificity	0.848	0.863	**0.885**
Precision	0.052	0.072	**0.151**
Fall out	0.151	0.136	**0.114**

3.3   Results

Figure 2 shows the comparison of the CAMs between our HR-CAM, Zhou's CAMs and Grad-CAM for the abnormal test cases. Table 1 and Fig. 3 provide the comparative quantitative analysis for the simulated CAMs. Table 1 provides the mean values for the evaluation quantifiers over all thresholds. It can be observed that HR-CAMs can accurately visualize the abnormalities than earlier techniques. For the PD dataset the HR-CAM model boosts the accuracy to 78.3% when compared to 76.2% with the ResNet50. Figure 4 demonstrates the heatmaps for PD test cases in comparison to Zhou's CAMs and Grad-CAM wherein it can be clearly seen that our method captures the SNc area (right and left separately) while the other two provide a very coarse activation map with the left-right SNc merged in a single activation blob. For the tumor data we demonstrate similar findings where the classification accuracy is boosted to 67.5% when compared to ResNet50–64.6%. Figure 5 demonstrates the CAMs computed for the tumor test cases. By employing the HR-CAM technique, we achieve higher classification accuracy as well as a detailed heatmap.

4   Conclusion

This work presented a novel CNN based technique named high resolution class activation mapping (HR-CAMs) that can generate precise maps of the most discriminative areas involved in distinguishing the groups under consideration. We demonstrated the accuracy of capturing the abnormalities through simulated data as well as through multiple applications. In summary, the presented framework is highly relevant to classification problems in medical imaging where the identification of discriminative regions is crucial for clinical rationalization as well as may aid in targeted therapy and treatment planning.

References

1. Krizhevsky, A., Sutskever, I., Hinton, G.E.: ImageNet classification with deep convolutional neural networks. In: Advances in Neural Information Processing Systems, vol. 25 (2012)
2. Kamnitsas, K., et al.: Efficient multi-scale 3D CNN with fully connected CRF for accurate brain lesion segmentation. Med. Image Anal. **36**, 61–78 (2017)
3. Zeiler, M.D., Fergus, R.: Visualizing and understanding convolutional networks. In: Fleet, D., Pajdla, T., Schiele, B., Tuytelaars, T. (eds.) ECCV 2014. LNCS, vol. 8689, pp. 818–833. Springer, Cham (2014). https://doi.org/10.1007/978-3-319-10590-1_53
4. Zhou, B., et al.: Learning deep features for discriminative localization. In: CVPR (2016)
5. Selvaraju, R.R., et al.: Grad-CAM: visual explanations from deep networks via gradient-based localization. In: Proceedings of the IEEE International Conference on Computer Vision (2017)
6. Zhao, G., Zhou, B., Wang, K., Jiang, R., Xu, M.: Respond-CAM: analyzing deep models for 3D imaging data by visualizations. In: Frangi, A.F., Schnabel, J.A., Davatzikos, C., Alberola-López, C., Fichtinger, G. (eds.) MICCAI 2018. LNCS, vol. 11070, pp. 485–492. Springer, Cham (2018). https://doi.org/10.1007/978-3-030-00928-1_55

7. Ahmad, A., et al.: Predictive and discriminative localization of IDH genotype in high grade gliomas using deep convolutional neural nets. In: IEEE 16th International Symposium on Biomedical Imaging (2019)

8. Chattopadhay, A., et al.: Grad-CAM++: generalized gradient-based visual explanations for deep convolutional networks. In: 2018 IEEE Winter Conference on Applications of Computer Vision (WACV). IEEE (2018)

9. Rosenfeld, A., Ullman, S.: Visual concept recognition and localization via iterative introspection. In: Lai, S.-H., Lepetit, V., Nishino, K., Sato, Y. (eds.) ACCV 2016. LNCS, vol. 10115, pp. 264–279. Springer, Cham (2017). https://doi.org/10.1007/978-3-319-54193-8_17

10. He, K., et al.: Deep residual learning for image recognition. In: Proceedings of the IEEE Conference on Computer Vision and Pattern Recognition 2016, pp. 770–778 (2016)

11. Shinde, S., et al.: Predictive markers for Parkinson's disease using deep neural nets on neuromelanin sensitive MRI. Neuroimage Clin. **22**, 101748 (2019)

Novel Iterative Attention Focusing Strategy for Joint Pathology Localization and Prediction of MCI Progression

Qingfeng Li[1,2], Xiaodan Xing[1,3], Ying Sun[2], Bin Xiao[1,4], Hao Wei[1,5],
Quan Huo[1], Minqing Zhang[1,6], Xiang Sean Zhou[1], Yiqiang Zhan[1],
Zhong Xue[1], and Feng Shi[1(✉)]

[1] Shanghai United Imaging Intelligence Co., Ltd., Shanghai, China
feng.shi@united-imaging.kcom
[2] School of Biomedical Engineering, Southern Medical University, Guangdong, China
[3] Medical Imaging Center, Shanghai Advanced Research Institute, Shanghai, China
[4] School of Biomedical Engineering, Med-X Research Institute,
Shanghai Jiaotong University, Shanghai, China
[5] School of Computer Science and Engineering,
Central South University, Hunan, China
[6] College of Software Engineering, Southeast University, Jiangsu, China

Abstract. Mild Cognitive Impairment (MCI) is the prodromal stage of Alzheimer's disease (AD), with a high incident rate converting to AD. Hence, it is critical to identify MCI patients who will convert to AD patients for early and effective treatment. Recently, many machine learning or deep learning based methods have been proposed to first localize the pathology-related brain regions and then extract respective features for MCI progression diagnosis. However, the intrinsic relationship between pathological region localization and respective feature extraction was usually neglected. To address this issue, in this paper, we proposed a novel iterative attention focusing strategy for joint pathological region localization and identification of progressive MCI (pMCI) from stable MCI (sMCI). Moreover, by connecting diagnosis network and attention map generator, the pathological regions can be iteratively localized, and the respective diagnosis performance is in turn improved. Experiments on 393 training subjects from the ADNI-1 dataset and other 277 testing subjects from the ADNI-2 dataset show that our method can achieve 81.59% accuracy for pMCI *vs.* sMCI diagnosis. Our results outperform those with the state-of-the-art methods, while additionally providing a focused attention map on specific pathological locations related to MCI progression, *i.e.*, left temporal lobe, entorhinal and hippocampus. This allows for more insights and better understanding of the progression of MCI to AD.

1 Introduction

As the most prevalent neurodegenerative disorder, Alzheimer's disease (AD) is characterized by the irreversible loss of neurons and progressive impairment of

© Springer Nature Switzerland AG 2019
D. Shen et al. (Eds.): MICCAI 2019, LNCS 11767, pp. 307–315, 2019.
https://doi.org/10.1007/978-3-030-32251-9_34

cognitive functions [4]. There is a continuous spectrum from normal cognition to AD, where mild cognitive impairment (MCI) is a prodromal stage. Hence, it is of vital importance to identify the MCI subjects who convert to AD after a period of time (progressive MCI, *i.e.*, pMCI) from those who remain stable cognitive functions (stable MCI, *i.e.*, sMCI).

Recently, dementia diagnosis strategies via deep learning approaches have achieved promising results over conventional machine learning methods, given that deep learning models can hierarchically extract discriminative feature representations and naturally combine features in different levels. For example, Liu et al. [9] reported 76.90% separation of 38 pMCI subjects from 239 sMCI subjects using patch-based CNN.

While extensive studies focus on the dementia diagnosis task, the localization of dementia-related anatomy are usually neglected. Liu et al. [9] used discriminative anatomical landmarks with certain distributions, *e.g.*, at bilateral temporal lobe and hippocampus. Lian et al. [7] modified their CNN diagnosis framework and got the class activation map [13], showing that hippocampus and both corners and boundaries of the ventricle are discriminative for pMCI against sMCI.

In our work, we propose a novel iterative attention focusing (IAF) strategy to simultaneously generate disease-related attention map and produce disease diagnosis result for pMCI. We observed that accurate localization of disease-related attention area can improve diagnosis performance, and the model with good diagnosis results can further generate better attention maps. Our specific contributions are summarized as follows: (1) Pathological region localization and identification tasks are jointly optimized; (2) A dedicated attention map generator is proposed to focus on the most disease-related discriminative anatomical locations; (3) Disease classification results outperform those with the state-of-the-art methods.

2   Method

2.1   Iterative Attention Focusing (IAF) Strategy

As shown in Fig. 1, we propose an iterative attention focusing (IAF) strategy for yielding disease-relevant attention map and predicting diagnosis result. There are two major components in IAF: (1) the full-size diagnosis network (FDN), and (2) the attention map generator (AMG). A FDN with corresponding AMG can be seen as a **sub-network**. Each sub-network takes inputs from (1) original intensity image and (2) attention maps generated by previous sub-networks. Multiple sub-networks connect with each other and iteratively optimize the classification performance and focus the attention on class activated regions. Details are described as follows.

FDN Component for Diagnosis. Most of previous CNN-based studies take 2D images or extract small size 3D image patches as input, which may cause the losing of global semantic information. Thus, we propose a FDN structure for

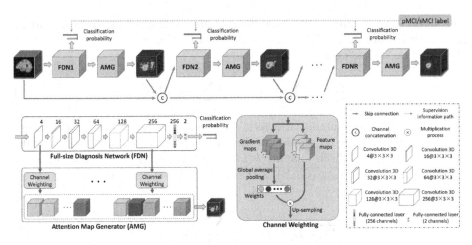

Fig. 1. Illustration of our purposed iterative attention focusing (IAF) strategy. Top row shows the pipeline where FDN and AMG form a subnetwork and multiple subnetworks connect each other and iteratively update to optimize the performance. Bottom row shows the details of FDN and AMG components.

extracting and processing disease-related feature representation from the input feature map, shown in Fig. 1. FDN is composed of 6 convolution layers and 2 fully-connected (FC) layers. Each convolution layer is followed by: (1) a batch normalization layer, which can normalize features by the computed mean and variance, (2) a dropout layer (with a ratio of 0.5), which helps prevent over-fitting, (3) a rectified linear unit (ReLU), which serves as activation function, and (4) a $2 \times 2 \times 2$ max pooling layer (except for the last convolution layer). After the last convolution layer, the obtained feature map group is compressed to a vector by a global average pooling layer, and the derived feature vector is then fed into a fully-connected layer to generate disease label prediction probability using softmax process.

AMG Component for Pathological Region Localization. Previous work [11] revealed an important observation that the feature maps from different layers of CNN possess hierarchies of information. Low (*i.e.*, near to the input layer) layers extract low-level features such as edges and lines, while deep (*i.e.*, near to the output layer) layers catch high-level semantic patterns. Therefore, the visualization results yielded from different layers complement one another and can be combined together to represent discriminative details. In addition, inspired by previous work [10], the gradient information flowing through each layer can produce the importance of each voxel in feature maps for a decision of interest.

In order to get high-resolution attention maps from current FDN, we propose AMG as a new design of class activation map generator, whose structure is shown in Fig. 1. Generally, AMG calculates the weighted feature maps for each convolution layer individually and then combines feature maps to one high-resolution feature map. Mathematically, AMG computes activation map A^c of class c by the following formula:

$$A^c = \frac{1}{L} \sum_l U p_l (ReLU(\sum_k \alpha_{k,l}^c M_{k,l})), \tag{1}$$

where L denotes the number of layers, $U p_l(\cdot)$ denotes the up-sampling process of l-th layer and $ReLU(\cdot)$ represents the rectified linear unit. $\alpha_{k,l}^c$ is the weight of feature map $M_{k,l}$ from channel k in convolutional layer l and is obtained by global average pooling (GAP) of the corresponding gradient map $G_{k,l}$ of y_c (score for class c):

$$\alpha_{k,l}^c = \frac{1}{W_l \times H_l \times D_l} \sum_{w \in W} \sum_{h \in H} \sum_{d \in D} G_{k,l}(w, h, d), \tag{2}$$

where W_l, H_l, D_l are the width, height and depth of a feature map of the l-th layer. $G_{k,l}(w, h, d)$ represents the gradient value generated via back-propagation on coordinate (w, h, d) of feature map $M_{k,l}$, which can be demonstrated as:

$$G_{k,l}(w, h, d) = \frac{\partial y^c}{\partial M_{k,l}(w, h, d)}, \tag{3}$$

where y^c is the classification score of class c before the soft-max process.

Connection Strategy Between Sub-networks. In Fig. 1, we connect sub-networks together to combine information generated in different iteration stages. Specifically, we first optimize FDN1 and compute attention maps from AMG. Then, FDN2 is updated and more focused attention maps are generated. Finally, other sub-networks are updated sequentially. We refer to this connection method as the "dense" connection, since the input of the r-th sub-network is a feature map concatenated by the original input image and the attention map generated from AMGs of previous sub-networks. The reason of such design is that the attention maps generated previously can provide guidance for separation task, and the improvement of FDN separation performance can be helpful for precise localization of disease-related regions. In the IAF strategy, we further modify the dense connection to a "partial dense connection", for the input of the r-th FDN only consists of: (1) the original input image, and (2) the attention maps generated by previous two sub-networks. We observed that the attention areas were coarse at first and relatively focused on a certain zone later, so previously generated coarse attention maps have little guidance to the performance of later sub-networks. The partial dense connection can be described as follows:

$$x_r = \begin{cases} x, & r = 1 \\ [x, Am_1, ..., Am_{r-1}], & r \in [2, 3], \\ [x, Am_{r-2}, Am_{r-1}], & r \geq 4 \end{cases} \tag{4}$$

where [·] refers to the concatenation operation, and Am_r is the attention map generated from the r-th sub-network. The framework with dense connection can *think globally and act locally* during iteration process, and the generated pathological regions can be iteratively localized and the respective diagnosis performance can also be improved.

2.2   Network Implementation

Our IAF strategy was implemented in the deep learning framework PyTorch. In the beginning of the iteration, we initialized the weights of FDNs with the strategy in [3], and the focal loss [8] was used as objective function. Adaptive moment estimation (Adam) [6] served as the optimizer with the learning rate of 10^{-4}, and the batch size was set to 10. Experiments were performed with a NVIDIA Tesla V100 32 GB GPU.

3   Experiments

3.1   Dataset and Preprocessing

Our analysis was based on public Alzheimer's Disease Neuroimaging Initiative (ADNI) [5] dataset. For better evaluation, we used the 1.5 T T1 MR images from ADNI-1 dataset for training and 3.0 T T1 images from ADNI-2 dataset for testing. It is worth noting that we followed previous studies [7,9] to use the exact same sMCI and pMCI data for easier comparison of results. In particular, the training set includes 226 sMCI and 167 pMCI subjects, and the testing set contains 239 sMCI and 38 pMCI subjects. sMCI and pMCI were defined according to whether MCI subjects converted to AD within 36 months after the baseline. All data in training and testing sets were processed using a standard pipeline, including image reorientation, resampling to voxel size of $1 \times 1 \times 1$ mm^3, bias correction and skull stripping.

3.2   Effectiveness of Iterative Attention Focusing Strategy

In Fig. 2, we reported the experimental results achieved in various iterative stages of IAF. In Fig. 2(a), diagnosis performance is described by four metrics: accuracy (ACC), sensitivity (SEN), specificity (SPE), and area under receiver operating characteristic curve (AUC); and from the figure we can have three observations. **First**, for FDNs in early stages of iteration, adding attention maps as guidance information significantly improves the performance. For instance, when FDN2 takes the original input and the attention maps generated from sub-network 1, the diagnosis accuracy improves from 0.6787 to 0.7978. At the same time, SEN, SPE and AUC also increase compared with FDN1. **Second**, when more iterations are added, the effectiveness of adding attention maps becomes smaller, characterized by the insignificance improvement of FDN performance, *e.g.*, AUC of FDN3 only improves 0.0079 compared to FDN2. **Third**, when the scale of

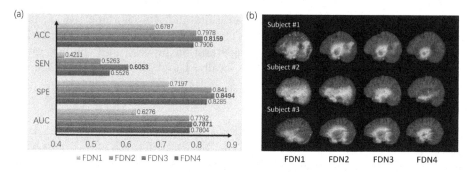

Fig. 2. Illustration of diagnosis performance and located attention area of different iteration stages in testing data. (a) shows the pMCI *vs.* sMCI separation performance of different FDNs. (b) shows the attention maps of three subjects generated in different stages, and warmer colors indicate that the location has better discriminative ability. All numerical results were done on testing data. (Color figure online)

IAF exceeds a certain degree, adding additional attention areas will no longer to provide useful guidance to subsequent FDNs. Figure 2(b) illustrates that the attention regions tend to focus, which provides evidences for the above inferences.

Note that, to generalize "stopping" criteria, in our experiments, the iteration number was determined by checking the validation data performance. In detail, our training set was randomly split into pure-training set (including 155 sMCI and 120 pMCI samples) and validation set (including 71 sMCI and 47 pMCI samples). As we trained our IAF on pure-training set, the best performance was obtained in FDN3. Thus we got the optimized iteration number as 3. For other datasets, the same approach could be applied and the parameter could be determined based on performance of validation data.

3.3   Disease Separation Performance

We compared our IAF method with 4 methods, including two conventional methods, *i.e.*, (1) region of interest-based method (ROI) [12] and (2) voxel-based morphometry (VBM) [1], and two deep learning-based methods, *i.e.*, (3) landmark-based deep multi-instance learning (LDMIL) [9] and (4) with-prior hierarchical fully convolutional network (wH-FCN) [7]. For ROI- and VBM-based methods, we used linear SVM (C = 1) classifier for feature processing. Results of pMCI *vs.* sMCI classification are presented in Table 1. From the table we can observe that: (1) Deep learning-based method generally outperforms other approaches in the pMCI *vs.* sMCI classification task. For example, in terms of the diagnosis accuracy, IAF achieves an 0.1553 and an 0.1733 improvement compared with VBM and ROI, respectively, which shows the outstanding feature extraction and process ability of CNN; (2) The performance of our purposed network-level dense structure outperform other state-of-the-art deep learning-based methods. It is worth noting that we achieved higher SEN, which indicates our method is more capable to identify possible MCI converters.

Table 1. Results of pMCI identification (i.e., pMCI *vs.* sMCI) using different methods.

Method	ACC	SEN	SPE	AUC
ROI	0.6606	0.4737	0.6904	0.6377
VBM	0.6426	0.3684	0.6862	0.5929
LDMIL	0.7690	0.4211	0.8243	0.7764
wH-FCN	0.8087	0.5263	**0.8536**	0.7813
IAF (ours)	**0.8159**	**0.6053**	0.8494	**0.7871**

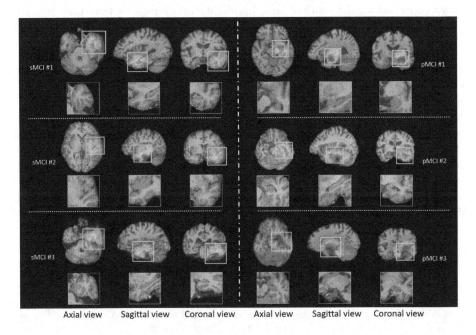

Axial view   Sagittal view   Coronal view   Axial view   Sagittal view   Coronal view

Fig. 3. Attention maps and corresponding local anatomic structure of 3 sMCI subjects and 3 pMCI subjects. We adjusted the transparency so that attention regions can be observed easily. Warmer colors indicate that the location has better discriminative ability. (Color figure online)

3.4 Attention Areas

In Fig. 3, attention maps of 6 subjects (including 3 sMCI subjects and 3 pMCI subjects) in the testing dataset, generated by AMG corresponding to FDN3, are shown in axial, sagittal and coronal views, and the corresponding local anatomic structures on T1 MRI images are also shown in the figure. From Fig. 3, one can reach the following conclusions: (1) Our method can provide a focused attention map on specific pathological locations related to MCI progression, with detailed anatomical patterns; (2) Generally, regions most relevant to MCI progression are mainly located at the left brain, including temporal lobe, entorhinal cortex, and hippocampus. These results are consistent with existing neurological studies like [2] and [9]. It is worth noting that the obtained attention areas were directly from the image itself with no prior knowledge involved. The agreement between our locations and the literature implies that our network grasps the essential diagnosis information; (3) The discriminative regions may differ among individuals. For instance, in pMCI group, pMCI #1 mainly focus on left hippocampus, while inferior temporal gyrus and entorhinal cortex are the most discriminative areas for pMCI #2; (4) The activated regions in sMCI group are relatively blurry than those of pMCI group, which may due to the fact that the pMCI subjects tend to have more pathology. From Fig. 2(b) one can observed that, in different stages of iteration, the method first highlights many regions that may related to AD progression, and then picks the regions that their changes may be subtle while contribute large to the diagnosis.

4 Conclusion

In this paper, we propose a novel iterative attention focusing strategy for joint pathological region localization and identification of pMCI from sMCI. Experiments on 277 testing subjects from ADNI-2 dataset show that our method can achieve 81.59% accuracy for pMCI vs. sMCI diagnosis, while yielding the focused attention maps on specific pathological locations related to MCI progression. This allows more insights and better understanding for progression of MCI to AD, compared to the state-of-the-art methods.

References

1. Ashburner, J., Friston, K.J.: Voxel-based morphometry-the methods. Neuroimage **11**(6), 805–821 (2000)
2. Galton, C.J., et al.: Differing patterns of temporal atrophy in Alzheimer's disease and semantic dementia. Neurology **57**(2), 216–225 (2001)
3. He, K., Zhang, X., Ren, S., Sun, J.: Delving deep into rectifiers: surpassing human-level performance on imagenet classification. In: Proceedings of the IEEE International Conference on Computer Vision, pp. 1026–1034 (2015)
4. Jagust, W.: Vulnerable neural systems and the borderland of brain aging and neurodegeneration. Neuron **77**(2), 219–234 (2013)
5. Jack Jr., C.R., et al.: The Alzheimer's disease neuroimaging initiative (ADNI): MRI methods. J. Magn. Reson. Imaging **27**(4), 685–691 (2010)
6. Kingma, D.P., Ba, J.: Adam: a method for stochastic optimization. arXiv preprint arXiv:1412.6980 (2014)
7. Lian, C., Liu, M., Zhang, J., Shen, D.: Hierarchical fully convolutional network for joint atrophy localization and Alzheimer's disease diagnosis using structural MRI. IEEE Trans. Pattern Anal. Mach. Intell. **PP**(99), 1 (2018)
8. Lin, T.Y., Goyal, P., Girshick, R., He, K., Dollár, P.: Focal loss for dense object detection. In: Proceedings of the IEEE International Conference on Computer Vision, pp. 2980–2988 (2017)
9. Liu, M., Zhang, J., Adeli, E., Shen, D.: Landmark-based deep multi-instance learning for brain disease diagnosis. Med. Image Anal. **43**, 157–168 (2018)

10. Selvaraju, R.R., Cogswell, M., Das, A., Vedantam, R., Parikh, D., Batra, D.: Grad-CAM: visual explanations from deep networks via gradient-based localization. In: Proceedings of the IEEE International Conference on Computer Vision, pp. 618–626 (2017)
11. Zeiler, M.D., Fergus, R.: Visualizing and understanding convolutional networks. In: Fleet, D., Pajdla, T., Schiele, B., Tuytelaars, T. (eds.) ECCV 2014. LNCS, vol. 8689, pp. 818–833. Springer, Cham (2014). https://doi.org/10.1007/978-3-319-10590-1_53
12. Zhang, D., Wang, Y., Zhou, L., Yuan, H., Shen, D.: Multimodal classification of Alzheimer's disease and mild cognitive impairment. Neuroimage **55**(3), 856–867 (2011)
13. Zhou, B., Khosla, A., Lapedriza, A., Oliva, A., Torralba, A.: Learning deep features for discriminative localization. In: Proceedings of the IEEE Conference on Computer Vision and Pattern Recognition, pp. 2921–2929 (2016)

Automatic Vertebrae Recognition from Arbitrary Spine MRI Images by a Hierarchical Self-calibration Detection Framework

Shen Zhao[1], Xi Wu[2(✉)], Bo Chen[1], and Shuo Li[1(✉)]

[1] Department of Medical Imaging and Medical Biophysics, Western University, London, ON, Canada
z-s-06@163.com, slishuo@gmail.com
[2] Chengdu University of Information Technology, Chengdu, Sichuan, China

Abstract. Automatic vertebrae recognition is crucial in spine diseases diagnosis, treatment planning, and response assessment. Although vertebrae detection has been studied for years, reliably recognizing vertebrae from arbitrary spine MRI images remains a challenge due to varying image characteristics, field of view (FOV) as well as vertebrae appearance. In this paper, we propose a Hierarchical Self-calibration Detection Framework (Hi-scene) to precisely recognize the labels and bounding boxes of all vertebrae in an arbitrary spine MRI image. Hi-scene is designed to first coarsely localize regions where vertebrae exist without the need of *a priori* knowledge about the scale, image characteristics and FOV; then accurately recognize vertebrae and automatically correct wrong recognitions by an elaborated self-calibration recognition network that embeds message passing into deep learning network. The method is trained and evaluated on a capacious and challenging dataset of 450 MRI scans, and the evaluation results show that our Hi-scene achieves high performance (testing accuracy reaches 0.933) from arbitrary input spine MRI and outperforms other state-of-the-art methods.

1 Introduction

Automatic vertebrae recognition (*i.e.*, label classification and bounding box localization) from magnetic resonance imaging (MRI) is an essential tool for spine diseases diagnosis, medical and surgical treatment planning, as well as postoperative response assessment [1]. Performing automatic vertebrae recognition accurately and reproducibly is crucial because incorrect recognition is the main cause of wrong-site surgery, which is one of five surgical Never Events in clinical practice [2].

However, as shown in Fig. 1, automatic vertebrae recognition in an arbitrary spine image is challenging because: (1) The field of view (FOV) varies unpredictably in input images, it is impossible to use some specifically-shaped vertebrae such as sacrum to classify the other ones [1]. (2) The MRI image

© Springer Nature Switzerland AG 2019
D. Shen et al. (Eds.): MICCAI 2019, LNCS 11767, pp. 316–325, 2019.
https://doi.org/10.1007/978-3-030-32251-9_35

Challenges of vertebrae detection in MRI images of different field of view (FOV)

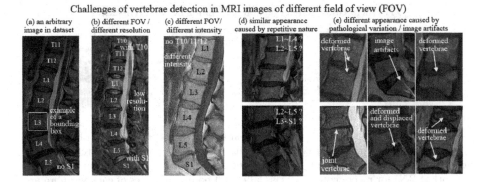

Fig. 1. Challenges of automatic vertebrae recognition in arbitrary spine images (classifying the labels and tight bounding boxes (*i.e..* the white box for L3 in Fig. 1 (a)) of each vertebrae). Figure 1(a–c) show the challenges caused by different field of view (FOV) and image characteristics (resolution, intensity, modality, and scales). Figure 1(d–e) show that the repetitive nature, pathological variation, and/or image artifacts make the problem more challenging.

characteristics (resolution, scales, and image intensity distribution) vary widely [3] and impose difficulty on learning representative features to distinguish vertebrae. (3) The appearances of different vertebrae are similar due to their repetitive nature (Fig. 1(d)); while the pathological variation and/or image artifacts alters the appearance of vertebrae in an unknown manner (Fig. 1(e)) [4,5].

While many methods have been proposed for vertebrae detection and nontrivial progress have been achieved, simultaneously recognizing the labels and bounding boxes of all vertebrae from arbitrary spine images remains a problem. Lootus [4] presents an accurate method using deformable part model, but it needs the sacrum to be present. Glocker [6] uses random forests and probabilistic graphical models to regress vertebrae centroid points using appearance-based features. [7–9] also use other methods such as snakes, multi-task learning and state-space approaches for detection and/or segmentation tasks. These universal methods can be modified to perform vertebrae detection. With the development of deep learning, [1,3,5] use convolutional neural network (CNN) as the basic method and use several advanced techniques (deep supervision, message passing, RNN, pairwise conditional dependency) to enhance the performance and accurately obtain pixel-wise probability maps for each vertebrae centroid. However, directly recognizing the labels and bounding boxes of the vertebrae (rather than the probability map of centroid points) may be more meaningful for clinical use because it reveals their relative sizes and positions; moreover, this strategy mitigates the problem of false positives [3,6].

We propose a two-stage hierarchical self-calibration recognition network (Hiscene) to recognize vertebrae from arbitrary spine MRI. As shown in Fig. 2, we first develop a hierarchical detection network (HDN) to coarsely detect regions containing vertebrae. HDN generates multi-scale anchors and extracts discrimi-

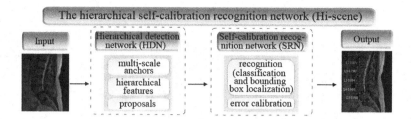

Fig. 2. Overview of Hi-scene, which is a two-stage network containing: (1) Hierarchical detection network (HDN) for coarsely localizing regions containing vertebrae (class-agnostic proposals) of different scales and resolutions. (2) Self-calibration recognition network (SRN) for recognizing the class label and bounding boxes of each vertebra and automatically calibrating the wrong detections using the message passing algorithm.

native hierarchical features to match the scales of different vertebrae, which deals with the multi-scale/resolution challenge. Then, we propose a self-calibration recognition network (SRN) to recognize each vertebra from the coarse detections. SRN creatively formulates message passing algorithm into deep learning network to calibrate the predicted class probabilities and correct the wrong recognitions, which deals with the appearance and FOV challenge.

Our contributions are: (1) We propose an accurate clinical tool to directly recognize vertebrae labels and bounding boxes from arbitrary MRI images. (2) For the first time, we formulate message passing into deep learning object recognition network for performance enhancement, which benefits other object recognition problems where the locations of the target objects have some certain internal spatial relationships.

2   Methodology

Our Hi-scene (Fig. 2) is composed of two stages: (1) The hierarchical detection network (HDN, Sect. 2.1, Fig. 3), which generates multi-scale anchors at different regular locations all over the input image and extracts hierarchical discriminative image features. This design requires no *a priori* knowledge of the input image; it simultaneously predicts the objectness scores and the coarse locations of regions containing vertebrae using the generated multi-scale anchors. (2) The self-calibration recognition network (SRN, Sect. 2.2, Fig. 4), which embeds message passing into multi-task recognition network to recognize vertebrae by predicting the class probabilities and refined bounding boxes based on the coarse locations obtained by HDN. The embedded message passing leverages the label relationship among different vertebrae to effectively calibrate the class probabilities of wrong recognitions caused by FOV variety and/or pathological deformation.

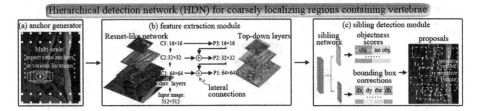

Fig. 3. The hierarchical detection network (HDN). The anchor generator (Fig. 3(a)) places anchors of different scales/aspect ratios at different locations. The feature extraction module (Fig. 3(b)) extracts discriminative features that are robust to resolution change. The sibling detection module (Fig. 3(c)) simultaneously predicts the objectness scores (OS) and bounding box corrections (BBC_1) of each anchor, and then the anchors are refined to multi-scale proposals by BBC_1's. The configuration of anchor scales, feature scales and anchor intervals are elaborately designed to approach multi-scale challenge.

2.1 Hierarchical Detection Network (HDN)

HDN coarsely localizes regions containing vertebrae and handles the scale/ resolution challenge through 3 carefully designed cascade modules:

The anchor generator (Fig. 3(a)) equidistantly samples grid points from the original input image and places boxes of different size and aspect ratio (namely, anchors) centered on the grid points. The sizes (16, 32 and 64 pixels in our work) and aspect ratios (1:1, 1:1.5, 1:2 in our work) are chosen to approximate the sizes and aspect ratios of vertebrae in the input images; and the sampling distance (8 pixels) is decided to ensure that the anchors are dense enough to cover all vertebrae. The elaborated configuration guarantees that vertebrae of all scales/aspect ratios at all possible locations can be detected by a similar-shaped anchor in its vicinity.

The feature extraction module (Fig. 3(b)) adopts a Resnet-like network as feature extractor with two careful designs: (1) The output size of each stage of Resnet (C1~C3 in Fig. 3(b)) is designed to be equal to that of one anchor scale (namely, 64, 32, and 16 for C1, C2, and C3). Redundant layers in the original Resnet [11] are deleted to reduce network parameters and computational cost. (2) Top-down layers are introduced to explicitly combine high- and low-level features. The features P2~P3 are up-sampled and merged with their lower level features using lateral connections [12]. This design preserves the inherent advantages of Resnet (e.g., shortcuts to prevent degradation problem in deeper networks, robustness to the resolution change), while guarantees that features of proper scales are associated with each anchor size.

The sibling detection module (Fig. 3(c)) sends the ablated features P1~P3 into a 3×3 convolutional layer and two sibling 1×1 convolutional layers to predict the objectness scores (probability of each anchor containing vertebra, OS) and first-stage bounding box corrections (BBC_1) of different anchors. Then, as inspired by Faster RCNN [10], the BBC_1's are applied to the anchors to obtain

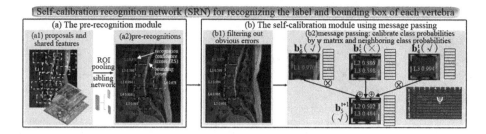

Fig. 4. The self-calibration recognition network (SRN). The pre-recognition module (Fig. 4(a)) classifies the proposals into class-aware labels and refines proposals to bounding boxes. The self-calibration module (Fig. 4(b)) filters out "easy" wrong recognitions and uses message passing to correct "hard" wrong detections. One iteration of message passing is shown in Fig. 4(b2), where the CPV of one pre-recognition ($\mathbf{b_5}^t$ in this figure) receives messages from its neighbors ($\mathbf{b_4}^t$ and $\mathbf{b_6}^t$) via the $\mathbf{\Psi}$ matrix. The messages contain CPV's of all other pre-recognitions and helps adjust the $\mathbf{b_5}^t$ to reach label compatibility. This self-calibration process corrects the recognition errors caused by appearance deformation in arbitrary FOVs. (Color figure online)

coarse detection boxes (called proposals as in [10]). Proposals with high OS are locations where vertebrae probably exist.

2.2   Self-calibration Recognition Network (SRN)

SRN recognizing the label/bounding box of each vertebra and handles the appearance/FOV challenges through two coherently integrated modules:

The pre-recognition module (Fig. 4(a)) adopts ROI-pooling [10] to choose one feature from P3~P1 according to the size of each proposal, then crops and resizes the feature to 32×32. The resized features are fed into a two-siblings network similar to that in HDN to pre-recognize class-aware labels and bounding boxes. This is implemented by predicting the class probability vectors (CPV) and second-stage bounding box corrections (BBC_2) for all classes. For each pre-recognition, the CPV is a vector whose elements are the probabilities of the pre-recognized vertebrae having different labels; the predicted label is the index of CPV's maximum, and the recognition confidence score (RS) is the maximum value (*i.e.*, if the kth element in CPV is maximum, this vertebra is predicted to have label k and its RS is the kth value in CPV). The BBC_2 corresponding to the predicted label is chosen and applied to the proposals to obtain the pre-recognition bounding boxes.

The self-calibration module (Fig. 4(b)) creatively formulates message passing [13] to correct wrong pre-recognitions by calibrating their CPV's. The essence of message passing is that, it adjusts the CPV of an arbitrary pre-recognition using the other CPV's by combining them with a label compatibility matrix $\mathbf{\Psi}$ and absorbing the combination to the target CPV (which will be detailed in Eq. 1); if the index of the maximum in the adjusted CPV alters, the

predicted label will thereupon alter. Thanks to our HDN and pre-recognize network, the majority of our pre-recognitions have acceptable CPV's with correct
labels and high RS values. Thus, the adjustments of the CPV's are in the correct
direction, *i.e.*, the undesired CPV's are calibrated and their maxima are urged
to appear at the correct indices. This calibration is performed in an iterative
manner [13]; we reformulate it into Eq. 1, which shows how an arbitrary CPV
absorbs messages (*i.e.*, combinations of CPV's) from the others:

$$\mathbf{b_i}^{t+1} = \frac{1}{Z}\mathbf{b_i}^t \prod_{j \in v(i)} \mathbf{m_{ji}}, \quad \text{where} \quad \mathbf{m_{ji}} = \sum_{label_j \in \mathcal{L}} \mathbf{b_j}^t \otimes \mathbf{\Psi} \otimes \prod_{k \in v(j) \setminus i} \mathbf{m_{kj}} \quad (1)$$

where: (1) The CPV of the ith pre-recognition ($\mathbf{b_i}^{t+1}$) is iteratively updated by
the product of its previous value ($\mathbf{b_i}^t$) and the message it receives from all its
neighbors $\{j\}$ ($\mathbf{m_{ji}}$); (2) The message from the jth to the ith pre-recognition
($\mathbf{m_{ji}}$) is a combination of the CPV's and the label compatibility matrix by
element wise product ($\otimes$) of: (i) the CPV of the jth pre-recognition ($\mathbf{b_j}^t$), (ii)
each row of the label compatibility matrix ($\mathbf{\Psi}$, a N×N trainable parameter), and
(iii) the message that flow into the jth pre-recognition from its neighbors except
the ith ($\mathbf{m_{kj}}$); (3) The notation $\sum_{label_j \in \mathcal{L}}$ means summing over labels, which
concerns all possible labels of the jth pre-recognition to form a comprehensive
message; (4) Z is a normalization constant to force the CPV's sum to 1.

In our vertebrae recognition work, the ith pre-recognition only neighbors the
$i-1$th and $i+1$th (*i.e.*, the CPV $\mathbf{b_i}^{t+1}$ in Eq. 1 is simplified to $\frac{1}{Z}\mathbf{b_i}^t\mathbf{m_{i-1,i}}\mathbf{m_{i+1,i}}$),
and $\mathbf{m_{i-1,i}}/\mathbf{m_{i+1,i}}$ is only dependent on the $i-2/i+2$th pre-recognition (*e.g.*,
$\mathbf{m_{i-1,i}} = \sum_{label_{i-1} \in \mathcal{L}} \mathbf{b_{i-1}}^t \otimes \mathbf{\Psi} \otimes \mathbf{m_{i-2,i-1}}$). Thus, by substituting the expression
of message $\mathbf{m}$ in turn, the CPV's of all pre-recognized vertebrae are combined
by the $\mathbf{\Psi}$ matrix and absorbed into $\mathbf{b_i}^{t+1}$, which means all other CPV's are used
to calibrate the ith CPV. After all CPV's exchange their messages and the iter-
ation reaches stability, the cross entropy loss ($\text{loss}_{mp} = -\sum_{i=1}^{N_o}\sum_{j=1}^{N} \mathbf{y_i}\text{ln}\mathbf{b_i}(j)$,
$\mathbf{y_i}$ is the one-hot ground truth label of the ith vertebrae) is calculated and mini-
mized together with the classification and localization loss of the pre-recognition
network to train SRN.

Our SRN reinforces mutual benefit of the pre-recognition network and the
message passing scheme. During training, the training label accuracy is very
high (near 100%) when the pre-recognition network (and also the HDN) reaches
stability, which provides reliable CPV's to train the $\mathbf{\Psi}$ matrix. There are no false
positives or wrong predictions to perturb the training. During testing, we first
filter out the "easy" false positives (*e.g.* those at wrong positions, as demonstrated by the yellow box in Fig. 4(a2)) using the predicted x coordinate. If the
predicted x coordinate of a vertebra is inappropriate, i.e., the deviations of the
x coordinates of one vertebra to those of its neighboring vertebrae are larger
than some threshold (one vertebrae width in our work), this pre-recognition is
judged as false positive. This procedure rejects the "easy" false positives, leav-
ing only the "hard" wrong pre-recognitions with approximately correct positions
but wrong labels (*e.g.*, the upper green box with label L3 in Fig. 4(a2)) to be

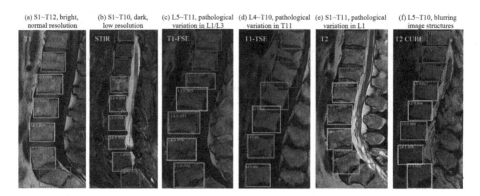

Fig. 5. The Hi-scene network achieves high vertebrae detection performance on a challenging dataset of different FOV, image characteristics and modalities. The dotted boxes are the detection boxes with confidence scores, and the solid boxes are ground truth boxes.

fed into the message passing scheme. Then, the wrong labels can be corrected by calibrating the CPV's using Eq. 1 (Fig. 4(b2)). Moreover, since BBC_2's are predicted for each class, the bounding boxes can be automatically refined by choosing the BBC_2 of the correct class.

3   Experiments and Results

Hi-scene has been intensively evaluated using a challenging dataset including 450 arbitrary MRI images of different image characteristics (such as vertebrae appearance, image resolution, intensity distribution) and FOV (containing S1~T12, S1~T11, S1~T10, L5~T11, L5~T10, L4~T10, each FOV has ~75 images). 2D slices (not necessarily the mid-sagittal slices) of each 3D MRI scan are automatically extracted and resized to 512×512. Hi-scene is implemented in Python 3.6 on Tensorflow 1.2 and trained using momentum optimizer with exponential learning rate decay. The initial learning rate is 1e–3, the decay factor is 0.96 per 10 epochs, and the learning momentum is 0.9. The training is implemented on an NVIDIA GTX1080 GPU for 20000 steps (~111 epochs). We use standard five-fold cross-validation for evaluation. The number of images of each FOV is kept approximately the same in the training/testing dataset in each fold. The five results from the folds are averaged to produce a single result. Four metrics are used to evaluate the detection performance: (1) Image accuracy, which means the ratio $\frac{correctly\ recognized\ images}{all\ images}$. This is a rather strict metric because an image is considered as correctly recognized only if all vertebrae in the image are correctly recognized. (2) Identification rate (IDR), which measures the accuracy of individual vertebra classification [3]. (3) mAP_{75}, which measures the mean AP (*average precision*) at IoU (*intersection over union*) threshold 0.75 for all images. This metric is detailed in [14] and is extensively used in object detection domain [10]; (4) mIoU, which is the average IoU of the detection and ground truth bounding boxes of all vertebrae in all images.

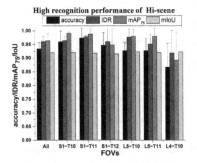

Fig. 6. Four evaluation metrics indicate that Hi-scene can accurately classify and localize vertebrae in images of different FOVs, image characteristics, and vertebrae appearances. (Color figure online)

Qualitative Demonstration. Figure 5 demonstrates that Hi-scene network achieves high vertebrae classification accuracy and bounding box localization precision. The detected boxes (dashed) have correct labels and high overlaps with their ground truth boxes (solid) despite the varied FOV and vertebrae appearance (for example, Fig. 5(c) and (d) both have 8 vertebrae, but their FOVs and vertebrae appearances are different) in arbitrary images.

Quantitative Analysis. As shown in Fig. 6, the average image accuracy reaches 0.933 (the first black bar), which means that all the vertebrae are correctly recognized in 93.3% of the input images without false positive/negatives. Image accuracies are high (the other six black bars) for individual FOV's; even the most difficult FOV (L4~T10, which tends to be confused with FOV L5~T11) has high accuracy (0.867). The mean IDR reaches 0.96 and shows high classification performance for individual vertebra. The mean mAP_{75}'s (the first blue bar) reaches 0.964, which shows that the recognition network has high precision at high recalls [14]. The mean mIoU (the first pink bar) reaches 0.919, which means the recognized bounding boxes have high overlaps with the ground truths. These indicate that our Hi-scene successfully approaches the challenge of vertebrae recognition from arbitrary spine MRI.

Comparison with the State-of-the-Art. Our approach is compared with three other methods in [1,3,10]. Since only [10] has published their code, we make our best effort to re-implement [3] and a 2D version of [1] and adjust their hyper-parameters for better performance. The re-implementation of [3] reaches the reported IDR using our dataset. However, probably because we lack the implementation details of their strategy (using cropped images to train CNN and then converting the CNN into FCN to process the whole image), the re-implementation of [1] does not reach the reported IDR. Quite some false positives occurs in the FCN results, which are not easy to distinguish and harm the successive training/inference of the LSTM. For comparison, as shown in Table 1, Hi-scene outperforms both the state-of-the-art methods and our baseline methods without message passing in all four metrics used in Fig. 6 as well as the localization error (Loc-Err). Particularly, the image accuracy of our method is significantly higher because only the minority of vertebrae are incorrect in most wrongly recognized images, which can be effectively corrected by message passing. Another interesting result is that although [3] and our work both use message passing, our work has a better performance because our HDN

Table 1. Comparison with the state-of-the-art. MP is the abbreviation of message passing.

Method	Loc-Err (pixel)	Image accuracy	IDR	mAP_{75}	mIoU
Our method	5.199 ± 3.063	0.933 ± 0.124	0.963 ± 0.036	0.964 ± 0.025	0.919 ± 0.036
Baseline method without MP	6.136 ± 4.108	0.844 ± 0.168	0.912 ± 0.068	0.866 ± 0.085	0.874 ± 0.155
FCN-LSTM [1]	7.923 ± 4.788	0.727 ± 0.231	0.816 ± 0.188	–	–
DI2IN [3]	6.891 ± 5.056	0.835 ± 0.183	0.904 ± 0.179	–	–
Faster-RCNN [10]	7.124 ± 3.259	0.831 ± 0.106	0.884 ± 0.098	0.829 ± 0.130	0.844 ± 0.162

and pre-recognition network in SRN successfully handles images of arbitrary scales/characteristics/FOVs; the pre-recognized vertebrae are more precise and contains less false positives compared with the predicted pixel-wise probability maps for vertebrae centroid, which gives play to the message passing algorithm to pass the correct probabilities for better CPV calibration performance.

4   Conclusion

In this paper, we develop Hierarchical Self-calibration Detection Framework to recognize vertebrae in arbitrary spine MRI images. It consists of two novel networks: a hierarchical detection network for detecting multi-scale/resolution regions containing vertebrae; and a self-calibration recognition network for recognizing the label and bounding box of each vertebra and automatically correcting wrong recognitions caused by FOV variety and pathological deformations. Its performance and effectiveness are demonstrated by extensive experiments.

References

1. Liao, H., Mesfin, A., Luo, J.: Joint vertebrae identification and localization in spinal CT images by combining short-and long-range contextual information. IEEE Trans. Med. Imaging **37**(5), 1266–1275 (2018)
2. Philip, F.: Patient Safety in Surgery. Springer, London (2014). https://doi.org/10.1007/978-1-4471-4369-7
3. Yang, D., et al.: Automatic vertebra labeling in large-scale 3D CT using deep image-to-image network with message passing and sparsity regularization. In: Niethammer, M., et al. (eds.) IPMI 2017. LNCS, vol. 10265, pp. 633–644. Springer, Cham (2017). https://doi.org/10.1007/978-3-319-59050-9_50
4. Lootus, M., Kadir, T., Zisserman, A.: Vertebrae detection and labelling in lumbar MR images. In: Yao, J., Klinder, T., Li, S. (eds.) Computational Methods and Clinical Applications for Spine Imaging. LNCVB, vol. 17, pp. 219–230. Springer, Cham (2014). https://doi.org/10.1007/978-3-319-07269-2_19
5. Chen, H., et al.: Automatic localization and identification of vertebrae in spine CT via a joint learning model with deep neural networks. In: Navab, N., Hornegger, J., Wells, W.M., Frangi, A.F. (eds.) MICCAI 2015. LNCS, vol. 9349, pp. 515–522. Springer, Cham (2015). https://doi.org/10.1007/978-3-319-24553-9_63

6. Glocker, B., Zikic, D., Konukoglu, E., Haynor, D.R., Criminisi, A.: Vertebrae localization in pathological spine CT via dense classification from sparse annotations. In: Mori, K., Sakuma, I., Sato, Y., Barillot, C., Navab, N. (eds.) MICCAI 2013. LNCS, vol. 8150, pp. 262–270. Springer, Heidelberg (2013). https://doi.org/10.1007/978-3-642-40763-5_33

7. Zhao, S., et al.: Robust segmentation of intima-media borders with different morphologies and dynamics during the cardiac cycle. IEEE J. Biomed. Health **22**(5), 1571–1582 (2018)

8. Zhao, R., Liao, W., Zou, B., Chen, Z., Li, S.: Weakly-supervised simultaneous evidence identification and segmentation for automated glaucoma diagnosis. In: AAAI (2019)

9. Gao, Z., et al.: Robust estimation of carotid artery wall motion using the elasticity-based state-space approach. Med. Image Anal. **37**, 1–21 (2017)

10. Ren, S., He, K., Girshick, R., Sun, J.: Faster R-CNN: towards real-time object detection with region proposal networks. In: NIPS, pp. 1–14 (2015)

11. He, K., Zhang, X., Ren, S., Sun, J.: Deep residual learning for image recognition. In: CVPR, pp. 770–778 (2016)

12. Lin, T., Dollar, P., Girshick, R., He, K., Hariharan, B., Belon, S.: Feature pyramid networks for object detection. In: CVPR, pp. 2117–2125 (2017)

13. Yedidia, J., Freeman, W., Weiss, Y.: Understanding belief propagation and its generalizations. Exploring Artif. Intell. New Millennium **8**, 236–239 (2003)

14. Everingham, M., Van, G., Williams, C., Winn, J., Zisserman, A.: The pascal visual object classes (VOC) challenge. Int. J. Comput. Vis. **88**(2), 303–338 (2010)

Machine Learning

Image Data Validation for Medical Systems

Pablo Márquez-Neila$^{(\boxtimes)}$ and Raphael Sznitman

ARTORG Center for Biomedical Engineering Research, University of Bern, Bern,
Switzerland
{pablo.marquez,raphael.sznitman}@artorg.unibe.ch

Abstract. Data validation is the process of ensuring that the input to
a data processing pipeline is correct and useful. It is a critical part of
software systems running in production. Image processing systems are
no different, whereby problems with data acquisition, file corruption or
data transmission, may lead to a wide range of unexpected issues in
the acquired images. Until now, most image processing systems of this
type involved a human in the loop that could detect these errors before
further processing. With the advent of powerful deep learning methods,
tools for medical image processing are becoming increasingly autonomous
and can go from data acquisition to final medical diagnosis without any
human interaction. However, deep networks are known for their inability
to detect corruption or errors in the input data. To overcome this, we
present a validation method that learns the appearance of images in the
training dataset that was used to train the deep network, and is able
to identify when an input image deviates from the training distribution
and therefore cannot be safely analyzed. We experimentally assess the
validity of our method and compare it with different baselines, reaching
an improvement of more than 10% points on all considered datasets.

1   Introduction

Over the last decade, the number of medical image scans acquired has steadily
grown and represents today over 90% of all medical data in hospitals worldwide [13]. Driven by widespread access to imaging devices, automated methods
dedicated to processing medical scans are becoming increasingly critical to cope
with the scale of images produced. Naturally, machine and deep learning play
key roles in filling this need. At the same time, it is well known that deep networks have very limited extrapolation capacities and that properly trained deep
networks behave unpredictably when presented with images that lie outside of
their training data distribution. Given that acquisition devices, data transmission systems and other softwares can all fail in unexpected ways and lead to

Electronic supplementary material The online version of this chapter (https://
doi.org/10.1007/978-3-030-32251-9_36) contains supplementary material, which is
available to authorized users.

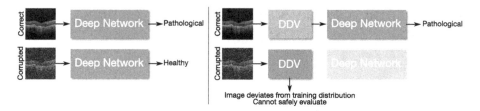

Fig. 1. Left: An automatic diagnosis method with no validation. The deep network correctly classifies a proper image as *pathological*. However, the presence of corruption—noise in this case—leads to an erroneous *healthy* prediction with potentially dangerous consequences for the patient. **Right:** Our DDV model learns the data distribution the network was trained on, and prevents any diagnosis when it detects an image outside the distribution.

corrupted images, any automatic medical diagnosis from such images should be prevented in fear of providing inaccurate results, if not, dangerously misleading ones (see Fig. 1). The fundamental problem however is that we typically do not know beforehand how and when a device will produce corrupted images.

To this end, we introduce a *deep data validation* (DDV) framework for images typically acquired by medical devices. We propose that every deep network, trained in a supervised manner for a dedicated medical task, be augmented with a DDV model that explicitly learns the training data distribution and rejects images that do not belong to it at test time. Be it for differential diagnosis or segmentation methods, each test time image should be validated with a DDV model first and only then analyzed by the intended method if approved by the DDV. If however the DDV detects a corrupted image, then the DDV interrupts the analysis and raises the attention of a human operator for further inspection.

As such, the contributions of this work are (1) introducing the concept of data validation for high resolution medical images, (2) proposing a non-parametric solution that is easy to train, stable and fast at test time, and (3) experimentally assessing the performance of our method and showing that it outperforms all baselines by a large margin in three different medical datasets.

Related Work: Despite its importance, the problem of image data validation has been overlooked in the medical imaging community. On the other hand, a great deal of research has focused on image quality control and assessment [9,15]. These methods focus on measuring the perceptual image quality to detect problems such as noise, compression artifacts or lens distortion. However, quality assessment methods are oblivious to the fact that modern analysis systems are trained with datasets of images and that perceptually correct images may still lead to misleading predictions when they do not belong to the training distribution.

Methods on anomaly detection have mainly focused on identifying abnormal or pathological structures using statistical shape analysis [8], clustering [7] and one-class learning [2]. However in this work, we are interested in validating incoming images meant to be processed by a method for which we know nothing except the data on which it was trained on. As such, our problem is much broader.

Perhaps the closest work to the one presented here is the one-class deep learning method presented in [12], where a neural network learns a low-dimensional ball to model the data and rejects outliers that fall outside of this ball. Autoencoders also allow data distributions to be learned, but typically only do so well for small images or patches, making them ill-suited for large medical images as considered here. Generative models, such as GANs or flow-based methods [3,6], do learn distributions of high-resolution images and seem appropriate to detect image corruption. However, we found and show in our experiments that they in fact perform poorly on this task.

2   Method

Problem Formulation: In this work, we assume that a task-specific algorithm has been trained with a dataset $\mathcal{X} = \{\mathbf{x}^{(i)}\}_{i=1}^N$, where $\mathbf{x} \in \mathcal{I}$ are images. For example, this may be a segmentation method tasked to outline brain tumors in MRIs and trained on a large dataset of examples. Given this, our aim is to learn a function that can identify *corrupted* images at test time, with the objective of stopping any subsequent method from processing them.

In particular, we would like to train a discriminative model, *e.g.*, a deep network, to learn the probability that a given input image is corrupted. Training such a model would be easy if we could acquire examples from the distribution of corrupted and valid images, $\mathcal{D}^+$ and $\mathcal{D}^-$, respectively. Unfortunately, the distribution of corrupted images $\mathcal{D}^+$ is extremely complex, containing modified versions of images in $\mathcal{D}^-$ with wide ranges of possible corruptions (*e.g.*, noise, occlusions, missing pixels, different zoom, alignment problems), as well as images that are completely unrelated to $\mathcal{D}^-$. For instance, if $\mathcal{D}^-$ is the distribution of chest X-rays, elements in D^+ would also include CT scans, MRIs and other real world photographs. In a sense, $\mathcal{D}^+$ is the complementary distribution of $\mathcal{D}^-$ in the space of all possible images. Therefore, the idea of obtaining a representative set of samples from $\mathcal{D}^+$ is simply hopeless.

To overcome this, we frame our problem in the context of one-class learning, where we assume that $\mathcal{X}$ is representative of the distribution of valid images $\mathcal{D}^-$. Our aim then is to learn a metric that measures the corruption level of a given image.

One approach would be to estimate the distribution $p(\mathbf{x})$ of $\mathcal{D}^-$ in the image space $\mathcal{I}$ itself. However, because medical images are typically of high dimension (*e.g.*, 1000×1000 pixels for a chest X-ray), doing so is difficult in practice. Taking this into consideration, our approach instead is to learn a projection from $\mathcal{I}$ to a manageable lower-dimensional latent space using a deep network, $f : \mathcal{I} \to \mathbb{R}^d$. In this projected space, we now define the likelihood $p(\mathbf{z})$, where $\mathbf{z} = f(\mathbf{x})$ corresponds to the latent vector of a valid image. Since we cannot assume any specific distribution of the data in the latent space, we use a kernel density estimation,

$$p(\mathbf{z}) = \frac{1}{N} \sum_{\mathbf{x}^{(j)} \in \mathcal{X}} K_h\left(\mathbf{z} - f(\mathbf{x}^{(j)})\right), \tag{1}$$

where $K_h(\mathbf{z}) \propto e^{-\frac{\|\mathbf{z}\|^2}{2h^2}}$ is the Gaussian kernel with bandwidth $h \in \mathbb{R}^+$. For simplicity of notation, we assume that $\int_{\mathbb{R}^d} K_h(\mathbf{z})d\mathbf{z} = 1$. As such, we represent our valid latent data distribution using a non-parametric representation.

Training: To train our DDV, we maximize the log-likelihood of the latent vectors of $\mathcal{X}$,

$$\arg\max_f \log \prod_{\mathbf{x}^{(i)} \in \mathcal{X}} p\left(f(\mathbf{x}^{(i)})\right), \tag{2}$$

which is done using standard stochastic-gradient-based methods with minibatches. However, solving Eq. (2) is computationally involved because the network f is used twice: once to define the density p and once to compute the image latent vectors from the minibatches,

$$\arg\max_f \sum_{\mathbf{x}^{(i)} \in \mathcal{X}} \log \sum_{\mathbf{x}^{(j)} \in \mathcal{X}} K_h\left(f(\mathbf{x}^{(i)}) - f(\mathbf{x}^{(j)})\right) - N \log N. \tag{3}$$

Hence optimizing over both f at the same time may lead to instability issues, as we are updating f to find the modes of the distribution p and simultaneously updating the distribution p. To avoid such instabilities, we freeze p by keeping a constant copy of the network, $\bar{f}$, which is updated $\bar{f} \leftarrow f$ at every epoch during training. This idea not only leads to more stable training, but also allows us to build acceleration structures, such as kd-trees, to efficiently compute the density p when the training dataset $\mathcal{X}$ is very large. Algorithm 1 summarizes our training procedure. This method performs iterative mode finding by moving the descriptor vectors $f(\mathbf{x})$ towards the closest modes. Unless the original distribution is unimodal, this method converges to a multimodal distribution, thus avoiding a degenerate convergence to a single point.

Algorithm 1. DDV training procedure. The operator $\leftarrow\!\!\!/$ indicates a detached assignment that disables gradient computation by blocking back-propagation through it.

Input: Training dataset $\mathcal{X}$, network f with parameters $\mathbf{w}$, optimizer $\mathcal{O}$, max_epochs
Output: Trained network f
    for epoch $\leftarrow 1$ **to** max_epochs **do**
        Create a frozen copy of the network: $\bar{f} \leftarrow\!\!\!/ f$
        Compute the latent vectors of training dataset: $\mathcal{Z} \leftarrow \{\bar{f}(\mathbf{x}^{(j)}) : \mathbf{x}^{(j)} \in \mathcal{X}\}$
        (Optional) Build a kd-tree with $\mathcal{Z}$ for efficient computation of p
        for all $\mathcal{M} \in$ minibatches of $\mathcal{X}$ **do**
            Compute log-likelihood of the minibatch: $\ell \leftarrow \sum_{\mathbf{x}^{(i)} \in \mathcal{M}} \log p(f(\mathbf{x}^{(i)}))$
            Back-propagate gradients: $\nabla_{\mathbf{w}} \ell$
            Update weights: $\mathbf{w} \leftarrow \mathcal{O}.\text{step}(\mathbf{w}, -\nabla_{\mathbf{w}} \ell)$
        end for
    end for

Test Time: To evaluate a new image at test time, we use the negative log-likelihood of the latent representation, $s(\mathbf{x}) = -\log p\left(f(\mathbf{x})\right)$, as the metric to measure the corruption level of the input image $\mathbf{x}$.

3   Experiments and Results

We now describe our experimental setup, as well as the datasets and the baselines used to evaluate our method. In particular, given that we do not have access to datasets of corrupted images, we validate our approach using synthetically corrupted images from the following datasets:

Retinal OCT: A collection of 1'201 retinal Optical Coherence Tomography (OCT) volumes obtained using a Heidelberg Spectralis device. Each volume consists of 49 slices for a total of 58'849 training images. For validation, we randomly sample images from a different collection of OCT scans that we use to build a testing dataset (see below).

ChestX-Ray8 [14]: Collection of 112'120 frontal-view X-ray images of 32'717 unique patients. We used the provided split of 85'524 images for training, and the remaining images are used to build the testing dataset.

BraTS 2017 [1,10]: Dataset of 750 multimodal MRI scans of the brain. Each scan consists of 155 slices from 4 modalities (FLAIR, t1gd, T1w and T2w) totaling $4{\times}116'250$ images. We trained our model with 484 t1gd scans (75'020 images). The remaining 266 scans are used to build the testing dataset.

Generating Corrupted Images: To evaluate the performance of our method and of the baselines, we build testing datasets by synthetically corrupting images from the test splits. We consider a wide range of possible corruptions working at different image levels. Some types of corruption (*e.g.*, additive noise, blurring) affect the local statistics of the image but keep the overall appearance unchanged. Other types (*e.g.*, rotation, random offset) preserve the local image statistics, but affect image-level statistics. Table 2 shows a few examples.

Baselines: We evaluate the following methods:

Ours: Our method as explained in Sect. 2. For the deep network f, we use a ResNet-50 architecture [4] initialized with pre-trained weights. The final layer is modified to provide d outputs and is randomly initialized. We train the network end-to-end using Adam [5] with a learning rate of 10^{-4} and no weight decay. The dimension of the latent space is set to $d = 16$ and the bandwidth of the Gaussian kernel, $h = 10^{-2}$.

SVDD [12]: A deep learning one-class learning method. For fair comparison, we use the same architecture, initialization procedure and image preprocessing as for **Ours**. Following [12], we remove the bias term of the final layer and train the network with weight decay 10^{-6}. We set the dimension of the latent space to $d = 16$.

Table 1. Experimental results. For **SVDD** and **Ours** values are averaged over 10 seeds with standard deviations in parenthesis.

		Retinal OCT	ChestX-Ray8	BraTS 2017
Ours $(d = 16, h = 10^{-2})$	AP	**96.17(0.73)**	**85.58(3.63)**	**98.93(0.16)**
	AUC	**96.31(0.65)**	**82.38(4.6)**	**98.43(0.3)**
SVDD $(d = 16)$	AP	83.35(7.87)	75.93(9.09)	95.43(0.98)
	AUC	77.38(10.56)	66.63(11.77)	92.1(1.9)
Glow $(K = 8, L = 5)$	AP	57.13	70.8	90.14
	AUC	44.83	54.62	85.73
Glow $(K = 32, L = 3)$	AP	55.70	70.19	88.27
	AUC	41.79	53.56	83.30

Glow [6]: A flow-based generative method that estimates the log-likelihood of data in the high-dimensional image space. We use the predicted negative log-likelihood as the measurement of corruption at test time. We use two different architectures with a depth of $K \in \{8, 32\}$ and $L \in \{5, 3\}$ levels. See [6] for details.

Results: We report the average precision (AP) and the area under the ROC curve (AUC) for all methods and datasets in Table 1. Our method outperforms all baselines by significant margins. Compared to **SVDD**, our method is not only superior but also more robust to initial conditions, as can be inferred from the standard deviations. Poor performance of **SVDD** may be explained by the relatively strong assumptions made about the distribution of the data, *i.e.*, the fact that the data falls in a ball in the latent space. To assess that this difference in performance is not due to the specific choice of hyperparemeters, we ran a grid search over the latent dimension d of both methods and the bandwidth h for **Ours**. Figure 2(left) shows the results. Our method is superior to **SVDD** for almost any combination of hyperparameters. The performance of **Ours** is high for a large range of d and h values, with a drop in performance only for extreme values $d = 2$ or $h = 10$. This stability over hyperparameters is a very desirable attribute in the problem of corruption detection, as a validation dataset is typically not available to perform proper model selection.

   Glow has a surprisingly low performance. According to our experience, this is the case with all generative models we tested, including autoencoders and GANs. While generative models are able to approximate the training data distribution, the high dimensionality of the latent space makes it possible to represent corrupted images with high-likelihood latent vectors. The probability of randomly sampling one of these invalid latent vectors is extremely low in practice, which makes generative models suitable to generate images of correct appearance but not to detect corruption of existing images. Furthermore, generative models commonly cannot capture the multimodal nature of the training data (in its most severe form, this problem is known as *mode collapse*). As a consequence, some correct images get low likelihood and are considered corrupted. Similar conclusions have been reported in [11].

For a more realistic analysis, we examine the performance of the medical diagnosis system of Fig. 1 under three different conditions: no image validation, validation using **SVDD** and validation with our method. The diagnosis method we consider here is tasked to detect the presence of fluid in retinal OCT scans. We train a ResNet-50 using a dataset of 51'401 OCT scans manually labeled as *fluid* or *no fluid* according to whether or not there is retinal fluid present in them. We also train our DDV model and **SVDD** with the same training images. To characterize the impact of our framework on this diagnosis task, we use a different set of 7'448 labeled images for testing and use additive Gaussian noise (with parameter σ) to corrupt images as it is common in OCT devices. We then measure the performance of the fluid classifier (*fluid* being the positive class) when we increase $\sigma = 0$ (no noise) to $\sigma = 60$.

Figure 2(right) shows the evolution of the AP as a function of the noise level σ for the three cases considered. To compute the performance, we assume that when an image is rejected by a data validation method, the device operator manages to fix the acquisition device and repeats the acquisition such that noise is no longer present. With no validation, the performance drops from 87.98% (no corruption) to 47.54% for $\sigma = 60$ (blue line). Our approach (orange line) detects far more corruptions than **SVDD** (green line), reaching a minimum performance of 76.13%. For $\sigma = 40$, DDV rejects 92.9% of the corrupted test data compared to 43.89% for **SVDD**. Figure 2(bottom) shows a few qualitative examples of accepted and rejected cases by our approach. Examples (a-d) are

Table 2. Classes of corruption in the testing datasets. Percentages indicate the proportion of elements with the corresponding corruption categories. The last three columns show example images.

Corruption class	Percentage	**Retinal OCT**	**ChestX-Ray8**	**BraTS 2017**
No corruption	50%			
Additive noise	4%			
Random offset	4%			
Misalignment	3%			
Different modality	5%			
Others	34%	**See supplementary material**		

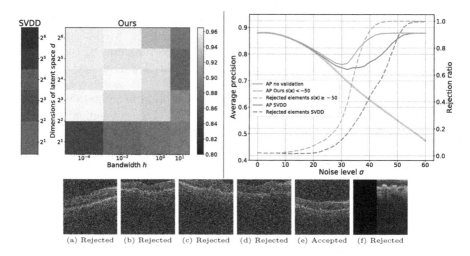

Fig. 2. Left: Average precision (AP) of **Ours** and **SVDD** with different hyperparameters on the **Retinal OCT** dataset. Values are averaged over 5 seeds. **Right:** Evolution of AP in the detection of retinal fluid vs. noise level σ using the medical system of Fig. 1. We also report the ratio of rejected elements at every σ. **Bottom:** Qualitative examples of accepted and rejected images using our method. See text for details. (Color figure online)

correctly rejected with $\sigma = 40$. The example (a) is a *no fluid* case predicted as *fluid* due to the noise. Similarly, examples (b) and (c) are *fluid* cases predicted as *no fluid*, meaning a misclassified pathology when no validation is present. The example (e) is also a misclassified pathology $\sigma = 40$, but wrongly accepted by our approach (a false negative). Finally, the example (f) is an image from the test dataset with no added noise ($\sigma = 0$) that was rejected. This image was supposed to be a false positive but upon inspection, we found that it was indeed a damaged image in our test set that we were not aware of.

4   Conclusion

We have presented a deep validation method that learns to estimate the corruption level of an image without needing to build a dataset of corrupted images. We have shown that our approach performs significantly better than state-of-the-art methods for one-class learning on a variety of datasets, and could potentially be used as a safety mechanism for medical imaging devices that automatically assess images using machine learning methods.

Acknowledgments. This work received partial financial support from the Innosuisse Grant #6362.1 PFLS-LS.

References

1. Bakas, S., et al.: Advancing the cancer genome atlas glioma MRI collections with expert segmentation labels and radiomic features. Sci. Data **4**, 170117 (2017)
2. Désir, C., Bernard, S., Petitjean, C., Heutte, L.: A random forest based approach for one class classification in medical imaging. In: Machine Learning in Medical Imaging, pp. 250–257 (2012)
3. Dinh, L., Sohl-Dickstein, J., Bengio, S.: Density estimation using Real NVP. In: International Conference on Learning Representations (2017)
4. He, K., Zhang, X., Ren, S., Sun, J.: Deep residual learning for image recognition. In: Computer Vision and Pattern Recognition, pp. 770–778 (2016)
5. Kingma, D.P., Ba, J.: Adam: a method for stochastic optimization. In: International Conference on Learning Representations (2014)
6. Kingma, D.P., Dhariwal, P.: Glow: generative flow with invertible 1x1 convolutions. In: Conference on Neural Information Processing Systems, pp. 10215–10224 (2018)
7. Lakovidis, D.K., Georgakopoulos, S.V., Vasilakakis, M., Koulaouzidis, A., Plagianakos, V.P.: Detecting and locating gastrointestinal anomalies using deep learning and iterative cluster unification. IEEE Trans. Med. Imaging **37**(10), 2196–2210 (2018)
8. Lekadir, K., Merrifield, R., Yang, G.: Outlier detection and handling for robust 3-D active shape models search. IEEE Trans. Med. Imaging **26**(2), 212–222 (2007)
9. Liu, Z., et al.: Quality control of diffusion weighted images. Soc. Photo Opt. Instrum. Eng. textbf7628 (2010). https://doi.org/10.1117/12.844748
10. Menze, B.H., et al.: The multimodal brain tumor image segmentation benchmark (BraTS). IEEE Trans. Med. Imaging **34**(10), 1993–2024 (2015)
11. Nalisnick, E., Matsukawa, A., Whye Teh, Y., Gorur, D., Lakshminarayanan, B.: Do deep generative models know what they don't know? In: International Conference on Learning Representations (2019)
12. Ruff, L., et al.: Deep one-class classification. In: International Conference on Machine Learning, vol. 80, pp. 4393–4402 (2018)
13. Stanford University: Stanford Medicine 2018 Health Trends Report (2018)
14. Wang, X., Peng, Y., Lu, L., Lu, Z., Bagheri, M., Summers, R.M.: ChestX-Ray8: hospital-scale chest X-ray database and benchmarks on weakly-supervised classification and localization of common thorax diseases. In: Computer Vision and Pattern Recognition (2017)
15. Woodard, J.P., Carley-Spencer, M.P.: No-reference image quality metrics for structural MRI. Neuroinformatics **4**(3), 243–262 (2006). https://doi.org/10.1385/NI:4: 3:243

Captioning Ultrasound Images Automatically

Mohammad Alsharid[1(✉)], Harshita Sharma[1], Lior Drukker[2], Pierre Chatelain[1],
Aris T. Papageorghiou[2], and J. Alison Noble[1]

[1] Institute of Biomedical Engineering, University of Oxford, Oxford, UK
`mohammad.alsharid@eng.ox.ac.uk`
[2] Nuffield Department of Women's and Reproductive Health, University of Oxford,
Oxford, UK

Abstract. We describe an automatic natural language processing
(NLP)-based image captioning method to describe fetal ultrasound video
content by modelling the vocabulary commonly used by sonographers
and sonologists. The generated captions are similar to the words spoken by a sonographer when describing the scan experience in terms of
visual content and performed scanning actions. Using full-length second-
trimester fetal ultrasound videos and text derived from accompanying
expert voice-over audio recordings, we train deep learning models consisting of convolutional neural networks and recurrent neural networks in
merged configurations to generate captions for ultrasound video frames.
We evaluate different model architectures using established general metrics (*BLEU, ROUGE-L*) and application-specific metrics. Results show
that the proposed models can learn joint representations of image and
text to generate relevant and descriptive captions for anatomies, such as
the spine, the abdomen, the heart, and the head, in clinical fetal ultrasound scans.

Keywords: Image description · Image captioning · Deep learning ·
Natural language processing · Recurrent neural networks · Fetal
ultrasound

1 Introduction

Automatic image captioning combines computer vision with natural language
processing to generate a textual statement, called a caption, to represent image
content. Image captioning has been widely explored for natural images with
benchmark datasets [1], however, most established image-captioning datasets do
not include medical images. Preparing medical image captioning benchmarks is

Electronic supplementary material The online version of this chapter (https://
doi.org/10.1007/978-3-030-32251-9_37) contains supplementary material, which is
available to authorized users.

© Springer Nature Switzerland AG 2019
D. Shen et al. (Eds.): MICCAI 2019, LNCS 11767, pp. 338–346, 2019.
https://doi.org/10.1007/978-3-030-32251-9_37

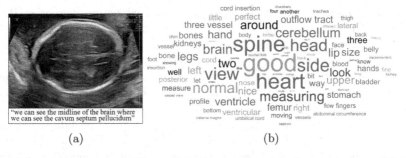

Fig. 1. (a) Example of a fetal ultrasound image with sonographer description. (b) Word cloud of most frequently occurring words in sonographer vocabulary. Red, green, and blue represent nouns, adjectives, and verbs, respectively. The size of a word in the word cloud is proportional to its frequency of use. (Color figure online)

challenging for two reasons: (a) describing medical images with specific terminology requires expert knowledge of medical professionals; and (b) the sensitive nature of medical images prevents wide-scale annotation, for instance, using crowd-sourcing services. Therefore, automatic image captioning has not been widely studied on ultrasound images before, the challenge being enhanced by the lack of readily available large datasets of ultrasound images with captions. To the best of our knowledge, this is the first attempt to perform automatic image captioning on fetal ultrasound video frames, using sonographer spoken words to describe their scanning experience.

As part of routine care, pregnant women are offered a detailed fetal anomaly ultrasound scan at approximately 20 weeks of gestation to identify any fetal malformations. While developing an ultrasound image-captioning model, we can analyse the vocabulary used by sonographers to describe the scans, reflecting their experience during the scan process in terms of visual content and performed scanning actions. The aim of our work is to learn joint image-text representations to describe ultrasound images with rich vocabulary consisting of nouns, verbs, and adjectives. The current work is application agnostic, but a potential application of the work is its use as an educational tool that communicates descriptions of anatomical views of interest to the subjects and sonography trainees. An example of an image and its caption is shown in Fig. 1a. The word cloud in Fig. 1b shows the most common spoken sonographer words used to describe fetal ultrasound scans in our work.

Related Work. There are currently two established ways to perform image captioning [1,20]: (a) text retrieval where descriptions are stored beforehand and retrieved using scores between stored and queried images [15]; and (b) text generation where novel text descriptions are generated. The latter is achieved using top-down or bottom-up approaches [23]. In the top-down approach, an image is described by translating visual representations to text, and in the bottom-up approach, constituent objects and concepts in an image are described with words that are then combined into sentences using language models [4]. In both cases, convolutional neural networks (CNNs) and recurrent neural networks (RNNs) are built from the images and text, respectively [20,22]. We are aware of only two previous ultrasound image captioning works [12,24]. In [12], captions are generated for the ImageCLEF dataset including other radiology images, which also uses a top down deep-learning based text generation approach. In our work, a reduced complexity is achieved using a merged configuration in which image feature vectors are not included as part of the input sequence to the recurrent network. In [24], the image captioning task is performed on adult abdominal ultrasound with a focus on diseases of the kidney and the gallbladder, where a structure and an associated disease are classified before generating a description with an RNN trained specifically on words of that structure. In contrast, we propose models where representations are jointly learned in a single step. Both [12] and [24] use text reports as a raw source of data. We use sonographer voice-over recordings to describe the videos in real-time, thereby providing a richer description of the spatio-temporal video content.

2   Methods

Data Acquisition and Processing. Full-length routine fetal anomaly ultrasound scan videos acquired by an expert sonographer were available for the research from the PULSE study [3]. We had the sonographer retrospectively record voice-overs in English for five anonymised videos with a mean duration of 37 min (range: 20–56 min). A total of 160 min of audiovisual content was recorded. From the full-length videos, freeze frames were automatically detected. The sonographers freeze a frame when they find a suitable view of interest for diagnostic examination, which are the anatomical standard planes. The display frame was automatically cropped to include only the anatomical view. The speech recordings were pre-processed for anonymisation and then transcribed using Google Cloud Speech (GCS) API [6]. GCS is designed for natural language, but the recordings contain additional medical vocabulary. The transcriptions contained a few errors which were corrected by manual post-processing. ELAN, a multimedia annotator for audiovisual content, was used to synchronize video contents with generated transcriptions and to correct erroneous text [19]. After the transcribed words were manually checked, grouped, and synced, a file containing the captions with start and end times was produced to automatically align video frames with captions. Figure 2 shows the process of creating image-caption pairs. The raw text was cleaned by removing punctuation, replacing numeric characters with their word equivalents, and removing stall words (e.g. 'so yeah', 'well'). Special tokens denoted a caption's start and end. The resulting caption length varied between 1–22 words, with a vocabulary of 158 unique words and distribution of adjectives, determiners, nouns, and verbs is 12.7%, 22.2%, 28.0%, and 16.0%, respectively. The remaining 21.1% are prepositions, pronouns, adverbs, and other parts-of-speech. Hence, the combined dataset was composed of real-world fetal anomaly ultrasound video freeze frames and their associated captions.

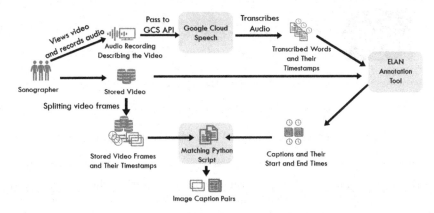

Fig. 2. Data acquisition and processing pipeline

Model Architecture. Image captioning often involves a CNN to encode image information followed by an RNN as a decoder to generate text [22]. However, to reduce computational complexity, an RNN was used solely as the textual feature extractor and the encoded image information from a CNN was combined with the textual features in merged configurations [20,21]. The model diagram is shown in Fig. 3. One branch of the model is a CNN based on the VGGNet16 [18] architecture, pre-trained on the ImageNet dataset and fine-tuned on fetal ultrasound standard planes of the abdomen, face, brain, femur, heart, spine, and placenta. The other branch represents the text encoding part of the model, including an embedding layer, which embeds the words in the sequence into a vector, followed by an RNN.

Features are extracted from the ultrasound video frames using the fine-tuned CNN. A textual caption is encoded by an embedding layer followed by a recurrent layer. The branches are merged, followed by a fully connected and decision-making layer. The model configurations generate the next word in a caption at every step as the probability distribution over the words in the vocabulary. We comparatively evaluated different embeddings, namely, word2vec embedding trained on the Google News corpus [7], GloVe embedding trained on Wikipedia-2014 corpus [17], and a plain random initialization. Word2vec is a shallow neural network trained to predict the context around a given word in a skip-gram model [14]. GloVe incorporates word co-occurrence probabilities with the idea that words occurring together often enough are likely to hold underlying semantic meaning. The embedded word vectors are learnt by an RNN consisting of a Long Short-Term Memory (LSTM) unit [9] or a Gated Recurrent Unit (GRU) [2]. GRUs have less trainable parameters than LSTMs and require fewer operations, which makes GRUs more efficient to train, scaling down well to smaller datasets. The two branches produce tensors of different lengths (200 and 300, respectively) that are joined together by merging. We compare two merge methods, namely, concatenation and addition. In concatenation configurations, text and image features vectors of unequal length are combined to deliberately force the model

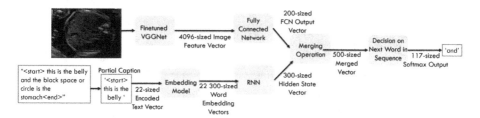

Fig. 3. Image captioning model (concatenation configurations)

towards relying more on the text branch when generating the next word in a sequence to have a textually well-structured generated caption. However, output vectors of an equal length of 300 are used in addition configurations.

Training Process. Sixty-five percent of the total data was used for training and thirty-five percent for testing. For training the deep learning models, we excluded captions that do not describe one of the four anatomical structures of highest interest, *i.e.*, head, heart, spine, and abdomen. These anatomical classes were selected due to having the most representation in the collected dataset compared to other anatomical classes, and they form 40%, 22%, 20%, and 18% of the data, respectively. From caption pre-processing, vocabularies of each of the four anatomical classes of interest were obtained. Lexical diversity scores, specifically MTLD [13], to measure word variety in each vocabulary were obtained as 21.2, 20.3, 17.9, and 21.8, respectively. To address class imbalance, an equal number of unique captions were included for each anatomical class, namely, abdomen, head, heart, and spine. In addition to class imbalance, caption imbalance is observed as some captions correspond to more than one video frame because sonographers spend a different amount of time looking at different fetal structures.

The training set consisted of 2,240 image-caption pairs and the validation set consisted of 560 image-caption pairs. The images were resized to 224 × 224 pixels. Each image in the dataset was augmented twice; first by rotating by an angle between −30° and 30°, and second by horizontally flipping the image. Pre-trained VGGNet16 was first fine-tuned on ultrasound images. During training of image captioning models, 'teacher forcing' was applied where the ground truth sequences of increasing length were used at every step rather than the sequence of the words generated by the model at previous steps [5]. The model was called in a recursive fashion with the sequence of generated words so far being iteratively fed into the model at every time-step, along with the corresponding image. This process continued until the model generated a special end token or the maximum caption length was reached. Adam optimization [10] and categorical cross-entropy loss were applied during training. Early stopping was used to stop training when validation loss did not improve for more than five epochs. Dropout (rate between 0.4 and 0.5) was used to reduce overfitting. During inference, the model relied on its previously generated words to generate the next word.

Evaluation Metrics. Different model configurations were compared using the established general metrics *BLEU* (Bilingual Evaluation Understudy) [16] and *ROUGE-L* (Recall-Oriented Understudy for Gisting Evaluation-Longest Common Subsequence) [11], a grammar score *GB* (GrammarBot) [8], a classification metric *Class. F1* (F1 score), and an anatomical description metric *ARS* (Anatomical Relevance Score). Objective metrics *BLEU* and *ROUGE-L* are calculated between the ground truth captions and the generated captions. These two metrics are commonly used when evaluating image captioning models but may lead to lower values when the pair of captions do not show exact matches. Hence, for our caption generation task, grammar-based, classification-based, description-based, and subjective metrics were additionally evaluated. To evaluate captions grammatically, the average number of grammatical mistakes in a generated caption was calculated. Classification F1 scores were calculated by determining the caption class as the class of the vocabulary that has the highest overlap with the predicted caption. We devised an anatomical relevance score (*ARS*) by matching words in a generated caption with the terminology of the anatomical class of interest. For example, an image of an abdomen may have a ground truth caption about the ribs, but if the generated caption describes the stomach, it is not an erroneous caption. *ARS* is calculated using Eqs. 1, 2 and 3

$$CS_k = \left(\sum_{i=1}^{L(W^c)} 1_{V_k}(w_i^c) \right)^{-1} \sum_{i=1}^{L(W^c)} 1_{V_k}(w_i^c) p_i \tag{1}$$

$$SS_c = \begin{cases} \max_{k \in K} CS_k & \text{if } \arg\max_{k \in K}(CS_k) = GT_c \\ 0 & \text{otherwise} \end{cases} \tag{2}$$

$$ARS = \frac{1}{C} \sum_{i=1}^{C} SS_c \tag{3}$$

where CS_k is a score that a caption has in relation to the anatomical class k, K is the set of four anatomical classes, V_k is the vocabulary set of class k, L is the length of a caption W^c consisting of words w_i^c with softmax probabilities p_i, $1_V(\cdot)$ is an indicator function which returns 1 if w_i is in V and 0 otherwise, SS_c is a score that only considers CS_k if it has the ground truth anatomical class GT_c, and C is the total number of captions in the set.

3   Results

Quantitative Evaluation. Table 1 presents quantitative evaluation results for different model configurations. An overall score is obtained by calculating the mean of the scores (*GB* was normalised and inverted). The overall best performing model was the Fine-tunable-Word2vec-LSTM-Concatenation configuration, which is used to demonstrate anatomical evaluation in Table 2 and Fig. 4. For a

Table 1. Evaluation results of model configurations

Word embedding	RNN	Merge mode	BLEU-4	ROUGE-L	GB↓	Class. F1	ARS	Overall
Fine-Tunable GloVe	LSTM	Concatenation	0.066	0.536	1.091	0.809	0.680	0.385
		Addition	0.081	0.580	0.9	0.948	0.686	0.397
	GRU	Concatenation	0.081	0.585	**0.889**	0.502	0.455	0.261
		Addition	0.094	0.561	0.923	0.529	0.449	0.268
Fine-Tunable Word2vec	LSTM	Concatenation	**0.105**	**0.594**	1.214	0.970	0.536	**0.427**
		Addition	0.045	0.546	0.929	0.679	0.506	0.297
	GRU	Concatenation	0.080	0.523	1.200	0.764	0.594	0.376
		Addition	0.086	0.539	1.077	0.609	0.476	0.307
Pretrained Word2vec	LSTM	Concatenation	0.085	0.574	1.200	0.921	0.567	0.413
		Addition	0.063	0.529	1.267	0.641	0.537	0.348
	GRU	Concatenation	0.066	0.530	1.100	0.768	**0.718**	0.385
		Addition	0.062	0.545	0.917	0.714	0.648	0.334
Random Initialisation	LSTM	Concatenation	0.075	0.560	1.222	**0.975**	0.564	0.422
		Addition	0.091	0.536	1.188	0.805	0.539	0.362
	GRU	Concatenation	0.067	0.507	1.308	0.763	0.632	0.394
		Addition	0.084	0.525	0.857	0.625	0.547	0.287

subjective measure, Likert Scale based evaluations are performed where a medical professional was asked to give a score of 0 ('No'), 1 ('Neutral'), or 2 ('Yes') in response to the following statements about a generated caption, namely it: (1) accurately describes the image; (2) has no incorrect information; (3) is grammatically correct; (4) is relevant for this image. For each caption, the responses were averaged. These scores are reported in Table 2 as *LSS* (Likert Scale Scores). Knowing the original image class and resulting caption classes, we plot the confusion matrix for the best performing configuration in Fig. 4.

Discussion. Table 1 shows that there is no clear superior configuration across the different metrics, but overall, the Fine-tunable-Word2vec-LSTM-Concatenation configuration performs the best across the different metrics. Its generated captions are shown in the supplementary material. It is marginally outperformed in anatomical classification scores by the Random-Initialisation-LSTM-Concatenation configuration but scores higher in *BLEU-4* and *ROUGE-L*, implying the usefulness of pre-trained embeddings to ensure superior caption structuring compared to randomly initialised vectors. Word2vec embeddings were found to be more effective than GloVe embeddings for the fetal ultrasound datasets. It is interesting to note that, in most cases, concatenation performed better than addition, and LSTM units outperformed GRUs, even for our limited datasets. Among the anatomical classes, from Table 2, abdomen and head show low scores in *BLEU-4* and *ROUGE-L* due to having the highest lexical diversity. Spine does well in *ROUGE-L* and *GB* because of its lower lexical diversity, however, *BLEU-4* is zero due to the absence of 4-gram overlaps but *BLEU-3*=0.319 is achieved. From *LSS*, we can see that the heart class is more

Table 2. Evaluation results for the different anatomical structures

Structure	BLEU-3	BLEU-4	ROUGE-L	GB↓	Class. F1	ARS	LSS
Abdomen	0.000	0.000	0.533	0.667	0.886	0.316	0.625
Head	0.122	0.058	0.479	2.000	**1.000**	0.213	0.625
Heart	0.252	**0.140**	0.581	0.857	0.993	**0.843**	0.500
Spine	**0.319**	0.000	**0.789**	**0.000**	1.000	0.771	**1.000**

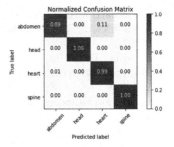

Fig. 4. Confusion matrix

challenging. In clinical practice, a fetal heart is typically identified by its beating motion (a video clip) rather than a still image. Further, the current captioning system is not trained to distinguish between the different heart views, but the textual description can be heart view specific. Adding more image-caption pairs of distinct heart views may solve this problem. In Fig. 4, it can be seen that all classes are accurately identified; however, the model struggles with 11% of abdomen images, misclassifying them as hearts. On investigation, it was found that for these specific images the stomach bubble has an elongated appearance, which has some resemblance to a heart view or heart chamber.

4 Conclusions

We proposed an automatic image captioning method to describe fetal ultrasound video content from four types of anatomical structures using real-world sonographer vocabularies. The Fine-tunable-Word2vec-LSTM-Concatenation performed best among the different evaluated model configurations. Richer vocabularies and extensions to spatio-temporal models will be considered in future work.

Acknowledgement. We acknowledge the ERC (ERC-ADG-2015 694 project PULSE), the EPSRC (EP/MO13774/1), the Rhodes Trust, and the NIHR BRC funding scheme.

References

1. Bernardi, R., et al.: Automatic description generation from images: a survey of models, datasets, and evaluation measures. In: IJCAI, pp. 4970–4974 (2017)
2. Cho, K., et al.: Learning phrase representations using RNN encoder-decoder for statistical machine translation. In: EMNLP, pp. 1724–1734. ACL (2014)
3. Department of Engineering Science, University of Oxford: PULSE. https://www.eng.ox.ac.uk/pulse/
4. Elliott, D., Keller, F.: Image description using visual dependency representations. In: EMNLP, pp. 1292–1302 (2013)
5. Goodfellow, I., et al.: Deep Learning (2016)
6. Google Cloud: Cloud Speech-to-Text. cloud.google.com/speech-to-text/
7. Google Code Archive: Word2Vec (2013). code.google.com/archive/p/word2vec/

8. GrammarBot: Grammar Check API. https://www.grammarbot.io/
9. Hochreiter, S., Schmidhuber, J.: Long short-term memory. NC **9**(8), 1735–1780 (1997)
10. Kingma, D.P., Ba, J.: Adam: a method for stochastic optimization. CoRR abs/1412.6980 (2015)
11. Lin, C.Y.: ROUGE: a package for automatic evaluation of summaries. Text Summarization Branches Out (2004)
12. Lyndon, D., et al.: Neural captioning for the Image CLEF 2017 medical image challenges. In: CEUR Workshop Proceedings, vol. 1866 (2017)
13. McCarthy, P.M., Jarvis, S.: MTLD, vocd-D, and HD-D: a validation study of sophisticated approaches to lexical diversity assessment. Behav. Res. Methods **42**(2), 381–392 (2010)
14. Mikolov, T., et al.: Distributed representations of words and phrases and their compositionality. In: Advances in Neural Information Processing Systems (2013)
15. Ordonez, V., et al.: Im2Text: describing images using 1 million captioned photographs. In: Advances in NIPS, pp. 1143–1151 (2011)
16. Papineni, K., et al.: BLEU: a method for automatic evaluation of machine translation. In: Proceedings of the 40th Annual Meeting on ACL, pp. 311–318. ACL (2002)
17. Pennington, et al.: GloVe: global vectors for word representation. In: EMNLP, pp. 1532–1543 (2014)
18. Simonyan, K., Zisserman, A.: Very deep convolutional networks for large-scale image recognition. In: International Conference on Learning Representations (2015)
19. Sloetjes, H., Wittenburg, P.: Annotation by category-ELAN and ISO DCR. In: LREC (2008)
20. Tanti, M., et al.: What is the role of recurrent neural networks (RNNs) in an image caption generator? ACL, pp. 51–60 (2017)
21. Tanti, M., et al.: Where to put the image in an image caption generator. Nat. Lang. Eng. **24**(3), 467–489 (2018)
22. Vinyals, O., et al.: Show and tell: a neural image caption generator. In: Proceedings of the IEEE conference on CVPR, pp. 3156–3164 (2015)
23. You, Q., et al.: Image captioning with semantic attention. In: Proceedings of the IEEE Conference on CVPR, pp. 4651–4659 (2016)
24. Zeng, X.H., et al.: Understanding and generating ultrasound image description. J. Comput. Sci. Technol. **33**(5), 1086–1100 (2018)

Feature Transformers: Privacy Preserving Lifelong Learners for Medical Imaging

Hariharan Ravishankar[(⊠)], Rahul Venkataramani, Saihareesh Anamandra, Prasad Sudhakar, and Pavan Annangi

Advanced Technology Group, GE Healthcare, Bangalore, India
{hariharan.ravishankar,rahul.venkataramani,saihareesh.anamandra, prasad.sudhakar,pavan.annangi}@ge.com

Abstract. Deep learning algorithms have achieved tremendous success in many medical imaging problems leading to multiple commercial healthcare applications. For sustaining the performance of these algorithms post-deployment, it is necessary to overcome catastrophic forgetting and continually evolve with data. While catastrophic forgetting could be managed using historical data, a fundamental challenge in Healthcare is data-privacy, where regulations constrain restrict data sharing. In this paper, we present a single, unified mathematical framework - *feature transformers*, for handling the myriad variants of lifelong learning to overcome catastrophic forgetting without compromising data-privacy. We report state-of-the-art results for lifelong learning on iCIFAR100 dataset and also demonstrate lifelong learning on medical imaging applications - X-ray Pneumothorax classification and Ultrasound cardiac view classification.

1 Introduction

Two major manifestations of lifelong learning are *domain adaptation* and *New task learning*. Despite the positive impact of deep learning on multiple healthcare applications, the highly diverse nature of medical imaging data owing to factors like imaging hardware, demographics, acquisition protocols, inter-subject variability, pathologies, etc necessitate frequent need for successful domain adaptation. In [3], authors report that the performance of MRI segmentation algorithms suffer when tested on data from a different protocol/vendor. New task Learning - the ability to augment existing neural networks with newer capabilities is critical to enable expert clinicians like radiologists to add new capabilities to existing applications and also to control explosion of number of models for different applications. For example, in [1] authors enable a model capable of performing brain structure segmentation to also perform white matter lesion segmentation.

Lifelong learning is trivial if the entire dataset is available during every episode. However, as access to past data is not practical and often impossible due to regulatory constraints, these algorithms are trained sequentially using

© Springer Nature Switzerland AG 2019
D. Shen et al. (Eds.): MICCAI 2019, LNCS 11767, pp. 347–355, 2019.
https://doi.org/10.1007/978-3-030-32251-9_38

only latest data. This leads to neural networks exhibiting a phenomenon known as *catastrophic forgetting* [4] - inability of models to retain past knowledge while learning from new data. To overcome this problem, researchers have attempted to retain past knowledge through proxy information, a technique dubbed as *pseudorehearsal*. Some of the popular methods of *pseudorehearsal* include the use of a knowledge distillation loss [5], rehearsal using exemplars [8,9] and the use of generative models for retaining knowledge from previous episodes [2,10,12]. Regularization [4,6] techniques are also used to constraint parts of network which are critical for the performance on previous tasks.

All these methods suffer from either of the two drawbacks rendering them unusable in medical imaging: (1) data privacy concerns arising from storage of exemplar images. (2) the ability of methods to work only on one of the variants of lifelong learning. In this paper, we propose one approach for all manifestations of lifelong learning to handle data privacy and catastrophic forgetting. We utilize an external memory to store only the features representing past data and *learn richer and newer representations incrementally* through transformation neural networks - *feature transformers*. Our major contributions are as follows:

- Formulate a generic mathematical framework - feature transformers to cater to domain adaptation and new task learning.
- Ensure data privacy by storing only features from previous episodes while successfully combating catastrophic forgetting.
- Demonstrate exemplary results on two challenging problems of cardiac ultrasound view classification and pneumothorax detection from X-ray images.

Section 2 describes our approach. Section 3 contains experiments and results.

2   Life-Long Learning via Feature Transformations

A neural network classifier, parameterised by $(\boldsymbol{\theta}, \boldsymbol{\kappa})$, is a composition of a feature extractor $\boldsymbol{\Phi}_\theta : \boldsymbol{X} \to \boldsymbol{F}$, and $\boldsymbol{\Psi}_\kappa$, a classifier $\boldsymbol{\Psi}_\kappa \circ \boldsymbol{\Phi}_\theta : \boldsymbol{X} \to [C]$, where $\boldsymbol{X}$ is the space of input data, and $\boldsymbol{F}$ is a space of low-dimensional feature vectors.

In the lifelong learning setup, at any time $t-1$, the model optimally classifies all the seen data $\cup_{t'=0}^{t-1} X^{(t')}$ into the classes $[C^{(t-1)}]$ and the corresponding features $\mathcal{F}^{(t-1)}$ are well separated. At t, when new training data $D^{(t)} = (X^{(t)}, Y^{(t)})$ is encountered, features extracted using the old feature extractor

$$\partial \mathcal{F}^{(t)} = \left(\boldsymbol{\Phi}_{\theta^{(t-1)}}(X^{(t)}) \right), \tag{1}$$

are not guaranteed to be optimized for classifying the new data and new classes. To alleviate this, we propose to change the feature representation at time t, just before the classification stage. We achieve this by defining a **feature transformer**

$$\boldsymbol{\Phi}_{\Delta\theta^{(t)}} : \boldsymbol{F}^{(t-1)} \to \boldsymbol{F}^{(t)}, \tag{2}$$

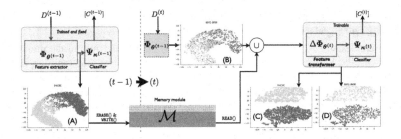

Fig. 1. Visual depiction of feature transformation process on new episodes.

parameterized by $\Delta\theta^{(t)}$, which maps any feature extracted by $\Phi_{\theta^{(t-1)}}$ to a new representation. The new feature extractor is now given by $\Phi_{\theta^{(t)}} \triangleq \Phi_{\Delta\theta^{(t)}} \circ \Phi_{\theta^{(t-1)}}$, where $\theta^{(t)} \triangleq \theta^{(t-1)} \cup \Delta\theta^{(t)}$. Practically, this is realized by augmenting the capacity of the feature extractor using dense layers[1].

Remembering History via Memory: The set of all extracted features $\mathcal{F}^{(t-1)}$ serves as a good abstraction of the model, for all the tasks and data encountered till $t-1$. We realize our psuedo-rehearsal strategy through the use of a finite memory module $\mathcal{M}$, equipped with READ(), WRITE() and ERASE() procedures, that can store a subset of $\mathcal{F}^{(t-1)}$ and retrieve the same at t.

Ensuring Class-Separation via Composite Loss: In all our training procedures, we augment classification loss with *center-loss* (described in [14]) : $J(\theta,\kappa) = classification\,loss_{(\theta,\kappa)} + \lambda \cdot centre\text{-}loss_{(\theta)}$. This composite loss explicitly forces the transformed features to have class-wise separation, in addition to classification performance. We train the feature transformer at any $t > 0$ by invoking TRAIN($\Delta\theta^{(t)}, \kappa^{(t)}; D^{(t)}$), with the combined set of features and obtain transformed features $\mathcal{F}^{(t)}$ which replace $\mathcal{F}^{(t-1)}$ in memory.

$$D^{(t)} = (\partial\mathcal{F}^{(t)} \cup \mathcal{F}^{(t-1)}, \cup_{t' \in [1,2,\cdots,t]} Y^{(t')}), \; \forall t > 0. \tag{3}$$

$$\mathcal{F}^{(t)} = \Phi_{\Delta\theta^{(t)}}(\partial\mathcal{F}^{(t)}) \cup \Phi_{\Delta\theta^{(t)}}(\mathcal{F}^{(t-1)}), \tag{4}$$

Figure 1 shows feature transformers in action using Pneumothorax classification (Sect. 3.2). A binary classifier is trained on 6000 images at time index $(t-1)$. As shown by the t-SNE plot (A), the feature extractor $\Phi_{\theta^{(t-1)}}$ produces features which are well-separated, and get stored in memory $\mathcal{M}$. However, at time t, when a set of 2000 new images is encountered, $\Phi_{\theta^{(t-1)}}$ produces features that are scattered (t-SNE plot (B)). Feature transformer learns a new representation using the (well-separated) features in $\mathcal{M}$ as well as poorly separated features (from new data). This ensures good class separation for all images encountered until time t(t-SNE plots (C) and (D)). This is repeated for all time indices t.

To enable practicality of the proposed approach, we ensure that the memory footprint is limited (Sect. 4.1) by storing only a subset of history selected by a sampling operator $\mathcal{S}$. Algorithm 1 presents the pseudocode for our framework.

---

[1] There is no restriction on the kind of layers to be used, but in this work we use only fully connected layers.

Input Training data $(X^{(t)}, Y^{(t)})$, $\forall t \geq 0$
Output $(\theta^{(t)}, \kappa^{(t)})$, $\forall t$
$t \leftarrow 0$, ERASE($\mathcal{M}$)   /* Set initial time, erase memory */
$D^{(0)} \leftarrow (X^{(0)}, Y^{(0)})$ /* Obtain initial tasks and training data */
TRAIN($\theta^{(0)}, \kappa^{(0)}$; $D^{(0)}$)   /* Train initial network */
$\mathcal{F}^{(0)} \leftarrow (\boldsymbol{\Phi}_{\theta^{(0)}}(X^{(0)}))$ /* Compute features */
WRITE($\mathcal{M}, \mathcal{S}(\mathcal{F}^{(0)}, Y^{(0)})$)   /* Write select features to memory */
while $TRUE$ **do**

> $t \leftarrow t + 1$, obtain $\mathcal{T}^{(t)}, (X^{(t)}, Y^{(t)})$ /* Obtain current tasks and data */
> Get $\partial \mathcal{F}^{(t)}$ using Eq. 1   /* Compute old model features on new data */
> $(\mathcal{F}^{(t-1)}, Y^{(t-1)}) \leftarrow$ READ($\mathcal{M}$)   /* Read previously computed features */
> Form $D^{(t)}$ using Eq. 3   /* Form composite training data */
> TRAIN($\Delta\theta^{(t)}, \kappa^{(t)}$; $D^{(t)}$)   /* Train feature transformer */
> $\boldsymbol{\Phi}_{\theta^{(t)}} \leftarrow \boldsymbol{\Phi}_{\Delta\theta^{(t)}} \circ \boldsymbol{\Phi}_{\theta^{(t-1)}}$ /* Obtain new feature extractor */
> Compute $\mathcal{F}^{(t)}$ using Eq. 4   /* Compute new features */
> ERASE($\mathcal{M}$)   /* Erase old features*/
> WRITE($\mathcal{M}, \mathcal{S}(\mathcal{F}^{(t)}, \cup_{t' \in [1,2,\cdots,t]} Y^{(t')})$)   /* Write new select features*/

end

Algorithm 1. The life-long learning framework

3   Experiments and Results

We first demonstrate our algorithm as a generic lifelong learner by conducting experiments on iCIFAR100 dataset. Then, we proceed to demonstrate the efficacy of feature transformers on two real world problems in medical imaging.

3.1   Conventional Continual Learning Paradigms on iCIFAR100

iCIFAR100 dataset contains images from 100 different classes and is a popular choice of study for comparing lifelong learning approaches [8]. The two conventional lifelong learning evaluation settings on iCIFAR100 are multi-task (MT) and single incremental task (SIT) [7], where the 100 class dataset is fed in a sequence of 20 tasks comprising 5 classes each. In MT setting, the algorithm is evaluated to learn an isolated set of new tasks while SIT entails learning all the classes incrementally. In our experiments, we used a basic CNN architecture inspired by the popular CIFAR architecture. Our feature transformer networks at every episode aims to transform features from dense layers using 2 additional dense layers of feature length 256 and were optimized for the composite loss $\lambda = 0.2$.

Multi Task Setting: We validate our algorithm against state-of-the-art methods [8] using 2 different metrics: accuracy and *backward transfer* (BWT). BWT is a quantitative metric that measures catastrophic forgetting on older tasks after learning new tasks. As shown in Fig. 2(a), Feature Transformers provide an improvement of >15% while showing negligible catastrophic forgetting and outperforms of all the methods reported in [8] by a big margin.

Single Incremental Task setting: Here, we compare our results to the two obvious life-long learners - *Naive* and *Cumulative learners*, which serve as the lower and upper bounds of performance respectively. Naive learner finetunes the entire network on the latest episode data while cumulative learner retrains the model from data accumulated over all the episodes seen so far. As seen in Fig. 2(b), after 20 episodes, naive learner performs very poorly, while feature transformer displays impressive performance numbers of 40% validation accuracy, while compared to cumulative learner at 50%. Our method significantly outperforms AR1 [7], iCaRL [9] achieves best-in-class performance close to gold-standard cumulative learner. We attribute it to iCaRL storing exemplar images while we only store features from previous episodes.

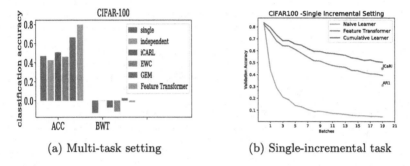

(a) Multi-task setting   (b) Single-incremental task

Fig. 2. Comparison with state-of-the-art methods - iCIFAR100 dataset

3.2   Lifelong Learning for Pneumothorax Classification

Our first medical imaging application for lifelong learning is Pneumothorax identification from X-ray images, which is a relevant as well as a challenging problem owing to diversity of disease manifestation. We utilize a subset of ChestXRay [13] dataset, which consists of chest X-rays labeled with corresponding diagnoses. We simulated incremental learning by providing the 8 k training images in incremental batches of 2 K and measured the performance on held-out validation set of ∼2 K images, which mimics a practical scenario of a model deployed to detect pneumothorax in a hospital with data arriving incrementally. Figure 3(a) establishes the baselines for the experiment. As in previous experiment, naive learner - which finetunes only on the latest episode and cumulative leaner - which retrains on the entire data seen so far define the performance bounds.

Experimental Details and Results: We used a pre-trained VGG-network [11] as the base network and explored the use of features from different layers of the VGG-network: post the two pooling layers and fully connected layers. Feature transformer network essentially had one additional dense layer per step.

Figure 3(a) captures the performance of feature transformer with the base features being extracted from first pooling layer - block3_pool. After fourth batch

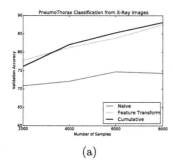

S.No	Base Feature Extraction Layer	Validation Accuracy
1	block3_pool	86.94%
2	block4_pool	85.84%
3	fc_1	84.6%
4	fc_2	83.2%

(a)   (b)

Fig. 3. (a) Performance comparison on validation dataset and (b) Comparison of feature transformers from different base layers

Table 1. Performance comparison on validation dataset

Episode No.	Episode definition	Naive learning accuracy (%)	Cumulative learner accuracy (%)	Feature transformer accuracy (%)
1	Adult 4ch + PLAX	97.2	97.2	97.2
2	Pediatric 4ch + PLAX	91	98.2	98
3	Adult 2ch + PSAX	55	96	87
4	Pediatric 2ch + PSAX	46	95.5	88

of data, performance of feature transformers almost matches the performance of cumulative training. This performance is achieved despite not having access to the full images but only the stored features. Figure 3b also presents the performance of feature transformer depending upon the base features used. It can be noted that performance is lowest for the layer that is closer to the classification layer - fc_2. This is intuitively satisfying because, the further layers in a deep neural network will be more finely tuned towards the specific task and deprives the feature transform of generic features.

3.3 Lifelong Learning for Cardiac View Classification

Cardiac Ultrasound (U/S) images exhibit a high degree of variability owing to the skill of the sonographer, acquisition parameters, types of probe, patient echogenicity and age. In this paper, we pursue classification of the four common views of standard cardiac study - 4chamber (4ch) and 2chamber (2ch), Paresternal Long Axis (PLAX) and Short Axis (PSAX). We set-up a series of lifelong episodes to investigate the proposed approach for domain adaptation and new task learning.

In the first episode, we train a classifier model to classify 2 views from adult subjects - 4ch and PLAX. To study domain adaptation, we demonstrate its performance on pediatric data for the same classes. As seen in Fig. 4, images

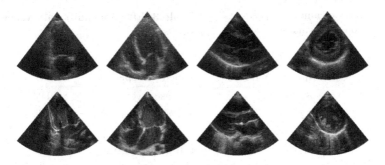

Fig. 4. Example images of 2ch, 4ch, PLAX and PSAX views (left to right) for adult (top row) and pediatric (bottom row) subjects

from pediatric subjects have higher contrast and smoother speckles compared to adult subjects primarily because of use of high frequency probes and lesser depth of penetration. In the next episode, we simulate new task learning by adding 2 additional views (2ch and PSAX) followed by the final episode where pediatric images of the new views are presented. The number of images per view was 5 K and was tested on a mutually exclusive set of 2 K images per view. Table 1 shows the comparison of proposed approach with naive and cumulative learners. It should be noted that fine-tuning on pediatric data in episode 2, results in a performance drop of 7%, while the cumulative learner and Feature transformer do not suffer from effects of domain change. The naive learner fails completely while presented with two new views in Episode 3, while Feature Transformer achieves a respectable 87% demonstrating new-task learning capabilities without catastrophic forgetting. This is further demonstrated in Episode 4, where domain adaptation on pediatric views are achieved with promising results.

4   Discussion

In the final section, we examine two important facets concerning the practicality of the proposed approach - (1) Memory management (2) Network capacity. We examine the amount of history necessary for successful lifelong learning and obtained satisfactory results by retaining only 25% of past samples in memory.

4.1   Memory Management

As discussed in Sect. 2, at every episode of lifelong learning we selectively retain only a small portion of history. There are two strategies that can be pursued for the same (1) Random sampling - where we randomly retain a percentage of the memory (2) Importance sampling - retain samples that are farther from cluster centroids, given that we optimize for center loss at every episode. For the Pneumothorax classification problem, Table 2 shows the effect of random sampling of features on the performance. We would also like to point out that storing low-dimensional features is economical than storing entire images.

Table 2. Effect of amount of features stored on performance

% of samples stored from history	Feature trans--former Val Acc
25	80.95%
50	82.95%
75	85.85 %
100	86.94 %

Table 3. Effect of additional layers on performance

Incremental capacity added per episode	Feature trans-former Val Acc
2 dense layers	86.94%
1 dense layers	86.43%
No additional capacity (after 3rd episode)	86.41%

4.2   Controlling the Growth of Network Capacity

Our framework can be formulated as a base feature extractor and feature transformer layers, adapting the features for new tasks. In order to check the growth of feature transformer layers, the base feature extractor remains fixed and only the base features are stored and not the latest updated features. This makes existing feature transformer layers reusable for future episodes. We varied the size of feature transformers and observed the difference in performance. Table 3 shows that halving the additional capacity retains the performance on pneumothorax dataset. These experiments (along with Sect. 4.1) clearly demonstrate that power of learning separable representations continually and make our proposed approach practically feasible.

4.3   Information Loss, Incremental Capacity, Data Privacy

As shown in Fig. 3(b), feature transformer becomes less effective if the base features do not contain enough relevant information. This also means that additional capacity that every feature transformer adds may not help or in-fact be counter-productive. If the base features are extracted from layers close to the input image, there will be problem of traceability which violates the data privacy requirement we want to accomplish. We feel this a potential trade-off between performance and data privacy which we will investigate in future.

5   Conclusion

In this work, we present Feature Transformers - privacy preserving lifelong learning framework that paves the way for practical lifelong learning for healthcare applications. In addition to achieving state-of-the-art performance on iCIFAR dataset, we demonstrate exemplary performance on two challenging medical imaging applications. Another major contributions include proposing a single framework to perform and switch between domain adaptation and new task learning, Future work would involve optimizing for limited memory budget, model growth and extending to applications like segmentation, regression, etc.

References

1. Baweja, C., Glocker, B., Kamnitsas, K.: Towards continual learning in medical imaging. arXiv preprint arXiv:1811.02496 (2018)
2. He, C., Wang, R., Shan, S., Chen, X.: Exemplar-supported generative reproduction for class incremental learning. In: 29th BMVC, 3–6 September 2018
3. Karani, N., Chaitanya, K., Baumgartner, C., Konukoglu, E.: A lifelong learning approach to brain MR segmentation across scanners and protocols. In: Frangi, A.F., Schnabel, J.A., Davatzikos, C., Alberola-López, C., Fichtinger, G. (eds.) MICCAI 2018. LNCS, vol. 11070, pp. 476–484. Springer, Cham (2018). https://doi.org/10.1007/978-3-030-00928-1_54
4. Kirkpatrick, J., et al.: Overcoming catastrophic forgetting in neural networks. In: Proceedings of the National Academy of Sciences (2017)
5. Li, Z., Hoiem, D.: Learning without forgetting. IEEE Trans. Pattern Anal. Mach. Intell. **40**, 2935–2947 (2017)
6. Liu, X., et al.: Rotate your networks: better weight consolidation and less catastrophic forgetting. arXiv preprint arXiv:1802.02950 (2018)
7. Lomonaco, V., Maltoni, D.: Core50: a new dataset and benchmark for continuous object recognition. arXiv preprint arXiv:1705.03550 (2017)
8. Lopez-Paz, D., et al.: Gradient episodic memory for continual learning. In: Advances in Neural Information Processing Systems, pp. 6467–6476 (2017)
9. Rebuffi, S.A., Kolesnikov, A., Lampert, C.H.: iCaRL: incremental classifier and representation learning. In: 2017 IEEE CVPR, pp. 5533–5542 (2017)
10. Shin, H., Lee, J.K., Kim, J., Kim, J.: Continual learning with deep generative replay. In: Advances in Neural Information Processing Systems, pp. 2990–2999 (2017)
11. Simonyan, K., Zisserman, A.: Very deep convolutional networks for large-scale image recognition. arXiv preprint arXiv:1409.1556 (2014)
12. Venkatesan, R., Venkateswara, H., Panchanathan, S., Li, B.: A strategy for an uncompromising incremental learner. arXiv preprint arXiv:1705.00744 (2017)
13. Wang, X., et al.: ChestX-ray8: hospital-scale chest x-ray database and benchmarks on weakly-supervised classification and localization of common thorax diseases. In: 2017 IEEE CVPR, pp. 3462–3471, July 2017
14. Wen, Y., Zhang, K., Li, Z., Qiao, Y.: A discriminative feature learning approach for deep face recognition. In: Leibe, B., Matas, J., Sebe, N., Welling, M. (eds.) ECCV 2016. LNCS, vol. 9911, pp. 499–515. Springer, Cham (2016). https://doi.org/10.1007/978-3-319-46478-7_31

As Easy as 1, 2... 4?
Uncertainty in Counting Tasks
for Medical Imaging

Zach Eaton-Rosen[1,2]([⊠]), Thomas Varsavsky[1,2], Sebastien Ourselin[2],
and M. Jorge Cardoso[2]

[1] Centre for Medical Imaging Computing, University College London, London, UK
`zach.eaton-rosen@kcl.ac.uk`
[2] Biomedical Engineering and Imaging Sciences, King's College London, London, UK

Abstract. Counting is a fundamental task in biomedical imaging and count is an important biomarker in a number of conditions. Estimating the uncertainty in the measurement is thus vital to making definite, informed conclusions. In this paper, we first compare a range of existing methods to perform counting in medical imaging and suggest ways of deriving predictive intervals from these. We then propose and test a method for calculating intervals as an output of a multi-task network. These predictive intervals are optimised to be as narrow as possible, while also enclosing a desired percentage of the data. We demonstrate the effectiveness of this technique on histopathological cell counting and white matter hyperintensity counting. Finally, we offer insight into other areas where this technique may apply.

1 Introduction

Counting is a common analysis task required in a wide range of medical imaging applications from histology (cell counting) to neuroradiology (lesion counting). For any of these clinical biomarkers, accurate quantification of the degree of uncertainty over the measurements is of high importance in deciding an appropriate course of action. In this paper, we demonstrate an improved method for quantifying the uncertainty for counting tasks.

Uncertainty can be broadly broken down into two constituent parts: model and data uncertainty. In the context of CNNs, 'model' or 'epistemic' uncertainty represents the uncertainty over the network (weights, hyperparameters, architecture) while 'data' or 'aleatoric' uncertainty represents the noise inherently associated with the data (noisy labels, measurement noise). Furthermore, out-of-distribution examples are likely to adversely affect the performance of machine-learning tools.

Electronic supplementary material The online version of this chapter (https://doi.org/10.1007/978-3-030-32251-9_39) contains supplementary material, which is available to authorized users.

© Springer Nature Switzerland AG 2019
D. Shen et al. (Eds.): MICCAI 2019, LNCS 11767, pp. 356–364, 2019.
https://doi.org/10.1007/978-3-030-32251-9_39

Epistemic uncertainty can be assessed through the comparison of several samples obtained from stochastic neural networks. If the stochasticity is induced by dropout, the sampling approximates full Bayesian inference [1], which has been employed in image segmentation applications [2]. When training deep learning models, the stochasticity inherent in minibatching makes it possible to compare different models trained on the same training dataset: differing predictions of these models can be attributed to model uncertainty. A network can be trained to output diverse predictions from m 'heads' [3] coming from a common network trunk: the m heads' differences are, again, due to model uncertainty.

Heteroscedastic models of the noise uncertainty have been used in image super-resolution [4] and also exploited for spatially adaptive task loss weighting in multi-task learning [5]. However, these parametric methods are restricted to unimodal, symmetric distributions, which are not necessarily realistic. Test-time augmentation has been used to perturb the data and thus infer the uncertainty from the differences in predictions [6, 7]. In these approaches, the estimated uncertainty will depend wholly on the model's lack of invariance to the chosen augmentations: this may suggest that the models are undertrained or lacking capacity.

While decomposing errors may be useful, other solutions exist. **Predictive Intervals** (PIs) estimate a lower and upper bound for an observation, such that the observation falls inside these bounds some chosen (high) percentage of the time: for a 95% PI, we would expect 95 of 100 observations to lie within the interval. PIs should satisfy the following properties: (a) to be as small as possible, while (b) still enclosing the appropriate fraction of results. This can be enforced through the loss function [8]. In this work, we propose an extension of this method for application to counting tasks. We first describe different methods to perform counting tasks and assess uncertainty over measurements before presenting the loss function. We then describe the proposed amendment which is more flexible and stabler to train.

2   Methods

2.1   Uncertainty in Counting

The overall aim of this work is to compute a predictive interval that (a) minimises the interval width, whilst (b) ensuring that the interval contains the appropriate percentage of results. Here we introduce several techniques to count cells and associated methods to calculate predictive intervals. While they present a novel contribution in their own right, these methods of counting are introduced here as a baseline against the method proposed in Sect. 2.3. These baseline methods do not explicitly regress a predictive interval. Instead, we use the multiple outputs from the models (e.g. MC samples or M-heads) to sample predictions of count. Although we could simply use percentiles of these results to calculate intervals, these perform badly (the true count is often not within the obtained bounds). In order to mitigate this issue and introduce a fair comparison, the predictive intervals for each method below are calibrated post hoc following [9]: we transform the bounds affinely until they encompass a fraction $f > 1 - \alpha$ on the validation data. This transformation is then applied to the test-set estimates.

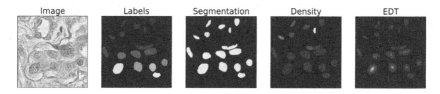

Fig. 1. An illustrative figure of the cell data. The image has ground-truth labels that we binarise for the segmentation targets. The density and Euclidean Distance Transform (EDT) are targets for regression.

Segmentation-Based: One counting method is to learn a segmentation of the input image and use connected-components analysis to determine the number of individual objects. To calculate uncertainty, we use three different approaches. We use Monte-Carlo samples of a network trained with dropout to produce N segmentation maps, counting the objects for each of the N. Secondly, we measure the number of objects at different thresholds of the output confidence map of the network. As the confidence threshold increases, fewer pixels will remain in the 'foreground' class. Finally, we also use M-heads [3], which produces M estimates of the segmentation with one forward pass of the network. This method produces a diverse mode-seeking ensemble, so higher variability in the heads may indicate that the model is more uncertain of the segmentation. For these methods, our target is the segmentation from Fig. 1.

Regressing the Euclidean Distance Transform: Naylor et al. [10] introduced a regression-based method for cell counting. Given an input image, the network learns to approximate the Euclidean Distance Transform of the cell segmentation maps (see Fig. 1). A non-maximum suppression is then used to count the cells. In order to calculate the uncertainty of the cell count, we use the MC-sampling paradigm described above, with a network with dropout trained.

Regressing the Pixel-Wise Cell Density: One popular technique for counting in computer-vision applications is to use a regression formulation to estimate a density-map from the raw image: summing over all pixels returns the count [11,12]. The density estimation function we use is a convolutional neural network. For these experiments, the ground truth density map has value 0 for background, and $\frac{1}{n_i}$ otherwise, where n_i is the number of pixels in the ith object. The network we use to estimate the density is a multi-task network with a shared backbone and two 'heads'. One head learns the segmentation while the other learns the density map. For uncertainty estimation, we use the M-heads paradigm to introduce variance in the output.

2.2 Distribution-Free Uncertainty Estimation

The previous examples all rely on sampling, followed by post-training calibration step which maps the sample uncertainty to the target predictive bounds. Conversely, the authors in [8] proposed to regress the predictive intervals directly from the data. They aim to estimate lower and upper confidence bounds for a desired quantity y, where b_l and b_u are the lower and upper bounds respectively. The hyper-parameter α determines the desired width of the interval: it is defined such that:

(i) $p\big(y \in [b_l, b_u]\big) = 1 - \alpha$, and
(ii) $p\big(y \in \cup\{(b_u, \infty], [-\infty, b_l)\}\big) = \alpha$.

Common choices for α include 0.10, 0.05 and 0.01, representing 90%, 95% and 99% confidence intervals respectively. In the original work, the authors propose a loss function $\mathcal{L}_{QD}$ to estimate 'Quality-Driven', distribution-free predictive intervals. For any given datapoint, x_i, the model returns b_{l_i} and b_{u_i}. For each input x_i we assess whether the observed corresponding datapoint y_i is in or out of the prediction bounds $[b_{l_i}, b_{u_i}]$. In order to provide useful information on the behaviour of the predictive interval estimates over multiple examples, the loss function is allowed to reason over an entire minibatch of size n. In this setup, an indicator variable is used to express if y_i within the predictive interval or not. The number of times y_i falls within the predictive interval is given by a binomial distribution Binomial$(n, (1 - \alpha))$, assuming i.i.d. data, which can be approximated by a normal distribution for large n. The loss, $\mathcal{L}_{QD}$, is then defined as the sum of a width term and the log-likelihood term.

$$\mathcal{L}_{QD} = \bar{W}_{captured} + \lambda \frac{n}{\alpha(1 - \alpha)} \max(0, (1 - \alpha) - q)^2 \tag{1}$$

where $\bar{W}_{captured}$ is the mean interval width for intervals that capture their associated ground truth, λ is a constant, n is the number in a batch, and q is the fraction of points that lie within their estimated predictive interval bounds.

2.3 Proposed Extension

In practice, we found $\mathcal{L}_{QD}$ difficult to optimise. We observed periodic instabilities in the training and attributed this, in part, to the one-sided nature of the second term; we sought to modify its formulation appropriately. With this in mind, let P_s be a discrete probability distribution function representing the probability of being 'in' or 'out' of the predicted interval, where the subscript s denotes 'state', i.e. $P_{in} = 1 - \alpha$, $P_{under} = \alpha/2$ and $P_{over} = \alpha/2$. For any minibatch, we define the observed proportions of 'over', 'under' and 'out' samples as Q_s, and use the Kullback-Leibler divergence (KL) to enforce similarities between the target P and the observed Q. With this framework, Q could be encouraged to match any desired distribution P (for instance, estimating several bounds to correspond to percentiles). Note that, in this proposed framework, and contrary to [8], P can represent any chosen distribution.

$$\mathcal{L}_{distribution} = KL(P||Q) = \sum_s P_s log\frac{P_s}{Q_s} = \sum_s \{P_s log(P_s) - P_s log(Q_s)\} \quad (2)$$

Since the target distribution P is constant, minimizing $L_{distribution}$ is identical to minimising the cross-entropy term with respect to the network weights; this means that we are simply promoting that the proportion of inliers in a given minibatch matches our desired distribution. As this loss function uses the categorical membership of the y_i to estimate Q, a soft membership function is used to make this operation differentiable and hence suitable for back-propagation.

We calculate the proportion inside the bounds as $Q_{in,soft} = \sigma\left(\xi\left(\mathbf{y} - \mathbf{b_l}\right)\right) \odot \sigma\left(\xi\left(\mathbf{b_u} - \mathbf{y}\right)\right)$. The minibatch of ground truth counts $\mathbf{y}$ is compared with the regressed bounds, $\mathbf{b_l}$ and $\mathbf{b_u}$, with σ representing the sigmoid function and ξ being a positive softening constant (set to $\xi = 2$). This formulation of the soft boundaries is as in [8], with the other soft memberships (over, under) being set analogously.

Our proposed loss is given by:

$$\mathcal{L}_{proposed} = \bar{W}_{captured} + \lambda \sum_s P_s log(Q_s) \quad (3)$$

In short, instead of using a one-sided data likelihood term, we used the cross-entropy calculated between the chosen P and Q. This reformulation has not only added flexibility, allowing for different state chosen P distributions, but we also found it easier to train than the model in Eq. 1.

2.4 Network Architectures and Implementation Details

The U-Net [13] forms the basis of all of our CNNs. The multi-task network has a U-Net backbone with the same parameters as for the single-task approaches. It then splits into separate branches (one for segmentation and one for density prediction).

For the proposed method of uncertainty prediction, we fit a regression network with three output quantities. First, it outputs a 'predicted count' which is trained with an $\mathcal{L}_2$ loss. The other two quantities are the upper and lower bounds, for a given α. In our experiments we choose $\alpha = 0.1$, making them 90% intervals. The architecture was chosen to have residual blocks as part of the arm to avoid vanishing gradients.

Due to the complexity of our network, we train it in stages. First, we train the U-Net part on the segmentation and density tasks. We then freeze the weights and train the predictive intervals, with a batch size of 64: as discussed, a large batch size to estimate good batch-wise statistics. In our experiments, we set $\lambda = 30$. The auxiliary L_2 loss is set to 1e-3. We parametrise the outputs of the network as such: the estimate for the mean value has no final activation. The upper and lower residuals go through a softplus activation function and are then

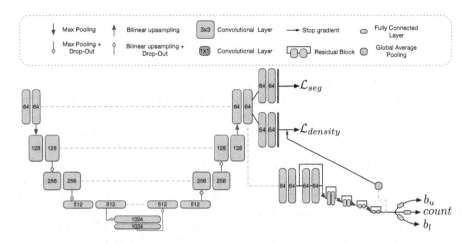

Fig. 2. Multi-task architecture for simultaneous segmentation and uncertainty prediction. All convolutions are 3×3 by the channel width, denoted in the diagram. The U-Net is complemented by an 'arm' which has residual blocks followed by max-pooling (maintaining 64 filters) until it reaches the output layer, where it returns an upper and lower bound. Dropout is enabled for methods that require MC-sampling where indicated in the diagram, with $p = 0.5$. The bounds are trained with the loss from Eq. 2.

added or subtracted, as appropriate, to the mean estimate. The segmentation has a sigmoid output, and the density a square function. Models are trained with early stopping as determined on the validation set, in NiftyNet [14].

2.5 Data

The proposed counting methods are applied to the counting of cells from histological slides [10]. This dataset has 33 labelled slides of dimension 512×512, taken from 7 different types of tissue, and each slide has an associated cell label map used here as the count ground truth. We separated this into 7 'test' images (21%), one from each cell type, and 4 'validation' images. To have larger batch sizes, we trained on images of size 256×256 and hence quartered each image while keeping the same fold label. Heavy augmentation is applied to the images in the training set (see figures in Supplementary Materials) using the 'imgaug' library [15].

We also fit to a white-matter hyperintensity (WMH) dataset [16]. In this task, we demonstrate a slightly different parameterisation of our bound prediction. We fitted an M-Heads model to the WMH segmentation and used the same model as a feature extractor to train the predictive bounds. In this data, of the 60 subjects, we used an 80/10/10 split for training/testing/validation respectively.

3   Results

We show the results in Table 1. All of the models exhibit good performance in counting, with the correlation between predicted and GT counts being above 0.8 for all models. The uncalibrated predictive intervals capture anything from 9% to 61% of the data. After calibrating these models, many achieved the correct percentage of inliers for the predictive intervals. Some (for example, the M-heads density regression with $f_{in} = 0.75$) did not: this may indicate that the calibration methods were overfitting (despite having few parameters—only an affine transformation). Our model predicted significantly smaller interval widths than for the baseline methods for both cells and lesions. While the baseline methods may seem to give large bounds, in the cases of cells, there may be a count of over 100 per image and in the lesions, up to 35. Because the EDT regression had the lowest MAE, we chose another, simple, baseline: we simply had a percentage count as the error. This method achieved a width of 18.6, compared to 12.20 (ours) in Fig. 3. It also does not capture the desired percentage of inliers, as it is too small. For the model fitted with $\mathcal{L}_{QD}$, we report the best results obtained after 3 independent model-fits, as we found the loss was unstable to fit—however, it still underperformed our proposed loss function.

Table 1. C_{EST} is the average estimated count. The ground truth counts were 25.71 for cells and 8.19 for lesions. MAE is the mean absolute error, $\pm$ standard deviation. ρ is the correlation coefficient between estimated and ground truth counts. f is the fraction of the ground truth points within the bounds and W is the mean width of the intervals—evaluated on both uncalibrated and calibrated intervals.

Method	Paradigm	C_{EST}	MAE $\pm$ STD	ρ	f_{uncal}	W_{uncal}	f_{cal}	W_{cal}
Segmentation	Thresholds	30.32	6.16 $\pm$ 5.43	0.90	0.61	15.33	0.86	23.42
	M-Heads	25.14	2.83 $\pm$ 3.34	0.95	0.46	2.80	0.96	102.22
	MC samples	31.36	6.70 $\pm$ 6.37	0.87	0.43	7.25	0.89	27.82
EDT regression	MC samples	26.16	2.85 $\pm$ 2.03	0.97	0.25	3.00	0.96	48.09
	% Errors	—	—		—	—	0.82	18.61
Density regression	M-Heads	26.42	3.53 $\pm$ 3.12	0.96	0.57	6.42	0.75	15.64
$\mathcal{L}_{QD}$	PI-estimate	26.01	3.04 $\pm$ 2.82	0.96	—	—	1.0	29.31
Ours	PI-estimate	26.23	2.93 $\pm$ 2.93	0.96	—	—	0.93	**12.20**
Lesions: segmentation	M-Heads	6.08	2.89 $\pm$ 2.96	0.83	0.09	0.63	0.96	24.1
Ours	PI-estimate	6.08	2.89 $\pm$ 2.96	0.83	—	—	0.89	**10.93**

4   Discussion

The aim of this work was to accurately predict intervals, such that they were of minimal width while containing the desired numbers of ground truth values. Our predictive bounds were over 20% smaller than the nearest competitor method while retaining the correct number of inliers; these smaller bounds are

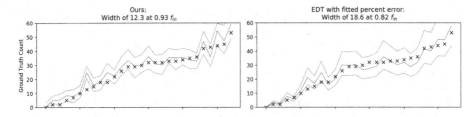

Fig. 3. Here we contrast our model (left) with the model with fitted percentage noise. The points represent the ground truths, and the lines represent the upper bound, mean and lower bound (note that the lines are for ease of visualisation: the x-axis is not continuous).

correspondingly more informative. We have demonstrated these results on a cell histology dataset and on WM lesions. For the cells, the next-best method was applying a constant percentage uncertainty to the counts of the EDT regression framework. Fitting this percentage is, in essence, optimising the same loss as we applied, but only using the predicted counts (and none of the image features). The fact that our model outperforms this baseline implies that the imaging features are being used to make an informed estimate of predictive error.

One limitation of this work is that it is not likely to generalise to samples drawn from outside of the training distribution. Domain-adaptation methods could help ameliorate this. It is also not an interpretable model and hence it would of interest to use model introspection methods to investigate how the network decides on its bounds. As the model we have presented can, in principle, be applied to any estimate derived from a machine-learning model, future work will investigate its applicability to 3D counting problems and a wider range of clinical biomarkers.

Acknowledgements. ZER is supported by the EPSRC Doctoral Prize. MJC & SO are supported by the Wellcome Flagship Programme (WT213038/Z/18/Z) and the Wellcome EPSRC CME (WT203148/Z/16/Z). We gratefully acknowledge NVIDIA Corporation for the donation of hardware.

References

1. Gal, Y., Ghahramani, Z.: Dropout as a Bayesian approximation: representing model uncertainty in deep learning. In: International Conference on Machine Learning, pp. 1050–1059 (2016)
2. Kendall, A., Badrinarayanan, V., Cipolla, R.: Bayesian SegNet: model uncertainty in deep convolutional encoder-decoder architectures for scene understanding. arXiv preprint arXiv:1511.02680 (2015)
3. Lee, S., Purushwalkam, S., Cogswell, M., Crandall, D., Batra, D.: Why M heads are better than one: training a diverse ensemble of deep networks. arXiv preprint arXiv:1511.06314 (2015)

4. Tanno, R., et al.: Bayesian image quality transfer with CNNs: exploring uncertainty in dMRI super-resolution. In: Descoteaux, M., Maier-Hein, L., Franz, A., Jannin, P., Collins, D.L., Duchesne, S. (eds.) MICCAI 2017. LNCS, vol. 10433, pp. 611–619. Springer, Cham (2017). https://doi.org/10.1007/978-3-319-66182-7_70
5. Bragman, F.J.S., et al.: Uncertainty in multitask learning: joint representations for probabilistic MR-only radiotherapy planning. In: Frangi, A.F., Schnabel, J.A., Davatzikos, C., Alberola-López, C., Fichtinger, G. (eds.) MICCAI 2018. LNCS, vol. 11073, pp. 3–11. Springer, Cham (2018). https://doi.org/10.1007/978-3-030-00937-3_1
6. Ayhan, M.S., Berens, P.: Test-time data augmentation for estimation of heteroscedastic aleatoric uncertainty in deep neural networks. In: MIDL (2018)
7. Wang, G., Li, W., Aertsen, M., Deprest, J., Ourselin, S., Vercauteren, T.: Aleatoric uncertainty estimation with test-time augmentation for medical image segmentation with convolutional neural networks. Neurocomputing 21, 34–45 (2019)
8. Pearce, T., Zaki, M., Brintrup, A., Neely, A.: High-quality prediction intervals for deep learning: a distribution-free, ensembled approach. arXiv preprint arXiv:1802.07167 (2018)
9. Eaton-Rosen, Z., Bragman, F., Bisdas, S., Ourselin, S., Cardoso, M.J.: Towards safe deep learning: accurately quantifying biomarker uncertainty in neural network predictions. In: Frangi, A.F., Schnabel, J.A., Davatzikos, C., Alberola-López, C., Fichtinger, G. (eds.) MICCAI 2018. LNCS, vol. 11070, pp. 691–699. Springer, Cham (2018). https://doi.org/10.1007/978-3-030-00928-1_78
10. Naylor, P., Laé, M., Reyal, F., Walter, T.: Segmentation of nuclei in histopathology images by deep regression of the distance map. IEEE Trans. Med. Imaging 38(2), 448–459 (2019)
11. Lempitsky, V., Zisserman, A.: Learning to count objects in images. In: Advances in neural information processing systems, pp. 1324–1332 (2010)
12. Xie, W., Noble, J.A., Zisserman, A.: Microscopy cell counting and detection with fully convolutional regression networks. Comput. Methods Biomech. Biomed. Eng. Imaging Vis. 6(3), 283–292 (2018)
13. Ronneberger, O., Fischer, P., Brox, T.: U-Net: convolutional networks for biomedical image segmentation. In: Navab, N., Hornegger, J., Wells, W.M., Frangi, A.F. (eds.) MICCAI 2015. LNCS, vol. 9351, pp. 234–241. Springer, Cham (2015). https://doi.org/10.1007/978-3-319-24574-4_28
14. Gibson, E., et al.: NiftyNet: a deep-learning platform for medical imaging. Comput. Methods Programs Biomed. 158, 113–122 (2018)
15. Jung, A.B.: imgaug. https://github.com/aleju/imgaug (2018)
16. Kuijf, H., et al.: Standardized assessment of automatic segmentation of white matter hyperintensities; results of the WMH segmentation challenge. IEEE Trans. Med. Imaging (2019, in press). https://www.ncbi.nlm.nih.gov/pubmed/30908194

Generalizable Feature Learning in the Presence of Data Bias and Domain Class Imbalance with Application to Skin Lesion Classification

Chris Yoon[1(✉)], Ghassan Hamarneh[2], and Rafeef Garbi[1]

[1] BiSICL, University of British Columbia, Vancouver, BC, Canada
yoon@alumni.ubc.ca, rafeef@ece.ubc.ca
[2] Medical Image Analysis Lab, Simon Fraser University, Burnaby, BC, Canada
hamarneh@sfu.ca

Abstract. Training generalizable data-driven models for medical imaging applications is especially challenging as acquiring and accessing sufficiently large medical datasets is often unfeasible. When trained on limited datasets, a high capacity model, as most leading neural network architectures are, is likely to overfit and thus generalize poorly to unseen data. Further aggravating the problem, data used to train models in medicine are typically collected in silos and from narrow data distributions that are determined by specific acquisition hardware, imaging protocols, and patient demographics. In addition, class imbalance within and across datasets is a common complication as disease conditions or subtypes have varying degrees of prevalence. In this paper, we motivate the need for generalizable training in the context of skin lesion classification by evaluating the performance of ResNet across 7 public datasets with dataset bias and class imbalance. To mitigate dataset bias, we extend the classification and contrastive semantic alignment (CCSA) loss that aims to learn domain-invariant features. As the CCSA loss requires labelled data from two domains, we propose a strategy to dynamically sample paired data in a setting where the set of available classes varies across domains. To encourage learning from underrepresented classes, the sampled class probabilities are used to weight the classification and alignment losses. Experimental results demonstrate improved generalizability as measured by the mean macro-average recall across the 7 datasets when training using the weighted CCSA loss and dynamic sampler.

1 Introduction

As deep learning pervades medical image computing, it is becoming critical to improve generalizability of deep neural networks (DNNs). Generalizability of such data-driven models is especially challenging in this field as availability and accessibility of large medical imaging datasets is usually strictly limited. Even when large datasets are available, medical conditions are diverse and unique

© Springer Nature Switzerland AG 2019
D. Shen et al. (Eds.): MICCAI 2019, LNCS 11767, pp. 365–373, 2019.
https://doi.org/10.1007/978-3-030-32251-9_40

with some having rare incidence, thus making the collection of comprehensive and representative data quite challenging. Privacy, security, and proprietary use regulations further complicate the aggregation and sharing of patient data. Additionally, data labelling costs by highly trained healthcare professionals are often prohibitive.

Medical image datasets used in research are also often collected in silos, sampled from narrow distributions determined by considerations such as imaging hardware (e.g., Siemens vs. Phillips MRI scanner), imaging protocol (e.g., choice of MRI pulse sequence, image resolution), and patient group bias (e.g., ethnicity, age). When trained on limited data, DNNs are likely to overfit due to their high capacity to learn irrelevant training data detail or noise. As such, when evaluated on new data with distribution shifts (e.g., change in patient ethnicity, scanning site), the overfit models perform poorly, failing to generalize to the new data.

We motivate generalizable training in the context of skin lesion classification where distribution shifts as well as inter and intra dataset class imbalance are prominent across 7 public datasets. In this setting, distribution shifts arise from the significant variability in photographic properties (e.g., camera resolution, angle, lighting), patient properties (e.g., skin tone, age, hairiness), and disease properties (e.g., location, disease stage). A number of convolutional neural network (CNN) architectures have been recently proposed for skin lesion classification. In a notably large scale study, Esteva et al. [4] trained Inception-v3 on 129,450 clinical dermatology images comprised of both public and private data. While this work reported performance measures comparable with dermatologists', the ability to aggregate extensive datasets is rare. In addition, even when training with extensive datasets, generalizable training may further improve performance by utilizing the notion of domains to learn more generalizable features. However, most generalizability methods [6,10,11,13,15] have been studied on data enjoying balanced classes within a domain (i.e., $P(class_i) \approx P(class_j)$), as well as having the same set of classes across domains. As with the 7 skin lesion datasets used in our work, this is often not the case in medical datasets, as certain conditions are more common than others.

In our work, we focus on a more realistic and common scenario where data is partitioned to multiple limited domains with inter and intra-domain class imbalance. We first expose and quantify poor generalizability of CNNs for skin lesion classification when trained on limited data by evaluating the performance of ResNet [8] architectures across the 7 public datasets. To improve generalizability, we extend the classification and constrastive semantic alignment (CCSA) loss [13] that encourages learning domain-invariant features to our class imbalanced setting. We chose to extend the CCSA loss for its simplicity to provide preliminary generalizability improvements in our setting. As the CCSA loss requires pairs of data from two domains, we propose a strategy to dynamically sample paired data, while considering the challenges arising from class imbalance such as unavailable classes. To encourage learning from underrepresented classes, we weight the CCSA loss by the sampled class probabilities. We evaluate our approach with varying amounts of training data available to demonstrate improved generalizability across different data assumptions.

2   Methods

Notation: Let $D_s = \{(x_i^s, y_i^s)\}$, $s \in \mathcal{S}$ denote the sth *source* domain where labelled samples $(x_i^s, y_i^s) \in (\mathcal{X}, \mathcal{Y})$ are realized from the domain distributions X^s and Y^s. Our goal is to train a classifier $f : \mathcal{X} \rightarrow \mathcal{Y}$ using source domains D_s that generalizes to a *target* domain realized from X^t and Y^t. Let $f = h \circ g$ be a composition of two function; $g : \mathcal{X} \rightarrow \mathcal{Z}$ is the mapping from the input space $\mathcal{X}$ to the feature space $\mathcal{Z}$ and $h : \mathcal{Z} \rightarrow \mathcal{Y}$ is the prediction function.

Summary of CCSA: The CCSA loss proposed by Motiian et al. [13] is defined as:

$$\mathcal{L}_{CCSA}(f) = \mathcal{L}_C(h \circ g) + \mathcal{L}_{SA}(g) + \mathcal{L}_S(g), \tag{1}$$

where $\mathcal{L}_C$ is a standard classification loss. For our multi-class classification task, we use the cross entropy loss. We evaluate the classification loss on data from both domains where

$$\mathcal{L}_C(h \circ g) = \mathcal{L}_{C1}(h \circ g) + \mathcal{L}_{C2}(h \circ g). \tag{2}$$

The semantic alignment loss, $\mathcal{L}_{SA}$, encourages features of the same class across two domains to map proximately in the feature space $\mathcal{Z}$, and is defined as:

$$\mathcal{L}_{SA}(g) = \sum_{a=1}^{C} d(p(g(X_a^s)), p(g(X_a^t))), \tag{3}$$

where C is the number of class labels, X_a^s is the domain distribution X^s for class a, $p(Z^s)$ is the probability distribution of embedded features in $\mathcal{Z}$, and d is a similarity metric between two distributions. In contrast, the separation loss, $\mathcal{L}_S$, encourages features of different classes across two domains to map distantly in the embedding space, and is defined as:

$$\mathcal{L}_S(g) = \sum_{a,b|a \neq b} k(p(g(X_a^s)), p(g(X_b^t))), \tag{4}$$

where k is a similarity metric that penalizes proximity between two distributions. When the paired data are from the same class ($y_1 = y_2$), Motiian et al. proposed

$$d(p(g(X_a^s)), p(g(X_a^t))) = \sum_{i,j} \|(g(x_i^s) - g(x_j^t)\|^2 \tag{5}$$

and when the paired data are from different classes ($y_1 \neq y_2$),

$$k(p(g(X_a^s)), p(g(X_b^t))) = \sum_{i,j} \max(0, m - \|(g(x_i^s) - g(x_j^t)\|)^2 \tag{6}$$

where m is the margin.

Dynamic Sampling: As the number of pairings grows quadratically with the size of the dataset, pairs are dynamically sampled. To ensure each image is sampled once per epoch, we set D_1 to be the aggregate of all the datasets. We then sample D_2 from the secondary domains with $P(D_s)$ set proportional to the size of the dataset N_s. With multiple classes, the probability of a positive match, $P(y_1 = y_2)$ for y_1, y_2 sampled from D_1 and D_2, becomes very small. In response, we follow the suggested strategy by Motiian et al. [13] by fixing the probability of positive matches to 0.25. After sampling (x_1, y_1) from D_1, with $P(y_1 = y_2) = 0.25$, we sample $(x_2, y_2 = y_1)$ from D_2. As we assume the presence of inter domain class imbalance, $P(x_2, y_2 = y_1)$ may be 0 when the second domain does not have class y_1. In such a case, we instead sample (x_2, y_2) from our primary dataset that contains all classes.

Weighted Loss: In the presence of class imbalance, the model may be biased towards predicting the more common classes, and in the extreme case, degenerate to predicting only the most probable classes. A possible solution is sampling each class with equal probability. However, we empirically observed slower convergence and worse performance with this strategy which is consistent with other works on training CNNs for skin lesion classification [5]. Therefore, given the dynamic sampling strategy, we propose weighting the classification losses $\mathcal{L}_{C_1}$ and $\mathcal{L}_{C_2}$ based on the probability of sampling classes c_i, c_j from D_1 and D_2, and weight the alignment losses based on the joint sampling probability $P(y_1 = c_i, y_2 = c_j)$ for every c_i, $c_j \in \mathcal{C}$, where $\mathcal{C}$ denotes the set of all classes. The sampled class probabilities can be computed directly based on the sampling policy or empirically by sampling for multiple epochs. We weight the losses by the inverse probability to encourage the model to learn from under-represented classes:

$$\mathcal{L}_C(class) = \frac{1}{P(y = class)}\mathcal{L}_C \tag{7}$$

$$\mathcal{L}_{CSA}(class_i, class_j) = \frac{1}{P(y_1 = class_i, y_2 = class_j)}\mathcal{L}_{CSA}. \tag{8}$$

3   Datasets and Implementation Details

We used 7 publicly available skin lesion datasets: HAM10000 [14], MSK [7], UDA [7], SONIC [7], Dermofit [1], Derm7pt [9], and PH2 [12]. Each dataset contained a subset of the following classes: melanocytic nevus (nv), melanoma (mel), basal cell carcinoma (bcc), dermatofibroma (df), benign keratosis (bkl), vascular lesion (vasc), and actinic keratosis (akiec). We partitioned each dataset into 50% training, 20% validation, and 30% test sets, where the relative class proportions were maintained across different partitions. HAM10000 was our primary dataset where the entire training data was accessible for all experiments. In HAM10000, in which the lesion IDs are known, we ensured that all images from the same lesion were in the same data partition. We removed data for classes beyond the 7 classes. Details regarding the class distribution is summarized in Table 1.

We implemented the weighted CCSA loss and dynamic sampler in PyTorch. When training the classifier, we used pretrained models available through PyTorch. We used AdamW with a base learning rate $= 10^{-4}$, weight decay $= 10^{-3}$, and batch size $= 32$. To simulate realistic training approaches, we augmented the data by resizing all images to 650×650, cropping the center 300×300, randomly resizing and cropping 224×224, and randomly flipping and rotating $[90°, 180°, 270°]$. We also used Cutout Regularization [3] with 1 cutout of size 64. The validation and test images were resized to 650×650 and the center 224×224 were cropped. We balanced the classification and alignment losses equally and used margin $m = 50$.

Table 1. Class distributions of the 7 public skin lesion datasets for the following 7 classes: melanocytic nevus (nv), melanoma (mel), basal cell carcinoma (bcc), dermatofibroma (df), benign keratosis (bkl), vascular lesion (vasc), and actinic keratosis (akiec).

	nv (%)	mel (%)	bcc (%)	df (%)	bkl (%)	vasc (%)	akiec (%)	total
HAM	6705 (67)	1113 (11)	514 (5.1)	115 (1.1)	1099 (11)	142 (1.4)	327 (3.3)	10015
DMF	331 (27)	76 (6.3)	239 (20)	65 (5.4)	257 (21)	121 (10)	123 (10)	1212
D7P	1150 (60)	504 (26)	82 (4.3)	40 (2.1)	90 (4.7)	58 (3.0)	0	1926
MSK	2241 (63)	826 (23)	32 (0.9)	452 (13)	0	0	0	3551
UDA	408 (68)	193 (32)	0	0	0	0	0	601
PH2	160 (80)	40 (20)	0	0	0	0	0	200
SON	9251 (100)	0	0	0	0	0	0	9251

4   Experiments and Results

Baselines: All models in the baseline experiments (Table 2. Exp $\mathcal{A}$–$\mathcal{E}$) were trained using only the cross-entropy loss for 135 epochs, starting with learning rate $= 10^{-4}$, reduced by a factor of 10 every 45 epochs. The best model was selected using the HAM10000 validation data. In Exp $\mathcal{A}$–$\mathcal{C}$, we train ResNet-18, ResNet-50, and ResNet-152 using only the HAM10000 dataset. The models performed well for the HAM10000 data with macro-average recall of at least 0.74, however, the scores across the other datasets were much worse, with macro-average recall lower than 0.10 in some cases. This result highlights the importance of generalizability in the training and validation of models for skin lesion classification and other medical imaging applications, as good performance in the training dataset may translate poorly to other datasets. We observe that larger models generalize more poorly, possibly due to having the capacity to overfit more to the training domain. For the remaining experiments, we train using ResNet-18.

Exp $\mathcal{D}$–$\mathcal{E}$ used additional n_{sec} samples per class across all datasets, with $n_{sec} = a$ and $n_{sec} = 5$. $n_{sec} = a$ refers to using the all samples per class. For experiments using additional data, the best model was selected based on the average validation score across only the datasets used for training. Even a few samples from each dataset greatly improved the scores, with a greater improvement when using more data.

CCSA: For the remaining experiments, we warm-start the model with the baseline model from Exp $\mathcal{A}$ and train for 20 epochs using the weighted CCSA loss, starting with learning rate $= 10^{-4}$, reduced by a factor of 10 after 10 epochs. As some data may be more useful than others, we use the same additional data in Exp $\mathcal{J}$ as in Exp $\mathcal{D}$. In addition, when incrementing n_{sec}, we append more samples to the existing n_{sec} dataset. Comparing Exp $\mathcal{E}$ and Exp $\mathcal{K}$ where $n_{sec} = a$, we observe improved scores across all datasets with an overall improvement from 64.9 to 71.2, suggesting generalizable training using separate domains may improve performance over aggregated training. As expected, using a smaller n_{sec} led to worse performance. However, even when we use a smaller $n_{sec} = 5$, comparing Exp $\mathcal{D}$ and Exp $\mathcal{J}$, we still observe an improvement from 57.4 to 63.6 when using generalizable training.

Weighting Ablations: In Exp $\mathcal{L}$–$\mathcal{N}$, we remove weighting the classification, alignment, or both losses. When compared to Exp $\mathcal{K}$, removing either loss lowered the performance with the greatest drop when both losses were removed.

Leave-1-Domain-Out: We evaluate domain generalizability by removing a secondary dataset from the additional data. We train using $n_{sec} = a$ and choose the best validations score using the remaining datasets. Scores for the removed datasets are reported with an asterisk in Exp $\mathcal{O}$–$\mathcal{T}$. Improvements to the removed domain appears to be dataset dependent. Compared to Exp $\mathcal{A}$, there are improvements in UDA, PH2, and D7P, similar performance in DMF and MSK, and even a drop in performance in SON.

Channel Pruning: Channel pruning, and model compression in general, is especially relevant as training lightweight models for mobile diagnostics can improve the accessibility and timeliness of skin lesion diagnosis. We use discrimination aware channel pruning [17] where channels are introduced until the difference in performance drops below a threshold. Compared to ResNet-18 with 11.1M parameters, the model pruned with threshold 1e−4 in Exp $\mathcal{U}$ used 8.5M parameters without an observable drop in performance. However, we observe that over-pruning may lead to a decay in performance in Exp $\mathcal{V}$, where the model pruned with threshold 1e−3 used 7.5M parameters.

Table 2. Experiments (Exp) are labeled $\mathcal{A}$–$\mathcal{V}$. ResNet (RN) architectures (Arch) were trained with the HAM data in addition to n_{sec} samples/class across other domains. $n_{sec} = a$ refers to all samples/class. Pr specifies the pruning threshold [17]. (–) denotes an unpruned model or an unused loss. Cl/Al refers to the classification/alignment losses, and can be (–), weighted (w) or unweighted (u).

	Experiment setup					Test dataset							
Exp	n_{sec}	Arch	*Cl*	*Al*	*Pr*	HAM	DMF	D7P	MSK	PH2	SON	UDA	*avg*
						Baselines							
$\mathcal{A}$	0	RN18	–	w	–	74.1	24.9	25.7	32.1	7.3	80.4	47.7	41.8
$\mathcal{B}$	0	RN50	–	w	–	75.6	26.3	27.8	28.3	9.4	53.6	43.8	37.8
$\mathcal{C}$	0	RN152	–	w	–	74.8	25.9	23.2	24.5	5.2	60.2	34.3	35.4
$\mathcal{D}$	5	RN18	–	w	–	71.9	52.4	41.6	46.5	61.5	70.5	57.5	57.4
$\mathcal{E}$	a	RN18	–	w	–	68.4	73.2	45.3	56.4	70.8	74.7	65.8	64.9
						CCSA w/Increasing n_{sec}							
$\mathcal{F}$	1	RN18	w	w	–	73.6	45.7	32.5	44.2	68.8	90.4	59.6	59.2
$\mathcal{G}$	2	RN18	w	w	–	75.0	48.7	36.2	41.8	71.9	96.2	64.4	62.0
$\mathcal{H}$	3	RN18	w	w	–	72.4	44.8	40.9	47.3	77.1	97.0	60.1	62.8
$\mathcal{I}$	4	RN18	w	w	–	74.0	54.6	40.6	43.9	68.8	94.5	60.0	62.3
$\mathcal{J}$	5	RN18	w	w	–	74.2	56.2	38.2	50.6	78.1	95.1	52.6	63.6
$\mathcal{K}$	a	RN18	w	w	–	72.3	74.3	44.4	58.9	82.3	99.6	66.7	71.2
						CCSA Weighting Ablations							
$\mathcal{L}$	a	RN18	u	w	–	68.8	67.1	37.8	54.6	69.8	99.9	68.7	66.7
$\mathcal{M}$	a	RN18	w	u	–	70.3	65.8	39.0	52.7	75.0	99.9	57.1	65.7
$\mathcal{N}$	a	RN18	u	u	–	59.1	54.5	32.4	43.8	69.8	100	57.6	59.6
						Leave-1-Domain-Out (* refers to the removed domain)							
$\mathcal{O}$	a	RN18	w	w	–	71.0	*27.0	48.3	60.0	82.3	99.9	58.6	63.9
$\mathcal{P}$	a	RN18	w	w	–	73.7	73.9	*33.7	58.1	72.9	99.5	64.1	68.0
$\mathcal{Q}$	a	RN18	w	w	–	71.1	75.6	43.9	*34.7	67.7	99.6	56.5	64.2
$\mathcal{R}$	a	RN18	w	w	–	71.8	73.0	48.5	60.9	*37.5	98.3	66.6	65.2
$\mathcal{S}$	a	RN18	w	w	–	73.9	73.9	49.8	61.5	64.6	*46.3	68.2	62.6
$\mathcal{T}$	a	RN18	w	w	–	70.1	75.2	45.5	55.6	76.0	99.5	*69.0	70.1
						Channel Pruning							
$\mathcal{U}$	a	RN18	w	w	1e–4	71.9	71.6	47.7	61.2	77.1	99.2	69.1	71.1
$\mathcal{V}$	a	RN18	w	w	1e–3	72.5	70.2	47.4	54.9	77.1	99.9	65.7	69.7

5 Discussion and Conclusion

In summary, we study generalizability in the context of skin lesion classification, which constitutes an ideal test-bed with multiple public heterogeneous datasets with inter and intra domain class imbalance. From our experiments, we affirm the importance of training and validating models to be generalizable across domains, which is critical in medical applications as incorrect predictions may lead to increased morbidity and mortality. Even when the performance in the trained domain is strong, the performance may be poor in domains unseen during training. Although additional data from each domain improves generalizability, training with the weighted CCSA loss shows greater improvements by better utilizing the additional data.

One limitation of our work is the imbalance in the overall sizes of each dataset. We think an interesting direction for future work is partitioning the domains into similar sizes based on semantics such as skin tone or resolution. We also found interpreting the results and isolating causal relationships in performance improvements to be challenging. Experimental results were sensitive to the experimental setup such as hyper-parameters and train/test partitioning policy. In addition, improvements may be due to a combination of the sampling policy and the alignment loss. We leave a more rigorous analysis to future work.

The intuition and motivation behind aligning features and dynamically sampling data are clear, and similar methods have been proposed in different contexts [2, 16]. Baur et al. [2] propose a similar alignment loss and dynamic sampler for multiple sclerosis lesion segmentation in a domain adaptation setting. While the core approach is similar, there are differences in the sampling policy arising from the unique nature of each problem such as missing classes. As the CCSA loss was chosen for simplicity, improvements, especially in the leave-1-out domain generalizability experiments, were modest. However, there are other methods that may provide greater improvements in generalizability [6,10,11,15]. This presents exciting opportunities for extending to settings with inter and intra domain class imbalance, improving the generalizability of models for problems such as skin lesion classification.

Acknowledgement. We thank NVIDIA for supporting our research through their GPU Grant Program by donating the GeForce Titan V used in this work.

References

1. Ballerini, L., Fisher, R., Aldridge, B., Rees, J.: A color and texture based hierarchical K-NN approach to the classification of non-melanoma skin lesions. In: Celebi, M., Schaefer, G. (eds.) Lecture Notes in Computational Vision and Biomechanics, vol. 6, pp. 63–86. Springer, Dordrecht (2013). https://doi.org/10.1007/978-94-007-5389-1_4
2. Baur, C., Albarqouni, S., Navab, N.: Semi-supervised deep learning for fully convolutional networks. In: MICCAI, pp. 311–319 (2017)
3. Devries, T., Taylor, G.W.: Improved regularization of convolutional neural networks with cutout. arXiv:abs/1708.04552 (2017)
4. Esteva, A., Kuprel, B., Novoa, R.A., Ko, J., Swetter, S.M., Blau, H.M., Thrun, S.: Dermatologist-level classification of skin cancer with deep neural networks. Nature **542**, 115–118 (2017)

5. Gessert, N., Sentker, T., Madesta, F., Schmitz, R., Kniep, H.C., Baltruschat, I.M., Werner, R., Schlaefer, A.: Skin lesion diagnosis using ensembles, unscaled multi-crop evaluation and loss weighting. arXiv:abs/1808.01694 (2018)
6. Ghifary, M., Kleijn, W.B., Zhang, M., Balduzzi, D.: Domain generalization for object recognition with multi-task autoencoders. In: ICCV, pp. 2551–2559 (2015)
7. Gutman, D., et al.: Skin lesion analysis toward melanoma detection: a challenge at the international symposium on biomedical imaging (ISBI) 2016, hosted by the international skin imaging collaboration (ISIC). arXiv:abs/1605.01397 (2016)
8. He, K., Zhang, X., Ren, S., Sun, J.: Deep residual learning for image recognition. In: CVPR, pp. 770–778 (2016)
9. Kawahara, J., Daneshvar, S., Argenziano, G., Hamarneh, G.: Seven-point checklist and skin lesion classification using multitask multimodal neural nets. IEEE J. Biomed. Health Inform. **23**(2), 538–546 (2019)
10. Li, D., Yang, Y., Song, Y.Z., Hospedales, T.M.: Learning to generalize: meta-learning for domain generalization. In: AAAI (2018)
11. Li, H., Pan, S.J., Wang, S., Kot, A.C.: Domain generalization with adversarial feature learning. In: CVPR, pp. 5400–5409 (2018)
12. Mendonca, T., Ferreira, P.M., Marques, J.S., Marcal, A.R., Rozeira, J.: PH2 - a dermoscopic image database for research and benchmarking. In: EMBS, pp. 5437–5440 (2013)
13. Motiian, S., Piccirilli, M., Adjeroh, D.A., Doretto, G.: Unified deep supervised domain adaptation and generalization. In: ICCV, pp. 5715–5725 (2017)
14. Tschandl, P., Rosendahl, C., Kittler, H.: The HAM10000 dataset, a large collection of multi-source dermatoscopic images of common pigmented skin lesions. Sci. Data **5**, 180161 (2018)
15. Tzeng, E., Hoffman, J., Saenko, K., Darrell, T.: Adversarial discriminative domain adaptation. In: CVPR, pp. 2962–2971 (2017)
16. Weston, J., Ratle, F., Mobahi, H., Collobert, R.: Deep learning via semi-supervised embedding. In: Montavon, G., Orr, G.B., Müller, K.-R. (eds.) Neural Networks: Tricks of the Trade. LNCS, vol. 7700, pp. 639–655. Springer, Heidelberg (2012). https://doi.org/10.1007/978-3-642-35289-8_34
17. Zhuang, Z., et al.: Discrimination-aware channel pruning for deep neural networks. In: NeurIPS, pp. 881–892 (2018)

Learning Task-Specific and Shared Representations in Medical Imaging

Felix J. S. Bragman[1,2]($\boxtimes$), Ryutaro Tanno[1,3,4], Sebastien Ourselin[2], Daniel C. Alexander[1,3], and M. Jorge Cardoso[2,1]

[1] Centre for Medical Image Computing, University College London, London, UK
f.bragman@ucl.ac.uk
[2] Artificial Medical Intelligence Group, Biomedical Engineering and Imaging Sciences, King's College London, London, UK
[3] Department of Computer Science, University College London, London, UK
[4] Machine Intelligence and Perception Group, Microsoft Research Cambridge, Cambridge, UK

Abstract. The performance of multi-task learning hinges on the design of feature sharing between tasks; a process which is combinatorial in the network depth and task count. Hand-crafting an architecture based on human intuitions of task relationships is therefore suboptimal. In this paper, we present a probabilistic approach to learning task-specific and shared representations in Convolutional Neural Networks (CNNs) for multi-task learning of semantic tasks. We introduce Stochastic Filter Groups; which is a mechanism that groups convolutional kernels into task-specific and shared groups to learn an optimal kernel allocation. They facilitate learning optimal shared and task specific representations. We employ variational inference to learn the posterior distribution over the possible grouping of kernels and CNN weights. Experiments on MRI-based prostate radiotherapy organ segmentation and CT synthesis demonstrate that the proposed method learns optimal task allocations that are inline with human-optimised networks whilst improving performance over competing baselines.

1 Introduction

The performance of predictive models is tied to the quality of the learned representations. This is important in medical image computing; where the learned low-dimensional embeddings [1] or features representing the spectrum of disease phenotypes [2] influence the utility of automated clinical tools. Multi-task learning (MTL) has been successful in medical image analysis [3,4] as it can enhance

---

F. J. S. Bragman and R. Tanno—Contributed equally.

Electronic supplementary material The online version of this chapter (https://doi.org/10.1007/978-3-030-32251-9_41) contains supplementary material, which is available to authorized users.

D. Shen et al. (Eds.): MICCAI 2019, LNCS 11767, pp. 374–383, 2019.
https://doi.org/10.1007/978-3-030-32251-9_41

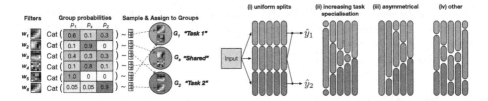

Fig. 1. (Left) Illustration of filter assignment in a SFG module. (Right) Possible grouping patterns learnable with the proposed method. The pink, green and blue blocks represent the ratio of filter groups G_1 (pink), G_s (green) and G_2 (blue), where (i) is the case a uniform kernel split, (ii) & (iii) where the networks becomes increasingly task-specific (iv) and an heterogeneous task split. (Color figure online)

learning efficiency and model performance by leveraging the inductive bias when jointly solving related tasks. [5]

A key factor for successful MTL models is the ability to determine when to share features within a network. A mechanism is needed to understand the commonalities and differences between tasks to effectively transfer information while optimising weights for individual tasks. The quality of this process is determined by the architectural design, where features or weights are either shared or task specific [6,7]. However, the space of possible architectures is combinatorially large whilst manual exploration of this space is inefficient and subject to bias on prior beliefs of task relationships. The number of kernels to allocate to each task or to a joint representation depends on the difficulty of individual tasks and the relationship between them [8]; neither of which are *a priori* known in most cases.

In an MTL setting, one would like to learn where to share network components across tasks to maximise performance. The main challenge lies in designing a mechanism that determines how and where to share CNN weights. There are broadly two categories for weight sharing in MTL networks. The first directly optimises weight sharing to maximise task-wise performance by learning a set a vectors that control which features are shared within a layer and how these are distributed across [6,7,9]. The second group of MTL methods focuses on weight clustering based on task-similarity, which can be performed by iteratively growing a tree-like deep architecture that clusters similar tasks hierarchically [10] or through maximising task's statistical dependency [11].

In this paper, we propose *Stochastic Filter Groups* (SFGs); a probabilistic mechanism that learns how to allocate kernels to task-specific and shared groups in each layer of MTL architectures (Fig. 1-Right). Specifically, the SFGs learn to allocate kernels in each convolutional layer into either "specialist" groups or a "shared" trunk, which are respectively specific to or shared across different tasks. The SFG equips the network with a mechanism to learn inter-layer connectivity and thus the structure of task-specific and shared representations. We evaluate the efficacy of SFGs on a joint semantic regression (i.e. image synthesis) and semantic segmentation (i.e. organ segmentation) problem applied to prostate data. Experiments show the proposed method achieves higher prediction accuracy than baselines with no mechanism to learn connectivity structures. Importantly, we also demonstrate that the learned representations are meaningful and specific towards each task.

2   Methods

We introduce a new approach for learning learn task-specific and shared representations in multi-task CNN architectures applied to medical imaging tasks i.e. modality transfer and organ segmentation. We propose *stochastic filter groups* (SFG), a probabilistic mechanism to partition kernels in each CNN layer into "specialist" groups or a "shared" group, which are specific to or shared across different tasks, respectively. We use variational inference to learn the distributions over the possible grouping of kernels and network weights that determines connectivity between layers and the shared and task-specific features. This naturally results in a learning algorithm that optimally allocates representation capacity across multi-tasks via gradient-based stochastic optimization.

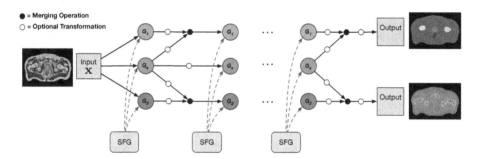

Fig. 2. Multi-task architecture based on SFG modules, where at each layer, kernels are stochastically assigned to task-specific and shared groups.

We consider the synthesis of a CT scan from MRI whilst simultaneously segmenting organs (Fig. 2). This is a significant challenge in MR-only radiotherapy treatment planning, which is attempting to eliminate CT acquisition for treatment planning. This is a complex task that can benefit from multi-task learning and disentangling anatomical rep)resentations since CT synthesis can exploit context from the segmentation whilst there are features specific to CT synthesis not necessarily useful for organ segmentation.

2.1   Stochastic Filter Groups

SFGs introduce a sparse connection structure into the architecture of CNN for multi-task learning to separate features into task-specific and shared components. Ioannou et al. [12] introduced *filter groups* to partition kernels in each convolution layer into groups, each of which acts only on a subset of the preceding features demonstrating that such sparsity reduces computational cost without compromising accuracy. We adapt the concept of filter groups to MTL and propose a mechanism for learning an optimal kernel grouping rather than pre-specifying them.

For simplicity, we describe SFGs for the case of two semantic tasks; image regression and object segmentation. At the lth convolution layer in a CNN architecture with K_l kernels $\{\mathbf{w}^{(l),k}\}_{k=1}^{K_l}$, the associated SFG performs two operations:

1 - Filter Assignment: each kernel $\mathbf{w}_k^{(l)}$ is stochastically assigned to either: (i) the "regression specific group" $G_{reg}^{(l)}$, (ii) "shared group" $G_s^{(l)}$ or (iii) "segmentation specific group" $G_{seg}^{(l)}$ with respective probabilities $\mathbf{p}^{(l),k} = [p_{reg}^{(l),k}, p_s^{(l),k}, p_{seg}^{(l),k}] \in [0,1]^3$. Convolving with the respective filter groups yields distinct sets of features $F_{reg}^{(l)}, F_s^{(l)}, F_{seg}^{(l)}$. Figure 1-Left illustrates this operation and Fig. 1-Right shows different learnable patterns.

2 - Feature Routing: the features $F_{reg}^{(l)}, F_s^{(l)}, F_{seg}^{(l)}$ are routed to the filter groups $G_{reg}^{(l+1)}, G_s^{(l+1)}, G_{seg}^{(l+1)}$ in the subsequent $(l+1)^{\text{th}}$ layer to respect the task-specificity and sharing of filter groups in the lth layer. Specifically, we perform the following routing for $l > 0$ where $F_{reg}^{(l+1)} = h^{(l+1)}([F_{reg}^{(l)}|F_s^{(l)}] * G_{reg}^{(l+1)})$, $F_s^{(l+1)} = h^{(l+1)}(F_s^{(l)} * G_s^{(l+1)})$, and $F_{seg}^{(l+1)} = h^{(l+1)}([F_{seg}^{(l)}|F_s^{(l)}] * G_{seg}^{(l+1)})$ and each $h^{(l+1)}$ defines the non-linear function, $*$ denotes convolution operation and $|$ denotes a merging operation of arrays (e.g. concatenation). At $l = 0$, input image $\mathbf{x}$ is simply convolved with the first set of filter groups to yield $F_i^{(1)} = h^{(1)}(\mathbf{x} * G_i^{(1)}), i \in \{reg, seg, s\}$.

Figure 2 provides a schematic of our architecture, in which each SFG module stochastically generates filter groups in each layer and the resultant features are sparsely routed as described above. The merging modules, denoted as black circles, combine the task-specific and shared features appropriately, i.e. $[F_i^{(l)}|F_s^{(l)}], i = reg, seg$ and pass them to the filter groups in the next layer. Each white circle denotes the presence of additional transformations (e.g. convolutions or fully connected layers) in each $h^{(l+1)}$, performed on top of the standard non-linearity (e.g. ReLU).

The proposed sparse connectivity is integral to ensure task performance and structured representations. In particular, one might argue that routing of "shared" features $F_s^{(l)}$ to the respective "task-specific" filter groups $G_{reg}^{(l+1)}$ and $G_{seg}^{(l+1)}$ is not necessary to ensure the separation of gradients across the task losses. However, this connection allows for learning more complex task-specific features at deeper layers in the network.

The varying dimensionality of feature maps is noteworthy. Specifically, the number of kernels in the respective filter groups $G_{reg}^{(l)}, G_s^{(l)}, G_{seg}^{(l)}$ can vary at each iteration of training, which influences the depth of the resultant feature maps $F_{reg}^{(l)}, F_s^{(l)}, F_{seg}^{(l)}$. To work with features maps of varying size, we implement the proposed architecture by defining $F_{reg}^{(l)}, F_s^{(l)}, F_{seg}^{(l)}$ as sparse tensors. At each SFG module, we first convolve the input features with all kernels, and generate the output features from each filter group by zeroing out the channels that root from the kernels in the other groups, resulting in $F_{reg}^{(l)}, F_s^{(l)}, F_{seg}^{(l)}$ that are sparse at non-overlapping channel indices. In the simplest form with no additional transformation (i.e. the grey circles in Fig. 2 are identity functions), we define the merging operation $[F_i^{(l)}|F_s^{(l)}], i = reg, seg$ as pixel-wise summation. In the presence of more complex transforms (e.g. residual blocks), we concatenate the output features in the channel-axis and perform a 1x1 convolution to ensure the number of channels in $[F_i^{(l)}|F_s^{(l)}]$ is the same as in $F_s^{(l)}$.

2.2   T + 1 Way "Drop-Out"

The CNN weights and grouping probabilities are simultaneously optimised by extending the variational interpretation of binary dropout [13] to the $(T+1)$-way assignment of each convolution kernel to the filter groups where T is the number of tasks. We consider the case $T = 2$ for CT synthesis and organ segmentation.

Suppose that the architecture consists of L SFG modules, each with K_l kernels where l is the index. As the posterior distribution over the convolution kernels in SFG modules $p(\mathcal{W}|\mathbf{X}, \mathbf{Y}^{(reg)}, \mathbf{Y}^{(seg)})$ is intractable, we approximate it with a simpler distribution $q_\phi(\mathcal{W})$ where $\mathcal{W} = \{\mathbf{w}^{(l),k}\}_{k=1,...,K_l,l=1,...,L}$. Assuming that the posterior distribution factorizes over layers and kernels up to group assignment, we defined the variational distribution as:

$$q_\phi(\mathcal{W}) = \prod_{l=1}^{L} \prod_{k=1}^{K_l} q_{\phi_{lk}}(\mathbf{w}^{(l),k}) = \prod_{l=1}^{L} \prod_{k=1}^{K_l} q_{\phi_{lk}}(\mathbf{w}_{reg}^{(l),k}, \mathbf{w}_s^{(l),k}, \mathbf{w}_{seg}^{(l),k})$$

where $\{\mathbf{w}_{reg}^{(l),k}, \mathbf{w}_s^{(l),k}, \mathbf{w}_{seg}^{(l),k}\}$ denotes the kth kernel in l^{th} layer after routing into task-specific $G_{reg}^{(l)}, G_{seg}^{(l)}$ and shared $G_s^{(l)}$ groups. Each $q_{\phi_{lk}}(\mathbf{w}_{reg}^{(l),k}, \mathbf{w}_{seg}^{(l),k}, \mathbf{w}_s^{(l),k})$ is defined as $\mathbf{w}_i^{(l),k} = z_i^{(l),k} \cdot \mathbf{w}^{(l),k}$ for $i \in \{reg, s, seg\}$, where $\mathbf{z}^{(l),k} = [z_{reg}^{(l),k}, z_{seg}^{(l),k}, z_s^{(l),k}] \sim \text{Cat}(\mathbf{p}^{(l),k})$. Here, $\mathbf{z}^{(l),k}$ is the sample one-hot encoding from the Categorical distribution over filter group assignments. The variational parameters ϕ_{lk} consists of pre-grouping convolution kernels $\mathbf{w}^{(l),k}$ and grouping probabilities $\mathbf{p}^{(l),k} = [p_{reg}^{(l),k}, p_s^{(l),k}, p_{seg}^{(l),k}]$.

We minimize the KL divergence between the approximate posterior $q_\phi(\mathcal{W})$ and $p(\mathcal{W}|\mathbf{X}, \mathbf{Y}^{(reg)}, \mathbf{Y}^{(seg)})$. Assuming likelihood factorisation over the two tasks, we have the following objective $\mathcal{L}_{MC}(\phi) = -\frac{N}{M} \sum_{i=1}^{M} \left[\log p(y_i^{(reg)}|\mathbf{x}_i, \mathcal{W}_i) + \log p(y_i^{(seg)}|\mathbf{x}_i, \mathcal{W}_i)\right] + \sum_{l=1}^{L} \sum_{k=1}^{K_l} \text{KL}(q_{\phi_{lk}}(\mathbf{w}^{(l),k})||p(\mathbf{w}^{(l),k}))$, where M is the size of the mini-batch, N is the total number of training data points, and $\mathcal{W}_i$ denotes a set of model parameters sampled from $q_\phi(\mathcal{W})$. The last KL term regularizes the deviation of the approximate posterior from the prior $p(\mathbf{w}^{(l),k}) = \mathcal{N}(0, \mathbf{I}/l^2)$ where $l > 0$. Adapting the approximation presented in [13] to our scenario, we obtain:

$$\text{KL}(q_{\phi_{lk}}(\mathbf{w}^{(l),k})||p(\mathbf{w}^{(l),k})) \propto \frac{l^2}{2}||\mathbf{w}^{(l),k}||_2^2 - \mathcal{H}(\mathbf{p}^{(l),k}) \tag{1}$$

where $\mathcal{H}(\mathbf{p}^{(l),k}) = -\sum_{i \in \{reg,seg,s\}} p_i^{(l),k} \log p_i^{(l),k}$ is the entropy of grouping probabilities. The first term performs the L2-weight norm and the second term pulls the grouping probabilities towards the uniform distribution. The overall loss is defined as:

$$\mathcal{L}_{MC}(\phi) = -\frac{N}{M} \sum_{i=1}^{M} \left[\log p\left(y_i^{(1)} | \mathbf{x}_i, \mathcal{W}_i\right) + \log p\left(y_i^{(2)} | \mathbf{x}_i, \mathcal{W}_i\right) \right]$$

$$+\lambda_1 \cdot \sum_{l=1}^{L} \sum_{k=1}^{K_l} ||\mathbf{w}^{(l),k}||_2^2 - \lambda_2 \cdot \sum_{l=1}^{L} \sum_{k=1}^{K_l} \mathcal{H}(\mathbf{p}^{(l),k}) \qquad (2)$$

where $\lambda_1 > 0, \lambda_2 > 0$ are regularization coefficients.

The discrete sampling operation during filter group assignment creates discontinuities, giving the first term in the objective function (Eq. 2) zero gradient with respect to the grouping probabilities $\{\mathbf{p}^{(l),k}\}$. We approximate each of the categorical variables $\text{Cat}(\mathbf{p}^{(l),k})$ by the Gumbel-Softmax distribution, $\text{GSM}(\mathbf{p}^{(l),k}, \tau)$ [14], a continuous relaxation which allows for sampling, differentiable with respect to the parameters $\mathbf{p}^{(l),k}$. The temperature term τ adjusts the bias-variance tradeoff of gradient approximation; as the value of τ approaches 0, samples from the GSM distribution become one-hot. while the variance of the gradients increases. We start at a high τ and anneal to a small but non-zero value as in [13].

3   Experiments

We tested *stochastic filter groups* (SFG) on the problem of simultaneous semantic image regression (synthesis) and segmentation on a prostate radiotherapy dataset. In radiotherapy treatment planning, a CT scan is necessary to allow dose propagation whilst an MRI is required for segmenting organs at risk of ionisation. Instead of acquiring both an MRI and a CT, algorithms can be used to synthesise a CT scan (task 1) and segment organs (task 2) given a single input MRI scan. We acquired 15 3D prostate cancer scans with respective CT and T2-weighted MRI scans with semantic 3D labels for organs (prostate, bladder, rectum and left/right femur heads) obtained from a trained radiologist. We created a training set of 10 patients, with the remaining 5 used for testing. We trained our networks on 2D slices; reconstructing the 3D volumes through patch aggregation.

Baselines: We compared our model against four baselines. They are: (1) single-task networks, (2) hard-parameter sharing multi-task network (MT-hard sharing), (3) SFG-networks with constant $1/3$ allocated grouping (MT-constant mask) as *per* Fig. 1-Right, and (4) SFG-networks with constant grouping probabilities (MT-constant **p**). We note that all four baselines can be considered special cases of the proposed SFG-network: single task networks have SFG shared grouping probability of kernels set to zero; *hard-parameter sharing networks* exists when all shared grouping probabilities are set to 'shared' up until the task-specific

Table 1. Model performance with best results in bold blue, and the second best results in red. Standard deviations are computed over the test subject cohort and shown in brackets.

(a) CT Synthesis (PSNR)

Method	Overall	Bones	Organs	Prostate	Bladder	Rectum
One-task (HighResNet) [15]	25.76 (0.80)	30.35 (0.58)	38.04 (0.94)	51.38 (0.79)	33.34 (0.83)	34.19 (0.31)
MT-hard sharing	26.31 (0.76)	31.25 (0.61)	39.19 (0.98)	52.93 (0.95)	34.12 (0.82)	34.15 (0.30)
MT-constant mask	24.43(0.57)	29.10(0.46)	37.24(0.86)	50.48(0.73)	32.29(1.01)	33.44(2.88)
MT-constant $\mathbf{p}$=[$^1/_3$,$^1/_3$,$^1/_3$]	26.64(0.54)	31.05 (0.55)	39.11 (1.00)	**53.20 (0.86)**	34.34 (1.35)	35.61 (0.35)
MT-SFG (ours)	**27.74 (0.96)**	**32.29 (0.59)**	**39.93 (1.09)**	53.01 (1.06)	**35.65 (0.44)**	**35.65 (0.37)**

(b) Segmentation (DICE)

Method	Overall	Left Femur Head	Right Femur Head	Prostate	Bladder	Rectum
One-task (HighResNet) [15]	0.848(0.024)	0.931 (0.012)	**0.917 (0.013)**	0.913 (0.013)	0.739 (0.060)	0.741 (0.011)
MT-hard sharing	0.829(0.023)	**0.933 (0.009)**	0.889 (0.044)	0.904 (0.016)	0.685 (0.036)	0.732 (0.014)
MT-constant mask	0.774(0.065)	0.908 (0.012)	0.911 (0.015)	0.806 (0.0541)	0.583 (0.178)	0.662 (0.019)
MT-constant $\mathbf{p}$=[$^1/_3$,$^1/_3$,$^1/_3$]	0.752(0.056)	0.917 (0.004)	0.917 (0.01)	0.729 (0.086)	0.560 (0.180)	0.639 (0.012)
MT-SFG (ours)	**0.852 (0.047)**	**0.935 (0.007)**	0.912 (0.013)	**0.923 (0.016)**	**0.750 (0.062)**	**0.758 (0.011)**

layers; and *MT-constant* $\boldsymbol{p}$ represents the situation where the grouping is non-informative and each kernel has equal probability of being specific or shared with probability $\mathbf{p}^{(l),k} = [^1/_3, ^1/_3, ^1/_3]$. We used HighResNet [15] as the baseline for CT synthesis and organ segmentation. In our model, we replace each convolutional layer with an SFG module. After the first SFG layer, three distinct repeated residual blocks are applied to $F_{reg}^{(l=0)}$, $F_{seg}^{(l=0)}$, $F_{s}^{(l=0)}$. These are then merged according to the feature routing methodology followed by a new SFG-layer and subsequent residual layers. Our model concludes with 2 successive SFG-layers followed by 1x1 convolutional layers applied to the merged features $F_{reg}^{(l=L)}$ and $F_{seg}^{(l=L)}$. Additional information on training details and dynamics can be found in the supplementary.

Results on CT synthesis and organ segmentation aredetailed in Table 1. Our method performed best overall in organ segmentation. Our method also obtained best synthesis performance across most anatomical regions; especially in the bone regions when compared against all the baselines. The bone voxel intensities are the most difficult to synthesise from an input MR scan as task uncertainty in the MR to CT mapping at the bone is often highest [3]. Our model was able to disentangle features specific to the bone intensity mapping (Fig. 3-Right) without supervision of the pelvic location, which allowed it to learn a more accurate mapping of an intrinsically difficult task.

3.1   Learned Architectures

Analysis of the grouping probabilities allows visualisation of network connectivity and the learned MTL architecture. To analyse the group allocation of kernels at each layer, we computed the sum of class-wise probabilities per layer. Learned grouping allocations are presented in presented in Fig. 3-Left. This illustrates increasing task specialisation in the kernels with network depth. At the first layer, all kernels are classified as shared ($\mathbf{p} = [0, 1, 0]$) as low-order features such as edge or contrast descriptors are generally learned earlier layers. In deeper layers, higher-order representations are learned, which describe various salient features specific to the tasks. This coincides with our network allocating kernels as task specific, as illustrated in Fig. 3. Notably, the learned connectivity of both models shows striking similarities to hard-parameter sharing architectures commonly used in MTL, where there is a set of shared layers aiming to learn a feature set common to both tasks. Task-specific branches then learn a mapping from this feature space for task-specific predictions. Our model learns this structure whilst allowing asymmetric allocation of task-specific kernels with no priors on network structure.

4   Discussion

We have proposed *stochastic filter groups* (SFGs) to disentangle *task-specific* and *generalist* features. SFGs define the grouping of kernels and the connectivity of features in a CNN. We used variational inference to estimate the distribution over connectivity given training data and sample over possible architectures during training. Our method can be considered as a probabilistic form of multi-task architecture search, as the learned posterior embodies the desired MTL architecture given the data.

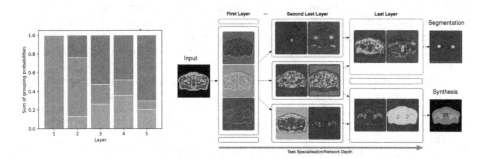

Fig. 3. (Left) Learned kernel grouping with 'CT synthesis', shared and 'organ segmentation' task allocations shown in blue, green and pink; (Right) Activation maps from low entropy (high "confidence") kernels in the learned task-specific and shared filter groups. (Color figure online)

The concept of disentangling features is important within medical image analysis where the goal is to develop automated tools of clinical utility. There is significant variability in human anatomy whilst many disease phenotypes are prevalent across multiple diseases. Our method offers the possibility to learn shared anatomical and pathological features common across the spectrum of health and disease whilst learning phenotype-specific features. Given a problem where one task consists of tumour segmentation and the second is subtype classification, the shared representation would represent anatomical information important across tasks whilst the subtype latent space may encode information specific across subtypes that can be investigated further for clinical research.

Our method can be exploited for transfer learning. Data scarcity is an issue in medical imaging where labelled data is expensive to acquire. Shared and task-specific representations can be learned on larger datasets and transferred to a new MTL problem with asymmetry in labelled data across tasks. This will be investigated in future work.

Acknowledgements. FB and MJC were supported by CRUK Grant A21993. RT was supported by Microsoft Scholarship. DA was supported by EU Horizon 2020 Research and Innovation Grant 666992, EPSRC Grant M020533, R014019, and R006032, and the NIHR UCLH BRC. We thank NVIDIA Corporation for hardware donation.

References

1. Singla, S., Gong, M., Ravanbakhsh, S., Sciurba, F., Poczos, B., Batmanghelich, K.N.: Subject2Vec: generative-discriminative approach from a set of image patches to a vector. In: Frangi, A.F., Schnabel, J.A., Davatzikos, C., Alberola-López, C., Fichtinger, G. (eds.) MICCAI 2018. LNCS, vol. 11070, pp. 502–510. Springer, Cham (2018). https://doi.org/10.1007/978-3-030-00928-1_57

2. Esteva, A., et al.: Dermatologist-level classification of skin cancer with deep neural networks. Nature **542**, 115–118 (2017)

3. Bragman, F., et al.: Uncertainty in multitask learning: joint representations for probabilistic MR-only radiotherapy planning. In: Frangi, A.F., Schnabel, J.A., Davatzikos, C., Alberola-López, C., Fichtinger, G. (eds.) MICCAI 2018. LNCS, vol. 11073, pp. 3–11. Springer, Cham (2018). https://doi.org/10.1007/978-3-030-00937-3_1

4. Tanno, R., et al.: AutoDVT: joint real-time classification for vein compressibility analysis in deep vein thrombosis ultrasound diagnostics. In: Frangi, A.F., Schnabel, J.A., Davatzikos, C., Alberola-López, C., Fichtinger, G. (eds.) MICCAI 2018. LNCS, vol. 11071, pp. 905–912. Springer, Cham (2018). https://doi.org/10.1007/978-3-030-00934-2_100

5. Caruana, R.: Multitask learning. Mach. Learn. **28**(1), 41–75 (1997)

6. Meyerson, E., Miikkulainen, R.: Beyond shared hierarchies: deep multitask learning through soft layer ordering. In: ICLR (2018)

7. Misra, I., Shrivastava, A., Gupta, A., Hebert, M.: Cross-stitch networks for multi-task learning. In: CVPR (2016)

8. Zamir, A.R., Sax, A., Shen, W.B., Guibas, L.J., Malik, J., Savarese, S.: Taskonomy: disentangling task transfer learning. In: CVPR, IEEE (2018)

9. Ruder, S., Bingel, J., Augenstein, I., Søgaard, A.: Latent multi-task architecture learning (2019)

10. Lu, Y., Kumar, A., Zhai, S., Cheng, Y., Javidi, T., Feris, R.S.: Fully-adaptive feature sharing in multi-task networks with applications in person attribute classification. In: CVPR (2017)

11. Mejjati, Y.A., Cosker, D., In Kim, K.: Multi-task learning by maximizing statistical dependence. In: CVPR (2018)
12. Ioannou, Y., Robertson, D., Cipolla, R., Criminisi, A., et al.: Deep roots: improving CNN efficiency with hierarchical filter groups (2017)
13. Gal, Y., Hron, J., Kendall, A.: Concrete dropout. In: NIPS, pp. 3581–3590 (2017)
14. Jang, E., Gu, S., Poole, B.: Categorical reparameterization with gumbel-softmax. arXiv preprint arXiv:1611.01144 (2016)
15. Li, W., Wang, G., Fidon, L., Ourselin, S., Cardoso, M.J., Vercauteren, T.: On the compactness, efficiency, and representation of 3D convolutional networks: brain parcellation as a pretext task (2017)

Models Genesis: Generic Autodidactic Models for 3D Medical Image Analysis

Zongwei Zhou[1], Vatsal Sodha[1], Md Mahfuzur Rahman Siddiquee[1],
Ruibin Feng[1], Nima Tajbakhsh[1], Michael B. Gotway[2], and Jianming Liang[1]([✉])

[1] Arizona State University, Scottsdale, AZ 85259, USA
{zongweiz,vasodha,mrahmans,rfeng12,ntajbakh,jianming.liang}@asu.edu
[2] Mayo Clinic, Scottsdale, AZ 85259, USA
Gotway.Michael@mayo.edu

Abstract. Transfer learning from *natural* image to *medical* image has established as one of the most practical paradigms in deep learning for medical image analysis. However, to fit this paradigm, 3D imaging tasks in the most prominent imaging modalities (*e.g.*, CT and MRI) have to be reformulated and solved in 2D, losing rich 3D anatomical information and inevitably compromising the performance. To overcome this limitation, we have built a set of models, called Generic Autodidactic Models, nicknamed Models Genesis, because they are created *ex nihilo* (with no manual labeling), self-taught (learned by self-supervision), and generic (served as source models for generating application-specific target models). Our extensive experiments demonstrate that our Models Genesis significantly outperform learning from scratch in all five target 3D applications covering both segmentation and classification. More importantly, learning a model from scratch simply in 3D may not necessarily yield performance better than transfer learning from ImageNet in 2D, but our Models Genesis consistently top any 2D approaches including fine-tuning the models pre-trained from ImageNet as well as fine-tuning the 2D versions of our Models Genesis, confirming the importance of 3D anatomical information and significance of our Models Genesis for 3D medical imaging. This performance is attributed to our unified self-supervised learning framework, built on a simple yet powerful observation: the sophisticated yet recurrent anatomy in medical images can serve as strong supervision signals for deep models to learn common anatomical representation automatically via self-supervision. As open science, all pre-trained Models Genesis are available at https://github.com/MrGiovanni/ModelsGenesis.

1 Introduction

Given the marked differences between *natural* images and *medical* images, we hypothesize that transfer learning can yield more powerful (application-specific)

Electronic supplementary material The online version of this chapter (https://doi.org/10.1007/978-3-030-32251-9_42) contains supplementary material, which is available to authorized users.

D. Shen et al. (Eds.): MICCAI 2019, LNCS 11767, pp. 384–393, 2019.
https://doi.org/10.1007/978-3-030-32251-9_42

Table 1. Target tasks.

Code[a]	Object	Modality	Source	Description
NCC	Lung nodule	CT	LUNA2016	Lung nodule false positive reduction
NCS	Lung nodule	CT	LIDC-IDRI	Lung nodule segmentation
ECC	Pulmonary embolism	CT	PE-CAD	Pulmonary embolism false positive reduction
LCS	Liver	CT	LiTS2017	Liver segmentation
DXC	Pulmonary diseases	X-ray	ChestX-ray8	Eight pulmonary diseases classification
IUC	CIMT RoI	Ultrasound	UFL MCAEL	RoI, bulb, and background classification
BMS	Brain tumor	MRI	BraTS2013	Brain tumor segmentation

[a] The first letter denotes the object of interest ("N" for lung nodule, "E" for pulmonary embolism, "L" for liver, etc.); the second letter denotes the modality ("C" for CT, "X" for X-ray, "U" for Ultrasound, etc.); the last letter denotes the task ("C" for classification, "S" for segmentation).

target models if the *source* models are built directly from medical images. To test this hypothesis, we have chosen chest imaging because the chest contains several critical organs, which are prone to a number of diseases that result in substantial morbidity and mortality and thus are associated with significant health-care costs. In this research, we focus on Chest CT, because of its prominent role in diagnosing lung diseases, and our research community has accumulated several Chest CT image databases, for instance, LIDC-IDRI[1] and NLST[2], containing a large number of Chest CT images. Therefore, we seek to answer the following question: *Can we utilize the large number of available Chest CT images without systematic annotation to train source models that can yield high-performance target models via transfer learning?*

To answer this question, we have developed a framework that trains generic, source models for 3D imaging. We call the models trained with our framework Generic Autodidactic Models, nicknamed Models Genesis, and refer to the model trained using Chest CT scans as Genesis Chest CT. As ablation studies, we have also trained a downgraded 2D version using 2D Chest CT slices, called Genesis Chest CT 2D. To demonstrate the effectiveness of Models Genesis in 2D applications, we have trained a 2D model based on ChestX-ray8[3], named as Genesis Chest X-ray.

Our extensive experiments detailed in Sect. 3 demonstrate that Models Genesis, including Genesis Chest CT, Genesis Chest CT 2D, and Genesis Chest X-ray, *significantly* outperform learning from scratch in all seven target tasks (see Table 1). As revealed in Table 4, learning from scratch simply in 3D may *not* necessarily yield performance better than fine-tuning state-of-the-art Ima-

---

[1] https://wiki.cancerimagingarchive.net/display/Public/LIDC-IDRI.

[2] https://biometry.nci.nih.gov/cdas/nlst/.

[3] https://nihcc.app.box.com/v/ChestXray-NIHCC.

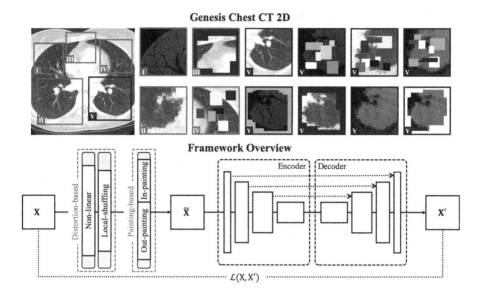

Fig. 1. Our unified self-supervised learning framework consolidates four novel transformations: (I) non-linear, (II) local-shuffling, (III) out-painting, and (IV) in-painting into a single image restoration task. Specifically, each arbitrarily-size patch X cropped at random location from an unlabeled image can undergo at most three of above transformations, resulting in a transformed patch X̃ (see I–V). Note that out-painting and in-painting are mutually exclusive. For simplicity and clarity, we illustrate our idea on a 2D CT slice, but our Genesis Chest CT is trained using 3D images directly. A Model Genesis, an encoder-decoder architecture, is trained to learn a common visual representation by restoring the original patch X (as ground truth) from the transformed one X̃ (as input), aiming to yield high-performance target models.

geNet models, but our Genesis Chest CT *consistently* top any 2D approaches including fine-tuning ImageNet models as well as fine-tuning our Genesis Chest X-ray and Genesis Chest CT 2D, confirming the importance of 3D anatomical information in Chest CT and significance of our self-supervised learning method in 3D medical image analysis.

This performance is attributable to the following key observation: medical imaging protocols typically focus on particular parts of the body for specific clinical purposes, resulting in images of similar anatomy. The sophisticated yet recurrent anatomy offers consistent patterns for self-supervised learning to discover common representation of a particular body part (the lungs in our case). The fundamental idea behind our unified self-supervised learning method as illustrated in Fig. 1 is to recover anatomical patterns from images transformed via various ways in a unified framework.

2 Models Genesis

Models Genesis learn from scratch on unlabeled images, with an objective to yield a common visual representation that is generalizable and transferable across diseases, organs, and modalities. In Models Genesis, an encoder-decoder, as shown in Fig. 1, is trained using a series of self-supervised schemes. Once trained, the encoder alone can be fine-tuned for target classification tasks; while the encoder and decoder together can be for target segmentation tasks. For clarity, we formally define a *training scheme* as the process that transforms patches with any of the transformations, as illustrated in Fig. 1, and trains a model to restore the original patches from the transformed counterparts. In the following, we first explain each of our self-supervised learning schemes with its learning objectives and perspectives, followed by a summary of the four unique properties of our Models Genesis. Along the way, we also contrast Models Genesis with existing approaches to show our **innovations** and **novelties**.

- **Learning appearance via non-linear transformation.** Absolute or relative intensity values in medical images convey important information about the imaged structures and organs. For instance, the Hounsfield Units in CT scans correspond to specific substances of the human body. As such, intensity information can be used as a strong source of pixel-wise supervision. To preserve relative intensity information of anatomies during image transformation, we use Bézier Curve, a smooth and monotonous transformation function, which assigns every pixel a unique value, ensuring a one-to-one mapping. Restoring image patches distorted with non-linear transformation focuses Models Genesis on learning organ appearance (shape and intensity distribution). Fig. 1–I shows examples of the transformed images. Due to limited space, we provide the implementation details in Appendix[4] Sect. B.

- **Learning texture via local pixel shuffling.** Given an original patch, local pixel shuffling consists of sampling a random window from the patch followed by shuffling the order of contained pixels resulting in a transformed patch. The size of the local window determines the task difficulty, but we keep it smaller than the model's receptive field, and also small enough to prevent changing the global content of the image. Note that our method is quite different from PatchShuffling [5], which is a regularization technique to avoid over-fitting. To recover from local pixel shuffling, Models Genesis must memorize local boundaries and texture. Examples of local-shuffling are illustrated in Fig. 1–II. We include the underlying mathematics and implementation details in Appendix (See footnote 4) Sect. C.

- **Learning context via out-painting and in-painting.** To realize the self-supervised learning via out-painting, we generate an arbitrary number of windows of various sizes and aspect ratios, and superimpose them on top of each other, resulting in a single window of a complex shape. We then assign a random value to all pixels outside the window while retaining the original intensities for the pixels within. As for in-painting, we retain the original

---

[4] Appendix can be found in the full version at tinyurl.com/ModelsGenesisFullVersion.

intensities outside the window and replace the intensity values of the inner pixels with a constant value. Unlike [6], where in-painting is proposed as a proxy task by restoring only the patch central region, we restore the entire patch in the output. Out-painting compels Models Genesis to learn global geometry and spatial layout of organs via extrapolating, while in-painting requires Models Genesis to appreciate local continuities of organs via interpolating. Examples of out-painting and in-painting are shown in Fig. 1–III and Fig. 1–IV, respectively. More visualizations can be found in Appendix (See footnote 4) Sects. D—E.

Models Genesis have the following four unique properties:

(1) Autodidactic—requiring no manual labeling. Models Genesis are trained in a self-supervised manner with abundant unlabeled image datasets, demanding *zero* expert annotation effort. Consequently, Models Genesis are very different from traditional *supervised* transfer learning from ImageNet [7,9], which offers modest benefit to 3D medical imaging applications as well as that from the pre-trained models of NiftyNet[5], which is ineffective (see Sect. 3 and Appendix (See footnote 4) Sect. I) due to the small datasets and specific applications (*e.g.,* brain parcellation and organ segmentation) these models are trained for.

(2) Eclectic—learning from multiple perspectives. Our unified approach trains Models Genesis from multiple perspectives (appearance, texture, context, etc.), leading to more robust models across all target tasks, as evidenced in Table 3, where our unified approach is compared with our individual schemes. This eclectic approach, incorporating multiple tasks into a single image restoration task, empowers Models Genesis to learn more comprehensive representation.

(3) Scalable—eliminating proxy-task-specific heads. Consolidated into a single image restoration task, our novel self-supervised schemes share the same encoder and decoder during training. Had each task required its own decoder, due to limited memory on GPUs, our framework would have failed to accommodate a large number of self-supervised tasks. By unifying all tasks as a single image restoration task, any favorable transformation can be easily amended into our framework, overcoming the scalability issue associated with multi-task learning [2], where the network heads are subject to the specific proxy tasks.

(4) Generic—yielding diverse applications. Models Genesis learn a general-purpose image representation that can be leveraged for a wide range of target tasks. Specifically, Models Genesis can be utilized to initialize the encoder for the target *classification* tasks and to initialize the encoder-decoder for the target *segmentation* tasks, while the existing self-supervised approaches are largely focused on providing encoder models only [4]. As shown in Table 2, Models Genesis can be generalized across diseases (*e.g.,* nodule, embolism, tumor), organs (*e.g.,* lung, liver, brain), and modalities (*e.g.,* CT, X-ray, MRI), a generic behavior that sets us apart from all previous works in the literature where the representation is learned via a specific self-supervised task; and thus lack generality. Such specific schemes include predicting the distance and 3D coordinates of two patches

---

[5] NiftyNet Model Zoo: https://github.com/NifTK/NiftyNetModelZoo.

randomly sampled from a same brain [8], identifying whether two scans belong to the same person, predicting the level of vertebral bodies [3], and finally the systematic study by Tajbakhsh *et al.* [10] where individualized self-supervised schemes are studied for a set of target tasks.

3   Experiments and Results

Experiment Protocol. Our Genesis CT and Genesis X-ray are self-supervised pre-trained from 534 CT scans in LIDC-IDRI (See footnote 1) and 77,074 X-rays in ChestX-ray8(See footnote 3), respectively. The reason that we decided not to use all images in LIDC-IDRI and in ChestX-ray8 for training Models Genesis is to avoid test-image leaks between proxy and target tasks, so that we can confidently use the rest images solely for testing Models Genesis as well as the target models, although Models Genesis are trained from *only* unlabeled images, involving *no* annotation shipped with the datasets. We evaluate Models Genesis in seven medical imaging applications including 3D and 2D image classification and segmentation tasks (codified as detailed in Table 1). For 3D applications in CT and MRI, we investigate the capability of both 2D slice-based solutions and 3D volume-based solutions; for 2D applications in X-ray and Ultrasound, we compare Models Genesis with random initialization and fine-tuning from ImageNet. 3D U-Net architecture[6] is used in five 3D applications; U-Net architecture with ResNet-18 encoder[7] is used in seven 2D applications. We utilize the L1-norm distance as the loss function in the image restoration tasks. Performances of target image classification and segmentation tasks are measured by the AUC (Area Under the Curve) and IoU (Intersection over Union), respectively, through at least 10 trials. We report the performance metrics with mean and standard deviation and further present statistical analysis based on the independent two-sample t-test.

Models Genesis Outperform 3D Models Trained from Scratch. We evaluate the effectiveness of Genesis Chest CT in five distinct 3D medical target tasks. These target tasks are selected such that they show varying levels of semantic distance to the proxy task, as shown in Table 2, allowing us to investigate the transferability of Genesis Chest CT with respect to the domain distance. Table 2 demonstrates that models fine-tuned from Genesis Chest CT consistently outperform their counterparts trained from scratch. Our statistical analysis show that the performance gain is significant for all the target tasks under study. Specifically, for NCC and NCS where the target and proxy tasks are in the same domain, initialization with Genesis Chest CT achieves 4 and 3 points increase in the AUC and IoU score, respectively, compared with training from scratch. For ECC, the target and proxy tasks are different in both the disease affecting the organ and the dataset itself; yet, Genesis Chest CT achieves a remarkable improvement over training from scratch, increasing the AUC by

---

[6] 3D U-Net Convolution Neural Network: https://github.com/ellisdg/3DUnetCNN.
[7] Segmentation Models: https://github.com/qubvel/segmentation_models.

Table 2. Fine-tuning models from our Genesis Chest CT (3D) significantly outper-forms learning from scratch in the five 3D target tasks ($p < 0.05$). The cells checked by ✗ denote the properties that are different between the proxy and target datasets. Our results show that our Genesis Chest CT generalizes across organs, diseases, datasets, and modalities. Footnotes show state-of-the-art performance for each target task.

Task	Metric	Disease	Organ	Dataset	Modality	Scratch (%)	Genesis (%)	p-value
NCC[a]	AUC					94.25 ± 5.07	$\mathbf{98.20 \pm 0.51}$	0.0180
NCS[b]	IoU					74.05 ± 1.97	$\mathbf{77.62 \pm 0.64}$	1.04e–4
ECC[c]	AUC	✗		✗		79.99 ± 8.06	$\mathbf{88.04 \pm 1.40}$	0.0058
LCS[d]	IoU	✗	✗	✗		74.60 ± 4.57	$\mathbf{79.52 \pm 4.77}$	0.0361
BMS[e]	IoU	✗	✗	✗	✗	90.16 ± 0.41	$\mathbf{90.60 \pm 0.20}$	0.0041

[a] LUNA winner holds an official score of 0.968 vs. 0.971 (ours)
[b] Wu *et al.* holds a Dice of 74.05% vs. 75.86% $\pm$ 0.90% (ours)
[c] Zhou *et al.* holds an AUC of 87.06% vs. 88.04% $\pm$ 1.40% (ours)
[d] LiTS winner w/postprocessing (PP) holds a Dice of 96.60% vs. 91.13% $\pm$ 1.51% (ours w/o PP)
[e] BraTS winner w/ensembling holds a Dice of 91.00% vs. 92.58% $\pm$ 0.30% (ours w/o ensembling)

Table 3. Comparison between our unified framework and each of the suggested self-supervised schemes on five 3D target tasks. The statistical analyses is conducted between the top-2 models in each column highlighted in bold and italic. While there is no clear winner, our unified framework is more robust across all target tasks, yielding either the best result or comparable performance to the best model ($p > 0.05$).

Approach	NCC (%)	NCS (%)	ECC (%)	LCS (%)	BMS (%)
Scratch	94.25 ± 5.07	74.05 ± 1.97	79.99 ± 8.06	74.60 ± 4.57	90.16 ± 0.41
Distortion (ours)	96.46 ± 1.03	$\mathit{77.08 \pm 0.68}$	$\mathbf{88.04 \pm 1.40}$	$\mathit{79.08 \pm 4.26}$	$\mathbf{90.60 \pm 0.20}$
Painting (ours)	$\mathbf{98.20 \pm 0.51}$	77.02 ± 0.58	87.18 ± 2.72	78.62 ± 4.05	90.46 ± 0.21
Unified (ours)	$\mathit{97.90 \pm 0.57}$	$\mathbf{77.62 \pm 0.64}$	$\mathit{87.20 \pm 2.87}$	$\mathbf{79.52 \pm 4.77}$	$\mathit{90.59 \pm 0.21}$
p-value	0.0848	0.0520	0.2102	0.4249	0.4276

8 points. Genesis Chest CT continues to yield significant IoU gain for LCS and BMS even though their domain distances with the proxy task are the widest. To our knowledge, we are the first to investigate cross-domain self-supervised learn-ing in medical imaging. Given the fact that Genesis Chest CT is pre-trained on Check CT only, it is *remarkable* that our model can generalize to different diseases, organs, datasets, and even modalities.

Models Genesis Consistently Top any 2D Approaches. A common tech-nique to handle limited data in medical imaging is to reformat 3D data into a 2D image representation followed by fine-tuning pre-trained ImageNet models [7,9]. This approach increases the training examples by an order of magnitude, but it scarifies the 3D context. It is interesting to compare how Genesis Chest CT compares to this *de facto* standard in 2D. For this purpose, we adopt the trained 2D models from an ImageNet pre-trained model[7] for the tasks of NCC, NCS, and ECC. The 2D representation is obtained by extracting axial slices from volumet-ric datasets. Table 4 compares the results for 2D and 3D models. Note that the

Table 4. Comparison between 3D solutions and 2D slice-based solutions on three 3D target tasks. Training 3D models from scratch does not necessarily outperform the 2D counterparts (see NCC). However, training the same 3D models from Genesis Check CT outperforms ($p < 0.05$) all 2D solutions, demonstrating the effectiveness of Genesis Chest CT in unlocking the power of 3D models.

Task	2D (%)			3D (%)			p-value[a]
	Scratch	ImageNet	Genesis	Scratch	ImageNet	Genesis	
NCC	96.03 ± 0.86	97.79 ± 0.71	97.45 ± 0.61	94.25 ± 5.07	N/A	98.20 ± 0.51	0.0213
NCS	70.48 ± 1.07	72.39 ± 0.77	72.20 ± 0.67	74.05 ± 1.97	N/A	77.62 ± 0.64	$<1e{-}8$
ECC	71.27 ± 4.64	78.61 ± 3.73	78.58 ± 3.67	79.99 ± 8.06	N/A	88.04 ± 1.40	$5.50e{-}4$

[a]These p-values are calculated between our Models Genesis vs. the fine-tuning from ImageNet, which always offers the best performance for all three tasks in 2D.

results for 3D models are identical to those reported in Table 2. As evidenced by our statistical analyses, the 3D models trained from Genesis Chest CT significantly outperform the 2D models trained from ImageNet, achieving higher average performance and lower standard deviation (see Table 4 and Appendix (See footnote 4) Sect. H). However, the same conclusion does not apply to the models trained from scratch —3D scratch models outperform 2D scratch models in only two out of the three target tasks and also exhibit undesirably larger standard deviation. We attribute the mixed results of 3D scratch models to the larger number of model parameters and limited sample size in the target tasks, which together impede the full utilization of 3D context. In fact, the undesirable performance of the 3D scratch models highlights the effectiveness of Genesis Chest CT, which unlocks the power of 3D models for medical imaging.

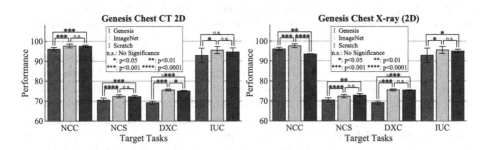

Fig. 2. Comparison of 2D solutions on four 2D target tasks. To investigate the same- and cross-domain transferability of Models Genesis, we have trained Genesis Chest CT 2D using 2D axial slices from LUNA dataset (left panel), and Genesis Chest X-ray (2D) trained using radiographs from ChestX-ray8 dataset (right panel). In same-domain target tasks (NCC and NCS in the left panel and DXC in the right panel), Models Genesis 2D outperform training from scratch and offer equivalent performance to fine-tuning from ImageNet. While in cross-domain target tasks (DXC and IUC in the left panel; NCS and IUC in the right panel), Models Genesis 2D also produce fairly robust performance.

Models Genesis (2D) Offer Equivalent Performances to Supervised Pre-trained Models. To compare our self-supervised approaches with those supervised pre-training from ImageNet [1], we deliberately downgrade our Models Genesis to 2D versions: Genesis Chest CT 2D and Genesis Chest X-ray (2D) (see visualization of Genesis 2D in Appendix (See footnote 4) Sects. F—G). The statistical analysis in Fig. 2 suggests that the downgraded Models Genesis 2D offer equivalent performance to state-of-the-art fine-tuning from ImageNet within modality, outperforming random initialization by a large margin, which is a significant achievement because ours comes at *zero* annotation cost. Meanwhile, the downgraded Models Genesis 2D are fairly robust in cross-domain transfer learning, although they tend to underperform when domain distance is large, which suggests same-domain transfer learning should be preferred where possible in medical imaging. For 3D applications, we also examine the effectiveness of fine-tuning from NiftyNet (See footnote 5), which is not designed for transfer learning but is the only available supervised pre-trained 3D model. Compared with training from scratch, fine-tuning NiftyNet suffers 3.37, 0.18, and 0.03 points decrease for NCS, LCS, and BMS tasks, respectively (detailed in Appendix (See footnote 4) Sect. I), suggesting that strong supervision with limited annotated data cannot guarantee good transferability like ImageNet. Conversely, Models Genesis benefit from both large scale unlabeled datasets and dedicated proxy tasks which are essential for learning general-purpose visual representation.

4   Conclusion and Future Work

A key contribution of ours is a collection of *generic source* models, nicknamed Models Genesis, built directly from *unlabeled* 3D image data with our novel unified self-supervised method, for generating powerful application-specific *target* models through transfer learning. While our empirical results are strong, surpassing state-of-the-art performances in most of the applications, an important future work is to extend our Models Genesis to modality-oriented models, such as Genesis MRI and Genesis Ultrasound, as well as organ-oriented models, such as Genesis Brain and Genesis Heart. In fact, we envision that Models Genesis may serve as a primary source of transfer learning for 3D medical imaging applications, in particular, with limited annotated data. To benefit the research community, we make the development of Models Genesis open science, releasing our codes and models to the public, and inviting researchers around the world to contribute to this effort. We hope that our collective efforts will lead to the Holy Grail of Models Genesis, effective across diseases, organs, and modalities.

Acknowledgments. This research has been supported partially by ASU and Mayo Clinic through a Seed Grant and an Innovation Grant, and partially by NIH under Award Number R01HL128785. The content is solely the responsibility of the authors and does not necessarily represent the official views of NIH.

References

1. Deng, J., et al.: ImageNet: A large-scale hierarchical image database. In: CVPR, 248–255 (2009)
2. Doersch, C., et al.: Multi-task self-supervised visual learning. In: ICCV **2051–2060**, (2017)
3. Jamaludin, A., Kadir, T., Zisserman, A.: Self-supervised learning for spinal MRIs. In: Cardoso, M.J., et al. (eds.) DLMIA/ML-CDS -2017. LNCS, vol. 10553, pp. 294–302. Springer, Cham (2017). https://doi.org/10.1007/978-3-319-67558-9_34
4. Jing, L., et al.: Self-supervised visual feature learning with deep neural networks: A survey. arXiv:1902.06162 (2019)
5. Kang, G., et al.: Patchshuffle regularization. arXiv:1707.07103 (2017)
6. Pathak, D., et al.: Context encoders: Feature learning by inpainting. In: CVPR, 2536–2544 (2016)
7. Shin, H.C., et al.: Deep convolutional neural networks for computer-aided detection: CNN architectures, dataset characteristics and transfer learning. TMI **35**(5), 1285–1298 (2016)
8. Spitzer, H., et al.: Improving cytoarchitectonic segmentation of human brain areas with self-supervised siamese networks. In: MICCAI, 663–671 (2018)
9. Tajbakhsh, N., et al.: Convolutional neural networks for medical image analysis: Full training or fine tuning? TMI **35**(5), 1299–1312 (2016)
10. Tajbakhsh, N., et al.: Surrogate supervision for medical image analysis: Effective deep learning from limited quantities of labeled data. In: ISBI, 1251–1255 (2019)

Efficient Ultrasound Image Analysis Models with Sonographer Gaze Assisted Distillation

Arijit Patra[✉], Yifan Cai, Pierre Chatelain, Harshita Sharma, Lior Drukker, Aris T. Papageorghiou, and J. Alison Noble

University of Oxford, Oxford OX3 7DQ, UK
{arijit.patra,yifan.cai}@eng.ox.ac.uk

Abstract. Recent automated medical image analysis methods have attained state-of-the-art performance but have relied on memory and compute-intensive deep learning models. Reducing model size without significant loss in performance metrics is crucial for time and memory-efficient automated image-based decision-making. Traditional deep learning based image analysis only uses expert knowledge in the form of manual annotations. Recently, there has been interest in introducing other forms of expert knowledge into deep learning architecture design. This is the approach considered in the paper where we propose to combine ultrasound video with point-of-gaze tracked for expert sonographers as they scan to train memory-efficient ultrasound image analysis models. Specifically we develop teacher-student knowledge transfer models for the exemplar task of frame classification for the fetal abdomen, head, and femur. The best performing memory-efficient models attain performance within 5% of conventional models that are 1000× larger in size.

Keywords: Model compression · Gaze tracking · Expert knowledge

1 Introduction

Current deep models for medical image analysis are recognized as having large memory footprints and inference costs, which are at odds with the increased focus on portability and low-resource usage [1]. While there have been studies on overparameterization of deep networks [2], efficient models have largely been defined empirically rather than using well-principled approaches. In this paper we explore efficient models using a combination of video and expert knowledge, defined by gaze tracking as a sonographer acquires an ultrasound (US) video.

A. Patra and Y. Cai—Both authors contributed equally.

Electronic supplementary material The online version of this chapter (https://doi.org/10.1007/978-3-030-32251-9_43) contains supplementary material, which is available to authorized users.

© Springer Nature Switzerland AG 2019
D. Shen et al. (Eds.): MICCAI 2019, LNCS 11767, pp. 394–402, 2019.
https://doi.org/10.1007/978-3-030-32251-9_43

We propose a novel approach called Perception and Transfer for Reduced Architectures (PeTRA), a teacher-student knowledge transfer framework in which human expert knowledge is combined with ultrasound video frames as input to a large *teacher* model, whose output and intermediate feature maps are used to condition compact *student* models. We define a compact model as one that has a significantly reduced number of parameters and lower memory requirement compared to state-of-the-art models. Our objective is to achieve competitive accuracies with such compact models for our ultrasound image analysis task.

Related Work. Model compression (or reduction) is a challenge in machine learning research due to both the interest in addressing over-parameterization [2] and for practical usage with reasonable computational resources. Model compression can be achieved through *pruning*, which consists in removing parameters based on feature importance [3]. However, pruning leads to compact models that are a sub-graph of the original model architecture, which unnecessarily constrains the architecture of the compact model. Knowledge transfer methods have been proposed that can transfer knowledge to an arbitrary compact model. Hinton et al. [4] introduce the concept of teacher-student knowledge distillation, which they define as a transfer of knowledge from the final layer of the large model to a compact model during the training of the latter. Romero et al. [5] extend the idea of knowledge transfer to include intermediate learnt feature maps in the training of the compact model as well. While model compression and teacher-student knowledge transfer have been studied in machine learning research, relatively few works deploy both concepts in ultrasound imaging settings despite research into ultrasound video understanding in terms of identification of standard fetal cardiac planes [6] and anatomy motion localisation [7] among others. Overcoming parameter redundancy is important to medical imaging as time required for diagnosis depends on model inference speeds, and memory footprint of algorithms come at the expense of storage space for other critical data. In a relevant study, [8] classify standard views in adult echocardiography by training traditional large deep learning models and use the method in [4] to train reduced versions of these models. In relation to using human knowledge in ultrasound video analysis, a related work concerns combining sonographer gaze and ultrasound video for fetal abdominal standard plane classification and gaze prediction [9]. Different from [8,9], we use a combination of distillation and intermediate feature adaptation along with human gaze priors for a fetal ultrasound anatomy classification task. Unlike [8], we do not use compact models derived from heavier models but those specifically proposed for low-compute situations.

Contributions. We propose a framework, Perception and Transfer for Reduced Architectures (PeTRA) which combines model knowledge transfer and expert knowledge cues. Our contributions are: (1) to train compact models using both final and intermediate knowledge distillation from large models for the exemplar task of anatomy classification of fetal abdomen, head, and femur frames from a free-hand fetal ultrasound sequence; (2) to incorporate sonographer knowledge in

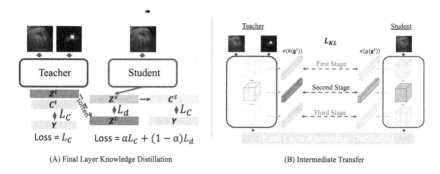

(A) Final Layer Knowledge Distillation   (B) Intermediate Transfer

Fig. 1. Schematic of our proposed knowledge-distillation pipeline. (A) Final layer knowledge distillation (B) Intermediate transfer. (Color figure online)

the form of gaze tracking data into a teacher model to enhance knowledge transfer. To our knowledge, this is the first attempt at model compression leveraging human visual attention with a teacher-student knowledge transfer approach.

2   Methods

Consider a K-class classification problem, which consists in finding the label $k \in [|1, K|]$ for an input $\mathbf{x}$. The output of a neural network can take the form $\mathbf{c} = \text{softmax}(\mathbf{z}) \in \mathbb{R}^K$, where $\mathbf{z} = f(\mathbf{x}) \in \mathbb{R}^K$ is the raw output of the last layer, or *logits*. We use a one-hot encoding for the classification target, such that, for a class $k \in [|1, K|]$, the corresponding target is $\mathbf{y} = (y_i)_1^K$ with $y_k = 1$ and $\forall i : i \neq k, y_i = 0$. The most commonly used loss function for multi-class classification is the categorical cross-entropy

$$L_c(\mathbf{y}, \mathbf{c}) = -\sum_{i=1}^{K} y_i \log c_i. \tag{1}$$

2.1   Knowledge Transfer

Let $\mathcal{T}$ be a large *teacher* model and $\mathcal{S}$ a smaller *student* model. Model compression by knowledge transfer, first introduced in [10], consists in using the representations learnt by $\mathcal{T}$ to guide the training of $\mathcal{S}$ (Fig. 1). The key principle is that it is easier to learn using the representation of the teacher than it is to learn from the original input in the first place.

Final Layer Knowledge Distillation. Let $\mathbf{z}^t$ and $\mathbf{z}^s$ be the logits of the final layer of $\mathcal{T}$ and $\mathcal{S}$, respectively. Following [4], we first incorporate teacher knowledge by adding a distillation loss to the cross-entropy loss as:

$$L = \alpha L_c + \beta L_d \tag{2}$$

where L_c is the cross-entropy loss defined in Eq. (1),

$$L_d = - \sum_{i=1}^{K} \text{softmax} \left(\frac{z_i^s}{E} \right) \log \left(\text{softmax} \left(\frac{z_i^t}{E} \right) \right) \tag{3}$$

is the distillation loss between teacher and student, and α, $\beta > 0$ are hyperparameters controlling the relative influence of both terms. E is a *temperature* term introduced by [4] as a form of relaxation to *soften* $\mathbf{z}^t$ and $\mathbf{z}^s$. Indeed, having been obtained by a cross-entropy objective in $\mathcal{T}$, $\mathbf{z}^t$ may be too close to the one-hot target vector $\mathbf{y}$. Softening provides more information about the relative similarity of classes rather than absolute maxima.

Intermediate Transfer (IT). To leverage knowledge contained in intermediate representations of the teacher model, we consider intermediate knowledge transfer, or *hint learning* [5], in conjunction with final layer knowledge distillation. Let $\mathbf{g}^t$ be the output of an intermediate layer of the teacher model. It is used to produce a *hint* $\sigma(h(\mathbf{g}^t))$, where σ is a sigmoid activation function and h is a fully-connected (FC) layer. Similarly, an intermediate layer of the student model (a *guided* layer) is used to produce a regularization output $\sigma(g(\mathbf{g}^s))$, where g is a FC layer with the same output dimension as h. The hint is used to train the guided layer with a Kullback-Leibler (KL) loss

$$L_{\text{KL}} = - \sum_j \sigma(g(\mathbf{g}^s))_j \log \left(\frac{\sigma(h(\mathbf{g}^t))_j}{\sigma(g(\mathbf{g}^s))_j} \right) \tag{4}$$

This creates a teacher model FC layer or *arm* (in purple, Fig. 1(B)) whose logits are associated with the student model FC *arm* (in orange, Fig. 1(B))in a KL divergence objective aimed at optimizing learned intermediate representations in the student model by supervising them with corresponding teacher model values (Fig. 1). Intermediate transfer essentially implements a regularization of the student learning using the most attentive intermediate features from the teacher. It is added to the optimization objective in Eq. (2) in training:

$$L = \alpha L_c + \beta L_d + \gamma L_{\text{KL}}, \tag{5}$$

where $\gamma > 0$ is a hyperparameter controlling the influence of IT.

After training, the FC arm is truncated. Resulting models have the same number of parameters as in the final layer knowledge distillation case, but with improved knowledge transfer from the teacher through intermediate layers.

2.2   Learning from Human Knowledge

We model the visual attention of a human expert looking at an image $\mathbf{I}$ through a gaze map $\mathbf{G}$. $\mathbf{G}$ is generated by recording the point-of-gaze of the human expert while looking at $\mathbf{I}$. To perform gaze-assisted knowledge distillation, we

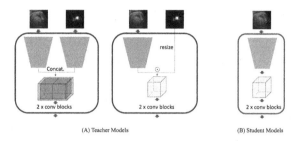

(A) Teacher Models   (B) Student Models

Fig. 2. Teacher and Student models used. (A) Teachers use concatenation or element-wise production to merge information from US image and visual attention map. (B) student only takes US image as input

train the *teacher* model $\mathcal{T}$ to perform a classification task using both $\mathbf{I}$ and $\mathbf{G}$ as input. The student models still only "sees" the image $\mathbf{I}$. Thus, the teacher model can transfer not only the knowledge learned through its high number of parameters, but also knowledge extracted from the human visual attention. We test two different architectures for learning from image and gaze: $\mathcal{T}_{+\text{gaze}}$ obtained by concatenation of extracted features of inputs (frame and gaze map) and $\mathcal{T}_{\times\text{gaze}}$ by computing the element-wise product between resized gaze maps (28×28) and feature maps extracted from US frames (Fig. 2).

2.3   Data and Training Details

Data. Clinical fetal ultrasound videos with simultaneously recorded sonographer gaze tracking data was available from the PULSE study [11]. Ethics approval was obtained for data recording and data stored as per local data governance rules. From this dataset we extracted 23016 abdomen, 24508 head, 12839 femur frames. Gaze tracking data was recorded using a Tobii Eye Tracker 4C (Tobii, Sweden) that records the point-of-gaze (relative x and y coordinates with corresponding timestamp) at a rate of 90 Hz, effectively recording 3 gaze points per frame. Gaze points less than $0.5°$ apart were merged as a single fixation point. A sonographer visual attention map G was generated for each image by adding a truncated Gaussian with width corresponding to a visual angle of $0.5°$ at the point of fixation.

Training Details. We tested different student models to demonstrate the utility of the PeTRA approach: *SqueezeNet* [12] (**S**), *MobileNet* (0.25 width multiplier) [13] (**M**), and *MobileNet* v2 (0.35 width multiplier) [14] (**MV**) modified to accept single channel inputs and include a joint loss objective in Eq. (5). These models are representative of the main types of compact architectures—squeeze-excite convolution blocks [12], group convolutions [13] and depthwise separable convolutions in groups [14]. Most other compact models proposed in computer vision literature derive from these basic architectures. For the teacher models we use a *VGG-16* feature extractor, modified to accept dual input of single-channel frames and gaze maps (with the depth of the first two fully connected

Table 1. Performance of MobileNetV2 (*MV*) with different configurations of knowledge distillation. IT indicates the level of intermediate transfer, if any.

Configuration			Validation accuracy				NetScore
Student	Teacher	IT	Abdomen	Head	Femur	Average	
MV	$\mathcal{T}$	–	0.63	0.67	0.69	0.66	60.16
$MV_{+\text{gaze}}$	$\mathcal{T}_{+\text{gaze}}$	–	0.71	0.73	0.68	0.71	61.43
$MV_{+\text{gaze}}^1$	$\mathcal{T}_{+\text{gaze}}$	1	0.73	0.74	0.70	0.72	61.67
$MV_{+\text{gaze}}^2$	$\mathcal{T}_{+\text{gaze}}$	2	**0.78**	**0.78**	0.76	0.77	62.84
$MV_{+\text{gaze}}^3$	$\mathcal{T}_{+\text{gaze}}$	3	**0.78**	0.77	**0.80**	**0.78**	63.06
$MV_{\times\text{gaze}}$	$\mathcal{T}_{\times\text{gaze}}$	–	0.84	0.84	0.79	0.82	63.93
$MV_{\times\text{gaze}}^1$	$\mathcal{T}_{\times\text{gaze}}$	1	0.80	0.83	0.79	0.81	63.72
$MV_{\times\text{gaze}}^2$	$\mathcal{T}_{\times\text{gaze}}$	2	0.86	**0.85**	0.83	**0.85**	**64.56**
$MV_{\times\text{gaze}}^3$	$\mathcal{T}_{\times\text{gaze}}$	3	**0.87**	**0.85**	**0.84**	**0.85**	**64.56**

layers changed from the original 4096 to 1024 and 512 to avoid overfitting). In a change to the standard VGG-16, for $\mathcal{T}_{\times\text{gaze}}$, the element-wise product after the fourth convolutional block is followed by the FC layers. In $\mathcal{T}_{+\text{gaze}}$, features are extracted by parallel convolutional blocks of the VGG16 and concatenated before FC layers. At inference, only one of the parallel blocks (processing single frame input, as gaze maps are not used at inference) and the following FC layers comprise the $\mathcal{T}_{\times\text{gaze}}$ model. This reflects in $\mathcal{T}_{\times\text{gaze}}$ having same number of parameters as $\mathcal{T}$ in Table 1. Data augmentation was performed using a 20 degrees rotational augmentation and horizontal flipping for both ultrasound and gaze map frames. Frames and corresponding gaze maps were resized to 224×224. All models were trained on 80% (71 subjects) and tested on 20% (18 subjects) of the dataset. Teacher models were trained for 100 epochs with learning rate of 0.005 and adaptive moment estimation (Adam) [15]. Students models were trained for 200 epochs over the *(N, image, label, logit)* set created for all N frames passed to the teacher model. The softening temperature value was set to 4.0 after a grid search for $E \in [|1, 10|]$. We investigated intermediate transfer at three different stages. First, second and third stage intermediate transfer was respectively applied from the 2nd, 4th, 5th maxpool layers in the teacher model to the FC arms after 2nd, 3rd, 5th maxpool layers of S and 3rd, 5th, 7th depthwise conv layer for M and MV. For experiments with intermediate transfer, such FC layer neurons were separately retained and appended to the set as *(N, image, label, logit,* $\text{IT}_1/../\text{IT}_m$*)*. α and β are set to 0.5 for equal influence of teacher knowledge and cross-entropy loss for the student model; γ is set at 1.

3   Results and Discussion

We report the classification accuracy MobileNetV2 (*MV*) in Table 1, and the accuracy of teacher models and compact models trained without knowledge

Table 2. Performance of teachers $T_{+gaze}/T_{\times gaze}$, student models (trained directly without teacher) and compared methods (T is teacher w/o gaze). No. of parameters are those in models used for inference.

Model						Validation accuracy			
Name	#parameters	Size (MB)	Time (ms)	MFLOP	NetScore	Abd	Head	Femur	Avg.
T	55,28,2178	221.24	336.23	110.55	36.67	0.76	0.74	0.69	0.73
T_{+gaze}	55,282,178	221.24	336.24	110.55	38.04	0.85	0.75	0.76	0.79
$T_{\times gaze}$	213,320,002	884.96	637.13	464.31	28.21	**0.92**	**0.90**	**0.87**	**0.90**
S_{direct}	619,644	0.22	127.43	82.65	51.21	0.48	0.53	0.52	0.51
M_{direct}	738,658	0.27	159.28	98.71	52.50	0.56	0.61	0.64	0.60
MV_{direct}	**284,850**	**0.12**	**79.64**	**64.20**	**59.63**	0.57	0.67	0.68	0.64

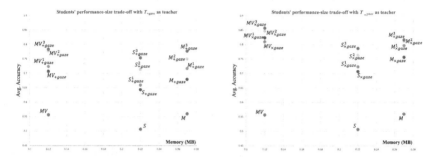

Fig. 3. Performance-size trade-off. Left: T_{+gaze}-trained students; Right: $T_{\times gaze}$-trained students (enlarged in Appendix). Accuracy is averaged across classes.

transfer in Table 2. We also report the number of parameters, memory requirement and inference time of models in Table 2. Complete overall results for the variants of students are shown in Fig. 3 and class-wise detailed results are in Supplementary Material. Student models are named X^l, X^l_{+gaze} and $X^l_{\times gaze}$ when trained using knowledge from T, T_{+gaze} and $T_{\times gaze}$, respectively. $X \in \{S, M, MV\}$ is the student architecture and $l \in \{1, 2, 3\}$ is the stage used for intermediate transfer.

Performance. Final layer knowledge distillation improves the accuracy of the compact model compared to training without knowledge transfer for all students. Compact models trained using gaze-assisted knowledge distillation reach a higher accuracy than the same models trained with image-only knowledge distillation (+0.05 for MV_{+gaze}, +0.16 for $MV_{\times gaze}$, compared to MV). Intermediate transfer further improves knowledge transfer over final layer distillation only, with transfers at 3rd level showing the best improvement in student model accuracy (+0.07 for MV^3_{+gaze}, +0.03 for $MV^3_{\times gaze}$, compared to MV_{+gaze}, $MV_{\times gaze}$). These trends are seen for all student models (S, M, MV). The baseline image-only knowledge distillation is analogous to prior work in [4,8].

Computational Complexity. We evaluated the computational complexity of the models by computing the number of floating point operations (FLOP) performed for inference (Table 2). We also report inference times for a batch of 100 frames from the test set using a 32 GB/Intel core i7-4940MX/3.1 GHz laptop. The inference speed-up compared to $\mathcal{T}_{\times\text{gaze}}$ is 5× for S, 8× for MV and 4× for M (Table 2). For the same student models, using human gaze in teacher training does not change the computational complexity, but the performance metrics of student models when distilled from gaze-trained teachers are superior (Table 1).

Memory Size. Student architectures (S, M, MV) show a 1000× to 7000× reduction of memory size compared to teachers (Table 2). The $MV^3_{+\text{gaze}}$ student with only 284,850 parameters achieves an average accuracy of 0.85, close to its teacher model $\mathcal{T}_{\times\text{gaze}}$ (0.90), and higher than $\mathcal{T}_{+\text{gaze}}$ (0.79) and $\mathcal{T}$ without gaze (0.73). Similar gains are seen for other students as well (Fig. 3). The MobileNet model M (738,658 parameters, 270 kB) trained with distillation from $\mathcal{T}_{\times\text{gaze}}$ attains accuracy (0.79) comparable to $\mathcal{T}_{+\text{gaze}}$ and higher than $\mathcal{T}$. Due to element-wise product operations, $\mathcal{T}_{\times\text{gaze}}$ has a higher number of parameters than $\mathcal{T}_{+\text{gaze}}$.

Model Efficiency. To evaluate model efficiency as a trade-off between accuracy a, number of parameters p and computational cost c, we estimated the *NetScore* metric $\Omega = 20 \log \left(a^\delta p^{-\epsilon} c^{-\phi}\right)$ proposed in [16]. We provide other model data in Table 2 for completeness. Based on [16] we set $\delta = 2$, $\epsilon = 0.5$ and $\phi = 0.5$. For computational cost c, we use the number of FLOP instead of multiply-accumulate (MAC) operations in [16] because FLOP includes overheads such as pooling and activation beyond dot product and convolution operations. We report MFLOP (million FLOP) and NetScore values in Table 2. The units of a, p, c in Ω are percent, millions of parameters and MFLOP. The best NetScore is obtained by $MV^3_{\times\text{gaze}}$, the most compact model with the highest accuracy.

The best performing reduced models achieve within 5% of the accuracy of full models with 1000× fewer parameters. The reduction of memory footprint and inference times make them very attractive for deployment in a clinical setting on equipments with lower computational power.

4   Conclusions

We proposed Perception and Transfer for Reduced Architectures as a general framework to train compact models with knowledge transfer from traditional large deep learning models using gaze tracking information to condition the solution without requiring such information at runtime. For the tasks of fetal abdomen, femur and head detection, compact model had an accuracy close to that of the large models, while having a much lower memory requirement. We found intermediate knowledge transfer to be more efficient when applied deeper in the networks. This is a proof-of-concept of human knowledge-assisted model compression for image analysis and the concept could be used for other modalities.

Acknowledgements. We acknowledge the ERC (ERC-ADG-2015 694581, project PULSE), the EPSRC (EP/GO36861/1, EP/MO13774/1, EP/R013853/1), the Rhodes Trust, and the NIHR Biomedical Research Centre funding scheme.

References

1. Becker, D.M., et al.: The use of portable ultrasound devices in low-and middle-income countries: a systematic review of the literature. Trop. Med. Int. Health **21**(3), 294–311 (2016)
2. Liu, B., et al.: Sparse convolutional neural networks. In: Proceedings of the IEEE Conference on Computer Vision and Pattern Recognition, pp. 806–814 (2015)
3. He, Y., et al.: Channel pruning for accelerating very deep neural networks. In: Proceedings of the IEEE International Conference on Computer Vision, pp. 1389–1397 (2017)
4. Hinton, G., Vinyals, O., Dean, J.: Distilling the knowledge in a neural network. In: NIPS 2014 Deep Learning Workshop (2014)
5. Romero, A., et al.: FitNets: Hints for thin deep nets. arXiv:1412.6550 (2014)
6. Patra, A., Huang, W., Noble, J.A.: Learning spatio-temporal aggregation for fetal heart analysis in ultrasound video. In: Cardoso, M.J., et al. (eds.) DLMIA/ML-CDS -2017. LNCS, vol. 10553, pp. 276–284. Springer, Cham (2017). https://doi.org/10.1007/978-3-319-67558-9_32
7. Patra, A., et al.: Sequential anatomy localization in fetal echocardiography videos. arXiv preprint arXiv:1810.11868 (2018)
8. Vaseli, H., et al.: Designing lightweight deep learning models for echocardiography view classification. In: SPIE Medical Imaging 2019: Image-Guided Procedures, Robotic Interventions, and Modeling, vol. 10951 (2019)
9. Cai, Y., et al.: SonoEyeNet: standardized fetal ultrasound plane detection informed by eye tracking. In: 15th IEEE ISBI, pp. 1475–1478. IEEE (2018)
10. Bucilă, C., et al.: Model compression. In: Proceedings of the 12th ACM SIGKDD International Conference on Knowledge Discovery and Data Mining, pp. 535–541 (2006)
11. PULSE: Perception ultrasound by learning sonographic experience (2018). www.eng.ox.ac.uk/pulse
12. Iandola, F.N., et al.: SqueezeNet: AlexNet-level accuracy with 50x fewer parameters and <0.5 MB model size. arXiv preprint arXiv:1602.07360 (2016)
13. Howard, A.G., et al.: MobileNets: efficient convolutional neural networks for mobile vision applications. arXiv preprint arXiv:1704.04861 (2017)
14. Sandler, M., et al.: MobileNetV2: inverted residuals and linear bottlenecks. In: CVPR (2018)
15. Kingma, D.P., Ba, J.: Adam: a method for stochastic optimization. arXiv:1412.6980 (2014)
16. Wong, A.: NetScore: towards universal metrics for large-scale performance analysis of deep neural networks for practical usage. arXiv:1806.05512 (2018)

Fetal Pose Estimation in Volumetric MRI Using a 3D Convolution Neural Network

Junshen Xu[1]($\boxtimes$), Molin Zhang[2], Esra Abaci Turk[3], Larry Zhang[4],
P. Ellen Grant[3,5], Kui Ying[2], Polina Golland[1,4], and Elfar Adalsteinsson[1,6]

[1] Department of Electrical Engineering and Computer Science, MIT,
Cambridge, MA, USA
junshen@mit.edu
[2] Department of Engineering Physics, Tsinghua University, Beijing, China
[3] Fetal-Neonatal Neuroimaging and Developmental Science Center,
Boston Children's Hospital, Boston, MA, USA
[4] Computer Science and Artificial Intelligence Laboratory, MIT,
Cambridge, MA, USA
[5] Harvard Medical School, Boston, MA, USA
[6] Institute for Medical Engineering and Science, MIT, Cambridge, MA, USA

Abstract. The performance and diagnostic utility of magnetic resonance imaging (MRI) in pregnancy is fundamentally constrained by fetal motion. Motion of the fetus, which is unpredictable and rapid on the scale of conventional imaging times, limits the set of viable acquisition techniques to single-shot imaging with severe compromises in signal-to-noise ratio and diagnostic contrast, and frequently results in unacceptable image quality. Surprisingly little is known about the characteristics of fetal motion during MRI and here we propose and demonstrate methods that exploit a growing repository of MRI observations of the gravid abdomen that are acquired at low spatial resolution but relatively high temporal resolution and over long durations (10–30 min). We estimate fetal pose per frame in MRI volumes of the pregnant abdomen via deep learning algorithms that detect key fetal landmarks. Evaluation of the proposed method shows that our framework achieves quantitatively an average error of 4.47 mm and 96.4% accuracy (with error less than 10 mm). Fetal pose estimation in MRI time series yields novel means of quantifying fetal movements in health and disease, and enables the learning of kinematic models that may enhance prospective mitigation of fetal motion artifacts during MRI acquisition.

Keywords: Pose estimation · Fetal magnetic resonance imaging
(MRI) · Deep learning · Convolutional neural network (CNN)

1 Introduction

Estimation of fetal pose from volumetric MRI in pregnancy has applications that include motion tracking and prospective artifact mitigation during diagnostic

---

J. Xu and M. Zhang—Equal contribution.

© Springer Nature Switzerland AG 2019
D. Shen et al. (Eds.): MICCAI 2019, LNCS 11767, pp. 403–410, 2019.
https://doi.org/10.1007/978-3-030-32251-9_44

imaging, retrospective analysis and evaluation of movement by the fetus, as well as the establishment of kinematic models of fetal movement during MRI. Prior work in fetal motion includes methods that rely on simple indices for fetal motion analysis and quantification, such as the angle of the fetal body axes with respect to the maternal body [1] and maternal perception of fetal movements [2].

Although pose estimation for the human (adult) body is an established domain in computer vision [3], to the best of our knowledge, no work has demonstrated fetal pose estimation over time in medical images by MRI. In contrast to human pose estimation from 2D photography, in fetal pose estimation we need to predict 3D pose from dense volumetric data, which increases the computational burden. Further complicating the task is the variable orientation of the fetus within the mother, rapid growth and change in fetal features over gestational age, and poor-quality observations of ground truth pose.

In pose estimation, handcrafted features such as graphical models and tree-based methods typically suffer from low accuracy and low processing speed while recent developments in deep learning have demonstrated great success in computer vision with acceleration by GPUs and the capability to learn high-level features from data. Consequently, deep convolution neural networks have also found their way into human pose estimation and achieved state-of-the-art results.

In an ongoing study of placental function by EPI BOLD imaging time series (see Fig. 1(a)), we have built an archive of over 70 subjects, each with 200–500 time frames of EPI volumes, imaged continuously over 10–30 min observation intervals and resulting in over 18,000 EPI volumes. By visual inspection, the fetal pose can be inferred from these data but manual labeling of keypoints for pose estimation (see Fig. 1(b)) across these volumes is prohibitive and here we propose a method based on deep neural networks to identify fetal key points.

We propose, demonstrate, and characterize the performance of a two-stage framework for fetal pose estimation in 3D MRI using deep learning, where we first generate heatmaps for each fetal keypoint using a convolution network and then infer fetal pose from heat maps using a Markov Random Field (MRF) that exploit anatomically rational information about connections between keypoints. Evaluation of performance shows that the proposed method achieves a mean error of 4.47 mm and a percentage of correct detection of 96.4%. Further, computation time of our pipeline is less than 1 s/volume, which potentially enables low-latency tracking of fetal pose during diagnostic MRI in pregnancy.

2   Methods

2.1   Pose Estimation Framework

Exploring the idea of heatmap prediction in human pose estimation [3], here we propose a two-stage framework for fetal pose estimation in 3D MRI using deep learning (see Fig. 2). In the first stage, a CNN is used to generate heatmaps from input MR volume, which produce per-pixel likelihoods for keypoints on the fetal skeleton. However, the generated heatmap may have multiple local maxima and simply using max activating location as prediction may lead to low accuracy.

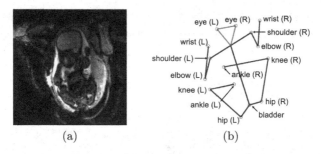

Fig. 1. (a) A representative slice from one MRI volume used in this study, and (b) an example of the associated 15 keypoints that characterize fetal pose in three dimensions at a single 3.5-s time frame extracted from a 30-min observation of the fetus by MRI.

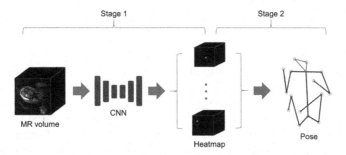

Fig. 2. The framework of fetal pose estimation in 3D MRI which consists of two stages. Stage 1: generate 3D heatmaps of each keypoint from the input MR volume. Stage 2: estimate keypoint locations from heatmaps.

To address this problem, a second stage is proposed to infer location from estimated heatmaps, exploiting the constraints of fetal pose to refine the results. We model the fetal pose as a MRF, where each keypoint of fetus is represented by a node in the graph and the states are the plausible locations of the keypoint. The final prediction is generated by performing inference on this MRF.

The following subsections describe the proposed framework in detail.

2.2 Heatmap Prediction Using CNN

Inspired by the successful application of hourglass networks in human pose estimation [3], we propose a 3D hourglass network for heatmap prediction of fetal keypoints. The overall architecture of the proposed network is shown in Fig. 3. The network is based on the encoder-decoder structure which is motivated by the idea of capturing multi-scale information. In pose estimation, while local evidence, e.g., local contrast, is important for identification of keypoint, global information can help resolve ambiguity, such as fetus' orientation and relative position of other joints or body parts. In each scale of the network, resblocks with 3D convolution layers are used to extract features. To recover loss of high resolution information in downscale-upscale structure, skipped connections with element-wise addition are adopted to connect symmetric scales.

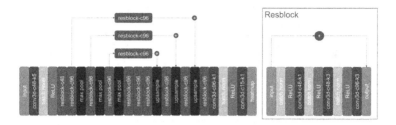

Fig. 3. Left: architecture of 3D hourglass network for heatmap prediction. Right: structure of resblock.

The CNN tries to learn a mapping from MR images to target heatmaps, which is generated by placing a Gaussian distribution with $\sigma = 2$ on the ground-truth position and stacking together. So the output heatmaps will be of the same spatial dimensions but have J channels, where J is the number of keypoints need to predict. The loss function used for training is the mean-squared error (MSE) between the predicted heatmap and target heatmap. Instead of using the whole volume, 3D patches with size of $64 \times 64 \times 64$ are used as input for training. This strategy can reduce GPU memory usage, enabling mini-batch training. Since the network is fully convolutional, in inference, the whole 3D MR volumes are fed into the network to generate heatmap of full scale.

2.3   Location Estimation from Heatmap

Given the output heatmap from CNN, the second stage of the pose estimation framework is to estimate location of each keypoint. Let x_i and H_i be the location and heatmap of the i-th keypoint, $i = 1, ..., J$. Let $x = (x_1, ..., x_J)$. Then one simple idea to infer keypoint positions from heatmaps is taking the max activating location of each heatmap However, this method handles each keypoint independently and does not make use of the connection between keypoints, e.g., the distance between two joints should be a constant if they are connected by bones. To exploiting these connections, we model the fetal pose as a MRF, where each keypoint correspond to a node in the graph and connections of keypoints are represented as edges in the graph. The states $\mathcal{S}_i = \{x_i^{(1)}, ..., x_i^{(L)}\}$ for node i is the top-L local maxima in heatmap i. Our prediction of fetal pose would be a particular configuration of the MRF, i.e., $\hat{x} \in \mathcal{S}_1 \times \cdots \times \mathcal{S}_J$. Each configuration is assigned an energy, $E(x)$, defined as

$$E(x) = \sum_{i=1}^{J} \varphi_i(x_i) + \sum_{(i,j) \in B} \phi_{i,j}(x_i, x_j) \tag{1}$$

where B is the set of connections. A low energy of a configuration implies high probability. Therefore, the inference is equivalent to finding the configuration with lowest energy

Since the heatmap can be considered as a surrogate for the probability distribution of the corresponding keypoint, the unary term in energy function F can be modeled as

$$\varphi_i(x_i) = -\log H_i(x_i) \tag{2}$$

As for the pairwise term, we define $\phi_{i,j}$ as a quadratic function of $\|x_i - x_j\|_2$, the distance between keypoint i and j.

$$\phi_{i,j}(x_i, x_j) = -\frac{\alpha(\|x_i - x_j\|_2/r_t - \mu_{ij})^2}{\sigma_{ij}^2}, \tag{3}$$

where r_t is the mean bone length at gestational age t, so that $\|x_i - x_j\|_2/r_t$ can be regarded as the distance of two keypoints normalized by gestational age. μ_{ij} and σ_{ij}^2 are the mean and variance of the normalized distance, which are estimated from training data. α is the regularization weight. The optimization problem is solved by a belief propagation algorithm [4].

3   Experiments and Results

3.1   Dataset

The data for this study consist of volumetric MRI time series from imaging of 70 mothers pregnant with singletons at a gestational age ranging from 25 to 35 weeks. MRIs were acquired on a 3T Skyra scanner (Siemens Healthcare, Erlangen, Germany). Multislice, single-shot, gradient echo EPI sequence was used for acquisitions with in-plane resolution of $3 \times 3\,\mathrm{mm}^2$, slice thickness of $3\,\mathrm{mm}$, mean matrix size $= 120 \times 120 \times 80$; TR $= 5\text{–}8\,\mathrm{s}$, TE $= 32\text{–}38\,\mathrm{ms}$, FA $= 90°$. Each subject was scanned for 10 to 30 min.

Similar to the task of adult human pose estimation, we model the pose of a fetus with a set of keypoints. We chose fifteen keypoints (ankles, knees, hips, bladder, shoulders, elbows, wrists and eyes) to capture pose and labeled manually, with a representative example shown in Fig. 1(b). These fifteen landmarks were selected as keypoints as they capture gross fetal anatomy that is critical in subsequent motion analysis, and they presented with adequate image contrast to be relatively robustly observed in the MR volumes, thus mitigating the error and noise in labelling. In total, 1705 MR volumes were labelled, 1028(~60%) for training, 240(~15%) for validation and 437(~25%) for testing, where the testing set consists of subjects different from training and validation sets.

In order to improve the generalization capacity and avoid overfitting, several data augmentation techniques were used, including intensity scaling, 3D rotation and flipping.

3.2 Experiments Setup

All experiments were performed on a server with an Intel Xeon E5-1650 CPU, 128 GB RAM and a NVIDIA TITAN X GPU. Neural networks were implemented with TensorFlow and for optimization we use Adam with an initial learning rate of 5×10^{-3}, weight decay of 1×10^{-4} and the restart strategy [5]. The networks are trained for 200 epochs. For the second stage, we set $L = 3$ and $\alpha = 1$.

3.3 Results

In this section, we evaluate the proposed pipeline for fetal pose estimation. First, we evaluate the proposed 3D hourglass network (HG) with max activating location of the heatmap as final prediction. For comparison, 3D UNet [6] is used in our experiment, which has been used for heatmap regression [7]. Finally, we examine the whole pipeline by combine the CNN-based heatmap regression and MRF. These models are denoted as UNet-M and HG-M respectively.

Several metrics are used for evaluation: (a) Percentage of Correct Keypoint (PCK), where a detected keypoint is considered correct if the distance between the predicted and the true keypoint is within a certain threshold, (b) mean error (in mm), i.e., the mean distance between the predicted and the ground-truth keypoint, and (c) median of error.

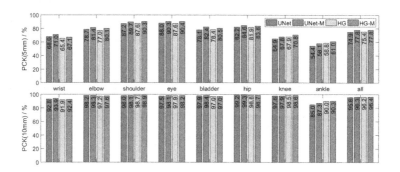

Fig. 4. PCK with two threshold, 5 mm (1.67 pixel) and 10 mm (3.33 pixel) for different keypoints.

Figure 4 shows PCK with two threshold, 5 mm (1.67 pixel) and 10 mm (3.33 pixel) while the mean and median of error of different models are illustrated in Table 1. Applying the proposed pipeline, 96.4% of the keypoints are located correctly (with error < 10 mm) and the mean distance between predicted and ground-truth keypoints is 4.47 mm (1.5 pixel). Besides, we see that, in average, the proposed 3D hourglass network has similar performance compared to 3D UNet. However, as illustrated in Table 2, the number of parameters of UNet is 6 times as large as that of hourglass network, indicating that the proposed network is more compact and efficient. The main reason is that the hourglass network use

Table 1. Mean and median of error of different models.

Metric	Method	Wrist	Elbow	Shoulder	Eye	Bladder	Hip	Knee	Ankle	All
Median (mm)	UNet	3.84	3.43	2.87	2.74	3.20	**3.12**	4.00	4.42	3.47
	UNet-M	3.84	3.43	2.87	2.73	**3.19**	**3.12**	3.99	4.36	3.46
	HG	**3.82**	3.42	**2.83**	**2.72**	3.37	3.16	3.87	**4.15**	**3.42**
	HG-M	**3.82**	**3.41**	**2.83**	**2.72**	3.36	3.16	**3.86**	**4.15**	**3.42**
Mean (mm)	UNet	7.34	4.06	4.27	3.96	4.48	3.33	5.19	10.2	5.41
	UNet-M	**5.64**	**3.81**	3.75	3.29	**3.52**	**3.23**	4.84	8.18	4.60
	HG	7.48	4.81	3.24	3.35	4.69	3.58	4.39	7.49	4.89
	HG-M	6.37	4.11	**3.10**	**3.28**	4.12	3.33	**4.19**	**7.07**	**4.47**

Table 2. Computation time and number of parameters of different networks.

Network	Computation time (ms/volume)	Number of parameters
UNet	271	22M
HG	225	3.5M

elementwise sum instead of concatenate in skip connection and fix the number of channels across different scales. We also notice that the second stage Markov network refinement improves the performance upon CNN heatmap regression, in terms of PCK as well as mean error. As illustrated in Fig. 5(b), fetal pose estimation based on max activating location of heatmap may result in irrational prediction. Such error is corrected in the MRF refinement by making a trade-off between prior information of keypoint connections and heatmaps generated by the CNN. As for computation time, the proposed 3D hourglass network runs at a speed of 225 ms/volume on a GPU and solving the optimization problem for inferring keypoint locations from heatmaps takes 290 ms/volume on CPU. Therefore, the end-to-end processing time of the whole pipeline is less than 1 s/volume and therefore shorter than the temporal resolution in the current fetal MR protocol, which potentially enables low latency tracking of fetal pose in fetal MR imaging.

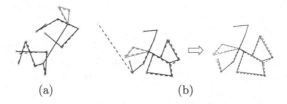

(a)   (b)

Fig. 5. (a) An example of fetal pose successfully predicted by the max activating location of heatmaps, where solid lines are the ground-truth pose and dashed lines are the predicted pose. (b) A failed case of fetal pose estimation with max activation (left), and the corresponding successful result after processed by MRF (right).

4   Conclusions

In this work, we proposed a two-stage deep learning framework for fetal pose estimation in 3D MRI. The proposed method achieves mean error of 4.47 mm (~1.5 pixels) and percentage of correct detection of 96.4%, which indicates that deep neural networks are able to identify key features for fetal pose estimation from time frames in low-resolution, volumetric EPI data from pregnant mothers. Further, the total processing time of the proposed framework is less than 1 s, potentially enabling low latency tracking of fetal pose in fetal MR imaging. Limitations of the current method include a pipeline that was only trained on singleton pregnancies. Also, the current pose detection was performed on each time frame in isolation without utilizing any form of temporal correlations in the MR series. In future work the proposed framework could be extended to work with multiplet pregnancies as well as exploit temporal correlations across volumes in a time sequence.

Overall, the proposed pipeline could be deployed for fetal motion estimation during MR scanning of pregnant mothers with applications to fetal health and disease, establishment of fetal kinetic motion models, and prospective motion correction with slice-prescription updates for more robust diagnostic fetal and maternal MRI.

Acknowledgements. This research was supported by NIH U01HD087211, NIH R01EB01733 and NIH NIBIB NAC P41EB015902.

References

1. Biglari, H., Sameni, R.: Fetal motion estimation from noninvasive cardiac signal recordings. Physiol. Meas. **37**(11), 2003 (2016)
2. Heazell, A.P., Frøen, J.: Methods of fetal movement counting and the detection of fetal compromise. J. Obstet. Gynaecol. **28**(2), 147–154 (2008)
3. Newell, A., Yang, K., Deng, J.: Stacked hourglass networks for human pose estimation. In: Leibe, B., Matas, J., Sebe, N., Welling, M. (eds.) ECCV 2016. LNCS, vol. 9912, pp. 483–499. Springer, Cham (2016). https://doi.org/10.1007/978-3-319-46484-8_29
4. Schmidt, M.: UGM: Matlab code for undirected graphical models (2012). http://www.di.ens.fr/mschmidt/Software/UGM.html
5. Loshchilov, I., Hutter, F.: Fixing weight decay regularization in adam. arXiv preprint arXiv:1711.05101 (2017)
6. Çiçek, Ö., Abdulkadir, A., Lienkamp, S.S., Brox, T., Ronneberger, O.: 3D U-Net: learning dense volumetric segmentation from sparse annotation. In: Ourselin, S., Joskowicz, L., Sabuncu, M.R., Unal, G., Wells, W. (eds.) MICCAI 2016. LNCS, vol. 9901, pp. 424–432. Springer, Cham (2016). https://doi.org/10.1007/978-3-319-46723-8_49
7. Payer, C., Štern, D., Bischof, H., Urschler, M.: Regressing heatmaps for multiple landmark localization using CNNs. In: Ourselin, S., Joskowicz, L., Sabuncu, M.R., Unal, G., Wells, W. (eds.) MICCAI 2016. LNCS, vol. 9901, pp. 230–238. Springer, Cham (2016). https://doi.org/10.1007/978-3-319-46723-8_27

Multi-stage Prediction Networks for Data Harmonization

Stefano B. Blumberg[1($\boxtimes$)], Marco Palombo[1], Can Son Khoo[1],
Chantal M. W. Tax[2], Ryutaro Tanno[1], and Daniel C. Alexander[1]

[1] Department of Computer Science and Centre for Medical Image Computing,
University College London (UCL), London, UK
`stefano.blumberg.17@ucl.ac.uk`
[2] Cardiff University Brain Research Imaging Centre (CUBRIC),
Cardiff University, Cardiff, UK

Abstract. In this paper, we introduce multi-task learning (MTL) to data harmonization (DH); where we aim to harmonize images across different acquisition platforms and sites. This allows us to integrate information from multiple acquisitions and improve the predictive performance and learning efficiency of the harmonization model. Specifically, we introduce the Multi Stage Prediction (MSP) Network, a MTL framework that incorporates neural networks of potentially disparate architectures, trained for different individual acquisition platforms, into a larger architecture that is refined in unison. The MSP utilizes high-level features of single networks for individual tasks, as inputs of additional neural networks to inform the final prediction, therefore exploiting redundancy across tasks to make the most of limited training data. We validate our methods on a dMRI harmonization challenge dataset, where we predict three modern platform types, from one obtained from an old scanner. We show how MTL architectures, such as the MSP, produce around 20% improvement of patch-based mean-squared error over current state-of-the-art methods and that our MSP outperforms off-the-shelf MTL networks. Our code is available [1].

Keywords: Data harmonization · Deep learning · Diffusion magnetic resonance imaging · Multi-task learning · Transfer learning

1 Introduction

Lack of standardization amongst imaging acquisitions is a long-standing problem, that confounds large scale multi-centre imaging studies. DH aims to remove differences arising from specifics of scanner, centre or acquisition protocol and increase the power of group studies. The problem aligns with the wider issue of

Electronic supplementary material The online version of this chapter (https:// doi.org/10.1007/978-3-030-32251-9_45) contains supplementary material, which is available to authorized users.

© Springer Nature Switzerland AG 2019
D. Shen et al. (Eds.): MICCAI 2019, LNCS 11767, pp. 411–419, 2019.
https://doi.org/10.1007/978-3-030-32251-9_45

estimating, from an image obtained from a particular subject and scanner, the image that would have been obtained from the same subject on another scanner. Various recent studies, such as Image Quality Transfer [2–4] and Modality Transfer [5], present solutions to this problem that may be repurposed for DH.

Current approaches used in practice, such as [6,7], generally register all images to a common template and align the mean and variances of image intensities from each platform (i.e. centre, scanner, and/or acquisition protocol), either voxelwise, regionally, or of whole images. Recently, deep learning has shown much promise, e.g. in the Multi-Shell Data Harmonization Challenge (MUSHAC) [8–10], outperforming statistical approaches. Methods to date include the Convolutional Neural Network with Rotationally Invariant Spherical Harmonics (CNN-RISH) [11] – a 5-layer CNN that harmonizes dMRI from 3 T to 7T; the Deeper Image Quality Transfer Network (DIQT) [4] – an extension of the FCSNet [8], which holds state-of-the-art results in dMRI super-resolution and the Spherical Harmonic Residual Network (SHResNet) [12] – A 7-layer CNN that processes different spherical harmonic (SH) coefficients separately. A common feature of all these methods is that they use a separate single CNN to estimate the target images from those of each individual platforms.

Multi-scanner or multi-centre studies often acquire traveling heads (TH) – a small number of subjects specifically scanned at each site, to support DH learning mappings from scanner to scanner. These learned mappings then transform other subjects to a common representation. However, acquiring TH data is expensive and typically the number of subjects is small (rarely more than 10). Therefore, single-network deep learning approaches easily overfit [4,12] and fail to exploit the synergy between multiple, often strongly related, prediction tasks.

MTL potentially offers a powerful solution to the paucity of training data in DH, by allowing the model to integrate information from acquisitions from multiple platforms. In contrast to single-network approaches, it exploits commonalities and differences across multiple tasks (in our case, predicting different acquisitions) to improve the predictive power of neural networks. Furthermore by incorporating predictions and loss functions into a single network, MTL approaches acquire additional regularisation [13]. There are a variety of existing approaches that cascade over multiple predictions of varying resolutions, that might be adapted to a MTL approach in DH. Examples include the Convolutional Pose Machine Networks (CPM) [14] comprising a sequential architecture of CNNs, to provide increasing refined estimates and the Holistically-Nested Edge Detection Network (HNED) [15] – a single-stream deep network with multiple side outputs to perform multi-scale and multi-level feature learning. However, these approaches process tasks sequentially, whilst the distinct tasks in DH differ in terms of resolution, contrast and noise patterns, with no simple notion of ordering. Furthermore it is unclear as to what might be the optimal subnetworks for such a larger network.

In this paper, we introduce a new MSP architecture designed to exploit, for the first time, MTL in DH. The MSP draws on sub-network structures from [14,15], but cascades across various estimation tasks, rather than assuming they

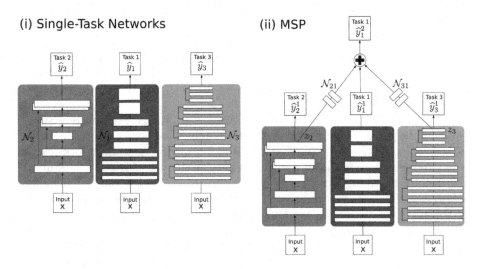

Fig. 1. We illustrate creating the MSP from three single networks, with input, target platforms $0, 1$ and other platforms $2, 3$. (i) Three trained neural networks $\mathcal{N}_i$, $i = 1, 2, 3$ separately predict patches $\widehat{y}_i$ $i = 1, 2, 3$, from input patch x. (ii) The MSP. We take $\mathcal{N}_2, \mathcal{N}_3$ and select their last features z_i $i = 2, 3$ as inputs to additional respective neural networks $\mathcal{N}_{21}, \mathcal{N}_{31}$. The first-stage predictions are $\widehat{y}_i^1$ $i = 1, 2, 3$, the second-stage prediction, a linear combination of $\widehat{y}_1^1, \mathcal{N}_{21}(z_2), \mathcal{N}_{31}(z_3)$, is $\widehat{y}_1^2$.

are sequentially structured. This avoids both duplicating features and allows us to use redundancy across tasks to make the most of limited training data. Furthermore the MSP allows us to incorporate pre-trained state-of-the art networks into a MTL framework, letting us explicitly use high-level features of multiple predictions, as network inputs to inform the final prediction.

We utilize the recent MUSHAC [8] data to evaluate various strategies. The specific task is to predict acquisitions of both low and high quality from different scanners, from data from the same subjects acquired on an ageing scanner. We compare performance of the state of the art, i.e. various single network approaches, with MTL frameworks, including the MSP, where the best performing single networks inform construction of a particular MSP architecture. The MSP outperforms both single networks and simple off-the-shelf MTL approaches. We expect this initial demonstration to motivate wider development and usage of MTL strategies for DH, therefore we release our implementation in [1].

2   Methods

In this section we outline the general DH problem with THs and setting from MUSHAC [8] with which we validate our methods. Then we construct the MSP.

In the typical DH setting, THs provide image data sets I_{ij} $i = 0, ..., P-1$ $j = 1, ..., N$ for each of N subjects imaged on each of P platforms (a scanner and imaging protocol combination). The challenge is to construct mappings M_{iT} $i =$

$0, ..., P - 1$ from images acquired on platform i to the corresponding image acquired on some target platform $T \in \{0, ..., P - 1\}$.

MUSHAC [8–10] tests the ability to predict multiple high quality targets (modern platforms) from a single low-quality input (an old out-of-date platform) thus concentrating on the most challenging aspect of DH. With the same notation as before, we predict images I_{ij} $i = 1, ..., P - 1$ $j = 1, ..., N$ from I_{0j} $j = 1, .., N$.

When predicting acquisitions from platform $T \in \{1, ..., P - 1\}$, current state-of-the-art deep learning approaches extract patch pairs $\{(x(k), y_T(k)), ...\}$ from respective I_{0j}, I_{Tj} $j = 1, ..., N$. These approaches train a neural network $\mathcal{N}_T$ on these patches, where for input patch x we denote the neural network's estimate (also denoted as prediction) of y_T i.e. $\hat{y}_T = \mathcal{N}_T(x)$ and the loss is calculated as $L(\hat{y}_T, y_T)$. This process is repeated for different T. In this paper we use CNN-RISH [11], DIQT [4], SHResNet [12] to represent this class of technique.

In Fig. 1 we contrast the MSP architecture that we propose, with the single network approach. The MSP integrates information from multiple platforms and utilizes high-level features from individual networks, to inform the final prediction with additional neural networks. In training we use the set of corresponding patches $\{(x(k), y_1(k), ..., y_T(k), ...), ...\}$ from all images. We first take the pre-trained networks $\mathcal{N}_i$ $i = 1, ..., P - 1$ as the state-of-the-art single-networks, which may have different architectures, that have already been optimized. We denote for input patch x, the predictions of these networks as the first-stage prediction of the MSP: $\hat{y}_i^1 = \mathcal{N}_i(x)$ $i = 1, ...T$. For networks $\mathcal{N}_i$ $i \neq T$, we denote its last feature map as z_i. We then create the new networks $\mathcal{N}_{iT}$ $i \neq T$, each taking input z_i, where $\mathcal{N}_{iT}$ informs the final prediction of platform T with information from platform $i \neq T$. The second-stage prediction of the MSP, is a linear combination of network outputs of $\mathcal{N}_{iT}(z_i)$ $i \neq T$, with the fist-stage prediction $\hat{y}_T^1$:

$$\hat{y}_T^2 = (1 - \alpha)\hat{y}_T^1 + \frac{\alpha}{P - 1}(\sum_{i \neq T} \mathcal{N}_{iT}(z_i) + \hat{y}_T^1) \quad \alpha \in [0, 1]. \tag{1}$$

We train the whole MSP in unison, using supervised loss functions calculated at both stage predictions: $L(\hat{y}_i^1, y_i), L(\hat{y}_T^2, y_T)$ $i = 1, ..., P - 1$, which are backprop-agated through the network. For $\alpha \in [0, 1]$, we manually increase α from 0 to 1 during training, to combine pre-trained $\mathcal{N}_T$ with the untrained $\mathcal{N}_{iT}$ as in [16].

We provide an example of the MSP in Fig. 1 for $P = 4, T = 1$ and code [1].

3   Experiments and Results

In this section we present an overview of our MUSHAC dMRI hamonization dataset [8]. We describe how to process the raw data to produce patches for our supervised neural network approach. We then illustrate how MTL approaches, such as the MSP, produce improved results over state-of-the-art methods.

Harmonization Data. Data are obtained from the MUSHAC [8]. 10 healthy volunteers were scanned on three different scanners, an ageing 3T General Electric Excite-HDx scanner (max. gradient $40\,\mathrm{mT/m}$), a modern but standard 3T

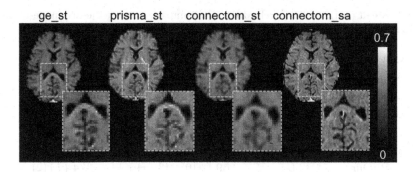

Fig. 2. Example of the normalized and direction-averaged dMRI image obtained from the same subject's brain using different acquisitions (st and sa) and different MRI scanners (GE, Prisma, Connectom).

Siemens Prisma scanner (max. gradient $80\,\mathrm{mT/m}$) and a state-of-the-art bespoke 3T Siemens Connectom scanner (max. gradient $300\,\mathrm{mT/m}$). dMRI images were acquired for $b = 1200\,\mathrm{s/mm^2}$ with two different manufacturer quality protocols: a standard (st) protocol – with voxel side 2.4 mm, 30 directions per b-value, TE $= 89\,\mathrm{ms}$ from all scanners; a state-of-the-art (sa) protocol on the Connectom – with voxel size 1.2 mm, 60 directions per b-value, TE $= 68\,\mathrm{ms}$. Note we excluded the sa protocol of the Prisma scanner, due to severe mis-alignments. For sa protocol, multiband-acquisition and stronger gradients shortened TE and improved both spatial and angular resolution per unit time. Additional $b = 0\,\mathrm{s/mm^2}$ images were acquired with TE and/or TR matching between protocols, as well as structural MPRAGEs for each scanner. The data were corrected for EPI and eddy-current distortions, subject motion and gradient non-linearity, as well as co-registered together as in [8]. In addition, brain masks excluding the skull and background were provided for each subject and each acquisition. The dataset size is representative of typical TH data-sets, where it is difficult to transport a large number of subjects from different centres and obtain multiple scans. See Fig. 2 for a visualisation.

Processing and Training. Raw data were pre-processed to extract signal features by SH deconvolution – variants of this technique are used as input-output common to the challenge and our comparison networks [4,11,12]. We employed [17,18] where the 28 coefficients of the 6th order real-and-symmetric SH deconvolution were estimated from the normalized raw signal considered as separate channels of our data. We first normalized the data, on each acquisition, per channel, to be mean 0 and standard deviation 1.

Neural-network data-harmonisation transformations work patch-by-patch on an input image. Each voxel within the brain mask of the input acquisition defines a patch with that voxel at the centre. The corresponding target patch comes from the corresponding location in the target image. For this paper we utilised input patch size as 11^3, with target patch size $11^3, 19^3$, depending on the target resolution. We then separated the patches into 90%, 10% training, test set.

Table 1. Mean (std), of 278 patch MSEs. We compare state-of-the-art single-network approaches, with MTL approaches, for three target platforms.

Model	Network type	prisma_st	connectom_st	connectom_sa
DIQT [4]	Single network	76 (±12)	59 (±14)	**463** (±123)
CNN-RISH [11]	Single network	78 (±11)	63 (±7)	532 (±144)
SHResNet [12]	Single network	**70** (±11)	**54** (±7)	524 (±112)
CPM [14]	MTL	67 (±12)	48 (±16)	417 (±102)
HNED [15]	MTL	71 (±12)	52 (±14)	406 (±98)
MSP (Ours)	MTL	**59** (±10)	**43** (±9)	**374** (±112)

Our implementation used PyTorch with Python, with a minibatch size of 12, ADAM optimizer, learning rate starting at $1E - 4$ and decaying by $\sqrt{2}$ per 15 or 25 epochs, for a minimum of 50 total epochs [1].

Comparison. We evaluate our approach via the tasks in MUSHAC [8]: to predict images from more modern platforms prisma_st, connectom_st, connectom_sa, from an older platform ge_st (see Fig. 2). Our evaluation was performed on a local scale, as in [8], we calculate the mean-squared-error (MSE) on the SH space. This metric is not based on the raw dMRI and encompasses all key aspects of the diffusion signal (anistropy, mean diffusivity, principle orientation).

We select three baselines, representing state-of-the-art approaches [9, 10], that predict each acquisition using separate neural networks: CNN-RISH [11], DIQT [4], SHResNet [12]. We also consider simple MTL sub-networks from CPM [14], HNED [15], illustrated in the supplementary material, which were formulated for different tasks and inspired the MSP. The super-resolution networks replaced a standard 3D convolution with a deconvolution/strided convolution layer, the connection networks are a stack of two 3D convolutions. We then constructed the MSP by combining the best single-network approaches (bold in Table 1).

Table 1 shows that MTL in general improves with respect to the single-network approaches, for all three target platforms. We use the Wilcoxon signed-rank test, a non-parametric statistical test, confirming that for all predicted platforms the differences in error scores are statistically significant, as p values obtained are all less than 10^{-5}, after Bonferroni correction.

Figure 3 shows qualitative results revealing differences in results from DIQT and MSP for connectom_sa, on a subject excluded from the training set. Improvements from MSP over DIQT are subtle but visible on both the SH and direction-encoded colour maps, e.g. MSP reduces errors directly underneath the left ventricle. Quantitatively in that figure, MSP improves the global SH MSE by 5% and the global direction-encoded colour MSE by 11%.

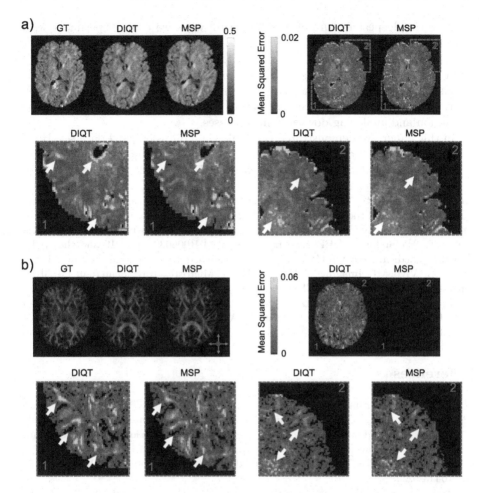

Fig. 3. A qualitative comparison of the DIQT – a single-network prediction, with our MSP network, compared to the Ground Truth (GT). (a) Comparison with the GT. The maps show the average of the first 6 SH coefficients. Quantitative maps of the MSE are also displayed in the second row. (b) Comparison with the reference GT. The maps show the colour-coded fractional anisotropy (FA) from diffusion tensor imaging computed using FSL [19]. Quantitative maps of the MSE are also displayed in the second row.

4   Conclusion and Future Work

In this paper we demonstrated how MTL approaches such as the MSP, increase the predictive power of deep learning in DH and improve over state-of-the-art single network approaches.

There are many potential directions of future work. Here we test just one MSP architecture, but many variations of deeper structures with more sophisticated connections between tasks are possible. For example, the MSP chooses

z_i to be the deepest feature of $\mathcal{N}_{iT}$, in future work we could experiment with connecting different layers.

One key problem in evaluating DH performance is residual misalignment of input and output images. This can mask strong performance when using simple global comparison metrics. It may be useful to devise alternative evaluation metrics that are robust to misalignment, or by moving away from direct image evaluation and analyzing downstream processes.

In this paper, we demonstrated the MSP via a diffusion MRI data set. However the same architecture extends naturally to harmonizing data between multiple different modalities, within or beyond MRI.

Acknowledgements. We thank: Tristan Clark and the HPC team (James O'Connor, Edward Martin) and the organizers of the 2017 MUSHAC challenge (Francesco Grussu, Enrico Kaden, Lipeng Ning, Jelle Veraart). This work was supported by an EPRSC and Microsoft scholarship and EPSRC grants M020533 R006032 R014019 and the NIHR UCLH Biomedical Research Centre. The data were acquired at the UK National Facility for In Vivo MR Imaging of Human Tissue Microstructure located in CUBRIC funded by the EPSRC (grant EP/M029778/1), and The Wolfson Foundation. Acquisition and processing of the data was supported by a Rubicon grant from the NWO (680-50-1527), a Wellcome Trust Investigator Award (096646/Z/11/Z), and a Wellcome Trust Strategic Award (104943/Z/14/Z).

References

1. Code. https://github.com/sbb-gh/. http://mig.cs.ucl.ac.uk/
2. Alexander, D.C., Zikic, D., Zhang, J., Zhang, H., Criminisi, A.: Image quality transfer via random forest regression: applications in diffusion MRI. In: Golland, P., Hata, N., Barillot, C., Hornegger, J., Howe, R. (eds.) MICCAI 2014. LNCS, vol. 8675, pp. 225–232. Springer, Cham (2014). https://doi.org/10.1007/978-3-319-10443-0_29
3. Tanno, R., et al.: Bayesian image quality transfer with CNNs: exploring uncertainty in dMRI super-resolution. In: Descoteaux, M., Maier-Hein, L., Franz, A., Jannin, P., Collins, D.L., Duchesne, S. (eds.) MICCAI 2017. LNCS, vol. 10433, pp. 611–619. Springer, Cham (2017). https://doi.org/10.1007/978-3-319-66182-7_70
4. Blumberg, S.B., Tanno, R., Kokkinos, I., Alexander, D.C.: Deeper image quality transfer: training low-memory neural networks for 3D images. In: Frangi, A.F., Schnabel, J.A., Davatzikos, C., Alberola-López, C., Fichtinger, G. (eds.) MICCAI 2018. LNCS, vol. 11070, pp. 118–125. Springer, Cham (2018). https://doi.org/10.1007/978-3-030-00928-1_14
5. Ye, D.H., Zikic, D., Glocker, B., Criminisi, A., Konukoglu, E.: Modality propagation: coherent synthesis of subject-specific scans with data-driven regularization. In: Mori, K., Sakuma, I., Sato, Y., Barillot, C., Navab, N. (eds.) MICCAI 2013. LNCS, vol. 8149. Springer, Heidelberg (2013). https://doi.org/10.1007/978-3-642-40811-3_76
6. Fortin, J.P., et al.: Harmonization of cortical thickness measurements across scanners and sites. NeuroImage **167**, 104–120 (2018)
7. Mirzaalian, H., et al.: Multi-site harmonization of diffusion MRI data in a registration framework. Brain Imaging Behav. **12**, 284–295 (2017)

8. Tax, C.M., et al.: Cross-scanner and cross-protocol diffusion MRI data harmonisation: a benchmark database and evaluation of algorithms. NeuroImage **195**, 285–299 (2019)
9. Ning, L., et al.: Cross-scanner and cross-protocol harmonisation of multi-shell diffusion MRI data: open challenge and evaluation results. In: ISMRM (2018)
10. Ning, L., et al.: Muti-shell diffusion MRI harmonisation and enhancement challenge (MUSHAC): progress and results. In: Bonet-Carne, E., Grussu, F., Ning, L., Sepehrband, F., Tax, C.M.W. (eds.) MICCAI 2018. MV, pp. 217–224. Springer, Cham (2019). https://doi.org/10.1007/978-3-030-05831-9_18
11. Cetin Karayumak, S., Kubicki, M., Rathi, Y.: Harmonizing diffusion MRI data across magnetic field strengths. In: Frangi, A.F., Schnabel, J.A., Davatzikos, C., Alberola-López, C., Fichtinger, G. (eds.) MICCAI 2018. LNCS, vol. 11072, pp. 116–124. Springer, Cham (2018). https://doi.org/10.1007/978-3-030-00931-1_14
12. Koppers, S., Bloy, L., Berman, J.I., Tax, C.M.W., Edgar, J.C., Merhof, D.: Spherical harmonic residual network for diffusion signal harmonization. In: Bonet-Carne, E., Grussu, F., Ning, L., Sepehrband, F., Tax, C.M.W. (eds.) MICCAI 2018. MV, pp. 173–182. Springer, Cham (2019). https://doi.org/10.1007/978-3-030-05831-9_14
13. Lee, C.Y., et al.: Deeply-supervised nets. In: AISTATS (2015)
14. Wei, S.E., et al.: Convolutional pose machines. In: CVPR (2016)
15. Xie, S., Tu, Z.: Holistically-nested edge detection. In: ICCV (2015)
16. Karras, T., et al.: Progressive growing of GANs for improved quality, stability, and variation. In: ICLR (2018)
17. Tournier, J.D., et al.: Direct estimation of the fiber orientation density function from diffusion-weighted MRI data using spherical deconvolution. NeuroImage **23**(3), 1176–1185 (2004)
18. Garyfallidis, E., et al.: DIPY, a library for the analysis of diffusion MRI data. Front. Neuroinformatics **8**, 8 (2014)
19. Jenkinson, M., et al.: Multi-site harmonization of diffusion MRI data in a registration framework. NeuroImage **62**, 782–790 (2012)

Self-supervised Feature Learning for 3D Medical Images by Playing a Rubik's Cube

Xinrui Zhuang[1,2], Yuexiang Li[2(✉)], Yifan Hu[2], Kai Ma[2], Yujiu Yang[1(✉)], and Yefeng Zheng[2]

[1] Graduate School at Shenzhen, Tsinghua University, Shenzhen, China
yang.yujiu@sz.tsinghua.edu.cn
[2] YouTu Lab, Tencent, Shenzhen, China
vicyxli@tencent.com

Abstract. Witnessed the development of deep learning, increasing number of studies try to build computer aided diagnosis systems for 3D volumetric medical data. However, as the annotations of 3D medical data are difficult to acquire, the number of annotated 3D medical images is often not enough to well train the deep learning networks. The self-supervised learning deeply exploiting the information of raw data is one of the potential solutions to loose the requirement of training data. In this paper, we propose a self-supervised learning framework for the volumetric medical images. A novel proxy task, i.e., Rubik's cube recovery, is formulated to pre-train 3D neural networks. The proxy task involves two operations, i.e., cube rearrangement and cube rotation, which enforce networks to learn translational and rotational invariant features from raw 3D data. Compared to the train-from-scratch strategy, fine-tuning from the pre-trained network leads to a better accuracy on various tasks, e.g., brain hemorrhage classification and brain tumor segmentation. We show that our self-supervised learning approach can substantially boost the accuracies of 3D deep learning networks on the volumetric medical datasets without using extra data. To our best knowledge, this is the first work focusing on the self-supervised learning of 3D neural networks.

Keywords: Self-supervised learning · Rubik's cube recovery · 3D medical images

1 Introduction

Compared with natural images, most medical images, e.g. computed tomography (CT) and magnetic resonance imaging (MRI), are volumetric which appear in a 3D form. A traditional diagnosis approach requires experienced physicians to manually browse the 3D volume data and search for the traits of abnormality,

---

This work was done when Xinrui Zhuang was an intern at YouTu Lab.

© Springer Nature Switzerland AG 2019
D. Shen et al. (Eds.): MICCAI 2019, LNCS 11767, pp. 420–428, 2019.
https://doi.org/10.1007/978-3-030-32251-9_46

which is laborious and suffers from the problem of inter-observer variation. Due to the development of deep learning, researchers proposed various 3D network architectures [1] to assist physicians in increasing the diagnosis accuracy. However, the training of deep learning models may require a large amount of training data. As the annotations of 3D medical images are difficult to acquire, i.e., each 3D volume requires experienced physicians to spend a couple of hours or even days for investigation, the performance of 3D deep learning frameworks suffers from the limited amount of annotated medical images.

To deal with the deficient annotated data, researchers attempted to exploit useful information from the unlabeled data with unsupervised approaches [10,12]. More recently, the self-supervised learning, as a new paradigm of unsupervised learning, attracts increasing attentions from the community. The pipeline consists of two steps: (1) pre-train a convolutional neural network (CNN) on a proxy task with a large non-annotated dataset. (2) fine-tune the pre-trained network for the specific target task with a small set of annotated data. The proxy task enforces neural networks to deeply mine useful information from the unlabeled raw data, which can boost the accuracy of the subsequent target task with limited training data. Various proxy tasks had been proposed, which include grayscale image colorization [5], jigsaw puzzle [8], object motion estimation [6] and rotation prediction [3].

For the applications with medical data, researchers took some prior-knowledge into account when formulating the proxy task. Zhang et al. [12] defined a proxy task that sorted the 2D slices extracted from the conventional 3D CT and MR volumes, to pre-train the neural networks for the fine-grained body part recognition (the target task). Spitzer et al. [10] proposed to pre-train neural networks on a self-supervised learning task, i.e., predicting the 3D distance between two patches sampled from the same brain, for the better segmentation of brain areas (the target task). However, all of the aforementioned self-supervised learning frameworks [10,12], including those for natural images [5,6,8], were proposed for 2D networks. As the 3D neural networks integrating the 3D spatial information usually outperform the 2D networks on volumetric medical data, a 3D-based self-supervised learning approach is worthwhile to develop.

In this paper, we propose a 3D-based self-supervised learning approach for volumetric medical data. We formulate a novel proxy task, namely Rubik's cube recovery, to deeply exploit the rich information from 3D medical data and loose the requirement of training data to well train a 3D deep learning model. Like playing a Rubik's cube, there are two operations in the process of our Rubik's cube recovery, i.e., cube rearrangement and cube rotation, which enforce the network to learn the features invariant to translation and rotation from the raw data. The pre-trained 3D network is then fine-tuned on two target tasks, i.e., brain hemorrhage classification and brain tumor segmentation. Experimental results show that the proposed approach can significantly improve accuracy of the 3D CNNs on target tasks, although the model is never explicitly pre-trained to exploit knowledge of brain hemorrhage and tumors. To our best knowledge, this is the first work focusing on the self-supervised learning of 3D CNNs.

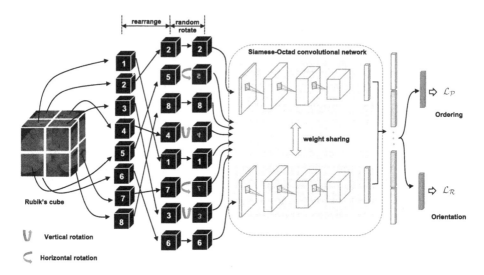

Fig. 1. Rubik's cube recovery. The proxy task has two operations, i.e., cube rearrangement and cube rotation.

2   Method

In this section, we introduce the proposed 3D self-supervised learning approach in details. The proposed approach aims to address the problem of deficient annotated 3D medical data by deeply exploiting the useful information from the limited training data. The approach first pre-trains a 3D CNN on the proxy task and then fine-tunes the pre-trained weights on the target tasks with manual annotations. Inspired by the jigsaw puzzle [8], a novel proxy task (Rubik's cube recovery), is proposed for the 3D neural networks. The pipeline of the proxy task is illustrated in Fig. 1.

2.1   Rubik's Cube Recovery

For a 3D medical volume, we first partition it into a grid (e.g., $2 \times 2 \times 2$) of cubes, and then permute the cubes with random rotations. Like playing a Rubik's cube, the proxy task aims to recover the original configuration, i.e., cubes are ordered and orientated.

Compared to the jigsaw puzzle, the Rubik's cube recovery task has two main differences: (1) The Rubik's cube recovery works on 3D volumetric data, while the jigsaw puzzle is proposed for 2D natural images; (2) The difficulty of recovering Rubik's cube is increased by adding the cube rotation operation, which encourages deep learning networks to leverage more spatial information.

Pre-processing. The neural networks are encouraged to learn and use high-level semantic features for Rubik's cube recovery rather than the texture information close to the cube boundaries. Therefore, we leave a gap (about 10 voxels) between two adjacent cubes during volume participation. The cube intensities are normalized to $[-1, 1]$ by using the mean and maximum intensity.

Network Architecture. As Fig. 1 shows, a Siamese network with M (which is the number of cubes) sharing weight branches, namely Siamese-Octad, is adopted to solve Rubik's cube. The backbone network for each branch can be any widely-used 3D CNN, e.g., 3D VGG [9]. The feature maps from the last fully-connected or convolution layer of all branches are concatenated and given as input to the fully-connected layer of separate tasks, i.e., cube ordering and orientating, which are supervised by permutation loss ($\mathcal{L}_P$) and rotation loss ($\mathcal{L}_R$), respectively.

Cube Ordering. The first step of our Rubik's cube recovery is the cube rearrangement. Taking a 2nd-order Rubik's cube, i.e., $2 \times 2 \times 2$ shown in Fig. 1, as an example, we first yield all the permutations ($\mathbb{P}$) of cubes, i.e., $\mathbb{P} = (P_1, P_2, ..., P_{8!})$. The permutations control the ambiguity of the task, if two permutations are too close to each other, the Rubik's cube recovery task becomes challenging and ambiguous for networks to learn. Therefore, we iteratively select the K permutations with the largest Hamming distance from $\mathbb{P}$. Then, for each time of Rubik's cube recovery, the eight cubes are rearranged according to one of the K permutations, e.g., $(2, 5, 8, 4, 1, 7, 3, 6)$ in Fig. 1. To properly reorder the cubes, the network is trained to identify the selected permutation from the K options, which can be seen as a classification task with K categories. Assuming the $1 \times K$ network prediction as p and the one-hot label as l, the permutation loss ($\mathcal{L}_P$) in this step can be defined as:

$$\mathcal{L}_P = -\sum_{j=1}^{K} l_j \log p_j. \tag{1}$$

Cube Orientation. The jigsaw puzzles only involve the translational motion of image tiles on a 2D plane, which makes the network only extract translational invariant features. In our 3D Rubik's cube task, we perform a new operation, i.e., random cube rotation, to encourage network to learn the rotational invariant features as well.

As the cubes often have a cuboid shape, free rotations result in 3 ($axes$) $\times$ 2 ($directions$) $\times$ 4 ($angles$) $= 24$ configurations. To reduce the complexity of the task, we limit the directions for cube rotation, i.e., only allowing 180° horizontal and vertical rotations. As Fig. 1 shows, the cubes (5, 7) and (4, 3) are horizontally and vertically rotated, respectively. To orientate the cubes, the network is required to recognize whether each of the input cubes has been rotated. It can be seen as a multi-label classification task using the $1 \times M$ (M is the number of cubes) ground truth (g) with 1 on the positions of rotated cubes and 0 vice versa. Hence, the predictions of this task are two $1 \times M$ vectors (r) indicating the possibilities of horizontal (hor) and vertical (ver) rotations for each cube.

The rotation loss ($\mathcal{L}_R$) can be written as:

$$\mathcal{L_R} = -\sum_{i=1}^{M}(g_i^{hor}\log r_i^{hor} + g_i^{ver}\log r_i^{ver}).\tag{2}$$

Objective. With the previously defined permutation loss ($\mathcal{L}_P$) and rotation loss ($\mathcal{L}_R$), the full objective ($\mathcal{L}$) for our 3D self-supervised CNN is summarized as:

$$\mathcal{L} = \alpha\mathcal{L}_P + \beta\mathcal{L}_R.\tag{3}$$

where α and β are loss weights, adjusting the relative influence of two tasks. We empirically find that equal weights $\alpha = \beta = 0.5$ leads to the best feature representations of pre-trained networks in the experiments.

2.2   Adapting Pre-trained Weights for Pixel-Wise Target Task

The CNN pre-trained on Rubik's cube recovery task can achieve a robust feature representation, which can then be transferred to the target tasks. For the classification task, the pre-trained CNN can be directly used for finetuning. For the segmentation of 3D medical images, the pre-trained weights can only be adapted to the encoder part of the fully convolutional network (FCN), e.g. U-Net [1]. The decoder of FCN still needs random initialization, which may wreck the pre-trained feature representation and neutralize the improvement generated by the pre-training. Inspired by the dense upsampling convolution (DUC) [11], we propose to apply convolutional operations directly on feature maps yield by the pre-trained encoder to get the dense pixel-wise prediction instead of the transposed convolutions. The DUC can significantly decrease the number of trainable parameters of the decoder and alleviate the influence caused by random initialization.

3   Experiment

In this section, we transfer the weights pre-trained on Rubik's cube recovery to two 3D medical image analysis tasks, i.e., pathological cause of brain hemorrhage classification and brain tumor segmentation. The datasets adopted in this study are randomly separated to training and test sets according to the ratio of 80:20.

3.1   Datasets

Brain Hemorrhage Dataset. We collected 1486 brain CT scan images from a collaborative hospital, which are used to analyze the pathological cause of brain hemorrhage. The 3D CT volumes containing brain hemorrhage can be classified to four pathological causes, i.e., aneurysm, arteriovenous malformation, moyamoya disease and hypertension. Each 3D CT volume is of size $230 \times 270 \times 30$

voxels. The weight pre-trained on Rubik's cube recovery can be directly transferred to this target task, i.e., brain hemorrhage classification. The cube size of Rubik's cube is $64 \times 64 \times 12$. The average classification accuracy (ACC) is adopted as metric for the performance evaluation.

BraTS-2018. The BraTS-2018 training set [7] consists of 285 brain tumor MR volumes, which have four modalities, i.e., native T1-weighted (T1), post-contrast T1-weighted (T1Gd), T2-weighted (T2), and T2 Fluid Attenuated Inversion Recovery (FLAIR). All MR images are co-registered to the same anatomical template, interpolated to the same resolution $(1\,\mathrm{mm}^3)$ and skull-stripped. The size of each volume is $240 \times 240 \times 155$ voxels. This dataset is widely-used to evaluate the accuracy of segmentation methods for brain tumors. The cube size of Rubik's cube is $64 \times 64 \times 64$. As the BraTS-2018 has four modalities, we concatenate the cubes from different modalities and send to each branch of Siamese-Octad network as input. The mean intersection over union (mIoU) [2] is adopted as the metric to evaluate the segmentation accuracy.

3.2   Performance on Solving Rubik's Cube

We evaluate the performance of the Siamese-Octad network on Rubik's cube recovery to verify whether the network can deal with the proxy task. The backbone of our Rubik's cube network (Siamese-Octad) is the 3D VGG [9], which is widely-used in self-supervised studies [8] and 3D medical image processing [1]. The test accuracies of $2 \times 2 \times 2$ Rubik's cube recovery on two datasets are listed in Table 1. As the random cube rotation increases the difficulty of solving Rubik's cube, the test accuracies of cube ordering degrade with -7.7% and -6.6% for brain hemorrhage dataset and BraTS-2018, respectively. On the other hand, the Rubik's cube network can achieve test accuracies of 93.1% and 82.1% for the cube orientation. The experimental results demonstrate that the cube rotation enables networks to develop the concept of rotated content, which means more structural information of brains is extracted compared to the rearrangement-only approach.

Table 1. The test accuracies of solving $2 \times 2 \times 2$ Rubik's cube on two datasets.

Dataset	Rearrange	Rotate	Accuracy (%)	
			Ordering	Orientation
Brain hemorrhage dataset	✓		99.7	-
Brain hemorrhage dataset	✓	✓	92.0	93.1
BraTS-2018	✓		99.5	-
BraTS-2018	✓	✓	92.9	82.1

Table 2. Test accuracies of models with different training strategies on target tasks.

	Brain hemorrhage cla. (ACC %)	Brain tumor seg. (mIoU %)	
	3D VGG [9]	U-Net [1]	3D DUC [11]
Train-from-scratch	72.6	73.3	74.0
Fine-tuned on UCF101	75.3	75.2	76.8
Cube ordering	81.1	73.9	75.0
Rubik's cube recovery (Ours)	**83.8**	**76.2**	**77.3**

3.3 Fine-Tuning Models on Target Tasks

We fine-tuned the networks pre-trained on the Rubik's cube recovery for the target tasks to evaluate the benefit produced by pre-trained weights. The training strategies, including train-from-scratch, fine-tuning with weights pre-trained on natural dataset (UCF101 [4]), are involved in comparison experiments. The test results are listed in Table 2.

Baselines. The train-from-scratch strategy is involved as the baseline. Furthermore, similar to the ImageNet pre-trained weights widely-used for 2D image processing, the action recognition dataset, i.e., UCF101, is adopted to pre-train our 3D CNNs. The UCF101 consists of 13320 videos, which can be classified to 101 action categories. We extract frames from videos to form a cube of $112 \times 112 \times 16$ to pre-train the 3D network. The pre-trained models are then transferred to the two target tasks for performance comparison. It is worthwhile to mention that our Rubik's cube pre-trained weights are generated by deeply exploiting useful information from limited training data without using any extra dataset.

Brain Hemorrhage Classification. As Table 2 shows, finetuning from the pre-trained weights can improve the accuracies of models for brain hemorrhage classification, compared to the train-from-scratch. Due to the gap between natural video and volumetric medical data, the improvement yielded by UCF101 pre-trained weights is limited, i.e., +2.7%. In comparison, our Rubik's cube pre-trained weights substantially boost the classification accuracy to 83.8%, which is 11.2% higher than that of train-from-scratch model.

Brain Tumor Segmentation. The mIoU of brain tumors yielded by models trained with different training strategies is also listed in Table 2. Two kinds of FCNs, i.e., U-Net [1] and DUC [11], are involved to evaluate the influence caused by random initialization of decoder. Compared to the models transferred from UCF101 pre-trained weights, the ones fine-tuned from our Rubik's cube recovery paradigm can generate more accurate segmentations for brain tumors, i.e., mIoUs of 76.2% and 77.3% are achieved by the U-Net and 3D DUC, respectively.

As the Rubik's cube recovery task only pre-trains the downsampling layers, the decoder (upsampling layers) of U-Net needs to be randomly initialized, which may wreck the feature representations learned by the pre-trained weights and consequently degrade the performance improvement. To alleviate the influence caused by random initialization, the DUC module, which significantly reduces the number of trainable parameters contained in the decoder, is more suitable for the transfer learning on pixel-wise prediction task. It can be observed from Table 2 that the 3D DUCs outperform the 3D U-Nets under all pre-training protocols, i.e., +1.6% and +1.1% for UCF101 and Rubik's cube pre-trained weights, respectively.

Comparison of Solving Different Rubik's Cubes. Table 2 shows the results of models fine-tuned from Rubik's cube without cube rotation as well. The models transferred from our Rubik's cube significantly outperform the ones only pre-trained with cube ordering task, i.e., +2.7% and +2.3% for brain hemorrhage classification and brain tumor segmentation, respectively. The experimental result reveals that the difficult Rubik's cube task may lead to the better generalization of models. Although the accuracy of cube ordering decreases by adding the cube rotation (as shown in Table 1), the 3D neural networks pre-trained on the multi-tasks, i.e., cube ordering and orientation, seem to exploit a more robustness feature representation, i.e., translational and rotational invariant, from the raw 3D data.

4   Conclusion

In this paper, we proposed a self-supervised learning framework for the volumetric medical images. A novel proxy task, i.e., Rubik's cube recovery, was formulated to pre-train 3D neural networks. The proxy task involved two operations, i.e., cube rearrangement and cube rotation, which enforced networks to learn translational and rotational invariant features from raw 3D data.

Acknowledgements. The work was supported by the National Key Research and Development Program of China (No. 2018YFB1601102), the Natural Science Foundation of China (No. 61702339), the Key Area Research and Development Program of Guangdong Province, China (No. 2018B010111001), and Shenzhen special fund for the strategic development of emerging industries (No. JCYJ20170412170118573).

References

1. Çiçek, Ö., Abdulkadir, A., Lienkamp, S.S., Brox, T., Ronneberger, O.: 3D U-Net: learning dense volumetric segmentation from sparse annotation. In: Ourselin, S., Joskowicz, L., Sabuncu, M.R., Unal, G., Wells, W. (eds.) MICCAI 2016. LNCS, vol. 9901, pp. 424–432. Springer, Cham (2016). https://doi.org/10.1007/978-3-319-46723-8_49

2. Garcia-Garcia, A., Orts-Escolano, S., Oprea, S., Villena-Martinez, V., Garcia-Rodriguez, J.: A review on deep learning techniques applied to semantic segmentation. arXiv e-print: arXiv:1704.06857 (2017)
3. Gidaris, S., Singh, P., Komodakis, N.: Unsupervised representation learning by predicting image rotations. In: ICLR (2018)
4. Khurram, S., Zamir, A.R., Shah, M.: UCF101: a dataset of 101 human actions classes from videos in the wild. arXiv e-print: arXiv:1212.0402 (2012)
5. Larsson, G., Maire, M., Shakhnarovich, G.: Colorization as a proxy task for visual understanding. In: CVPR, pp. 840–849 (2017)
6. Lee, H.Y., Huang, J.B., Singh, M., Yang, M.H.: Unsupervised representation learning by sorting sequences. In: ICCV, pp. 667–676 (2017)
7. Menze, B.H., Jakab, A., Bauer, S., et al.: The multimodal brain tumor image segmentation benchmark (BRATS). IEEE Trans. Med. Imaging $34(10)$, 1993–2024 (2015)
8. Noroozi, M., Vinjimoor, A., Favaro, P., Pirsiavash, H.: Boosting self-supervised learning via knowledge transfer. In: CVPR, pp. 9359–9367 (2018)
9. Simonyan, K., Zisserman, A.: Very deep convolutional networks for large-scale image recognition. In: ICLR (2015)
10. Spitzer, H., Kiwitz, K., Amunts, K., Harmeling, S., Dickscheid, T.: Improving cytoarchitectonic segmentation of human brain areas with self-supervised siamese networks. In: Frangi, A.F., Schnabel, J.A., Davatzikos, C., Alberola-López, C., Fichtinger, G. (eds.) MICCAI 2018. LNCS, vol. 11072, pp. 663–671. Springer, Cham (2018). https://doi.org/10.1007/978-3-030-00931-1_76
11. Wang, P., et al.: Understanding convolution for semantic segmentation. In: WACV, pp. 1451–1460 (2018)
12. Zhang, P., Wang, F., Zheng, Y.: Self supervised deep representation learning for fine-grained body part recognition. In: ISBI, pp. 578–582 (2017)

Bayesian Volumetric Autoregressive Generative Models for Better Semisupervised Learning

Guilherme Pombo[1]([✉]), Robert Gray[1], Thomas Varsavsky[1,2], John Ashburner[1], and Parashkev Nachev[1]

[1] Institute of Neurology, UCL, London, UK
rmapgcp@ucl.ac.uk
[2] School of Biomedical Engineering and Imaging Sciences, Kings College London, London, UK

Abstract. Deep generative models are rapidly gaining traction in medical imaging. Nonetheless, most generative architectures struggle to capture the underlying probability distributions of volumetric data, exhibit convergence problems, and offer no robust indices of model uncertainty. By comparison, the autoregressive generative model PixelCNN can be extended to volumetric data with relative ease, it readily attempts to learn the true underlying probability distribution and it still admits a Bayesian reformulation that provides a principled framework for reasoning about model uncertainty.

Our contributions in this paper are two fold: first, we extend Pixel-CNN to work with volumetric brain magnetic resonance imaging data. Second, we show that reformulating this model to approximate a deep Gaussian process yields a measure of uncertainty that improves the performance of semi-supervised learning, in particular classification performance in settings where the proportion of labelled data is low. We quantify this improvement across classification, regression, and semantic segmentation tasks, training and testing on clinical magnetic resonance brain imaging data comprising T1-weighted and diffusion-weighted sequences.

Keywords: Generative · Semi-supervised · Bayesian · Autoregressive

1 Introduction

There are two common problems with discriminative learning: class imbalance and sparse labels. These problems are particularly prevalent in medical imaging, due to the essential nature of clinical data. Semi-supervised learning provides a partial solution to these problems. Semi-supervised learning can be improved by using deep generative models, to learn better representations of the data, where generalisable decision boundaries are easier to identify [7].

© Springer Nature Switzerland AG 2019
D. Shen et al. (Eds.): MICCAI 2019, LNCS 11767, pp. 429–437, 2019.
https://doi.org/10.1007/978-3-030-32251-9_47

Variational autoencoders (VAEs), generative adversarial networks (GANs), and autoregressive (AR) models are the leading architectures for deep generative modelling. Unfortunately, their application to volumetric data has so far proved challenging, owing to poor convergence and distribution mode dropping, in the case of GANs [8], or to potentially inaccurate error bounds and inappropriate independence assumptions, in the case of VAEs [8]. The use of generative modelling with high resolution 3D data is still only tentatively explored.

Our contributions are as follows: in Sect. 3 we show how the 2D generative model PixelCNN [10] can be extended to work efficiently with volumetric data. We call the resulting model 3DPixelCNN. Furthermore, we incorporate the architectural changes suggested in [4] so that we can compute voxel-wise measures of uncertainty with little computational overhead. In Sect. 4 we show the benefits of using these uncertainty measures and 3DPixelCNN's hidden layer activations, in semi-supervised scenarios where labelled data is limited. Our evaluation incorporates three tasks: semantic segmentation of acute stroke lesions on diffusion weighted imaging (DWI) and age regression and sex classification on grey matter tissue compartments extracted from T1-weighted magnetic resonance imaging (MRI). Code available at https://github.com/guilherme-pombo/3DPixelCNN.

2   Related Work

2.1   Generative Models for Brain Imaging

We are interested in modelling $p(\boldsymbol{x})$, the probability distribution for the stochastic process that generates our brain volumes. In the context of brain imaging, we have a likelihood model p_θ, where the parameters θ are found by maximising the following objective:

$$\mathcal{L}(\theta) = \frac{1}{N} \sum_{i=1}^{N} \log p_\theta\left(x_i\right) \sim \int p(\boldsymbol{x}) \log p_\theta(\boldsymbol{x}) d\boldsymbol{x}; \tag{1}$$

here, $x_1, ..., x_N$ are the training volumes, which we assume have been sampled i.i.d from $p(\boldsymbol{x})$. In medical imaging it is common to process volumes as 2D slices to reduce processing time and memory consumption. However, in order to utilise all of the information in x_i, and to demonstrate the feasibility 3DPixelCNN, we use a fully 3D model.

To the best of our knowledge, [11] is the only work prior to ours to train a generative model on high-resolution 3D brain imagery. They model the (relatively low-detail) computed tomography (CT) modality using an approximation to a deep Gaussian process (c.f. Sect. 2.3) and an Autoencoder (AE). In the present article we also use this approximation but with a generative model that has increased representational power. We describe this model in the following section.

2.2   PixelRNN

In [10], the authors show how to model $p(\boldsymbol{x})$ autoregressively, by modelling the joint distribution of pixels in an image using recurrent neural networks. They treat their (2D) images, with dimensions $M \times N$, as a one-dimensional sequence of length MN, and they write the product of the conditional distributions over pixels as:

$$p(\boldsymbol{x}) = \prod_{i=1}^{MN} p\left(x_i | x_1, \ldots, x_{i-1}\right).$$

This model is comparatively slow due to RNNs' difficulty in parallelising, so the authors approximate it with much faster standard convolutional networks. To ensure the receptive field of each convolution around each pixel only includes the pixels on which its probability is conditioned (thus, avoiding seeing the future context) they add masks to the convolutions. However, the bounded nature of this 'masked' convolutional architecture causes a significant part of the input image to be ignored: a triangular pattern of omitted voxels they call the 'blind spot'. To remedy this, the authors of [9] use two masks instead of one, which they call 'stacks': the first one is conditioned on the row so far (the 'horizontal' stack) and the second one conditions on all rows above (the 'vertical' stack).

The greater computational efficiency of PixelCNN compared with PixelRNN carries a cost in reconstruction quality. However, it has been shown [9] that this can be ameliorated by replacing the rectified linear units between the convolutional stacks with a gated activation unit. This results in a better emulation of a long short-term memory (LSTM) gate. This use of both the convolutional stacks and the gated unit has enabled PixelCNN to match PixelRNN's reconstruction quality, whilst maintaining computational feasibility.

2.3   Dropout as a Bayesian Approximation

Unlike VAEs, AR models are not Bayesian by construction, and they do not produce implicit or explicit estimates of model uncertainty. In [4], Gal and Ghahramani show that simply incorporating Dropout [13] in every layer of any given neural network makes it capable of doing Bayesian inference, without harming performance. Once these changes are made, the standard deviation of a large-enough batch of forward passes yields a robust measure of uncertainty.

In [14] it is shown that since natural images exhibit strong spatial correlation, the feature map activations are strongly correlated - so applying standard Dropout to the kernels of the convolution operators is ill advised. Hence, they purpose a new dropout method, SpatialDropout, whereby for a given convolution feature tensor of size $H \times W \times D \times$ channels, a mask of size $1 \times 1 \times 1 \times$ channels is applied.

3   Methods

To extend the PixelCNN solution to volumetric data we must first solve the blind spot problem for 3D (c.f. Sect. 2.2). Consider our model processing an $M \times N \times K$

volume, and currently calculating the conditional distribution of the voxel with coordinates (R, C, D), which we denote $x_{R,C,D}$. We must now use three stacks (c.f. Sect. 2.2): horizontal, depth and vertical.

The **Horizontal stack** conditions on the current depth channel and takes as input the output of the previous horizontal stack gate, as well as the output of the depth and vertical stacks. The set of voxels it considers is $\{x_{R,C,d}|d \in \{1, \ldots, D-1\}\}$. In turn the **Depth stack** conditions on all the entries to the left of the current voxel, but does not go up any rows. It takes as input the output of the previous depth gate, as well as the output of the vertical stack. Its receptive field grows in 2D rectangular fashion, defined by the set $\{x_{R,c,d}|c \in \{1, \ldots, C-1\}, d \in \{1, \ldots, K\}\}$. Finally, the **Vertical Stack** conditions on all the rows and columns in the level above the current voxel. It does not have any masking. Its output is fed into the horizontal and depth stacks and its receptive field grows as a cuboid, defined by the set $\{x_{r,c,d}|r \in \{1, \ldots, R-1\}, c \in \{1, \ldots, N\}, d \in \{1, \ldots, K\}\}$.

These stacks ensure our convolution operations have the correct receptive fields. To reiterate, using just regular convolutions would lead to a bounded receptive field, which in turn would have led to the omission of several voxels from calculations of the conditional distribution (a pyramidal 'blind spot'). These stacks are represented in Fig. 1. We use the gated activation unit from [9] to efficiently combine the information of different stacks. We first add the stacks together and do a channel-wise split. If the tensor has N channels, then we now have tensor W_1 with the first $N/2$ channels and tensor W_2 with the remaining channels. The gated activation unit is calculated as $\tanh(W_1) \odot sigmoid(W_2)$, where $\odot$ is the Hadamard product. After each gate we have a skip shortcut [5] to the next stack in the model. After the first layer, as in [12] we also add a residual connection [5] from a Gated unit to the next one. SpatialDropout is applied after every convolution operator so that we can approximate a deep Gaussian process (see Sect. 2.2). Model statistics are derived at test time from batches of multiple forward passes with dropout enabled. We denote the mean and standard deviation of these batches by μ and σ respectively.

We train our 3DPixelCNN models using continuous negative log likelihood (NLL), and evaluate using log likelihood. We used continuous rather than discrete NLL as it has been shown [12] that treating pixel intensities as emission probabilities performs poorly for large images, resulting in noisy and speckly reconstructions. We trained for 20 epochs using the Adam optimiser [6]. The initial learning rate was 0.001, the batch size was 1 and the dropout rate was 0.15 (dropout rates between 0.1 and 0.2 are recommended in [4]). Our model has five layers with the structure depicted in Fig. 1. We use kernel sizes of $3 \times 3 \times 3$ for all non-masked convolutions in the network. We could have incorporated downsampling as in [12], but we leave this for future work.

4   Experiments and Results

Data: We use two separate datasets. One is a collection of routinely acquired DWI from patients evaluated for acute stroke at our clinic. This comprises 1333 scans with evidence of an acute ischaemic lesion, and 982 scans with no evidence of an acute lesion but variable presence of chronic vascular disease. The volumes we use consist of the b1000 sequence non-linearly registered to MNI space with unified segmentation [1]. A manually-curated binary mask delineating the area of ischaemic damage is our ground truth for lesion semantic segmentation [15]. We also use a manually curated mask to remove any voxels outside of the brain.

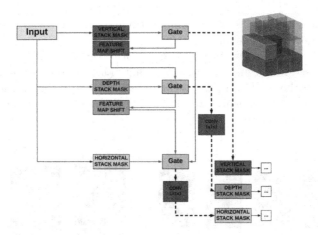

Fig. 1. The two figures show how the vertical (blue), depth (orange) and horizontal(green) stacks, are used to get the conditional distributions over the pixels, for the pixel in consideration (red) (Cube upside down for easier visualisation) (Color figure online)

The second dataset consists of 13287 SPM Grey Matter (GM) tissue compartments from MRIs obtained from UK Biobank, and routinely acquired clinical imaging at UCLH. The GM segmentations were derived using methods from [1]. Sex and age are known for all patients and were used to evaluate models on classification and regression tasks. For both modalities we reduced the computational burden (due to time constraints) by downsampling the volumes, using bilinear resampling, to 3 mm resolution $52 \times 64 \times 52$ volumes.

Image Reconstructions: For each volume in the DWI and GM datasets, we produce its reconstruction, and then generate μ and σ by performing $T = 20$ forward passes with dropout left on (c.f. Sect. 2.3).

We use a train/validation/test split of 80/10/10. The best log likelihood obtained by the model in the task of volume reconstruction on the test sets at 3 mm, are **0.360** for the DWI data and **0.105** for the GM data. Our model outperforms the Bayesian AE from [11] which achieves 0.378 on DWI and 0.222 on GM. Notice that on the more detailed modality (T1-GM) our model performs 111% better.

In order to produce uncertainty estimates (σ) for DWI, we trained our 3DPixelCNN only on data with no evidence of stroke lesion, i.e. from the distribution

$p(\boldsymbol{x}|\text{no lesion})$. Therefore, when producing $\boldsymbol{\sigma}$ for lesioned data, the uncertainty masks provide a measure of the distance from the lesioned brain to the expected distribution of non-lesioned brains. We use a simple classification strategy on the volumes - thresholding the average intensity of the volume, x_i, which we denote as $\tau(x_i)$. On the DWI ischemic stroke lesion test set, applying this classification strategy on regular volumes yields Dice coefficients of 14.7%, whereas on $\boldsymbol{\sigma}$ it yields Dice coefficients of 23.7%. This same strategy on the Bayesian AE, $|x_i - AE(x_i)|$ (see [11] for more details) yields a performance of 17.3%. This provides early confirmation that uncertainty estimates of generative models capture useful task-independent signal.

Figure 2 shows a representative selection of reconstructions of GM volumes and unsupervised lesion masks produced using $\tau(x_i)$. Notice on the MRI reconstruction, when the original image is corrupted, the 3DPixelCNN model acts as a super resolution mechanism, further showing the model has learnt $p(\boldsymbol{x})$ and is not simply memorising the training set.

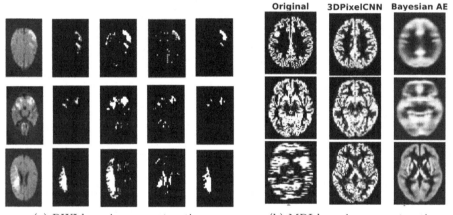

(a) DWI bayesian reconstructions   (b) MRI bayesian reconstructions

Fig. 2. (a): From left to right: (1) The slice through the axial plane with the greatest area of lesion, (2) The stroke label map, (3) $\tau(x_i)$ (4) $|x_i - AE(x_i)|$ (5) $\tau(\boldsymbol{\sigma})$. $\boldsymbol{\sigma}$ helps capture the tightest bound on the lesion (b) Axial slices of (1) The original volume, (2) The 3DPixelCNN reconstruction and (3) The Bayesian AE reconstruction (On the last volume there was a capture problem and we use it to test 3DPixelCNN's ability to super resolve)

Semi-supervised Learning: To experiment with using our uncertainty measures to improve supervised tasks, we use our DWI dataset for evaluating models on the task of **semantic segmentation** and our GM dataset to evaluate **regression** and **classification** tasks.

For the segmentation task we use a 3D U-Net [2] as the **baseline**. As the DWI dataset is not yet public, there are no state of the art results to which we can compare our results. For the age regression and sex classification tasks we use the architecture from [3] as our baseline, which we'll call ASC, adding only L2 regularisation and Dropout to ensure better generalisation. All models are trained with early stopping using the validation set, the criterion being 20 successive epochs without a drop in validation error. The models are trained in 5-fold fashion (80/10/10 split) for added statistical resilience. We compare the models' Dice scores on a semantic segmentation task, their mean absolute errors on an age regression task and their binary accuracy on a sex classification task, all evaluated on the test set.

Figure 3 shows mean model performance with error bars for three different types of inputs into both the 3D-UNet and ASC classifiers: (1) using just the original volumes as input (red- χ); (2) using original data concatenated with μ and σ (blue - ξ). For the case Bayesian AE we concatenate μ and $|x_i - AE(x_i)|$; (3) using the activations of the penultimate convolutional layer of the 3DPixelCNN. (black/green - ψ). For the Bayesian AE we use its latent space.

When using 3DPixelCNN, we notice that performance with ξ was significantly better than with χ, for all dataset sizes tested and classification tasks. For sex classification and age regression, using ψ results in better performance than both χ and ξ. We speculate that this is because the embeddings, which are higher-dimensional (10 vs 3 channels), comprise a decomposition of the data from which useful decision boundaries can be more readily identified, although this extra dimensionality comes at the cost of greater GPU memory requirements. On the other hand, for lesion segmentation, using ξ performs better than using either χ or ψ.

For semantic segmentation using ξ, the increase is most noticeable at smaller N with an improvement of 0.082 (25.6%) in Dice coefficient for $N < 500$ and an average increase of 0.056 (15.2%) for all N. Using ψ provides less of a performance gain, with an average increase in Dice of 0.025 (6.9%). For age regression and sex classification, we notice a steady increase in performance when using ξ, with an average error reduction of 0.30 years (3.98%) and accuracy increase of 1.87%, respectively. Using ψ, on the other hand, results in an average error reduction of 0.68 years (9.09%) for age regression and accuracy increase of 3.36%, for sex classification. Using the Bayesian AE's ξ results in a performance degradation of at least 2% for all tasks, compared to using the original volume. We suspect this is because here ξ is relatively noisy, as can be seen in Fig. 2. On the other hand, using the latent space, ψ, results in an average 5.6% increase for the age regression task and a 2.2% increase for sex classification. The Bayesian AE's latent space degraded performance for the semantic segmentation task.

Clearly, 3DPixelCNN's uncertainty measures help most with semantic segmentation. They seem to be most useful for tasks with more localised signal (lesion segmentation) as opposed to global signal. We speculate this is because in the lesioned brains σ is more focused on the lesion, since we had the generative model learn $p(x|\text{no lesion})$, whereas the uncertainty maps are much noisier for volumes with less obvious abnormalities, since the 3DPixelCNN learnt only $p(x)$. We hypothesize these uncertainty measures are also helpful in the presence of artifacts (as can be seen in Fig. 2), which is why they also helped for tasks with less abnormal brains.

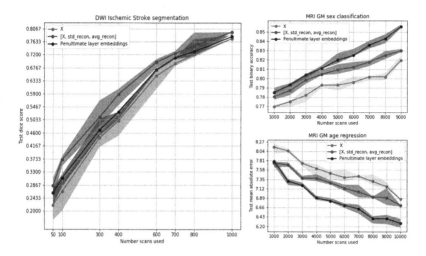

Fig. 3. From left to right: Comparison of DWI segmentation performance, Comparison of GM sex classification performance and age regression performance (Color figure online)

5   Conclusion

We have presented the first implementation of a volumetric neural network-based autoregressive model. We have shown that it is a method that can capture the richness of a complicated 3D probability distribution and is therefore well-suited to medical imaging. By augmenting labelled data with measures of uncertainty derived from unsupervised models, we saw improved performance in every supervised task we carried out. For tasks on brains without gross abnormalities, we found it was better to use 3DPixelCNN's penultimate layer activations than the uncertainty estimates. For lesion detection, we found that the uncertainty measures provided a bigger performance increase, which is of more utility in the medical imaging domain.

Acknowledgments. This research has been conducted using the UK Biobank Resource under Application Number 16273. This work is supported by the EPSRC-funded UCL CDT in Medical Imaging (EP/L016478/1), the Department of Health's NIHR-funded BRC at UCLH and the Wellcome Trust.

References

1. Ashburner, J., et al.: Unified segmentation. Neuroimage **26**(3), 839–851 (2005)
2. Çiçek, Ö., Abdulkadir, A., Lienkamp, S.S., Brox, T., Ronneberger, O.: 3D U-Net: learning dense volumetric segmentation from sparse annotation. In: Ourselin, S., Joskowicz, L., Sabuncu, M.R., Unal, G., Wells, W. (eds.) MICCAI 2016. LNCS, vol. 9901, pp. 424–432. Springer, Cham (2016). https://doi.org/10.1007/978-3-319-46723-8_49

3. Cole, J.H., et al.: Predicting brain age with deep learning from raw imaging data results in a reliable and heritable biomarker. NeuroImage **163**, 115–124 (2017)
4. Gal, Y., Ghahramani, Z.: Dropout as a Bayesian approximation: representing model uncertainty in deep learning. In: ICML, pp. 1050–1059 (2016)
5. He, K., et al.: Deep residual learning for image recognition. CoRR (2015)
6. Kingma, D.P., et al.: Adam: a method for stochastic optimization. arXiv preprint arXiv:1412.6980 (2014)
7. Kingma, D.P., et al.: Semi-supervised learning with deep generative models. In: NIPS, pp. 3581–3589 (2014)
8. Kingma, D.P., et al.: Glow: generative flow with invertible 1x1 convolutions. In: NIPS, pp. 10236–10245 (2018)
9. van den Oord, A., et al.: Conditional image generation with PixelCNN decoders. In: NIPS, pp. 4790–4798 (2016)
10. van den Oord, A., et al.: Pixel recurrent neural networks. arXiv preprint arXiv:1601.06759 (2016)
11. Pawlowski, N., et al.: Unsupervised lesion detection in brain CT using Bayesian convolutional autoencoders (2018)
12. Salimans, T., et al.: PixelCNN++. In: ICLR (2017)
13. Srivastava, N., et al.: Dropout: a simple way to prevent neural networks from overfitting. J. Mach. Learn. Res. **15**, 1929–1958 (2014)
14. Tompson, J., et al.: Efficient object localization using convolutional networks. In: CVPR, pp. 648–656 (2015)
15. Xu, T., et al.: High-dimensional therapeutic inference in the focally damaged human brain. Brain **141**, 48–54 (2017)

Hydranet: Data Augmentation for Regression Neural Networks

Florian Dubost[1](✉), Gerda Bortsova[1], Hieab Adams[1,2], M. Arfan Ikram[1,2,3],
Wiro Niessen[1,4], Meike Vernooij[1,2], and Marleen de Bruijne[1,5]

[1] Department of Radiology and Nuclear Medicine,
Erasmus MC - University Medical Center Rotterdam, Rotterdam, The Netherlands
floriandubost1@gmail.com, marleen.debruijne@erasmusmc.nl
[2] Department of Epidemiology, Erasmus MC, Rotterdam, The Netherlands
[3] Department of Neurology, Erasmus MC, Rotterdam, The Netherlands
[4] Department of Imaging Physics, Faculty of Applied Science,
TU Delft, Delft, The Netherlands
[5] Department of Computer Science, University of Copenhagen,
Copenhagen, Denmark

Abstract. Deep learning techniques are often criticized to heavily depend on a large quantity of labeled data. This problem is even more challenging in medical image analysis where the annotator expertise is often scarce. We propose a novel data-augmentation method to regularize neural network regressors that learn from a single global label per image. The principle of the method is to create new samples by recombining existing ones. We demonstrate the performance of our algorithm on two tasks: estimation of the number of enlarged perivascular spaces in the basal ganglia, and estimation of white matter hyperintensities volume. We show that the proposed method improves the performance over more basic data augmentation. The proposed method reached an intraclass correlation coefficient between ground truth and network predictions of 0.73 on the first task and 0.84 on the second task, only using between 25 and 30 scans with a single global label per scan for training. With the same number of training scans, more conventional data augmentation methods could only reach intraclass correlation coefficients of 0.68 on the first task, and 0.79 on the second task.

1 Introduction

Deep learning techniques are getting increasingly popular for image analysis but are often dependent on a large quantity of labeled data. In case of medical images, this problem is even stronger as data acquisition is administratively and technically more complex, as data sharing is more restricted, and as the annotator expertise is scarce.

To address biomarker (e.g. number or volume of lesions) quantification, many methods propose to optimize first a segmentation problem and then derive the

© Springer Nature Switzerland AG 2019
D. Shen et al. (Eds.): MICCAI 2019, LNCS 11767, pp. 438–446, 2019.
https://doi.org/10.1007/978-3-030-32251-9_48

target quantity with simpler methods. These approaches require expensive voxel-wise annotations. In this work, we circumvent the segmentation problem by opti-mizing our method to directly regress the target quantity [1–5]. Therefore we need only a single label per image instead of voxel-wise annotations. Our main contribution is that we push this limit even further by proposing a data augmen-tation method to reduce the number of training images required to optimize the regressors. The proposed method is designed for global image-level labels that represent a countable quantity. Its principle is to combine *real* training samples to construct many more *virtual* training samples. During training, our model takes as input random sets of images and is optimized to predict a single label for each of these sets that denotes the sum of the labels of all images of the set. This is motivated by the idea that adding a large quantity of virtual samples with weaker labels may reduce the over-fitting to training samples and improve the generalization to unseen data.

1.1 Related Work

Data augmentation can act as a regularizer and improve the generalization per-formance of neural networks. In addition to simple data-augmentations such as rotation, translation and flipping, the authors of Unet [6] stress for instance that random elastic deformations significantly improved the performance of their model. Generative adversarial networks have for instance also been used to gen-erate training samples, and hence reduce the over-fitting [7].

Recently, data augmentation methods using combinations of training sam-ples have been published. Zhang et al. [8] proposed to construct virtual training samples by computing a linear combination of pairs of real training samples. The corresponding one-hot labels are summed with the same coefficients. The authors evaluated their method on classification datasets from computer vision and on a speech dataset, and demonstrate that their method improves the gener-alization of state-of-the-art neural networks. Simultaneously, Inoue et al. [9] and Tokozume et al. [10] reached similar conclusions. In case of grayscale volumetric inputs, summing image intensity values could overlay the target structures, con-fuse discriminative shapes, and thus harm the performance of the network. With our method, training samples can be combined without overlaying the intensity values. The other difference with the above-mentioned approaches is that our method is also not designed for classification, but for regression of global labels, such as volume or count in an image. With the proposed combination of samples, our method computes plausible augmentation.

2   Methods

The principle of the proposed data augmentation method is to create many new (and weaker) training samples by combining existing ones (see Fig. 1). In the remainder, the original samples are called *real samples*, and the newly created samples are called *virtual samples*.

2.1   Proposed Data Augmentation.

During training, the model is not optimized on single real samples I with label y, but on sets S of n random samples $I_1, I_2, ..., I_n$ with label $y_s = \sum_{i=1}^{n} y_i$, with y_i the label of sample I_i. These sets S with labels y_s are the virtual samples. Consequently, the loss function L is computed directly on these virtual samples S and not anymore the individual real samples I_i. This approach is designed for labels describing a quantitative element in the samples, such as volume or count in an image.

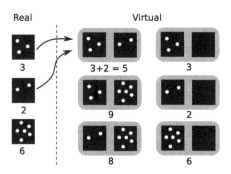

Fig. 1. Creating virtual training samples by recombining real training samples for regression tasks. The real training samples are displayed on the left, and the virtual samples on the right. The label is indicated under each sample, and corresponds to the number of white blobs. By recombining samples, we can significantly increase the size of the training dataset. For example, by recombining the real samples with labels 3 and 2, we can create a new sample with label 5 (arrows). All possible combinations are shown in blue. For the illustration, we show only combinations of two samples, but any number of samples can be combined. In our experiments, we used combinations of maximum 4 samples. (Color figure online)

To create the sets S, the samples I_i are drawn without replacement from the training set at each epoch. To create more combinations of samples, and to allow the model to use the real samples for its optimization, the size of the sets S can randomly vary in $\{1, n\}$ during training. If the training set contains m samples, with our method, we can create $\sum_{i=1}^{n} \binom{m}{i}$ possible different combinations (the order of the samples I_i in S has no effect on the optimization).

Difference with Mini-batch Stochastic Gradient Descent (SGD). In mini-batch SGD, the model is also optimized on sets of random samples, but the loss function L is computed individually for each sample of the batch, and then summed (averaged). For the proposed method, the predictions are first summed, and the loss function is then computed a single time. For non-linear loss functions, this is not equivalent: $\sum_{i=1}^{n} L(\hat{y}_i, y_i) \neq L(\sum_{i=1}^{n} \hat{y}_i, \sum_{i=1}^{n} y_i)$, with $\hat{y}_i$ the model's prediction for sample I_i.

Regularization Strength. The regularization strength can usually be modulated by at least one parameter, for instance the degree of rotation applied to the input image, or the percentage of neurons dropped in Dropout [14]. In the proposed method, the regularization effect can be controlled by varying the average number of samples used to create combinations.

2.2 Implementation

We optimize a regression neural network with a 3D image for input, and global label representing a volume or count for output. There are at least two possible implementations of the proposed method. The first implementation could consist of modifying the computation of the loss function across samples in a mini-batch, and provide mini-batches of random size. Alternatively the model's architecture could be adapted to receive the set of images. We opted for the second approach.

Base Regressor. Figure 2 left shows the architecture of the base regression neural network. It is both simple (196 418 parameters) and flexible to allow fast prototyping. There is no activation function after the last layer. The output $\hat{y}$ can therefore span $\mathbb{R}$ and the network is optimized with the mean squared error (MSE). We call this regression network f, such that $f(x) = \hat{y}$, with x the input image.

Combination of Samples. To process several images simultaneously, we replicate n times the regressor f during training (Fig. 2 right), resulting in n different branches $f_1, f_2, ..., f_n$ that receive the images $I_1, I_2, ..., I_n$. The weights of each head f_i are shared such that $f_i = f$. A new network g is constructed as:

$$g(S) = g(I_1, I_2, ..., I_n) = \sum_{i=1}^{n} f_i(I_i) = \sum_{i=1}^{n} f(I_i) = \sum_{i=1}^{n} \hat{y}_i. \tag{1}$$

To allow the size of the sets S to randomly vary in $\{1, n\}$ during training, each element of S has a chance p to be a black image B of zero intensities only (Fig. 1 right column). With $f(B) = 0$, the following situation becomes possible:

$$g(S) = f(I_j) + \sum_{i=1, i \neq j}^{n} f_i(B) = f(I_j) + (n-1)f(B) = f(I_j). \tag{2}$$

For this implementation, the batch size b has to be a multiple of the number of branches n. We chose $b = n$ due to constraints in GPU memory. The regularization strength is controlled by the averaged number of samples used to create combinations, hence depends on n and p. During inference, to predict the label for a single input image, the input of all other branches is set to zero.

3   Experiments

Enlarged perivascular spaces (PVS) and white matter hyperintensities (WMH) are two types of brain lesions associated with small vessel disease. The method is evaluated for the estimation of number PVS in the basal ganglia, and estimation of WMH volume. We compare the performance of our method to that of the base regressor f with and without and Dropout, and for different sizes of training set.

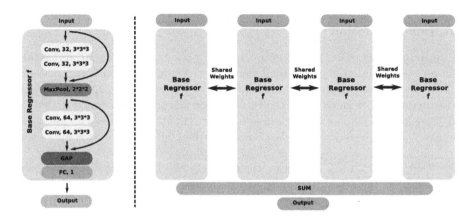

Fig. 2. Architectures. On the left, architecture of the base regressor f. 'Conv' stands for 3D convolutions, followed by the number of feature maps, and the kernel size. After each convolution, there is a ReLU activation. The round arrows are skip connections with concatenated feature maps. GAP stands for Global Average Pooling layer, and FC for Fully Connected layer. On the right, example of our data augmentation method with $n = 4$ replications. Each replication f_i is a copy of the base regressor f on the left. Once the training is done, all f_i but one can be removed, and the evaluation is performed using the original architecture.

The PVS dataset contains T2-weighted scans, from 2017 subjects, acquired from a 1.5T GE scanner. The scans were visually scored by an expert rater who counted the PVS in the basal ganglia in a single slice. The WMH dataset is the training set of the MICCAI2017's WMH challenge [11]. We use the available 2D multi-slice FLAIR-weighted MRI scans as input to the networks. Scans were acquired from 60 participants from 3 centers: 20 scans from Amsterdam (GE scanner), 20 from Utrecht (Philips) and 20 from Singapore (Siemens). Although the ground truths of the challenge are pixel-wise, we only used the number of WMH voxels as ground truth during training.

For the regression of PVS in the basal ganglia, a mask of the basal ganglia is created with the subcortical segmentation algorithm from FreeSurfer [12], and smoothed with a gaussian filter (standard deviation of 2 voxels) before being applied the image. The result is subsequently cropped around the basal ganglia.

For the WMH dataset, we only crop each image around its center of mass, weighted by the voxel intensities. For both tasks the intensities are then rescaled between 0 and 1.

During training, for all methods, the images are randomly augmented on-the-fly with standard methods. The possible augmentations are flipping in x, y or z, 3D rotation from -0.2 to 0.2 rad and random translations in x, y or z from -2 to 2 voxels. Adadelta [13] is used as optimizer. The networks are trained with batch-size $b = 4$. For the proposed method, the network's architecture has then four branches ($n = b = 4$). During an epoch, the proposed method gets as input m/n different combinations of n training samples, were m is the total number of training images. During the same epoch, the base regressor f simply gets the m images separately (in batches of size $b = 4$). For the proposed method p was set to 0.1. In some experiments with Dropout [14] we included a dropout layer after each convolution and after the global pooling layer. The code is written in Keras with Tensorflow as backend, and the experiments were run on a Nvidia GeForce GTX 1070 GPU.

For the PVS dataset, we experiment with varying size of training set, between 12 and 25 scans. The validation set always contains the same 5 scans. All methods are evaluated on the same separated test set of 1977 scans. For the WMH dataset, the set is split into 30 training scans and 30 testing scans. Six scan from the training set are used as validation scans. In both cases, the dataset is randomly (uniform distribution) split into training and testing sets. For the PVS dataset, once the dataset has been split into 30 training scans and 1977 testing scan, we manually sample scans to keep a pseudo-uniform distribution of the lesion count when decreasing the number of training scans.

To compare the automated predictions to visual scoring (for PVS) or volumes (for WMH), we use two evaluation metrics: the mean squared error (MSE), and the intraclass correlation coefficient (ICC).

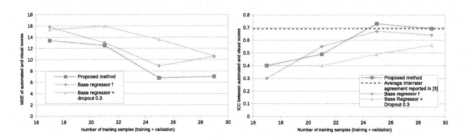

Fig. 3. Comparison between the proposed method with $n = 4$ and the base regressor on the PVS dataset. MSE is displayed on the left, and ICC on the right.

3.1   Results

Enlarged Perivascular Spaces (PVS). Figure 3 compares the proposed method to the base regressor f on the PVS datasets, and for an increasing number of training samples. Their performance is also compared to the average interrater agreement computed for the same problem and reported in [2]. The proposed method always reaches a better MSE than the conventional methods for all training set sizes. The proposed method also significantly outperforms the base regressor in ICC (Williams' test p-value < 0.001) when averaging the predictions of the methods across the four points of their learning curve.

Table 1. Results on the WMH dataset. We conducted three series of experiments with different training set sizes and loss functions. In the two first rows, we repeated the experiments with three random initializations of the weights (on the same split), and report mean and standard deviation. MAE is an acronym for mean absolute error.

Method	Training scans	Testing scans	Loss	Performance (ICC)
Base network f	30	30	MSE	0.79 ± 0.12
Proposed method	30	30	MSE	**0.84 ± 0.02**
Base network f	30	30	MAE	0.78
Proposed method	30	30	MAE	**0.87**
Base network f	40	20	MSE	**0.89**
Proposed method	40	20	MSE	0.86

White Matter Hyperintensities (WMH). We conducted three series of experiments, and trained in total five neural networks (Table 1). When using small training sets, the proposed method outperforms the base network f, when optimized either for MSE or for mean absolute error. With larger training sets, the difference of performance reduces, and the base regressor performs slightly better on the ICC.

4   Discussion and Conclusion

With the proposed data augmentation method, we could reach the inter-rater agreement performance on PVS quantification reported by Dubost et al. [2] with only 25 training scans, and without pretraining.

Dubost et al. [2] also regressed the number of PVS in the basal ganglia with a neural network. We achieve a similar result (0.73 ICC) while training on 25 scans instead of 1000. Zhang et al. [8] also proposed to combine training samples as a data augmentation method. In their experiments, combining more than $n = 2$ images does not bring any improvement. With the proposed method, training with combinations of four images brought improvement over only using pairs of images. We did not experiment with values of n larger than 4 due to GPU memory constraints. Contrary to the expected gain in generalization, on both PVS (Fig. 3) and WMH datasets, using Dropout [14] worsened the results when training on very little data, even with low dropout rates such as 0.3. As dropout already did not improve the performance of the baseline, we do not expect improvement by including dropout in the proposed method.

To create combination of images for the proposed method, images where drawn without replacement for the sake of implementation simplicity. The regularization strength could be increased by drawing samples with replacement, which could be beneficial for small training sets. We also mentioned two possible implementations of the proposed method: (1) changing the computation of the loss over mini-batches, (2) replicating the architecture of network. In this work we used the second approach, as it was simpler to implement with our library (Keras). However with this approach, all samples used in a given the combination have to be simultaneously processed by the network, which can cause GPU memory overload in case of large 3D images or large values of n. The first approach does not suffer from this overload, as the samples can be successively loaded, while only saving the individual scalar predictions in the GPU memory. In case of large 3D images, we would consequently recommend implementing the first approach.

Acknowledgments. This research was funded by the Netherlands Organisation for Health Research and Development (ZonMw) Project104003005, with additional support of Netherlands Organisation for Scientific Research (NWO), project NWO-EWVIDI 639.022.010 and project NWO-TTW Perspectief Programme P15-26. This work was partly carried out on the Dutch national e-infrastructure with the support of SURFCooperative.

References

1. Cole, J.H., et al.: Predicting brain age with deep learning from raw imaging data results in a reliable and heritable biomarker. NeuroImage **163**, 115–124 (2017)
2. Dubost, F., et al.: 3D regression neural network for the quantification of enlarged perivascular spaces in Brain MRI. Medical Image Analysis (2019)
3. González, G., Washko, G.R., Estépar, R.S.J.: Deep learning for biomarker regression: application to osteoporosis and emphysema on chest CT scans. In: Medical Imaging 2018: Image Processing, vol. 10574, p. 105741H. International Society for Optics and Photonics (2018)
4. Wang, J., et al.: Grey Matter age prediction as a biomarker for risk of dementia: a population-based study. BioRxiv, p. 518506 (2019)
5. Lee, J.H., Kim, K.G.: Applying deep learning in medical images: the case of bone age estimation. Healthc. Inform. Res. **24**(1), 86–92 (2018)
6. Ronneberger, O., Fischer, P., Brox, T.: U-Net: convolutional networks for biomedical image segmentation. In: Navab, N., Hornegger, J., Wells, W.M., Frangi, A.F. (eds.) MICCAI 2015. LNCS, vol. 9351, pp. 234–241. Springer, Cham (2015). https://doi.org/10.1007/978-3-319-24574-4_28

7. Sixt, L., Wild, B., Landgraf, T.: RenderGAN: generating realistic labeled data. Front. Robot. AI **5**, 66 (2018)
8. Zhang, H., Cisse, M., Dauphin, Y.N., Lopez-Paz, D.: MIXUP: beyond empirical risk minimization. In: ICLR 2018 (2017)
9. Inoue, H.: Data augmentation by pairing samples for images classification. arXiv preprint arXiv:1801.02929 (2018)
10. Tokozume, Y., Ushiku, Y., Harada, T.: Learning from between-class examples for deep sound recognition. In: ICLR (2018)
11. Kuijf, H.J., et al.: Standardized assessment of automatic segmentation of white matter hyperintensities; results of the WMH segmentation challenge. IEEE Trans. Med. Imaging (2019)
12. Desikan, R.S., et al.: An automated labeling system for subdividing the human cerebral cortex on MRI scans into gyral based regions of interest. Neuroimage **31**(3), 968–980 (2006)
13. Zeiler, M.D.: ADADELTA: an adaptive learning rate method. arXiv preprint arXiv:1212.5701 (2012)
14. Srivastava, N., Hinton, G., Krizhevsky, A., Sutskever, I., Salakhutdinov, R.: Dropout: a simple way to prevent neural networks from overfitting. J. Mach. Learn. Res. **15**(1), 1929–1958 (2014)

A Dirty Multi-task Learning Method for Multi-modal Brain Imaging Genetics

Lei Du[1(✉)], Fang Liu[1], Kefei Liu[2], Xiaohui Yao[2], Shannon L. Risacher[3], Junwei Han[1], Lei Guo[1], Andrew J. Saykin[3], Li Shen[2], and for the Alzheimer's Disease Neuroimaging Initiative

[1] School of Automation, Northwestern Polytechnical University, Xi'an, China
dulei@nwpu.edu.cn
[2] Perelman School of Medicine, University of Pennsylvania, Philadelphia, PA, USA
Li.Shen@pennmedicine.upenn.edu
[3] Indiana University School of Medicine, Indianapolis, IN, USA

Abstract. Brain imaging genetics is an important research topic in brain science, which combines genetic variations and brain structures or functions to uncover the genetic basis of brain disorders. Imaging data collected by different technologies, measuring the same brain distinctly, might carry complementary but different information. Unfortunately, we do not know the extent to which phenotypic variance is shared among multiple imaging modalities, which might trace back to the complex genetic mechanism. In this study, we propose a novel dirty multi-task SCCA to analyze imaging genetics problems with multiple modalities of brain imaging quantitative traits (QTs) involved. The proposed method can not only identify the shared SNPs and QTs across multiple modalities, but also identify the modality-specific SNPs and QTs, showing a flexible capability of discovering the complex multi-SNP-multi-QT associations. Compared with the multi-view SCCA and multi-task SCCA, our method shows better canonical correlation coefficients and canonical weights on both synthetic and real neuroimaging genetic data. This demonstrates that the proposed dirty multi-task SCCA could be a meaningful and powerful alternative method in multi-modal brain imaging genetics.

This work was supported by NSFC [61602384]; NSFC of Shaanxi [2017JQ6001]; CPSF [2017M613202]; PSF of Shaanxi [2017BSHEDZZ81]; Fundamental Research Funds for Central Universities [3102018zy029] at Northwestern Polytechnical University. This work was also supported by the National Institutes of Health [R01 EB022574, R01 LM011360, U01 AG024904, P30 AG10133, R01 AG19771, R01 AG 042437, R01 AG046171, R01 AG040770 and NSF IIS 1837964] at University of Pennsylvania and Indiana University.
Data used in preparation of this article were obtained from the Alzheimer's Disease Neuroimaging Initiative (ADNI) database (adni.loni.usc.edu). As such, the investigators within the ADNI contributed to the design and implementation of ADNI and/or provided data but did not participate in analysis or writing of this report. A complete listing of ADNI investigators can be found at: http://adni.loni.usc.edu/wp-content/uploads/how_to_apply/ADNI_Acknowledgement_List.pdf.

D. Shen et al. (Eds.): MICCAI 2019, LNCS 11767, pp. 447–455, 2019.
https://doi.org/10.1007/978-3-030-32251-9_49

Keywords: Brain imaging genetics · Multi-task sparse canonical correlation analysis · Multi-modal brain imaging

1   Introduction

Imaging genetics gains more and more attention recently. The primal aim of imaging genetics is to uncover the genetic basis of brain disorders [6]. Hence the genetic variations such as the single nucleotide polymorphisms (SNPs) and neuroimaging quantitative traits (QTs) are usually analyzed together. The imaging QTs obtained by different image technologies, measuring the brain from different perspectives, might carry complementary but different information. Therefore, combining multi-modal imaging QTs, and using them to study the modality-consistent biomarkers as well as the modality-dependent biomarkers could be beneficial to exploit meaningful genetic mechanism for brain disorders.

Both regression-based multi-task learning (MTL) and sparse canonical correlation analysis (SCCA) are widely used in brain imaging genetics [7]. The MTL methods only select features for the predicting variables [5,8], thereby are insufficient if we pursue a simultaneous feature selection for both SNPs and imaging QTs. SCCA improves the MTL methods, and yields a pair of canonical weights showing the relevance of SNPs and QTs simultaneously [2,10]. However, they could not load multi-modal imaging QTs in a unified model, resulting in the lack of the identification ability. The multi-view/multi-set SCCA studies the relationship among multiple sets of data, thereby could handle multi-modal imaging genetics. Unfortunately, similar to the multi-task SCCA (MTSCCA) [1,3], it could not identify diverse imaging genetic patterns such as the modality-consistent and modality-dependent associations.

In this paper, we propose a novel multi-modal imaging data oriented imaging genetic learning method. Our method takes advantage of MTL and parameters decomposition. The MTL modeling strategy makes it easier and reasonable to incorporate multiple modalities of imaging QTs, and the parameters decomposition accommodates a flexible regularization. We call it the *dirty* MTSCCA following the terminology in [4]. The proposed dirty method decomposes the canonical weights into two parts, i.e. the task-consistent component which is shared among all tasks, and the task-dependent component which is close related to a specific task. By penalizing both components distinctly, the proposed method is able to identify both SNPs and imaging QTs that are revealed by all imaging technologies, as well as SNPs and QTs that could be only revealed using a specific imaging technology. We propose an efficient algorithm to solve the dirty MTSCCA which converges to a local optimum. The results on the real neuroimaging genetics data from the Alzheimer's Disease Neuroimaging Initiative (ADNI) database [9] show that, the dirty MTSCCA learns improved bi-multivariate associations, the modality-shared SNPs and brain areas, as well as the modality-specific SNPs and brain areas, exhibiting a flexible and meaningful identification capability. Therefore, our dirty MTSCCA model is quite suitable to multi-modal imaging genetics, and further a significant addition to the existing method library.

2   The Dirty Multi-task SCCA

The Model. In this paper, we denote scalars as italic letters, column vectors as boldface lowercase letters, and matrices as boldface capitals. The i-th row and j-th column of $\mathbf{X} = (x_{ij})$ is denoted as $\mathbf{x}^i$ and $\mathbf{x}_j$ respectively. $\|\mathbf{x}\|_2$ denotes the Euclidean norm, $\|\mathbf{X}\|_F = \sqrt{\sum_i \sum_j x_{ij}^2}$ denotes the Frobenius norm, and $\|\mathbf{X}\|_{2,1}$ denotes the $\ell_{2,1}$-norm. $\mathbf{X} \in \mathbb{R}^{n \times p}$ loads the genetic data with n subjects and p SNPs, and $\mathbf{Y}_c \in \mathbb{R}^{n \times q}(c = 1, \cdots, C)$ loads the c-th modality of phenotype data with q imaging QTs, where C is the number of imaging modalities (tasks).

To discover the flexible imaging genetic patterns in a multi-modal scene, we propose the dirty multi-task SCCA as follows

$$\min_{\mathbf{S}, \mathbf{W}, \mathbf{B}, \mathbf{Z}} \sum_{c=1}^{C} -(\mathbf{s}_c + \mathbf{w}_c)^\top \mathbf{X}^\top \mathbf{Y}_c (\mathbf{b}_c + \mathbf{z}_c)$$

$$+ \lambda_s \|\mathbf{S}\|_{G_{2,1}} + \beta_s \|\mathbf{S}\|_{2,1} + \lambda_w \|\mathbf{W}\|_1 + \beta_b \|\mathbf{B}\|_{2,1} + \lambda_z \|\mathbf{Z}\|_1$$

$$s.t. \quad \|\mathbf{X}(\mathbf{s}_c + \mathbf{w}_c)\|_2^2 \leq 1, \|\mathbf{Y}_c(\mathbf{b}_c + \mathbf{z}_c)\|_2^2 \leq 1, \ \forall c. \tag{1}$$

In this model, the conventional canonical weights $\mathbf{U}$ and $\mathbf{V}$ are decomposed as $\mathbf{U} = \mathbf{S} + \mathbf{W}$ and $\mathbf{V} = \mathbf{B} + \mathbf{Z}$. The $\mathbf{S}$ and $\mathbf{W}$ are associated with the SNP data, where $\mathbf{S}$ is the task-consistent component shared by multiple tasks, and $\mathbf{W}$ is the task-dependent component only associated with a single task. Similarly, $\mathbf{B}$ is the task-consistent component and $\mathbf{Z}$ is the task-dependent component for imaging QTs. The λ_s, β_s, λ_w, β_b, λ_z are nonnegative tuning parameters.

The model above encourages the modality-shared sparsity [4] and modality-dependent sparsity via distinct regularization terms. It penalizes the task-consist-ent component jointly by the block-sparse regularization, such as the $G_{2,1}$-norm (definition is in [8]) and $\ell_{2,1}$-norm for SNPs and $\ell_{2,1}$-norm for QTs. This could help identify the shared SNPs and imaging QTs repeated by different imaging technologies. In addition, the task-dependent component is penalized differently by the ℓ_1-norm to induce element-wise sparsity for both SNPs and imaging QTs. This might uncover the SNPs and QTs that could only be identified using a specific imaging technology. Owing to this decomposition strategy, the proposed method is able to facilitate joint feature selection while allowing disparities as well. Since simultaneously demanding features being task-consistent and task-dependent is conflicting, the proposed dirty model is flexible and thus practical.

The Optimization Algorithm. The Eq. (1) is not a jointly convex function and thus can not be solved directly. Fortunately, it is convex in $\mathbf{S}$ if we fix $\mathbf{W}$, $\mathbf{B}$ and $\mathbf{Z}$. Likewise, Eq. (1) is also convex in $\mathbf{W}$, $\mathbf{B}$ and $\mathbf{Z}$ alternately with those remaining weight matrices being fixed. On this account, the dirty multi-task SCCA problem can be solved using the alternative iteration algorithm.

Updating **S** *and* **W***:* When **B** and **Z** are fixed to constants, the objective with respect to **S** and **W** can be rewritten as

$$\min_{\mathbf{S},\mathbf{W}} \sum_{c=1}^{C} -(\mathbf{s}_c + \mathbf{w}_c)^\top \mathbf{X}^\top \mathbf{Y}_c(\mathbf{b}_c + \mathbf{z}_c) + \lambda_s \|\mathbf{S}\|_{G_{2,1}} + \beta_s \|\mathbf{S}\|_{2,1} + \lambda_w \|\mathbf{W}\|_1, \quad s.t. \|\mathbf{X}(\mathbf{s}_c + \mathbf{w}_c)\|_2^2 \le 1, \tag{2}$$

which can be solved by the following theorem.

Theorem 1. *The solution of Eq. (2) is given by* $\mathbf{s}_c^* = \frac{\hat{\mathbf{s}}_c}{\|\mathbf{X}(\hat{\mathbf{s}}_c + \hat{\mathbf{w}}_c)\|_2}$ *and* $\mathbf{w}_c^* = \frac{\hat{\mathbf{w}}_c}{\|\mathbf{X}(\hat{\mathbf{s}}_c + \hat{\mathbf{w}}_c)\|_2}$, *where* $\hat{\mathbf{s}}_c$ *is the solution of*

$$\min_{\mathbf{S}} \sum_{c=1}^{C} \frac{1}{2} \|\mathbf{X}\mathbf{s}_c - \mathbf{Y}_c(\mathbf{b}_c + \mathbf{z}_c)\|_2^2 + \lambda_s \|\mathbf{S}\|_{G_{2,1}} + \beta_s \|\mathbf{S}\|_{2,1}, \tag{3}$$

and $\hat{\mathbf{w}}_c$ *is the solution of*

$$\min_{\mathbf{W}} \sum_{c=1}^{C} \frac{1}{2} \|\mathbf{X}\mathbf{w}_c - \mathbf{Y}_c(\mathbf{b}_c + \mathbf{z}_c)\|_2^2 + \lambda_w \|\mathbf{W}\|_1. \tag{4}$$

Theorem 1 can be proved following the same procedure in [10] (Appendix A.2). Now Eq. (3) becomes a multi-task regression, and can be solved using the off-the-shelf methods. Given that $\mathbf{s}_c$'s can be solved jointly, we take the derivative of the objective of Eq. (3) with respect to **S**, and then let it be zero, i.e.

$$(\mathbf{X}^\top \mathbf{X} + \lambda_s \tilde{\mathbf{D}} + \beta_s \mathbf{D})\mathbf{S} = \mathbf{X}^\top [\mathbf{Y}_1(\mathbf{b}_1 + \mathbf{z}_1) \quad \cdots \quad \mathbf{Y}_C(\mathbf{b}_C + \mathbf{z}_C)], \tag{5}$$

where $\tilde{\mathbf{D}}$ is a block diagonal matrix with the k-th block being $\frac{1}{\|\mathbf{S}^k\|_F}\mathbf{I}_k$, and $\mathbf{I}_k$ is an identity matrix of size equaling to the size of the k-th group. The grouping information could be previously defined according to the linkage disequilibrium (LD) structure of SNPs. **D** is a diagonal matrix with the i-th diagonal element being $\frac{1}{\|\mathbf{s}^i\|_2}(i = 1, \cdots, p)$. Then we can easily obtain $\hat{\mathbf{S}}$ from Eq. (5), which can be efficiently solved via the iterative algorithm [8].

Due to the ℓ_1-norm regularization, $\mathbf{w}_c$'s are not coupled and thus can be updated separately. By first taking the derivative of Eq. (4) regarding each $\mathbf{w}_c$, and letting it be zero, we arrive at

$$(\mathbf{X}^\top \mathbf{X} + \lambda_w \breve{\mathbf{D}}_c)\mathbf{w}_c = \mathbf{X}^\top \mathbf{Y}_c(\mathbf{b}_c + \mathbf{z}_c), \tag{6}$$

with $\breve{\mathbf{D}}_c$ being a diagonal matrix whose i-th element is $\frac{1}{|w_{ic}|}(i = 1, \cdots, p)$.

Updating **B** *and* **Z***:* Once we obtain **S** and **W**, we can fix them to solve **B** and **Z**. Since each $\mathbf{b}_c$ and $\mathbf{z}_c$ are associated with each modality of imaging QTs, i.e. $\mathbf{Y}_c$, they are not closely coupled too. Thus $\mathbf{b}_c$ and $\mathbf{z}_c$ for different task can be solved separately.

With this observation, we follow the same procedure to that of updating $\mathbf{w}_c$ according to Theorem 1. Taking the derivative of the objective with respect to every $\mathbf{b}_c$, we easily obtain

$$(\mathbf{Y}_c^\top \mathbf{Y}_c + \beta_b \mathbf{Q})\mathbf{b}_c = \mathbf{Y}_c^\top \mathbf{X}(\mathbf{s}_c + \mathbf{w}_c), \tag{7}$$

with $\mathbf{Q}$ being a diagonal matrix and the j-th element is $\frac{1}{\|\mathbf{b}^j\|_2}(j = 1, \cdots, q)$.

Similarly, we have

$$(\mathbf{Y}_c^\top \mathbf{Y}_c + \lambda_z \check{\mathbf{Q}}_c)\mathbf{z}_c = \mathbf{Y}_c^\top \mathbf{X}(\mathbf{s}_c + \mathbf{w}_c), \tag{8}$$

where $\check{\mathbf{Q}}_c$ is a diagonal matrix whose j-th diagonal element is $\frac{1}{|z_j|}(j = 1, \cdots, q)$.

Equations (5)–(8) pave the way to solve the problem Eq. (1), and then we present the pseudo-code in Algorithm 1. The algorithm iteratively updates $\mathbf{S}$, $\mathbf{W}$, $\mathbf{B}$ and $\mathbf{Z}$ till the predefined stopping conditions are satisfied. Further, this algorithm is guaranteed to converge to a local optimum since Eqs. (5–8) converge according to the Theorem 1 in [8].

Algorithm 1. The Dirty Multi-task SCCA Algorithm

Require:

$\quad \mathbf{X} \in \mathcal{R}^{n \times p}, \mathbf{Y}_c \in \mathcal{R}^{n \times q}, c = 1, \cdots, C, \lambda_s, \beta_s, \lambda_w, \beta_b, \lambda_z$

Ensure:

$\quad$ Output $\mathbf{S}, \mathbf{W}, \mathbf{B}, \mathbf{Z}$.

1: Initialize $\mathbf{S} \in \mathcal{R}^{p \times C}, \mathbf{W} \in \mathcal{R}^{p \times C}, \mathbf{B} \in \mathcal{R}^{q \times C}$ and $\mathbf{Z} \in \mathcal{R}^{q \times C}$;

2: **while** not convergence **do**

3: $\quad$ Update $\hat{\mathbf{S}}$ according to Eq. (5), and update $\hat{\mathbf{w}}_c$ according to Eq. (6);

4: $\quad$ Compute $\mathbf{S}^*$ and $\mathbf{W}^*$ according to Theorem 1;

5: $\quad$ Update $\hat{\mathbf{b}}_c$ according to Eq. (7), and update $\hat{\mathbf{z}}_c$ according to Eq. (8);

6: $\quad$ Compute $\mathbf{B}^*$ and $\mathbf{Z}^*$ according to $\mathbf{b}_c^* = \frac{\hat{\mathbf{b}}_c}{\left\|\mathbf{Y}_c(\hat{\mathbf{b}}_c + \hat{\mathbf{z}}_c)\right\|_2}$, and $\mathbf{z}_c^* = \frac{\hat{\mathbf{z}}_c}{\left\|\mathbf{Y}_c(\hat{\mathbf{b}}_c + \hat{\mathbf{z}}_c)\right\|_2}$;

7: **end while**

---

3 Experiments

We choose the most related MTSCCA (multi-task SCCA) [1] and mSCCA (multi-view/multi-set SCCA) [10] as benchmarks. The experiments are conducted via a nested 5-fold cross-validation method where the inner loop is for parameter tuning. In this study, all methods run on the same platform and data partition, and employ the same stopping condition, i.e. both $\max_c |(\mathbf{s}_c + \mathbf{w}_c)^{t+1} - (\mathbf{s}_c + \mathbf{w}_c)^t| \leq 10^{-5}$ and $\max_c |(\mathbf{b}_c + \mathbf{z}_c)^{t+1} - (\mathbf{b}_c + \mathbf{z}_c)^t| \leq 10^{-5}$.

Real Neuroimaging Genetics Data. The genotying and brain imaging data used in this article were obtained from the Alzheimer's Disease Neuroimaging Initiative (ADNI) database (adni.loni.usc.edu). One primary goal of ADNI has been to test whether serial magnetic resonance imaging (MRI), positron emission tomography (PET), other biological markers, and clinical and neuropsychological assessment can be combined to measure the progression of mild cognitive impairment (MCI) and early Alzheimer's disease (AD). For up-to-date information, see www.adni-info.org. The SNP, MRI and PET data were downloaded from the LONI website (adni.loni.usc.edu). Table 1 shows the details of 755 non-Hispanic Caucasian participants, including 281 AD, 292 MCI and 182 healthy control (HC). There were three modalities of imaging data, i.e. the 18-F florbetapir PET (AV45) scans, fluorodeoxyglucose positron emission tomography (FDG) scans, and structural MRI (sMRI) scans. These multi-modality imaging data had been aligned to every participant's same visit. The sMRI data were processed with voxel-based morphometry (VBM) via SPM. These scans were aligned to a T1-weighted template image, segmented into gray matter (GM), white matter (WM) and cerebrospinal fluid (CSF) maps, normalized to the standard MNI space, and smoothed with an 8 mm FWHM kernel. The FDG and AV45 scans were also registered into the same MNI space. Then a subsample step was conducted and 116 regions of interest (ROI) level measurements were generated based on the MarsBaR automated anatomical labeling (AAL) atlas. These imaging QTs were pre-adjusted to remove the effects of the baseline age, gender, education, and handedness by the regression weights generated from HCs. We investigated 1011 SNPs from chromosome 19 including the well-known AD risk genes such as *APOE*. The LD block information is also used as prior knowledge. Our goal was to examine correlations between the multiple modalities of QTs (GM densities for sMRI scans, amyloid values for AV45 scans and glucose utilization for FDG scans) and SNPs.

Table 1. Participant characteristics.

	HC	MCI	AD
Num	182	292	281
Gender(M/F, %)	47.16/52.84	54.52/45.48	47.37/52.63
Handedness(R/L, %)	90.91/9.09	87.35/12.65	91.50/8.50
Age (mean±std)	72.97±6.00	71.81±7.62	72.38±7.31
Education (mean±std)	16.52±2.58	15.97±2.78	16.14±2.78

Bi-multivariate Associations. Table 2 contains both training and testing canonical correlation coefficients (CCCs), showing the identified bi-multivariate associations. There are three CCCs for each method since we have three imaging modalities, thereby three SCCA tasks. The proposed method obtains better CCCs than both mSCCA and MTSCCA, which is further confirmed by the p-values (p-values for SNP-AV45 on testing set look strange, but are normal due to the directionality of the paired t-test) between our method and benchmarks. This demonstrates that, by decomposing the canonical weights and penalizing them distinctly, our method has the superior modeling capability in multi-modal scenes, thereby exhibits improved bi-multivariate associations.

Table 2. CCCs (mean±std.) between SNP and three modalities of imaging QTs. p-values between our method and benchmarks are also shown in parentheses.

	Training CCCs			Testing CCCs		
	SNP-AV45	SNP-FDG	SNP-VBM	SNP-AV45	SNP-FDG	SNP-VBM
mSCCA	0.44 ± 0.01	0.33 ± 0.01	0.25 ± 0.02	0.41 ± 0.07	0.29 ± 0.07	0.21 ± 0.07
	(8.69E$-$09)	(1.80E$-$07)	(2.60E$-$05)	(1.4E$-$01)	(3.2E$-$01)	(4.1E$-$01)
MTSCCA	0.47 ± 0.01	0.35 ± 0.01	0.29 ± 0.01	0.43 ± 0.07	0.30 ± 0.06	0.19 ± 0.08
	(3.50E$-$09)	(1.4E$-$01)	(1.09E$-$02)	(1.02E$-$03)	(2.00E$-$01)	(2.90E$-$02)
Our method	0.48 ± 0.01	0.36 ± 0.01	0.29 ± 0.01	0.44 ± 0.07	0.30 ± 0.06	0.21 ± 0.07

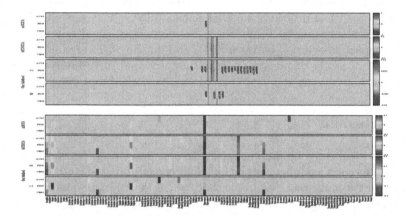

Fig. 1. Comparison of canonical weights. The weights for SNPs are shown on top, and those of imaging QTs are on bottom. Row 1–4: (1) mSCCA; (2) MTSCCA; (3) our method. Our method has two weights for SNPs and QTs owing to the parameter decomposition. Within each panel, there are three rows corresponding to three type of imaging QTs, i.e. AV45, FDG and VBM.

Task-Consistent and Task-Dependent Feature Selection. Now we investigate the identified SNPs and imaging QTs based on the absolute values of the estimated canonical weights. The upper half part of Fig. 1 shows the feature selection for SNPs while that of imaging QTs is presented on the lower half part. Since our model has two separate components for SNPs, i.e. the task-consistent component **S** and the task-dependent **W**, we show both of them here. mSCCA yields one canonical weight vector other than a weight matrix for SNPs, and thus we repeatedly stack its canonical weight vector three times to make its heat map available. We observe that all SNPs with nonzero values of our method have been shown to be relevant to the progression of AD. For example, rs429358 is identified by both **S** and **W**, demonstrating its strong association with AD. In addition, the proposed dirty MTSCCA shows a clear task-consistent pattern, indicating that these SNPs, e.g. rs12721051, rs56131196, rs438811, rs483082, rs56131196, rs5117 etc., could be correlated with AD no matter which imaging technology is employed. Our method and MTSCCA identify more AD-related loci than mSCCA, demonstrating the multi-task modeling possesses comprehensive feature selection capacity. The heat maps of imaging QTs exhibit interesting task-consistent and task-dependent profiles. Our method shows that the left hippocampus, the left olfactory sulcus, the inferior parietal lobule and the left amygdala show clearly task-consistent patterns, indicating that these brain areas could be revealed by all imaging technologies, i.e. the sMRI, FDG and AV45 scans. Besides, task-dependent Z shows that the right medial orbitofrontal cortex and the left medial frontal gyrus are highlighted using the AV45-PET scans. The left and right angular gyrus, and the cingulum are identified by using the FDG-PET scans. Both left and right of the eighth cerebelum are highlighted when using the VBM measures of sMRI scans. MTSCCA and mSCCA can also identify several meaningful brain areas, however, they could not uncover the diverse complex association between SNPs and imaging QTs of multiple modalities. This real study demonstrates that our proposed dirty multi-task SCCA could be very promising and meaningful in multi-modal brain imaging genetics.

4   Conclusions

Imaging data collected by different technologies, measuring the same brain distinctly, might carry complementary but different information. In this paper, we propose a dirty multi-task SCCA method which incorporates multiple modalities of imaging data into a unified model. By decomposing the SCCA's canonical weights into the task-consistent component and the task-dependent component, and penalizing them distinctly, our method has the ability of identifying diverse meaningful bi-multivariate associations between SNPs and imaging QTs. We derive an efficient optimization algorithm to solve the dirty model. The neuroimaging genetics study demonstrates that the proposed method obtains better canonical correlation coefficients and canonical weights than multi-view SCCA and multi-task SCCA. A future direction is to extend this flexible model to be guided by the diagnosis status since currently it is unsupervised.

References

1. Du, L., et al.: Fast multi-task SCCA learning with feature selection for multi-modal brain imaging genetics. In: BIBM, pp. 356–361 (2018)
2. Du, L., et al.: A novel SCCA approach via truncated ℓ_1-norm and truncated group lasso for brain imaging genetics. Bioinformatics **34**(2), 278–285 (2018)
3. Du, L., et al.: Identifying progressive imaging genetic patterns via multi-task sparse canonical correlation analysis: a longitudinal study of the adni cohort. Bioinformatics **35**(14), i474–483 (2019)
4. Jalali, A., Ravikumar, P., Sanghavi, S.: A dirty model for multiple sparse regression. IEEE Trans. Inf. Theory **59**(12), 7947–7968 (2013)
5. Lee, S., Zhu, J., Xing, E.P.: Adaptive multi-task lasso: with application to eQTL detection. In: NIPS, pp. 1306–1314 (2010)

6. Potkin, S.G., et al.: Genome-wide strategies for discovering genetic influences on cognition and cognitive disorders: methodological considerations. Cogn. Neuropsychiatry **14**(4–5), 391–418 (2009)
7. Shen, L., Thompson, P.M., Potkin, S.G., Bertram, L., Farrer, L.A., et al.: Genetic analysis of quantitative phenotypes in AD and MCI: imaging, cognition and biomarkers. Brain Imaging Behav. **8**(2), 183–207 (2014)
8. Wang, H., et al.: Identifying quantitative trait loci via group-sparse multitask regression and feature selection: an imaging genetics study of the ADNI cohort. Bioinformatics **28**(2), 229–237 (2012)
9. Weiner, M.W., et al.: The Alzheimer's disease neuroimaging initiative: progress report and future plans. Alzheimer's Dement. **6**(3), 202–211 (2010)
10. Witten, D.M., Tibshirani, R., Hastie, T.: A penalized matrix decomposition, with applications to sparse principal components and canonical correlation analysis. Biostatistics **10**(3), 515–34 (2009)

Robust and Discriminative Brain Genome Association Study

Xiaofeng Zhu[1] and Dinggang Shen[2(✉)]

[1] University of Electronic Science and Technology of China, Chengdu, Sichuan, China
[2] University of North Carolina at Chapel Hill, Chapel Hill, NC, USA
dgshen@med.unc.edu

Abstract. Brain Genome Association (BGA) study, which investigates the associations between brain structure/function (characterized by neuroimaging phenotypes) and genetic variations (characterized by Single Nucleotide Polymorphisms (SNPs)), is important in pathological analysis of neurological disease. However, the current BGA studies are limited as they did not explicitly consider the disease labels, source importance, and sample importance in their formulations. We address these issues by proposing a robust and discriminative BGA formulation. Specifically, we learn two transformation matrices for mapping two heterogeneous data sources (*i.e.,* neuroimaging data and genetic data) into a common space, so that the samples from the same subject (but different sources) are close to each other, and also the samples with different labels are separable. In addition, we add a sparsity constraint on the transformation matrices to enable feature selection on both data sources. Furthermore, both sample importance and source importance are also considered in the formulation via adaptive parameter-free sample and source weightings. We have conducted various experiments, using Alzheimer's Disease Neuroimaging Initiative (ADNI) dataset, to test how well the neuroimaging phenotypes and SNPs can represent each other in the common space.

1 Introduction

Brain Genome Association (BGA) study is an emergent field of research that investigates the influence of genetic variations on brain structure and function. This field is advancing rapidly due to the vast availability of high resolution neuroimaging and whole-genome sequencing data, as well as the growing needs to utilize the respective findings in the pathological study of neurological illness. In particular, many machine learning approaches have been proposed to identify the subsets of neuroimaging phenotypes (*e.g.,* a subset of Region-Of-Interests

This work was supported in part by NIH grants (AG053867, AG041721, and AG042599). X. Zhu was supported in part by the National Natural Science Foundation of China (61876046 and 61573270), the Guangxi High Institutions Program of Introducing 100 High-Level Overseas Talents, the Strategic Research Excellence Fund at Massey University, and the Marsden Fund of New Zealand (MAU1721). The authors thank the Alzheimer's Disease Neuroimaging Initiative for providing the data sets.

© Springer Nature Switzerland AG 2019
D. Shen et al. (Eds.): MICCAI 2019, LNCS 11767, pp. 456–464, 2019.
https://doi.org/10.1007/978-3-030-32251-9_50

(ROIs) of Magnetic Resonance Image (MRI)) and genetic variations (*i.e.,* a subset of Single Nucleotide Polymorphism (SNP) of the entire brain of human being) that are associated with each other [2,13].

Based on the scale of neuroimaging features, there are two approaches for the BGA study. The first approach uses the extremely high-dimensional voxel-based neuroimaging features as phenotypes [7,9]. For example, Stein *et al.* [7] and Vounou *et al.* [9], used the t-test technique and a reduced-rank regression model, respectively, to conduct association study between the voxel-based neuroimaging features and SNPs. Due to the high-dimensionality and small-sample-size issue, this approach can result in overfitting if all the data (*i.e.,* voxels and SNPs) are analyzed simultaneously; while, if each voxel or a SNP is analyzed separately, the correlations among data are ignored. The second approach significantly reduces the dimensionality of neuroimaging data by first partitioning the whole brain into ROIs, and using ROI-based neuroimaging features as phenotypes.

Many machine learning methods have modeled the BGA study as a feature selection problem, *i.e.,* to select informative neuroimaging features (*i.e.,* ROIs in this paper) that are associated with SNPs, and/or vice versa.

To further reduce the computational complexity, earlier BGA studies limit the number of SNPs or neuroimaging features in their analyses. For example, Brun *et al.* selected a subset of brain-wide neuroimaging features that are associated with a small set of SNPs [1], while Wang *et al.* selected a subset of genome-wide SNPs that associated with a small set of neuroimaging features [10]. Recent BGA studies (*e.g.,* the low-rank feature selection model in [18]) removed this limitation, by considering brain-wide neuroimaging features and genome-wide SNPs in their analyses. To address the high dimensionality issue, the most recent strategy of the current BGA study, commonly known as data harmonization, is to map the two high-dimensional heterogenous data sources (*i.e.,* ROIs and SNPs) into a lower-dimensional common space, so that two corresponding samples from both data sources are comparable (*i.e.,* close to each other) in this space. During this mapping process, a subset of useful ROIs and SNPs can be identified.

In this paper, we address the above issues by proposing a data harmonization approach that is guided by disease diagnostic labels, constrained by feature sparsity, and adaptively weighted by sample and source importance (without introducing extra tuning parameters). We achieve this by (1) learning two transformation matrices to map the ROIs and SNPs into a common space spanned by the label space, (2) using $\ell_{2,1}$-norm regularizers on the transformation matrices to select discriminative and associated ROIs and SNPs, and (3) using square-root $\ell_{2,1}$-norm on the loss functions to impose adaptive and parameter-free sample weighting and source weighting.

2   Method

Let $\mathbf{X} \in \mathbb{R}^{n \times p}$, $\mathbf{Y} \in \mathbb{R}^{n \times q}$, and $\mathbf{Z} \in \mathbb{R}^{n \times c}$ denote the ROI-based neuroimaging features, and the corresponding SNP data and disease diagnostic labels, respectively, where n, p, q, and c denote the numbers of samples, ROIs, SNPs, and classes, respectively. We propose to find the associations between $\mathbf{X}$ and $\mathbf{Y}$ with the help of $\mathbf{Z}$. We achieve this by transforming $\mathbf{X}$ and $\mathbf{Y}$ to a common space associated with $\mathbf{Z}$, by learning two transformation matrices, *i.e.*, $\mathbf{A} \in \mathbb{R}^{p \times c}$ for $\mathbf{X}$, and $\mathbf{B} \in \mathbb{R}^{q \times c}$ for $\mathbf{Y}$.

2.1   Data Harmonization and Data Sparsity

The neuroimaging phenotypes ($\mathbf{X}$) and SNP geneotypes ($\mathbf{Y}$) are two heterogeneous data that describes the current state of the brain structure and the underlying genetics that characterize the brain structure, respectively. To make both data comparable, many of the current BGA studies utilize data harmonization approach to map these heterogeneous data sources into a common space [2,18]. In this paper, we also perform data harmonization on $\mathbf{X}$ and $\mathbf{Y}$, but with extra sparsity constraint on the transformation matrices, considering that not all of the given SNPs and ROIs are associated with each other. Assuming linear transformation matrices, $\mathbf{A}$ and $\mathbf{B}$, for $\mathbf{X}$ and $\mathbf{Y}$, respectively, the data harmonization process that minimizes the difference between $\mathbf{XA}$ and $\mathbf{YB}$, with sparsity constraints on $\mathbf{A}$ and $\mathbf{B}$, is given as

$$\min_{\mathbf{A},\mathbf{B}} \|\mathbf{XA} - \mathbf{YB}\|_F^2 + \alpha\|\mathbf{A}\|_{2,1} + \beta\|\mathbf{B}\|_{2,1}, \tag{1}$$

where $\|\cdot\|_F$ and $\|\cdot\|_{2,1}$ indicate the Frobenius norm and the $\ell_{2,1}$-norm, respectively, while α and β are the tuning parameters. The first term of Eq. (1) is the data harmonization term, which transforms $\mathbf{X}$ and $\mathbf{Y}$ to a common pace spanned by $\mathbf{XA}$ and $\mathbf{YB}$, so that each pair of corresponding samples in $\mathbf{X}$ and $\mathbf{Y}$ are comparable in the transformed space, *i.e.*, $\{\mathbf{x}_i\mathbf{A} \approx \mathbf{y}_i\mathbf{B}, i = 1, ..., n\}$, where $\mathbf{x}_i$ and $\mathbf{y}_i$ indicate the i-th sample of $\mathbf{X}$ and $\mathbf{Y}$, respectively. This term is also equivalent to the least square version of Canonical Correlation Analysis (CCA) [2]. The $\ell_{2,1}$-norm regularizers of the second and third terms of Eq. (1), on the other hand, are used to impose row sparsity constraint on $\mathbf{A}$ and $\mathbf{B}$, so that only certain columns of $\mathbf{X}$ (*i.e.*, ROIs) and $\mathbf{Y}$ (*i.e.*, SNPs) are involved in the transformation. Thus, by checking the non-zero-rows of $\mathbf{A}$ and $\mathbf{B}$, we can locate the corresponding ROIs and SNPs as the associated phenotypes and genotypes.

However, as shown in Fig. 1, using Eq. (1) without the consideration of neurological disease diagnostic labels will result in serious drawback. Figure 1(b) shows that, though data harmonization can successfully make two data sources (*i.e.*, ROI and SNP) of the same samples comparable in the common space, the separability of different diagnostic labels is not guaranteed in this space. We argue that the common space in Fig. 1(c) is more meaningful and accurate, as the corresponding points from two data sources are not only harmonized (*i.e.*, close to each other in the common space), but also separable in terms of diagnostic labels. Furthermore, from the optimization point of view, Eq. (1) may result in a trivial solution, *i.e.*, $\mathbf{A}$ and $\mathbf{B}$ are both equivalent to zero matrices, if there is no other constraint on $\mathbf{A}$ and $\mathbf{B}$.

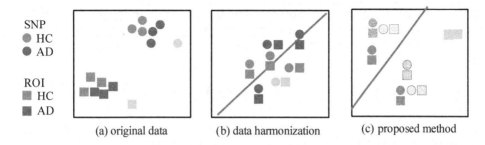

Fig. 1. An illustration of the difference between (b) the current data harmonization method [2, 18] based on Eq. (1), and (c) our proposed data harmonization method which considers diagnostic label information, sample importance, and source importance. The circles and squares represent samples from SNPs and ROIs, respectively; the blue, red and yellow colors denote Healthy Control (HC), Alzheimer's Disease (AD) and outlier, respectively; the green solid line denotes the separation hyperplane between HC and AD, while different shades in (c) denote the variations in sample and source importance. (Color figure online)

2.2 Discriminative Ability

Different from the conventional data harmonization approach of the current BGA study (*e.g.,* [2,6,10,13,18]) which is not label-guided, we include diagnostic label information in the formulation of data harmonization, so that the samples from the same class are close to each other in the common space. Specifically, we assume that the common space is also spanned by the corresponding label matrix $\mathbf{Z}$, *i.e.,*

$$\min_{\mathbf{A},\mathbf{B}} \|\mathbf{Z} - \mathbf{XA}\|_F^2 + \eta\|\mathbf{Z} - \mathbf{YB}\|_F^2 + \gamma\|\mathbf{XA} - \mathbf{YB}\|_F^2 + \alpha\|\mathbf{A}\|_{2,1} + \beta\|\mathbf{B}\|_{2,1}, \quad (2)$$

where α, β, γ, and η are the tuning parameters. The first two terms of Eq. (2) are the discriminative terms, which respectively map $\mathbf{X}$ and $\mathbf{Y}$ into the label space. Using these two new terms, the trivial solution in Eq. (1) is overcome, and the samples with different class labels are discriminative in the common space, as shown in Fig. 1(c).

2.3 Parameter-Free Sample and Source Weighting

Lastly, we also consider sample noises and source importance in our formulation via parameter-free sample weighting and source weighting. In this study, the ROI-based neuroimaging data may be prone to different sources of noises such as scanning device variations, inconsistent image quality, image preprocessing errors (*e.g.,* segmentation and registration inaccuracies), etc. For genetic data, not all SNPs are equally importance in determining the values of phenotypes and disease status. Furthermore, the phenotype data and the genotype data may have different contributions/importance to the class labels. These observations suggest that either different samples or different sources may have different level of importance/reliability and should contribute differently in the BGA study. In addition, we would also like to compute the parameter η in Eq. (2) automatically from the data, as less tuning parameters is always more preferable. Considering the above criteria, our final objective function is given as

$$\min_{\mathbf{A},\mathbf{B}} \sqrt{\|\mathbf{Z} - \mathbf{XA}\|_{2,1}} + \sqrt{\|\mathbf{Z} - \mathbf{YB}\|_{2,1}} + \gamma\|\mathbf{XA} - \mathbf{YB}\|_F^2 + \alpha\|\mathbf{A}\|_{2,1} + \beta\|\mathbf{B}\|_{2,1},$$

(3)

where we employ the square root of the $\ell_{2,1}$-norm instead of the conventional Frobenius-norm (*i.e.*, least square) as the loss functions for the first two terms in Eq. (3). We will show sooner that the $\ell_{2,1}$ loss function is robust against outliers, while the squared root of a loss function is equivalent to adaptive weighting of this loss function during the optimization process. To the best of our knowledge, no study has been reported to simultaneously consider both sample importance and source importance in a framework.

To prove our points, we perform derivative on the first term of Eq. (3) *w.r.t.* $\mathbf{A}$ using chain rule, yielding $\frac{1}{2\sqrt{\|\mathbf{Z}-\mathbf{XA}\|_{2,1}}} \frac{\delta\|\mathbf{Z}-\mathbf{XA}\|_{2,1}}{\delta\mathbf{A}}$. Then by letting $\omega_1 = \frac{1}{\sqrt{\|\mathbf{Z}-\mathbf{XA}\|_{2,1}}}$ and $\omega_2 = \frac{1}{\sqrt{\|\mathbf{Z}-\mathbf{YB}\|_{2,1}}}$, it is not difficult to show that Eq. (3) is equivalent to:

$$\min_{\mathbf{A},\mathbf{B}} \omega_1\|\mathbf{Z}-\mathbf{XA}\|_{2,1} + \omega_2\|\mathbf{Z}-\mathbf{YB}\|_{2,1} + \gamma\|\mathbf{XA}-\mathbf{YB}\|_F^2 + \alpha\|\mathbf{A}\|_{2,1} + \beta\|\mathbf{B}\|_{2,1},$$ (4)

where ω_1 and ω_2 can be regarded as the source weights for $\mathbf{X}$ and $\mathbf{Y}$, respectively, resulting in parameter-free source weightings. Further analysis on ω_1 shows that whenever $\sqrt{\|\mathbf{Z} - \mathbf{XA}\|_{2,1}}$ is small (*i.e.*, when $\mathbf{XA}$ is a good estimation of $\mathbf{Z}$), ω_1 is assigned with a large weight, and vice versa. On the other hand, it can be shown that $\|\mathbf{Z} - \mathbf{XA}\|_{2,1} = tr((\mathbf{Z} - \mathbf{XA})^T\mathbf{D}(\mathbf{Z} - \mathbf{XA}))$, where $tr(\cdot)$ is a trace operator, $\mathbf{D}$ is the diagonal matrix with its i-th diagonal element given as $\frac{1}{2\|\mathbf{z}_i-\mathbf{x}_i\mathbf{A}\|}$, and $\mathbf{z}_i$ indicates the label of i-th sample (*i.e.*, i-th row of $\mathbf{Z}$). This implies that a good sample which is characterized by a small prediction loss (*i.e.*, $\|\mathbf{z}_i - \mathbf{x}_i\mathbf{A}\|$) is assigned with a large weight, while a noisy sample with high prediction loss will be assigned with a small weight [5,12,14]. Equation 4 consists of two parts, (1) using labels to conduct brain genome association (BGA) study to overcome the issue of weak genotype-phenotype relations in existing BGA study, *e.g.*, all comparison methods in this paper, and (2) adding the term of BGA to improve the diagnostic accuracy compared to existing classification study. Moreover, we tuned γ in Eq. 4 to obtain the trade-off between discriminative ability and association.

We employed the alternating optimization strategy [11,15,17] to solve Eq. (3), *i.e.*, variables $\mathbf{A}$ and $\mathbf{B}$ as our proposed Eq. (3) is non-convex for two variables but is convex for each variable while fixing the other. Specifically, the value of ω_1 is adaptively obtained if conducting the derivative on $\mathbf{A}$ to obtain $\mathbf{A}$. The value of ω_2 will be adaptively obtained if conducting the derivative on $\mathbf{B}$ to optimize $\mathbf{B}$. In this way, the optimization of Eq. (3) is transferred to Eq. (4) without tuning ω_1 and ω_2. By contrast, the optimization of Eq. (4) should tune different values of ω_1 and ω_2 with expensive time cost to obtain their best combination.

3   Experimental Analysis

We conducted various experiments using ADNI dataset ('www.adni-info.org') to compare our method with the state-of-the-art methods.

We used baseline MRI images of 737 subjects, including 171 AD, 362 MCIs, and 204 HCs. We preprocessed the MRI images by sequentially applying distortion correction, skull-stripping, cerebellum removal, tissue segmentation, and template registration. Finally, we acquired 90 ROI features (gray matter volumes) for each MRI image.

The genotype data of all participants were first obtained from the ADNI1 and then genotyped using the Human 610-Quad BeadChip. In our experiments, 2,098 SNPs, from 153 AD candidate genes (boundary: 20 KB) listed on the AlzGene database (www.alzgene.org) as of 4/18/2011, were selected by the standard quality control (QC) and imputation steps. The imputation step imputed the QCed SNPs using the MaCH software.

3.1   Experiment Setting

The comparison methods include sparse feature selection with an $\ell_{2,1}$-norm regularizer (L21 for short) [3], Group sparse Feature Selection (GFS) [10], sparse Canonical Correlation Analysis (sCCA) [6], sparse Reduced-Rank Regression (sRRR) [8], and Low-Rank Group Sparse Regression (LRGSR) [18].

We conducted grid search to select the best parameters for all the methods, and used the average of 10 repetitions of 5-fold cross-validation results as the final result. We set the parameter search range for all the methods so that this range would output best sparse results for all the methods, e.g., $\alpha \in \{10^{-2}, ..., 10^1, 10^3\}$, $\beta \in \{10^{-3}, ..., 10^0, 10^1\}$, and $\gamma \in \{10^{-2}, ..., 10^1, 10^2\}$ for our proposed method.

For each experiment, we ran all methods to select SNPs, from which we picked up the top $\{50, 100, ..., 500\}$ SNPs to predict the ROI values of the test data, following the pipeline in [10,18]. The performance of each experiment was assessed by Root-Mean-Square Error (RMSE). We also included 'Relative Frequency' as another evaluation metric, which is the percentage of SNPs (or ROIs) selected in 50 experiments.

We conducted two BGA studies, i.e., the two-class BGA study, which includes 171 AD and 204 healthy subjects (total 381 subjects), and the three-class BGA study, which includes 737 subjects.

3.2   Experimental Results

Figures 2 and 3 summarize the performances in terms of RMSE, the 'Relative Frequency' of the top 10 selected SNPs, and the 'Relative Frequency' of the top 10 selected ROIs, for two-class and three-class BGA studies, respectively.

The following is observed from the RMSE performance curves (where error bar denotes standard deviation). First, the proposed method achieved the best performance, e.g., on average of 10.25% improvement, than the best comparison

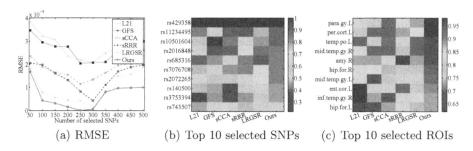

(a) RMSE   (b) Top 10 selected SNPs   (c) Top 10 selected ROIs

Fig. 2. The results using 381 AD-HC subjects in the two-class BGA study. The top 10 selected ROIs include parahippocampal gyrus left, perirhinal cortex left, temporal pole left, middle temporal gyrus right, amygdala right, hippocampal formation right, middle temporal gyrus left, entorhinal cortex left, inferior temporal gyrus right, and hippocampal formation left.

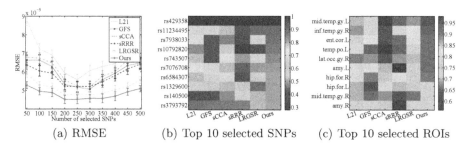

(a) RMSE   (b) Top 10 selected SNPs   (c) Top 10 selected ROIs

Fig. 3. The results using all 737 subjects in the three-class BGA study. The top 10 selected ROIs include middle temporal gyrus left, inferior temporal gyrus right, entorhinal cortex left, temporal pole left, lateral occipitotemporal gyrus right, amygdala left, hippocampal formation right, hippocampal formation left, middle temporal gyrus right, and amygdala right.

method *i.e.*, LRGSR. This showed that our method can more accurately estimate the neuroimaging features from SNPs, thanks to the consideration of (1) the label information and (2) the sample and sources weightings in the BGA study. Further paired t-tests between our method and each of the comparison methods also showed that the p-values were less than 0.001 on both studies, which statistically verified the superiority of the proposed method. Second, for all the methods, the RMSE values were first decreased to their minimum at about 200–300 SNPs (out of 2098 SNPs) before being increased afterward. This indicated that too many SNPs may introduce noises, thus confirming the necessity to conduct SNP selection for the BGA study.

Both the top 10 selected SNPs and selected ROIs are shown to be related to AD in the literatures. For example, the selected SNPs came from the genes PICALM, SORL1, and APOE, which have been reported as the top 40 genes at AlzGene database that are related to AD, while the selected ROIs (*e.g.*, hippocampus and temporal lobe) have also been frequently reported to undergo significant shrinkage in AD [4,10].

Finally, we conducted a binary classification task (AD vs. HC) and a multi-class classification task (AD vs. HC vs. MCI), compared to a purely classification-based study [16], and all comparison methods in this paper. Specifically, we first used all methods including ours to select features, and then used the selected features to conduct classification tasks by the SVM classifier with the best parameter combination for all the methods. As a result, our method improved on average by 3.6% and 7.1%, compared to [16] and the best comparison method, *i.e.,* LRGSR for two classification works. Moreover, our method in the multi-class classification task achieved more improvement than its binary classification task, compared to all comparison methods. This implied the advantages of our method on the classification, *i.e.,* discriminative ability.

4   Conclusion

This paper has proposed a BGA study that took into considerations of the disease labels, sample importance, and source importance. Our selected ROIs and SNPs are more meaningful, as they are not only associated with each other but also discriminative to the disease diagnostic labels. Our model is also robust to sample noise and source importance, by the introduction of adaptive sample and source weightings in our formulation.

References

1. Brun, C.C., et al.: Mapping the regional influence of genetics on brain structure variability: a tensor-based morphometry study. NeuroImage **48**(1), 37–49 (2009)
2. Du, L., et al.: A novel structure-aware sparse learning algorithm for brain imaging genetics. In: Golland, P., Hata, N., Barillot, C., Hornegger, J., Howe, R. (eds.) MICCAI 2014. LNCS, vol. 8675, pp. 329–336. Springer, Cham (2014). https://doi.org/10.1007/978-3-319-10443-0_42
3. Evgeniou, A., Pontil, M.: Multi-task feature learning. NIPS **19**, 41–48 (2007)
4. Hao, X., Yu, J., Zhang, D.: Identifying genetic associations with MRI-derived measures via tree-guided sparse learning. In: Golland, P., Hata, N., Barillot, C., Hornegger, J., Howe, R. (eds.) MICCAI 2014. LNCS, vol. 8674, pp. 757–764. Springer, Cham (2014). https://doi.org/10.1007/978-3-319-10470-6_94
5. Lei, C., Zhu, X.: Unsupervised feature selection via local structure learning and sparse learning. Multimed. Tools Appl. **77**(22), 29605–29622 (2018)
6. Lin, D., et al.: Sparse models for correlative and integrative analysis of imaging and genetic data. J. Neurosci. Methods **237**, 69–78 (2014)
7. Stein, J.L., et al.: Voxelwise genome-wide association study (vGWAS). NeuroImage **53**(3), 1160–1174 (2010)
8. Vounou, M., et al.: Discovering genetic associations with high-dimensional neuroimaging phenotypes: a sparse reduced-rank regression approach. NeuroImage **53**(3), 1147–1159 (2010)

9. Vounou, M., et al.: Sparse reduced-rank regression detects genetic associations with voxel-wise longitudinal phenotypes in Alzheimer's disease. NeuroImage **60**(1), 700–716 (2012)

10. Wang, H., et al.: Identifying quantitative trait loci via group-sparse multitask regression and feature selection: an imaging genetics study of the ADNI cohort. Bioinformatics **28**(2), 229–237 (2012)

11. Zheng, W., Zhu, X., Wen, G., Zhu, Y., Yu, H., Gan, J.: Unsupervised feature selection by self-paced learning regularization. Pattern Recogn. Lett. https://doi.org/10.1016/j.patrec.2018.06.029 (2018)

12. Zheng, W., Zhu, X., Zhu, Y., Hu, R., Lei, C.: Dynamic graph learning for spectral feature selection. Multimed. Tools Appl. **77**(22), 29739–29755 (2018)

13. Zhu, H., et al.: Bayesian generalized low rank regression models for neuroimaging phenotypes and genetic markers. J. Am. Stat. Assoc. **109**(507), 977–990 (2014)

14. Zhu, X., Li, X., Zhang, S.: Block-row sparse multiview multilabel learning for image classification. IEEE Trans. Cybern. **46**(2), 450–461 (2016)

15. Zhu, X., Li, X., Zhang, S., Xu, Z., Yu, L., Wang, C.: Graph PCA hashing for similarity search. IEEE Trans. Multimed. **19**(9), 2033–2044 (2017)

16. Zhu, X., Suk, H.I., Wang, L., Lee, S.W., Shen, D., Alzheimer's Disease Neuroimaging Initiative: A novel relational regularization feature selection method for joint regression and classification in AD diagnosis. Med. Image Anal. **38**, 205–214 (2017)

17. Zhu, X., Zhang, S., Hu, R., He, W., Lei, C., Zhu, P.: One-step multi-view spectral clustering. IEEE Trans. Knowl. Data Eng. (2018). https://doi.org/10.1109/TKDE.2018.2873378

18. Zhu, X., Suk, H.-I., Huang, H., Shen, D.: Structured sparse low-rank regression model for brain-wide and genome-wide associations. In: Ourselin, S., Joskowicz, L., Sabuncu, M.R., Unal, G., Wells, W. (eds.) MICCAI 2016. LNCS, vol. 9900, pp. 344–352. Springer, Cham (2016). https://doi.org/10.1007/978-3-319-46720-7_40

Symmetric Dual Adversarial Connectomic Domain Alignment for Predicting Isomorphic Brain Graph from a Baseline Graph

Alaa Bessadok[1,2], Mohamed Ali Mahjoub[1], and Islem Rekik[2(✉)]

[1] LATIS Lab, ISITCOM, University of Sousse, Sousse, Tunisia
[2] BASIRA Lab, Faculty of Computer and Informatics, Istanbul Technical University, Istanbul, Turkey
irekik@itu.edu.tr
http://basira-lab.com

Abstract. Medical image synthesis techniques can circumvent the need for costly clinical scan acquisitions using different modalities such as functional Magnetic Resonance Imaging (MRI). Recently, deep learning frameworks were designed to predict a target medical modality from a source one (e.g., MRI from Computed Tomography (CT)). However, such methods which work well on images might fail when handling *geometric* brain data such as graphs (or connectomes). To the best of our knowledge, learning how to predict brain graph from a source graph based on geometric deep learning remains unexplored [1]. Given a set of isomorphic source and target brain graph (i.e., derived from the same parcellation brain template so their topology is similar), learning how to predict target brain graph from a source graph has two major challenges. The first one is that the source and target domains might have different distributions, which causes a domain fracture. The second challenge can be viewed as a limitation of existing image synthesis methods which address the domain fracture and multimodal data prediction independently. To address both limitations, we *unprecedentedly* propose a Symmetric Dual Adversarial Domain Alignment (SymDADA) framework for predicting target brain graph from a source graph. SymDADA aligns source and target domains by learning their shared embedding while alternating two regularization constraints: (i) adversarial regularization matching the distribution of the learned shared embedding with that of the source graphs using training and testing data, and (ii) adversarial regularization enforcing the embedded source distribution to match the distribution of the predicted target graphs using only the training samples. In this way, we are optimally adapting the source to the target space as we are *jointly* predicting the target graph when learning the graph embedding. Our proposed SymDADA framework outperformed its variants for predicting a target brain graph from a source graph in healthy and autistic subjects.

This work was supported by Bilimsel Araştırma Projeleri (BAP) fund from Istanbul Technical University.

D. Shen et al. (Eds.): MICCAI 2019, LNCS 11767, pp. 465–474, 2019.
https://doi.org/10.1007/978-3-030-32251-9_51

1 Introduction

Medical image synthesis is becoming an active research topic in medical imaging due to the high cost of medical modalities such as magnetic resonance imaging (MRI). Most of the existing data imputation frameworks adopted deep learning (DL) algorithms to predict a medical imaging modality from another. For instance, [2] used Generative Adversarial Network (GAN), originally proposed by [3], to generate Magnetic Resonance Angiography (MRA) from T1- and T2-weighted MRI images. More recently, [4] combined a fully convolutional network with a conditional GAN to predict positron emission tomography (PET) from computerized tomography (CT). However, these works focus on synthesizing imaging modalities rather than geometric data types such as brain representations encoded in graphs (e.g., connectomes) or manifolds (e.g., cortical surfaces). [5] is a recent application of geometric deep learning, where a Graph Convolution Network (GCN) was adopted to learn a similarity metric between functional brain graphs for autism spectrum disorder (ASD) diagnosis. Another recent work [6] proposed a graph-based classification framework where the disease state (healthy or affected) of a subject was predicted from a partially labeled graph. However, existing DL methods trained on brain connectomes overlooked the problem of 'graph synthesis'. Specifically, predicting a target brain graph from a source graph using *geometric deep learning* remains unexplored. Undoubtedly, there is a need to develop predictive learners on such non-Euclidean geometric data for clinical applications.

However, to make such a cross-domain (i.e., source to target) prediction there is even a more pressing need to handle the domain shift (or fracture) between source and target data. There has been extensive work to overcome the fracture issue between two domains [7]. For example, [8] relied on image-to-image translation techniques, where cycle-consistent GAN was leveraged to estimate PET images from MRI data. The domain shift was bridged by learning bi-directional domain mapping where MRI source domain was mapped to the PET target domain, then a reverse mapping was learned from the synthesized PET data back to MRI space for early Alzheimer's Disease diagnosis. However, these GAN-based methods were mainly devised for synthesizing *image* data [9], which might fail in handling geometric medical data such as brain graphs. A second major limitation of the majority of these existing image synthesis works lies in solving the data shift issue and multimodal image prediction task *independently*.

To overcome these limitations, we unprecedentedly propose a Symmetric Dual Adversarial Domain Alignment (SymDADA) framework for predicting a target brain graph from a source graph. Both brain graphs are considered as isomorphic as they are derived from the same parcellation brain template which enforces their coherence in topology. Specifically, we leverage the adversarially-regularized generative autoencoder (ARGA) proposed in [10], which extended the concept of autoencoder and GAN to graphs. ARGA comprises a generator G defined as a Graph Convolution Network (GCN) [11] and a discriminator D defined as a multi layer perceptron. However, ARGA was not designed for graph prediction and domain alignment but for simple graph embedding. We extend it to our aim

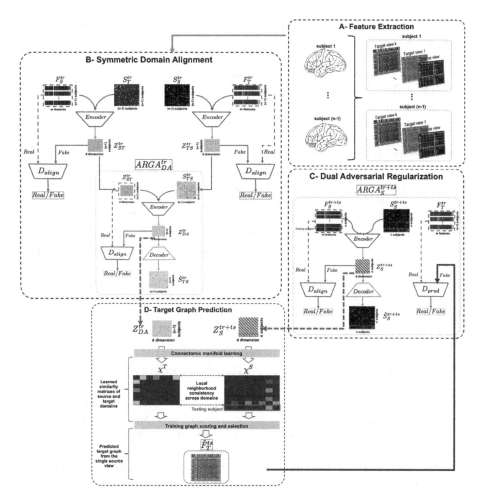

Fig. 1. *Proposed framework of Symmetric Dual Adversarial Domain Alignment (Sym-DADA) for target brain graph prediction from a single source graph.* **(A) Feature extraction.** Extraction of feature vectors from isomorphic brain graphs for each subject in both source and target domains. **(B) Symmetric Domain Alignment.** We train three separate ARGA models. The first one aims to move the source to the target domain while the second one moves the target to the source domain and the third one aims to learn the latent representation of both aligned spaces. These three models are regularized by a discriminator D_{align}. **(C) Dual Adversarial Regularization.** We regularize the source embedding of training and testing graphs by alternating between two discriminators: the D_{align} and D_{pred}. **(D) Target graph prediction.** We first propose to learn a *source* manifold capturing the similarities between the encoded source graphs of both training and testing subjects, and a *symmetrically aligned target* manifold capturing the similarities between the symmetrically aligned target graphs of the training subjects. Next, to predict the target graph for a testing subject, we identify its most similar source training samples that have consistent local neighbourhoods which largely overlap across both manifolds. By averaging the target graphs of the selected training samples, we predict the testing target brain graph.

for *jointly solving the domain shift problem along with isomorphic brain graph prediction from a baseline source graph.*

Our SymDADA framework has three main contributions: (i) the symmetric adversarial domain alignment, (ii) the *dual* adversarial regularization and (iii) the target brain graph prediction. In the first step, we propose to align the source brain domain to the target domain, and simultaneously learn the inverse mapping that moves the target to the source. Next, we propose to learn the inherent representation of both resulting embedded aligned graphs. This symmetric alignment is regularized using one discriminator, which maps the distribution of one domain (e.g., source) to the distribution of a second domain (e.g., target). In the second step, we propose an alternating optimization for dual discriminators: the first one enforces the embedded source distribution to match the distribution of the original source data, and the second one matches the distribution of the learned shared embedding of the source graphs with the distribution of the *predicted* target graphs of training subjects. In the final step, we learn a connectomic manifold of training and testing subjects using the embeddings of the aligned target and source graphs. Next, by searching the nearest neighbors to the testing subject in the source domain we average their corresponding target graphs in each target domain to ultimately predict the target graph for the testing subject.

2   Proposed SymDADA for Graph Prediction

In this section, we detail the steps of our joint brain graph domain alignment and prediction framework from a source graph. In Fig. 1, we present a flowchart of the four proposed steps including: (1) extraction of source and target brain graph features, (2) embedding source and target graphs into a low-dimensional space while symmetrically aligning their respective domains, (3) dual adversarial regularization of the source graph embedding, and (4) prediction of target brain graph.

A- Source and target brain graph feature extraction. Each subject i in our dataset has a source brain graph and a target brain graph. Since each brain graph can be encoded in a symmetric matrix, we only extract the upper-diagonal part (Fig. 1–A). Next, we stack these feature vectors of all disordered and healthy subjects vertically to get $\mathbf{F}_S$ matrix for source graphs of size $(n \times m)$, where n is the number of training and testing subjects and m denotes the number of features. $\mathbf{F}_T$ is the matrix for target graphs of size $((n-1) \times m)$ having the same feature's dimension m and $(n-1)$ training subjects since the testing subject have a missed target graph.

B- Symmetric adversarial domain alignment of source and target domains. In this step, we propose to first move the source domain to the target domain while learning the inherent representation (i.e., embedding) of the aligned source graphs. Second, we move the target domain to the source domain to learn the inherent representation of the aligned target graphs. Next, we learn a new graph embedding using the aligned source to the target domain and the aligned target to source domain, respectively. In this way, we are learning a *symmetric alignment* of source and target domains which is jointly optimized with deep representation learning of both embeddings. This is achieved by learning a GAN-based method dedicated to graph embedding called ARGA, that is a graph convolutional autoencoder regularized by a discriminator. We aim to use a GCN as an encoder to learn the latent representation of the brain graphs. In addition to taking the input graph, GCN inputs the adjacency matrix capturing the topological structure of the graph. Basically, our domain alignment strategy comprises three major learning steps (Fig. 1–B):

(i) To align the source to the target space, our generator $G(\mathbf{F}, \mathbf{S})$ takes as input training brain graph features from the source domain $\mathbf{F}_S^{tr}$ and their target adjacency matrix $\mathbf{S}_T^{tr}$ that encodes the similarities between training subjects using their target graphs. Instead of predefining the adjacency matrix as in the conventional ARGA [10], we further propose to learn it by leveraging multiple kernel manifold learning (MKML) algorithm proposed in [12] which uses multiple kernels (e.g., Euclidian distance) to learn the similarity between data points with high dimensionality and heterogeneous distribution. Such data might not be well represented with ordinary distance metric (e.g., Euclidean distance) [12] that might fail to capture heterogeneous data distribution.

(ii) To align the target to the source space, we train another encoder that takes as input training brain graph features from the target domain $\mathbf{F}_T^{tr}$ and their source adjacency matrix $\mathbf{S}_S^{tr}$ that encodes the similarities between training subjects using their source graphs.

(iii) Our proposed symmetric domain alignment consists in training an $ARGA_{DA}^{tr}$ that encodes the latent representation $\mathbf{Z}_{ST}^{tr}$ of the aligned source to the target and the adjacency matrix between training subjects using their aligned target to source embeddings $\mathbf{Z}_{TS}^{tr}$.

Specifically, each GCN encoder used in the overall framework is constructed with two layers defined as follows:

$$\mathbf{Z}^{(1)} = f_{ReLU}(\mathbf{F}, \mathbf{S}|\mathbf{W}^{(0)}); \qquad \mathbf{Z}^{(2)} = f_{linear}(\mathbf{Z}^{(1)}, \mathbf{S}|\mathbf{W}^{(1)}),$$

$\mathbf{W}^{(l)}$ is a weight matrix used as a filter to learn the convolution in the GCN for each layer l. Rectified Linear Unit, $ReLU(.)$ is the activation function of the first layer and a linear function is used for the second layer. $\mathbf{Z}^{(1)}$ and $\mathbf{Z}^{(2)}$ are the results of computing the first and the second layers, respectively. $\mathbf{Z}^{(2)}$ represents the desired embedded graphs. $f_{(.)}$ function is defined as follows:

$$f_\phi(\mathbf{F}^{(l)}, \mathbf{S}|\mathbf{W}^{(l)}) = \phi(\widetilde{\mathbf{D}}^{-\frac{1}{2}}\widetilde{\mathbf{S}}\widetilde{\mathbf{D}}^{-\frac{1}{2}}\mathbf{F}^{(l)}\mathbf{W}^{(l)})$$

ϕ is the activation function ($ReLU$ or $linear$) we choose for a specific layer (l). $\widetilde{\mathbf{S}} = \mathbf{S} + \mathbf{I}$ where $\mathbf{I}$ is the identity matrix, and $\widetilde{\mathbf{D}}_{ii} = \sum_j \widetilde{\mathbf{S}}_{ij}$ is a diagonal matrix. As suggested in [10], we propose to decode the embedded graph $\mathbf{Z}$ by reconstructing the adjacency matrix which is achieved by computing the weight (similarity) of the edge existing between the node i and j. Specifically, we measure it by computing the sigmoid function of the embedded graphs z_j of the subject j and the transposed embedded graphs $z_i^\top$ of the subject i. The decoder energy is written as follows:

$$Dec(\hat{S}|Z) = \text{sigmoid}(z_i^\top, z_j)$$

The key idea in this step is conditioning the embedded graphs by a prior distribution. We model this by an adversarial regularizer D_{align} that enforces the latent representation to match the prior distribution. Particularly, D_{align} is a multilayer perceptron that aims to minimize the error in discriminating between real data distribution and fake one generated from our encoder. We formulate the adversarial symmetric alignment of source and target domains as a cost function to minimize as follows:

$$\min_{G_{DA}} \max_{D_{align}} \mathbf{E}_{p(real)}[\log D_{align}(\mathbf{Z}_{DA}^{tr})] + \mathbf{E}_{p(fake)}[\log(1 - D_{align}(G_{DA}(\mathbf{Z}_{ST}^{tr}, \mathbf{S}_{TS}^{tr})))]$$

where $\mathbf{E}$ is the cross-entropy cost, $G_{DA}(\mathbf{Z}_{ST}^{tr}, \mathbf{S}_{TS}^{tr})$ is the graph encoder and D_{align} is the binary classifier with maximum log likelihood objective to maximize.

C- Dual adversarial regularization for source graph latent representation. To predict the target brain graph of a testing subject, we propose to search its nearest training neighbors in the *embedded* source domain then average their corresponding *symmetrically-aligned* target graphs. The resulting graph represents the predicted target graph of our testing subject. Following the symmetric alignment domain (**B**), we learn in this step a source graph embedding of both training and testing subjects. To do so, we learn a source ARGA for source graph embedding of training and testing subjects $ARGA_S^{tr+ts}$. Specifically, we stack the source feature vector of a testing subject below those of the training samples, then we generate their latent representation using the graph encoder $G_S(\mathbf{F}_S^{tr+ts}, \mathbf{S}_S^{tr+ts})$. The encoded source domain is regularized by alternating two discriminators: *at each epoch, we activate only one discriminator*:

(1) the discriminator D_{align} that aims to regularize the generation of $\mathbf{Z}_S^{tr+ts}$ by distinguishing between the real source feature vectors and the embedded source domain (Fig. 1–C). We define the cost of optimizing $ARGA_S^{tr+ts}$ when training the first discriminator as follows:

$$\min_{G_S} \max_{D_{align}} \mathbf{E}_{p(real)}[\log D_{align}(\mathbf{Z}_S^{tr+ts})] + \mathbf{E}_{p(fake)}[\log(1 - D_{align}(G_S(\mathbf{F}_S^{tr+ts}, \mathbf{S}_S^{tr+ts})))]$$

The resulting embedded source domain is then fed to the block of target graph prediction illustrated in (Fig. 1–D) to predict the target graphs of the training subjects. Specifically, we predict for each source graph its target graph using nested leave-one-out cross-validation on the training set. The predicted target brain graphs are fed to a second discriminator D_{pred} that will regularize, in the next epoch, the source graph embedding of the training and testing subjects.

(2) the discriminator D_{pred} regularizes $ARGA_S^{tr+ts}$ by distinguishing between the real target graphs of the training samples $\mathbf{F}_T^{tr}$ and their predicted target graphs $\hat{\mathbf{F}}_T^{tr}$. In the epoch following the optimization of D_{align} and G_S, we then activate the second discriminator D_{pred}, which is optimized as follows:

$$\max_{D_{pred}} \mathbf{E}_{p_{(real)}}[\log D_{pred}(\mathbf{F}_T^{tr})] + \mathbf{E}_{p_{(fake)}}[\log(1 - D_{pred}(\hat{\mathbf{F}}_T^{tr}))]$$

D- Target graph prediction for the training subjects. For the final prediction step, we aim to find the most similar training subjects to the testing subject using their learned source embeddings. We further propose to enforce a local consistency in source and target neighborhoods for the selected training source neighbors. Basically, we select source training graphs that have a large overlap in nearest neighbors across the embedded symmetrically aligned source and target domains. A selected training source sample becomes more reliable with larger local neighborhood overlaps across both domains. To do so, we leverage MKML [12] to learn connectomic manifolds χ^S (testing + training) and χ^T (only training) for each symmetrically-aligned source and target embeddings, respectively (Fig. 1–D). Next, we (1) identify in χ^S the top K-closest training subjects to the testing subject tst, (2) find for each of these K selected training samples, its nb nearest neighbors in both manifolds χ^S and χ^T, (3) assign a weighted similarity score $w(k)$ for each training subject k by extracting the list $\mathbf{L}_S$ of its top m closest neighbors in χ^S and $\mathbf{L}_T$ in χ^T then compute their overlap as follows: $\mathbf{w}(k) = \exp((\frac{\mathbf{L}_S \cap \mathbf{L}_T}{m}) \times \chi^S(tst, k))$. Finally, we average the target graphs of the selected m neighbors with the highest w scores to predict the testing target graph.

3   Results and Discussion

Connectomic Dataset and Parameter Setting. We evaluated our framework on 150 subjects (75 ASD and 75 NC) from Autism Brain Imaging Data Exchange (ABIDE[1]) using leave-one-out cross-validation. Each subject has two morphological brain graphs constructed using the following measurements in a cortical hemisphere: one source brain graph derived from the mean sulcal depth and one target brain graph derived from the average curvature. Specifically, each brain graph was derived from left and right cortical hemispheres, meshed by applying FreeSurfer to T1-w MRI of each subject. Each hemisphere was parcellated into 35 anatomical regions using Desikan-Killiany atlas, defining the nodes of a brain graph and encoded in a symmetric matrix that quantifies morphological dissimilarity between pairs of cortical regions using a specific measurement [13–15]. Our graph convolution encoder comprises two layers: the hidden and the embedding layers. We set the number of neurons for each layer to 32. We construct both discriminators D_{align} and D_{pred} with 64 and 32-neurons hidden layers. Both encoder and discriminator learning rates are set as 0.001 as in [10].

---

[1] http://fcon_1000.projects.nitrc.org/indi/abide/.

For MKML [12], we empirically set the number of kernels $K = 10$ for Sym-DADA. For the prediction step **(D)**, used a nested grid search to identify the optimal combination of the number of clusters c ($1 \leq c \leq 5$) and neighbors n_b ($3 \leq n_b \leq 50$). The same parameters are used for all comparison methods.

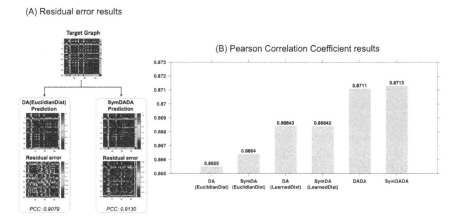

Fig. 2. *Comparison between the original and the predicted target graph of a representative subject.* We display in **(A)** the residual error matrix computed using mean absolute error (MAE) between the ground truth and predicted target brain graph. We plot in **(B)** the Pearson Correlation Coefficient (PCC) results for each of the six baseline methods and our proposed SymDADA.

Evaluation and Comparison Methods. We compare the performance of our SymDADA framework with different baseline methods: **(1) DADA:** is a variant of SymDADA where symmetric alignment illustrated in (Fig. 1–B) is replaced with a domain alignment in one direction moving the source to the target domain. **(2) DA+EuclidianDist and DA+LearnedDist:** we use for these two methods a domain alignment in one direction and remove the dual regularization illustrated in (Fig. 1–C) so that we regularize the source embedding of the training and testing subjects using only one discriminator (D_{align}). We propose to compute the adjacency matrix between subjects using Euclidian distance and learned distance by MKLM for both methods, respectively. **(3) SymDA+EuclidianDist and SymDA+LearnedDist:** similar to (2) but with symmetric domain alignment. Fig. 2–B shows the average Pearson Correlation Coefficient (PCC) between the ground truth and predicted target graphs for all methods. Our SymDADA achieved the best prediction performance. This demonstrates that our proposed symmetric domain alignment and the integration of predicted target graphs into the source embedding regularization boost brain graph prediction accuracy from a source graph. We display in Fig. 2–A the residual prediction error computed using mean absolute error (MAE) between the ground truth and predicted brain graphs for a representative subject. This clearly shows that our method leads to a low residual (dark colors) in comparison to its simpler variant.

4 Conclusion

In this work, we introduced a geometric deep learning framework for predicting a brain graph from a single source graph. We proposed: (i) a *symmetric domain alignment* of both source and target domains while learning their respective latent representations, and (ii) a *dual adversarial regularization* that learns a source embedding of training and testing brain graphs while alternating two discriminators enforcing the embedded source distribution to simultaneously match (a) the distribution of the original source brain graphs, and (2) the distribution of the nested predicted target graphs, alternatingly. Our framework clearly outperformed comparison methods on a relatively large dataset. Inspired by [10], we will develop in our future work a *geometric* Cycle-DADA which performs cyclic domain alignment while leveraging our proposed dual discriminators and simultaneously predicting multiple target brain graphs from one source graph.

References

1. Soussia, M., Rekik, I.: A review on image-and network-based brain data analysis techniques for Alzheimer's Disease diagnosis reveals a gap in developing predictive methods for prognosis. arXiv preprint arXiv:1808.01951 (2018)
2. Olut, S., Sahin, Y.H., Demir, U., Unal, G.: Generative adversarial training for MRA image synthesis using multi-contrast MRI. arXiv preprint arXiv:1804.04366 (2018)
3. Goodfellow, I., Pouget-Abadie, J., et al.: Generative adversarial nets. In: Advances in Neural Information Processing Systems, pp. 2672–2680 (2014)
4. Ben-Cohen, A., et al.: Cross-modality synthesis from CT to PET using FCN and GAN networks for improved automated lesion detection. Eng. Appl. Artif. Intell. **78**, 186–194 (2019)
5. Ktena, S.I., et al.: Distance metric learning using graph convolutional networks: application to functional brain networks. In: Descoteaux, M., Maier-Hein, L., Franz, A., Jannin, P., Collins, D.L., Duchesne, S. (eds.) MICCAI 2017. LNCS, vol. 10433, pp. 469–477. Springer, Cham (2017). https://doi.org/10.1007/978-3-319-66182-7_54
6. Parisot, S., et al.: Spectral graph convolutions for population-based disease prediction. In: Descoteaux, M., Maier-Hein, L., Franz, A., Jannin, P., Collins, D.L., Duchesne, S. (eds.) MICCAI 2017. LNCS, vol. 10435, pp. 177–185. Springer, Cham (2017). https://doi.org/10.1007/978-3-319-66179-7_21
7. Moreno-Torres, J.G., Raeder, T., Alaiz-RodríGuez, R., Chawla, N.V., Herrera, F.: A unifying view on dataset shift in classification. Pattern Recogn. **45**, 521–530 (2012)
8. Pan, Y., Liu, M., Lian, C., Zhou, T., Xia, Y., Shen, D.: Synthesizing missing PET from MRI with cycle-consistent generative adversarial networks for Alzheimer's disease diagnosis. In: Frangi, A.F., Schnabel, J.A., Davatzikos, C., Alberola-López, C., Fichtinger, G. (eds.) MICCAI 2018. LNCS, vol. 11072, pp. 455–463. Springer, Cham (2018). https://doi.org/10.1007/978-3-030-00931-1_52
9. Yi, X., Walia, E., Babyn, P.: Generative adversarial network in medical imaging: a review. arXiv preprint arXiv:1809.07294 (2018)

10. Pan, S., Hu, R., Long, G., Jiang, J., Yao, L., Zhang, C.: Adversarially regularized graph autoencoder. arXiv preprint arXiv:1802.04407 (2018)
11. Kipf, T.N., Welling, M.: Semi-supervised classification with graph convolutional networks. arXiv preprint arXiv:1609.02907 (2016)
12. Wang, B., Ramazzotti, D., De Sano, L., Zhu, J., Pierson, E., Batzoglou, S.: SIMLR: a tool for large-scale single-cell analysis by multi-kernel learning. bioRxiv (2017) 118901
13. Mahjoub, I., Mahjoub, M.A., Rekik, I.: Brain multiplexes reveal morphological connectional biomarkers fingerprinting late brain dementia states. Sci. Rep. **8**, 4103 (2018)
14. Soussia, M., Rekik, I.: Unsupervised manifold learning using high-order morphological brain networks derived from T1-w MRI for autism diagnosis. Front. Neuroinform. **12** (2018)
15. Dhifallah, S., Rekik, I., Initiative, A.D.N., et al.: Clustering-based multi-view network fusion for estimating brain network atlases of healthy and disordered populations. J. Neurosci. Methods **311**, 426–435 (2019)

Harmonization of Infant Cortical Thickness Using Surface-to-Surface Cycle-Consistent Adversarial Networks

Fenqiang Zhao[1,2], Zhengwang Wu[2], Li Wang[2], Weili Lin[2], Shunren Xia[1],
Dinggang Shen[2], Gang Li[2(✉)], and the UNC/UMN Baby Connectome Project
Consortium

[1] Key Laboratory of Biomedical Engineering of Ministry of Education,
Zhejiang University, Hangzhou, China
[2] Department of Radiology and BRIC, University of North Carolina at Chapel Hill,
Chapel Hill, NC, USA
gang_li@med.unc.edu

Abstract. Increasing multi-site infant neuroimaging datasets are facilitating the research on understanding early brain development with larger sample size and bigger statistical power. However, a joint analysis of cortical properties (e.g., cortical thickness) is unavoidably facing the problem of non-biological variance introduced by differences in MRI scanners. To address this issue, in this paper, we propose cycle-consistent adversarial networks based on spherical cortical surface to harmonize cortical thickness maps between different scanners. We combine the spherical U-Net and CycleGAN to construct a surface-to-surface CycleGAN (S2SGAN). Specifically, we model the harmonization from scanner X to scanner Y as a surface-to-surface translation task. The first goal of harmonization is to learn a mapping $G_X : X \rightarrow Y$ such that the distribution of surface thickness maps from $G_X(X)$ is indistinguishable from Y. Since this mapping is highly under-constrained, with the second goal of harmonization to preserve individual differences, we utilize the inverse mapping $G_Y : Y \rightarrow X$ and the cycle consistency loss to enforce $G_Y(G_X(X)) \approx X$ (and vice versa). Furthermore, we incorporate the correlation coefficient loss to guarantee the structure consistency between the original and the generated surface thickness maps. Quantitative evaluation on both synthesized and real infant cortical data demonstrates the superior ability of our method in removing unwanted scanner effects and preserving individual differences simultaneously, compared to the state-of-the-art methods.

Keywords: Spherical U-Net · CycleGAN · Harmonization

1 Introduction

In recent years, large-scale multi-site infant neuroimaging datasets are increasingly facilitating the research on understanding early brain development with

© Springer Nature Switzerland AG 2019
D. Shen et al. (Eds.): MICCAI 2019, LNCS 11767, pp. 475–483, 2019.
https://doi.org/10.1007/978-3-030-32251-9_52

larger sample size and bigger statistical power [3,7]. However, directly combining neuroimaging data across scanners will unavoidably introduce the non-biological variance to the data, typically due to differences in imaging acquisition protocol (e.g., field of view, coil channels, gradient directions, etc.) and hardware (e.g., manufacturer, magnetic field strengths, etc.). Such unwanted sources of bias and variability are referred as "site effects" in [1] that are non-biological in nature and associated with different scanning parameters. Herein, we also use different sites to represent different scanners. In previous studies, the site effects have been long understood to hinder the accurate detection of imaging features [2] and preclude joint analysis of multi-site data [9]. Therefore, harmonizing neuroimaging data to both remove site effects and preserve biological associations is imperative for joint analysis of the multi-site data.

Several harmonization techniques have been developed for adult diffusion MRI [4,8]. However, there are very few published methods for harmonizing brain morphological properties from structural MRI, e.g., cortical thickness, which are highly associated with brain development and disorders. Fortin et al. [1] proposed a statistical data pooling tool that uses Combat (a batch-effect correction tool used in genomics) for adult cortical thickness harmonization. Combat estimates a linear model with additive and multiplicative site-effect coefficient at each cortical region, thus accounting for site differences. However, this method has several limitations. First, a linear model at the region level might not be able to account for the complex mapping between multi-site data. Second, their optimization procedure assumes that the site-effect parameters follow a particular parametric prior distribution (Gaussian and Inverse-gamma), which might not hold well in many scenarios of cortical property harmonization. Third, as a statistical tool, the major drawback of Combat is the weak generalization ability, because Combat processes all data at one time and treat them equally, making it sensitive to outliers. Forth, Combat is designed for harmonizing two sites into one intermediate site, which is not applicable for mapping one less reliable site (with low-quality data) to another more reliable site (with high-quality data).

While not developed explicitly for harmonization, a number of recently developed deep learning techniques [11,12] could potentially be adapted to address these issues. First, the spherical U-Net architecture [11] provides an effective Direct Neighbor (DiNe) filter to extend conventional convolutional neural network (CNN) to the cortical surface with an inherent spherical topology. It was originally designed for cortical surface parcellation [10] and achieves state-of-the-art performance, which could be used as a generator for site-to-site cortical surface property map translation. Second, since most neuroimaging studies do not have paired data across sites, the popular image generation technique Cycle-GAN [12] could be leveraged for the unpaired surface translation. Therefore, we propose to extend the conventional CycleGAN to cortical surface data based on spherical U-Net termed S2SGAN. Specifically, we model harmonization from site X to site Y as a surface-to-surface translation task. A preliminary goal of harmonization is to learn a mapping $G_X : X \rightarrow Y$ such that the distribution of $G_X(X)$ is indistinguishable from the distribution of Y. Since this mapping is highly under-constrained, with the second goal of harmonization to preserve biological variance, we utilize the inverse mapping $G_Y : Y \to X$ and the cycle consistency loss to enforce $G_Y(G_X(X)) \approx X$ (and vice versa). Furthermore, we incorporate the correlation coefficient loss to guarantee the structure consistency between the original surface thickness maps and the generated maps.

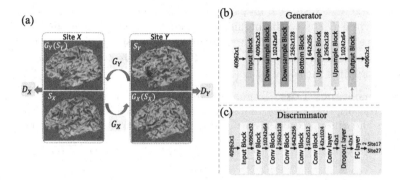

Fig. 1. The framework of our proposed S2SGAN. (a) Two generators (G_X and G_Y) learn cross-site mappings of surface maps (herein, cortical thickness maps). Two discriminators (D_X and D_Y) distinguish generated surface maps and real surface maps. (b) In generators, each block contains repeated DiNeConv+BN+ReLU with input size and output size denoted before and after the block, and one more spherical pooling layer for each downsample block, one more spherical transposed convolution layer for upsample block to deal with the skip concatenated feature maps (grey arrows). (c) In discriminators, each block is DiNeConv+BN+ReLU+Pooling, except for the input block without pooling.

2   Method

2.1   Loss Design

As shown in Fig. 1(a), suppose we have two cortical surface datasets obtained from two sites, site X and site Y. Our goal is to learn the cross-site mapping functions of cortical surface property (e.g., cortical thickness) maps G_X and G_Y for $X \to Y$ and $Y \to X$ mapping, respectively. In addition, discriminator D_X is used to distinguish real and generated site X surface maps, and discriminator D_Y is similarly for site Y. All the mapping and discrimination functions can be approximated by spherical neural networks. The objective of optimizing the whole model includes three types of losses: (1) an adversarial loss for matching the distribution of generated surface maps to the distribution in the target site; (2) a cycle-consistency loss to prevent generators from producing surface maps that are irrelevant to the inputs; and (3) a correlation coefficient loss to constrain structure consistency between original and generated surface maps.

Adversarial Loss. We apply adversarial loss to both mapping functions $G_X : X \rightarrow Y$ and $G_Y : Y \rightarrow X$. For the mapping function G_X and its discriminator D_Y, the objective function is expressed as:

$$\mathcal{L}_{GAN}(G_X, D_Y) = E_{x \sim p_{data}(X)}[(1 - D_Y(G_X(x)))^2] + E_{y \sim p_{data}(Y)}[D_Y(y)^2],$$

where $x \sim p_{data}(X)$ and $y \sim p_{data}(Y)$ denotes the data distribution of X and Y. G_X aims to generate surface maps $G_X(x)$ close to the real target surface maps in site Y, while D_Y is to distinguish between generated surface maps and real surface maps of site Y. Therefore, the optimization of this minimax two-player game can be written as: $min_{G_X} max_{D_Y} \mathcal{L}_{GAN}(G_X, D_Y)$. A similar adversarial loss is also applied for G_Y and D_X.

Cycle-Consistency Loss. To guarantee the generated surface maps are meaningful to the original surface maps, an additional cycle consistency loss [12] is defined as the difference between original and reconstructed surface maps:

$$\mathcal{L}_{cyc}(G_X, G_Y) = E_{x \sim p_{data}(X)}[\|G_Y(G_X(x)) - x\|_1] + E_{y \sim p_{data}(Y)}[\|G_X(G_Y(y)) - y\|_1].$$

Correlation Coefficient Loss. For cortical surface property maps, it is crucial to preserve local structural information in the mapping functions. To further reduce the ambiguity of indirect cycle-consistency loss between the original and generated surface maps, we adopt the correlation coefficient loss to enforce structure consistency between input and generated surface maps:

$$\mathcal{L}_{cc}(G_X, G_Y) = -E_{x \sim p_{data}(X)}\left[\frac{\text{cov}(G_X(x), x)}{\sigma_{G_X(x)} \sigma_x}\right] - E_{y \sim p_{data}(Y)}\left[\frac{\text{cov}(G_Y(y), y)}{\sigma_{G_Y(y)} \sigma_y}\right],$$

where cov denotes the covariance, σ denotes the standard deviation.

(Optional) Paired Loss. In our method, we don't require any paried data from different sites for training, which are typically hard to acquire. However, if we have paired data, we can add an additional paired loss to directly constrain the vertex-wise similarity between the generated surface maps and the corresponding groundtruth surface maps:

$$\mathcal{L}_{pair}(G_X, G_Y) = E_{x \sim p_{data}(X)}[\|G_X(x) - gt(x)\|_1] + E_{y \sim p_{data}(Y)}[\|G_Y(y) - gt(y)\|_1],$$

where $gt(x)$, $gt(y)$ represent the groundtruth of x and y in the paired dataset.

Full Objective. Finally, the full objective of our model is written as: $\mathcal{L}(G_X, G_Y, D_X, D_Y) = \mathcal{L}_{GAN}(G_X, D_Y) + \mathcal{L}_{GAN}(G_Y, D_X) + \alpha \mathcal{L}_{cyc}(G_X, G_Y) + \beta \mathcal{L}_{cc}(G_X, G_Y) + \lambda \mathcal{L}_{pair}(G_X, G_Y)$, where α, β, and λ control the relative importance of the loss terms. Note that the last loss term will be removed when having no paired data.

2.2   Network Architecture

We use the spherical U-Net [11] architecture as our generative network. Leveraging the spherical topology of cortical surfaces, the spherical U-Net first extends convolution, pooling, and upsampling operations to the spherical space using DiNe filter on regularly resampled spherical surfaces, and then constructs U-Net using corresponding spherical operations. We modified the spherical U-Net with half feature channels and 4 resolution steps, first 3 of which are concatenated with skip connections; see Fig. 1(b) for more detailed information. For the discriminator network, we extend a VGG style classification CNN to spherical surfaces. It consists of 7 DiNe convolution layers, 5 spherical pooling layers, a dropout layer with probability 0.2, and 1 fully connected layer, as shown in Fig. 1(c). Note all the DiNe convolution layers are followed by batch normalization (BN) and leaky rectified linear unit (ReLU) with negative slope of 0.2.

3 Experiments and Results

3.1 Validation on Synthetic Paired Surface Data

To better evaluate the performance of our method for harmonizing cortical thickness maps across sites, we synthesized a paired dataset to simulate cortical surfaces reconstructed from images scanned at different resolutions, which is a typical occurrence in harmonization task. Specifically, we used the BCP dataset [3] from one scanner, with 360 MRI scans from 183 infants and age from 0 to 2 years, named site X. Both T1w and T2w images were acquired at the resolution of $0.8 \times 0.8 \times 0.8$ mm^3. We resampled all T1w and T2w images in site X to $1 \times 1 \times$ mm^3 to form another dataset, site Y. All MR images were processed using an infant-dedicated computational pipeline [6]. All cortical surfaces were mapped onto the spherical space, nonlinearly aligned, and further resampled.

In our experiment, for S2SGAN model without paired data, we set α as 15, β as 1, and λ as 0; for S2SGAN model with paired data, we set α as 15, β as 1, and λ as 100. We trained both models using Adam optimizer to alternately update G and D with an initial learning rate 0.0001 for the first 20 epochs and linearly-reduced rate to 0 for the next 180 epochs. We used 70% of the data as the training set and remaining 30% as the testing set using stratified sampling. We used two well accepted metrics of mean absolute error (MAE) and peak signal-noise ratio (PSNR) for quantitatively evaluating the results.

We compare the harmonization results from site Y with low quality data to site X with high quality data. On average, our S2SGAN achieves MAE 0.0928 $\pm$ 0.0109 mm, PSNR 31.48 $\pm$ 1.116 (the standard deviation is between scans). The S2SGAN (paired) model achieves MAE 0.082 $\pm$ 0.0178 mm and PSNR 33.09 $\pm$ 1.727, which represents the best that a S2SGAN can achieve. For comparison, the Combat [1] results were obtained by using the official code with age and gender as biological covariates, achieving MAE 0.124 $\pm$ 0.0137 mm and PSNR 29.00 $\pm$ 1.019. In all, our S2SGAN achieves better performance than Combat in both MAE and PSNR and also produces closer results to S2SGAN (paired). Figure 2 shows the harmonization results of different methods on a testing subject.

3.2 Validation on Real Unpaired Surface Data

To demonstrate the practical ability of our method in harmonizing cortical thickness across sites, we employed two real longitudinal infant datasets with matched

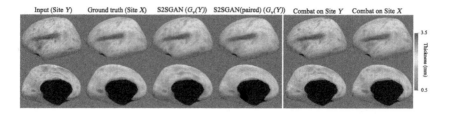

Fig. 2. Comparison of harmonization results using different methods on a testing subject. The first four columns show the S2SGAN model results. The last two columns show the Combat results. Note that Combat harmonizes two sites into one intermediate site, thus should generate two identical surfaces in the last two columns.

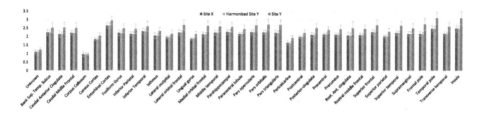

Fig. 3. Comparison of cortical thickness value across sites for each ROI.

demographics. Site X is the same dataset in Sect. 3.1. Site Y has 251 longitudinal scans from 50 infants, acquired at the resolution of $1 \times 1 \times 1$ mm³, from a different scanner. We trained our S2SGAN model using the same experimental configuration as in Sect. 3.1.

Validation on Removing Site Effects. For unpaired data, we use the same evaluation method in [5] to perform ROI-based analysis to estimate if the site effects are removed. With matched demographics, we aim to achieve the same average ROI thickness values as the target site after harmonization. In Fig. 3, we show the 36 mean ROI thickness values of site X, site Y, and harmonized site Y. We observed that statistical differences of ROI thickness are significant prior to harmonization and are successfully removed after harmonization. Same as in [1], we also performed unsupervised dimension reduction on all vertex-wise thickness data: site X + site Y + harmonized Y, using PCA. The data projected into the first two principal components are presented in Fig. 4. Figure 5 shows the boxplots of vertex-wise thickness for stratified sampled 100 subjects from site X, site Y and harmonized Y, sorted by age. We note that our method *not only* achieves similar distribution as the target site, *but also* well preserves the individual differences.

Validation on Preserving *Group* Differences. Same as in [5], we adopted Cohen's d for evaluating age group differences preservation. Cohen's d is defined

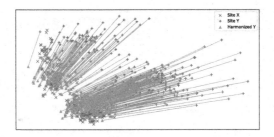

Fig. 4. Dimension reduction results of site X + site Y + harmonized site Y using PCA. The x-axis is the first principal component and y-axis is the second principal component. The grey lines represent the correspondences of the same scans before and after harmonization.

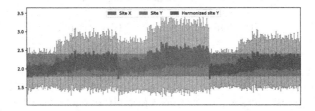

Fig. 5. Boxplots of vertex-wise thickness for different sites. Each boxplot represents a scan. Stratified sampled 100 scans are presented for each site and are sorted by age within the site.

as the group differences: $d_{ij} = \frac{1}{N_r} \sum_r \left| (M_{ir} - M_{jr}) / \sqrt{\frac{(n_i - 1)s_{ir}^2 + (n_j - 1)s_{jr}^2}{n_i + n_j - 2}} \right|$, where i and j represent two groups, r represents each ROI feature, N_r is the number of ROIs, M is the mean cortical thickness, s is the standard deviation and n is the number of subjects in the group. Cohen's d is thus free of data value size and generally ranges from 0.1 to 2.0, proportional to the effect sizes between groups. We divided all the data into 6 groups separated by 45, 135, 225, 315, and 450 days of age and compute Cohen's d for each two of them. The Δd is then computed as the mean absolute deviation of Cohen's d before and after harmonization: $\Delta d = \frac{1}{N_g(N_g - 1)} \sum_{i=1}^{N_g} \sum_{j \neq i}^{N_g} \left| d_{ij}^{before} - d_{ij}^{after} \right|$, where N_g is the number of groups and d_{ij}^{before}, d_{ij}^{after} represent the Cohen's d before and after harmonization, respectively. Thus a smaller Δd generally represents a better difference preservation. For comparison, we adopted Combat using the official code with age as biological covariate. On average, our S2SGAN achieves Δd 0.0683 $\pm$ 0.0520 and Combat achieves Δd 0.2069 $\pm$ 0.1467 (the standard deviation is between group pairs). With a smaller Δd, we can conclude that our method better preserves the group differences in brain development.

Validation on Preserving *Individual* Differences. Instead of using median values in [4], we use ROI feature values to compute Euclidean distances between

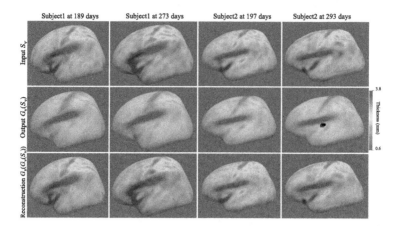

Fig. 6. Visualization of harmonization results on two age-matched testing subjects.

any two scans, thus forming a distance matrix, denoted as $\mathbf{E}_{ij}^{n \times n} = \|F_i - F_j\|_2$, where n is the number of scans, and F is the feature vector. The goal is to estimate how the distances are preserved relatively to each other before and after harmonization. Therefore, we compute the correlation Cor of the two distance matrices before and after harmonization. We also adopted Combat with age and gender as biological covariates for comparison. Our S2SGAN achieves Cor 0.9766, and Combat achieves Cor 0.9606. With a higher Cor, we can conclude that our method better preserves the individual differences. Figure 6 shows two age-matched subjects' harmonization results. We can see that the differences both between subjects and ages are well preserved.

4   Conclusion

In this paper, we propose a novel cortical thickness harmonization method, based on spherical U-Net to learn the inherent complex mapping from one site to another site in a CycleGAN manner. Our proposed method, S2SGAN, has been validated on both synthetic paired data and real unpaired data of infant brain MRI. Both visual and quantitative results demonstrate its superior capability to reduce inter-site variance, while preserving individual variance simultaneously.

Acknowledgements. This work was partially supported by NIH grants: MH107815, MH116225, and MH117943. This work utilizes approaches developed by an NIH grant (1U01MH110274) and the efforts of the UNC/UMN Baby Connectome Project Consortium.

References

1. Fortin, J.P., et al.: Harmonization of cortical thickness measurements across scanners and sites. Neuroimage **167**, 104–120 (2018)

2. Han, X., et al.: Reliability of mri-derived measurements of human cerebral cortical thickness: the effects of field strength, scanner upgrade and manufacturer. Neuroimage **32**(1), 180–194 (2006)
3. Howell, B.R., et al.: The UNC/UMN baby connectome project (BCP): an overview of the study design and protocol development. NeuroImage **185**, 891–905 (2019)
4. Huynh, K.M., et al.: Multi-site harmonization of diffusion mri data via method of moments. IEEE Trans. Med. Imaging **38**, 1599–1609 (2019)
5. Karayumak, S.C., et al.: Retrospective harmonization of multi-site diffusion MRI data acquired with different acquisition parameters. Neuroimage **184**, 180–200 (2019)
6. Li, G., et al.: Construction of 4D high-definition cortical surface atlases of infants: methods and applications. Med. Image Anal. **25**(1), 22–36 (2015)
7. Li, G., et al.: Computational neuroanatomy of baby brains: a review. Neuroimage **185**, 906–925 (2019)
8. Mirzaalian, H., et al.: Harmonizing diffusion MRI data across multiple sites and scanners. In: MICCAI, pp. 12–19 (2015)
9. Takao, H., et al.: Effect of scanner in longitudinal studies of brain volume changes. J. Magn. Reson. Imaging **34**(2), 438–444 (2011)
10. Zhao, F., et al.: Spherical U-Net for infant cortical surface parcellation. In: ISBI, pp. 1882–1886 (2019)
11. Zhao, F., et al.: Spherical U-Net on cortical surfaces: methods and applications. In: IPMI, pp. 855–866 (2019)
12. Zhu, J.Y., et al.: Unpaired image-to-image translation using cycle-consistent adversarial networks. In: ICCV, pp. 2223–2232 (2017)

Quantifying Confounding Bias in Neuroimaging Datasets with Causal Inference

Christian Wachinger[1(✉)], Benjamin Gutierrez Becker[1], Anna Rieckmann[2], and Sebastian Pölsterl[1]

[1] Artificial Intelligence in Medical Imaging (AI-Med), KJP, LMU München, Munich, Germany
christian@ai-med.de
[2] Department of Radiation Sciences, Umeå University, Umeå, Sweden

Abstract. Neuroimaging datasets keep growing in size to address increasingly complex medical questions. However, even the largest datasets today alone are too small for training complex machine learning models. A potential solution is to increase sample size by pooling scans from several datasets. In this work, we combine 12,207 MRI scans from 15 studies and show that simple pooling is often ill-advised due to introducing various types of biases in the training data. First, we systematically *define* these biases. Second, we *detect* bias by experimentally showing that scans can be correctly assigned to their respective dataset with 73.3% accuracy. Finally, we propose to tell causal from confounding factors by *quantifying* the extent of confounding and causality in a single dataset using causal inference. We achieve this by finding the simplest graphical model in terms of Kolmogorov complexity. As Kolmogorov complexity is not directly computable, we employ the minimum description length to approximate it. We empirically show that our approach is able to estimate plausible causal relationships from real neuroimaging data.

1 Introduction

As neuroimaging is joining the ranks of a "big data" science with more and larger datasets becoming available [22], the issue of dataset bias is becoming apparent. Usually, neuroimaging datasets are collected with a particular research question in mind, and inclusion criteria are tailored to answering this particular question. With the advancement of machine learning, in particular deep learning, researchers require large sample sizes for training their models. However, pooling data from studies that have been designed with different research questions in mind, will likely lead to bias in the learned model. For the same reason, an estimate of a statistic from one dataset, will likely differ from the estimate in another dataset. In general, bias refers to an estimate of a statistic that is systematically different from its population value. If estimates would be truly unbiased

© Springer Nature Switzerland AG 2019
D. Shen et al. (Eds.): MICCAI 2019, LNCS 11767, pp. 484–492, 2019.
https://doi.org/10.1007/978-3-030-32251-9_53

on a population level, models would naturally generalize to other datasets. However, in practice, neuroimaging datasets are subject to various types of biases, including subject selection, acquisition method, and processing biases [9,13].

Selection bias stems from the fact that subjects included in the study do not represent the overall population. Examples are: (i) the recruitment of particular target groups, e.g., young adults; (ii) the recruitment of a particular disease group; or (iii) an over-representation of more educated participants in convenience samples. While the first two are potentially related to the study objective and can be controlled for, the third one is more difficult to control and also seems to appear in epidemiological studies [22]. A second bias stems from the image acquisition, where magnetic field strength, manufacturer, gradients, pulse sequences and head positioning cause variations in the images. While standardization efforts are undertaken for instance by the ADNI [11], variations related to the scanner remain [13], and it is even questionable if a further standardization is in the manufacturer's interest. In addition, there is processing bias in image segmentation and registration, which is in part related to acquisition bias, because of motion artifacts, voxel sizes, and image noise that can cause bias in segmentation results. Moreover, different segmentation algorithms and different choices for their hyper-parameters often lead to varying segmentation results. Finally, an association between an image-derived measure and an outcome is subject to confounding bias, if both variables are affected by a third latent random variable.

Table 1. Overview of neuroimaging datasets used in this study.

Dataset	Diagnosis	N	Age (mean)	Age (SD)	Males %	Sites	Diseased
ABIDE I	Autism	1,095	17.1	8.1	85.2	24	526
ABIDE II	Autism	1,032	15.2	9.4	76.1	17	477
ADHD200	ADHD	965	12.1	3.3	61.8	8	384
ADNI	Alzheimer's	1,682	73.6	7.2	55.0	62	1,144
AIBL	Alzheimer's	262	72.9	7.6	47.3	2	91
COBRE	Schizophrenia	146	37.0	12.8	74.7	1	72
CORR		1,476	25.9	15.4	50.0	32	0
GSP		1,563	21.5	2.8	42.3	5	0
HBN	Psychiatric	689	10.7	3.6	59.7	2	497
HCP		1,113	28.8	3.7	45.6	1	0
IXI		561	48.6	16.5	44.6	3	0
MCIC	Schizophrenia	194	33.1	11.5	71.6	3	104
NKI	Psychiatric	624	38.4	22.5	39.1	1	268
OASIS	Alzheimer's	415	52.8	25.1	38.6	1	100
PPMI	Parkinson's	390	61.2	10.0	62.6	-	284

In this paper, we study bias in neuroimaging data. To this end, we combine data from 15 large-scale studies. We propose, (i) to predict the dataset that a subject is part of as a means to detect inter-dataset bias; (ii) to distinguish between causal and confounded statistical relationships; (iii) to quantify the extent of confounding and causality in a single dataset using causal inference. To this end, we use the algorithmic Markov condition to determine the simplest model in terms of Kolmogorov complexity to determine the true causal model.

Related Work: Correcting confounding factors in neuroimaging have to date been mainly studied within datasets [4,15,21], but not across datasets. The focus of these studies has primarily been on age and sex as confounders. The harmonization of cortical thickness across datasets was studied in [7]. An instance reweighting approach for domain adaptation in Alzheimer's prediction was proposed in [25]. In contrast to prior work, note that our proposed approach aims to detect and quantify bias using causal inference, but not to remove bias.

2   Data

We work on MRI T1 brain scans from 15 large-scale public datasets: ABIDE I+II [3], ADHD200 [19], ADNI [11], AIBL [5], COBRE [18], CORR [26], GSP [2], HBN [1], HCP [24], IXI[1], MCIC [8], NKI [20], OASIS [16], and PPMI [17]. All datasets were processed with FreeSurfer [6] version 5.3. We keep only one scan per subject from longitudinal or test-retest datasets. After exclusion of scans with processing errors and incomplete meta data, scans from 12,207 subjects (6,827 male; 8,126 controls; mean age: 33.5 ± 23.9) remained. We present an overview of demographics per dataset in Table 1.

3   Name That Dataset

In order to evaluate the impact of dataset bias, we play the game *Name That Dataset* on neuroimaing data that was originally proposed by Torralba and Efros [23] on natural images. The task is to predict the dataset an MRI scan is coming from solely based on image-derived measures, where we use volume and thickness. We mainly focus on healthy controls to exclude disease-specific effects that would ease classification. Figure 1 illustrates the performance for classifying the 15 datasets for different combinations of image features. A random forest classifier with default settings was used for the prediction. When splitting data into training and testing sets, we take the dataset membership into account to ensure each dataset is accordingly represented.

If dataset bias would be absent, we would expect a prediction accuracy close to random chance (6.7% for 15 datasets). As not all datasets have the same size and have different distributions of age and sex, we compare to results of a classifier trained on age and sex alone as baseline. With only 0.1% of the data used for

_____

[1] http://brain-development.org/ixi-dataset/.

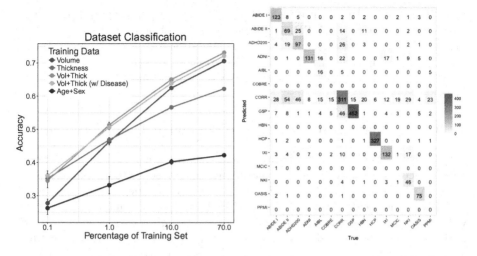

Fig. 1. Left: Dataset classification accuracy for age and sex, volume, thickness, and their combination. The percentage of the data used for training is shown in log-scale. Lines show the average score over 50 repetitions, error bars show the standard deviation. Right: Confusion matrix for volume and thickness with 70% training data.

training, volume measures perform similar to prediction with age and sex. As we increase the amount of training data to 70%, the accuracy increases to 73.3% for the combination of volume and thickness features, which perform better than each of them alone. The classifier with age and sex has 42.2% accuracy, which is well above random and therefore hints at selection bias. But compared to the 73.3% accuracy for image features, there must be another source of bias that cannot be explained by basic demographics, such as confounding bias. Figure 1 also shows similar results after including diseased patients, denoted by '(w/ Disease)'.

From the confusion matrix in Fig. 1, we can see that datasets with a similar population result in higher confusion, e.g., between ABIDE I+II, and ADHD200. Single-site datasets, like HCP, that have strict inclusion criteria and imaging protocols show almost no confusion with any of the other datasets. In contrast, multi-site datasets like CORR that also cover a wide age range, show high confusion with other datasets. Overall, the high classification accuracy (diagonal elements) indicates that datasets possess unique, identifiable characteristics.

The lesson learned from this experiment is that even when working with image-derived values that represent physical measures (volume, thickness), substantial bias in datasets remains, despite techniques like atlas renormalization [10] were employed to improve consistency across scanners. Of course, much of the bias can be attributed to the different goals of the studies, like the inclusion of subjects from different age groups. However, even when focusing on datasets that cover a similar age range, we observe a high accuracy, e.g., ABIDE I and II. While we are not aware of previous attempts to *Name That Dataset*, our results echo concerns raised in previous studies. In an ENIGMA study with over 15,000 subjects on brain asymmetry [9], it was reported that dataset heterogeneity explained over 10% of the total observed variance per structure. In ADNI, which has an optimized MPRAGE imaging protocol across all sites [11], the intra-subject variability of compartment volumes for scans on different scanners was roughly 10 times higher than repeated scans on the same scanner [13]. Similarly, [25] reported a drop in accuracy when training and testing on different datasets.

4   Telling Causal from Confounded with Causal Inference

In the previous section, we have established that there is correlation between a feature vector $\mathbf{y}$, derived from MRI scans, and the dataset D the scan belongs to, by estimating the probability $P(D = d \mid Y = \mathbf{y})$ via a random forest classifier. While this has yielded useful insights, it is flawed: (i) it cannot be used with MRI scans from a single dataset only, and (ii) it only provides a measure of statistical dependence, which alone is insufficient to determine causal structures of confounding bias. Here, we want to study bias in a more principal manner by looking at confounding bias in a causal inference framework. Given one particular dataset, we want to quantify to what extent the correlation between biological factors $\mathbf{X} = \{X_1, \ldots, X_m\}$ and a single image-derived measure Y_j is due to $\mathbf{X}$ influencing Y_j, i.e., an underlying neurobiological cause, and to what extent it is due to other common causes, i.e., confounders $\mathbf{Z} = \{Z_1, \ldots, Z_k\}$. In the purely causal setting, where there is no confounding, there is a causal relationship between biological variables $\mathbf{X}$ and image-derived measure Y_j, which we denote as $\mathbf{X} \rightarrow Y_j$. On the other end of the spectrum, the correlation between $\mathbf{X}$ and Y_j is entirely due to other measured or unmeasured causes that have an effect on both the biological factors *and* image-derived measures. This would constitute a purely confounded relationship: $\mathbf{X} \leftarrow \mathbf{Z} \rightarrow Y_j$. Figure 2 illustrates the different scenarios, where the statistical dependency between $\mathbf{X}$ and Y_j is due confounding (middle), a causal relationship (right), or a mixture of both (left).

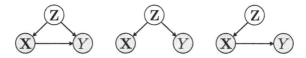

Fig. 2. Probabilistic graphical models for observed variables $\mathbf{X}$, Y and unobserved confounders $\mathbf{Z}$. The statistical relationship between $\mathbf{X}$ and Y is due to confounder $\mathbf{Z}$ and due to the influence of $\mathbf{X}$ on Y (left). Limiting cases are pure confounding (middle) and pure causality (right).

4.1   Causal Inference by Minimum Description Length

Inferring causal relations from observational data is challenging and is only attainable under specific model assumptions. We use an approach that incorporates the algorithmic Markov condition [12], which states that the simplest factorization of the joint distribution $P(X, Y)$, in terms of Kolmogorov complexity, corresponds to the true generative process. As Kolmogorov complexity is not directly computable, we employ the minimum description length to approximate it. Here, we consider two factorizations of $P(X, Y)$ as depicted in Fig. 2: (i) the causal model $P(X, Y) = P(Y|X)P(X|Z)P(Z)$ is represented by a linear regression model, and (ii) the confounded model $P(X, Y) = P(Y|Z)P(X|Z)P(Z)$ by probabilistic PCA. Thus, the complexity under the causal model can be estimated by minimum description length $L_{ca}(\mathbf{X}, Y_j)$ via:

$$L_{ca}(\mathbf{X}, Y_j) = -\log P(\mathbf{X}) \int P(Y_j|\mathbf{X}, \mathbf{w})P(\mathbf{w})d\mathbf{w},$$
$$X_i \sim \mathcal{N}(0, \sigma_x^2 I), \qquad \mathbf{w} \sim \mathcal{N}(0, \sigma_w^2 I), \qquad Y_j|\mathbf{X}, \mathbf{w} \sim \mathcal{N}(\mathbf{w}^\top \mathbf{X}, \sigma_y^2 I).$$

(1)

The complexity of the confounded model can be estimated by

$$L_{co}(\mathbf{X}, Y_j) = -\log \int P(\mathbf{X}, Y_j|\mathbf{Z}, \mathbf{W})P(\mathbf{Z})P(\mathbf{W})d\mathbf{W}d\mathbf{Z},$$
$$Z_i \sim \mathcal{N}(0, \sigma_z^2 I), \qquad W_i \sim \mathcal{N}(0, \sigma_w^2 I), \qquad \mathbf{X}|\mathbf{Z}, \mathbf{W} \sim \mathcal{N}(\mathbf{W}^\top \mathbf{Z}, \sigma_x^2 I),$$

(2)

where the confounders $\mathbf{Z}$ and the principal axes $\mathbf{W}$ are estimated using probabilistic PCA as in [12]. Note that we do not require that the confounders are known or measured; since we marginalize over $\mathbf{Z}$, we only need to specify its dimensionality k. To compare the causal $(\mathbf{X} \to Y_j)$ and the confounded model $(\mathbf{X} \leftarrow \mathbf{Z} \to Y_j)$, we just need to compute $\Delta(\mathbf{X}, Y_j) = L_{co}(\mathbf{X}, Y_j) - L_{ca}(\mathbf{X}, Y_j)$. If the causal model better describes the data than the confounded model, we obtain $\Delta(\mathbf{X}, Y_j) > 0$ – the more positive, the more confident we are. If instead $\Delta(\mathbf{X}, Y_j) < 0$, the roles are reversed. We estimate the complexity of both models with automatic differentiation variational inference [14], efficiently implemented in PyMC3, and use $k = 1$ as the dimensionality of $\mathbf{Z}$ throughout our experiments.

4.2   Results

Based on neurobiology, we use age, age^2, and sex as presumed causes $(\mathbf{X})$ of the volume of one brain structure (Y_j), where j denotes one of 22 brain structures. We estimate the complexity of the causal and confounded model across all brain structures and datasets, where we only select healthy subjects to facilitate comparison. Figure 3 (left) shows the mean difference between confounded and causal models (Δ) across volumes of all brain structures. Positive values indicate evidence for a predominantly causal relationship (age, sex) $\to$ volume, whereas negative values indicate a predominantly confounded relationship. The average relationship is most causal in HCP; or in other words, the estimated impact of confounders is low. This is not surprising, considering all MRI scans in HCP have been acquired on a single, dedicated scanner that was customized for this project. In contrast, COBRE, HBN, PPMI, MCIC, and AIBL have zero or negative mean difference. While we do not know the actual source of confounding, the result seems plausible, because these datasets comprise diverse scans from various sites

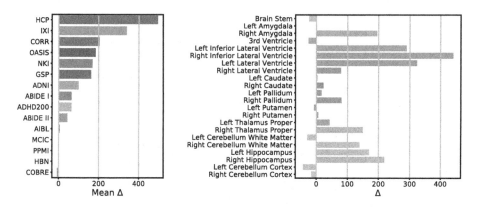

Fig. 3. Left: Mean difference Δ across brain structures for all datasets. Higher values indicate datasets where age and sex have a stronger causal effect on volume. Right: Differences Δ for all brain structures on the ADNI dataset.

and scanners (cf. Table 1), which likely constitute sources of confounding. Consequently, we are unable to reliably attribute the relationship between age, sex, and volume to either model in these datasets. We also note that these datasets have among the lowest accuracy in the classification experiment in Fig. 1. ABIDE I+II and ADHD200 pooled previously collected data from independent sites, yielding fairly heterogeneous datasets. Nevertheless, their estimated causal effect is weaker compared to ADNI, GSP, and IXI, which put more effort into standardizing imaging protocols. Harmonization across sites may strengthen the causal relationship in multi-site data.

In Fig. 3 (right), we focus on individual differences Δ for each brain structure in the ADNI dataset, due to its prominent role in the community. Our estimate is most causal for lateral and inferior lateral ventricles, which is consistent with the characteristic expansion of ventricular spaces in older ages. We observed the strongest confounding bias for cerebellum cortex, suggesting the association between age, sex and cerebellum cortex is more likely due to confounders.

5   Conclusion

We defined various forms of bias common to neuroimaging data. Based on a dataset with more than 12,000 individuals, we have demonstrated that simply pooling scans from distinct studies can introduce substantial bias that would be passed on to a machine learning model trained on the pooled data. Next, we introduced a novel approach for differentiating causal from confounded relationships based on causal inference. We estimated the strength of the neurobiological causal model – age and sex influence a brain structure's volume – versus the confounded model – age, sex, and volume are influenced by latent confounders – for 15 datasets and 22 brain structures. Results yielded large differences in the causal strength across datasets and brain structures. These results are specific to our assumptions for causal and confounding model, where other choices are possible and may yield different conclusions. Overall, we believe that the growing amount of neuroimaging data necessitates to quantify bias in datasets and image-derived features, for which we have proposed a causal model in this work. Finally, we note that our approach is not restricted to a biology-derived causal model, but could also be used to estimate the causal effect for other relationships, such as the effect of magnetic field strength on signal-to-noise ratio.

Acknowledgements. This research was partially supported by the Bavarian State Ministry of Science and the Arts in the framework of the Centre Digitisation.Bavaria (ZD.B).

References

1. Alexander, L.M., Escalera, J., et al.: An open resource for transdiagnostic research in pediatric mental health and learning disorders. bioRxiv, p. 149369 (2017)
2. Buckner, R., et al.: The brain genomics superstruct project. HDN (2012)
3. Di Martino, A., Yan, C., et al.: The autism brain imaging data exchange: towards a large-scale evaluation of the intrinsic brain architecture in autism. Mol. Psychiatry **19**(6), 659–667 (2014)
4. Dukart, J., Schroeter, M.L., Mueller, K.: Age correction in dementia-matching to a healthy brain. PLoS ONE **6**(7), e22193 (2011)
5. Ellis, K., Bush, A., Darby, D., et al.: The australian imaging, biomarkers and lifestyle (AIBL) study of aging. Int. Psychogeriatr. **21**(04), 672–687 (2009)
6. Fischl, B., Salat, D.H., et al.: Whole brain segmentation: automated labeling of neuroanatomical structures in the human brain. Neuron **33**(3), 341–355 (2002)
7. Fortin, J.P., Cullen, N., et al.: Harmonization of cortical thickness measurements across scanners and sites. Neuroimage **167**, 104–120 (2018)
8. Gollub, R.L., et al.: The MCIC collection: a shared repository of multi-modal, multi-site brain image data from a clinical investigation of schizophrenia. Neuroinformatics **11**(3), 367–388 (2013)
9. Guadalupe, T., Mathias, S.R., Theo, G., et al.: Human subcortical brain asymmetries in 15,847 people worldwide reveal effects of age and sex. Brain Imaging Behav. **11**(5), 1497–1514 (2017)
10. Han, X., Fischl, B.: Atlas renormalization for improved brain MR image segmentation across scanner platforms. IEEE TMI **26**(4), 479–486 (2007)
11. Jack, C.R., Bernstein, M.A., Fox, N.C., Thompson, P., et al.: The Alzheimer's disease neuroimaging initiative (ADNI): MRI methods. J. Magn. Reson. Imaging **27**(4), 685–691 (2008)
12. Kaltenpoth, D., Vreeken, J.: We are not your real parents: telling causal from confounded by MDL. In: SIAM International Conference on Data Mining (2019)
13. Kruggel, F., Turner, J., Muftuler, L.T.: Impact of scanner hardware and imaging protocol on image quality and compartment volume precision in the ADNI cohort. Neuroimage **49**(3), 2123–2133 (2010)
14. Kucukelbir, A., Tran, D., et al.: Automatic differentiation variational inference. J. Mach. Learn. Res. **18**(1), 430–474 (2017)
15. Linn, K.A., Gaonkar, B., Doshi, J., Davatzikos, C., Shinohara, R.T.: Addressing confounding in predictive models with an application to neuroimaging. Int. J. Biostatistics **12**(1), 31–44 (2016)

16. Marcus, D.S., Wang, T.H., Parker, J., Csernansky, J.G., Morris, J.C., Buckner, R.L.: Open access series of imaging studies (OASIS): cross-sectional mri data in young, middle aged, nondemented, and demented older adults. J. Cognitive Neurosci. **19**(9), 1498–1507 (2007)
17. Marek, K., et al.: The parkinson progression marker initiative (PPMI). Progress Neurobiol. **95**(4), 629–635 (2011)
18. Mayer, A., et al.: Functional imaging of the hemodynamic sensory gating response in schizophrenia. Hum. Brain Mapp. **34**(9), 2302–2312 (2013)
19. Milham, M.P., Fair, D., Mennes, M., Mostofsky, S.H., et al.: The ADHD-200 consortium: a model to advance the translational potential of neuroimaging in clinical neuroscience. Front. Syst. Neurosci. **6**, 62 (2012)
20. Nooner, K.B., et al.: The NKI-rockland sample: a model for accelerating the pace of discovery science in psychiatry. Front. Neurosci. **6**, 152 (2012)
21. Rao, A., Monteiro, J.M., Mourao-Miranda, J.: Predictive modelling using neuroimaging data in the presence of confounds. NeuroImage **150**, 23–49 (2017)
22. Smith, S.M., Nichols, T.E.: Statistical challenges in "big data" human neuroimaging. Neuron **97**(2), 263–268 (2018)
23. Torralba, A., Efros, A.A.: Unbiased look at dataset bias. In: Computer Vision and Pattern Recognition (CVPR), pp. 1521–1528 (2011)
24. Van Essen, D.C., et al.: The WU-Minn human connectome project: an overview. Neuroimage **80**, 62–79 (2013)
25. Wachinger, C., Reuter, M.: Domain adaptation for Alzheimer's disease diagnostics. Neuroimage **139**, 470–479 (2016)
26. Zuo, X.N., Anderson, J.S., Bellec, P., et al.: An open science resource for establishing reliability and reproducibility in functional connectomics. Sci. Data **1**, 140049 (2014)

Computer-Aided Diagnosis

Multi Scale Curriculum CNN for Context-Aware Breast MRI Malignancy Classification

Christoph Haarburger[1(✉)], Michael Baumgartner[1], Daniel Truhn[1,2],
Mirjam Broeckmann[2], Hannah Schneider[2], Simone Schrading[2],
Christiane Kuhl[2], and Dorit Merhof[1]

[1] Institute of Imaging and Computer Vision, RWTH Aachen University,
Aachen, Germany
christoph.haarburger@lfb.rwth-aachen.de
[2] Department of Diagnostic and Interventional Radiology,
University Hospital Aachen, Aachen, Germany

Abstract. Classification of malignancy for breast cancer and other cancer types is usually tackled as an object detection problem: Individual lesions are first localized and then classified with respect to malignancy. However, the drawback of this approach is that abstract features incorporating several lesions and areas that are not labelled as a lesion but contain global medically relevant information are thus disregarded: especially for dynamic contrast-enhanced breast MRI, criteria such as background parenchymal enhancement and location within the breast are important for diagnosis and cannot be captured by object detection approaches properly.

In this work, we propose a 3D CNN and a multi scale curriculum learning strategy to classify malignancy globally based on an MRI of the whole breast. Thus, the global context of the whole breast rather than individual lesions is taken into account. Our proposed approach does not rely on lesion segmentations, which renders the annotation of training data much more effective than in current object detection approaches.

Achieving an AUROC of 0.89, we compare the performance of our approach to Mask R-CNN and Retina U-Net as well as a radiologist. Our performance is on par with approaches that, in contrast to our method, rely on pixelwise segmentations of lesions.

Keywords: Breast cancer · Lesion detection · Lesion classification

1 Introduction

Detection of anatomical structures or lesions in medical images is mostly solved by object detection algorithms that rely on pixelwise segmentations of individual objects. However, there is not always a clear consensus among clinicians on which object is considered a suspicious lesion that should be segmented. Moreover, segmentations are subject to high inter-rater variability [19]. Both of these aspects

© Springer Nature Switzerland AG 2019
D. Shen et al. (Eds.): MICCAI 2019, LNCS 11767, pp. 495–503, 2019.
https://doi.org/10.1007/978-3-030-32251-9_54

limit the quality of training data and a reliable and meaningful evaluation. The degree of natural variation cannot be captured by interpreting tumors as objects with hard boundaries. The latter does make sense in classical computer vision, but for biomedical applications, a more holistic approach that takes the global *context* of a lesion into account is crucial. Another limitation of the detection and instance segmentation approach lies in the high cost associated with labeling large datasets. As a consequence, most datasets are rather small, preventing that deep learning algorithms unfold their full potential and limiting the power of evaluation results. Finally yet importantly, clinicians demand a decision support at patient-level rather than a classification of individual objects/regions of interest to efficiently integrate computer-aided diagnosis algorithms into clinical workflow.

Related Work. A naive approach to incorporating global context would be a classification of whole axial slices instead of detecting individual objects. However, this approach has produced poor results so far because it is a needle-in-haystack kind of problem [18]. Other works have adapted object detection algorithms such as Mask R-CNN [4] and RetinaNet [13] for lesion detection and classification [9]. In [8], diffusion-weighted breast magnetic resonance (MR) images are classified for malignancy by setting all voxels outside the lesion segmentation to zero. Lotter et al. [14] proposed a curriculum learning strategy for mammogram classification that concatenates features maps from patch level for a global breast malignancy classification. In a similar approach Koshravan et al. [10] propose a detection and malignancy classification algorithm for lung nodules by superimposing a grid on CT scans and by classifying each grid cell as benign or malignant. Maicas et al. [17] proposed a reinforcement learning approach for breast MRI lesion detection using bounding boxes. Several other authors have proposed methods for lesion classification based on bounding boxes [1,2,22]. In [16], a curriculum learning strategy is proposed and extended to classification of whole volumes in [15] showing promising results. Zhu et al. [23] propose a multiple instance learning loss for whole mammogram classification. In [21], a multi scale convolutional neural network (CNN) for detection of lesions in breast ultrasound images is proposed. Finally Jäger et al. [7] proposed Retina U-Net, which advances RetinaNet [13] by leveraging segmentation supervision for breast lesions. We introduce a CNN that is trained on several scales in a curriculum learning strategy, which is highly efficient for small datasets. Moreover, our 3D CNN does not rely on pixelwise segmentations or bounding boxes but rather lesion center points. This allows for efficient annotation and leverages the whole lesion context for classification at patient level.

Contributions. We introduce a simple 3D CNN for breast cancer malignancy classification that does not need to detect lesions individually and does not rely on pixelwise segmentations or bounding boxes. Moreover, we propose a multi scale curriculum learning strategy that efficiently trains the network on two scales, starting on patch scale and continuing training on the whole breast including all global context. We provide a comparison with other state of the art methods: Naive whole breast classification, Mask-R-CNN and Retina U-Net. Finally, in order to maximize reproducibility, comparisons and adaption, we provide all code[1] including implementations of network architectures, preprocessing and curriculum training in PyTorch and Delira [3].

2   Image Data

Our dataset consists of dynamic contrast-enhanced (DCE) MR images of 408 patients from clinical routine at our institution. Images were acquired on a 1.5 T Philips Scanner using a standardized protocol consisting of a T2-weighted turbo spin echo sequence and a T1-weighted gradient echo sequence acquired as a dynamic series [11]. DCE T1-weighted images were acquired before and every 70 s after injection of contrast agent (gadobutrol) for four post-contrast agent time points. The acquisition matrix was 512×512, yielding an in-plane resolution of 0.6×0.6 mm and slice thickness was 3 mm. In order to allow a comparison of our approach with approaches that rely on an auxiliary segmentation such as Mask R-CNN and Retina U-Net, all lesions were manually segmented on every slice by a radiologist with 13 years of experience in breast MRI.

Out of the 408 patients, 305 had malignant and 103 had benign findings. Malignancy was determined by biopsy; diagnoses of benign lesions were validated by follow up for 24 months. Since many of the malignant findings were only present in one breast, the overall ratio of malignant and benign samples at breast level (rather than patient level) in the whole dataset is 40.4%/59.6%. All images were resampled to $512 \times 512 \times 32$ voxels. No bias field correction was performed. Finally, we cropped all images by removing voxels that only contain air or tissue from the thorax, leading to images of a spatial resolution of $512 \times 256 \times 32$ voxels.

3   Methods

3.1   Multi Scale Curriculum Network

The network architecture we propose consists of two basic components as depicted in Fig. 1: (1) A Backbone network that consists of a 3D CNN to generate feature maps. (2) Classification head that performs a classification based on the aggregated feature maps provided by the two previous components. For the Backbone we initially evaluated many different architectures including ResNets [5] and DenseNets [6] of different depths, U-Net [20] and Feature Pyramid Network [12]. Since choice of the backbone architecture did not have a significant impact on the overall performance for the final model, we focus on ResNet18 in this work, because of its efficiency.

---

[1] https://github.com/haarburger/multi-scale-curriculum.

Multi Scale Curriculum Training. Training is conducted in two stages:

- Stage 1: Classification of 3D lesion *patches* with size $64 \times 64 \times 4$, where each patch contains at least one lesion as determined by the location of the lesion centerpoints. If at least one malignant lesion is contained in the patch, the patch label is set to malignant and benign otherwise.
- Stage 2: Classification of 3D volumes containing a whole breast with size $256 \times 256 \times 32$. To account for the changed input size, the network architecture is modified by introducing an additional adaptive average pooling layer between the original average pooling and fully-connected layer. All network parameters are trained during Stage 2.

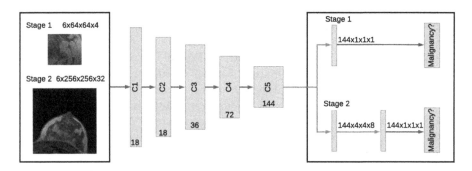

Fig. 1. Network architecture: residual blocks are named C_i as in [5] with channel dimensions indicated at the bottom of each block. Convolutions are indicated in blue, pooling operations in red. (Color figure online)

From all MRI scans, left and right breast were fed into the network separately. The five time points from the dynamic T1-weighted series and the T2-weighted series were fed into the CNN in the channel dimension, which leads to an input volume of $6 \times 256 \times 256 \times 32$ (channels, x, y, z). The network was trained with batch size 4, Adam optimizer with default parameters, instance normalization, leaky ReLU activation functions and a learning rate of 10^{-4} and 10^{-5} for Stages 1 and 2, respectively.

For data augmentation, we mirrored all images and rotated around the z axis by $\pm 15°$. Training, hyperparameter tuning and testing were performed in a 5-fold cross validation, using 261 patients (64%), 65 patients (16%) and 82 patients (20%) of the data for training, validation and testing, respectively. Since each single breast is fed into the network separately, splitting at patient level guarantees that both breasts of a single patient are exclusively contained in only one of the three data subsets.

3.2   Comparison Methods

Naive ResNet. In this approach, we naively train a vanilla 3D ResNet18 to directly predict malignancy globally without multi scale curriculum learning.

Since only a very small fraction of voxels belongs to a lesion, this approach is a needle-in-a-haystack kind of problem. It serves as a baseline for the multi scale curriculum learning approach.

Mask R-CNN. Mask R-CNN [4] is a widely used two-stage detection framework that leverages supervision information from a segmentation auxiliary task.

Retina U-Net. Based on the RetinaNet one stage detection framework [13], Retina U-Net combines RetinaNet with enhanced segmentation supervision using the U-Net architecture.

The Mask R-CNN and Retina U-Net approaches were trained as implemented in the medical detection toolkit [7]. We adjusted the patch size to $128 \times 128 \times 16$ and set the batch size to 2 in order to fit the images into the GPU memory. The learning rate was tuned using grid search to allow a fair comparison with our methods.

4 Results

On a Nvidia GeForce 2080 Ti GPU, training of Stage 1 and 2 takes about 4 and 6 h, respectively. Prediction of a single breast can be performed in under 100 ms.

In order to show the benefit of multi scale curriculum learning, we evaluated Mask R-CNN and Retina U-Net as described above as well as a naive 3D ResNet18 without curriculum training (Stage 2 only) and the proposed approach with multi scale curriculum learning. In addition, a radiologist with 2 years of experience in breast MRI rated the images with respect to malignancy. Test performance is provided in Table 1. The highest area under the receiver operating characteristic (AUROC) is achieved by the radiologist, followed by ResNet18 Curriculum and Retina U-Net. Mask R-CNN performs slighly worse. The naive 3D image classification approach achieved a very poor performance that is not significantly different from random guessing.

Table 1. Test performance of the comparison methods and proposed approach over a 5-fold cross validation.

	AUROC	Accuracy	#Parameters
Mask R-CNN [4]	0.88 ± 0.01	0.77 ± 0.03	3.91M
Retina U-Net [7]	0.89 ± 0.01	0.82 ± 0.02	3.90M
ResNet18 Naive	0.50 ± 0.04	0.45 ± 0.05	2.66M
ResNet18 Curriculum	0.89 ± 0.01	0.81 ± 0.02	2.66M
Radiologist	0.93	0.93	–

In Fig. 3, class activation maps for ResNet18 Curriculum are shown. Regions with high activations for malignancy are marked in red, in order to provide clinicians with enhanced guidance by our algorithm.

5   Discussion

Our proposed multi scale curriculum training enabled successful training of the relatively simple 3D ResNet18 from an AUROC of 0.5 to 0.89. In other experiments that are out of the scope of this work, we found that the particular choice of the backbone architecture had negligible effect on the performance. On our dataset, the performance of our approach is on par with Retina U-Net [7] and even exceeds the performance of Mask R-CNN [4]. Since we did not tune our models extensively with respect to ensembling, the performance in comparison with the reported results in [7] seem reasonable to us. We hypothesize that the high performance of our model at least partly arises from the high amount of context and global information that is provided. Both Retina U-Net and Mask R-CNN incorporate more model parameters and hyperparameters such as the IoU threshold. Most importantly, these approaches rely on pixelwise segmentations for all individual lesions. Our approach on the other hand only needs a coarse localization (i.e. coordinate) for Stage 1 training and only one global label per breast for Stage 2. Since in most clinical sites performing breast MRI, a global BIRADS classification per breast is assessed and provided along with the image data, global labels are relatively cheap to generate. This would allow a Stage 2 training with much more training data and more thorough evaluation with much more test data in the future. Curriculum learning on a series of tasks as proposed in [16] achieved very similar performance on a breast MRI dataset. Our approach has some similarities with [14]: Stage 1 training is very similar, yet

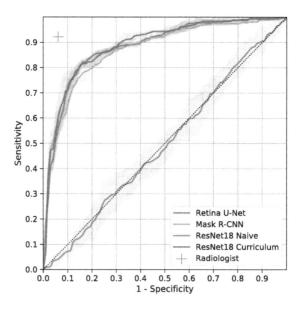

Fig. 2. Receiver operating characteristic. Means and standard deviations over the 5-fold cross validation are encoded as lines and contiguous areas, respectively.

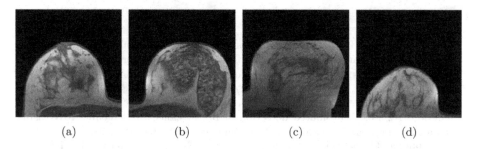

(a)   (b)   (c)   (d)

Fig. 3. Class activation maps for (a): Malignant case that was correctly classified by our algorithm and the radiologist. (b): Benign case that was classified correctly by the CNN and incorrectly by the radiologist. (c): Malignant case that was classified incorrectly by both CNN and radiologist. (d): Malignant case that was classified incorrectly by the CNN and correctly by the radiologist. Images have been masked. (Color figure online)

performed in 3D in our case. In Stage 2, Lotter et al. [14] concatenate and pool feature vectors of individual (2D) regions while we perform direct predictions of whole images in 3D (Fig. 1).

Our work has several limitations: Firstly, our dataset is monocentric and even though to our best knowledge it is the largest breast MRI dataset for computer aided diagnosis, it is limited in size. However, extension is relatively easy since only global labels are required for Stage 2 training and assessment of test performance. For Stage 1 a coarse localization that has to be marked manually is still required. In comparison to the diagnostic performance of a breast radiologist, our model is inferior to human performance.

For future work, we will expand the size of our Stage 2 dataset. Since breast MRI experts are rare, it would be interesting to assess whether our algorithm (including the activation maps) can be applied to teach radiologists with limited experience. Moreover, it would be interesting to assess whether a combination of an expert rater with our algorithm could further improve the overall performance.

6   Conclusion

We presented a simple 3D CNN architecture that is able to perform breast cancer malignancy classification based on magnetic resonance images using a multi scale curriculum learning strategy. The network architecture predicts malignant breast cancer globally for a whole 3D volume *without* scoring individual lesions. This approach provides the whole spatial context of a breast to the network, yielding state of the art performance and without the need for lesion segmentations.

Acknowledgements. The authors thank Paul Jäger for making Medical Detection Toolkit [7] publicly available, which was a great help when comparing our method with Mask R-CNN and Retina U-Net.

References

1. Amit, G., et al.: Hybrid mass detection in breast MRI combining unsupervised saliency analysis and deep learning. In: Descoteaux, M., Maier-Hein, L., Franz, A., Jannin, P., Collins, D.L., Duchesne, S. (eds.) MICCAI 2017. LNCS, vol. 10435, pp. 594–602. Springer, Cham (2017). https://doi.org/10.1007/978-3-319-66179-7_68
2. Dalmış, M.U., Vreemann, S., Kooi, T., Mann, R.M., Karssemeijer, N., Gubern-Mérida, A.: Fully automated detection of breast cancer in screening MRI using convolutional neural networks. J. Med. Imaging 5(01), 014502 (2018)
3. Haarburger, C., Schock, J., Baumgartner, M., Rippel, O., Merhof, D.: Delira: a high-level framework for deep learning in medical image analysis. J. Open Source Softw. 4, 1488 (2019). https://doi.org/10.21105/joss.01488
4. He, K., Gkioxari, G., Dollár, P., Girshick, R.: Mask R-CNN. In: ICCV, pp. 2961–2969 (2017)
5. He, K., Zhang, X., Ren, S., Sun, J.: Deep residual learning for image recognition. In: (CVPR) (2016)
6. Huang, G., Liu, Z., Weinberger, K.Q., van der Maaten, L.: Densely connected convolutional networks. In: CVPR, pp. 4700–4708 (2017)
7. Jaeger, P.F., et al.: Retina U-Net: embarrassingly simple exploitation of segmentation supervision for medical object detection (2018). http://arxiv.org/abs/1811.08661
8. Jäger, P.F., et al.: Revealing hidden potentials of the q-space signal in breast cancer. In: Descoteaux, M., Maier-Hein, L., Franz, A., Jannin, P., Collins, D.L., Duchesne, S. (eds.) MICCAI 2017. LNCS, vol. 10433, pp. 664–671. Springer, Cham (2017). https://doi.org/10.1007/978-3-319-66182-7_76
9. Jung, H., et al.: Detection of masses in mammograms using a one-stage object detector based on a deep convolutional neural network. PLoS ONE 13(9), 1–16 (2018)
10. Khosravan, N., Bagci, U.: S4ND: single-shot single-scale lung nodule detection. In: Frangi, A.F., Schnabel, J.A., Davatzikos, C., Alberola-López, C., Fichtinger, G. (eds.) MICCAI 2018. LNCS, vol. 11071, pp. 794–802. Springer, Cham (2018). https://doi.org/10.1007/978-3-030-00934-2_88
11. Kuhl, C.K.: The current status of breast MR imaging part I. Choice of technique, image interpretation, diagnostic accuracy, and transfer to clinical practice. Radiology 244(2), 356–378 (2007)
12. Lin, T.Y., Dollár, P., Girshick, R., He, K., Hariharan, B., Belongie, S.: Feature pyramid networks for object detection. In: CVPR, pp. 2117–2125 (2017)
13. Lin, T.Y., Goyal, P., Girshick, R., He, K., Dollár, P.: Focal loss for dense object detection. In: ICCV, pp. 2980–2988 (2017)
14. Lotter, W., Sorensen, G., Cox, D.: A multi-scale CNN and curriculum learning strategy for mammogram classification. In: Cardoso, M.J., et al. (eds.) DLMIA/ML-CDS -2017. LNCS, vol. 10553, pp. 169–177. Springer, Cham (2017). https://doi.org/10.1007/978-3-319-67558-9_20
15. Maicas, G., Bradley, A.P., Nascimento, J.C., Reid, I., Carneiro, G.: Pre and post-hoc diagnosis and interpretation of malignancy from breast DCE-MRI (2018). http://arxiv.org/abs/1809.09404
16. Maicas, G., Bradley, A.P., Nascimento, J.C., Reid, I., Carneiro, G.: Training medical image analysis systems like radiologists. In: Frangi, A.F., Schnabel, J.A., Davatzikos, C., Alberola-López, C., Fichtinger, G. (eds.) MICCAI 2018. LNCS, vol. 11070, pp. 546–554. Springer, Cham (2018). https://doi.org/10.1007/978-3-030-00928-1_62

17. Maicas, G., Carneiro, G., Bradley, A.P., Nascimento, J.C., Reid, I.: Deep reinforcement learning for active breast lesion detection from DCE-MRI. In: Descoteaux,
M., Maier-Hein, L., Franz, A., Jannin, P., Collins, D.L., Duchesne, S. (eds.) MIC-
CAI 2017. LNCS, vol. 10435, pp. 665–673. Springer, Cham (2017). https://doi.
org/10.1007/978-3-319-66179-7_76
18. Maier-Hein, K. http://on-demand.gputechconf.com/gtc-eu/2018/video/e8481/.
Accessed 06 Mar 2019
19. Menze, B.H., Jakab, A., et al.: The multimodal brain tumor image segmentation
benchmark (BRATS). IEEE TMI **34**(10), 1993–2024 (2015)
20. Ronneberger, O., Fischer, P., Brox, T.: U-Net: convolutional networks for biomedical image segmentation. In: Navab, N., Hornegger, J., Wells, W.M., Frangi, A.F.
(eds.) MICCAI 2015. LNCS, vol. 9351, pp. 234–241. Springer, Cham (2015).
https://doi.org/10.1007/978-3-319-24574-4_28
21. Wang, N., et al.: Densely deep supervised networks with threshold loss for cancer detection in automated breast ultrasound. In: Frangi, A.F., Schnabel, J.A.,
Davatzikos, C., Alberola-López, C., Fichtinger, G. (eds.) MICCAI 2018. LNCS,
vol. 11073, pp. 641–648. Springer, Cham (2018). https://doi.org/10.1007/978-3-
030-00937-3_73
22. Yan, K., Bagheri, M., Summers, R.M.: 3D context enhanced region-based convolutional neural network for end-to-end lesion detection. In: Frangi, A.F., Schnabel, J.A., Davatzikos, C., Alberola-López, C., Fichtinger, G. (eds.) MICCAI 2018.
LNCS, vol. 11070, pp. 511–519. Springer, Cham (2018). https://doi.org/10.1007/
978-3-030-00928-1_58
23. Zhu, W., Lou, Q., Vang, Y.S., Xie, X.: Deep multi-instance networks with sparse
label assignment for whole mammogram classification. In: Descoteaux, M., Maier-
Hein, L., Franz, A., Jannin, P., Collins, D.L., Duchesne, S. (eds.) MICCAI 2017.
LNCS, vol. 10435, pp. 603–611. Springer, Cham (2017). https://doi.org/10.1007/
978-3-319-66179-7_69

Deep Angular Embedding and Feature Correlation Attention for Breast MRI Cancer Analysis

Luyang Luo[1], Hao Chen[2(✉)], Xi Wang[1], Qi Dou[3], Huangjing Lin[1],
Juan Zhou[4], Gongjie Li[5], and Pheng-Ann Heng[1]

[1] Department of Computer Science and Engineering,
The Chinese University of Hong Kong, Hong Kong, China
lyluo@cse.cuhk.edu.hk
[2] Imsight Medical Technology, Co., Ltd., Shenzhen, China
hchen@cse.cuhk.edu.hk
[3] Department of Computing, Imperial College London, London, UK
[4] Department of Radiology, The Fifth Medical Center of Chinese PLA General
Hospital, Beijing, China
[5] Beijing Image Diagnostic Center of Rimag, Beijing, China

Abstract. Accurate and automatic analysis of breast MRI plays a vital role in early diagnosis and successful treatment planning for breast cancer. Due to the heterogeneity nature, precise diagnosis of tumors remains a challenging task. In this paper, we propose to identify breast tumor in MRI by Cosine Margin Sigmoid Loss (CMSL) with deep learning (DL) and localize possible cancer lesion by COrrelation Attention Map (COAM) based on the learned features. The CMSL embeds tumor features onto a hyper-sphere and imposes a decision margin through cosine constraints. In this way, the DL model could learn more separable inter-class features and more compact intra-class features in the angular space. Furthermore, we utilize the correlations among feature vectors to generate attention maps that could accurately localize cancer candidates with only image-level labels. We build the largest breast cancer dataset involving 10,290 DCE-MRI scan volumes for developing and evaluating the proposed methods. The model driven by CMSL achieved a classification accuracy of 0.855 and AUC of 0.902 on the testing set, with sensitivity and specificity of 0.857 and 0.852, respectively, outperforming competitive methods overall. In addition, the proposed COAM accomplished more accurate localization of the cancer center compared with other state-of-the-art weakly supervised localization method.

1 Introduction

Breast cancer is the most common malignancy affecting women worldwide [1]. Early diagnosis of breast cancer is essential for successful treatment planning, where Magnetic Resonance Imaging (MRI) plays a vital role in screening high-risk populations [2]. Clinically, radiologists use the Breast Imaging-Reporting

© Springer Nature Switzerland AG 2019
D. Shen et al. (Eds.): MICCAI 2019, LNCS 11767, pp. 504–512, 2019.
https://doi.org/10.1007/978-3-030-32251-9_55

and Data System (BI-RADS) to categorize breast lesions into various levels according to their phenotypic characteristics presented in MRI images, indicating different degrees of cancer risk. However, such assessment suffers from inter-observer variance and often subjectively relies on the radiologists' experience. Moreover, due to the heterogeneity nature, tumors of the same pathological result (malignant or benign) could have diverse patterns and hence result in different BI-RADS assessments. In other words, tumors could possess ambiguous inter-class difference and large intra-class variance, which poses a severe challenge to accurate diagnosis of breast cancer.

Generally, there are two major tasks regarding breast MRI tumor analysis: identification of tumors and localization of cancer candidates. Recently, Deep Learning (DL) based approaches have demonstrated great potential in assisting the diagnosis of breast cancer in an automatic and efficient manner. Previous studies manually annotated tumors and deliberately extracted the corresponding slices or patches for classification [3,4]. Such methods depended on careful anno-tations both for training and testing and could not easily be adapted to clinical application. Meanwhile, Guy et al. [5] proposed to first automatically localize the lesions and then classify cancer candidates at the second stage. Although the inference stage thereby was free of lesion delineation, it still required anno-tations for model training. To get rid of manual lesion extraction, Gabriel et al. [6] proposed to meta-train a breast MRI cancer classifier with only image-level labels. However, all the mentioned studies were limited to small size datasets and consequently lack of generalization validation. More importantly, the relatively low precision or specificity reported in these works implied that the problem of inter-class difference and intra-class variance has not been addressed yet.

To this end, we propose a Cosine-Margin Sigmoid Loss (CMSL) to tackle the heterogeneity problem for breast tumor classification and COrrelation Attention Map (COAM) for precise cancer candidates localization, both with image-level labels only. The CMSL is extended from the cosine loss originally designed for face verification [7]. It embeds the deep feature vectors onto a hyper-sphere and learns a decision margin between classes in the angular feature space. As a result, the learned features possess more compact intra-class variance and more separable intra-class difference. In addition, we observe a Region of Interest (RoI) shifting problem of localizing cancer by class activation map [8]. Hence, we propose a novel weakly supervised method, i.e., COAM, to localize cancer candidates more accurately by leveraging deep feature correlations based on the Gram matrix. Furthermore, we build the largest breast DCE-MRI dataset, including 10,290 volume scans from 1715 subjects to develop and evaluate our methods.

2 Methods

Our framework of breast MRI tumor analysis consists of two parts, as illustrated in Fig. 1. One is tumor classification by deep-angular-embedding-driven DL net-work. The other is weakly supervised cancer candidates localization with feature correlation attention map.

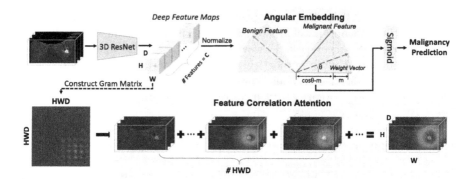

Fig. 1. The framework of breast MRI cancer analysis. A 3D ResNet is first trained with CMSL by embedding the deep features onto hyper-sphere. In the testing stage, the deep features are used to construct the Gram matrix to obtain correlation attention map. Best viewed in color. (Color figure online)

2.1 Cosine Margin Sigmoid Loss for Tumor Classification

The phenotype of tumors has ambiguous inter-class difference and large intra-class variance. Accordingly, the features learned by the DL model could inherit these characteristics. To address this issue, we start by revisiting the traditional sigmoid loss for the binary classification problem. Given the input feature vector x of the last fully connected (FC) layer and its corresponding label y, the binary sigmoid loss is as follows:

$$\mathcal{L}(w; x) = -y \cdot \log(p(y \mid x)) - (1 - y) \cdot \log(1 - p(y \mid x)) \tag{1}$$

$$= -y \cdot \log(\frac{1}{1 + e^{-w^T x}}) - (1 - y) \cdot \log(1 - \frac{1}{1 + e^{-w^T x}}) \tag{2}$$

where w is the weight parameter of the FC layer, and $p(y \mid x)$ represents the probability of x being classified to y. To distinguish different classes, the DL model is expected to give different predictions by adjusting the value of $w^T x$. Notice that $w^T x = \|w\|\|x\|cos\theta$, where θ is the angle between feature vector x and weight vector w, and $\|\cdot\|$ is the L_2 norm operation. Generally, the DL model would implicitly alter $\|w\|$ and $\|x\|$ in the Euclidean space and $cos\theta$ in the angular space. However, the aforementioned heterogeneity issue could lead to ambiguous features that are quite hard to discriminate. To this end, constraints on feature distances are considered to regulate the DL model for more separable inter-class features and more compact intra-class features [7]. Since Euclidean distance is not bounded and hence difficult to constrain, we prefer to add regularization on the angular distance which is bounded by $-1 \leq cos\theta \leq 1$. Specifically, we eliminate the influence of the norms $\|x\|$ and $\|w\|$ by modifying the computation of $p(y \mid x)$ to:

$$p(y \mid x) = \frac{1}{1 + e^{-s\frac{w^T x}{\|w\|\|x\|}}} = \frac{1}{1 + e^{-s \cdot cos\theta}} \tag{3}$$

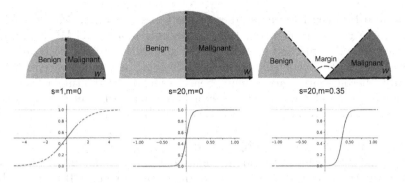

Fig. 2. The illustration of NSL with $s = 1$, NSL with $s = 20$ and CMSL with $s = 20$ and $m = 0.35$. The first row is the geometric interpretation of feature projection on a 2D sphere. Dashed arrows represent the decision boundaries. The second row is the plot of corresponding sigmoid functions. Dashed curves represent the values out of range.

where s is a hyper-parameter adjusting the slope of the sigmoid function and controlling the back propagated gradient values. If s is too small, the loss cannot converge to 0 because the sigmoid function is not able to reach its saturation area, given that $-1 \leq cos\theta \leq 1$. On the contrast, if s is set to a large value, the sigmoid function could easily reach the saturation area and result in small gradients, which prevents the network from learning sufficient knowledge. Following [7], we refer to the loss with modified p in Eq. (3) as Normalized Sigmoid Loss (NSL), which focuses on separating features in the angular space with the decision boundary $cos\theta = 0$ for both classes. Geometrically, we embed the feature vector and the weight vector onto a hyper-sphere whose radius is tuned by s. However, the ambiguous features can still distribute near this boundary. Therefore we add explicit guidance to NSL as follows:

$$\mathcal{L}(w; x) = -y \cdot \log(\frac{1}{1 + e^{-s \cdot (cos\theta - I(y) \cdot m)}}) - (1 - y) \cdot \log(1 - \frac{1}{1 + e^{-s \cdot (cos\theta - I(y) \cdot m)}})$$
(4)

where $I(\cdot)$ is an indicator function. $I(y) = 1$ if $y = 1$ and $I(y) = -1$ otherwise. m is a hyper-parameter that changes the decision boundaries for separating two classes (0 and 1 for benign and malignant) to: $B_0 : cos\theta + m < 0$ and $B_1 : cos\theta - m > 0$. Hence a decision margin is imposed by m in the angular space to make the learned inter-class features more separable. Consequently, the distribution space of features shrinks, which eventually leads to more compact intra-class features. Figure 2 shows a comparison among different sigmoid functions and the corresponding geometric illustrations.

2.2 Feature Correlation Attention for Cancer Localization

With highly informative deep features learned by the network, localization of cancer candidates can provide further clinical references. To this end, our secondary goal is to localize possible cancer out of other lesion mimics. Generally, it is natural for deep learning studies to use Class Activation Map (CAM) [8] for obtaining region of interests (RoIs) when only image-level labels are available. However, this method cannot be well generalized to our case due to an observed RoI shifting problem. With the CNN going deeper, the reception fields of neurons become larger accordingly, hence neighbors of the tumor feature are also able to capture views over the tumor patch. Since the deep features could still be ambiguous, the classifier layer would possibly tend to find discriminative patterns in the neighbors. As a consequence, the corresponding RoI generated by CAM would shift from the originally desired target.

To tackle this problem, we further figure out two insights of our task. First, the feature vectors of the same semantic (malignant or normal) ought to have higher correlations with each other than with those of different semantic. Second, through a series of rectified linear units, the network would implicitly learn larger activation values for features related to suspicious cancer patch (with the label "1") and smaller activation values for features related to normal patch (with the label "0"). Based on these two intuitions, we propose to leverage the Gram matrix [9] to find out the RoI. Given the deep feature map $X \in \mathbb{R}^{H \times W \times S \times C}$ generated from the last activation layer, where H, W, S and C are the height, width, number of slices and number of channels, respectively, we first reshape X to $X' \in \mathbb{R}^{N \times C}$, where $N = H \times W \times S$. Afterwards, we compute an attention vector $M \in \mathbb{R}^N$ as follows:

$$M_i = \sum_{j=1}^{N} G_{i,j} = \sum_{j=1}^{N} \sum_{k=1}^{C} X'_{i,k} X'_{j,k} \tag{5}$$

where $G \in \mathbb{R}^{N \times N}$ is the Gram matrix over the set of deep feature vectors in X'. Each entry $G_{i,j}$ is the inner product of X'_i and X'_j, representing the correlation between i-th and j-th vector. Then the columns of the Gram matrix are summed over to form the attention vector M. Because our network is trained for binary classification, it enables the gap between large and small activation values of feature vector related to suspicious cancer and normal patches. Correspondingly, the correlation value would also be relatively large or small according to the activation values of the features. Inspired by [10], each column G_i of the Gram matrix can be interpreted as a sub-attention map implying the network's attention of the class that i-th vector belongs to. Thus, Eq. (5) is actually an element-wise summation over all sub-attention maps. Moreover, since G is symmetric, the operation is also the same as summing over G_i to be the value of M_i. Essentially, $\sum_{j=1}^{N} G_{i,j}$ indicates the *importance* of i-th feature determined by the sub-attention of the feature map at its i-th position. Finally, we simply reshape M to size $H \times W \times S$ to obtain an attention map purely based on the feature correlations. We refer to this method as COrrelation Attention Map (COAM). It is worth mentioning that COAM is related to the self-attention mechanism [10] and the stationary feature space representation [9]. However, our work is characterized that the Gram matrix is not involved in any optimization stage and is directly used for attention generation.

3   Experiments and Results

3.1   Implementation Details

Dataset. We built the largest breast tumor Dynamic Contrast Enhanced (DCE) MRI dataset involving 10,290 scans from 1715 subjects, with 1137 cases containing malignant tumors and 578 cases containing benign tumors. All of the scans were conducted with a 1.5-T Siemens system. We collected 6 DCE-MRI subtraction scans and 1 non-fat suppressed T1 scan from each subject. BI-RADS categories were assessed by 3 radiologists. Pathological labels were given by biopsy or surgery diagnosis. The data were randomly divided into training, validation, and testing sets with 1204, 165, and 346 subjects, respectively.

Preprocessing. Frangi's approach [11] was first applied on the slices of each non-fat suppressed T1 scan to detect evident edges. Next, thresholding, small connected component removal, and hole filling were employed to obtain coarse breast region masks. The 2D masks were then stacked into volumes and smoothed by Gaussian smooth. The 3D masks were used to segment the DCE-MRI scans. Note the two modalities were already registered in the scanning machine. Finally, we clipped and normalized the intensity values, concatenated six subtractions, and fixed the image size to $340 \times 220 \times 128$ by cropping or padding.

Training Strategy. We used 3D ResNet34 [12] as the base model and replaced the global average pooling layer and FC layer with a $1 \times 1 \times 1$ convolutional layer appended by a pooling layer. The hyper-parameter s and m were set to 20 and 0.35, respectively, similar to [7]. The learning rate was initially set to 10^{-4} and decreased ten times when the training error stagnated. The base model is trained until convergence and then employed to initialize all other methods.

3.2   Evaluation and Comparison

Tumor Classification. We conducted comparison among several deep learning methods: (1)*2D MIL*: a multi-instance method aggregating features from 2D slices by 2D ResNet34 [13]; (2)*3D ResNet*: a 3D implementation of ResNet34; (3)*3D Sparse MIL*: a sparse label assign method [14]; (4)*3D DK-MT*: a domain knowledge driven multi-task learning network [15]; (5)*3D ResNet+NSL*: Normalized sigmoid loss based on (2); (6)*3D ResNet+CMSL*: our proposed CMSL based on (2). We computed the accuracy, specificity, sensitivity, F1 score, and AUC as the evaluation metrics. Experimental results are reported in Table 1.

Compared with 2D methods, 3D models achieved better results by utilizing information from one more dimension. Both *3D Sparse MIL* and *3D DK-MT* adopted additional knowledge, leading to better performance than vanilla *3D ResNet*. Noticeably, *3D DK-MT* showed a poor specificity, which may be due to imbalanced auxiliary knowledge (more BI-RADS 4 and 5 than 3) dominating the learning process. For *3D ResNet+NSL* based on deep angular embedding, simply

Table 1. Comparison of different methods on cancer classification.

Method	Accuracy	Sensitivity	Specificity	F1	AUC
2D MIL [13]	0.789	0.870	0.626	0.846	0.842
3D ResNet [12]	0.821	0.840	0.783	0.862	0.880
3D Sparse MIL [14]	0.832	0.857	0.783	0.872	0.885
3D DK-MT [15]	0.824	**0.896**	0.643	0.864	0.883
3D ResNet+NSL	0.821	0.840	0.783	0.862	0.874
3D ResNet+CMSL (ours)	**0.855**	0.857	**0.852**	**0.888**	**0.902**

taking the features into angular space without the margin constraint caused certain performance decay. It indicated that the network could not learn sufficient knowledge if s is too large. Moreover, our proposed *3D ResNet+CMSL* significantly improved the results with imposed cosine margin forcing the network to learn more underlying discriminative patterns. Our method achieved the highest specificity, with over 7.9% better than all other methods and kept a competitive sensitivity in the meantime. It exceeded other methods with over 2% in AUC, over 3% in accuracy and over 1.5% in F1 score, proving that addressing the inter- and intra-class problem can improve performance of breast tumor classification.

Cancer Localization. We invited the radiologists to annotate 85 samples that were classified as malignant by our model. COAM and CAM were obtained and resized by interpolation to be the same size as original inputs. We then compared these two methods by computing the Euclidean distance between the center point of the annotation and the voxel position with the highest value in the attention maps. Then the distance is multiplied by the voxel spacing, i.e., 1.1 mm, as the final measurement. The criterion is reported in the form

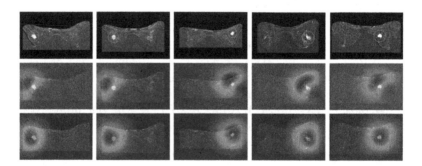

Fig. 3. Comparison between CAM and COAM with typical slices from different subjects. First row: DCE-MRI subtraction slice; second row: visualization of CAM; third row: visualization of COAM. Cancer lesions are circled in red. Best viewed in color. (Color figure online)

of *mean* ± *std*, where *mean* and *stdv* represent the mean value and standard deviation of the center distances over 85 samples, respectively. Compared to the distance of 39.84 ± 8.82 mm by CAM, COAM showed a significant advantage with 18.26 ± 13.65 mm. Figure 3 showed a qualitative comparison with the two methods.

4   Conclusion

In this paper, we propose the cosine margin sigmoid loss for breast tumor classification and correlation attention map for weakly supervised cancer candidates localization based on MRI scans. First, we use CMSL-driven deep network to learn more separable inter-class features and more compact intra-class features which effectively tackle the heterogeneity problem of tumors. In addition, the proposed COAM leverages correlations among deep features to localize ROIs in a weakly supervised manner. Extensive experiments on our large-scale dataset demonstrate the efficacy of our methods, which outperform other state-of-the-art approaches significantly on both tasks. Our methods are general and can be extended to many other fields. Our future work would involve more cases without lesion when training the classification task to suppress false positives in the localization stage.

Acknowledgement. This work was supported by Research Grants Council of Hong Kong Special Administrative Region under Project No. CUHK14225616 and Hong Kong Innovation and Technology Fund under Project No. ITS/426/17FP.

References

1. DeSantis, C.E., et al.: Breast cancer statistics, racial disparity in mortality by state. CA Cancer J. Clin. **67**(6), 439–448 (2017)
2. Kuhl, C., et al.: Prospective multicenter cohort study to refine management recommendations for women at elevated familial risk of breast cancer: the EVA trial. J. Clin. Oncol. **28**(9), 1450–1457 (2010)
3. Zheng, H., Gu, Y., Qin, Y., Huang, X., Yang, J., Yang, G.-Z.: Small lesion classification in dynamic contrast enhancement MRI for breast cancer early detection. In: Frangi, A.F., Schnabel, J.A., Davatzikos, C., Alberola-López, C., Fichtinger, G. (eds.) MICCAI 2018. LNCS, vol. 11071, pp. 876–884. Springer, Cham (2018). https://doi.org/10.1007/978-3-030-00934-2_97
4. Amit, G., et al.: Classification of breast MRI lesions using small-size training sets: comparison of deep learning approaches. In: Medical Imaging 2017: Computer-Aided Diagnosis, vol. 10134. International Society for Optics and Photonics (2017)
5. Amit, G., et al.: Hybrid mass detection in breast MRI combining unsupervised saliency analysis and deep learning. In: Descoteaux, M., Maier-Hein, L., Franz, A., Jannin, P., Collins, D.L., Duchesne, S. (eds.) MICCAI 2017. LNCS, vol. 10435, pp. 594–602. Springer, Cham (2017). https://doi.org/10.1007/978-3-319-66179-7_68

6. Maicas, G., Bradley, A.P., Nascimento, J.C., Reid, I., Carneiro, G.: Training medical image analysis systems like radiologists. In: Frangi, A.F., Schnabel, J.A., Davatzikos, C., Alberola-López, C., Fichtinger, G. (eds.) MICCAI 2018. LNCS, vol. 11070, pp. 546–554. Springer, Cham (2018). https://doi.org/10.1007/978-3-030-00928-1_62

7. Wang, H., et al.: CosFace: large margin cosine loss for deep face recognition. In: Proceedings of the IEEE Conference on Computer Vision and Pattern Recognition (2018)

8. Zhou, B., et al.: Learning deep features for discriminative localization. In: Proceedings of the IEEE Conference on Computer Vision and Pattern Recognition (2016)

9. Gatys, L., Ecker, A.S., Bethge, M.: Texture synthesis using convolutional neural networks. In: Advances in Neural Information Processing Systems, pp. 262–270 (2015)

10. Fu, J., et al.: Dual attention network for scene segmentation. arXiv preprint arXiv:1809.02983 (2018)

11. Frangi, A.F., Niessen, W.J., Vincken, K.L., Viergever, M.A.: Multiscale vessel enhancement filtering. In: Wells, W.M., Colchester, A., Delp, S. (eds.) MICCAI 1998. LNCS, vol. 1496, pp. 130–137. Springer, Heidelberg (1998). https://doi.org/10.1007/BFb0056195

12. He, K., et al.: Deep residual learning for image recognition. In: Proceedings of the IEEE Conference on Computer Vision and Pattern Recognition, pp. 770–778 (2016)

13. Wu, J., et al.: Deep multiple instance learning for image classification and auto-annotation. In: Proceedings of the IEEE Conference on Computer Vision and Pattern Recognition (2015)

14. Zhu, W., Lou, Q., Vang, Y.S., Xie, X.: Deep multi-instance networks with sparse label assignment for whole mammogram classification. In: Descoteaux, M., Maier-Hein, L., Franz, A., Jannin, P., Collins, D.L., Duchesne, S. (eds.) MICCAI 2017. LNCS, vol. 10435, pp. 603–611. Springer, Cham (2017). https://doi.org/10.1007/978-3-319-66179-7_69

15. Liu, J., et al.: Integrate domain knowledge in training CNN for ultrasonography breast cancer diagnosis. In: Frangi, A.F., Schnabel, J.A., Davatzikos, C., Alberola-López, C., Fichtinger, G. (eds.) MICCAI 2018. LNCS, vol. 11071, pp. 868–875. Springer, Cham (2018). https://doi.org/10.1007/978-3-030-00934-2_96

Fully Deep Learning for Slit-Lamp Photo Based Nuclear Cataract Grading

Chaoxi Xu[1,2,3], Xiangjia Zhu[4], Wenwen He[4], Yi Lu[4], Xixi He[3],
Zongjiang Shang[5], Jun Wu[5], Keke Zhang[4], Yinglei Zhang[4], Xianfang Rong[4],
Zhennan Zhao[4], Lei Cai[4], Dayong Ding[3], and Xirong Li[1,2,3(✉)]

[1] MOE Key Lab of DEKE, Renmin University of China, Beijing, China
`xirong@ruc.edu.cn`
[2] AI & Media Computing Lab, School of Information,
Renmin University of China, Beijing, China
[3] Vistel AI Lab, Visionary Intelligence Ltd., Beijing, China
[4] Eye and ENT Hospital of Fudan University, Shanghai, China
[5] School of Electronics and Information, Northwestern Polytechnical University,
Xi'an, China

Abstract. Age-related cataract is a priority eye disease, with nuclear cataract as its most common type. This paper aims for automated nuclear cataract grading based on slit-lamp photos. Different from previous efforts which rely on traditional feature extraction and grade modeling techniques, we propose in this paper a fully deep learning based solution. Given a slit-lamp photo, we localize its nuclear region by Faster R-CNN, followed by a ResNet-101 based grading model. In order to alleviate the issue of imbalanced data, a simple batch balancing strategy is introduced for improving the training of the grading network. Tested on a clinical dataset of 157 slit-lamp photos from 39 female and 31 male patients, the proposed solution outperforms the state-of-the-art, reducing the mean absolute error from 0.357 to 0.313. In addition, our solution processes a slit-lamp photo in approximately 0.1 s, which is two order faster than the state-of-the-art. With its effectiveness and efficiency, the new solution is promising for automated nuclear cataract grading.

Keywords: Nuclear cataract grading · Slit-lamp photos · Deep learning

1 Introduction

This paper studies automated *nuclear cataract grading* based on slit-lamp photos. A cataract is clouding of the lens in the eye. As the lens is to focus light rays onto the retina, such clouding leads to decrease in vision including blurry vision, faded colors halos around light, trouble seeing at night, *etc.* The most common factor of cataract is ageing [13]. Age-related cataract is reported to be

---

C. Xu, X. Zhu, W. He, Y. Lu—Equal contributions.

© Springer Nature Switzerland AG 2019
D. Shen et al. (Eds.): MICCAI 2019, LNCS 11767, pp. 513–521, 2019.
https://doi.org/10.1007/978-3-030-32251-9_56

responsible for over 50% of world blindness, and thus considered as a priority eye disease by the World Health Organization[1]. Nuclear cataract, which involves the central or *nuclear* area of the lens, is the most common type of age-related cataracts [1].

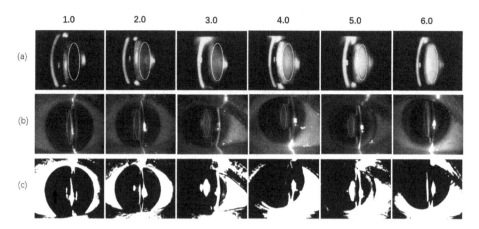

Fig. 1. **Slit-lamp photos showing nuclear cataract of six scales**, with scale 1.0 as the mildest and scale 6.0 as the severest. (a) Reference photos specified by the LOCS III [3], with the nuclear area in each photo marked out by a white ellipse. (b) Slit-lamp photos collected from a clinical scenario, with their nuclear areas (white ellipses) labeled by ophthalmologists. (c) Intensity-based binarization on (b), required by previous works [5,7,10,15] as a prerequisite step to localize a region of interest. Note that the white of the eye and specular highlights in the background make this step ineffective. By contrast, we train Faster R-CNN [12], a state-of-the-art object detection network, to directly localize the nuclear zone, see the yellow bounding boxes with dotted borders in (b). Best viewed in digital format. (Color figure online)

In clinical practice, nuclear cataract is diagnosed by an eye examination, where an ophthalmologist uses a slit-lamp to obtain a magnified view of the eye structures including the nuclear area in detail. Based on the opacification of the nuclear area, the cataract is further graded on a scale from 1.0 to 6.0. In particular, given a slit-lamp photo, a grade is manually estimated by comparing the photo against exemplars provided by the lens opacities classification system LOCS III [3], see Fig. 1(a). Apparently, the manual grading process not only requires well-trained eyes and is also time-consuming.

While automating the grading process is much in demand, challenges exist. The first challenge is how to reliably localize the nuclear region in a relatively complex background. Slit-lamp photos collected from a clinical scenario contain the eyelids, the sclera and the cornea with spectral highlights, as exemplified in Fig. 1(b). Previous works [5,7,10,15] share an initial step, where a region of

---

[1] https://www.who.int/blindness/causes/priority/en/index1.html.

interest (ROI) is roughly localized by thresholding 20% to 30% of the brightest pixels in a gray-scale photo. However, such an intensity-based binarization cannot cope with the background noise, as Fig. 1(c) shows. One might argue the necessity of nuclear region localization. Indeed, we notice an early study by Fan *et al.* [4] where the whole image is used. Considering that the nuclear region contributes less than 3% of the pixels in a slit-lamp photo, grading based on the whole image is suboptimal.

Table 1. An overview of recent methods for nuclear catatract grading. Different from the previous works, our method is based on fully deep learning.

Method	Region detection	ROI	ROI representation	Grading
Li *et al.* [10]	Intensity-based binarlization + active shape model [9]	Lens	21-d intensity and color feature	SVM regression
Huang *et al.* [7]		Lens	6-d intensity and color feature	Nearest neighbor
Xu *et al.* [15]		Central part of lens	12,600-d bag-of-quantized color moment feature	Group sparsity regression
Gao *et al.* [5]		Central part of lens	32,768-d CRNN feature	SVM regression
This paper	Faster R-CNN	Nuclear region	ResNet-101	

Given the ROI successfully localized, the second challenge is how to derive a vectorized representation of the ROI, upon which a grading (or regression) model will be built. Due to variance in slit-lamp photography including the lighting condition, the skill of the technician, and the eye condition of the subject, both intra-grade divergence and inter-grade similarity exists in the photometric appearance of the nuclear area. Good features are thus needed. Earlier works rely on handcrafted features. To describe the intensity and color statistics in the lens, Li *et al.* [10] extract a 21-dim feature, while a shorter 6-dim feature is used in Huang *et al.* [7]. Xu *et al.* [15] represent the central part of the lens by a 12,600-dim bag-of-quantized color moment feature. The latest work by Gao *et al.* [5] employ convolutional-recursive neural networks (CRNN) [14] to extract a 32,768-dim deep feature. The authors then train an RBF-kernel SVM regression model for nuclear cataract grading. In all the above works (Table 1), feature extraction and the grading are separated and thus cannot be optimized jointly.

For answering the two challenges in nuclear cataract grading, this paper makes the following contributions:

1. We propose a fully deep learning based solution, which is the first work of its kind. In particular, we localize the nuclear region by Faster R-CNN [12]. With the nuclear region as input, a ResNet-101 [6] based grading model is trained. In contrast to the previous works, the use of ResNet-101 allows us to naturally

achieve feature extraction and grading in a unified framework. Hence, the proposed solution is not only more effective and also computationally more efficient.

2. Tested on a clinical dataset of 157 slit-lamp photos from 39 female and 31 male patients, our solution outperforms the state-of-the-art [5], reducing the mean absolute error (MAE) from 0.357 to 0.313.

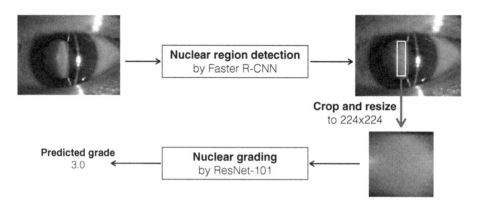

Fig. 2. An illustration of the proposed fully deep learning based solution for slit-lamp based nuclear cataract grading.

2 Proposed Solution

Given a slit-lamp photo from a specific patient having nuclear cataract, our goal is to automatically grade the severity level of the cataract in terms of the photometric appearance of the nuclear area. We propose a two-step solution. As shown in Fig. 2, the nuclear region is localized by Faster R-CNN, a state-of-the-art CNN for object detection. The second step is grading, where the detected region is fed to a grading model with ResNet-101, a state-of-the-art CNN for image classification, as its backbone. We use x to indicate a given photo, x_{nuc} for the sub-image corresponding to the nuclear area, and $y \in [1.0, 6.0]$ as the predicted grade. Accordingly, the above solution is expressed as follows,

$$\begin{cases} x_{nuc} \leftarrow \text{Faster R-CNN}(x), \\ \quad y \leftarrow \text{ResNet-101}(x_{nuc}). \end{cases} \tag{1}$$

2.1 Nuclear Region Localization by Faster R-CNN

Faster R-CNN by Ren *et al.* [12] consists of two subnetworks, *i.e.*, a region proposal network (RPN) followed by a detection network. The RPN proposes a number of bounding boxes that have the highest probability of containing ROIs. The detection network is responsible for discriminating foreground from background and refining the predicted location and size of the ROIs. Since a slit-lamp photo has one nuclear region, we select the top-ranked ROI as x_{nuc}.

To train Faster R-CNN for nuclear region localization, we adopt an SGD [2] optimizer with its default hyper-parameters setup except for the learning rate which is empirically set to 0.001. The mini-batch size is set to 4. The iteration is set to 100K batches and the learning rate is decayed by 0.1 at the 60K and the 80K batch. We set three anchor scales, i.e., 3, 8 and 16 and two aspect ratios, i.e., 1:1 and 1:4. The input image is sized to 500×500. Nuclear regions are well localized, with an IoU of 0.763 on average.

Note that Faster R-CNN cannot be directly used to grade a detected nuclear region. We therefore develop a grading model as follows.

2.2 ResNet-101 Based Grading

According to the LOCS III [3], the estimated grade y shall have a precision of one decimal place. In other words, the value of y can be 1.3, 2.8, 5.3 etc. Therefore, we formulate the grading task as a regression problem. We depart from ResNet-101 pretrained on ImageNet [6], which requires an input size of 224×224. So we resize x_{nuc} accordingly. We substitute a regression layer for the original classification layer. We use the mean square error (MSE), a common loss function for regression. We minimize the MSE loss by the Adam [8] optimizer with its default hyper-parameters setup except for the learning rate, which is initially set to 0.0001, and decayed by 0.1 every 30 epochs. An early stop occurs if the performance on a validation set does not increase in 15 consecutive epochs. We perform data augmentation on the detected regions, changing brightness, saturation and contrast by a factor uniformly sampled from $[0, 2]$ respectively. The three operations are executed in a randomized order.

Batch Balancing. The grades, ranging from 1.0 to 6.0, are not uniformly distributed. In our experimental data, the amount of photos graded between 3.0 and 4.0 is the largest. When constructing a mini-batch at random, the grading model will learn from unbalanced instances and thus become biased. To alleviate the issue, we introduce a simple batch balancing strategy. In particular, we quantize the grades into five groups, i.e., $[1, 2)$, $[2, 3)$, $[3, 4)$, $[4, 5)$ and $[5, 6]$. When constructing a mini-batch, we randomly select the same amount of instances, which is 25, from each group, making the batch fully balanced.

3 Experiments

3.1 Experimental Setup

Dataset. As we have noted, there is no public dataset available for training and evaluating models for nuclear cataract grading. Our experiment data, provided by our hospital partner, consists of 847 slit-lamp photos from 214 female and 141 male patients with nuclear cataract. As shown in the second row of Fig. 1, these photos have complex background showing pupil, sclera, eyelid *etc.* , which are irrelevant with respect to the task and thus noisy. The photos have been graded collectively by six experienced ophthalmologists based on the LOCS III criteria [3]. Besides, the experts mark out the nuclear area in each photo.

We make a patient-based data partition, dividing randomly the dataset into three disjoint subsets, *i.e.,* training, validation and test, at a ratio of 7:1:2. A profile of the three subsets is shown in Table 2.

Performance Metrics. Nuclear cataract grading is essentially a regression problem, so we report the mean absolute error (MAE), a common regression error metric. As an absolute error smaller than 0.5 is considered acceptable in the clinical practice, we report Accuracy, defined as the percentage of test photos that meet this criterion.

Table 2. Profile of slit-lamp photos used in this work. In order to avoid over-fitting, a specific patient is exclusively assigned to the training, validation or test sets, so images from the same patient appear only in one dataset. For the purpose of approximately showing the grade distribution, we quantize the grades into five groups.

Dataset	Patients	Ages	Photos	Photos per group				
				$[1,2)$	$[2,3)$	$[3,4)$	$[4,5)$	$[5,6]$
Training	155 females + 94 males	17–95	587	73	152	209	108	45
Validation	20 females + 16 males	50–94	103	13	22	41	20	7
Test	39 females + 31 males	39–87	157	24	22	67	37	7

Table 3. Evaluating the choice of input and the influence of batch balancing for the grading model. Lower MAE and higher Accuracy are better.

Input	Batch balancing	MAE	Accuracy(%)
Whole image	✗	0.482	67.5
	✓	0.362	79.6
Nuclear region	✗	0.357	81.5
	✓	**0.313**	**84.7**

Table 4. Group-based evaluation. Lower MAE is better.

Input	Batch balancing	MAE per group				
		$[1,2)$	$[2,3)$	$[3,4)$	$[4,5)$	$[5,6]$
Whole image	✗	**0.325**	0.459	0.476	0.422	1.457
	✓	0.513	0.423	0.279	**0.186**	1.386
Nuclear region	✗	0.654	0.423	**0.260**	0.305	**0.343**
	✓	0.454	**0.309**	0.313	0.197	0.443

3.2   Experiment 1. Ablation Study

Choice of the Input for Grading. As Table 3 shows, using the detected nuclear region as input outperforms the whole image. Class activation maps are shown at Fig. 3, where red colors indicate highly activated regions. For the grading model with the whole image as input, the nuclear region is activated, suggesting that the model can indeed focus on the correct region. However, the relatively small ROI makes the model less effective. These results justify the necessity of nuclear region localization.

The Influence of Batch Balancing. As Tables 3 and 4 show, batch balancing is beneficial, regardless of the input.

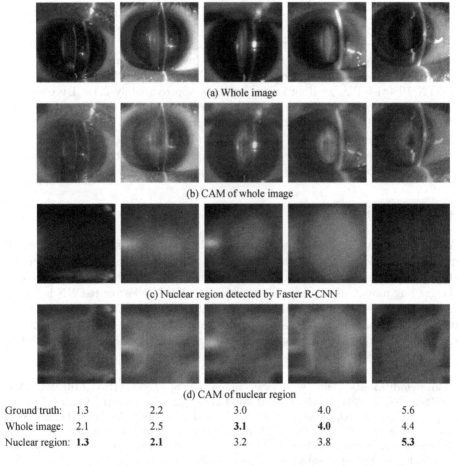

(a) Whole image

(b) CAM of whole image

(c) Nuclear region detected by Faster R-CNN

(d) CAM of nuclear region

Ground truth:	1.3	2.2	3.0	4.0	5.6
Whole image:	2.1	2.5	**3.1**	**4.0**	4.4
Nuclear region:	**1.3**	**2.1**	3.2	3.8	**5.3**

Fig. 3. Visualizing the discriminative locations of an input image for nuclear cataract grading by class activation mapping (CAM) [16]. Each column indicates a specific test image. The second row and the last row are CAMs obtained when using the whole image and the detected nuclear as the input to the grading model, respectively. Red regions show high activations. Decimals in **bold font** means they are more close to the ground truth. (Color figure online)

3.3   Experiment 2. Comparison with the State-of-the-Art

We compare with Gao *et al.* [5], the current state-of-the-art. As aforementioned, their ROI detection method mostly fails on the new dataset. So for a more fair comparison, our implementation of [5] uses the ROI found by Faster R-CNN as a candidate region and crops it as specified in [5].

Table 5. Comparison with SOTA. Lower MAE and higher Accuracy are better.

Method	MAE	Accuracy (%)
Gao *et al.* [5]	0.357	82.2
This paper	**0.313**	**84.7**

As Table 5 shows, the proposed method surpasses Gao *et al.* [5] in terms of both MAE and Accuracy. Moreover, our method is computationally more efficient. On a normal computer with a 3.6 GHz six-core CPU, 64 GB RAM and a GTX 1080ti GPU, grading an image costs approximately 0.1 s. By contrast, the grading process of [5] takes 17 s per image, tested on a PC with a four-core 2.4 GHz CPU and 24 GB RAM. While our machine is more powerful, the efficiency is largely due to the fully deep learning property of our method.

The proposed method is general and can, in principle, be applied to recognizing other types of cataracts, *e.g.,* pediatric cataract [11].

4   Conclusions

A fully deep learning based solution for slit-lamp photo based nuclear cataract grading is developed. A test set of 157 slit-lamp photos from 70 patients verifies the effectiveness of the proposed solution. Concerning the choice of the input of the grading model, using the nuclear region localized by Faster R-CNN is better than using the whole image, with the mean absolute error (MAE) from 0.482 to 0.357. The proposed batch balancing strategy is also helpful, with MAE reduced to 0.313. Consequently, the new solution surpasses the state-of-the-art which has MAE of 0.357.

Acknowledgments. This work was supported by NSFC (No. 61672523, No. 81870642, No. 81670835), the Fundamental Research Funds for the Central Universities and the Research Funds of Renmin University of China (No. 18XNLG19), Special Research Project of Intelligent Medicine, Shanghai Municipal Health Commission (2018ZHYL0220), National Key R&D Program of China (No. 2018YFC0116800) and CSC State Scholarship Fund (201806295014).

References

1. Asbell, P.A., Dualan, I., Mindel, J., Brocks, D., Ahmad, M., Epstein, S.: Age-related cataract. Lancet **365**(9459), 599–609 (2005)
2. Bottou, L.: Large-scale machine learning with stochastic gradient descent. In: Lechevallier, Y., Saporta, G. (eds.) COMPSTAT 2010, pp. 177–186. Springer, Heidelberg (2010). https://doi.org/10.1007/978-3-7908-2604-3_16
3. Chylack, L.T., et al.: The lens opacities classification system III. Arch. Ophthalmol. **111**(6), 831–836 (1993)
4. Fan, S., Dyer, C.R., Hubbard, L., Klein, B.: An automatic system for classification of nuclear sclerosis from slit-lamp photographs. In: Ellis, R.E., Peters, T.M. (eds.) MICCAI 2003. LNCS, vol. 2878, pp. 592–601. Springer, Heidelberg (2003). https://doi.org/10.1007/978-3-540-39899-8_73
5. Gao, X., Lin, S., Wong, T.Y.: Automatic feature learning to grade nuclear cataracts based on deep learning. IEEE Trans. Biomed. Eng. **62**(11), 2693–2701 (2015)
6. He, K., Zhang, X., Ren, S., Sun, J.: Deep residual learning for image recognition. In: CVPR (2016)
7. Huang, W., Chan, K.L., Li, H., Lim, J.H., Liu, J., Wong, T.Y.: A computer assisted method for nuclear cataract grading from slit-lamp images using ranking. IEEE Trans. Med. Imaging **30**(1), 94–107 (2011)
8. Kingma, D.P., Ba, J.: Adam: a method for stochastic optimization (2014)
9. Li, H., Chutatape, O.: Boundary detection of optic disk by a modified ASM method. Pattern Recogn. **36**(9), 2093–2104 (2003)
10. Li, H., et al.: A computer-aided diagnosis system of nuclear cataract. IEEE Trans. Biomed. Eng. **57**(7), 1690–1698 (2010)
11. Liu, X., et al.: Localization and diagnosis framework for pediatric cataracts based on slit-lamp images using deep features of a convolutional neural network. PLoS ONE **12**(3), e0168606 (2017)
12. Ren, S., He, K., Girshick, R., Sun, J.: Faster R-CNN: towards real-time object detection with region proposal networks. In: NIPS (2015)
13. Robman, L., Taylor, H.: External factors in the development of cataract. Eye **19**(10), 1074 (2005)
14. Socher, R., Huval, B., Bath, B., Manning, C.D., Ng, A.Y.: Convolutional-recursive deep learning for 3D object classification. In: NIPS (2012)
15. Xu, Y., et al.: Automatic grading of nuclear cataracts from slit-lamp lens images using group sparsity regression. In: Mori, K., Sakuma, I., Sato, Y., Barillot, C., Navab, N. (eds.) MICCAI 2013. LNCS, vol. 8150, pp. 468–475. Springer, Heidelberg (2013). https://doi.org/10.1007/978-3-642-40763-5_58
16. Zhou, B., Khosla, A., Lapedriza, A., Oliva, A., Torralba, A.: Learning deep features for discriminative localization. In: CVPR (2016)

Overcoming Data Limitation in Medical Visual Question Answering

Binh D. Nguyen[1], Thanh-Toan Do[2(✉)], Binh X. Nguyen[1], Tuong Do[1],
Erman Tjiputra[1], and Quang D. Tran[1]

[1] AIOZ Pte Ltd., Singapore, Singapore
{binh.duc.nguyen,binh.xuan.nguyen,tuong.khanh-long.do,erman.tjiputra,
quang.tran}@aioz.io
[2] University of Liverpool, Liverpool, UK
thanh-toan.do@liverpool.ac.uk

Abstract. Traditional approaches for Visual Question Answering (VQA) require large amount of labeled data for training. Unfortunately, such large scale data is usually not available for medical domain. In this paper, we propose a novel medical VQA framework that overcomes the labeled data limitation. The proposed framework explores the use of the unsupervised Denoising Auto-Encoder (DAE) and the supervised Meta-Learning. The advantage of DAE is to leverage the large amount of unlabeled images while the advantage of Meta-Learning is to learn meta-weights that quickly adapt to VQA problem with limited labeled data. By leveraging the advantages of these techniques, it allows the proposed framework to be efficiently trained using a small labeled training set. The experimental results show that our proposed method significantly outperforms the state-of-the-art medical VQA. The source code is available at https://github.com/aioz-ai/MICCAI19-MedVQA.

Keywords: Visual Question Answering · Auto-Encoder · Meta-Learning

1 Introduction

Visual Question Answering (VQA) aims to provide a correct answer to a given question such that the answer is consistent with the visual content of a given image. In medical domain, VQA could benefit both doctors and patients. For example, doctors could use answers provided by VQA system as support materials in decision making, while patients could ask VQA questions related to their medical images for better understanding their health. However, one major problem with medical VQA is the lack of large scale labeled training data which usually requires huge efforts to build. The first attempt for building the dataset for medical VQA is by ImageCLEF-Med [6]. In particular in [6], images were automatically captured from PubMed Central articles. The questions and answers were automatically generated from corresponding captions of images. By that

© Springer Nature Switzerland AG 2019
D. Shen et al. (Eds.): MICCAI 2019, LNCS 11767, pp. 522–530, 2019.
https://doi.org/10.1007/978-3-030-32251-9_57

construction, the data has high noisy level, i.e., the dataset includes many images that are not useful for direct patient care and it also contains questions that do not make any sense. Recently, in [10], the authors released the first manually constructed dataset VQA-RAD for medical VQA. Unfortunately, it contains only 315 images, which prevents to directly apply the powerful deep learning models for the VQA problem. One may think about the use of transfer learning in which the pretrained deep learning models [7,18] that are trained on the large scale labeled dataset such as ImageNet [16] are used for finetuning on the medical VQA. However, due to difference in visual concepts between ImageNet images and medical images, finetuning with very few medical images is not sufficient, which is confirmed by our experiments in Sect. 4. Therefore it is necessary to develop a new VQA framework that can improve the accuracy while still only needs a small labeled training data.

The motivation for our approach to overcome the data limitation of medical VQA comes from two observations. Firstly, we observe that there are large scale unlabeled medical images available. These images are from same domain with medical VQA images. Hence if we train an unsupervised deep learning model using these unlabeled images, the trained weights may be easier to be adapted to the medical VQA problem than the pretrained weights on ImageNet images. Another observation is that although the labeled dataset VQA-RAD in [10] is primarily designed for VQA, by spending a little effort, we can extract the new class labels[1] for that dataset. The new class labels allow us to apply the recent meta-learning technique [4] for learning meta-weights, that can be quickly adapted to the VQA problem later.

From these two observations, we propose a novel medical VQA framework as presented in Fig. 1, in which the Model-Agnostic Meta-Learning (MAML) [4] and the Convolutional Denoising Auto-Encoder (CDAE) [12] are used to initialize the model weights for the image feature extraction.

2   Literature Review

Medical Visual Question Answering. Most approaches for medical VQA [1, 10,13,20] are to directly apply the state-of-the-art general VQA models to medical domain. The 2018 ImageCLEF-Med challenge [6] provides a good overview about the approaches and their results. Typically, in [1,13,20], the authors use the state-of-the-art attention mechanisms in general VQA (e.g., MCB [5], SAN [19]) to learn a join representation between an image and a question. Note that in the mentioned approaches, the models pretrained on ImageNet such as VGG [18] or ResNet [7] are directly finetuned on medical VQA images for image feature extraction. However, directly finetuning those models on medical VQA images is not effective due to the limited medical VQA data.

Meta-Learning. Traditional machine learning algorithms, especially deep learning based approaches, require large scale labeled training set when learning

---

[1] The descriptions of new defined classes are presented in Sect. 4.1.

Algorithm 1. Overview of the meta-training procedure

1: **procedure** META-TRAIN($\mathcal{D}$, model f_θ)
2:     Initialize model parameters θ
3:     **for** $h = 1$ *to* H **do**   ▷ Meta-update Loop
4:         **Create** meta-batch of tasks $\{\mathcal{T}_1, \mathcal{T}_2, ..., \mathcal{T}_m\}$
5:         **for** each task $\mathcal{T}_i$ **do**
6:             Sample data $\{\mathcal{D}_i^{tr}, \mathcal{D}_i^{val}\}$ of task $\mathcal{T}_i$
7:             Update task models with Eq. (1) using samples from $\mathcal{D}_i^{tr}$
8:         **Update** meta-model θ with Eq. (2) using $\{\mathcal{D}_1^{val}, \mathcal{D}_2^{val}, ..., \mathcal{D}_m^{val}\}$

---

a new task, even when the model is pretrained on other classification problems [2,11]. Contrasting with traditional machine learning algorithms, meta-learning approach [17] targets to deal with the problem of data limitation when learning new tasks. Recently, in [4] the authors proposed a new approach for meta-learning, i.e., Model-Agnostic Meta-Learning (MAML), which helps to learn a meta-model (e.g. network weights) from current tasks that is broadly suitable for many tasks. Hence, the model can be quickly adapted to new tasks that have a small number of training images.

Denoising Auto-Encoder. In medical domain, the lack of labeled data makes training process become inefficiency. Thus, unlabeled data, which is easy to achieve, is encouraged to use for training. Auto-Encoder [12,15], which helps to extract high-level features without any label information, is a typical solution to take the advantage of unlabeled data. Besides, medical images such as MRI, CT, X-ray may contain various degree of noises, which might happen during transmission and acquisition [8]. Hence, it requires a feature extraction model that is robust to noise, i.e., it can still extract useful information from the noisy input image. In this work, to leverage the benefit of large scale unlabeled datasets and also to make the model robust to the noise in input images, we propose to use the Convolutional Denoising Auto-Encoder (CDAE) [12] as one of image feature extraction components in our framework.

3 Methodology

The proposed medical VQA framework is presented in Fig. 1. In our framework, the image feature extraction component is initialized by pretrained weights from MAML and CDAE. After that, the VQA framework will be finetuned in an end-to-end manner on the medical VQA data. In the following sections, we detail the architectures of MAML, CDAE, and our framework.

3.1 Model-Agnostic Meta-Learning – MAML

The MAML classification model is represented by a parametrized function f_θ with meta-parameters θ. When adapting to a new task $\mathcal{T}_i$, the model's parameters θ become θ_i'. Let $\mathcal{D} = \{x_i, y_i\}_{i=1}^N$ be the dataset for training MAML. N is the number of samples. $\{x_i, y_i\}$ is a pair of image (x_i) and its class label (y_i). A task in MAML is defined as a "**k**-shot **n**-way" classification problem. The dataset for each task is defined as $\mathcal{D}' = \{x'_i, y'_i\}_{i=1}^{N'}$; samples in $\mathcal{D}'$ come from n different classes which are a subset of classes in $\mathcal{D}$. The task dataset $\mathcal{D}'$ is split equally into two sets $\mathcal{D}^{tr}$ – training set and $\mathcal{D}^{val}$ – validation set; in $\mathcal{D}^{tr}$, each class contains k training images. The training procedure is described in the Algorithm 1. In each iteration h, m tasks are generated forming a meta-batch for MAML training. For each task $\mathcal{T}_i$, the corresponding adapted parameters θ'_i are calculated as follows

$$\theta'_i = \theta - \alpha \nabla_\theta L_{\mathcal{T}_i}(f_\theta(\mathcal{D}_i^{tr})) \tag{1}$$

where $L_{\mathcal{T}_i}$ is the classification loss of task i. After all adapted parameters of m tasks are calculated, the meta-model's parameters θ are updated via *stochastic gradient descent* (SGD) as follows

$$\theta \leftarrow \theta - \beta \nabla_\theta \sum_{\mathcal{T}_i} L_{\mathcal{T}_i}(f_{\theta'_i}(\mathcal{D}_i^{val})) \tag{2}$$

We follow [4] to design MAML. It consists of four 3×3 convolutional layers with stride 2 and is ended with a mean pooling layer; each convolutional layer has 64 filters and is followed by a ReLu layer. The detail training of MAML is presented in Sect. 4.2. After training, the weights of the meta-model are used for finetuning in the VQA framework as presented in Fig. 1.

3.2 Convolutional Denoising Auto-Encoder – CDAE

The encoder maps an image x', which is the noisy version of the original image x, to a latent representation z which retains useful amount of information. The decoder transforms z to the output y. The training algorithm aims to minimize the reconstruction error between y and the original image x as follows

$$L_{rec} = \|x - y\|_2^2 \tag{3}$$

In our design, the encoder is a stack of convolutional layers; each of them is followed by a max pooling layer. The decoder is a stack of deconvolutional and convolutional layers. The noisy version x' is achieved by adding Gaussian noise to the original image x. The detail training of CDAE is presented in Sect. 4.2. After training, the trained weights of both encoder and decoder are used for finetuning in the VQA framework as presented in Fig. 1.

3.3 The Proposed Medical VQA Framework

VQA Detail. Each input question is trimmed to a 12-word sentence. The question is zero-padded in case its length is less than 12. Each word is represented by a 600-D vector which is a concatenation of the 300-D GloVe word embedding [14] and the augmenting embedding from the VQA-RAD training data [9].

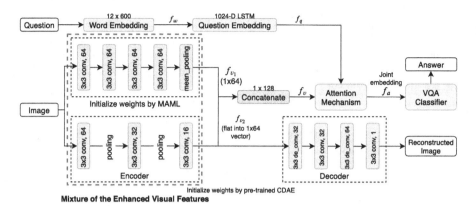

Fig. 1. The proposed medical VQA. The image feature extraction is denoted as "Mixture of Enhanced Visual Features (MEVF)" and is marked with the red dashed box. The weights of MEVF are intialized by MAML and CDAE. Best view in color (Color figure online.

The word embedding is fed into a 1024-D LSTM in order to produce the question embedding, denoted as f_q in Fig. 1. Each input image is passed through the Mixture of Enhanced Visual Features (MEVF) component, which produces two 64-D vectors f_{v1} and f_{v2}. Those vectors are concatenated to form an 128-D enhanced image feature, denoted as f_v in Fig. 1.

Image feature f_v and question embedding f_q are fed into an attention mechanism (BAN [9] or SAN [19]) to produce a joint representation f_a. This feature f_a is used as input for a multi-class classifier (over the set of predefined answer classes [10]). To train the proposed model, we introduce a multi-task loss function to incorporate the effectiveness of the CDAE to VQA. Formally, our loss function is defined as follows

$$L = \alpha_1 L_{vqa} + \alpha_2 L_{rec} \tag{4}$$

where L_{vqa} is a Cross Entropy loss for VQA classification and L_{rec} stands for the reconstruction loss of CDAE (Eq. 3). The whole VQA model is finetuned in an end-to-end manner using VQA-RAD dataset as presented in Sect. 4.2.

4   Experiments

4.1   Dataset

The VQA-RAD [10] dataset contains 315 images and 3,515 corresponding questions. Each image is associated with more than one question. The questions are divided into 11 categories which are "Abnormality", "Attribute", "Color", "Count", "Modality", "Organ", "Other", "Plane", "Positional reasoning", "Object/Condition Presence", "Size". We use exactly the same training set and test set described in [10]. The test set contains 451 questions and the rest is for training. The questions can be close-ended questions, i.e. the questions in which the answers are "yes/no" and other limited choices, or open-ended questions, i.e., the questions do not have a limited structure and could have multiple correct answers. The dataset has 458 answers. The VQA is posed as a classification over the set of answers.

4.2   Training MAML, CDAE, and the Whole VQA Framework

MAML. We create the dataset for training MAML by *manually reviewing* around three thousand question-answer pairs from the training set of VQA-RAD dataset. In our annotation process, images are split into three parts based on its *body part* labels (head, chest, abdomen). Images from each body part are further divided into three subcategories based on the interpretation from the question-answer pairs corresponding to the images. These subcategories are: (1) *normal* images in which no pathology is found; (2) *abnormal present* images in which there are the existence of fluid, air, mass, or tumor; (3) *abnormal organ* images in which the organs are large in size or in wrong position. Thus, all the images are categorized into 9 classes: *head normal, head abnormal present, head abnormal organ, chest normal, chest abnormal organ, chest abnormal present, abdominal normal, abdominal abnormal organ, and abdominal abnormal present.* For every iteration of MAML training (line 3 in Algorithm 1), 5 tasks are sampled per iteration. For each task, we randomly select 3 classes (from 9 classes). For each class, we randomly select 6 images in which 3 images are used for updating task models and the remaining 3 images are used for updating meta-model.

CDAE. To train CDAE, we collect $11,779$ unlabeled images available online which are brain MRI images [3], chest X-ray images[2] and CT abdominal images[3]. The dataset is split into train set with $9,423$ images and test set with $2,356$ images. We use Gaussian noise to corrupt the input images before feeding them to the encoder.

VQA. After training MAML and CDAE, we use their trained weights to initialize the MEVF image feature extraction component in the VQA framework. We then finetune the whole VQA model using the training set of VQA-RAD dataset. In order to make a fair comparison to [10], we evaluate our framework on 300 free-form questions of the test set. The proposed framework is implemented using PyTorch. The experiments are conducted on a single NVIDIA 1080Ti with 11 GB RAM. The VQA accuracy is computed as the percentage of the total correct answers over the number of testing questions.

4.3   Ablation Study

We evaluate the effectiveness of different image feature extraction methods in the VQA model when using only MAML, using only CDAE, and their combination

---

[2] https://www.kaggle.com/paultimothymooney/chest-xray-pneumonia.
[3] https://www.synapse.org/#!Synapse:syn3193805/wiki/217753.

MEVF. For each extraction method, we present results when training the VQA model using only VQA-RAD training set (i.e. *from scratch*) or when pretraining as described in Sect. 4.2 and then finetuning using VQA-RAD training set (i.e. *finetuning*). We also present the results when the pretrained VGG model (on ImageNet) is finetuned on VQA-RAD for image feature extraction.

Table 1 presents VQA accuracy in both VQA-RAD open-ended and close-ended questions on the test set. The results show that for both MAML and CDAE, by firstly pretraining as described in Sect. 4.2, then finetuning, the fine-tuning significantly improves the performance over the training from scratch using only VQA-RAD. In addition, the results also show that our pretraining and finetuning of MAML and CDAE give better performance than the finetuning of VGG-16 which is pretrained on the ImageNet dataset. Our proposed image feature extraction MEVF which leverages both pretrained weights of MAML and CDAE, then finetuning them give the best performance. This confirms the effectiveness of the proposed MEVF for dealing with the limitation of labeled training data for medical VQA.

Table 1. VQA results on VQA-RAD test set. All reference methods differ at the image feature extraction component. Other components are similar. The Stacked Attention Network (SAN) [19] is used as the attention mechanism in all methods.

Reference methods	VQA accuracy (%)	
	Open-ended	Close-ended
VGG-16 (finetuning) [10]	24.2	57.2
MAML (from scratch)	6.5	68.6
MAML (finetuning)	**38.2**	**69.7**
CDAE (from scratch)	13.8	69.2
CDAE (finetuning)	**36.7**	**70.8**
MEVF (from scratch)	15.4	70.8
MEVF (finetuning)	**40.7**	**74.1**

Table 2. Performance comparison on VQA-RAD test set. The results of SAN framework (fw.) and MCB framework (fw.) are cited from the paper [10].

	SAN fw. [10,19] (baseline)	MCB fw. [5,10] (baseline)	BAN fw. [9] (baseline)	SAN + proposal	BAN + proposal
Open-ended	24.2	25.4	27.6	40.7	**43.9**
Close-ended	57.2	60.6	66.5	74.1	**75.1**

The results also show that for all MAML, CDAE, and MEVF, the accuracy on close-ended questions (CEQ) are higher than those on the open-ended questions (OEQ). Furthermore, the improvements of the finetuning over the training from scratch are more significant on OEQ. We found that OEQ are usually difficult to answer than CEQ, i.e., OEQ mainly ask about the detail description and require long answers, while CEQ mainly ask about the confirmation (i.e., "yes/no") and usually have short answers. That observation implies that the description answers which need more information from input images take more benefits from the proposed image feature extraction.

4.4 Comparison with the State of the Art

We compare our framework (Fig. 1) with the baselines in [10]. In [10], the authors report the results when applying the general VQA frameworks, i.e., SAN framework [19], MCB framework [5][4] and finetuning on VQA-RAD dataset. We also report another strong baseline when finetuning the state-of-the-art BAN framework [9]. For our framework, we report results when using SAN [19] or BAN [9] as the attention mechanisms, although other attention mechanisms are straightforward to use in our framework.

Table 2 presents comparative results between methods. Note that for the image feature extraction, the baselines use the pretrained models (VGG or ResNet) that have been trained on ImageNet and then finetune on the VQA-RAD dataset. For the question feature extraction, all baselines and our framework use the same pretrained models (i.e., Glove [14]) and finetuning on VQA-RAD. The results show that when BAN or SAN is used as the attention mechanism in our framework, it significantly outperforms the baseline frameworks BAN [9] and SAN [10,19]. Our best setting, i.e. the one with BAN as the attention, achieves the state-of-the-art results and it significantly outperforms the best baseline framework BAN [9], i.e., the improvements are 16.3% and 8.6% on open-ended and close-ended VQA, respectively.

5   Conclusion

In this paper, we proposed a novel medical VQA framework that leverages the meta-learning MAML and denoising auto-encoder CDAE for image feature extraction in order to overcome the limitation of labeled training data. Specifically, CDAE helps to leverage information from the large scale unlabeled images, while MAML helps to learn meta-weights that can be quickly adapted to the VQA problem. We establish new state-of-the-art results on VQA-RAD dataset for both close-ended and open-ended questions.

---

[4] Those frameworks are completed VQA models in which the core components in those frameworks are SAN and MCB attentions. We refer the reader to the corresponding papers [5,19] for the detail of those models.

References

1. Abacha, A.B., Gayen, S., Lau, J.J., Rajaraman, S., Demner-Fushman, D.: NLM at ImageCLEF 2018 visual question answering in the medical domain. In: CEUR Workshop Proceedings (2018)
2. Bar, Y., Diamant, I., Wolf, L., Greenspan, H.: Deep learning with non-medical training used for chest pathology identification. In: Medical Imaging: Computer-Aided Diagnosis (2015)
3. Clark, K., Vendt, B., Smith, K., Freymann, J., et al.: The cancer imaging archive (TCIA): maintaining and operating a public information repository. J. Digit. Imaging **26**(6), 1045–1057 (2013)
4. Finn, C., Abbeel, P., Levine, S.: Model-agnostic meta-learning for fast adaptation of deep networks. In: ICML (2017)
5. Fukui, A., Park, D.H., Yang, D., Rohrbach, A., Darrell, T., Rohrbach, M.: Multimodal compact bilinear pooling for visual question answering and visual grounding. In: EMNLP (2016)
6. Hasan, S.A., Ling, Y., Farri, O., Liu, J., Lungren, M., Müller, H.: Overview of the ImageCLEF 2018 medical domain visual question answering task. In: CEUR Workshop Proceedings (2018)
7. He, K., Zhang, X., Ren, S., Sun, J.: Deep residual learning for image recognition. In: CVPR (2016)
8. Jifara, W., Jiang, F., Rho, S., Cheng, M., Liu, S.: Medical image denoising using convolutional neural network: a residual learning approach. J. Supercomputing **75**, 1–15 (2017). https://doi.org/10.1007/s11227-017-2080-0
9. Kim, J.H., Jun, J., Zhang, B.T.: Bilinear attention networks. In: NIPS (2018)
10. Lau, J.J., Gayen, S., Abacha, A.B., Demner-Fushman, D.: A dataset of clinically generated visual questions and answers about radiology images. Nature **5**, 180251 (2018)
11. Maicas, G., Bradley, A.P., Nascimento, J.C., Reid, I., Carneiro, G.: Training medical image analysis systems like radiologists. In: MICCAI (2018)
12. Masci, J., Meier, U., Cireşan, D., Schmidhuber, J.: Stacked convolutional autoencoders for hierarchical feature extraction. In: ICANN (2011)
13. Peng, Y., Liu, F., Rosen, M.P.: UMass at ImageCLEF medical visual question answering (MeD-VQA) 2018 task. In: CEUR Workshop Proceedings (2018)
14. Pennington, J., Socher, R., Manning, C.D.: Glove: global vectors for word representation. In: EMNLP (2014)
15. Rumelhart, D.E., Hinton, G.E., Williams, R.J.: Learning internal representations by error propagation. Tech. rep. (1985)
16. Russakovsky, O., Deng, J., Su, H., et al.: Imagenet large scale visual recognition challenge. In: IJCV, pp. 211–252 (2015)
17. Schmidhuber, J.: Evolutionary principles in self-referential learning (1987)
18. Simonyan, K., Zisserman, A.: Very deep convolutional networks for large-scale image recognition. In: ICLR (2015)
19. Yang, Z., He, X., Gao, J., Deng, L., Smola, A.J.: Stacked attention networks for image question answering. In: CVPR (2016)
20. Zhou, Y., Kang, X., Ren, F.: Employing inception-Resnet-v2 and Bi-LSTM for medical domain visual question answering. In: CEUR Workshop Proceedings (2018)

Multi-Instance Multi-Scale CNN for Medical Image Classification

Shaohua Li[1,2(✉)], Yong Liu[1], Xiuchao Sui[2], Cheng Chen[1], Gabriel Tjio[1], Daniel Shu Wei Ting[3], and Rick Siow Mong Goh[1]

[1] Institute of High Performance Computing, A*STAR, Singapore, Singapore
shaohua@gmail.com
[2] Artificial Intelligence Initiative, A*STAR, Singapore, Singapore
[3] Singapore Eye Research Institute, Singapore, Singapore

Abstract. Deep learning for medical image classification faces three major challenges: (1) the number of annotated medical images for training are usually small; (2) regions of interest (ROIs) are relatively small with unclear boundaries in the whole medical images, and may appear in arbitrary positions across the x, y (and also z in 3D images) dimensions. However often only labels of the whole images are annotated, and localized ROIs are unavailable; and (3) ROIs in medical images often appear in varying sizes (scales). We approach these three challenges with a Multi-Instance Multi-Scale (MIMS) CNN: (1) We propose a multi-scale convolutional layer, which extracts patterns of different receptive fields with a shared set of convolutional kernels, so that scale-invariant patterns are captured by this compact set of kernels. As this layer contains only a small number of parameters, training on small datasets becomes feasible; (2) We propose a "top-k pooling" to aggregate the feature maps in varying scales from multiple spatial dimensions, allowing the model to be trained using weak annotations within the multiple instance learning (MIL) framework. Our method is shown to perform well on three classification tasks involving two 3D and two 2D medical image datasets.

1 Introduction

Training a convolutional neural network (CNN) from scratch demands a massive amount of training images. Limited medical images encourage people to do transfer learning, i.e., fine-tune 2D CNN models pretrained on natural images [10]. A key difference between medical images and natural images is that, regions of interest (ROIs) are relatively small with unclear boundaries in the whole medical images, and ROIs may appear multiple times in arbitrary positions across the x, y (and also z in 3D images) dimensions. On the other hand, annotations for medical images are often "weak", in that only image-level annotations are available, and there are no localized ROIs. In this setting, we can view each ROI

Electronic supplementary material The online version of this chapter (https://doi.org/10.1007/978-3-030-32251-9_58) contains supplementary material, which is available to authorized users.

as an instance in a bag of all image patches, and the image-level classification falls within the Multiple-Instance Learning (MIL) framework [2,6,11].

Another challenge with medical images is that ROIs are often *scale-invariant*, i.e., visually similar patterns often appear in varying sizes (scales). If approached with vanilla CNNs, an excess number of convolutional kernels with varying receptive fields would be required for full coverage of these patterns, which have more parameters and demand more training data. Some previous works have attempted to learn scale-invariant patterns, for example [8] adopted image pyramids, i.e. resizing input images into different scales, processing them with the same CNN and aggregating the outputs. However, our experiments show that image pyramids perform unstably across different datasets and consume much more computational resources than vanilla CNNs.

This paper aims to address all the challenges above in a holistic framework. We propose two novel components: (1) a *multi-scale convolutional layer* (MSConv) that further processes feature maps extracted from a pretrained CNN, aiming to capture scale-invariant patterns with a shared set of kernels; (2) a *top-k pooling* scheme that extracts and aggregates the highest activations from feature maps in each convolutional channel (across multiple spatial dimensions in varying scales), so that the model is able to be trained with image-level labels only.

The MSConv layer consists of a few resizing operators (with different output resolutions), and a shared set of convolutional kernels. First a pretrained CNN extracts feature maps from input images. Then the MSConv layer resizes them to different scales, and processes each scale with the same set of convolutional kernels. Given the varying scales of the feature maps, the convolutional kernels effectively have varying receptive fields, and therefore are able to detect scale-invariant patterns. As feature maps are much smaller than input images, the computation and memory overhead of the MSConv layer is insignificant.

The MSConv layer is inspired by ROI-pooling [1], and is closely related to Trident Network [5]. Trident Network uses shared convolutional kernels of different dilation rates to capture scale-invariant patterns. Its limitations include: (1) the receptive fields of dilated convolutions can only be integer multiples of the original receptive fields; (2) dilated convolutions may overlook prominent activations within a dilation interval. In contrast, the MSConv interpolates input feature maps to any desired sizes before convolution, so that the scales are more refined, and prominent activations are always retained for further convolution. [3] proposed a similar idea of resizing the input multiple times before convolution and aggregating the resulting feature maps by max-pooling. However we observed that empirically, activations in larger scales tend to dominate smaller scales and effectively mask smaller scales. MSConv incorporates a batchnorm layer and a learnable weight for each scale to eliminate such biases. In addition, MSConv adopts multiple kernel sizes to capture patterns in more varying scales.

A core operation in an MIL framework is to aggregate features or predictions from different instances (pattern occurrences). Intuitively, the most prominent patterns are usually also the most discriminative, and thus the highest activations could summarize a set of feature maps with the same semantics (i.e., in the same channel). In this regard, we propose a top-k pooling scheme that selects the highest activations of a group of feature maps, and takes their weighted average as the aggregate feature for downstream processing. The top-k pooling extends [9] with learnable pooling weights (instead of being specified by a hyperparameter as in [9]) and a learnable magnitude-normalization operator.

The MSConv layer and the top-k pooling comprise our Multi-Instance Multi-Scale (MIMS) CNN. To assess its performance, we evaluated 12 methods on three classification tasks: (1) classifying Diabetic Macular Edema (DME) on three Retinal Optical Coherence Tomography (OCT) datasets (two sets of 3D images); (2) classifying Myopic Macular Degeneration (MMD) on a 2D fundus image dataset; and (3) classifying Microsatellite Instable (MSI) against microsatellite stable (MSS) tumors of colorectal cancer (CRC) patients on histology images. In most cases, MIMS-CNN achieved better accuracy than five baselines and six ablated models. Our experiments also verified that both the MSConv layer and top-k pooling make important contributions.

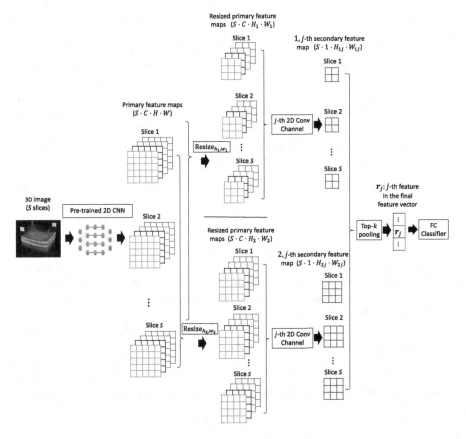

Fig. 1. The Multi-Instance Multi-Scale CNN on a 3D input image. For clarity, only the j-th convolutional channel of the MSConv layer is shown.

2   Multi-Instance Multi-Scale CNN

The architecture of our Multi-Instance Multi-Scale CNN is illustrated in Fig. 1. It consists of: (1) a pretrained 2D CNN to extract primary feature maps, (2) a multi-scale convolutional (MSConv) layer to extract scale-invariant secondary feature maps, (3) a top-k pooling operator to aggregate secondary feature maps, and (4) a classifier.

2.1   Multi-Scale Convolutional Layer

Due to limited training images, a common practice in medical image analysis is to extract image features using 2D CNNs pretrained on natural images. These features are referred as the *primary feature maps*. Due to the domain gap between natural images and medical images, feeding primary feature maps directly into a classifier does not always yield good results. To bridge this domain gap, we propose to use an extra convolutional layer to extract more relevant features from primary feature maps. This layer produces the *secondary feature maps*.

In order to capture scale-invariant ROIs, we resize the primary feature maps into different scales before convolution. Each scale corresponds to a separate pathway, and weights of the convolutional kernels in all pathways are tied. In effect, this convolutional layer has multiple receptive fields on the primary feature maps. We name this layer as a *multi-scale convolutional (MSConv) layer*.

More formally, let x denote the primary feature maps, $\{F_1, \cdots, F_N\}$ denote all the output channels of the MSConv layer[1], and $\{(h_1, w_1), \cdots, (h_m, w_m)\}$ denote the scale factors of the heights and widths (typically $\frac{1}{4} <= h_i = w_i <= 2$) adopted by the m resizing operators. The combination of the i-th scale and the j-th channel yields the ij-th secondary feature maps:

$$\boldsymbol{y}_{ij} = F_j\left(\text{Resize}_{h_i, w_i}(\boldsymbol{x})\right), \tag{1}$$

where in theory $\text{Resize}_{h_i, w_i}(\cdot)$ could adopt any type of interpolation, and our choice is bilinear interpolation.

For more flexibility, the convolutional kernels in MSConv could also have different kernel sizes. In a setting of m resizing operators and n different sizes of kernels, effectively the kernels have at most $m \times n$ different receptive fields. The multiple resizing operators and varying sizes of kernels complement each other and equip the CNN with scale-invariance.

Among $\{\boldsymbol{y}_{1j}, \boldsymbol{y}_{2j}, \cdots, \boldsymbol{y}_{mj}\}$, feature maps in larger scales contain more elements and tend to have more top k activations, hence dominate the aggregate feature and effectively mask out the feature maps in smaller scales. In order to remove such biases, the feature maps in different scales are passed through respective magnitude normalization operators. The magnitude normalization

---

[1] Each convolutional kernel yields multiple channels with different semantics, so output channels are indexed separately, regardless of whether they are from the same kernel.

operator consists of a batchnorm operator BN_{ij} and a learnable scalar multiplier sw_{ij}. The scalar multiplier sw_{ij} adjusts the importance of the j-th channel in the i-th scale, and is optimized with back-propagation.

The MSConv layer is illustrated in Fig. 1 and the left side of Fig. 2.

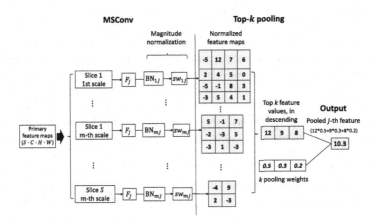

Fig. 2. The MSConv and Top-k pooling (on the j-th channel only) in m scales.

2.2 Top-k Pooling

Multiple Instance Learning (MIL) views the whole image as a bag, and each ROI as an instance in the bag. Most existing MIL works [6,11] were *instance-based MIL*, i.e., they aggregate label predictions on instances to yield a bag prediction. In contrast, [2] adopted *embedding-based MIL*, which aggregates features (embeddings) of instances to yield bag features, and then do classification on bag features. [2] showed that embedding-based MIL methods outperformed instance-based MIL baselines. Here we propose a simple but effective *top-k pooling* scheme to aggregate the most prominent features across a few spatial dimensions, as a new embedding-based MIL aggregation scheme.

Top-k pooling works as follows: given a set of feature maps with the same semantics, we find the top k highest activation values, and take a weighted average of them as the aggregate feature value. Intuitively, higher activation values are more important than lower ones, and thus the pooling weight should decrease as the ranking goes lower. However it may be sub-optimal to specify the weights manually as did in [9]. Hence we adopt a data-driven approach to learn these weights automatically. More formally, given a set of feature maps $\{x_i\}$, top-k pooling aggregates them into a single value:

$$\text{Pool}_k(\{x_i\}) = \sum_{r=1}^{k} w_r a_r, \tag{2}$$

where $a_1, \cdots, a_k$ are the highest k activations within $\{\boldsymbol{x}_i\}$, and $w_1, \cdots, w_k$ are nonnegative pooling weights to be learned, subject to a normalization constraint $\sum_r w_r = 1$. In practice, $w_1, \cdots, w_k$ is initialized with exponentially decayed values, and then optimized with back-propagation.

An important design choice in MIL is to choose the spatial dimensions to be pooled. Similar patterns, regardless of where they appear, contain similar information for classification. Correspondingly, features in the same channel could be pooled together. On 2D images, we choose to pool activations across the x, y-axes of the secondary feature maps, and on 3D images we choose to pool across the x, y and z (slices) axes. In addition, feature maps in the same channel but different scales (i.e., through different $\text{Resize}_{h_i, w_i}(\cdot)$ and the same F_j) encode the same semantics and should be pooled together. Eventually, all feature maps in the j-th channel, $\{\boldsymbol{y}_{\cdot j}\} = \boldsymbol{y}_{1j}, \boldsymbol{y}_{2j}, \cdots, \boldsymbol{y}_{mj}$ are pooled into a single value $\text{Pool}_k(\{\boldsymbol{y}_{\cdot j}\})$. Then following an N-channel MSConv layer, all feature maps will be pooled into an N-dimensional feature vector to represent the whole image. As typically $N < 100$, the downstream FC layer doing classification over this feature vector has only a small number of parameters and less prone to overfitting.

Figure 2 illustrates the top-k pooling being applied to the j-th channel feature maps in m scales.

3   Experiments

3.1   Datasets

Three classification tasks involving four datasets were used for evaluation.

DME classification on OCT images. The following two 3D datasets acquired by Singapore Eye Research Institute (SERI) were used:

(1) **Cirrus** dataset: 339 3D OCT images (239 normal, 100 DME). Each image has 128 slices in 512 * 1024. A 67–33% training/test split was used;

(2) **Spectralis** dataset: 197 3D OCT images (60 normal, 137 DME). Each image has 25 ∼ 31 slices in 497 * 768. A 50–50% training/test split was used;

MMD classification on fundus images:

(3) **MMD** dataset (acquired by SERI): 19,272 2D images (11,924 healthy, 631 MMD) in 900 * 600. A 70–30% training/test split was used.

MSI/MSS classification on CRC histology images:

(4) **CRC-MSI** dataset [4]: 93,408 2D training images (46,704 MSS, 46,704 MSI) in 224 * 224. 98,904 test images (70,569 MSS, 28,335 MSI) also in 224 * 224.

3.2   Compared Methods

MIMS-CNN, 5 baselines and 6 ablated models were compared. Unless specified, all methods used the ResNet-101 model (without FC) pretrained on ImageNet for feature extraction, and top-k pooling ($k = 5$) for feature aggregation.

MI-Pre. The ResNet feature maps are pooled by top-k pooling and classified.

Pyramid MI-Pre. Input images are scaled to $\{\frac{i}{4} | i = 2, 3, 4\}$ of original sizes, before being fed into the MI-Pre model.

MI-Pre-Conv. The ResNet feature maps are processed by an extra convolutional layer, and aggregated by top-k pooling before classification. It is almost the same as the model in [6], except that [6] does patch-level classification and aggregates patch predictions to obtain image-level classification.

MIMS. The MSConv layer has 3 resizing operators that resize the primary feature maps to the following scales: $\{\frac{i}{4}|i = 2,3,4\}$. Two groups of kernels of different sizes were used.

MIMS-NoResizing. It is an ablated MIMS-CNN with all resizing operators removed. This is to evaluate the contribution of the resizing operators.

Pyramid MIMS. It is an ablated MIMS-CNN with all resizing operators removed, and the multi-scaledness is pursued with input image pyramids of scales $\{\frac{i}{4}|i = 2,3,4\}$. The MSConv kernels is configured identically as above.

MI-Pre-Trident [5]. It extends MI-Pre-Conv with dilation factors $1, 2, 3$.

SI-CNN [3]. It is an ablated MIMS-CNN with the batchnorms and scalar multipliers removed from the MSConv layer.

FeatPyra-4,5. It is a feature pyramid network [7] that extracts features from conv4_x and conv5_x in ResNet-101, processes each set of features with a respective convolutional layer, and classifies the aggregate features.

ResNet34-scratch. It is a ResNet-34 model trained from scratch.

MIMS-patchcls and **MI-Pre-Conv-patchcls.** They are ablated MIMS and MI-Pre-Conv, respectively, evaluated on 3D OCT datasets. They classify each slice, and average slice predictions to obtain image-level classification.

3.3 Results

Table 1 lists the AUROC scores (averaged over three independent runs) of the 12 methods on the four datasets. All methods with an extra convolutional layer on top of a pretrained model performed well. The benefits of using pretrained models are confirmed by the performance gap between ResNet34-scratch and others. The two image pyramid methods performed significantly worse on some datasets, although they consumed twice as much computational time and GPU memory as other methods. MIMS-CNN almost always outperformed other methods.

The inferior performance of the two *-patchcls models demonstrated the advantages of top-k pooling for MIL. To further investigate its effectiveness, we trained MIMS-CNN on Cirrus with six MIL aggregation schemes: average-pooling (**mean**), max-pooling (**max**), top-k pooling with $k = 2, 3, 4, 5$, and an instance-based MIL scheme: max-pooling over slice predictions (**max-inst**).

As can be seen in Table 2, the other three aggregation schemes fell behind all top-k schemes, and when k increases, the model tends to perform slightly better. It confirms that embedding-based MIL outperforms instance-based MIL.

Table 1. Performance (in AUROC) of 12 methods on four image datasets.

Methods	Cirrus	Spectralis	MMD	CRC-MSI	Avg.
MI-Pre	0.574	0.906	0.956	0.880	0.829
Pyramid MI-Pre	0.638	0.371	0.965	0.855	0.707
MI-Pre-Conv	0.972	0.990	0.961	0.870	0.948
MIMS-NoResizing	0.956	0.975	0.961	0.879	0.942
Pyramid MIMS	0.848	0.881	0.966	0.673	0.842
MI-Pre-Trident	0.930	**1.000**	0.966	0.897	0.948
SI-CNN	0.983	**1.000**	**0.972**	0.880	0.959
FeatPyra-4,5	0.959	0.991	0.970	0.888	0.952
ResNet34-scratch	0.699	0.734	0.824	0.667	0.731
MIMS	**0.986**	**1.000**	**0.972**	**0.901**	**0.965**
MIMS-patchcls	0.874	0.722	/	/	/
MI-Pre-Conv-patchcls	0.764	0.227	/	/	/

Table 2. Performance of seven MIL aggregation schemes on the Cirrus dataset.

Methods	mean	max	max-inst	$k = 2$	$k = 3$	$k = 4$	$k = 5$
AUROC on Cirrus	0.829	0.960	0.975	0.980	0.980	0.986	0.986

4   Conclusions

Applying CNNs on medical images faces three challenges: datasets are of small sizes, annotations are often weak and ROIs are in varying scales. We proposed a framework to address all these challenges. This framework consists of two novel components: (1) a multi-scale convolutional layer on top of a pretrained CNN to capture scale-invariant patterns, which contains only a small number of parameters, (2) a top-k pooling operator to aggregate feature maps in varying scales across multiple spatial dimensions to facilitate training with weak annotations within the Multiple Instance Learning framework. Our method has been validated on three classification tasks involving four image datasets.

Acknowledgments. We gratefully acknowledge the support of NVIDIA Corporation with the donation of the Titan Xp used for this research.

References

1. Girshick, R.: Fast R-CNN. In: Proceedings of the 2015 IEEE International Conference on Computer Vision (ICCV). ICCV 2015, pp. 1440–1448 (2015)
2. Ilse, M., Tomczak, J.M., Welling, M.: Attention-based deep multiple instance learning. In: Proceedings of the 35th International Conference on Machine Learning ICML, ICML 2018, pp. 2132–2141 (2018)

3. Kanazawa, A., Sharma, A., Jacobs, D.W.: Locally scale-invariant convolutional neural networks. In: NIPS Workshop on Deep Learning and Representation Learning (2014)
4. Kather, J.N.: Histological images for MSI vs. MSS classification in gastrointestinal cancer, FFPE samples. https://doi.org/10.5281/zenodo.2530835
5. Li, Y., Chen, Y., Wang, N., Zhang, Z.: Scale-aware trident networks for object detection. arXiv e-prints arXiv:1901.01892 (2019)
6. Li, Z., et al.: Thoracic disease identification and localization with limited supervision. In: The IEEE Conference on Computer Vision and Pattern Recognition (CVPR), June 2018 (2018)
7. Lin, T.Y., Dollár, P., Girshick, R., He, K., Hariharan, B., Belongie, S.: Feature pyramid networks for object detection. In: Proceedings of the IEEE Conference on Computer Vision and Pattern Recognition, pp. 2117–2125 (2017)
8. Rasti, R., Rabbani, H., Mehridehnavi, A., Hajizadeh, F.: Macular OCT classification using a multi-scale convolutional neural network ensemble. IEEE Trans. Med. Imaging 37(4), 1024–1034 (2018)
9. Shi, Z., Ye, Y., Wu, Y.: Rank-based pooling for deep convolutional neural networks. Neural Networks 83, 21–31 (2016)
10. Tajbakhsh, N., et al.: Convolutional neural networks for medical image analysis: full training or fine tuning? IEEE Trans. Med. Imaging 35(5), 1299–1312 (2016)
11. Zhu, W., Lou, Q., Vang, Y.S., Xie, X.: Deep multi-instance networks with sparse label assignment for whole mammogram classification. In: Medical Image Computing and Computer Assisted Intervention - MICCAI 2017, pp. 603–611 (2017)

Improving Uncertainty Estimation in Convolutional Neural Networks Using Inter-rater Agreement

Martin Holm Jensen[(✉)], Dan Richter Jørgensen, Raluca Jalaboi,
Mads Eiler Hansen, and Martin Aastrup Olsen

LEO Innovation Lab, København, Denmark
{martin.holm,dan.joergensen,raluca.jalaboi,meiler,
martin.olsen}@leoilab.com
https://www.leoilab.com

Abstract. Modern neural networks are pushing the boundaries of medical image classification. For some tasks in dermatology, state of the art models are able to beat human experts in terms of accuracy and type I/II errors. However, in the domain of medical applications, models should also be evaluated on how well they capture uncertainty in samples and labels. This aspect is key to building trust in computer-assisted systems, otherwise largely considered to be black boxes by their users. A common practice in supervised learning is to collect multiple evaluations per sample, which is particularly useful when inter-rater agreement is expected to be low. At the same time, model training traditionally uses label fusion, such as majority voting, to produce a single label for each sample. In this paper, we experimentally show that models trained to predict skin conditions become overconfident when this approach is used; i.e. the probability estimates of the model exceeds the true correctness likelihood. Additionally, we show that a better calibrated model is obtained when training with a label sampling scheme that takes advantage of inter-rater variability during training. The calibration improvements come at no cost in terms of model accuracy. Our approach is combined and contrasted with other recent techniques in uncertainty estimation. All experiments are evaluated on a proprietary dataset consisting of 31017 images of skin, where up to 12 experts have diagnosed each image.

Keywords: Supervised deep learning · Model calibration · Dermatology

1 Introduction

Diagnosing skin conditions is a difficult, yet crucial process for the well-being of patients. One study found that diagnoses provided by general practitioners were

M. H Jensen, D. R. Jørgensen, R. Jalaboi, M. E. Hansen, M. A. Olsen—Equal contribution

© Springer Nature Switzerland AG 2019
D. Shen et al. (Eds.): MICCAI 2019, LNCS 11767, pp. 540–548, 2019.
https://doi.org/10.1007/978-3-030-32251-9_59

concordant with those of dermatologists in 57% of the cases [15], while another study showed that agreement between dermatologists can be as low as 71.3% [8]. In order to deal with the inter-rater variability, classification systems trained in a supervised manner often use some form of label fusion, e.g. majority voting or weighted voting.

In recent years, deep learning diagnosis models have been shown to achieve classification performance comparable to that of dermatologists [5,8,18]. However, such modern architectures have a tendency to become overconfident in their predictions [7]. We posit that a well-calibrated model, where confidence scores reflect likelihood of correctness, is important to establish trust in automated solutions. Recently proposed methods [1,2,6,12,17] are used to improve uncertainty estimates of neural networks, which can be used for calibration. When multiple evaluations are available for a sample, training time label sampling can improve model certainty and thus calibration [11].

We state two primary contributions based on experiments conducted on a proprietary dataset of 31017 images of skin conditions that were evaluated by up to 12 dermatologists. First, we show that training with the label sampling technique of [11] over plurality label fusion leads to better calibrated models with no cost to the overall model accuracy. Second, we evaluate the effect of label sampling in combination with recently proposed methods for uncertainty estimations and show that only one method [17] improves our baseline in terms of expected calibration error.

2   Materials and Methods

In this section, we describe model calibration, label fusion, and recent methods in deep learning for uncertainty estimation. To this end, let X denote a set of input samples with size N, each associated with one of K classes. We define a ground truth label by $y_x \in \{1, \ldots, K\}$ for each sample $x \in X$. We consider a neural network (or simply model) h given by a function $h : X \to [0,1]^K$, where $h(x)$ outputs a confidence score vector $\mathbf{z}_x$ of length K. We use $\hat{y}_x = \text{argmax}_k \mathbf{z}_x^{(k)}$ to denote the class prediction, and $\hat{p}_x = \max_k \mathbf{z}_x^{(k)}$ the confidence score, where $\mathbf{z}_x^{(k)}$ is the confidence score of class k.

2.1   Model Calibration

A well-calibrated model reports a prediction certainty that reflects the actual probability of a correct prediction [3], e.g. when the model outputs a certainty of 75% on 100 samples it is correct on 75 of the samples. To quantify model calibration, we follow [16] and partition samples into M bins of size $1/M$ based on the confidence score. For $m \in \{1, \ldots, M\}$, let $I_m = \left(\frac{m-1}{M}, \frac{m}{M}\right]$ and denote by $B_m = \{x \in X \mid \hat{p}_x \in I_m\}$ the set of samples with size b_m whose confidence score falls within I_m. Our focus is on the expected calibration error (ECE), a summary statistic given by

$$\text{acc}(B_m) = \frac{1}{b_m} \sum_{x \in B_m} \mathbf{1}\,(y_x = \hat{y}_x)$$

$$\text{conf}(B_m) = \frac{1}{b_m} \sum_{x \in B_m} \hat{p}_x$$

$$\text{ECE} = \sum_{m=1}^{M} \frac{b_m}{N} \mid \text{acc}(B_m) - \text{conf}(B_m) \mid \tag{1}$$

The accuracy and calibration error of each I_m is illustrated through reliability diagrams. A model is considered overconfident when $\text{acc}(B_m) - \text{conf}(B_m)$ is negative and underconfident when it is positive.

2.2   Methods for Uncertainty Estimation

To improve model calibration, we consider four methods shown to behave as uncertainty estimators: ensembles [12], test-time augmentation [1], Monte Carlo batch normalization [17], and Monte Carlo dropout [6]. Each method involves multiple forward passes to calculate a confidence score vector. To obtain $\mathbf{z}_x^{(k)}$, the confidence score of class k, we take the arithmetic mean over $\mathbf{z}_x^{(k),1}, \ldots, \mathbf{z}_x^{(k),I}$ for I forward passes.

Ensembles. In classical machine learning and deep learning, ensembles of models have been shown to improve the predictive performance. Recently, they have also been applied to the task of capturing prediction uncertainty by using the training time variance in deep networks. To produce $\mathbf{z}_x^{(k),i}$, we do a forward pass using the i'th network in the ensemble. In our experiments, we use an ensemble of 25 networks, each trained in the same manner.

Test-Time Augmentation (TTA). Data augmentation allows for uncertainty estimation by exploring the locality of each sample x. A perturbation x' is constructed, and a forward pass of the network on the i'th random pertubation of x produces $\mathbf{z}_x^{(k),i}$. In our experiments, we use the same types of transformations as during training with 25 pertubations per sample.

Monte Carlo Batch Normalization (MCBN). Many modern neural networks use Batch Normalization (BN) and these layers can be used for uncertainty estimation [17]. To use BN as an uncertainty estimator, a single training step is conducted for a randomly selected mini-batch $X' \subseteq X$ from the training set, during which only μ and σ, the moving moments of the BN layers, are updated. We construct I models with a variation in the moving moments by randomly selecting I mini-batches from the training set, and produce $\mathbf{z}_x^{(k),i}$ by a forward pass of the i'th model. We use 100 randomly selected mini-batches in our experiments.

Monte Carlo Dropout (MCD). Prior to MCBN, a Monte Carlo dropout method was suggested where dropout is turned on at inference time, instead of only acting as a regulariser during training [6]. The difference in confidence scores between forward passes is therefore determined by which units are dropped. Our implementation drops the same units for each combination of mini-batch X' and forward pass i to produce $\mathbf{z}_x^{(k),i}$, where $x \in X'$. In our experiments, we use a dropout rate of 0.5 and 25 forward passes per sample.

2.3 Dataset

We use a dataset of 31017 skin images collected via a smartphone app, in compliance with GDPR and HIPAA standards. Board certified dermatologists label images with ICD-10 codes[1] through a web-based annotation tool. If no evidence of a skin disease is found in an image, the expert can classify it as Clinically Normal Skin (CNS). All images are evaluated by between 2 and 12 dermatologists, with an average of 4.8 ± 1.9 evaluations per image. We group individual evaluations into one of the four classes: psoriasis, dermatitis, other-lesion, and CNS.

Following [13] we compute the average agreement rate (AAR) for each dermatologist as their pairwise accuracy against every other dermatologist. The mean AAR on our dataset is $76.8\% \pm 3.7\%$.

After removing ties, our dataset consists of 11254 (36%) CNS images, 8847 (28%) psoriasis images, 6409 (21%) other-lesion images and 4507 (15%) dermatitis images. Using plurality label fusion, we define three disjunct subsets based on expert agreement: Unanimous, when all dermatologists agree on the class; Majority, if more than half of all evaluations are of the same class; and Plurality, when one class has more votes than the others, but does not reach majority. We form a test set from approximately 19% of the samples.

2.4 Label Sampling

Uncertainty estimation for segmentation is explored in [11] on a synthetic 2D dataset and on a post-operative brain tumor MRI dataset (30 samples, 3 raters). The results in [11] show that combining MCD and Label Sampling (LS) outperforms MCD combined with either of four other label fusion schemes. A significant shortcoming in plurality label fusion is that label uncertainty, represented as inter-rater variability, is not captured. LS takes advantage of inter-rater variability by randomly selecting, at each epoch, one of the evaluation labels for each sample during the training phase. LS is agnostic to model architecture, requires no modification to the model itself, and allows for a variable number of labels on each sample. We contrast LS with plurality label fusion on our classification task.

---

[1] World Health Organization - http://www.who.int/iris/handle/10665/37958.

2.5   Model Training and Experimental Setup

Our Baseline configuration is ResNet50 [9], pre-trained on the ImageNet [4] dataset. This choice is motivated by [10], who shows that pre-trained models are more robust and better calibrated than networks trained from scratch.

The final dense layer is replaced to output the classes in our dataset. Training is done in two phases: (1) the final dense layer is fine-tuned for 9 epochs; (2) both the final dense layer and the final convolution block are trained for another 9 epochs. We use the Adam optimiser with warm restarts [14] (cycle length 3, multiplier 2, and maximum learning rate 0.001), mini-batch size of 96, categorical cross-entropy loss, and weighted classes. Training time data augmentation consists of vertical and horizontal flips, rotations, and scaling.

We refer to the configurations Ensemble, TTA, MCBN and MCD as the Baseline configuration enhanced with one of the methods described in Sect. 2.2. In the case of MCD, a dropout layer is added in front of the final dense layer. Each configuration is trained using all evaluations of a sample with either LS as detailed in Sect. 2.4, or plurality label fusion (LF).

3   Results

We proceed to examine what impact the choice of LS/LF and method for uncertainty estimation has on accuracy and model calibration. We take the ground truth y_x for a test sample x to be the plurality label fusion over all evaluations of x. The ECE ($M = 10$) and accuracy are calculated for each experiment on the entire test set, as well as each of the disjoint test subsets with unanimous, majority, or plurality agreement.

Table 1. The accuracy (%) of each experiment on the test set and on the unanimous, majority, and plurality subsets.

Method	Test set	Unanimous	Majority	Plurality
Baseline LF	73.9	85.1	62.5	40.8
Ensemble LF	74.5	85.2	63.7	41.2
TTA LF	76.6	87.3	65.9	42.7
MCD LF	73.8	84.8	62.3	43.1
MCBN LF	73.8	85.8	61.8	40.4
Baseline LS	75.3	86.8	63.4	43.6
Ensemble LS	76.0	87.3	64.9	41.7
TTA LS	**77.7**	**88.9**	**66.5**	**48.3**
MCD LS	75.4	86.3	64.2	43.1
MCBN LS	74.1	85.9	61.8	44.9

3.1   Effects on Accuracy

Table 1 shows that the accuracy of the baseline configuration is slightly higher (1.4%) when trained using label sampling instead of label fusion. The choice of LS over LF slightly improves accuracy for all configurations across all test subsets (unanimous, majority, and plurality). We see that the accuracy improves when confidence scores are produced using either an ensemble or TTA, yet this effect is not present for MCD and MCBN. The accuracy across all experiments is highest on the unanimous subset, and drops significantly on the majority and plurality subsets.

Table 2. The ECE (%) of each experiment on the test set and on the unanimous, majority, and plurality subsets.

Method	Test set	Unanimous	Majority	Plurality
Baseline LF	7.7	2.2	14.1	30.2
Ensemble LF	5.1	**1.3**	10.9	27.3
TTA LF	3.0	2.2	7.7	23.1
MCD LF	6.7	1.7	13.6	25.0
MCBN LF	7.7	1.7	14.7	30.4
Baseline LS	1.9	6.7	3.8	15.5
Ensemble LS	3.6	8.2	**2.5**	16.5
TTA LS	3.9	7.3	2.7	9.3
MCD LS	2.4	6.5	3.3	20.4
MCBN LS	1.4	5.0	5.4	18.0

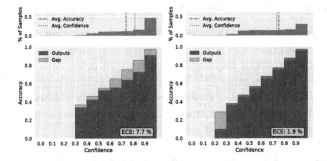

Fig. 1. Training using label sampling (right) improves ECE of baseline (left) by more than a factor of four. We show sample histograms (top) and reliability diagrams with $M = 10$ (bottom). Within a confidence interval, blue is sample accuracy, red or purple gaps show the distance to a perfectly calibrated model (Color figure online).

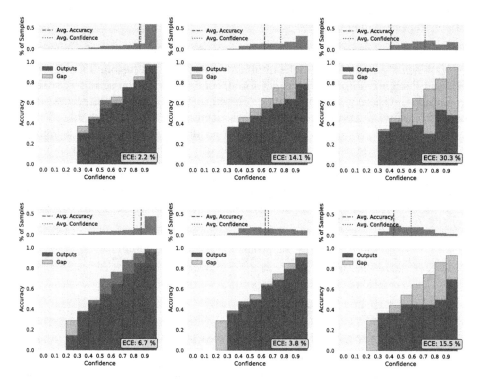

Fig. 2. Reliability diagrams for Baseline LF (top) and Baseline LS (bottom), on test subsets unanimous (left), majority (center), plurality (right). Within a confidence interval, blue is sample accuracy, red or purple gaps show the distance to a perfectly calibrated model. (Color figure online)

3.2   Effects on Model Calibration

The ECE in Table 2 shows that while the choice of training scheme only has a slight effect on accuracy, it has a large impact on model calibration. On the complete test set, the ECE improves by a factor of more than four when comparing Baseline LS to Baseline LF. This difference is illustrated in Fig. 1 which shows that training using label fusion leads to a poorly calibrated model with over-confident predictions. In contrast, training using label sampling results in a well-calibrated, albeit slightly under-confident model.

Additionally, Table 2 shows that for samples in the unanimous subset, all models trained using label sampling have a worse ECE than models trained with label fusion. In Fig. 2, we see that label sampling causes models to be under-confident on this subset. However, on the majority and plurality subsets, the ECE when using label sampling is significantly lower than when using label fusion.

Moreover, even the best calibrated model trained using label fusion (TTA LF) has a higher ECE than any of the models trained using label sampling. In particular, the combination of label sampling and TTA performs well on samples in the plurality subset with an ECE of 9.3% (compared to TTA LF with an ECEs of 23.1%). In addition, the TTA LS method has the highest accuracy across the board.

4 Conclusion

In this work, we have shown that fine-tuning a modern CNN using label fusion can lead to models that are over-confident in their predictions. We have demonstrated how a label sampling scheme can be used to create models that are better calibrated. The label sampling methods gave small but consistent improvements in terms of model accuracy when compared like-to-like with models trained using label fusion. The method can be combined with other methodologies such as ensembles or TTA to increase the accuracy, although our results indicate that this may have a slightly negative effect on model calibration. Finally, our results suggest that for datasets where multiple labels per sample are not available, using TTA can lead to models that are reasonably well calibrated.

Acknowledgement. We're thankful to our reviewers and area chairs for their relevant feedback, and to the MICCAI program committee for organizing the review process. This paper was made possible by all of the LEO Innovation Lab members who have labelled images and/or have contributed to the Imagine project and the Core services underpinning it.

References

1. Ayhan, M.S., Berens, P.: Test-time data augmentation for estimation of heteroscedastic aleatoric uncertainty in deep neural networks. In: MIDL (2018)
2. Blundell, C., Cornebise, J., Kavukcuoglu, K., Wierstra, D.: Weight uncertainty in neural networks. In: ICML (2015)
3. DeGroot, M.H., Fienberg, S.E.: The comparison and evaluation of forecasters. Statistician: J. Inst. Statisticians **32**, 12–22 (1983)
4. Deng, J., Dong, W., Socher, R., et al.: ImageNet: a large-scale hierarchical image database. In: CVPR (2009)
5. Esteva, A., Kuprel, B., Novoa, R.A., et al.: Dermatologist-level classification of skin cancer with deep neural networks. Nature **542**, 115–118 (2017)
6. Gal, Y., Ghahramani, Z.: Dropout as a Bayesian approximation: representing model uncertainty in deep learning. In: ICML (2016)
7. Guo, C., Pleiss, G., Sun, Y., Weinberger, K.Q.: On calibration of modern neural networks. In: ICML (2017)
8. Haenssle, H.A., Fink, C., Schneiderbauer, R., et al.: Man against machine: diagnostic performance of a deep learning convolutional neural network for dermoscopic melanoma recognition in comparison to 58 dermatologists. Ann. Oncol. **29**(8), 1836–1842 (2018)

9. He, K., Zhang, X., Ren, S., Sun, J.: Deep residual learning for image recognition. In: CVPR (2016)
10. Hendrycks, D., Lee, K., Mazeika, M.: Using pre-training can improve model robustness and uncertainty (2019)
11. Jungo, A., Meier, R., Ermis, E., et al.: On the effect of inter-observer variability for a reliable estimation of uncertainty of medical image segmentation. In: MICCAI (2018)
12. Lakshminarayanan, B., Pritzel, A., Blundell, C.: Simple and scalable predictive uncertainty estimation using deep ensembles. In: NIPS, pp. 6402–6413 (2017)
13. Laserson, J., Lantsman, C.D., Cohen-Sfady, M., et al.: TextRay: mining clinical reports to gain a broad understanding of chest x-rays. In: MICCAI (2018)
14. Loshchilov, I., Hutter, F.: SGDR: stochastic gradient descent with warm restarts. In: ICLR (2017)
15. Lowell, B.A., Froelich, C.W., Federman, D.G., Kirsner, R.S.: Dermatology in primary care: prevalence and patient disposition. J. Am. Acad. Dermatol. **45**(2), 250–255 (2001)
16. Niculescu-Mizil, A., Caruana, R.: Predicting good probabilities with supervised learning. In: ICML (2005)
17. Teye, M., Azizpour, H., Smith, K.: Bayesian uncertainty estimation for batch normalized deep networks. In: ICML (2018)
18. Yang, J., Sun, X., Liang, J., Rosin, P.L.: Clinical skin lesion diagnosis using representations inspired by dermatologist criteria. In: CVPR (2018)

Improving Skin Condition Classification with a Visual Symptom Checker Trained Using Reinforcement Learning

Mohamed Akrout[1,2(✉)], Amir-massoud Farahmand[2,3], Tory Jarmain[1], and Latif Abid[1]

[1] Triage, 1, Adelaide St. E., Suite 3001, Toronto M5C1J4, Canada
makrout@cs.toronto.edu
[2] Department of Computer Science, University of Toronto, Toronto, Canada
[3] Vector Institute, Toronto, Canada

Abstract. We present a visual symptom checker that combines a pretrained Convolutional Neural Network (CNN) with a Reinforcement Learning (RL) agent as a Question Answering (QA) model. This method increases the classification confidence and accuracy of the visual symptom checker, and decreases the average number of questions asked to narrow down the differential diagnosis. A Deep Q-Network (DQN)-based RL agent learns how to ask the patient about the presence of symptoms in order to maximize the probability of correctly identifying the underlying condition. The RL agent uses the visual information provided by CNN in addition to the answers to the asked questions to guide the QA system. We demonstrate that the RL-based approach increases the accuracy more than 20% compared to the CNN-only approach, which only uses the visual information to predict the condition. Moreover, the increased accuracy is up to 10% compared to the approach that uses the visual information provided by CNN along with a conventional decision tree-based QA system. We finally show that the RL-based approach not only outperforms the decision tree-based approach, but also narrows down the diagnosis faster in terms of the average number of asked questions.

Keywords: Skin condition classification · Question answering model · Reinforcement Learning · Deep Q-Learning

M. Akrout—Research conducted while working at Triage.
A. Farahmand—AMF would like to acknowledge funding from the Canada CIFAR AI Chairs Program.

Electronic supplementary material The online version of this chapter (https://doi.org/10.1007/978-3-030-32251-9_60) contains supplementary material, which is available to authorized users.

D. Shen et al. (Eds.): MICCAI 2019, LNCS 11767, pp. 549–557, 2019.
https://doi.org/10.1007/978-3-030-32251-9_60

1 Introduction

Doctors often ask their patients a series of questions in order to narrow down the set of plausible conditions matching the observed symptoms. By asking relevant questions, they can diagnose their patients more efficiently. We are interested in designing an automatic system that diagnoses patients based on an image and a sequence of questions and their corresponding answers.

Given an initial set of symptoms, a QA system such as a symptom checker enables the emulation of this conventional approach by asking the relevant questions in order to refine the differential diagnosis. Some work has been done to formulate the symptom checker using Bayesian networks [11] and recurrent neural networks [3]. All these symptom checkers, however, rely only on clinical descriptions without leveraging the visual information usually available in several domains such as dermatology and radiology.

The recent work of Akrout et al. [1] makes use of the visual information by combining a CNN and a decision tree QA model to improve the skin condition classification task. Their proposed decision tree-based approach picks the best symptom to ask by maximizing the information gain $IG(\mathcal{S}, \mathcal{C})$ between symptoms $\mathcal{S}$ and conditions $\mathcal{C}$. Since decision trees are learned by heuristic methods such as greedy search, they only consider immediate information gain at the current splitting node and often result in sub-optimal solutions in a constrained search space. The RL framework overcomes this problem by searching for splitting strategies in the global search space based on the evaluation of long-term payoff.

Designing QA systems has already been successfully formulated as an RL task for Query Reformulation [5], search engine querying [2], and automatic diagnosis [10]. The latter one is the closest work to ours, in which the authors formulate the problem of learning a QA system for differential diagnoses problems as an RL problem. A major difference with our work is that they do not use visual information as a prior for the QA system, while this work does, as will be explained in Sect. 2. Additionally, they use a different action space, where actions are *inform, request, deny, confirm, thanks* and *close_dialogue*, which is unlike our action space consisting of the presence of the symptoms themselves. Moreover, they use a reward function with hard-coded discrete values based on whether they find the right diagnosis or not, whereas ours is a dense reward given to the agent at each step and is defined based on the probability of choosing the true condition given the sequence of actions taken so far. In this work, we extend the study in [1] by formulating the symptom checking problem as a Markov Decision Process (MDP). We show that the RL agent learns using DQN to ask the best symptom and outperforms the decision tree approach while asking fewer questions. This paper makes the following contributions:

- We formulate the visual symptom checking problem as an MDP problem, and propose an RL-based approach to solve it.
- We show a significant accuracy improvement compared with the decision tree approach.

- We illustrate how the RL approach not only significantly improves the accuracy of the skin disease classification compared to the decision tree approach but also decreases the average number of asked questions.

2   A Visual Symptom Checker as an MDP

A visual symptom checker interacts with the patient by asking symptoms and receiving the patient's answer. In this section, we show how the visual symptom checking problem can be formulated as an MDP [6,8].

2.1   MDP Definition

An MDP is a tuple $(\mathcal{X}, \mathcal{A}, \mathcal{P}, \mathcal{R}, \gamma)$ where $\mathcal{X}$ is the set of states, $\mathcal{A}$ is a finite set of actions from which the agent can choose, $\mathcal{P} : \mathcal{X} \times \mathcal{A} \times \mathcal{X} \rightarrow [0, 1]$ is a transition probability in which $\mathcal{P}(x, a, x')$ defines the probability of observing state x' after executing action a in the state x, $\mathcal{R} : \mathcal{X} \times \mathcal{A} \rightarrow \mathbb{R}$ is the expected reward after being in state x and taking action a, and $\gamma \in [0, 1)$ is the discount factor.

An RL agent continually makes value judgments in order to select the right action. The action selection mechanism of an RL agent is called its policy, which is a mapping $\pi : \mathcal{X} \rightarrow \mathcal{A}$ from the state space to the action space. Given a policy π, the action-value function $Q^\pi : \mathcal{X} \times A \rightarrow \mathbb{R}$ is

$$Q^\pi(x, a) = \mathbb{E}\left[\sum_{k=0}^{\infty} \gamma^k r_{t+k+1} \mid X_t = x, A_t = a \right]. \tag{1}$$

The action-value function Q^π at state-action pair (x, a) is the expected discounted reward that the RL agent receives if it starts from state x at time t, chooses action a, and afterwards selects actions according to policy π, i.e., $A_{t+k} = \pi(X_{t+k})$ for $k = 1, 2, \ldots$. The goal of an RL agent is to find a policy π that maximizes this value for all state-action pairs. Such a policy is called the optimal policy π^*, and its corresponding action-value function is called the optimal action-value function Q^*. If the agent has access to the optimal action-value function, the optimal policy π^* can be computed as $\pi^*(x) \leftarrow \arg\max_{a \in \mathcal{A}} Q^*(x, a)$. Many RL algorithms, including Deep Q-Network (DQN) [4] that we briefly describe in Sect. 2.3, try to estimate Q^*. For more information, refer to [8].

We show how the MDP framework can be applied to the symptom checking problem in two steps: we first describe in Sect. 2.2 how $\mathcal{X}$, $\mathcal{A}$, $\mathcal{P}$ and $\mathcal{R}$ are designed for the symptom checker. Afterwards, we describe in Sect. 2.3 the agent's algorithm that improves the skin condition classification.

2.2   MDP Formulation

Let $\mathcal{S}$ be the symptom space. Some examples are rash, redness and pigmented lesion. Let $\mathcal{C}$ be the condition space. Some examples are cellulitis, psoriasis and melanoma, to name a few. We denote any symptom by s_i and any condition by c_j where $1 \leq i \leq |\mathcal{S}|$, $1 \leq j \leq |\mathcal{C}|$, and $|\cdot|$ refers to the cardinality operator. Let $\mathcal{S}^a \subset \mathcal{S}$ be the set of asked symptoms and s^a any asked symptom among $\mathcal{S}^a$.

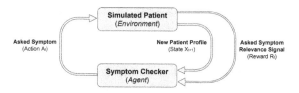

Fig. 1. The agent-patient interaction in an MDP.

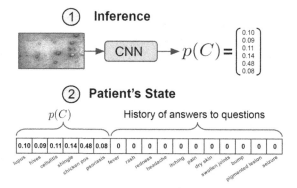

Fig. 2. State design of the simulated patient's environment: (1) CNN inference on the patient's image to compute $p(C)$ which is a vector of $|\mathcal{C}|$ elements. Here $|\mathcal{C}| = 6$, (2) The state of the simulated patient is a concatenation of $p(C)$ with the history of answers to questions, which is a vector of $|\mathcal{S}|$ elements. Here $|\mathcal{S}| = 11$.

A symptom checker agent learns which symptom $s \in \mathcal{S}$ to ask for an environment of a simulated patient having a condition $c^* \in \mathcal{C}$. Figure 1 summarizes pictorially how a symptom checker can be viewed as an RL agent finding an optimal policy for an MDP. We define the MDP parameters as follows:

- **Action space** $\mathcal{A}$: It corresponds to the symptom space $\mathcal{S}$ where each action $a \in \mathcal{A}$ is a possible symptom s to ask.
- **State space** $\mathcal{X}$: Each state $x \in \mathcal{X}$ corresponds to a patient state. A state x is the concatenation of the patient's history of all answers and the pretrained CNN's output probabilities of the patient's image (see Fig. 2).
- **Transition probability** $\mathcal{P}$: For an asked question, $+1$ or -1 are put at the question's position if the answer is respectively "yes" or "no" (see Fig. 3). For each new random patient simulation, its condition $c_i = c^*$ is known. The simulated patient answers the asked symptom s^a by referring to the

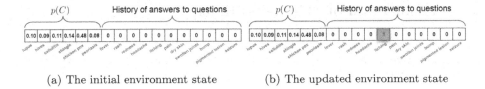

(a) The initial environment state   (b) The updated environment state

Fig. 3. An example of the update of environment state: (a) the vector of history answers is set to 0, (b) the environment state gets updated by putting +1 in the "itching" position after answering "yes" to the asked symptom "itching".

health knowledge matrix $\mathcal{M}$ [7] computed from electronic medical records of 273,174 patients. It represents a matrix of condition-symptom relationships where each cell (i, j) represents the conditional probability $p(s_j|c_i)$ of a symptom s_j given a condition c_i. The simulated environment answers s^a by generating a random number k from a uniform distribution between 0 and 1. If $k \leq p(s^a|c^*)$, the answer is "yes", and "no" otherwise.

- **Reward** $\mathcal{R}$: This function is equal to $p(c^*|S^a)$, the probability of correct condition c^* given the asked questions S^a. This design of the reward function is mainly based on the intuition that we want to keep the probability of the true condition of the simulated patient as high as possible. At each interaction, when the simulated patient answers s^a, we update the conditional probability $p(c_i|S^a)$ $\forall i$ using the Bayes rule as described in the Appendix A.

2.3   Deep Q-Learning

The visual symptom checker agent learns an estimate of the optimal action-value function Q^*. Mnih et al. [4] introduced the Deep Q-Network (DQN), a CNN approximating the action-value function $Q(x, a; \omega) \approx Q^*(x, a)$, where ω represents the network's parameters. The DQN squared error loss function $L(\omega)$ is defined as:

$$L(\omega) = \mathbb{E}\left[\left(r + \gamma \max_{a'} Q_{\text{target}}(x', a'; \omega^-) - Q_{\text{net}}(x, a; \omega) \right)^2 \right], \qquad (2)$$

where x is the current state, x' is the next-state, and γ is the discount factor. DQN uses $Q_{\text{target}}(\omega^-)$, a fixed version of $Q_{\text{net}}(\omega)$ with parameters ω^- that are periodically updated in order to stabilize rapid policy changes, due to the quick variations in Q-values. Another trick used in [4] to avoid divergence because of successive data sampling is the experience replay buffer. It stores transitions of (x, a, r, x') and is randomly sampled to create the mini-batches used for training.

3   Classification of Skin Conditions

In this section, we describe both the training and inference setting of the visual symptom checker. In our setting, we consider $|\mathcal{S}| = 330$, $|\mathcal{C}| = 9$, and the discount factor $\gamma = 0.99$.

3.1   The Training Step

We initially train an Inception-v3 network [9] on a dataset consisting of 5,841 images that are equally divided into 9 skin conditions: atopic dermatitis, lupus, shingles, cellulitis, chickenpox, hives, psoriasis, gout and melanoma. We have used a data split of 70%–15%–15% for training, validation and testing the CNN, respectively. For a given patient image, we run inference on the pretrained CNN to get the CNN's output probabilities which, concatenated with the history of answers initialized at zero, form the environment's state of the simulated patient. The RL agent interacts with this environment until either a predefined maximum number of questions to ask is reached or one of the 9 condition probabilities $p(c_i|S^a)$ exceeds a predefined threshold.

3.2   The Inference Step

We run inference on our visual symptom checker using annotated test images (i.e. a labeled image with a paragraph describing the patient's symptoms). The image description, commonly called a *vignette*, does not include the true condition of the patient, but rather their symptoms. We answer the asked questions of the trained RL agent with "yes" if the symptom is present in the vignette and with "no" otherwise. The Appendix B provides 9 examples of vignettes, one for each condition.

4   Experiments and Results

All the experiments have been performed within the simulated patient environment described in Sect. 2.2. We fix the maximum number of questions to ask at 10 and the confidence threshold to 95% respectively.

4.1   Architecture of the Q-Network (DQN)

The Q network has 5 layers: an input layer of 339 units (a vector of $|\mathcal{S}| = 330$ elements representing the history of answers concatenated with a vector of $|\mathcal{C}| = 9$ probabilities from the CNN output), 3 hidden fully connected layers consisting of 350 ReLu units and an output layer composed of $|\mathcal{S}| = 330$ linear units.

4.2 Evaluation

We have evaluated our visual symptom checker using 600 annotated test images. The evaluation metric chosen to compare the system before and after the visual symptom checker is the top-K accuracy, which is well known in medical imaging scenarios to successfully assess the differential diagnosis cases. Additionally, we compare the average number of asked questions between the RL approach and the decision tree approach in [1].

Top-K Accuracy. Table 1 shows how the RL agent that learns from a simulated patient environment increases the rank and the probability of the correct condition compared to the classification performance of the CNN alone. Here we show five-fold cross-validation classification accuracy for the CNN model. In each fold, a different fifth of the dataset is used for validation, with the rest of the dataset used for training. For the CNN model, reported values are the mean and standard deviation of the validation accuracy across all $n = 5$ folds.

Table 1. The CNN individual and combined classification performance with two QA models: RL and decision tree.

	CNN model	CNN + QA model	
		Decision tree	RL
Top-1	49.75 ± 0.2%	57.64 ± 0.3%	**70.41 ± 0.2%**
Top-2	63.55 ± 0.6%	73.01 ± 0.5%	**82.45 ± 0.1%**
Top-3	80.29 ± 0.5%	85.62 ± 0.5%	**91.22 ± 0.2%**

The results of the decision tree QA model are those of [1]. For the RL approach, 5 independent agents were trained on one of the 5 CNNs corresponding to a specific cross-validation fold. Reported values are the mean and standard deviation of the evaluation accuracy across all the 5 environments. These results demonstrate that the proposed RL approach can significantly improve the classification performance across a multiclass classification task and outperform the decision tree approach used in [1].

By sampling many times, the RL agent asymptotically learns, as the number of simulated patients increases, the conditional probabilities between symptoms and conditions. For instance, given two specific symptom s_0 and condition c_0, if $p(s_0|c_0) = 60\%$, the environment will answer 60% of the times "yes". Therefore, 60% of the data collected by the agent from a simulated patient with a condition c_0 will have s_0 included. The fact that the training data is balanced proportionally to the symptoms' occurrences allows the agent to learn the probabilistic relationships which is one reason explaining why the RL approach can outperform greedy approaches like decision trees. Another reason is that RL sequentially backtracks rewards unlike decision trees which search through the space of possible branches with no backtracking.

Average Number of Asked Questions. While the reported number of Table 1 are obtained after a maximum number of 10 questions, we examined the evolution of the top-K accuracy after answering each asked question by both the proposed RL-based QA model and the decision tree model studied in [1] on the same dataset. Figure 4 shows the evolution of the top-K accuracy with the number of asked questions for both approaches. One can see that both top-K accuracy and top-K rate of the RL approach are higher compared to the decision tree approach.

Additionally, the RL agent achieves its highest performance with fewer questions compared to the decision tree approach where top-K accuracy keeps increasing with a lower top-K accuracy rate as the number of questions increases. This suggests that the RL agent succeeds not only to narrow down the differential diagnosis with a better performance, but also quickly as compared with the decision tree approach.

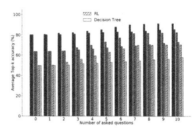

Fig. 4. Evolution of the top-3 (■), top-2 (■) and top-1 (□) accuracy with the number of asked questions. The top-K accuracy with a decision tree as QA model keeps increasing slowly. The top-K accuracy rate of the RL agent as a QA model is not only higher than the decision tree method but also converges quicker in around 7 questions (Color figure online).

5   Conclusion

The results of the visual symptom checker formulated as an RL problem demonstrate that the proposed methodology can effectively not only learn the probabilistic relationships between symptoms and conditions, but also find the most relevant questions to ask for improving the final predictions across the nine skin conditions considered. Future work remains as to extend the symptom checker to support more conditions and symptoms and to further look into ways to evaluate its performance against doctors and other diagnostic systems.

Acknowledgements. We thank the rest of the Triage team for assisting with infrastructure and evaluation, as well as with providing feedback and helpful discussions. We acknowledge Mitacs Accelerate program for the funding they provide.

References

1. Akrout, M., Farahmand, A.M., Jarmain, T.: Improving skin condition classification with a question answering model. In: Medical Imaging Meets NeurIPS Workshop (2018). https://arxiv.org/abs/1811.06165
2. Chali, Y., Hasan, S.A., Mojahid, M.: A reinforcement learning formulation to the complex question answering problem. Inf. Process. Manage. **51**(3), 252–272 (2015)
3. Choi, E., Bahadori, M.T., Schuetz, A., Stewart, W.F., Sun, J.: Doctor AI: predicting clinical events via recurrent neural networks. In: Machine Learning for Healthcare Conference, pp. 301–318 (2016)
4. Mnih, V., et al.: Human-level control through deep reinforcement learning. Nature **518**(7540), 529 (2015)
5. Nogueira, R., Cho, K.: Task-oriented query reformulation with reinforcement learning. In: Proceedings of the 2017 Conference on Empirical Methods in Natural Language Processing, Copenhagen, Denmark, September 2017, pp. 574–583. Association for Computational Linguistics (2017)
6. Puterman, M.L.: Markov Decision Processes: Discrete Stochastic Dynamic Programming. Wiley, New York (1994)
7. Rotmensch, M., Halpern, Y., Tlimat, A., Horng, S., Sontag, D.: Learning a health knowledge graph from electronic medical records. Sci. rep. **7**(1), 5994 (2017)
8. Sutton, R.S., Barto, A.G.: Reinforcement Learning: An Introduction, 2nd edn. MIT Press, Cambridge (2018)
9. Szegedy, C., Vanhoucke, V., Ioffe, S., Shlens, J., Wojna, Z.: Rethinking the inception architecture for computer vision. In: Proceedings of the IEEE Conference on Computer Vision and Pattern Recognition, pp. 2818–2826 (2016)
10. Wei, Z., et al.: Task-oriented dialogue system for automatic diagnosis. In: Proceedings of the 56th Annual Meeting of the Association for Computational Linguistics, vol. 2: Short papers, pp. 201–207 (2018)
11. Zagorecki, A., Orzechowski, P., Holownia, K.: A system for automated general medical diagnosis using Bayesian networks. In: MedInfo, pp. 461–465 (2013)

DScGANS: Integrate Domain Knowledge in Training Dual-Path Semi-supervised Conditional Generative Adversarial Networks and S3VM for Ultrasonography Thyroid Nodules Classification

Wenkai Yang[1], Juanjuan Zhao[1], Yan Qiang[1(✉)], Xiaotang Yang[2],
Yunyun Dong[1], Qianqian Du[1], Guohua Shi[1],
and Muhammad Bilal Zia[1]

[1] Taiyuan University of Technology, No.79 West Street Yingze, Taiyuan,
Shanxi, China
qiangyan@tyut.edu.cn
[2] Department of Radiology, Shanxi Province Cancer Hospital,
Shanxi Medical University, Taiyuan 030013, China

Abstract. Semi-supervised learning can reduce the burden of manual label data and improve classification performance by learning with unlabelled data. However, due to the absence of label constraints, unlabelled data is usually ambiguous, which typically results in requiring large datasets to learn the correct feature space distribution. The inherently small sample characteristics of medical image datasets may make semi-supervised learning unstable, which may lead to mixed results and even degrade performance. The domain knowledge (DK) of the physician is of great value for disease diagnosis. In this paper, we propose to promote semi-supervised learning with DK and develop a DScGANS model (DScGAN (dual-path semi-supervised conditional generative adversarial networks) and S3VM (semi-supervised support vector machine)) to diagnose ultrasound thyroid nodules. DScGAN uses DK as a condition and multimodal ultrasound data for training. We concatenate the image representation of DScGAN learning and use it as the input of S3VM. DK will be used as a condition to constrain S3VM for thyroid nodule classification. The experimental results show that our proposed model can effectively avoid mixed results that may occur in semi-supervised learning with a small medical dataset with insufficient labels. Additionally, our model provides stable and advanced diagnostic performance and is potentially integrated into the thyroid ultrasound system.

Keywords: Domain knowledge · Semi-supervised · Generative adversarial networks · Ultrasound · Thyroid nodules classification

1 Introduction

Ultrasonography has become the preferred method for clinical diagnosis of thyroid nodules [1]. The Thyroid Imaging Reporting and Data System (TI-RADS) [2] provides standardised terminology that describes thyroid nodule features in ultrasound B-mode

© Springer Nature Switzerland AG 2019
D. Shen et al. (Eds.): MICCAI 2019, LNCS 11767, pp. 558–566, 2019.
https://doi.org/10.1007/978-3-030-32251-9_61

images, including boundary, calcification, echo pattern, etc. Ultrasound elastography reflects the hardness of lesion tissue by using the colour distribution ratio [3]. In clinical diagnosis, radiologists generally consider these two kinds of information together and then give diagnostic results. However, manual diagnostics not only have a large workload but also have subjective differences. Therefore, reducing the workload and misdiagnosis rate of radiologists by computer-aided diagnosis is important.

Recently, deep learning has become greatly successful in the diagnosis of ultrasound thyroid nodules. Among them, semi-supervised learning has been receiving increasingly more attention because it can greatly reduce the burden of manually annotating data by using unlabelled data for learning [4, 5]. Wang et al. [4] proposed a semi-supervised learning model based on weak label data for the diagnosis of thyroid nodules. Ding et al. [5] used the MIL (multiple-instance learning) method to extract pre-designed features of ultrasound B-mode and elasticity data and applied SVM for classification. Although these methods produce commendable results, the inherently small sample characteristics of medical image datasets may make the semi-supervised learning process unstable, which will lead to mixed results and even degrade the performance of the model. Therefore, how to ensure stable and advanced diagnostic performance when performing semi-supervised learning on a small medical dataset with insufficient labels remains a challenging issue.

To address these challenges, we propose the DScGANS model (DScGAN (dual-path semi-supervised conditional generative adversarial networks) and the S3VM (semi-supervised support vector machine)), which is built by combining semi-supervised generative adversarial networks (sGAN) [6], conditional generative adversarial networks (cGAN) [7] and S3VM [8]. The uniqueness of our model includes the following: (1) We quantify the features of thyroid nodules in the B-mode ultrasound image described by TI-RADS and the hardness information of lesion tissue in the elasticity image and use them as domain knowledge (DK) to promote semi-supervised learning; (2) DK acts as a conditional constraint generator to produce higher quality images. When DK connects with deep features of labelled data in the discriminant network, correlation information between DK, deep features and class labels will be learned. The correlation information can be used as a condition constraint for the unlabelled data when DK is connected with deep features of unlabelled data. Thus, the ambiguity of unlabelled data will significantly reduce, which will enable DScGAN to use unlabelled data for stable and high-performing feature extraction; (3) DK is used as a condition to constrain S3VM for thyroid nodule classification. As S3VM combines powerful regularization-based SVMs with the cluster assumption [9], when concatenating DK and the deep features learned by DScGAN as the input of S3VM, the conditional constraint DK will make the different class of unlabelled data more inclined to their own cluster, which greatly improves the classification results. The experimental results show that our proposed model can provide a stable 90.5% accuracy and 91.4% AUC using only 35% of labelled data by semi-supervised learning and potentially integrated into the thyroid ultrasound system.

2 Datasets

We collected 3090 fully anonymous thyroid nodule lesion images of 1030 different age stages (the age older than 18 years) patients from the co-operative hospital and ensured that different sizes of nodules were included. The average size of the nodules is 2.4 cm. Each lesion image includes two types of images, B-mode and elasticity, which correspond to the same lesion area. In 3090 pairs of images, including 1601 pairs of benign nodules and 1489 pairs of malignant nodules. Each pair of images is labelled as benign or malignant by two senior radiologists based on pathological examination results. Finally, a total of 6180 images are obtained, with each type of image accounting for 50%.

3 Methods

Our proposed DScGANS model is shown in Fig. 1. The model has three steps: (1) image pre-processing and augmentation, (2) acquiring DK, and then use the B-mode and elastic data as input to train the DScGAN component (DScGAN-A/B) under the constraints of DK, (3) saving the discriminator network as a feature extraction network and concatenating the output image representation of a penultimate fully connected layer (the output result includes both deep features and DK) as input to S3VM for thyroid nodule classification.

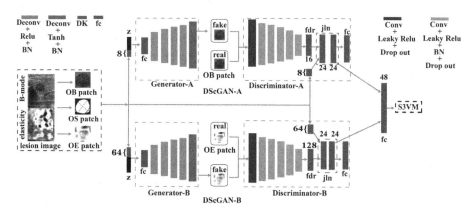

Fig. 1. Framework of our proposed DScGANS model, where fc denotes a fully connected layer, fdr denotes a feature dimension reduction layer, and jln denotes a joint learning network.

3.1 Image Preprocessing and Augmentation

From each B-mode image, we obtain square regions of interest (ROI) by using the method in [10] and define the ROI as an OB patch. We also obtain an elasticity ROI according to the B-mode ROI position and define it as the OE patch. To characterise the shape of the nodule, we use the live-wire algorithm [11] to semi-automatically segment the nodule area in the OB patch with the help of an experienced radiologist; then, we set the pixel value of the nodule region to 255 and that of the non-nodule region to 0 and define it as an OS patch. Then, the OB patch, OE patch, and OS patch are resized to 128 × 128. We applied data augmentation (including random rotation and horizontal and vertical flipping) to enlarge each patch and apply them to form three datasets. Note that the OS patch is only used to automatically extract DK, while the OB and OE patches are the inputs of DScGAN-A and DScGAN-B.

3.2 Automatic Acquisition of Domain Knowledge

According to TI-RADS [2] and the elastography score [3] and after discussing with experienced radiologists, we calculated the following DK.

1. **Dimension.** First, the OS patch is fitted using an ellipse [12]. For two axes of the fitting ellipse, the axis closer to the horizontal is defined as the horizontal axis, and its length is represented by L_h. The other axis is defined as the vertical axis, and its length is represented by L_v. L_h and L_v are used as the values of dimension.
2. **Orientation.** Growth direction is important for reflecting the shape of the nodule. We use the rotation angle of the fitting ellipse as the values of orientation.
3. **Aspect ratio.** The aspect ratio of malignant nodules is likely to be greater than 1 [2]. The ratio of L_v to L_h is used as the aspect ratio.
4. **Boundary feature.** It can be described as clear or unclear. According to the nodule area (pixel value is 255) and surrounding tissue (pixel value is 0) in the OS patch, we use acutance [13] to calculate the nodule boundary feature in the OB patch.
5. **Echo pattern.** This pattern can be described as hypoechoic, hyperechoic, or isoe-choic. Locate the nodule area with the OS patch. We calculated the ratio of the gray value of the nodule area to the gray value of the surrounding tissue area in the OB patch and used it as the value of the echo pattern.
6. **Cystic or Solid.** A cystic nodule is more likely to be benign. Locate the nodule area with the OS patch. We calculated the average gray value of the nodule area in the OB patch and used the result to determine if the value represents cystic or solid.
7. **Calcification.** The calcification can be described as coarse or micro-calcification. Locate the nodule area with the OS patch. We calculated the calcification infor-mation of the nodule area in the OB patch using the method in [13].
8. **Elastography colour distribution.** The colour distribution is quantised by calcu-lating the RGB colour histogram inside the image [14]. For each OE patch, a 1 × 64-dimensional vector is obtained as values of elastography colour distribution.

Finally, the DK dimensions of the B-mode and elasticity patches are 1 × 8 and 1 × 64.

3.3 DScGAN Component

The DScGAN component is built by combining sGAN [6] and cGAN [7].

Generator: We use G to indicate, which consists of a fully connected layer and five deconvolution layers, the parameter is θ_g. Each input random noise vector z has a corresponding DK as condition $\boldsymbol{Dk}$, which is obtained from the real image corresponding to a fake image. G can use both to generate image patch $G((z, \boldsymbol{Dk}); \theta_g)$.

Discriminator: We use D to indicate, which consists of six convolutional layers, a feature dimension reduction layer (fdr), a joint learning network (jln) and a fully connected layer; the parameter is θ_d. The fdr layer is a fully connected layer that has 16 neurons (DScGAN-B has 128 neurons) and is used to reduce the dimension of deep features before concatenating the DK and deep features. Our experimental results demonstrate that high-dimensional deep features will overwhelm low-dimensional DK if they are connected directly. After the DK and deep features are concatenated, they are fed into the jln. The jln consists of two fully connected layers to learn the correlation information between DK, deep features and class labels of labelled data. Assuming that the real image patch has k classes, we define the image patch generated by G as the $(k+1)$-th class. Thus, the last fully connected layer has $(k+1)$ neurons, of which the first k are softmax neurons, and the $(k+1)$-th is a sigmoid neuron. An input image patch I may come from a real image with a label $data(x, y)$, a real image without a label $data(x)$, or a generated fake image $G((\boldsymbol{z}, \boldsymbol{Dk}); \theta_g)$. We use the first k neurons to calculate the class probability that the input $I \sim data(x, y)$ belongs to class j as follows:

$$P_D(y = j|(I, \boldsymbol{Dk})) = D^{(j)}((I, \boldsymbol{Dk}); \theta_d) \tag{1}$$

where y is the class label of input I. We use the $(k+1)$-th neuron to calculate the probability that the input I is from the real image $data(x)$ or the fake image $G((\boldsymbol{z}, \boldsymbol{Dk}); \theta_g)$. We define the output of th e $(k+1)$-th neuron as $D^{(k+1)}((I, \boldsymbol{Dk}); \theta_d)$ as follows:

$$P_D(l = 0|(I, \boldsymbol{Dk})) = D^{(k+1)}((I, \boldsymbol{Dk}); \theta_d) \tag{2}$$

If I is from a fake image, the value of variable l is 0; otherwise the value is 1.

3.4   Training

To train the DScGAN component, we use a variety of loss functions during the training process. For the input random noise vector z, the generator loss function is:

$$L_G = -E_{I \sim G((\boldsymbol{z}, \boldsymbol{Dk}), \theta_g)} \log\{P_D(l = 1|(I, \boldsymbol{Dk}))\} \tag{3}$$

The loss function of the discriminator consists of two parts: the supervised loss function L_{D_su} and the unsupervised loss function L_{D_un}. We use L_{D_un} as the loss of distinguishing whether input I is from the real or fake image and L_{D_su} as the loss of distinguishing whether input I belongs to class j. Given an input I, the loss function of the discriminator is:

$$L_D = L_{D\_su} + L_{D\_un} \tag{4}$$

$$\text{where,}\quad L_{D\_su} = -E_{I \sim data(x,y)} \log\{P_D(y = j|(I, \boldsymbol{Dk}))\} \tag{5}$$

$$L_{D\_un} = -E_{l \sim data(x)} \log\{P_D(l = 1|(I, Dk))\} - E_{l \sim G((z,Dk),\theta_g)} \log\{P_D(l = 0|(I, Dk))\}$$

(6)

S3VM Classifier. S3VM [8] is used as a classifier, given its good application in the two-category classification task. We denote F_α and F_β as the outputs of the penultimate fully connected layer of DScGAN-A and DScGAN-B, which contain their own deep features and DK. We concatenate F_α with F_β, and define them as feature vector $F_{\alpha*\beta}$. Thus, DK will be used as a conditional constraint for unlabelled data during the classification process of S3VM. Assuming that $F_{\alpha*\beta}^{(i)}$ represents the i-th vector in $F_{\alpha*\beta}$, $L = \left\{ \left(F_{\alpha*\beta}^{(1)}, y_1 \right), \ldots, \left(F_{\alpha*\beta}^{(m)}, y_m \right) \right\}$ denote the labelled dataset, y_m is the benign or malignant label, $U = \left\{ F_{\alpha*\beta}^{(m+1)}, \ldots, F_{\alpha*\beta}^{(m+n)} \right\}$ denote the unlabelled dataset, and $f\left(F_{\alpha*\beta}^{(i)} \right) = \left\langle \omega, \varphi\left(F_{\alpha*\beta}^{(i)} \right) \right\rangle + b$ is the discriminating hyperplane. ω is the hyperplane normal vector, b is the offset term, and φ is a transformation function from an input space to a high-dimensional reproducing kernel Hilbert space. The S3VM discriminator optimisation problem is as follows:

$$min_{\omega, b} \frac{1}{2} \langle \omega, \omega \rangle + C \sum_{i=1}^{m} H\left(y_i f\left(F_{\alpha*\beta}^{(i)} \right) \right) + C^* \sum_{i=m+1}^{m+n} \tilde{H}\left(\left| f\left(F_{\alpha*\beta}^{(i)} \right) \right| \right) \quad (7)$$

where $H(t)$ is the hinge loss of labelled data, $\tilde{H}(t)$ is the symmetric hinge loss of unlabelled data, C is the regularization parameter, and C^* is the penalization parameter of unlabelled data. When $C^* = 0$, Eq. (7) will degenerate into the standard SVM.

4 Experiments and Results

In our experiments, we randomly divide the dataset in a mutually exclusive way: 80% for training, and 20% as an independent test set. To mitigate the problem that labelled data are usually too few to perform effective cross-validation, 5-fold cross-validation is thus used at each stage to increase the number of labelled data in each fold and tested on an independent test set for evaluation. Since more than one ultrasound image can be collected from each patient, we ensure that the image patches from the same patient are assigned to the same folding.

Table 1 shows the mean and standard deviation (std) of the predictive capability of the DScGANS model on the test set. Specifically, 25% means that 25% of data in the training set are labelled, which are obtained by random selection. FSL (fully supervised learning) indicates that the training set is composed entirely of labelled data. We applied ten experiments on the training set independently (ensuring that all samples were used as labelled and unlabelled data to form the training set at least once), with 5-fold cross-validation, and calculated the average test result on the test set. The results indicate that regardless of the proportion of labelled data being used, the standard deviation of the obtained performance is smaller when using DK. This result clearly shows that DK tremendously improves the stability of semi-supervised learning. Furthermore, with the help of DK, our proposed model can achieve stable and advanced diagnostic performance that is almost on par with that of FSL, using only approximately 30%–35% of labelled data. Subsequently, we continue to increase the amount of labelled data without significant performance gains.

Table 1. The mean ± std of the predictive capability of the proposed DScGANS model using different amounts of labelled data with or without DK on the test set

	DScGANS						
	DK (No)				DK (Yes)		
	25%	30%	35%	FSL	25%	30%	35%
Acc (%)	79.2 ± 0.16	80.5 ± 0.13	81.6 ± 0.12	90.8 ± 0.05	88.3 ± 0.10	90.2 ± 0.07	**90.5 ± 0.06**
Sen (%)	75.7 ± 0.31	76.7 ± 0.25	78.8 ± 0.20	88.5 ± 0.09	85.6 ± 0.13	87.8 ± 0.09	**88.1 ± 0.08**
Spe (%)	80.6 ± 0.23	83.2 ± 0.18	84.1 ± 0.14	92.9 ± 0.05	91.2 ± 0.11	92.5 ± 0.07	**92.6 ± 0.07**
AUC (%)	78.5 ± 0.13	80.5 ± 0.11	81.2 ± 0.10	91.7 ± 0.03	88.6 ± 0.05	91.2 ± 0.04	**91.4 ± 0.04**

5 Discussion

Comparison of Deep Features and DK Combinations in Different Dimensions:
Figure 2 shows the ROC curve and AUC value obtained when the original deep feature (without dimensionality reduction) and the reduced dimensional feature size are 3, 2, or 1 times that of DK, using 35% of the labelled data (given this situation, almost optimal performance is obtained with minimal labelled data). When the dimension of the deep features was twice that of DK, the proposed model obtained an optimal AUC value. Plausibly, the deep learning model can capture more valuable implied information than can human experts, and when the dimension of deep features is too high, DK will be overwhelmed, which will degrade the performance of the DScGANS model.

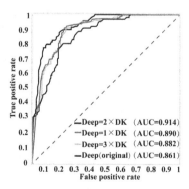

Fig. 2. ROC curve and AUC value of the proposed DScGANS model when using different dimensional deep features and DK combinations.

S3VM Kernel Function and Parameter C and C* Setting: In Table 2, we compare the test results of using the linear kernel and the Gaussian kernel (based on libsvm in sklearn[1]) on different proportions of labelled data. Specifically, 25% means that 25% of the data in the training set are labelled. To mitigate the possible negative effect of unlabelled data on the results, we set C^* to begin with a small value and reach the same value as C when the model converges and define $C^* = C_p \times C$, where C_p is the proportionality factor of C. Note that C^* is 0 in FSL. The grid search strategy was adopted to find optimal parameters. Finally, we use the Gaussian kernel and $C = 10$, $C_p = 0.2$ and $\gamma = 2$ with 35% of labelled data and obtain stable and advanced diagnostic performance that is almost on par with that of FSL.

Table 2. Two kernel functions and optimal parameters obtained using the grid search strategy

	Linear			Gaussian		
	25%	30%	35%	25%	30%	35%
	(C, C_p)	(C, C_p)	(C, C_p)	(C, C_p, γ)	(C, C_p, γ)	(C, C_p, γ)
	(5, 0.5)	(5, 0.4)	(5, 0.25)	(5, 0.4, 4)	(10, 0.25, 2)	(10, 0.2, 2)
Acc (%)	86.4	87.2	88.6	88.3	90.2	**90.5**
AUC (%)	84.6	85.8	86.7	88.6	91.2	**91.4**

6 Conclusion

We propose the DScGANS model for the diagnosis of ultrasound thyroid nodules based on multimodal ultrasound data. The experimental results suggest that with the help of DK, our proposed model can effectively avoid mixed results that may occur when learning with a small medical dataset with insufficient labels and can provide stable and advanced diagnostic performance; this model can be potentially integrated into the thyroid ultrasound system. In future works, we aim to achieve automatic segmentation of the nodules and integrate more types of DK to train the proposed model and extend our model to real medical environments.

Acknowledgements. This work is partly supported by the National Natural Science Foundation of China (Grant number 61872261), the Funding Project of State Key Laboratory of Virtual Reality Technology and Systems, Beihang University (Grant No. 2018-VRLAB2018B07), Shanxi Scholarship Council of China (201801D121139) and the Department of Radiology, Shanxi Province Cancer Hospital.

---

[1] https://scikit-learn.org/stable/modules/svm.html#svm-kernels

References

1. Acharya, U.R., Faust, O., Sree, S.V., et al.: ThyroScreen system: high resolution ultrasound thyroid image characterization into benign and malignant classes using novel combination of texture and discrete wavelet transform. Comput. Methods Programs Biomed. **107**(2), 233–241 (2012)
2. Park, J.Y., Lee, H.J., Jang, H.W., et al.: A proposal for a thyroid imaging reporting and image system for ultrasound features of thyroid carcinoma. Thyroid **19**(11), 1257–1264 (2009)
3. Hong, Y., et al.: Real-time ultrasound elastography in the differential diagnosis of benign and malignant thyroid nodules. J. Ultrasound Med. **28**(7), 861–867 (2009)
4. Wang, J., Li, S., Song, W., et al.: Learning from weakly-labelled clinical image for automatic thyroid nodule classification in ultrasound images. In: 2018 25th IEEE International Conference on Image Processing (ICIP), pp. 3114–3118. IEEE (2018)
5. Ding, J., Cheng, H., Huang, J., et al.: Multiple-instance learning with global and local features for thyroid ultrasound image classification. In: 2014 7th International Conference on Biomedical Engineering and Informatics, pp. 66–70. IEEE (2014)
6. Odena, A.: Semi-supervised learning with generative adversarial networks. arXiv preprint arXiv:1606.01583 (2016)
7. Mirza, M., Osindero, S.: Conditional generative adversarial nets. arXiv preprint arXiv:1411.1784 (2014)
8. Gu, B., Yuan, X.T., Chen, S., et al.: New incremental learning algorithm for semi-supervised support vector machine. In: Proceedings of the 24th ACM SIGKDD International Conference on Knowledge Discovery & Data Mining, pp. 1475–1484. ACM (2018)
9. Chapelle, O., Zien, A.: Semi-supervised classification by low density separation. In: AISTATS 2005, pp. 57–64 (2005)
10. Koundal, D., Vishraj, R., Gupta, S., et al.: An automatic ROI extraction technique for Thyroid Ultrasound image. In: 2015 2nd International Conference on Recent Advances in Engineering & Computational Sciences (RAECS), pp. 1–5. IEEE (2015)
11. Falcão, A.X., Udupa, J.K., Samarasekera, S., et al.: User-steered image segmentation paradigms: live wire and live lane. Graph. Models Image Process. **60**(4), 233–260 (1998)
12. Fitzgibbon, A., Pilu, M., Fisher, R.B.: Direct least square fitting of ellipses. IEEE Trans. Pattern Anal. Mach. Intell. **21**(5), 476–480 (1999)
13. Wang, H., Yang, Y., Peng, B., et al.: A thyroid nodule classification method based on TI-RADS. In: Ninth International Conference on Digital Image Processing (ICDIP 2017), vol. 10420, pp. 1042041. International Society for Optics and Photonics (2017)
14. Zhou, J.X., Liu, X., Xu, T.W., et al.: A new fusion approach for content-based image retrieval with color histogram and local directional pattern. Int. J. Mach. Learn. Cybernet. **9**(4), 677–689 (2018). https://doi.org/10.1007/s13042-016-0597-9

Similarity Steered Generative Adversarial Network and Adaptive Transfer Learning for Malignancy Characterization of Hepatocellualr Carcinoma

Hanqiu Ju[1], Wanwei Jian[1], Xiaoping Cen[1], Guangyi Wang[2], and Wu Zhou[1(✉)]

[1] School of Medical Information Engineering,
Guangzhou University of Chinese Medicine, Guangzhou, China
zhouwu@gzucm.edu.cn
[2] Department of Radiology, Guangdong General Hospital, Guangzhou, China

Abstract. Deep learning with Convolutional Neural Network (CNN) has exhibited high diagnostic performance for lesion characterization. However, it is still challenging to train powerful deep learning systems for lesion characterization, because there are often limited samples in different malignancy types and there exist considerable variabilities across images from multiple scanners in clinical practice. In this work, we propose a similarity steered generative adversarial network (SSGAN) coupled with pre-train and adaptive fine-turning of data from multiple scanners for lesion characterization. Specifically, SSGAN is based on adding a similarity discriminative measure in the conventional generative adversarial network to effectively generate more discrepant samples, while the adaptive fine-tune strategy is adopted to optimally make decisions on whether to use the pre-train layers or the fine-tune layers. Experimental results of pathologically confirmed malignancy of clinical hepatocellular carcinoma (HCCs) with MR images acquired by different scanners (GE, Philips and Siemens) demonstrate several intriguing characteristics of the proposed end-to-end framework for malignancy characterization of HCC as follows: (1) The proposed SSGAN remarkably improves the performance of lesion characterization and outperforms several recently proposed methods. (2) The adaptive fine-tuning combined with the proposed SSGAN can further improve the performance of lesion characterization in the context of limited data. (3) Clinical images acquired by one MR scanner for pre-train can be used to improve the characterization performance of images acquired by another MR scanner, outperforming the pre-train with ImageNet.

1 Introduction

Preoperative malignancy differentiation of hepatocellular carcinoma (HCC) is important for establishing treatment strategies and predicting treatment outcomes and prognosis [1]. Computer-aided methods combined with machine learn-

© Springer Nature Switzerland AG 2019
D. Shen et al. (Eds.): MICCAI 2019, LNCS 11767, pp. 567–574, 2019.
https://doi.org/10.1007/978-3-030-32251-9_62

ing techniques have shown great potential for providing radiologists with a second opinion on the visual diagnosis of diseased malignancies [2]. In particular, the deep features obtained from sample learning based on data-driven methods show excellent ability to describe tumor features [3]. Although deep features based on deep learning techniques have been shown to be promising for lesion characterization, it is still challenging to train powerful deep learning systems for lesion characterization, because there are often limited samples in different malignancy types in addition to the variability across images from multiple scanners in clinical practice [4].

Generative Adversarial Network (GAN) has been widely applied for data augmentation to improve the performance of deep learning [5]. Salimans et al. proposed a semi-supervised learning model by simply adding samples generated by GAN to the actual data to improve the performance of classification [6]. Subsequently, Shams et al. used a similar semi-supervised learning to combine CNN and GAN for breast cancer screening and diagnosis [7]. Mahapatra et al. proposed a content loss combined with GAN and CNN, which encourages the generated samples to have a different appearance than the real data, where the content loss is measured by the mutual information (NMI), the L2 distance and the intensity mean square error between the generated image and the real image [8]. However, these similarity measures in content loss are closely related to the nature of the image and may not be suitable for processing diverse images and also subject to image artifacts and noise. In addition, due to the expensive calculation of NMI, the calculation of content loss is very time consuming. Therefore, it is desirable to develop new methods to accurately and efficiently improve the discrepancy of generated samples.

Furthermore, the technique of transfer learning has been expected to mitigate the problem of variability of images across multiple scanners in the society of Radiology [9]. Previous studies have shown that CNN models pre-trained with a typical computer vision database (ImageNet) have been shown to improve the classification performance of medical image analysis [10]. Since the features of ImageNet are significantly different from those of specific medical images, it can be anticipated that a CNN model pre-trained using data from different MR scanners may be superior to pre-training with ImageNet to improve the performance of lesion characterization. In addition, a recent study shows that fine-tuning with the final fully connected layer can improve classification performance [11]. Meanwhile, another recently proposed study proposes an adaptive fine-tuning strategy in computer vision based on a policy network, which makes the optimal decision on which layer is frozen and which layer is fine-tuned [12]. Inspired by the concept of the policy network, it is expected that the adaptive fine-tuning strategy may be effective to simulate the image variability of multiple scanners, thereby mitigating image variation problems between multiple scanners. Therefore, we hypothesize that pre-training and adaptive fine-tuning of data from different MR scanners may improve the performance of lesion characterization in clinical practice.

In this work, we propose a similarity steered generative adversarial network (SSGAN) coupled with pre-train and adaptive fine-turning of data from multiple scanners for lesion characterization. Specifically, we introduce a similarity discriminative network to make the GAN efficiently generate more discrepant samples, while we adopt an adaptive fine-tune strategy to optimally make decisions on whether to use the pre-train layers or the fine-tune layers. Finally, we devise hybrid loss functions to embed the similarity discriminative network, GAN, policy network and CNN into the proposed end-to-end framework for malignancy characterization of HCC.

2 Method

The architecture of our proposed method is shown in Fig. 1. The network is comprised of several components: generator, discriminator, policy network and similarity discriminative network, where the generator, the similarity discriminative network and the discriminator jointly constitute the end-to-end similarity steered GAN based classification network (SSGAN). The generator is trained to generate images that cannot be distinguished by the discriminator, the discriminator is trained adversarially to figure out whether the input images are real or fake, the policy network is trained jointly with the discriminator and to decide which layer is frozen and which layer is fine-tuned, and the similarity discriminative network is trained to measure the similarity between the generated images and the real images to increase the discrepancy of the generated images. We will illustrate the details of the proposed framework in the following sections.

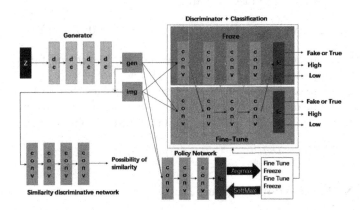

Fig. 1. The architecture of our proposed method.

2.1 Similarity Steered Generative Adversarial Network

Inspired by GAN [5], the similarity discrimination is performed on the generated patch and the real patch, which is implemented by the fully convolutional network (FCN). The detailed architecture of the proposed similarity discriminative network is shown in the bottom left of Fig. 1, which consists of four downsampling convolutional blocks. Note that the last convolutional layer is activated by sigmoid function. Let $\{X_i, y_i\}_{i=1}^N$ represent a set of N input patches, where X_i and y_i denote the patch and its label, respectively. The generator takes the random noise as input and outputs the generated patch. Let G denote the generator and θ_g denote its parameters. Let z denote a random noise, the generated patch can be denoted as $G(z; \theta_g)$. Considering that a standard classifier classifies an input patch into one of k possible classes, the number of neurons of the last fully connected layer is increased from k to $k+1$. The output of the first k neurons are activated by Softmax function and the output of the $(k+1)^{th}$ neuron is activated by sigmoid function.

As the discriminator both discriminates real patches from those generated patches and performs lesion classification, there are two loss functions for the discriminator. The loss for discriminating real patches from generated patches is:

$$L_d(z, X) = -logP(r = 1|X) - logP(r = 0|G(z; \theta_g)) \tag{1}$$

where r is the output value of the $(k+1)^{th}$ neuron and takes value 1 if the patch is from a real patch and 0 otherwise. For the lesion classification loss, we adopt cross-entropy as the loss function. The loss function for lesion classification is:

$$L_c(X, y) = -\sum_i y^{(i)} logP(y = y^{(i)}|X) \tag{2}$$

Finally, the loss function of the similarity discriminative network is similar to the loss function for the discriminator:

$$L_s(z, X) = -logP(r' = 1|X) - logP(r' = 0|G(z; \theta_g)) \tag{3}$$

where r' is the output value of the last convolutional layer and takes value 1 if the patch is completely similar to a real patch and 0 otherwise.

As the purpose of the generator is to generate patches that look like the real one and meanwhile different from the real one, the loss function of the generator contains the real-looking part and the similarity discriminative part:

$$L_g(z) = -logP(r = 1|G(z; \theta_g)) - logP(r' = 0|G(z; \theta_g)) \tag{4}$$

2.2 GAN-Based Adaptive Fine-Tuning

We first pre-train the discriminator with pre-trained data in the SSGAN, and then their parameters are transferred to the frozen part and fine-tune part as shown in Fig. 1. The mechanism of the adaptive fine-tuning for the CNN model used in the present work is inspired by the recently proposed work of spot-tune in the residual network [12]. It is evident that the initial parameters of the frozen part and fine-tune part are the same. Let $F_l(x_{l-1})$ and $F'_l(x_{l-1})$ denote the output of the lth layer of the frozen part and the output of the lth layer of the fine-tune part, respectively, where x_{l-1} denotes the output of the $l - 1^{th}$ layer of the discriminator. The output of the lth layer of the discriminator is:

$$x_l = I_l(x_l)F_l'(x_{l-1}) + (1 - I_l(x_l))F_l(x_{l-1}) \qquad (5)$$

where $I_l(x_l)$ is a binary random variable, which indicates whether the parameter of the lth layer should be frozen or fine-tuned, conditioned on the input image. $I_l(x)$ is sampled from a discrete distribution with two categories (freeze or fine-tune), which is parameterized by the output of the policy network depicted in Fig. 1. However, $I_l(x_l)$ is discrete, which makes the optimization of the network non-differentiable. The Gumbel-Max trick [13] can draw samples from a categorical distribution parameterized by $\alpha_1, \alpha_2, ..., \alpha_z$, where α_i are scalars not confined to the simplex, and z is the number of categories. In the present work, we just consider two categories, namely froze or fine-tune. As a result, z is 2. A random variable G is said to have a standard Gumbel distribution if $G = -log(-log(U))$ with U sampled from a uniform distribution, i.e. $U \sim Unif[0, 1]$. Based on the Gumbel-Max trick, samples can be drawn from a discrete distribution parameterized by α_i in the following way: we first draw samples $G_i, ..., G_z$ from Gumbel $(0, 1)$ and then generate the discrete sample as follows:

$$A = argmax_i[log\alpha_i + G_i] \qquad (6)$$

The argmax operation is non-differentiable. However, the Gumbel Softmax distribution can be used [12,14], which adopts Softmax as a continuous relaxation to argmax. Let A represent a one-hot vector where the index of the non-zero entry of the vector is equal to A, and the one-hot encoding of A is relaxed to a z-dimensional real-valued vector Y using Softmax:

$$Y_i = \frac{exp((log\alpha_i + G_i)/\tau)}{\sum_{j=1}^{z} exp((log\alpha_i + G_i)/\tau)} \qquad for \quad i = 1, 2, \cdots, z \qquad (7)$$

where τ is a temperature parameter, which controls the discreteness of the output vector Y. During the forward pass, the fine-tuning policy $I_l(x)$ is sampled using Eq. (5) for the lth layer. During the backward pass, the gradient of the discrete samples is approximated by computing the gradient of the continuous Softmax relaxation in Eq. (7).

2.3   The Implementation and Training

The proposed framework was implemented by an open source deep learning framework "Tensorflow". Date augmentation based on image resampling is first adopted to generate more 2D real patches (e.g., 125 patches for each tumor) within each tumor for training the deep learning framework. We first train the discriminator, the policy network and the similarity discriminative network, and then train the generator. Note that the policy network is jointly trained with the discriminator. The optimization of each loss is based on stochastic gradient descent (SGD). The training and testing process were conducted on the platform of GeForce GTX1080 8G. The convolution layer is performed by convolving patches with a 5×5 convolutional filter with stride 2. The max pooling layer is the size of kernels 2×2 with stride 2. The parameter of dropout was 0.5. The learning rate is initialized by $1e - 4$ with the decay value 0.98.

3   Results

3.1   Clinical Data

The performance of the proposed end-to-end framework was assessed by 154 clinical HCCs with T1-weighted MR images, in which 77 HCCs were acquired by the GE scanner, 37 HCCs were acquired by the Philips scanner and 40 HCCs were acquired by the Siemens scanner. The MR images of HCCs from the Philips scanner and the Siemens scanner were separately used for the pre-train, and the MR images of HCCs from the GE scanner were used for the fine-tuning and independent test. Of the 77 HCCs acquired by the GE scanner, 37 HCCs were used for the fine-tuning and the left 40 HCCs were used for the independent test. Accuracy, sensitivity and specificity were calculated to assess the performance of differentiating the high-grade and low-grade HCCs. Receiver operating characteristic curve (ROC) and area under the curve (AUC) were also used to assess the characterization performance. The output probability of the deep learning model for differentiating the low-grade and high-grade in the test set were also assessed by the student's t-test for statistical analysis. $P < 0.05$ was considered statistically significant. The training and testing were repetitively performed five times in order to assess the stability of the deep learning framework and reduce the measurement error.

3.2   Performance Comparison of CNN, GAN+CNN, NMI+L2+MSE, Similarity Steered GAN

Table 1 showed the characterization performance of the proposed method and other methods using the 37 HCCs of GE for training and the left 40 HCCs of GE for independent test. The GAN+CNN method [6] is superior to the traditional CNN method due to the increase of effective training data. This finding is consistent with the previous study [6], indicating that the combination of real data and data generated by GAN can further improve the performance of lesion characterization. The recently proposed NMI+MSE+L2 method [8] yields slightly better results than that of the GAN+CNN method as the discrepancy of the generated data has been considered. It can be clearly found that the proposed similarity steered GAN method obtained best results due to the superiority of the proposed similarity discriminative measure. Furthermore, it should be noted that our proposed similarity steered method consumes much less time (20 min) than the recently proposed NMI+L2+MSE method (4 h) with the same task of increasing the discrepancy of generated data for malignancy characterization of HCC.

Table 1. Characterization performance of different methods assessed by the independent test set (%).

Methods	Accuracy	Sensitivity	Specificity	AUC	P-value
CNN	65.53 ± 2.08	65.92 ± 2.77	65.00 ± 3.16	69.02 ± 2.01	0.02
GAN+CNN	69.36 ± 1.04	68.89 ± 1.81	70.00 ± 3.16	73.23 ± 1.54	0.01
NMI+MSE+L2	71.49 ± 1.04	71.11 ± 1.48	$\mathbf{72.00 \pm 2.45}$	75.81 ± 1.36	0.00
SSGAN	$\mathbf{73.61 \pm 1.04}$	$\mathbf{74.82 \pm 1.48}$	$\mathbf{72.00 \pm 2.45}$	$\mathbf{77.32 \pm 1.25}$	0.00

3.3 Performance Comparison of Pre-train with ImageNet, Philips and Siemens and Fine-Tuning with All Layers, One Last Layer and Adaptive Fine-Tuning Coupled with Proposed SSGAN

Table 2 showed the characterization performance of the proposed method with different pre-train methods and different fine-tuning methods in the train and test set. For recently proposed different fine-tuning methods, it can be found that the method of fine-tuning the last layer [11] yields better performance than that of fine-tuning all the layers [10], which is consistent with the previous finding [11]. It can be clearly found that the adaptive fine-tuning coupled with the proposed SSGAN yields the best performance. Furthermore, results of different pre-train methods demonstrates that pre-train with multiple scanners can improve the performance of lesion characterization using data from other scanners, slightly outperforming the pre-train with ImageNet [10].

Table 2. Characterization performance assessed by Pre-train with ImageNet/Philips/Siemens and Fine-tuning with all layers, last layer and adaptive fine-tuning based on our proposed SSGAN (%).

Pre-train	Fine-tuning	Accuracy	Sensitivity	Specificity	AUC	P-value
ImageNet	All layers	68.09 ± 1.90	65.19 ± 3.78	70.00 ± 3.16	71.63 ± 1.62	0.02
	Last layer	70.64 ± 0.85	71.11 ± 2.77	70.00 ± 3.16	77.42 ± 1.04	0.01
	Adaptive	73.19 ± 1.70	73.33 ± 1.48	73.00 ± 2.45	77.52 ± 1.07	0.00
Philips	All layers	70.64 ± 1.59	69.63 ± 2.77	72.00 ± 2.45	73.98 ± 1.61	0.01
	Last layer	72.77 ± 1.59	74.07 ± 2.34	71.00 ± 2.00	76.45 ± 1.78	0.01
	Adaptive	$\mathbf{75.32 \pm 1.04}$	74.81 ± 1.48	$\mathbf{76.00 \pm 2.00}$	79.31 ± 1.14	0.00
Siemens	All layers	71.49 ± 1.04	71.85 ± 1.81	71.00 ± 2.00	76.10 ± 1.22	0.01
	Last layer	72.34 ± 1.35	72.59 ± 2.96	72.00 ± 2.45	76.46 ± 1.13	0.01
	Adaptive	74.47 ± 1.35	$\mathbf{74.82 \pm 1.48}$	74.00 ± 2.00	$\mathbf{79.45 \pm 1.02}$	0.00

4   Conclusion

We proposed a similarity steered generative adversarial network (SSGAN) coupled with pre-train and adaptive fine-turning of data from multiple scanners for malignancy characterization of HCC. Our experimental results showed that the proposed similarity steered GAN outperformed conventional GAN and a recently proposed study. Furthermore, we also showed that the proposed SSGAN coupled with the adaptive fine-tuning yielded significantly improved performance. Finally, our study suggested that pre-train with multiple scanners has considerable contribution to improve the performance, outperforming the pre-train with ImageNet.

Acknowledgment. This research is supported by the grant from National Natural Science Foundation of China (NSFC: 81771920).

References

1. Jonas, S., Bechstein, W.O., Steinmuller, T., et al.: Vascular invasion and histopathologic grading determine outcome after liver transplantation for hepatocellular carcinoma in cirrhosis. Hepatology **33**(5), 1080–1086 (2001)
2. Miles, K.A., Ganeshan, B., Griffiths, M.R., Young, R.C., Chatwin, C.R.: Colorectal cancer: texture analysis of portal phase hepatic CT Images as a potential marker of survival. Radiology **250**(2), 444–452 (2009)
3. Litjens, G., Kooi, T., Bejnordi, B.E., et al.: A survey on deep learning in medical image analysis. Med. Image Anal. **42**(7), 60–88 (2017)
4. Parmar, C., Barry, J.D., Hosny, A., et al.: Data analysis strategies in medical imaging. Clin. Cancer Res. **24**(15), 3492–3499 (2018)
5. Goodfellow, I., Pouget-Abadie, J., Mirza, M., et al.: Generative adversarial nets. In: NIPS (2014)
6. Frid-adar, M., Klang, E., Amitai, M., Goldberger, J., Greenspan, H.: Synthetic data augmentation using GAN for improved liver lesion classification. In: IEEE 15th International Symposium on Biomedical Imaging, pp. 289–293(2018)
7. Salimans, T., Goodfellow I., Zaremba, W., et al.: Improved techniques for training GANs. In: NIPS (2016)
8. Shams, S., Platania, R., Kim, J., Park, S.: Deep generative cancer screening and diagnosis. In: MICCAI, pp. 859–867 (2018)
9. Yasaka, K., Akai, H., Kunimatsu, A., Kiryu, S., Abe, O.: Deep learning with convolutional neural network in radiology. Japan. J. Radiol. **36**, 257–272 (2018)
10. Carneiro, G., Nascimento, J., Bradley, A.P.: Unregistered multiview mammogram analysis with pre-trained deep learning models. In: MICCAI, pp. 652–660 (2015)
11. Shermin, T., Murshed, M.M., Lu, G., et al.: An efficient transfer learning technique by using final fully-connected layer output features of deep networks. arXiv : Computer Vision and Pattern Recognition (2018)
12. Guo, Y., Shi, H., Humar, A., et al.: SpotTune: transfer learning through adaptive fine-tuning. arXiv:1811.08737v1 [cs CV] (2018)
13. Maddison, C.J., Mnih, A., Teh, Y.W.: The concrete distribution: a continuous relaxation of discrete random variables. arXiv: 1801.06519 (2016)
14. Jang, E., Gu, S., Poole, B.: Categorical reparameterization with gumbel-softmax. arXiv:1611.01144v5 [stat. ML] (2017)

Unsupervised Clustering of Quantitative Imaging Phenotypes Using Autoencoder and Gaussian Mixture Model

Jianan Chen[1,3], Laurent Milot[2,3], Helen M. C. Cheung[2,3], and Anne L. Martel[1,3(✉)]

[1] Department of Medical Biophysics, University of Toronto, Toronto, ON, Canada
anne.martel@sri.utoronto.ca
[2] Department of Medical Imaging, University of Toronto, Toronto, ON, Canada
[3] Sunnybrook Research Institute, Toronto, ON, Canada

Abstract. Quantitative medical image computing (radiomics) has been widely applied to build prediction models from medical images. However, overfitting is a significant issue in conventional radiomics, where a large number of radiomic features are directly used to train and test models that predict genotypes or clinical outcomes. In order to tackle this problem, we propose an unsupervised learning pipeline composed of an autoencoder for representation learning of radiomic features and a Gaussian mixture model based on minimum message length criterion for clustering. By incorporating probabilistic modeling, disease heterogeneity has been taken into account. The performance of the proposed pipeline was evaluated on an institutional MRI cohort of 108 patients with colorectal cancer liver metastases. Our approach is capable of automatically selecting the optimal number of clusters and assigns patients into clusters (imaging subtypes) with significantly different survival rates. Our method outperforms other unsupervised clustering methods that have been used for radiomics analysis and has comparable performance to a state-of-the-art imaging biomarker.

Keywords: MRI · Radiomics · Unsupervised clustering · Liver metastases · Probabilistic generative modeling

1 Introduction

Quantitative medical image computing, known as radiomics, has been an emerging field in medical image analysis. The goal of radiomics is to extract hundreds of features that are mathematical summarizations of the volume-of-interest (VOI) from computed tomography (CT), magnetic resonance imaging (MRI) or positron emission tomography (PET), for the purpose of disease characterization and patient stratification. Imaging biomarkers built on radiomic features have demonstrated great performance in predicting patients outcome [1,5,7]. However, there are two critical issues in radiomics analysis.

© Springer Nature Switzerland AG 2019
D. Shen et al. (Eds.): MICCAI 2019, LNCS 11767, pp. 575–582, 2019.
https://doi.org/10.1007/978-3-030-32251-9_63

First, there is always the possibility of overfitting. Building statistically powerful models at medically meaningful effect sizes using hundreds of radiomic features would at least require thousands of samples [9], while such datasets are rarely available for research in medical settings. Even with generalization techniques such as feature reduction and cross-validation, overfitting remains a primary concern.

Second, conventional radiomics analysis does not necessarily consider the heterogeneity of the disease of interest. Breast cancer imaging subtypes identified using a radiomics approach are distinct from established breast cancer molecular and pathological subtypes [13]. This suggests that tumors in different subtypes or genotypes may have similar appearances. However, radiomic models are usually trained with either linear or deterministic models such as logistic regression or support vector machines for subtype prediction. These approaches are not ideal for the modeling of overlapping distributions.

Unsupervised clustering can be leveraged to alleviate these problems. Consensus clustering (CC), for example, has been used with radiomic features extracted from the tumor and surrounding parenchyma to define imaging subtypes in breast cancer [8,13]. However, it is difficult to glean further insights of the imaging subtypes through clustering without additional analyses, and often non-trivial to select the optimal number of clusters.

In this paper, we alleviated the issues of overfitting and non-distinct feature distributions using a radiomics pipeline that identifies imaging subtypes based on radiomic features using a probabilistic generative model with minimum supervision. We made use of an autoencoder to reduce the dimensions of our radiomic features and find representations with minimal correlations. We incorporated a Gaussian mixture model (GMM) with minimum message length criterion (MML) to cluster patient MRIs into imaging subtypes using the learned representations of features [3]. We compared the performance of other clustering algorithms with our approach and investigated the clinical value of the defined imaging subtypes. In addition, we demonstrated that the imaging subtypes derived from our pipeline have comparable prognostic ability to state-of-the-art clinical and imaging biomarkers.

2   Method

The workflow of our unsupervised clustering radiomics analysis includes five steps (Fig. 1). First, quantitative imaging features are extracted from MRI scans. Then an autoencoder is applied to learn feature representations for the purpose of dimension reduction. Next, the learned representations from the latent space are clustered using a GMM. Finally, the significance and clinical value of the learned imaging subtypes (clusters) are evaluated. Clinical outcome is held out during model training and only used in evaluation stage.

Radiomic Feature Extraction. The first step of our pipeline was MRI tumour lesion segmentation and radiomic features extraction. The MRIs were resampled

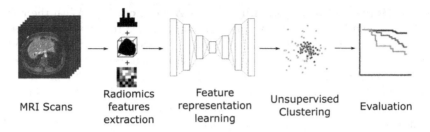

MRI Scans | Radiomics features extraction | Feature representation learning | Unsupervised Clustering | Evaluation

Fig. 1. Workflow of the proposed unsupervised radiomics pipeline

to isotropic spacing [3, 3, 3] using B-spline transformation. A Z-score transformation was applied to normalize the resampled images and rescale their intensities to range from 0 to 100. Outliers with extreme intensity values were capped in normalization. Image discretization was performed using a bin width of 5 to simplify computation. Finally, 100 features from three categories describing the characteristics (intensity, shape and texture) of the volume of interest, *e.g.* tumour lesions, were extracted using pyradiomics [11].

Quantile Normalization. We observed that radiomic features extracted from medical images frequently included outliers, *i.e.* samples with extreme feature values. However, in order to be able to reconstruct features from very few latent features in autoencoders, extreme values should be avoided. Experimentally we found that Z-normalization and capping did not work well for this problem. Hence, we used a quantile normalization approach with thresholds designed for radiomic features. We transform feature quantiles: 0–5% (min), 5–25%, 25%–50%, 50%–75%, 75%–95%, 95%–100% (max) to floats: 0, 1/6, 2/6, 3/6, 4/6, 5/6, 1, respectively. The quantile thresholds were empirically determined based on experiments.

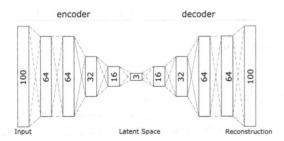

Fig. 2. Network architecture of the autoencoder with fully-connected layers used for feature representation learning. The numbers in the blocks denote number of hidden units in each layer.

Feature Representation Learning (with Autoencoder). With the transformed radiomic features, we leveraged an autoencoder to learn feature representations *i.e.* features in low dimensional latent space that best summarize the data. The input for the autoencoder was the 100-element radiomic feature vector previously mentioned (Fig. 2). There were five layers for both the encoder and the decoder. A relatively deep structure compared to the size of input was used to add non-linearity. The autoencoder was blinded to all clinical information to prevent overfitting. All layers were fully connected with SELU activation [6]. We chose three as the number of latent features because there were three categories of radiomic features. The latent features were used as the input for subsequent unsupervised clustering.

Unsupervised Clustering (with GMM-MML). Given the known extant of heterogeneity in cancer, imaging phenotypes of tumors with different genotypes/subtypes cannot be expected to be discrete. This motivated the choice of a probabilistic model instead of a deterministic one for tumor image clustering across known molecular and pathological categories. Therefore, we used a GMM for the unsupervised discovery of imaging subtypes.

Gaussian mixtures are weighted linear combinations of c-component Gaussians that are used to model a probability density. The optimum number of components c and parameters θ are estimated using minimum message length criterion (MML) [3]. The idea of MML is to simplify estimation of GMM parameters by minimization of encoding length. Consider a dataset $\mathcal{Y}$ which is generated from a probabilistic distribution $p(\mathcal{Y}|\theta)$, the message length required to encode and transmit $\mathcal{Y}$ is:

$$\mathcal{L}(\theta, \mathcal{Y}) = \mathcal{L}(\theta) + \mathcal{L}(\mathcal{Y}|\theta)) \tag{1}$$

where θ is the prior and $\mathcal{L}$ is the encoding message length.

Then θ and c can be simultaneously estimated using the following equation:

$$\hat{\theta} = arg\min_{\theta}\{-\log p(\theta) - \log p(\mathcal{Y}|\theta) + \frac{1}{2}\log|I(\theta)| + \frac{c}{2}(1 + \log\frac{1}{12})\} \tag{2}$$

where $|I(\theta)|$ is the determinant of the expected Fisher information matrix [3].

3   Experiments and Results

3.1   Experimental Design

Data Description. The dataset we used is an institutional retrospective cohort of 108 patients with colorectal cancer liver metastases (CRCLM). The number of slices for each volume is between 57 and 170 (mean = 100). Institutional Review Board approved the study and waived informed consent. Gadobutrol-enhanced liver MRIs, specifically 10-minute-delayed T1 MRIs were acquired after chemotherapy and prior to hepatic resection, with 1.5/3T MR systems. Tumor segmentation was performed by a single reader with 6 years of experience. The reader was blinded to all clinical information expect patient history of CRCLM. Patient mortality right-censored at three years were available.

Implementation Details. Radiomic feature extraction was implemented using packages pyradiomics (v2.0.0) [11], numpy (v1.14.3) and SimpleITK (v1.1.0) in Python (v2.7.15).

An autoencoder was trained with Keras on a NVIDIA TITAN Xp Graphics Card (with 12 G memory). The loss function was set to binary cross entropy loss. We used adam optimization with a mini-batch size of 64. Default parameters were used, specifically initial learning rate of 0.001, decay rates of 0.9 and 0.999. The model was trained for 400 epochs.

GMM with MML was implemented using Python package gmm-mml (v0.11). Initial number of clusters k_max was set to 25. Maximum iteration of 100 and convergence threshold of 10^{-5} was used.

Evaluation Metrics. In radiomic subtype classification tasks, there is no "ground truth". Thus, instead of using normalized mutual information and Rand index, which are typically used for evaluating the performances of unsupervised clustering methods, we evaluated the clinical value of our imaging clusters according to their association with patient outcome. Cox proportional hazard models were built for comparing different unsupervised clustering methods, in terms of concordance index (CI), hazard ratio (HR) and p-value. A cluster number of three was automatically selected by both GMM-MML and the heuristic algorithms provided in SIMLR (v1.8.1) [12], so we compared the methods by the maximum pair-wise HR produced from their clustering results.

Evaluation. The resulting clusters from our pipeline and their clinical values were demonstrated using a kaplan-meier plot and results from a log-rank test. We also compared our approach with other unsupervised clustering methods that have been used to cluster radiomic features, including baseline consensus clustering [8,13] and state-of-the-art SIMLR [12]. Further, we compared our approach to validated clinical and imaging biomarkers for prognostic ability [2,4].

Table 1. Comparison of unsupervised learning algorithms for imaging phenotype clustering. Numbers in parentheses are confidence intervals. "*" denotes significant p value.

Method	Concordance index↑	Hazard ratio↑	P value
CC [8]	0.531 ± 0.046	2.90 (0.75−14.45)	0.113
SIMLR [12]	0.582 ± 0.047	3.20 (0.73−13.93)	0.122
AE + GMM + MML	$\mathbf{0.623 \pm 0.052}$	**3.32 (1.35−8.18)**	**0.009***

3.2 Results

We estimated Gaussian mixtures of latent representations of radiomic features from liver MRIs using our pipeline. Three Gaussian distributions were learned, each representing an imaging subtype (Fig. 3a–b). We compared the raw radiomic feature distributions of the three tumor subtypes. We found subtype II tumors to be larger but otherwise very similar to subtype I tumors. In contrast, tumors in subtype III were drastically different from the other two, mostly with higher heterogeneity in texture and were more elongated. There are 46, 41 and 21 patients in cluster I-III, respectively. Patients in subtype III had significantly worse survival rates than patients in the other two subtypes (Fig. 3c).

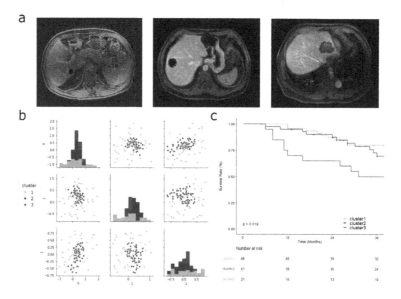

Fig. 3. Image subtypes defined by our pipeline (a) from left to right, example images that are representative of cluster I, II and III tumors, respectively. Tumor regions of interest are marked in red. (b) latent features and the estimated Gaussian mixtures. The x- and y-axis of each subplot are latent features values (indexed 0–2). (c) 3-year survival rates for patients assigned to different subtypes. (Color figure online)

We compared our approach and other unsupervised clustering algorithms for defining imaging subtypes (Table 1). Our approach achieved the highest CI and the only statistically significant HR of 3.32 [1.35–8.18]. Therefore our approach was uniquely able to produce imaging subtypes predictive of patient survival. In addition, the estimated GMM components can be used to model theoretical distributions of CRCLM tumor appearance and be expanded to a validated training-testing model, while the subtypes defined by SIMLR and consensus clustering are hard to interpret and cannot be expanded to incorporate new samples.

We also compared the prognostic ability of our approach to other biomarkers for CRCLM (Table 2). The Fong score is a clinical risk score based on five independent preoperative risk factors built to predict patient prognosis [4]. Target-tumor-enhancement (TTE) is an imaging biomarker specifically designed for stratifying CRCLM patients with late-gadolinium-enhanced MRI [2]. The comparison was based on a subset of 99 patients who had all three biomarkers available. Our approach outperformed the Fong score and had comparable performance to TTE in predicting 3-year survival rates for CRCLM patients.

Table 2. Comparison of our approach with clinical and imaging biomarkers for CRCLM. The methods are adjusted for age and sex. Numbers in parentheses are confidence intervals. "*" denotes significant p value.

Method	Hazard ratio↑	P value
Fong score [4]	2.28 [0.96−5.42]	0.060
Target tumor enhancement[2]	**4.06 [1.73−9.51]**	**0.001***
AE + GMM + MML	**3.98 [1.60−9.89]**	**0.003***

4   Discussion and Conclusion

Probabilistic generative modeling for unsupervised clustering can alleviate the issues of overfitting and overlapping feature distributions in radiomics analysis. We proposed an unsupervised pipeline composed of an autoencoder and a GMM-MML for identifying imaging subtypes from radiomic features that achieved clinically meaningful results. Experiments showed that our approach outperformed other unsupervised algorithms typically used in radiomics by finding imaging subtypes that were associated with patient survival. We also demonstrated that our unsupervised model outperformed a clinical prognostic biomarker and had comparable performance to a state-of-the-art imaging biomarker designed for this specific tumor type and contrast agent.

Due to the modest sample size, we didn't perform a train-test split for feature representation learning and Guassian mixture modeling. However, since the prediction of patient survival rate was independent of radiomic feature encoding and clustering, the survival difference between imaging subtypes were not due to overfitting in this respect. Also, our study was based on manual segmentations of tumor lesions. In future work, we will apply convolutional neural network structures which can extract features directly from MRI scans and remove the need of manual segmentations.

The underlying biological mechanisms of the identified imaging clusters can be elucidated further using pathway enrichment analysis [10,13]. Investigations into targetable recurrent mutational or expressional changes in the subtypes may also open the way to guided personalized treatments for colorectal cancer liver metastases patients based on imaging analysis.

Acknowledgements. The authors would like to thank The Natural Sciences and Engineering Research Council of Canada (NSERC) for funding, and acknowledge the contribution of Drs. Karanicolas, Law and Coburn in helping to create the patient cohort for this study.

References

1. Aerts, H.J., et al.: Decoding tumour phenotype by noninvasive imaging using a quantitative radiomics approach. Nat. Commun. **5** (2014). https://doi.org/10.1038/ncomms5006

2. Cheung, H.M., et al.: Late gadolinium enhancement of colorectal liver metastases post-chemotherapy is associated with tumour fibrosis and overall survival post-hepatectomy. Eur. Radiol. **28**(8), 1–8 (2018)

3. Figueiredo, M.A.T., Jain, A.K.: Unsupervised learning of finite mixture models. IEEE Trans. Pattern Anal. Mach. Intell. **3**, 381–396 (2002)

4. Fong, Y., Fortner, J., Sun, R.L., Brennan, M.F., Blumgart, L.H.: Clinical score for predicting recurrence after hepatic resection for metastatic colorectal cancer: analysis of 1001 consecutive cases. Ann. Surg. **230**(3), 309 (1999)

5. Ha, S., Park, S., Bang, J.I., Kim, E.K., Lee, H.Y.: Metabolic radiomics for pre-treatment 18 F-FDG PET/CT to characterize locally advanced breast cancer: histopathologic characteristics, response to neoadjuvant chemotherapy, and prognosis. Sci. Rep. **7**(1), 1556 (2017)

6. Klambauer, G., Unterthiner, T., Mayr, A., Hochreiter, S.: Self-normalizing neural networks. In: Advances in Neural Information Processing Systems, pp. 971–980 (2017)

7. Kontos, D., et al.: Radiomic phenotypes of mammographic parenchymal complexity: toward augmenting breast density in breast cancer risk assessment. Radiology **290**(1), 41–49 (2018)

8. Monti, S., Tamayo, P., Mesirov, J., Golub, T.: Consensus clustering: a resampling-based method for class discovery and visualization of gene expression microarray data. Mach. Learn. **52**(1–2), 91–118 (2003)

9. Napel, S., Mu, W., Jardim-Perassi, B.V., Aerts, H.J., Gillies, R.J.: Quantitative imaging of cancer in the postgenomic era: Radio(geno)mics, deep learning, and habitats. Cancer, 4633–4649 (2018). https://doi.org/10.1002/cncr.31630

10. Reimand, J., et al.: Pathway enrichment analysis and visualization of omics data using g: Profiler, GSEA, cytoscape and enrichmentmap. Nat. Protoc. **14**, 1 (2019)

11. Van Griethuysen, J.J., et al.: Computational radiomics system to decode the radiographic phenotype. Cancer Res. **77**(21), e104–e107 (2017)

12. Wang, B., Ramazzotti, D., De Sano, L., Zhu, J., Pierson, E., Batzoglou, S.: SIMLR: a tool for large-scale genomic analyses by multi-kernel learning. Proteomics **18**(2), 1700232 (2018)

13. Wu, J., et al.: Unsupervised clustering of quantitative image phenotypes reveals breast cancer subtypes with distinct prognoses and molecular pathways. Clin. Cancer Res. **23**(13), 3334–3342 (2017). https://doi.org/10.1158/1078-0432.CCR-16-2415

Adaptive Sparsity Regularization Based Collaborative Clustering for Cancer Prognosis

Hangfan Liu[1], Hongming Li[1], Yuemeng Li[1], Shi Yin[1],
Pamela Boimel[2], James Janopaul-Naylor[2], Haoyu Zhong[2],
Ying Xiao[2], Edgar Ben-Josef[2], and Yong Fan[1(✉)]

[1] Center for Biomedical Image Computing and Analysis,
University of Pennsylvania, Philadelphia, PA 19104, USA
yong.fan@pennmedicine.upenn.edu
[2] Department of Radiation Oncology, University of Pennsylvania,
Philadelphia, PA 19104, USA

Abstract. Radiomic approaches have achieved promising performance in prediction of clinical outcomes of cancer patients. Particularly, feature dimensionality reduction plays an important role in radiomic studies. However, conventional feature dimensionality reduction techniques are not equipped to suppress data noise or utilize latent supervision information of patient data under study (*e.g.* difference in patients) for learning discriminative low dimensional representations. To achieve feature dimensionality reduction with improved discriminative power and robustness to noisy radiomic features, we develop an adaptive sparsity regularization based collaborative clustering method to simultaneously cluster patients and radiomic features into distinct groups respectively. Our method is built on adaptive sparsity regularized matrix tri-factorization for simultaneous feature denoising and dimension reduction so that the noise is adaptively isolated from the features, and grouping information of patients with distinctive features provides latent supervision information to guide feature dimension reduction. The sparsity regularization is grounded on distribution modeling of transform-domain coefficients in a Bayesian framework. Experiments on synthetic data have demonstrated the effectiveness of the proposed approach in data clustering, and empirical results on an FDG-PET/CT dataset of rectal cancer patients have demonstrated that the proposed method outperforms alternative methods in terms of both patient stratification and prediction of patient clinical outcomes.

Keywords: Sparsity · Collaborative clustering · Unsupervised learning · Radiomics

1   Introduction

Rectal cancer is a major cause of tumor-related deaths in the US. Chemoradiation therapy (CRT) is one of the most widely-used treatments for rectal cancer. However, only 15–20% rectal tumors treated by CRT attain pathologic complete response (pCR), and most of the others achieve different degrees of partial response [1]. Patients with pCR expect optimistic outcomes, whereas those without pCR have a high risk of

© Springer Nature Switzerland AG 2019
D. Shen et al. (Eds.): MICCAI 2019, LNCS 11767, pp. 583–592, 2019.
https://doi.org/10.1007/978-3-030-32251-9_64

developing local recurrences and distant metastasis. For better treatment planning and patient management, it is desired to early predict treatment response of individual patients.

Radiomic approaches have obtained promising results on cancer staging and prognosis [2, 3]. The typical components of radiomic approaches include radiomic feature extraction, feature selection, dimension reduction, and prediction modeling [4, 5]. Particularly, feature selection and dimension reduction are often used to identify a compact set of informative features for building robust prediction models in radiomic studies where a small number of samples are characterized by high dimensional features.

Typical feature selection methods identify informative features in a supervised learning framework [6], and tend to overfit the data when the sample size is small. In contrast, feature dimension reduction techniques, such as principal component analysis (PCA), learn low dimensional feature presentations in an unsupervised setting [7]. However, conventional unsupervised learning approaches fail to consider latent discriminative information of the data, which may provide weak supervision in dimension reduction.

Noise in radiomic features remains underexplored in radiomic studies, although the extraction of radiomic features inevitably introduces noise during the processes of image acquisition and tumor segmentation. It is non-trivial to learn robust and informative feature representations from noisy radiomic features. Therefore, it is helpful to suppress the influence of noise while keeping the fidelity of feature data.

In this paper, we propose to integrate *feature denoising* and *unsupervised collaborative clustering* within a single framework for radiomic analysis. Specifically, a robust collaborative clustering method is developed to learn discriminative low dimensional features by utilizing latent supervision information derived via simultaneously grouping patients with distinctive radiomic features in a sparse learning framework. The noise in features is suppressed by adaptively applying sparsity regularization to the collaborative clustering of patients and radiomic features in a Bayesian framework, leading to improved feature dimensionality reduction.

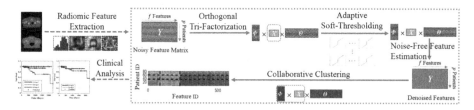

Fig. 1. Illustration of the proposed robust collaborative clustering for radiomic analysis.

2   Sparsity Regularization Based Collaborative Clustering

This study focuses on feature dimension reduction to enhance discriminative power of radiomic features and subsequently improve prediction modeling in a radiomic system, as illustrated by Fig. 1. We develop a sparsity regularized matrix tri-factorization method for robust collaborative clustering of patients and features. Particularly, the collaborative clustering is enhanced by sparsity regularization for simultaneous denoising and dimension reduction. Differences between patients with distinctive features are utilized to obtain discriminative low dimensional features via collaboratively clustering the features and the samples. Meanwhile, sparsity regularization is used to suppress noise, so that improved feature representation and patient stratification are achieved.

Given radiomic features of all the patients under study as a matrix $Y \in \mathbb{R}^{p \times f}$, where p is the number of patients and f denotes the number of features, we decompose matrix Y into three matrices Φ, X, and Θ via solving:

$$\{\Phi, X, \Theta\} = \arg \min_{\phi, X, \Theta \geq 0} \|\Lambda \cdot X\|_1 + \|Y - \Phi X \Theta\|_F^2 \text{ s.t. } \Phi^T \Phi = I_{k_P}, \Theta \Theta^T = I_{k_F}, \quad (1)$$

where I_{k_P} and I_{k_F} are identity matrices, $\Phi \in \mathbb{R}_+^{p \times k_P}$ encodes a mapping between the patients and k_P patient clusters, $\Theta \in \mathbb{R}_+^{k_F \times f}$ encodes a mapping between the features and k_F feature clusters, $X \in \mathbb{R}_+^{k_P \times k_F}$ reflects the magnitude of the mappings and the interactions between Φ and Θ, $\cdot$ is element-wise multiplication, and $\Lambda \in \mathbb{R}_+^{k_P \times k_F}$ contains coefficient-adaptive regularization parameters. Given a noisy observation Y, Eq. (1) aims to find a noise-free sparse representation X. In Eq. (1), $\|Y - \Phi X \Theta_F^2\|$ is the data fidelity term, and $\|\Lambda \cdot X\|_1$ is the ℓ_1-norm sparsity regularization, *i.e.*

$$\|\Lambda \cdot X\|_1 = \sum_{i=1}^{k_P} \sum_{j=1}^{k_F} \lambda_{ij} |x_{ij}|, \quad (2)$$

where λ_{ij} is a regularization parameter assigned to $x_{ij} \in X$. Particularly, Φ and Θ can be seen as a pair of orthonormal dictionaries used to decompose the feature matrix, and X contains the corresponding coefficients. Once Φ, X, and Θ are obtained, it is straightforward to compute a low-dimensional representation of the radiomic features, referred to as meta-features, $M \in \mathbb{R}_+^{p \times k_F}$. The meta-features in M are weighted combinations of the radiomic features in the same feature clusters, *i.e.* $M = \Phi X$. They can be used in prediction modeling to predict clinical outcomes. The patient grouping results could be used to stratify patients into groups with distinctive radiomic features.

Since many radiomic features are correlated with each other, especially when a large number of features are extracted in both original image domain and wavelet domains [8], the coefficients in X are relatively sparse and discriminative information might be contained in only a few of them. In contrast, since noise is randomly introduced and roughly uncorrelated, it is roughly uniformly distributed among different coefficients and cannot be sparsely represented by the learned dictionaries, hence the noise can be isolated from the feature components [9, 10]. As a result, the sparsity regularization helps suppress the noise and thus facilitates learning of more effective dictionaries that could be used to simultaneously cluster the subjects and radiomic features.

We solve the optimization problem (1) by decomposing it into 3 sub-problems, each of which can be tackled efficiently. Since the proposed collaborative clustering method is robust to noise, we dub it robust collaborative clustering (RCC).

2.1 Preliminary Dictionary Learning

The best way to learn a pair of dictionaries Φ and Θ is applying the tri-factorization to a noise-free feature matrix, which is unavailable in practice. Instead, we learn a preliminary pair of dictionaries Φ and Θ from the noisy feature matrix Y by optimizing

$$\{\Phi, \Theta\} = \arg \min_{\Phi \geq 0, X \geq 0, \Theta \geq 0,} \|Y - \Phi X \Theta\|_F^2, \text{ s.t. } \Phi^T \Phi = I, \Theta \Theta^T = I \quad (3)$$

via an alternative optimization method [11]. To solve Eq. (3), we need to decide hyperparameters k_F and k_p. The optimal number of feature clusters k_F can be chosen based on gap criterion [12], which is formulated as $G_f(k_F) = E_n^*[\log(W_{k_F})] - \log(W_{k_F})$, where $E_n^*[\cdot]$ is an expectation estimated using Monte Carlo sampling from a reference distribution (typically a uniform distribution), and $W_{k_F} = \sum_{r=1}^{k_F} D_r/2n_r$ is a measure of pooled within-cluster dispersion, where r is an index of feature clusters, n_r is the number of radiomic features in a cluster r, and D_r is the sum of the pairwise distances for all radiomic feature samples in the cluster r. We use correlation between the feature samples as the distance metric to compute D_r. The number of patient clusters k_p could be empirically chosen to stratify the patients in to high, intermediate, or low risk groups.

2.2 Adaptive Soft-Thresholding in Bayesian Framework

With Φ and Θ fixed, the optimization problem of Eq. (1) becomes

$$\tilde{X} = \arg \min_{X \geq 0} \|Y - \Phi X \Theta\|_F^2 + \|\Lambda \cdot X\|_1. \quad (4)$$

Due to non-differentiability of the ℓ_1 norm, a straightforward solution to Eq. (4) is not available. Since Φ and Θ are orthonormal, $i.e.$ $\Phi^T \Phi = I$ and $\Theta \Theta^T = I$, we have

$$\|Y - \Phi X \Theta\|_F^2 = \|\Phi^T(Y - \Phi X \Theta)\Theta^T\|_F^2 = \|\Phi^T Y \Theta^T - X\|_F^2 \quad (5)$$

Let $V = \Phi^T Y \Theta^T$ be the coefficient matrix of Y, we transform Eq. (4) into

$$\tilde{X} = \arg \min_{X \geq 0} \|V - X\|_F^2 + \|\Lambda \cdot X\|_1 \quad (6)$$

A closed form solution to Eq. (6) is a simple soft-thresholding operation [13]:

$$\tilde{X} = \text{soft}(V, \Lambda) \triangleq \max(|V| - \Lambda, 0) \cdot \text{sgn}(V) \quad (7)$$

where $\cdot$ is an element-wise multiplication operator. Since there is a one-to-one correspondence between Λ and X, such a soft-thresholding operation leads to an adaptive denoising of the coefficients. We pursuit the optimal parameters $\lambda_{ij} \in \Lambda$ in a Bayesian framework. From the Bayesian point of view, Eq. (4) is derived from maximum a posteriori estimation: $\tilde{X} = \arg \max_{X \geq 0} P(X|Y) = \arg \max_{X \geq 0} P(Y|X)P(X)/P(Y)$, or equivalently $\tilde{X} = \arg \max_{X \geq 0} \log P(Y|X) + \log P(X)$, where $\log P(Y|X)$ is the log-likelihood of X, and $\log P(X)$ reflects prior knowledge of the coefficients. We use Gaussian white noise to approximate errors introduced in the observed features Y, and consider the coefficients in X conform to Laplace distributions that are good at ruling out outliers, *i.e.*

$$P(Y|X) \propto \exp\left(-\|Y - \Phi X \Theta\|_2^2 / 2\sigma_n^2\right), \; P(X) \propto \exp\left(-\sqrt{2}\|X/\Sigma\|_1\right), \quad (8)$$

where σ_n^2 is the variance of noise, $\Sigma \in \mathbb{R}_+^{k_P \times k_F}$ is the standard deviations of corresponding coefficients in X, and the division calculation of Eq. (8) is element-wise. It is worth noting that coefficients in X could have different variances under the assumption of Laplacian distributions, which could better model the features than an assumption of i.i.d. distribution because the statistics of the coefficients can be significantly different, which is analogous to the difference between high- and low-frequency coefficients in classic orthonormal transforms [13]. Then, Eq. (6) evolves into

$$\tilde{X} = \arg \min_{X \geq 0} \frac{1}{2\sigma_n^2} \|Y - \Phi X \Theta\|_F^2 + \sqrt{2}\left\|\frac{X}{\Sigma}\right\|_1. \quad (9)$$

Comparing Eq. (4) with Eq. (9), we can see that each element in Λ is calculated as

$$\lambda_{ij} = 2\sqrt{2}\sigma_n^2/\sigma_{ij}, \quad (10)$$

where σ_{ij} is the standard deviation of $x_{ij} \in X$.

It is noteworthy that the strength of sparsity regularization is proportional to the noise level and inversely proportional to the uncertainty of feature coefficients. Specifically, Eqs. (7) and (10) indicate that the strength of the soft thresholding is inversely proportional to the standard deviation of the coefficient under consideration. This is because coefficients with larger variance contain more information, which should be preserved rather than shrunk. On the contrary, coefficients with small variance typically has little information, hence should be shrunk more to remove the noise. Furthermore, the equations indicate that the regularization strength is proportional to noise variance, which is reasonable because heavier noise needs stronger shrinkage for denoising.

Another problem is that the standard deviations of noise-free coefficients in Σ are unknown because the radiomic features are noisy. Since the additive noise can be considered to be evenly distributed over the subspaces spanned by the pair of dictionaries Φ and Θ, we can estimate the variances of coefficients via the element-wise calculation:

$$\Sigma^2 = \max\left(V^2 - c\sigma_n^2, 0\right), \tag{11}$$

where c is a constant, and noise variance σ_n^2 can be estimated from the observations.

2.3   Final Collaborative Clustering

After the soft-thresholding operations are applied to the coefficients of radiomic features, the denoised version of Y can be computed as $\tilde{Y} = \Phi \tilde{X} \Theta$ based on which more effective collaborative clustering can be performed by solving the optimization problem (3), and better meta-features M can be obtained via Eq. (2).

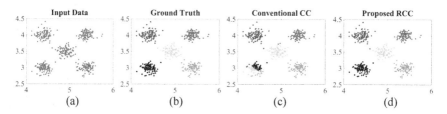

Fig. 2. (a) 2D synthetic data points from 5 clusters; (b) Corresponding ground-truth clustering labeled by colors; (c) Clustering results of conventional CC; (d) Results of the proposed RCC. Points in the same color belong to the same cluster obtained by the clustering algorithm. (Color figure online)

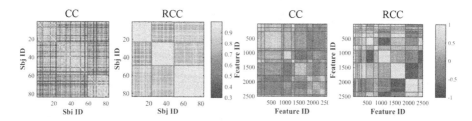

Fig. 3. Visualization of CC and RCC. From left to right: The Pearson correlation matrix between patients obtained by CC and RCC; the Pearson correlation matrix between features obtained by CC and RCC. Different sub-clusters are separated by red lines.

3   Experiments on Synthetic Data

Before applying the proposed approach to real-world clinical data, we tested it on synthetic data to provide a straightforward view of the improvement over the conventional collaborative clustering (CC) using tri-matrix decomposition [11]. In order to better visualize the clustering results, we obtain synthetic 2-dimensional (2D) data with 500 vectors distributed in 5 Gaussian clusters from [14] to perform the methods under comparison (see Fig. 2(a)). Each dimension of the 2D data points was treated as one feature, and 5 clusters of data points and 2 clusters of features were obtained.

For the clustering results, we labeled the data points in the same cluster by the same color, and matched the color labeling with that of the ground-truth clustering in Fig. 2 (b) by majority matching. As shown in Fig. 2(c), some elements of the cluster in black were wrongly assigned to the cluster in cyan by the CC, while the clustering results obtained by the RCC was largely consistent with the ground truth.

4 Experiments on Patient Stratification and Survival Prediction

4.1 Data

The proposed method was further evaluated in terms of patient stratification and survival prediction in a radiomic study of rectal cancer based on a dataset of 83 rectal cancer patients treated by CRT for locally advanced rectal cancer. All the patients had pre-treatment FDGPET/CT scans, and 8 patients deceased within a median follow-up of 3 years. The tumors were manually contoured by professional radiologists. Standardized uptake value (SUV) was computed for the PET scans. We computed both non-texture features and texture features from the CT scan and SUV map respectively using a radiomic method, which is capable of extracting multimodal imaging features [8]. The number of CT radiomic features was 1249, and that of PET features was 1254. All these features were pooled together for patient stratification and prediction modeling.

4.2 Patient Stratification and Survival Prediction Based on Clustering Results

The clustering result with 3 patient sub-clusters and 11 feature sub-clusters obtained by basic collaborative clustering (CC) [15] and RCC are shown in Fig. 3. The correlation coefficients within the same cluster (diagonal blocks) of the patients and the features obtained by the RCC was higher than that obtained by the CC, indicating that the RCC obtained better clustering results in terms of both patient stratification and the clustering of the features since highly-correlated features and patients with similar features should to be grouped together respectively.

To evaluate the patient stratification performance, we used k-means [16] as a baseline method, and adopted Kaplan-Meier estimation [17] to generate a survival function for each group of patients in terms of survival. The differences between the 3 patient groups were measured by log-rank test [18] with results summarized in Table 1. The proposed RCC achieved better log-rank results, and the difference between Group 3 and Group 2 was statistically significant, with a p-value of 0.0016.

To predict the risk of mortality for each patient, we built prediction models with the meta features using three survival modeling methods, *i.e.* Cox proportional hazard regression (Cox) [19], Cox with LASSO (CoxL) [20], and random survival forests (RSF) [21]. We used PCA [7] based feature extraction as a baseline to evaluate the effectiveness of low-dimensional representation obtained by RCC. We repeated the cross-validation procedures 100 times and report the average scores. The sparsity parameter in CoxL was decided by a nested 3-fold cross validation. Table 2 summarizes the prediction

Table 1. Comparison of p-values between different groups.

Group	K-Means	CC	RCC
1 vs. 2	0.0701	0.0711	**0.0429**
3 vs. 2	0.0032	0.0032	**0.0016**
1 vs. 3	0.8624	0.8624	0.8533

Table 2. Prediction performance (C-index) comparison.

–	PCA	CC	RCC
Cox	0.6322	0.6291	0.6731	**0.7103**
CoxL	0.6086	0.5827	0.6663	**0.7273**
RSF	0.5378	0.4978	0.5486	0.6300

performance measured by concordance index (C-index) [22]. The first column of C-indices are results of Cox, CoxL, and RSF without feature extraction. For the PCA based prediction, the best results with the number of extracted features ranging from 5–13 were obtained. Evidently, prediction models based on meta features produced by RCC remarkably outperformed those built upon features generated by the PCA and meta features obtained by the CC [15]. The best performance was achieved by the CoxL model built on meta features obtained by the RCC, with a gain of **15.6%** over the best performance achieved by PCA, and **8.1%** over the best performance attained by CC.

5   Discussion and Conclusions

In order to predict clinical outcomes based on radiomic features, this paper presents an adaptive sparsity regularization based robust collaborative clustering approach to compute low dimensional, informative meta features. The adaptive sparsity regularization and the collaborative clustering benefit from each other. The collaborative clustering effectively utilizes the discriminative information of feature data so that the obtained sparse representation is more informative after denoising. In contrast, due to lack of relevant guidance, such discriminative information is prone to being removed along with noise by conventional techniques. Meanwhile, the adaptive sparsity regularization makes the method robust to noise, yielding better meta features for clinical analysis. Compared with supervised learning, the proposed method does not rely on any clinical measures, thus can circumvent problems like overfitting brought by limited samples. The experiments on synthetic data have demonstrated the effectiveness of the proposed approach, and empirical results on clinical analysis have shown that the method groups highly-correlated features in the same clusters, leading to more effective low-dimensional representation and better patient stratification. Quantitative evaluation measures of both patient stratification and survival prediction have further demonstrated the superiority of the proposed approach over existing methods.

Acknowledgement. This study was supported in part by National Institutes of Health grants [CA223358, CA189523, EB022573]. The funding sources were not involved in the study design, in the collection, analysis and interpretation of data, in the writing of the report, or in the decision to submit the article for publication.

References

1. Maas, M., et al.: Long-term outcome in patients with a pathological complete response after chemoradiation for rectal cancer: a pooled analysis of individual patient data. Lancet Oncol. **11**, 835–844 (2010)
2. Li, H., et al.: Deep convolutional neural networks for imaging data based survival analysis of rectal cancer. In: IEEE International Symposium on Biomedical Imaging, pp. 846–849. (2019)
3. Li, H., Galperin-Aizenberg, M., Pryma, D., Simone, C.B., Fan, Y.: Unsupervised machine learning of radiomic features for predicting treatment response and overall survival of early stage non-small cell lung cancer patients treated with stereotactic body radiation therapy. Radiother. Oncol. **129**, 218–226 (2018)
4. Gillies, R.J., Kinahan, P.E., Hricak, H.: Radiomics: images are more than pictures, they are data. Radiology **278**, 563–577 (2015)
5. Kumar, V., et al.: Radiomics: the process and the challenges. Magn. Reson. Imaging **30**, 1234–1248 (2012)
6. Peng, H., Fan, Y.: Feature selection by optimizing a lower bound of conditional mutual information. Inf. Sci. **418**, 652–667 (2017)
7. Jolliffe, I.T., Cadima, J.: Principal component analysis: a review and recent developments. Philos. Trans. Roy. Soc. Math. Phys. Eng. Sciences **374**, 20150202 (2016)
8. Vallières, M., Freeman, C.R., Skamene, S.R., El Naqa, I.: A radiomics model from joint FDG-PET and MRI texture features for the prediction of lung metastases in soft-tissue sarcomas of the extremities. Phys. Med. Biol. **60**, 5471 (2015)
9. Liu, H., Zhang, X., Xiong, R.: Content-adaptive low rank regularization for image denoising. In: IEEE International Conference on Image Processing, pp. 3091–3095 (2016)
10. Liu, H., Xiong, R., Liu, D., Wu, F., Gao, W.: Low rank regularization exploiting intra and inter patch correlation for image denoising. In: IEEE Visual Communications and Image Processing. IEEE (2017)
11. Ding, C., Li, T., Peng, W., Park, H.: Orthogonal nonnegative matrix tri-factorizations for clustering. In: ACM SIGKDD International Conference on Knowledge Discovery and Data Mining, pp. 126–135 (2006)
12. Tibshirani, R., Walther, G., Hastie, T.: Estimating the number of clusters in a data set via the gap statistic. J. Roy. Stat. Soc. Ser B (Stat Methodol) **63**, 411–423 (2001)
13. Liu, H., Xiong, R., Zhang, J., Gao, W.: Image denoising via adaptive soft-thresholding based on non-local samples. In: IEEE Conference on Computer Vision and Pattern Recognition, pp. 484–492 (2015)
14. Rezaei, M., Fränti, P.: Set matching measures for external cluster validity. IEEE Trans. Knowl. Data Eng. **28**, 2173–2186 (2016)
15. Liu, H., et al.: Collaborative clustering of subjects and radiomic features for predicting clinical outcomes of rectal cancer patients. In: IEEE International Symposium on Biomedical Imaging (2019)
16. Coates, A., Ng, A.Y.: Learning feature representations with k-means. In: Montavon, G., Orr, Geneviève B., Müller, K.-R. (eds.) Neural Networks: Tricks of the Trade. LNCS, vol. 7700, pp. 561–580. Springer, Heidelberg (2012). https://doi.org/10.1007/978-3-642-35289-8_30
17. Kaplan, E.L., Meier, P.: Nonparametric estimation from incomplete observations. J. Am. Stat. Assoc. **53**, 457–481 (1958)
18. Mantel, N.: Evaluation of survival data and two new rank order statistics arising in its consideration. Cancer Chemother. Rep. **50**, 163–170 (1966)

19. Fox, J.: Cox proportional-hazards regression for survival data. An R and S-PLUS Companion to Applied Regression 2002 (2002)
20. Tibshirani, R.: The lasso method for variable selection in the Cox model. Stat. Med. **16**, 385–395 (1997)
21. Ishwaran, H., Kogalur, U.B., Blackstone, E.H., Lauer, M.S.: Random survival forests. Ann. Appl. Stat. **2**, 841–860 (2008)
22. Harrell Jr., F.E., Lee, K.L., Califf, R.M., Pryor, D.B., Rosati, R.A.: Regression modelling strategies for improved prognostic prediction. Stat. Med. **3**, 143–152 (1984)

Coronary Artery Plaque Characterization from CCTA Scans Using Deep Learning and Radiomics

Felix Denzinger[1,2(✉)], Michael Wels[2], Nishant Ravikumar[1],
Katharina Breininger[1], Anika Reidelshöfer[3], Joachim Eckert[4],
Michael Sühling[2], Axel Schmermund[4], and Andreas Maier[1]

[1] Pattern Recognition Lab, Friedrich-Alexander-Universität Erlangen-Nürnberg,
Erlangen, Germany
`felix.denzinger@siemens-healthineers.com`
[2] Computed Tomography, Siemens Healthcare GmbH, Forchheim, Germany
[3] University Clinic Frankfurt, Frankfurt am Main, Germany
[4] Cardioangiological Centrum Bethanien, Frankfurt am Main, Germany

Abstract. Assessing coronary artery plaque segments in coronary CT angiography scans is an important task to improve patient management and clinical outcomes, as it can help to decide whether invasive investigation and treatment are necessary. In this work, we present three machine learning approaches capable of performing this task. The first approach is based on radiomics, where a plaque segmentation is used to calculate various shape-, intensity- and texture-based features under different image transformations. A second approach is based on deep learning and relies on centerline extraction as sole prerequisite. In the third approach, we fuse the deep learning approach with radiomic features. On our data the methods reached similar scores as simulated fractional flow reserve (FFR) measurements, which - in contrast to our methods - requires an exact segmentation of the whole coronary tree and often time-consuming manual interaction. In literature, the performance of simulated FFR reaches an AUC between 0.79–0.93 predicting an abnormal invasive FFR that demands revascularization. The radiomics approach achieves an AUC of 0.84, the deep learning approach 0.86 and the combined method 0.88 for predicting the revascularization decision directly. While all three proposed methods can be determined within seconds, the FFR simulation typically takes several minutes. Provided representative training data in sufficient quantities, we believe that the presented methods can be used to create systems for fully automatic non-invasive risk assessment for a variety of adverse cardiac events.

Keywords: Plaque characterization · Computer aided diagnosis · Coronary CT angiography · Radiomics · Deep learning

© Springer Nature Switzerland AG 2019
D. Shen et al. (Eds.): MICCAI 2019, LNCS 11767, pp. 593–601, 2019.
https://doi.org/10.1007/978-3-030-32251-9_65

1   Introduction

Cardiovascular diseases (CVDs) have persisted to be the leading cause of death across all developed countries [10]. Most CVDs are related to atherosclerotic plaques in the associated arteries [11]. Two types of high risk plaque segments exist: functionally significant plaques, which narrow the lumen and immediately lead to cardiac ischemia, and vulnerable plaques, which can rupture and cause thrombus formation and adverse coronary syndromes (ACS) such as stroke or cardiac infarction.

The reference standard measure to judge whether a plaque segment is functionally significant and the corresponding vessel needs to be revascularized is the fractional flow reserve (FFR) value. FFR is defined as the pressure after a lesion relative to the pressure before the lesion, and is measured invasively [3]. As interventional procedures involving the heart have the risk of inducing adverse cardiac events, a non-invasive assessment of the type of plaque for further patient selection is highly desirable. A non-invasive approach for this task is simulated FFR, which aims to simulate the FFR values from coronary computed tomography angiography (CCTA) data using a fluid dynamics approach [14], which requires an exact segmentation of the whole coronary tree and computational mesh generation [16]. Sufficient segmentation quality can often only be achieved with time-consuming manual interaction.

Previously, radiomics have been proposed to represent quantitative image information which is inherent in the data but hard to interpret for human readers [8]. They include multiple intensity-, texture-, shape- and transformation-based metrics extracted from a lesion segmentation and have been shown to be able to characterize coronary plaques [6]. More recently, deep learning has been investigated to detect lesions with a high stenosis degree and to categorize the calcification grade of coronary plaques using a recurrent convolutional neural network (RCNN) [18]. In their work, they first extract multi planar reformatted (MPR) slices orthogonally to each centerline point. Next, they cut the resulting image stack into multiple overlapping cubes from which features are extracted using a 3D convolutional neural network (CNN). Finally, classification is achieved using a sequence analysis network.

In this work, we propose a fully automatic method to directly predict the clinical decision of revascularization based on single plague segments. We investigate three machine-learning approaches for classification: radiomic feature analysis, deep learning and a combination of both. For the first variant, radiomic features are extracted from each vessel segment based on the vessel segmentation in the region of interest. Contrary to the approach in [6], we do not perform data mining since it neglects cross-feature correlations. Instead, we train a bagging classifier, namely the XGBoost algorithm [1], which automatically detects relevant features and uses all information from the features. For the deep learning approach, we extend the approach presented in [18] by improving the data representation using a transformation of the image stack into a cylindrical coordinate system which allows for a more effective training of the network and reduce the risk of overfitting by using 2D instead of 3D convolutions. Thirdly, we propose a novel combination of both aforementioned approaches. After extracting a sequence of cubes along the centerline, we calculate the radiomic features of each cube using a plaque segmentation mask extracted a priori. The resulting sequence of radiomic features is then recombined with a multi-layer perceptron (MLP) and subsequently analyzed using a sequence analysis network based on gated recurrent units (GRUs). We evaluate all variants on CCTA scans of 95 patients with a total of 345 plague segments using ten-fold cross validation and compare our results with simulated FFR.

2   Data

The data collection contains CCTA scans of 95 patients taken within a time span of 2 years with the same system. The decision for revascularization or further invasive assessment was based on different clinical indications, e.g., functional tests including cardiac stress MRI or MIBI SPECT, and was made by trained cardiologists. In some cases, identification of culprit lesions was additionally based on ECG abnormalities if these indicated a bad perfusion of a specific part of the heart muscle. In total, the data contained 345 lesions, which were annotated by defining their start and end centerline point and segmenting their inner and outer vessel wall using a fully automatic approach [9]. For all data sets, automatic centerline extraction was performed as described in [17]. For each main branch of the coronaries a label indicated whether it was revascularized or not. To obtain reliable labels on the segment level, we propagated a positive revascularization decision only to the segment with the highest stenosis grade. In order to allow for an comparison with the results in [18], we additionally assessed for all segments whether the stenosis grade was below or above 50%. With this procedure 85 (24.64 %) lesions were labeled as having a high stenosis grade and 93 (26.97 %) as requiring revascularization.

3   Methods

3.1   Radiomic-Based Classification

As mentioned, a multitude of shape-, intensity- and texture-based features is extracted under different image transformations from the lesion segmentation as radiomics. A detailed description of all radiomic features can be found in [7]. The extracted feature vector has a high dimensionality. Therefore, direct classification is hard to achieve due to the curse of dimensionality. To overcome this we used the XGBoost classifier [1], which calculates its prediction based on an ensemble of decision trees while minimizing a loss function based on the total ensemble prediction. Since new leaves are added based on greedy search, only relevant non-redundant features are selected during training. Features were calculated using the open source PyRadiomics library [5] selecting all possible features under all transformations.

3.2   Deep Learning-Based Classification

The second approach is based on deep learning and can be separated into several steps: data extraction, local feature extraction and sequence analysis. An overview of the workflow is shown in Fig. 1. First, MPR slices are extracted orthogonally to each point of the centerline in the segment. Then, the resulting image stack is cut into multiple overlapping cubes. The extracted cubes are transformed to polar coordinates to allow for a better representation for the neural network. The motivation behind this lies in the assumption that features that characterize lesions are formed radially to the centerline and vary along the centerline direction. The slices of each transformed cube are then used as input to a 2D-CNN that performs a slice-wise feature extraction. This is followed by 1×1 convolutions in centerline direction that recombine and fuse the information across a cube to perform a local feature extraction. The architecture of the feature extraction network is depicted in Fig. 2, alongside the 3D-CNN network proposed in [18] that we evaluate for comparison. To obtain a final classification, we perform a sequence analysis using a two layer recurrent neural network (RNN) using gated recurrent units [2] on the features extracted from the cubes with the centerline direction as "temporal" dimension. Based on the assumption that information about the plaque composition is contained in both directions of the centerline, we perform the sequence analysis in a bidirectional fashion.

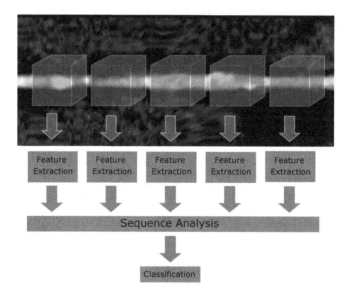

Fig. 1. Algorithm overview: extraction of a sequence of cubes along the centerline is followed up by a feature extraction method – either with a convolutional neural network or the PyRadiomics module. The resulting sequence of features is then analyzed by a sequence analysis neural network.

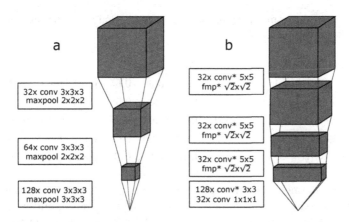

Fig. 2. Feature extraction model overview: (a) model as described in [18]. (b) our proposed model. * denotes a slice-wise operation, and fmp denotes fractional max pooling [4], which allows a pooling size smaller than 2 which enables feature extraction from intermediate scales.

3.3 Combined Approach

A common way to train neural networks with a limited amount of data is to use pretrained models, which comprise relevant image features already learned on different data sets. However, this is difficult when dealing with medical data, since data of different organs, modalities and use cases are often not correlated and three-dimensional. To overcome this, non-deep learning feature extraction methods can be used and combined with deep learning. Therefore, we combine the above mentioned radiomic and deep learning approaches. Again, the vessel was sliced in a sequence of overlapping volume cubes, but now the feature extraction was performed using the PyRadiomics library and the vessel segmentation of the plaque segment. Since preliminary experiments suggested the shape-based feature group to be the most important for estimating both the revascularization decision and the stenosis degree, we focused on these features. The resulting sequence of radiomic feature vectors was further evaluated using a three layer MLP before analyzing the sequence with bidirectional GRUs.

4   Experiments and Results

We evaluate the proposed approach for binary stenosis grade classification (high-degree stenosis > 50%, low-degree stenosis < 50%) to allow for a direct comparison with [18] and for the prediction of clinical revascularization decisions. For all experiments, evaluations were performed using ten-fold cross validation with patient-wise stratified splitting. For the neural network based methods, 20% of the training data was set aside as validation set in each fold. For each fold, the networks were trained for 50 epochs and the model that performed best on the validation set was selected for evaluation on the test set. For the CNN-based

Table 1. Evaluation results for stenosis degree prediction on lesion-level. The results in the first row are copied from [18].

Model/metric	AUC	Acc	F1	PPV	NPV	Sens	Spec	MCC
3D-RCNN [18] (orig data)	–	0.94	0.64	0.65	0.97	0.63	0.97	0.60
3D-RCNN [18] (our data)	0.89	0.85	0.67	0.58	**0.94**	0.79	0.86	0.59
2D-RCNN + polar transform	0.86	0.87	0.64	0.68	0.91	0.60	**0.93**	0.56
Radiomics + XGBoost	0.89	0.84	0.69	0.69	0.90	0.68	0.90	0.58
Radiomics + GRUs	**0.96**	**0.92**	**0.95**	**0.94**	0.82	**0.96**	0.75	**0.74**

methods, data augmentation was performed in form of random rotation, mirroring along the x-axis, translation and additive Gaussian noise, and we resampled the data during batch generation to achieve class balance. In order to normalize our data, histogram equalization was performed for each approach before feature extraction. To evaluate our approaches, we computed the area under the receiver operating characteristic curve (AUC), accuracy (Acc), F1-score, positive predictive value (PPV), negative predictive value (NPV), sensitivity, specificity and the Matthews correlation coefficient (MCC).

4.1 Stenosis Grade Classification

The classification results of the stenosis grade classification for the proposed methods and the 3D-CNN approach proposed in [18] are shown in Table 1. Compared to the results reported in [18], the performance of the 3D-RCNN approach on our dataset is lower. The main reason for this is likely the size of the respective data set, which was much smaller in our case. The proposed 2D-RCNN and radiomics approach achieved results on par with the 3D-RCNN. However, our combined approach outperformed all three other methods by a large margin (AUC 0.96 vs. 0.89 for 3D-RCNN/Radiomics+XGBoost and 0.86 for 2D-RCNN).

4.2 Classification of Revascularization Decision

The metrics for the revascularization prediction can be seen in Table 2. Since there exists a lot of variance with respect to the reference standard simulated

Table 2. Evaluation results for revascularization decision prediction on lesion-level.

Model/metric	AUC	Acc	F1	PPV	NPV	Sens	Spec	MCC
Simulated FFR best [13][a]	0.93	0.86	–	0.61	0.95	0.84	0.86	–
Simulated FFR worst [12][a]	0.79	0.69	–	0.56	0.84	0.61	0.89	–
3D-RCNN [18] (our data)	0.80	0.76	0.55	0.45	**0.91**	0.72	0.77	0.42
2D-RCNN + polar transform	0.84	0.82	0.57	0.60	0.88	0.54	0.91	0.46
Radiomics + XGBoost	0.86	0.86	0.62	0.69	0.89	0.56	**0.94**	0.54
Radiomics + GRUs	**0.88**	**0.87**	**0.92**	**0.90**	0.74	**0.95**	0.61	**0.60**

[a]Simulated FFR is compared to abnormal invasive FFR instead of revascularization decision

FFR, we compare our approaches to the best [13] and worst [12] results reported in the review paper of [15]. Note that simulated FFR is compared to an abnormally high invasive FFR value rather than the revascularization decision in the referenced publications, with both targets being highly correlated. The experiments in [12, 13] were performed on different non-publicly available data sets. Comparing the two RCNN networks, our proposed method performed slightly better. This indicates that features other than the stenosis degree are relevant for the revascularization decision, and that transforming the image data into the polar space was beneficial. The radiomics approach outperformed both deep learning methods, while our combined approach again performed best.

5   Discussion and Conclusion

Identifying functionally significant stenosis in a non-invasive setup is an important task to improve clinical outcomes. We presented and compared three machine-learning methods for the prediction of stenosis degree and clinical revascularization decision based on CCTA scans: Radiomics combined with boosting trees, a convolutional recurrent neural network, and an approach that combines shape-based radiomics and recurrent neural networks. We were able to show that all methods were able to differentiate stenosis grade $> 50\%$ and $< 50\%$, and reliably identify plaque lesion that were later revascularized. Across both tasks, the combined approach performed best, also compared to results reported in literature. The combined approach comes at a cost of a higher computation time of up to 2 s compared to only milliseconds for the RCNN approaches and requires a prior segmentation of the vessel lumen in the region of the plague segment. Still, the additional computation time does not pose a clinical limitation and the lumen segmentation is easily obtainable in an automated fashion. In contrast to this, simulated FFR requires an exact segmentation of the whole coronary tree and computation times of several minutes. For classification of revascularization, we showed that the performance of the proposed methods lies well within the range of prediction performance obtained by FFR simulation in literature. Given data with appropriate annotations, we believe that our methods would also perform well in identifying so-called culprit lesions that cause adverse cardiac events. Interestingly, the performance difference between the combined approach and the RCNN methods leads to the conclusion that extracting the shape-based features is highly relevant for differentiating lesions, but is harder to achieve for a completely data driven CNN-based feature extractor and may require a larger training data set. If only limited data is available, the combined approach proposed here seems to be promising, as predefined features and data-driven learning are fused. A limitation of the current study is that no simulated FFR values for the data set under investigation were available, which will be subject of future work. Additionally, the results will be validated on additional data collections that also include the invasive FFR measurements for comparison.

Disclaimer. The methods and information here are based on research and are not commercially available.

References

1. Chen, T., Guestrin, C.: XGBoost: a scalable tree boosting system. In: Proceedings of the 22nd ACM SIGKDD International Conference on Knowledge Discovery and Data Mining, pp. 785–794. ACM (2016)
2. Cho, K., et al.: Learning phrase representations using RNN encoder-decoder for statistical machine translation. arXiv preprint arXiv:1406.1078 (2014)
3. Cury, R.C., et al.: Coronary artery disease-reporting and data system (CAD-RADS): an expert consensus document of SCCT, ACR and NASCI: endorsed by the ACC. JACC: Cardiovasc. Imaging **9**(9), 1099–1113 (2016)
4. Graham, B.: Fractional max-pooling. arXiv preprint arXiv:1412.6071 (2014)
5. van Griethuysen, J., et al.: Computational radiomics system to decode the radiographic phenotype. Cancer Res. **77**(21), e104–e107 (2017)
6. Kolossváry, M., et al.: Radiomic features are superior to conventional quantitative computed tomographic metrics to identify coronary plaques with napkin-ring signclinical perspective. Circ. Cardiovasc. Imaging **10**(12), e006843 (2017)
7. Kolossváry, M., et al.: Cardiac computed tomography radiomics: a comprehensive review on radiomic techniques. J. Thorac. Imaging **33**(1), 26–34 (2018)
8. Lambin, P., et al.: Radiomics: extracting more information from medical images using advanced feature analysis. Eur. J. Cancer **48**(4), 441–446 (2012)
9. Lugauer, F., Zheng, Y., Hornegger, J., Kelm, B.M.: Precise lumen segmentation in coronary computed tomography angiography. In: Menze, B., et al. (eds.) MCV 2014. LNCS, vol. 8848, pp. 137–147. Springer, Cham (2014). https://doi.org/10.1007/978-3-319-13972-2_13
10. Mendis, S., Davis, S., Norrving, B.: Organizational update: the World Health Organization global status report on noncommunicable diseases 2014. Stroke **46**(5), e121–e122 (2015)
11. Naghavi, M.: From vulnerable plaque to vulnerable patient: a call for new definitions and risk assessment strategies. Part II. Circulation **108**, 1772–1778 (2003)
12. Nakazato, R., et al.: Noninvasive fractional flow reserve derived from computed tomography angiography for coronary lesions of intermediate stenosis severity: results from the DeFACTO study. Circ. Cardiovasc. Imaging **6**(6), 881–889 (2013)
13. Nørgaard, B.L., et al.: Diagnostic performance of noninvasive fractional flow reserve derived from coronary computed tomography angiography in suspected coronary artery disease: the NXT trial (analysis of coronary blood flow using CT angiography: next steps). J. Am. Coll. Cardiol. **63**(12), 1145–1155 (2014)
14. Taylor, C.A., Fonte, T.A., Min, J.K.: Computational fluid dynamics applied to cardiac computed tomography for noninvasive quantification of fractional flow reserve: scientific basis. J. Am. Coll. Cardiol. **61**(22), 2233–2241 (2013)
15. Tesche, C., et al.: Coronary CT angiography-derived fractional flow reserve. Radiology **285**(1), 17–33 (2017)
16. Wels, M., Lades, F., Hopfgartner, C., Schwemmer, C., Sühling, M.: Intuitive and accurate patient-specific coronary tree modeling from cardiac computed-tomography angiography. In: The 3rd Interactive Medical Image Computing Workshop, Athens, pp. 86–93 (2016)

17. Zheng, Y., Tek, H., Funka-Lea, G.: Robust and accurate coronary artery centerline extraction in CTA by combining model-driven and data-driven approaches. In: Mori, K., Sakuma, I., Sato, Y., Barillot, C., Navab, N. (eds.) MICCAI 2013. LNCS, vol. 8151, pp. 74–81. Springer, Heidelberg (2013). https://doi.org/10.1007/978-3-642-40760-4_10

18. Zreik, M., et al.: Automatic detection and characterization of coronary artery plaque and stenosis using a recurrent convolutional neural network in coronary CT angiography. arXiv preprint arXiv:1804.04360 (2018)

Response Estimation Through Spatially Oriented Neural Network and Texture Ensemble (RESONATE)

Jeffrey E. Eben[1]([⊠]), Nathaniel Braman[1], and Anant Madabhushi[1,2]

[1] Case Western Reserve University, Cleveland, OH, USA
{jee50,nmb60,axm788}@case.edu
[2] Louis Stokes Cleveland Veterans Administration Medical Center,
Cleveland, OH, USA

Abstract. Neoadjuvant chemotherapy (NAC) is considered to be the standard treatment for locally advanced breast cancer, but less than half of all recipients achieve pathological complete response (pCR), necessitating a way to predict pCR prior to NAC. Previous work has shown that pCR prediction is viable via either radiomic or deep learning classification methods when applied to the tumoral region on breast MRI. Others have shown that analysis within the peritumoral region directly outside of the tumor can contribute unique value to pCR prediction. In this work we present Response Estimation through Spatially Oriented Neural Network and Texture Ensemble (RESONATE): an approach to spatially invoke different types of analytic representations in different tumor compartments to create a multi-representation based prediction of response to NAC in breast cancer. A total of 114 NAC recipients with pre-treatment MRI were retrospectively analyzed, with 80 of the patients used for training and 34 held out as an independent testing set. Deep learning and radiomic classifiers were trained separately within the tumor and the peritumoral region, with separate classifier predictions then being fused

J. E. Eben and N. Braman—Equal contribution.

Research reported in this publication was supported by the National Cancer Institute of the National Institutes of Health under award numbers 1F31CA221383-01, 1U24CA199374-01, R01CA202752-01A1, R01CA208236-01A1, R01 CA216579-01A1, R01 CA220581-01A1, 1U01 CA239055-01, National Center for Research Resources under award number 1 C06 RR12463-01, VA Merit Review Award IBX004121A from the United States Department of Veterans Affairs Biomedical Laboratory Research and Development Service, the DOD Prostate Cancer Idea Development Award (W81XWH-15-1-0558), the DOD Lung Cancer Investigator-Initiated Translational Research Award (W81XWH-18-1-0440), the DOD Peer Reviewed Cancer Research Program (W81XWH-16-1-0329), the Ohio Third Frontier Technology Validation Fund, the Wallace H. Coulter Foundation Program in the Department of Biomedical Engineering and the Clinical and Translational Science Award Program (CTSA) at Case Western Reserve University. The content is solely the responsibility of the authors and does not necessarily represent the official views of the National Institutes of Health, the U.S. Department of Veterans Affairs, the Department of Defense, or the United States Government.

D. Shen et al. (Eds.): MICCAI 2019, LNCS 11767, pp. 602–610, 2019.
https://doi.org/10.1007/978-3-030-32251-9_66

together via a logistic regression classifier. In the testing set, individual radiomics and deep learning classifiers achieved area under the curve (AUC) values of 0.69 and 0.75 within the tumor, respectively, and 0.69 and 0.66 within the peritumoral region. A weighted fusion of these four classifiers, however, best predicted pCR with an AUC of 0.79. This approach also outperformed fusions incorporating radiomic (AUC = 0.77) or deep learning (AUC = 0.75) only, as well as combinations of representations only within (AUC = 0.78) or outside (AUC = 0.70) the tumor.

1   Introduction

Neoadjuvant chemotherapy (NAC) is the standard treatment for locally advanced breast cancer [1]. Favorable response to NAC is best measured by pathological complete response (pCR), where the patient has no residual invasive disease in the breast and lymph nodes following treatment [2]. Only 10–50% of patients receiving NAC will experience pCR, leading to many unnecessary side effects and detriments to quality of life for non-responsive patients [3]. However, a growing body of work has suggested the potential of computational medical image analysis to enable the prediction of response to NAC from dynamic contrast-enhanced (DCE) MRI. Radiomics, the high-throughput extraction and analysis of algorithmically defined features from radiology, has been shown to predict response on pre-treatment DCE-MRI through attributes such as image texture [4]. Deep learning, involving the training of a convolutional neural network to identify novel predictive image patterns, has successfully been applied to response prediction prior to treatment [5].

An emerging trend is that prediction of response to NAC is not only a matter of selecting the right computational tools, but also where they are deployed. For instance, previous work has shown that supplementing radiomic features extracted from the tumor itself with texture features computed within the peritumoral region - the tumor's surrounding environment - enables improved prediction of pCR from pre-treatment DCE-MRI [4] and the ability to identify genotypes associated with response to targeted therapy [6]. A related study, using deep learning for predicting response to esophageal cancer based on the tumor and peritumoral region on PET, was reported in [7].

While several studies have investigated the fusion of radiomics and deep learning, a large portion employ naive ensembling strategies [8,9] that weight each equally without consideration of their relative strengths and weaknesses. However, it is not clear that the different types of representations are ideally suited uniformly across the different parts of the region of interest (ROI). For instance, in the case of a lung nodule on CT, while CNNs might capture unique heterogeneity patterns pertaining to ground glass opacity within the nodule, radiomic edge operators might accentuate unique attributes relating to margin spicularity. In other words, spatially invoking specific representations might be a better mechanism for feature fusion compared to combining multiple representations within the same ROI.

In this work, we present Response Estimation through Spatially Oriented Neural Network and Texture Ensemble (RESONATE): a novel approach for the fusion of radiomic and deep learning data streams by invoking them in the spatial regions at which they are most discriminative.

2 Previous Works and Novel Contributions

Despite the individual promise of radiomics and deep learning approaches, relatively few have explored how these approaches can be combined. Antropova et al. [8] and Paul et al. [9] averaged the outputs and predictions of deep learning and radiomic based classifiers for diagnostic problems relating to breast and lung cancer, respectively. Others have explored more complex fusion strategies that attempt to account for differences in model performance through training a model across ensembled classifiers and data streams [10,11]. A common theme of these approaches is the fact that they leverage CNNs and radiomics as ways of providing different types of representations from within the same region to boost classifier performance.

The approach presented in this work, RESONATE, is unique from these previous approaches by using a spatial preference to invoke different types of representations, radiomics and deep learning, within different tumor subcompartments. The approach differentially weights representations based on their relative regional strengths within a fused regression model.

3 Methodology

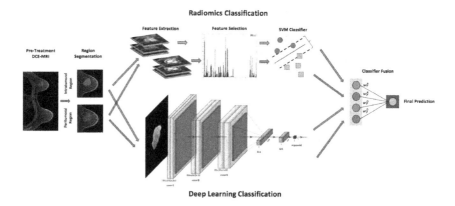

Fig. 1. RESONATE Workflow – Image segmentation (left) separates the patient's tumor into intratumoral (red) and peritumoral (blue) regions. Deep learning (bottom) and radiomic (top) classification is then performed separately within each region, with the predictions of each classifier being fused with a logistic regression classifier (right) to create a final prediction. (Color figure online)

3.1   Spatial Localization of Tumor Habitat

We define an image scene $\mathcal{I}$ as a 3-dimensional spatial grid of voxels, corresponding to one phase of a DCE-MRI volume. Let $\mathcal{T}$ represent a sub-volume of $\mathcal{I}$ corresponding to a segmentation of a tumor. From $\mathcal{T}$ we further define a peri-tumoral volume, $\mathcal{P}$, which corresponds to the region surrounding the tumor, originating at the tumor border, and extending out to all voxels within some user-specified maximum physical distance.

3.2   Spatial-Specific Model Representation

The spatial regions, $\mathcal{T}$ and $\mathcal{P}$, were separately analyzed using deep learning and radiomic classification methods. For each $\mathcal{I}$, let y indicate an accompanying binary outcome to treatment, where a value of 1 indicates successful response.

Deep Learning. Two models were created, one for each region $\mathcal{S} \in \{\mathcal{T}, \mathcal{P}\}$, using the following procedure. We define $\mathcal{I}_\mathcal{S}$ as a volumetric box, which is a sub-volume of $\mathcal{I}$ large enough to contain all points of $\mathcal{S}$. To isolate the ROI, the intensity value of all voxels contained within $\mathcal{I}_\mathcal{S}$ but not in $\mathcal{S}$ are set equal to the mean intensity within $\mathcal{S}$ in order to prevent deep learning models from relying too heavily on annotation boundaries. A convolutional neural network, $\mathcal{D}_\mathcal{S}$ is then trained using $\mathcal{I}_\mathcal{S}$ from a number of different image volumes to predict a probability of response $p_\mathcal{S}^\mathcal{D}$ as close as possible to y, as measured by some loss function $L(y, p_\mathcal{S}^\mathcal{D})$.

Radiomics. Radiomic models were created for each region $\mathcal{S} \in \{\mathcal{T}, \mathcal{P}\}$. For every voxel within $\mathcal{S}$, a set of unique radiomic descriptors is computed. The distribution of each radiomic descriptor across all voxels of $\mathcal{S}$ are statistically summarized into a feature vector, and a feature selection algorithm is applied to the feature vector to create an optimal reduced set of features. A classifier $\mathcal{R}_\mathcal{S}$ accepts this reduced set of features and outputs a response prediction $p_\mathcal{S}^\mathcal{R}$.

3.3   Model Fusion

A logistic regression classifier, $\mathcal{L}$, was designed to fuse the predictions of classifiers $\mathcal{C}_\mathcal{S}$, where $\mathcal{C} \in \{\mathcal{D}, \mathcal{R}\}$, $\mathcal{S} \in \{\mathcal{T}, \mathcal{P}\}$. Each classifier, $\mathcal{C}_\mathcal{S}$ is first trained independently, with $\mathcal{L}$ then being trained using the predictions of each individual classifier as

$$\ln(\frac{p_\mathcal{L}}{1 - p_\mathcal{L}}) = W_0 + \sum_{n=1}^{N} W_n p_\mathcal{S}^\mathcal{C} \tag{1}$$

where $p_\mathcal{S}^\mathcal{C}$ represents a prediction output for classifier $\mathcal{C}$ in region $\mathcal{S}$. This model fusion approach allows $\mathcal{L}$ to learn a weighted combination between per-patient predictions from each classifier based on the relative strengths of representation and location, giving the ability for a stronger ensemble prediction.

4 Experimental Design

4.1 Data Description

The dataset used consists of axial-plane breast DCE-MRIs of 114 patients with biopsy-proved breast cancer, collected prior to administration of neoadjuvant chemotherapy with a 1.5 or 3 T magnet [4,12]. DCE-MRI acquisitions were collected across six separate contrast enhancement sequences for each patient, and three-frame intratumoral masks were annotated at the peak-enhancement sequence by a trained radiologist. Peritumoral masks were generated by expanding the intratumoral mask 3 mm outward. For all experiments, the patients were divided into a training (N = 80) and held out testing (N = 34) cohort. The training cohort was further stratified into three training (N = 53) and validation (N = 27) folds for cross-validation.

4.2 Implementation Details

Deep Learning: CNN inputs, of size $150 \times 110 \times 3 \times 3$ for the peritumoral network and $146 \times 104 \times 3 \times 3$ for the tumoral network, consist of 3-dimensional blocks centered at the region of interest with a fourth, temporal dimension corresponding to different phases of DCE-MRI acquisition. The network (depicted in Fig. 1) consists of three convolutional blocks, with a block containing two convolutional layers with ReLU activation, followed by a batch normalization and max pooling layer. Each block sequentially widens the network by increasing the number of filters used in the convolutional layers, going from 8 to 16 to 32 filters, all with kernels of size $3 \times 3 \times 1$. After flattening the final convolutional outputs, a small dense block consisting of two dense layers (with 128 and 64 filters, respectively), each followed by ReLU activation and 50% dropout. A final sigmoid layer computes final probability output. Data augmentation was performed, applying random rotations and spatial zooming, as well as random sampling preserving temporal order from 5 available DCE-MRI post-contrast acquisitions to include with the pre-contrast scan as input for training. Training was performed using a binary cross-entropy loss function, and a stochastic gradient descent optimizer with a nesterov momentum of 0.9, a learning rate of 0.0005, and a learning rate decay of 0.01. Visual attention with guided back-propogation [13], via keras-vis [14], was implemented post-hoc for evaluation of image regions corresponding to a prediction of response.

Radiomics Classifier: Within the tumor and peri-tumoral region, a total of 99 radiomic texture features were extracted voxelwise on the DCE-MRI phase of peak contrast enhancement, including 25 Laws, 48 Gabor, 13 gray level co-occurrence matrix (GLCM), and 13 co-occurrence of local anisotropic gradient orientation (CoLlAGe) features. See [4] for greater description on the radiomic feature set explored. Five first order statistics - mean, median, standard deviation (SD), skewness, and kurtosis - were computed to describe the distribution of features within each region. A set of top features were chosen with a two-part feature selection scheme. First, the feature set was pruned to eliminate correlated features based on a minimum allowable spearman correlation between features (with the retained feature chosen by wilcoxon rank sum test). Second, two rounds of minimum redundancy maximum relevance (mRMR) feature selection were used to identify between 1–20 top features optimized over 1000 iterations in cross-validation [4]. Top features within each fold were used to train several classifiers: naive bayes, support vector machine (SVM), and diagonal linear discriminant analysis (DLDA). The optimal combination of correlation threshold for pruning, number of top features, and type of classifier was chosen based on cross-validated AUC within the training set, then applied to the testing set.

Model Fusion: The fused model was developed in the following fashion:

1. *Tuning individual models:* Region-specific radiomic and deep learning classifiers were optimized via 3-fold cross-validation within the training set. Specific hyper-parameter details are provided in Sect. 5.1.
2. *Evaluating model fusion by cross-validation:* For each optimized model, validation fold predictions were accumulated into a set of predicted response probabilities for the full training set. Cross-validation was repeated, this time training logistic regression model weights based on predictions from the training fold and evaluating on predictions from the validation fold.
3. *Creating and testing final fusion models:* The final regression model was trained on accumulated cross-validation predictions from each of the 3 folds. A final version of each individual model was retrained using the full training set with the optimal hyper-parameters discovered in cross-validation. Fusion model predictions were then collected by passing in the prediction outputs of each individual final model to the logistic regression classifier.

5   Results and Discussion

5.1   Individual pCR Prediction Models

Deep Learning: Final deep learning models were trained on the full training set for 67 epochs, based on average convergence time observed in cross-validation. Two variants of the deep learning classifier were trained, one using intratumoral segmentations and the other using peritumoral segmentations. The deep learning model focused on the tumor outperformed the peritumoral model in both the training and testing set (Table 1).

Radiomics: Best performance was achieved in cross-validation of the training set when using a SVM classifier, initially pruning features with correlation higher than 90%, and choosing a final set of 11 features via mRMR feature selection. Two variants of the SVM classifier, $\mathcal{R}_T$ and $\mathcal{R}_P$, were trained within each region. Performance between tumoral and peri-tumoral models was found to be comparable (Table 1).

Table 1. Classification results for single model and multi-model fusion

	Deep Learning	
	Tumor	*Peri*
CV, AUC (SD)	0.688 (0.104)	0.620 (0.057)
Testing, AUC	0.750	0.663
Radiomics	**Merged**	
Tumor	**Representations**	
CV, AUC (SD)	0.733 (0.057)	0.776 (0.106)	0.748 (0.078)
Testing, AUC	0.692	0.779	0.697
Peri		
CV, AUC (SD)	0.744 (0.046)	0.775 (0.0371)	0.750 (.046)
Testing, AUC	0.692	0.784	0.697

5.2 Experiment 2: Multi-region, Multi-representation Response Prediction via RESONATE

A fusion of predictions from all spatially-oriented classifiers, $\mathcal{L}(\mathcal{D}_T, \mathcal{D}_P, \mathcal{R}_T, \mathcal{R}_P)$, was found to best identify pCR, achieving an AUC of 0.78 ± 0.05 in cross-validation and 0.79 in the testing set. Confidence intervals (CI) and p-values were computed on the test set AUC via 50,000 iteration permutation testing [15], giving a 95% testing set CI $= .62 - .96$, p $= .003$. Note that, for the full RESONATE model, as well as some individual models, performance increased in the testing set relative to the training set: likely a result of using the full training set to derive final models, as compared to models evaluated in cross-validation which leveraged only a portion of the training data. We found that, based on the weights of $\mathcal{L}$, the ensemble prediction relied primarily on $\mathcal{R}_P$, $\mathcal{R}_T$, and $\mathcal{D}_T$, which had weights of 0.80, 0.99, and 0.77 respectively. The difference in these representations between patients identified as pCR, as compared to non-responders, are depicted visually in Fig. 2. Meanwhile, the peritumoral deep learning model, $\mathcal{D}_P$, was found to contribute the least to pCR prediction relative to other models, with a weight of -0.08.

5.3 Experiment 3: Comparative Strategies - Pairwise Fusion

Each pairwise combination of classifiers was similarly combined into a fused model for comparison against the full RESONATE model (Table 1), none of which matched its performance. A radiomics model combining information from both the tumor and peritumoral region, previously shown to be an effective pCR prediction strategy [4], was found to under-perform relative to the model also incorporating multi-region deep learning, with an AUC of 0.75 ± 0.04 in the training set and 0.77 in the testing set (95% CI $= .58 - .97$, p $= .006$). Likewise, fusion of deep learning models from both regions achieved AUC of 0.73 ± 0.07 in the training set and 0.75 in the test set (95% CI $= .50 - .99$, p $= .026$).

Similarly, fusion of representations in a single region was found to less effectively predict pCR, with combinations of models fusing deep learning and radiomic representations only inside or outside the tumor achieving AUCs of 0.78

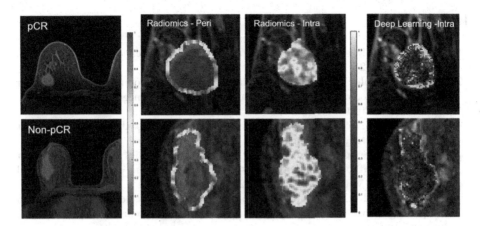

Fig. 2. Middle, radiomics feature maps: Increased expression of mid frequency Gabor features within the peri-tumoral region and CoLlAGe entropy features within the tumor distinguished non-response (right). Visual attention maps for the intra-tumoral CNN emphasize tumor border and core in patients who achieved pCR (Right).

(95% CI = .55 − 1.00, p = .012) and 0.70 (95% CI = .45 − .94, p = .052) within the testing set, respectively. Of all pairwise combinations, the best performance was observed when combining the tumoral deep learning model and the peritumoral radiomics model (AUC = 0.78, 95% CI = .55 − 1.00, p = .014). This finding emphasizes the value of considering both multiple representations and multiple regions of analysis in pre-treatment response prediction.

6   Conclusion

Our results show that an ensemble of classifiers oriented spatially in the tumor habitat is a viable method for predicting favorable response to NAC in patients with biopsy-proven breast cancer. We applied deep learning and radiomic classifiers with attention focused in either the intratumoral or peritumoral regions of the breast, with individual classifier predictions being further boosted by a logistic regression ensemble model and achieving an AUC of 0.79 in a held out test set. This work is the first to present a methodology for the fusion of radiomics and deep learning approaches across multiple regions of biological significance and emphasizes the importance of multi-region, multi-representation in the pre-treatment determination of which patients will benefit from therapeutic intervention.

References

1. Thompson, A.M., et al.: Neoadjuvant treatment of breast cancer. Ann. Oncol. **23**, x231–x236 (2012)
2. Kong, X., et al.: Meta-analysis confirms pathological complete response after neoadjuvant chemotherapy predicts favourable breast cancer prognosis. Eur. J. Canc. **47**(14), 2084–2090 (2011)
3. Earl, H., et al.: Neoadjuvant trials in early breast cancer: pathological response at surgery and correlation to longer term outcomes. BMC Med. **13**(1), 234 (2015)
4. Braman, N.M., et al.: Intratumoral and peritumoral radiomics for the pretreatment prediction of pathological complete response to neoadjuvant chemotherapy based on breast DCE-MRI. BCR **19**(1), 57 (2017)
5. Ravichandran, K., et al.: A deep learning classifier for prediction of pathological complete response to neoadjuvant chemotherapy from baseline breast DCE-MRI. In: SPIE (2018)
6. Braman, N., et al.: Association of peritumoral radiomics with tumor biology and pathologic response to preoperative targeted therapy for HER2 (ERBB2)-positive breast cancer. JAMA Netw. Open **2**(4), e192561–e192561 (2019)
7. Amyar, A., et al.: 3-D RPET-NET: development of a 3-D pet imaging convolutional neural network for radiomics analysis and outcome prediction. IEEE TRPMS **3**(2), 225–231 (2019)
8. Antropova, N., et al.: A deep feature fusion methodology for breast cancer diagnosis demonstrated on three imaging modality datasets. Med. Phys. **44**(10), 5162–5171 (2017)
9. Paul, R., et al.: Predicting nodule malignancy using a CNN ensemble approach. In: Proceedings of the International Joint Conference on Neural Networks (2018)
10. Bizzego, A., et al.: Integrating deep and radiomics features in cancer bioimaging. bioRxiv (2019)
11. Liu, S., et al.: Pulmonary nodule classification in lung cancer screening with three-dimensional convolutional neural networks. J. Med. Imaging **4**(4), 041308 (2017)
12. Braman, N., Prasanna, P., Alilou, M., Beig, N., Madabhushi, A.: Vascular network organization via hough transform (VaNgOGH): a novel radiomic biomarker for diagnosis and treatment response. In: Frangi, A.F., Schnabel, J.A., Davatzikos, C., Alberola-López, C., Fichtinger, G. (eds.) MICCAI 2018. LNCS, vol. 11071, pp. 803–811. Springer, Cham (2018). https://doi.org/10.1007/978-3-030-00934-2_89
13. Springenberg, J.T., et al.: Striving for simplicity: the all convolutional net. In: ICLR (2015)
14. Kotikalapudi, R., et al.: keras-vis (2017). https://github.com/raghakot/keras-vis
15. Pauly, M., et al.: Permutation based inference for the AUC: a unified approach for continuous and discontinuous data. Biometrical **58**(6), 1319–1337 (2016)

STructural Rectal Atlas Deformation (StRAD) Features for Characterizing Intra- and Peri-wall Chemoradiation Response on MRI

Jacob Antunes[1], Zhouping Wei[1], Charlems Alvarez-Jimenez[2],
Eduardo Romero[2], Marwa Ismail[1], Anant Madabhushi[1,3], Pallavi Tiwari[1],
and Satish E. Viswanath[1(✉)]

[1] Case Western Reserve University, Cleveland, USA
sev21@case.edu
[2] Universidad Nacional de Colombia, Bogota, Colombia
[3] Louis Stokes VA Medical Center, Cleveland, USA

Abstract. Radiomic features which quantify morphologic texture and shape of tumor regions on imaging have found wide success in characterizing treatment response *in vivo*. A more detailed interrogation of intra- and peri-tumoral regions for response-related cues could be achieved by capturing subtle structural deformations that occur due to tumor shrinkage or growth. In this work, we present a novel suite of STructural Rectal Atlas Deformation (StRAD) features to quantify tumor-related deformations in rectal cancers via a cohort of 139 patient MRIs. In flexible non-rigid organs such as the rectum, inter-patient differences complicate evaluation of tumor-related deformations that may occur within the rectal wall or in the peri-rectal environment; necessitating construction of a canonical rectal imaging atlas. Using 63 pelvic MRIs where healthy rectums could be clearly visualized, we built the first structural atlas for the healthy rectal wall. This atlas was used to compute structural deformations within and around locations in the rectal wall of patients where tumor was present, resulting in intra- and peri-wall StRAD descriptors. We evaluated the efficacy of our StRAD features in 2 different tasks: (a) predicting which rectal tumors will or will not respond to therapy via baseline MRIs (n = 42), and (b) identifying which

J. Antunes and Z. Wei—Joint first authors.
Research supported by NCI (U24CA199374-01, R01CA202752-01A1, R01CA208236-01A1, R01CA216579-01A1, R01CA220581-01A1, U01CA239055-01, F31CA216935-01A1), NCRR (1C06RR12463-01), DOD/CDMRP (W81XWH-15-1-0558, W81XWH-16-10329, W81XWH-18-0404, W81XWH-18-1-0440), NIDDK (1P30DK09794 Pilot Award), NBIB (T32EB00750912), VA (IBX004121A Merit Review Award), the Dana Foundation David Mahoney Neuroimaging Program, the Ohio Third Frontier Technology Validation Fund, the Wallace H. Coulter Foundation Program in the Department of Biomedical Engineering and the Clinical and Translational Science Award Program at CWRU. Content solely responsibility of the authors and does not necessarily represent the official views of the NIH, USDVA, DOD, or the United States Government.

D. Shen et al. (Eds.): MICCAI 2019, LNCS 11767, pp. 611–619, 2019.
https://doi.org/10.1007/978-3-030-32251-9_67

rectal tumors were exhibiting regression on post-chemoradiation MRIs (n = 34). Using a linear discriminant analysis classifier in a three-fold cross-validation scheme, we found that intra-wall deformations were significantly lower for responders to chemoradiation; both on baseline MRIs (AUC = 0.73±0.05) as well as on post-therapy MRIs (AUC = 0.87±0.03). By comparison, radiomic texture features for both intra- and peri-wall locations yielded significantly worse classification performance in both tasks.

1 Introduction

The advent of radiomics has demonstrated great success for predicting and evaluating treatment response via imaging in different cancers [1]. Radiomic approaches have typically extracted morphologic texture or shape descriptors of the tumor region, which have been related to underlying pathologic or molecular heterogeneity that drive therapy response [2]. As an example, prediction of response to chemoradiation in rectal cancers via pre- or post-treatment MRI [3, 4] has been limited to morphologic radiomic descriptors for image appearance alone. Unlike deep learning approaches (which are data-driven solutions to lesion segmentation, localization, or detection [5]), radiomics also leverages "handcrafted" descriptors to quantify specific imaging characteristics both within and around the tumor [6]. For instance, new classes of features that quantify tissue deformations or surface distentions on imaging have been linked to aggressive tumor growth [7] as well as tumor recurrence [8] (based on available reference atlas representations in solid organs such as the brain or the prostate). Quantifying such structural changes in more flexible organs such as the rectum requires construction of a healthy rectal wall atlas (i.e. rectal anatomy without tumor). We hypothesized that constructing a healthy rectal atlas could allow for unique quantification of disease-specific structural changes in the rectal environment (wall/tumor, peri-wall/tumor) that may be closely related to tumor response to therapy. The novel contributions of this work are:

- Development of the first structural atlas representation for healthy rectal wall anatomy, via a multi-stage registration scheme using pelvic MRIs (from other cancers) where normal rectums are visible.
- The first attempt at relating subtle structural deformations occurring within and around rectal wall regions against chemoradiation-related tumor growth or shrinkage *in vivo*.

Our novel STructural Rectal Atlas Deformation (StRAD) features were evaluated in the context of 2 distinct clinical problems in rectal cancer: (a) prediction of pathologic non-responders to chemoradiation via baseline treatment-naïve MRI, and (b) assessment of pathologic responders on post-chemoradiation MRI. Together, these represent the major clinical challenges facing personalization of patient management in rectal cancers.

2   Methodology

Quantifying structural deformations within and around the rectum involves 3 major steps: (i) building a structural atlas for normal rectal wall anatomy on imaging [9], (ii) computing structural deformations of the rectal wall in patients with tumors with respect to this atlas [10], and (iii) extracting tumor-related structural deformation descriptors within the rectal wall and peri-rectal environment. The steps to extract StRAD features are illustrated in Fig. 1.

2.1   Construction of Structural Rectal Atlas

A set of N MRI scenes depicting the healthy rectum is utilized, denoted $\mathcal{X} = (C, f)$, where C is a 3-dimensional spatial grid and $f(c)$ represents the MRI intensity at each voxel $c \in C$. The primary anatomic region defined within this MRI scene is the healthy rectal wall, denoted $\mathcal{X}^r = (C, f^r)$, where $f^r(c) = 1$ within the rectal wall and zero in the rest of the scene. $\mathcal{X}^r$ can be identified and annotated by experts on all $\mathcal{X}$, and is depicted via the color green in Fig. 1.

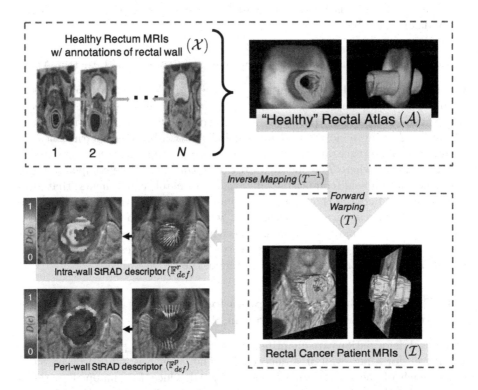

Fig. 1. Overall workflow for extracting StRAD descriptors including construction of healthy rectal atlas, computing deformations within and around the rectal wall in rectal cancer patients (with respect to the atlas), and extracting structural deformation features for intra- and peri-wall regions.

The final output of this step is the healthy rectal wall atlas, denoted $\mathcal{A} = (C, g^r)$. We define $g^r(c) \in [0, 1]$, as the frequency of a particular location $c \in C$ where $f^r(c) = 1$ (i.e. corresponding to rectal wall); across N different input subject scenes. These N different subject scenes are aligned to a registration template for projection into a canonical space to construct $\mathcal{A}$, via the following 3 transformations [9]:

1. A simple transformation, τ_ρ, is used to map N different subject scenes $\mathcal{X}$ such that they are all centered and isotropically scaled in X, Y, and Z axes. The resulting initial atlas, $\mathcal{A}_\rho$, is therefore not dependent on selecting a specific subject as the template and is constructed such that $A_\rho = (C, g^r)$, where $g^r(c) = \frac{1}{N} \sum_N f^r(c)$, for every location $c \in C$, across all N studies after τ_ρ has been applied (i.e. $g^r(c)$ is the frequency of a location corresponding to the rectal wall).
2. Affine registration is used to compute τ_α for projecting all $\mathcal{X}$ onto $\mathcal{A}_\rho$. The affinely transformed subject scenes are used to construct $A_\alpha = (C, g^r)$ (based on re-computing $g^r(c) \ \forall c \in C$, across all N studies).
3. Deformable registration is used to align $\mathcal{X}$ to $\mathcal{A}_\alpha$. The final structural rectal atlas $A = (C, g^r)$, is constructed based on re-computing $g^r(c) \ \forall c \in C$, across N deformed subject scenes.

2.2   Computing Structural Deformations with Respect to the Atlas

Given a patient MRI scene, denoted $\mathcal{I}$, structural deformations in the rectal environment are quantified [10] with respect to the healthy atlas $\mathcal{A}$. The rectal wall within the patient MRI scene is denoted $\mathcal{I}^r$. First, $\mathcal{A}$ is non-rigidly registered to $\mathcal{I}$ using a normalized mutual information-based similarity measure within a b-spline registration scheme. This non-rigid alignment is formulated as $(\mathcal{I}^r, \mathcal{I}) = T(\mathcal{A})$, where T is the forward transformation of the composite voxel-wise deformation field (comprising affine and deformable components) that maps the rectal wall between the reference $(\mathcal{I}^r)$ and floating $(\mathcal{A})$ volumes. This transformation is then inverted to yield T^{-1}, which is used to map $\mathcal{I}$ into the $\mathcal{A}$ space. This 2-stage mapping process is designed to compute structural deformations within $\mathcal{I}$ with respect to $\mathcal{A}$ at every $c \in C$, hypothesized to occur as a result of tumor-related growth or shrinkage of the rectal wall.

2.3   Extracting StRAD Descriptors for Subregions Within Rectal Wall and Peri-rectal Environment

Structural deformations are quantified for each rectal cancer patient scene within $\mathcal{I}^r$, as well for a peri-wall area denoted $\mathcal{I}^p$. The latter was defined based on $\mathcal{I}^r$ within each of the experiments later conducted. Once $\mathcal{I}$ is mapped to the $\mathcal{A}$ space, all voxel positions (c_x, c_y, c_z) are assumed to be displaced by $[\delta x, \delta y, \delta z]$, to result in $(c'_x, c'_y, c'_z) = (c_x, c_y, c_z) + (\delta x, \delta y, \delta z)$. Based on this displacement vector, the deformation magnitude is computed as $D(c) = \sqrt{(\delta x)^2 + (\delta y)^2 + (\delta z)^2}$, for every $c \in C$. The descriptor $\mathbb{F}^r_{def}$ for intra-wall deformations comprises first order statistics (i.e. mean, median, standard deviation, skewness, and kurtosis) of $D(c)$ for all the voxels c within the rectal wall $\mathcal{I}^r$. Similarly, the peri-wall deformation descriptor $\mathbb{F}^p_{def}$ can be computed based on first-order statistics of the deformation magnitudes in $\mathcal{I}^p$.

3   Experimental Design

3.1   Data Description

Healthy Rectum Cohort (S_1): A cohort of 63 patients who had been diagnosed with prostate cancer and had undergone an axial pelvic MRI scan were curated. As no endorectal coil had been used during the MRI scans, these images provided a clear *in vivo* visualization of the healthy rectal wall.

Baseline RCa Cohort (S_2): A cohort of 42 patients who had been diagnosed with rectal cancer were identified, all of whom had undergone axial 3 Tesla (T) T2w MR imaging <u>before</u> standard-of-care chemoradiation. The goal was to predict non-responders to chemoradiation using this baseline MRI scan. Pathologic tumor stage (T-stage, based on excised rectal specimens) was used as a marker of response, where ypT3-4 corresponded to extensive tumor being present in the specimen despite chemoradiation. Based on this pathologic classification, $n = 22$ patients were identified as being non-responsive to chemoradiation (ypT3-4), and the remainder as responders to chemoradiation (ypT0-2, $n = 20$).

Post-therapy RCa Cohort (S_3): A separate cohort of 34 RCa patients was curated, where patients had axial 3 T T2w MRIs available <u>after</u> undergoing standard-of-care chemoradiation but prior to excision surgery. In this cohort, the goal was to identify which patients exhibited marked tumor regression (based on pathologic T-stage) via the post-therapy MRI scan. With ypT0-2 indicating minimal or dying tumor within the rectal wall after chemoradiation, $n = 17$ patients were assessed as being responders and the remaining $n = 17$ were classified as exhibiting minimal or no response to chemoradiation (ypT3-4).

3.2   Implementation Details

For all 139 MRI scans in cohorts S_{1-3}, the entire length of the visible rectal wall from the anus to the peritoneal reflection was annotated by an expert radiologist. For the 76 RCa cases in S_2 and S_3, the slices most suspicious for tumor presence were also identified by the radiologist (using anatomic information from pathology reports). The healthy atlas $\mathcal{A}$ was constructed using $N = 63$ MRI pelvic scans in S_1 using the approach from Sect. 2.1. Evaluation of the atlas in terms of overlap in annotated rectal wall as well as internal lumen regions (across all patients in S_1 after deformable mapping) yielded a Dice similarity coefficient of 0.87, indicating $\mathcal{A}$ was a relatively accurate representation.

Deformation fields for the remaining 79 RCa scans in S_2 and S_3 (with respect to $\mathcal{A}$) were then computed to yield intra-wall and peri-wall StRAD descriptors,

$\mathbb{F}^r_{def}$ and $\mathbb{F}^p_{def}$ respectively (each a 5×1 vector). The peri-wall region was empirically defined as an 8 pixel band along the outer wall boundary for S_2 and S_3. All registration steps were implemented using *elastix* [11], with a grid spacing of $9 \times 9 \times 9$ when computing b-spline deformations. Radiomic texture features were also extracted to characterize the appearance of intra- and peri-wall areas on all 79 RCa scans [1], yielding $\mathbb{F}^r_{tex}$ and $\mathbb{F}^p_{tex}$ (each a 825×1 vector). Both deformation and texture features were extracted from 3 consecutive slices comprising the largest wall area suspicious for tumor, assuming that this region was most likely to exhibit signatures related to tumor growth or shrinkage on MRI.

Separate experiments were conducted using each of S_2 and S_3 in a cross-validation setting, with the goal of distinguishing between the 2 patient groups in each cohort. Following feature extraction, minimum redundancy maximum relevance feature selection [12] (mRMR) was used to identify the 3 most relevant features within each of $\mathbb{F}^r_{def}$, $\mathbb{F}^p_{def}$, $\mathbb{F}^r_{tex}$, and $\mathbb{F}^p_{tex}$. The most relevant set of features from each vector was then evaluated via a Linear Discriminant Analysis (LDA) classifier. A total of 50 iterations of a three-fold (one fold held-out for testing), patient-stratified, cross-validation scheme were utilized to ensure robustness of feature selection and classifier evaluation steps; with ROC analysis for evaluation. These steps were repeated for each of S_2 and S_3, and the area under the ROC curve (AUC) across all cross-validation runs was used to compare each of $\mathbb{F}^r_{def}$, $\mathbb{F}^p_{def}$, $\mathbb{F}^r_{tex}$, and $\mathbb{F}^p_{tex}$ (via Wilcoxon ranksum testing) to determine which feature set was most relevant for treatment response characterization.

4   Results and Discussion

4.1   Experiment 1: Predicting Non-responders to Chemoradiation via Baseline MRIs

The most relevant StRAD descriptors identified in experimental evaluation of S_2 were the skewness and standard deviation of intra-wall deformation magnitudes, the former of which is visualized in Fig. 2. Higher deformation magnitudes are shown in red in Fig. 2(b) and (d), while lower magnitudes are in blue. Our results indicate that non-responders to chemoradiation may be associated with significantly higher structural deformations within the rectal wall on baseline MRI scans (Fig. 2(e), positive skew associated with non-responders), when compared to the healthy rectal atlas. This resonates with previous findings where it has been reported that smaller rectal tumors tend to respond favorably to chemoradiation [13], which would result their being associated with less pronounced wall deformations (with reference to a healthy atlas). Further, the intra-wall StRAD descriptor ($\mathbb{F}^r_{def}$) also yielded the best overall AUC in this classification task (blue bar in Fig. 2(f), 0.73 ± 0.05). This was significantly higher ($p < 0.001$) than the AUCs for each of $\mathbb{F}^p_{def}$, $\mathbb{F}^r_{tex}$, and $\mathbb{F}^p_{tex}$.

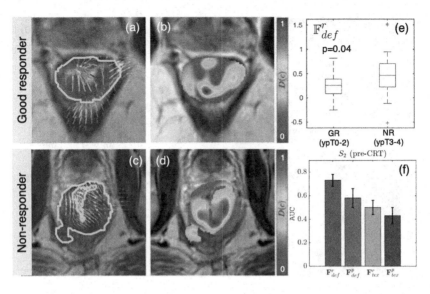

Fig. 2. (a), (c) Representative baseline T2w MRI scans from S_2 for two different patients showing deformation field as colored arrows within the rectal wall (annotated in yellow). (b), (d) Corresponding intra-wall deformation magnitudes visualized as a heatmap, where red corresponds to higher $D(c)$. (e) Boxplots of skewness in deformation magnitudes reveal intra-wall deformations in non-responders to chemoradiation are positively skewed (i.e. larger magnitudes in NR patients, ypT3-4), compared to responders (GR). (f) Bar plot of AUC values for different feature descriptors, where $\mathbb{F}_{def}^r$ (blue) resulted in a significantly higher performance than $\mathbb{F}_{def}^p$ (red), $\mathbb{F}_{tex}^r$ (ochre), and $\mathbb{F}_{tex}^p$ (purple). (Color figure online)

4.2 Experiment 2: Identifying Responders After Chemoradiation via Post-therapy MRIs

In S_3, the median and standard deviation of the intra-wall deformation magnitude were identified as the most relevant StRAD descriptors. Figure 3 visualizes representative heatmaps of intra-wall deformation magnitudes on post-therapy MRIs, indicating that responders are associated with significantly lower and less variable structural intra-wall deformations (Fig. 3(e), blue corresponds to lower magnitude in heatmaps). As non-responders (i.e. ypT3-4) are likely to have more tumor extent outside the rectal wall despite chemoradiation [14], this would be reflected in the rectal wall being more deformed with respect to the healthy rectal atlas. The intra-wall StRAD descriptor ($\mathbb{F}_{def}^r$) significantly outperformed all of $\mathbb{F}_{def}^p$, $\mathbb{F}_{tex}^r$, and $\mathbb{F}_{tex}^p$ in terms of AUC values for this classification task (0.87 ± 0.03, $p < 0.001$, note blue bar in Fig. 3(f)).

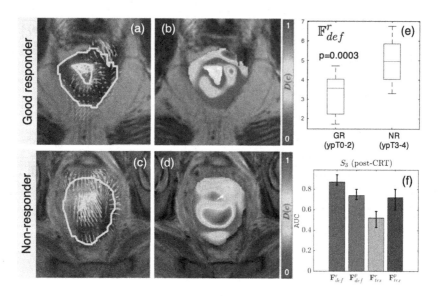

Fig. 3. Representative post-therapy T2w MRI scans from S_3 for two different patients showing deformation field (visualized as colored arrows) within yellow outline of rectal wall. (b), (d) Corresponding intra-wall deformation magnitudes for these patients visualized as heatmaps (red corresponds to higher $D(c)$). (e) Boxplots of standard deviation of deformation magnitudes within the rectal wall reveal significantly less variable deformations associated with responders to chemoradiation (GR, ypT0-2), compared to non-responders (NR). (f) Barplot of AUCs for different feature descriptors, where $\mathbb{F}_{def}^r$ (blue) resulted in a significantly higher performance than $\mathbb{F}_{def}^p$ (red), $\mathbb{F}_{tex}^r$ (ochre), and $\mathbb{F}_{tex}^p$ (purple). (Color figure online)

5   Concluding Remarks

In this study, we presented novel STructural Rectal Atlas Deformation (StRAD) features for characterizing intra- and peri-wall response to chemoradiation on rectal MRIs. Our study involved construction of a reference healthy rectal wall atlas, which was then applied to compute tumor-related deformations on baseline and post-chemoradiation MRIs separately. StRAD features from within the rectal wall were found to be most effective for characterizing tumor treatment response on MRI. Non-responder RCa patients in both pre- and post-therapy settings were found to be associated with significantly higher and more variable intra-wall deformations; likely occurring as a result of more aggressive tumor growth. By contrast, morphologic texture features performed significantly worse both for predicting as well as evaluating response to therapy via MRI. Future work will include validation of StRAD features on a larger, multi-site cohort of data as well as evaluation of parameter sensitivity. Additionally, we will integrate StRAD features with morphologic descriptors and clinical variables to reliably predict and assess treatment response for rectal cancers *in vivo*.

References

1. Yip, S., Aerts, H.: Applications and limitations of radiomics. Phys. Med. Biol. **61**(13), R150 (2016)
2. Grossman, P., et al.: Defining the biological basis of radiomic phenotypes in lung cancer. Elife **6**, e23421 (2017)
3. Sun, Y., et al.: Radiomic features of pretreatment MRI could identify T stage in patients with rectal cancer: preliminary findings. J. Magn. Reson. Imaging **48**, 615–621 (2018)
4. Horvat, N., et al.: MR imaging of rectal cancer: radiomics analysis to assess treatment response after neoadjuvant therapy. Radiology **287**(3), 833–843 (2018)
5. Litjens, G., et al.: A survey on deep learning in medical image analysis. Med. Image Anal. **42**, 60–88 (2017)
6. Rathore, S., et al.: Radiomic signature of infiltration in peritumoral edema predicts subsequent recurrence in glioblastoma: implications for personalized radiotherapy planning. J. Med. Imaging **5**(2), 021219 (2018)
7. Davatzikos, C., et al.: A framework for predictive modeling of anatomical deformations. IEEE Trans. Med. Imaging **20**(8), 836–843 (2001)
8. Ghose, S., et al.: Prostate shapes on pre-treatment MRI between prostate cancer patients who do and do not undergo biochemical recurrence are different: preliminary findings. Nat. Sci. Rep. **7**, 15829 (2017)
9. Rusu, M., et al.: Prostatome: a combined anatomical and disease based MRI atlas of the prostate. Med. Phys. **41**, 072301 (2014)
10. Prasanna, P., et al.: Mass Effect Deformation Heterogeneity (MEDH) on Gadolinium-contrast T1-weighted MRI is associated with decreased survival in patients with right cerebral hemisphere Glioblastoma: a feasibility study. Nat. Sci. Rep. **9**(1), 1145 (2017)
11. Klein, S., et al.: elastix: a toolbox for intensity based medical image registration. IEEE Trans. Med. Imaging **29**(1), 196–205 (2010)
12. Peng, H., et al.: Feature selection based on mutual information: criteria of max-dependency, max-relevance, and min-redundancy. IEEE Trans. Pattern Anal. Mach. Intell. **27**(8), 1226–1238 (2005)
13. Yoon, S., et al.: Clinical parameters predicting pathologic tumor response after preoperative chemoradiotherapy for rectal cancer. Int. J. Radiat. Oncol. Biol. Phys. **69**(4), 1167–1172 (2007)
14. Jessup, J., et al.: Colon and rectum. AJCC Cancer Staging Manual (2018)

Dynamic Routing Capsule Networks for Mild Cognitive Impairment Diagnosis

Zhicheng Jiao[1], Pu Huang[1,2], Tae-Eui Kam[1], Li-Ming Hsu[1], Ye Wu[1], Han Zhang[1(✉)], and Dinggang Shen[1(✉)]

[1] Department of Radiology and BRIC,
University of North Carolina at Chapel Hill, Chapel Hill, NC, USA
{hanzhang, dgshen}@med.unc.edu
[2] Shandong Normal University, Jinan, China

Abstract. Alzheimer's disease (AD) is a chronic neurodegenerative disease that could cause severe cognitive damage to the patients. Diagnosis of AD at its preclinical stage, i.e., mild cognitive impairment (MCI), could help to prevent or slow down AD progression. With machine learning, automatic MCI diagnosis could be achieved. Most of the previous studies mainly share a similar framework, i.e., building a classifier based on the features extracted from static or dynamic functional connectivity. Recently, inspired by the great successes achieved by deep learning in other areas of medical image analysis, researchers have introduced neural network models for MCI diagnosis. In this paper, we propose dynamic routing capsule networks for MCI diagnosis. Our proposed methods are based on a novel neural network fashion of *capsule net*. Two variants of capsule net are designed and discussed, which respectively uses the intra-ROIs and inter-ROIs dynamic routing to obtain functional representation. More importantly, we design a learnable dynamic functional connectivity metric in our inter-ROIs dynamic model, in which the functional connectivity is dynamically learned during network training. To the best of our knowledge, it's the first time to propose dynamic routing capsule networks for MCI diagnosis. Compared with other machine learning methods and deep learning model, our method can achieve superior performance from various aspects of evaluations.

Keywords: Alzheimer's disease · Mild cognitive impairment · Deep learning · Capsule networks · Computer-aided diagnosis

1 Introduction

As a chronic neurodegenerative disease, Alzheimer's disease (AD) usually starts slowly and gradually worsens over time [1]. The preclinical stage of AD is mild cognitive impairment (MCI), and the early intervention in this stage is of great importance to slow the progression of AD and relieve the suffering of the patients. Resting-state functional MRI (RS-fMRI) is a non-invasive functional imaging method widely used in MCI studies. With the development of machine learning and computer-aided diagnosis (CAD) technology, some studies started focusing on designing CAD methods for distinguishing MCI patients from normal control (NC) subjects. Most of these methods share a two-step workflow: (1) extracting adequate feature representation from

© Springer Nature Switzerland AG 2019
D. Shen et al. (Eds.): MICCAI 2019, LNCS 11767, pp. 620–628, 2019.
https://doi.org/10.1007/978-3-030-32251-9_68

RS-fMRI; (2) designing a classifier or a series of boosted classifiers to categorize the obtained features into NC and MCI. In the first step, static functional connectivity (SFC) and dynamic functional connectivity (DFC) are calculated to construct brain networks the static and time-varying functional connectomics properties of the brain. For SFC, Pearson's correlation coefficient (PCC) matrix of full-length BOLD signals is usually chosen as functional connectivity. When it comes to DFC, the functional connectivity features are obtained via high-order mining of SFCs with sliding windows at different time points of fMRI. Then, classifiers such as support vector machine (SVM) and Gaussian process regression (GPR) are applied to perform the classification of NC *vs* MCI [2, 3]. In recent years, deep learning methods have made breakthroughs in medical image analysis [4]. For the image-based AD diagnosis, deep neural network models [5, 6] are also reported to achieve competitive results. More recently, researchers propose a bidirectional long short-term memory (BiLSTM) model (a representative recurrent neural network (RNN) model) for MCI diagnosis [7]. Although the calculation of functional connectivity and classification are integrated into a network, the functional connectivity is not learnable during the training process.

Recently, a novel deep learning fashion named capsule network (CapsNet) was proposed [8]. Being different from existed neural networks, each node (capsule) within capsule layers contains a series of neurons. The activity of each capsule is represented by an activation vector (activation values of a series of neurons in it). The norm of this vector stands for the probability that an object exists in it. The key operation of CapsNet is called *"dynamic routing by agreement"*, which means capsules in lower-level layers predict the outcomes of that in higher-level layers, and the higher-level capsules get activated only if these predictions agree with each other. Some researchers have applied CapsNets to medical image analysis tasks to obtain competitive results [9–11]. Inspired by the dynamic routing strategy of CapsNet, we propose two dynamic routing CapsNet models for MCI diagnosis. To the best of our knowledge, it is the first time to introduce this novel deep learning model to fMRI-based MCI diagnosis. There are two variants of our CapsNet for MCI diagnosis: (1) *Intra-ROIs dynamic CapsNet*; (2) *Inter-ROIs dynamic CapsNet*. Compared with both traditional machine learning methods and the state-of-the-art deep learning model, the *Intra-ROIs dynamic CapsNet* obtains comparable diagnosis results while the *Inter-ROIs dynamic CapsNet* achieves superior performance. More importantly, our *Inter-ROIs dynamic CapsNet* provides a novel and learnable strategy to capture DFC during training of deep neural networks.

2   Method

The input to our CapsNet are timeseries of BOLD signal from the automated anatomical labeling (AAL) [12] template, which contains 116 brain ROIs. Since there are two variants of proposed CapsNet, which respectively mines intra-ROIs dynamic representation and inter-ROIs dynamic representation for MCI diagnosis, we detail network structures of them in the following subsections.

2.1   Intra-ROIs Dynamic CapsNet

Structures of our *Intra-ROIs dynamic CapsNet* are illustrated in Fig. 1. Before being fed into the *Intra-ROIs dynamic CapsNet*, the fMRI signals of different brain regions are computed from the AAL atlas template to obtain ROI-wise fMRI $X = [x_1, \ldots, x_2, \ldots, x_N]$, $N = 116$ represents the number of ROIs. X is the input to *Intra-ROIs dynamic representation layers* which consist of two 1D convolution layers in the temporal dimension. $F = [f_1, \ldots, f_i, \ldots, f_M]$ (*M* is the number of capsules in F) is the output of these layers. Then, F is fed into two capsule layers (*High-order dynamic combination* and *Dynamic diagnosis* in Fig. 1), successively obtaining high-order combination representation $F_{com} = [f_{1c}, \ldots, f_{ic}, \ldots, f_{Mc}]$ and the diagnosis result $F_d = [f_{MCI}, f_{NC}]$ (f_{MCI} and f_{NC} represent output of *MCI* capsule and *NC* capsule).

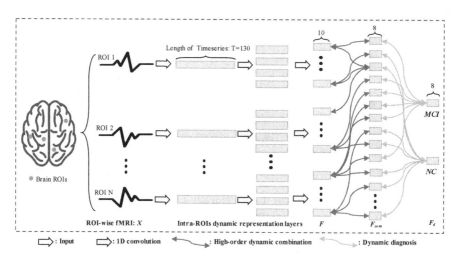

Fig. 1. Illustration of our *Intra-ROIs dynamic CapsNet*. According to the AAL template, there are 116 ROIs in the preprocessed fMRI. The length of timeseries is 130. The ROI-wise input is successively propagated through *Intra-ROIs dynamic representation layers* and *Dynamic diagnosis layer*. Operations of these layers are listed in the bottom of this figure, and details of the network parameters are described in the *Experiments and results* section.

Capsules in these capsule layers (*High-order dynamic combination* and *Dynamic diagnosis*) are connected and optimized via "dynamic routing by agreement" algorithm [8]. Considering that μ_i is the output of capsule i in a capsule layer (For Intra-ROIs dynamic representation layers, μ_i is set as f_i. For High-order dynamic combination layers, μ_i is set as f_{ic}), the related prediction for its parent capsule j in next layer is:

$$\mu_{j|i} = W_{ij}\mu_i \tag{1}$$

where W_{ij} are learnable weights in the form of a matrix. The coupling c_{ij} between these two capsules is defined as Eq. 2:

$$c_{ij} = \frac{exp(b_{ij})}{\sum_k exp(b_{ik})} \tag{2}$$

where b_{ij} represents the probability that capsule i is coupled with capsule j, and it is initialized as 0 at the beginning of routing. So, s_j which stands for the input to capsule j can be computed as Eq. 3:

$$s_j = \sum_i c_{ij} \mu_{j|i} \tag{3}$$

Then, a squashing function is used to limit the norm of output value v_j from capsule j to [0, 1], which can make sure that the norm of this vector can act as a probability.

$$v_j = \frac{\| s_j \|^2}{1 + \| s_j \|^2} \frac{s_j}{\| s_j \|} \tag{4}$$

For the *High-order dynamic combination layer*, v_j is calculated as f_{jc}, and the norm of v_j represents the probability that a weighted combination of brain ROIs signals exist in capsule j; while for the *Diagnosis capsule layer*, v_j is calculated as f_{MCI} or f_{NC}, and the norm of v_j represents the probability that a scan belongs to *MCI* or *NC*.

The agreement a_{ij} between capsule i and its parent capsule j can be calculated in the form of inner product as Eq. 5:

$$a_{ij} = v_j \cdot \mu_{j|i} \tag{5}$$

In the next iteration of dynamic routing, a_{ij} will be added to the b_{ij} to enhance the coupling between the capsule i and capsule j.

The dynamic routing strategy described above is performed in both the *High-order dynamic combination* and *Dynamic diagnosis* layers illustrated in Fig. 1. L_D is the loss function of the CapsNet, which is in the form of a margin loss as Eq. 6:

$$L_D = T_c \max(0, m^+ - \| v_c \|)^2 + \lambda(1 - T_c)\max(0, \| v_c \| - m^-)^2 \tag{6}$$

$T_c = 1$ *iff* an instance from class c (*MCI* or *NC*) is present to the network, v_c is the output of the capsule which represent class c, and λ is a weight that is set as 0.5. $m^+ = 0.9$ and $m^- = 0.1$ are the margins which are set as the recommended values in capsule net paper [8].

2.2 Inter-ROIs Dynamic CapsNet

Majority of traditional MCI diagnosis methods are based on the Inter-ROIs functional connectivity feature representation. Even though our Intra-ROIs dynamic CapsNet combines information from different ROIs in the *High-order representation capsule layer*, it cannot make full use of the rich information of inter-ROIs correlations. Thus, we further propose an *inter-ROIs dynamic CapsNet* which can capture the inter-ROIs dynamic representation for more superior diagnosis performance. Structures of *Inter-ROIs CapsNet* are illustrated in Fig. 2, which consist of *Inter-ROIs dynamic representation* layers and *Dynamic diagnosis layer*.

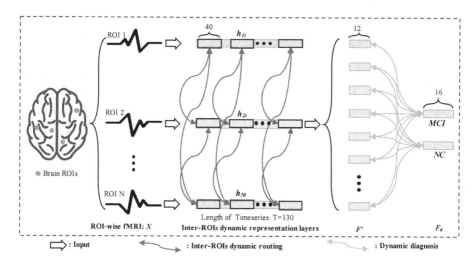

Fig. 2. Illustration of our *Inter-ROIs dynamic CapsNet*. According to the AAL template, there are 116 ROIs in the preprocessed fMRI. The length of timeseries is 130. The ROI-wise input is successively propagated through *Inter-ROIs dynamic representation layers* and *Dynamic diagnosis layer*. Operations of these layers are listed in the bottom of this figure, and details of the network parameters are described in the *Experiments and results* section.

The *Inter-ROIs dynamic representation layers* can dynamically calculate correlations between ROIs. The dynamic correlation is defined as a weighted agreement f_{ijt} which is shown as Eq. 7. For each two brain ROIs, the agreement value of them at timepoint t is defined as a weighted inner product, $\boldsymbol{h}_{it}$ and $\boldsymbol{h}_{jt}$ are fMRI signal of *i-th* and *j-th* ROIs in temporal slide windows. Across the whole timeseries, there is an agreement vector $\boldsymbol{f}_{ij} = [f_{ij1}, f_{ij2}, \dots f_{ijt}, \dots f_{ijN_t}]$, N_t is the total number of sliding windows, all agreement vectors form the input $\boldsymbol{F}'$ to *Dynamic diagnosis* layers, $\boldsymbol{F}' = [\boldsymbol{f}_{12}, \boldsymbol{f}_{13}, \dots \boldsymbol{f}_{ij}, \dots \boldsymbol{f}_{N-1N}]$.

$$f_{ijt} = w_{ijt}\boldsymbol{h}_{it} \cdot \boldsymbol{h}_{jt} \tag{7}$$

According to the number of ROIs $N = 116$, there are total $N \times (N-1)/2 = 6670$ nodes in $\boldsymbol{F}'$ which stands for the output of these *Inter-ROIs dynamic representation layers*. Then, dynamic routings are performed between $\boldsymbol{F}'$ and capsules in the *diagnosis capsule layer*. The dynamic routing strategy between these two layers is the same as that described in Sect. 2.1. Loss function of the *Inter-ROIs dynamic CapsNet* is also in the same form as Eq. 6.

3 Experiments and Results

In this section, we first describe the preprocessing of fMRI data, settings of experiments, and details of network structures. Then, we compare the proposed models with other diagnosis methods.

3.1 Data Preprocessing and Experiments

In this study, we use the ADNI dataset (http://adni.loni.usc.edu/) for training and testing the proposed methods. The RS-fMRI data are preprocessed by AFNI software package (1) According to a well-accepted pipeline, we performed first ten volumes removal, head motion correction, normalization, nuisance signals regression, detrend and bandpass filtering. (2) To minimize artifacts due to excessive motion, subjects with an average frame displacement greater than 0.5 mm were removed. Finally, RS-fMRI data were smoothed with 6 mm full width at half maximum Gaussian kernel.

Via the preprocess above, a dataset containing 395 scans of MCI patients and 485 scans of NC subjects is built. The number of scans for each subject varies from 1 to 8. The whole dataset is split to form the training set and testing set for 5 times. In each split, there are 25% of total scans (220 scans) in the testing set, while there are 75% of total scans (660 scans) in the training set. Since some subjects are scanned for more than once, scans of the same subject are split into either training set or test set to make the strict separation at the subject level. For training of our model, the optimizer is set as Adam, and the weights of network are initialized by Xavier. 20% instances in training set are used for validation to monitor the performance. Once the validation loss and validation error stop declining, the trained network parameters are applied to obtain diagnosis results on testing set. Our experiments are based on Pytorch [13].

3.2 Results and Analysis

We compare the proposed models with state-of-the-art traditional machine learning methods and deep learning model. The classification *accuracy, sensitivity, specificity,* and related *standard deviations* are listed in Table 1.

Table 1. Diagnosis performance of comparison methods and ours.

Method	Accuracy(std)	Sensitivity(std)	Specificity(std)
Static SVM	0.630(0.021)	0.621(0.035)	0.636(0.029)
Dynamic SVM	0.651(0.030)	0.672(0.032)	0.639(0.033)
Static GPR	0.673(0.021)	0.570(0.044)	0.772(0.047)
Dynamic GPR	0.705(0.042)	0.641(0.038)	0.756(0.062)
Bi-LSTM	0.726(0.017)	0.725(0.039)	0.727(0.057)
Intra-ROIs CapsNet	0.729(0.023)	**0.799(0.042)**	0.673(0.065)
Inter-ROIs CapsNet	**0.773(0.022)**	0.771(0.027)	**0.774(0.040)**

In this table, *Static SVM* and *Static GPR* represent traditional methods based on SFC which is calculated by Pearson's correlation between full-length BOLD signals. After building SFC matrix, the SVM or GPR are trained to classify the SFC matrix. *Dynamic SVM* and *Dynamic GPR* stand for dynamic connectivity methods in which dynamic representations are obtained from high-order analysis of functional connectivity at different slide windows [2, 3]. Construction of FC and selection of classifiers of these compared methods follow that in related studies. All these mentioned above are widely used and competitive traditional machine learning based MCI diagnosis methods.

In the other hand, Bi-LSTM is a recently proposed deep learning model for MCI diagnosis, which is in the form of bidirectional long short-term memory, and it has achieved competitive performance for diagnosing MCI. Besides, it is also based on dynamic functional connectivity. *Intra-ROIs CapsNet* and *Inter-ROIs CapsNet* stand for our CapsNet models. Network structures of Bi-LSTM follow the optimal ones which are chosen in the related MCI diagnosis study [7].

For *Intra-ROIs CapsNet* shown in Fig. 1, parameters of these two 1D convolution layers are set as (1) *Conv1*: kernel size = 1 × 20, number of kernels is 4, stride = 4; (2) *Conv2*: kernel size = 1 × 10, number of kernels is 4, stride = 2. Parameters of *High-order representation capsule layer* are set as: length of input = 10, length of output = 8; Parameters of *diagnosis capsule layer* are set as: length of input = 8, length of output = 16. For *Inter-ROIs CapsNet* shown in Fig. 2, parameters of *inter-ROIs dynamic representation layer* are set as *width of slide window* = 40, stride of slide window = 8; for the *diagnosis capsule layer,* length of input = 12, length of output = 16. Parameters of the proposed models are selected according to both experiments and optimal values in capsule net paper [8].

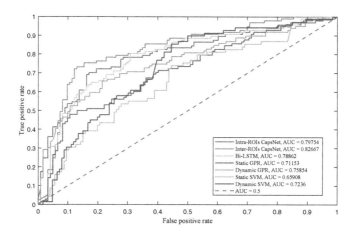

Fig. 3. ROC curves and related AUC values of different diagnosis methods

As could be seen, according to the listed evaluations (Table 1), the inter-ROIs dynamic connectivity methods (Dynamic SVM, Dynamic GPR, BiLSTM, and Inter-ROIs CapsNet) can achieve superior performance than static ones and Inra-ROIs dynamic method (Static SVM, Dynamic GPR, Intra-ROIs CapsNet). The deep learning models (BiLSTM, Intra-ROIs CapsNet, and Inter-ROIs CapsNet) are more competitive than traditional machine learning based methods. The dynamic routing networks proposed in this paper outperformed both state-of-the-art traditional machine learning methods and deep learning model.

For further analysis, we also compare the receiver operating characteristic (ROC) curves and area under the curve (AUC) values of different methods in Fig. 3. Specifically, MCI is the positive class while NC is the negative class. As could be seen, our dynamic routing networks can achieve superior ROC performance and higher AUC values than other methods. Results in this figure can further demonstrate the efficiency of our CapsNets for MCI diagnosis.

4 Conclusions

In this study, we propose both two variants of CapsNet for MCI diagnosis. In the intra-ROIs model, temporal-dynamic representation of fMRI is first represented by ROI-wise convolutional networks. Then, high-order combinations of intra-ROIs representations are dynamically routed to obtain the diagnosis results. In the improved inter-ROIs dynamic variant, a novel weighted agreement metric is designed to capture the DFC across ROIs. With the help of our DFC metric, our *Inter-ROIs dynamic CapsNet* can achieve competitive diagnosis performance for MCI.

Acknowledgement. This work was supported in part by NIH grants EB022880, AG053867, AG041721, AG049371 and AG042599.

References

1. Alzheimer's Association: 2018 Alzheimer's disease facts and figures. Alzheimer's Dement. **14**(3), 367–429 (2018)
2. Chen, X., et al.: High-order resting-state functional connectivity network for MCI classification. Hum. Brain Mapp. **37**(9), 3282–3296 (2016)
3. Challis, E., et al.: Gaussian process classification of Alzheimer's disease and mild cognitive impairment from resting-state fMRI. NeuroImage **112**, 232–243 (2015)
4. Shen, D., et al.: Deep learning in medical image analysis. Ann. Rev. Biomed. Eng. **19**, 221–248 (2017)
5. Suk, H.-I., et al.: Hierarchical feature representation and multimodal fusion with deep learning for AD/MCI diagnosis. NeuroImage **101**, 569–582 (2014)
6. Liu, S., et al.: Early diagnosis of Alzheimer's disease with deep learning. In: ISBI. IEEE (2014)
7. Yan, W., Zhang, H., Sui, J., Shen, D.: Deep chronnectome learning via full bidirectional long short-term memory networks for MCI diagnosis. In: Frangi, A.F., Schnabel, J.A., Davatzikos, C., Alberola-López, C., Fichtinger, G. (eds.) MICCAI 2018. LNCS, vol. 11072, pp. 249–257. Springer, Cham (2018). https://doi.org/10.1007/978-3-030-00931-1_29
8. Sabour, S., et al.: Dynamic routing between capsules. In: NeurIPS (2017)
9. Mobiny, A., Van Nguyen, H.: Fast CapsNet for lung cancer screening. In: Frangi, A.F., Schnabel, J.A., Davatzikos, C., Alberola-López, C., Fichtinger, G. (eds.) MICCAI 2018. LNCS, vol. 11071, pp. 741–749. Springer, Cham (2018). https://doi.org/10.1007/978-3-030-00934-2_82

10. Pal, A., Chaturvedi, A., Garain, U., Chandra, A., Chatterjee, R., Senapati, S.: CapsDeMM: capsule network for detection of munro's microabscess in skin biopsy images. In: Frangi, A. F., Schnabel, J.A., Davatzikos, C., Alberola-López, C., Fichtinger, G. (eds.) MICCAI 2018. LNCS, vol. 11071, pp. 389–397. Springer, Cham (2018). https://doi.org/10.1007/978-3-030-00934-2_44
11. Afshar, P., et al.: Brain tumor type classification via capsule networks. In: ICIP. IEEE (2018)
12. Tzourio-Mazoyer, N., et al.: Automated anatomical labeling of activations in SPM using a macroscopic anatomical parcellation of the MNI MRI single-subject brain. Neuroimage **15** (1), 273–289 (2002)
13. Paszke, A., et al.: Automatic differentiation in PyTorch (2017)

Deep Multi-modal Latent Representation Learning for Automated Dementia Diagnosis

Tao Zhou[1], Mingxia Liu[2(✉)], Huazhu Fu[1], Jun Wang[3], Jianbing Shen[1(✉)], Ling Shao[1], and Dinggang Shen[2(✉)]

[1] Inception Institute of Artificial Intelligence, Abu Dhabi, UAE
jianbing.shen@inceptioniai.org
[2] Department of Radiology and BRIC, University of North Carolina,
Chapel Hill, USA
{mxliu,dgshen}@med.unc.edu
[3] Shanghai Institute for Advanced Communication and Data Science,
School of Communication and Information Engineering, Shanghai University,
Shanghai, China

Abstract. Effective fusion of multi-modality neuroimaging data, such as structural magnetic resonance imaging (MRI) and fluorodeoxyglucose positron emission tomography (PET), has attracted increasing interest in computer-aided brain disease diagnosis, by providing complementary structural and functional information of the brain to improve diagnostic performance. Although considerable progress has been made, there remain several significant challenges in traditional methods for fusing multi-modality data. *First,* the fusion of multi-modality data is usually independent of the training of diagnostic models, leading to suboptimal performance. *Second,* it is challenging to effectively exploit the complementary information among multiple modalities based on low-level imaging features (*e.g.,* image intensity or tissue volume). To this end, in this paper, we propose a novel Deep Latent Multi-modality Dementia Diagnosis (DLMD^2) framework based on a deep non-negative matrix factorization (NMF) model. Specifically, we integrate the feature fusion/learning process into the classifier construction step for eliminating the gap between neuroimaging features and disease labels. To exploit the correlations among multi-modality data, we learn latent representations for multi-modality data by sharing the common high-level representations in the last layer of each modality in the deep NMF model. Extensive experimental results on the Alzheimer's Disease Neuroimaging Initiative (ADNI) dataset validate that our proposed method outperforms several state-of-the-art methods.

© Springer Nature Switzerland AG 2019
D. Shen et al. (Eds.): MICCAI 2019, LNCS 11767, pp. 629–638, 2019.
https://doi.org/10.1007/978-3-030-32251-9_69

1 Introduction

The Alzheimer's Disease Neuroimaging Initiative (ADNI) was launched in 2003 by the National Institute on Aging, which collected data from multiple modalities, such as structural magnetic resonance imaging (MRI) [13] and fluorodeoxyglucose positron emission tomography (PET) [2]. The goal of ADNI is to better understand the pathological progression of AD and to identify the most related biomarkers using multi-modality data. Since different modalities provide complementary information, it is critical to effectively fuse multi-modality data to boost diagnostic performance [19,20].

Recently, several approaches [15] towards multi-view learning(or multi-modality fusion) have been developed and also applied for brain disease diagnosis [6,18]. As the most straightforward strategy, a simple fusion method is used to pool features from multi-modalities together [5], followed by the training of a classifier (*e.g.*, support vector machine, SVM). However, such a strategy cannot effectively exploit the correlation among multi-modalities, thus leading to sub-optimal diagnostic performance. To effectively fuse multi-modality data, the model in [3] uses Multiple Kernel Learning (MKL) to fuse the data by learning optimal linearly-combined kernels for classification. Additionally, a multi-task learning based feature selection method is proposed in [6], using an inter-modality relationship preserving constraint. Then, Liu *et al.* [7] uses a zero-masking strategy for data fusion to extract complementary information from multi-modality data. Besides, several multi-view learning methods have been recently proposed for multi-modality fusion, where each modality is treated as a specific view. For example, the Multi-View Dimensionality Co-Reduction (MDCR) method [16] adopts the kernel matching to regularize the dependence across multiple views and projects each view into a low-dimensional space. The Multi-view Learning with Adaptive Neighbours (MLAN) method [8] performs clustering/semi-supervised classification and local structure learning simultaneously. The Deep Matrix Factorization (DMF) method [17] conducts deep semi-nonnegative matrix factorization (NMF) to seek a common representation for the multi-view clustering task. Although considerable progress has been made, there are still several challenges for effective fusion of multi-modality data. *First*, the fusion of multi-modality data is usually independent of the training of diagnostic models, leading to a sub-optimal performance. *Second*, it is challenging to effectively exploit the complementary information among multiple modalities based on low-level imaging features.

To address these issues, we propose a Deep Latent Multi-modality Dementia Diagnosis (DLMD²) model to jointly perform high-level feature learning and classifier construction (as shown in Fig. 1). The key idea is to develop a deep NMF model to learn high-level shared latent representations for multi-modality data, whose learned features could have strong interpretability to help uncover the complex structure of the brain. We also reconstruct the original features using the latent representations, making the learned representations to effectively preserve critical and useful information. In addition, the feature learning/fusion of multi-modality data and classification model training are

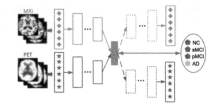

Fig. 1. Overview of the proposed DLMD² model. It performs deep NMF in a layer-wise manner to learn shared latent representations for multi-modality data, and then projects the new representations into the label space for diagnosis model training. Our method also uses the learned latent representations to reconstruct the original features of multi-modality data, encouraging the new representations to effectively preserve critical and useful information.

integrated into a unified framework for automated dementia diagnosis. Experimental results on the ADNI dataset show the effectiveness of our DLMD² model against other state-of-the-art methods, for several brain disease diagnosis tasks.

In summary, the key contributions of this study are *three-fold*. (1) A deep NMF model is built using a layer-wise decomposition strategy to effectively uncover the hidden information of multi-modal neuroimaging data. (2) Our model exploits the correlations among multi-modality data by learning shared latent representations for different modalities. (3) Both multi-modality fusion and classification model training are seamlessly integrated into a unified framework for automated dementia diagnosis.

2   Method

Overview of Standard NMF. Consider a non-negative data matrix $\mathbf{X} = [\mathbf{x}_1, \mathbf{x}_2, \ldots, \mathbf{x}_n] \in \mathbb{R}^{d \times n}$ with n samples, where $\mathbf{x}_i$ $(i = 1, \cdots, n)$ denotes the i-th sample and d is the feature dimension. NMF aims to seek two non-negative matrices $\mathbf{B}$ and $\mathbf{H}$, and its objective function is given as

$$\min_{\mathbf{B} \geq 0, \mathbf{H} \geq 0} \|\mathbf{X} - \mathbf{B}\mathbf{H}\|_F^2, \tag{1}$$

where $\mathbf{B} \in \mathbb{R}^{d \times h}$ denotes the basis matrix, $\mathbf{H} \in \mathbb{R}^{h \times n}$ is regarded as the new representation of the original data $\mathbf{X}$, and h is the dimension of the new feature representation.

2.1   Proposed Method

Suppose we have a multi-modality neuroimaging dataset $\{\mathbf{X}^{(1)}, \mathbf{X}^{(2)}, \ldots, \mathbf{X}^{(V)}\}$, where $\mathbf{X}^{(v)} \in \mathbb{R}^{d_v \times n}$ denotes the v-th $(v = 1, \cdots, V)$ modality, d_v is the dimension of the v-th modality, n is the number of samples, and V is the number of data modalities. The formulation of the multi-modal NMF model can be written as follows

$$\min_{\{\mathbf{B}^{(v)}\geq 0,\mathbf{H}^{(v)}\geq 0\}_{v=1}^{V}} \sum\nolimits_{v=1}^{V} \|\mathbf{X}^{(v)} - \mathbf{B}^{(v)}\mathbf{H}^{(v)}\|_F^2, \tag{2}$$

where $\mathbf{B}^{(v)}$ and $\mathbf{H}^{(v)}$ denote the basis and representation matrices for the v-th modality, respectively. Using Eq. (2), the new representation can be learned for each modality independently, but the underlying correlation among multiple modalities cannot be captured explicitly. To address this issue, another model can be developed as follows:

$$\min_{\{\mathbf{B}^{(v)}\geq 0\}_{v=1}^{V},\mathbf{H}\geq 0} \sum\nolimits_{v=1}^{V} \|\mathbf{X}^{(v)} - \mathbf{B}^{(v)}\mathbf{H}\|_F^2, \tag{3}$$

where $\mathbf{H}$ can be considered as the shared representation for different modalities, and can thus be used to exploit the correlation among multiple modalities. In the dementia diagnosis task, we can construct a unified multi-modal feature learning and classifier training framework, defined as

$$\min_{\{\mathbf{B}^{(v)}\geq 0\}_{v=1}^{V},\mathbf{H}\geq 0,\mathbf{W}} \sum\nolimits_{v=1}^{V} \|\mathbf{X}^{(v)} - \mathbf{B}^{(v)}\mathbf{H}\|_F^2 + \lambda\|\mathbf{W}\mathbf{H} - \mathbf{Y}\|_F^2, \tag{4}$$

where $\mathbf{W}$ denotes a projection matrix, and $\mathbf{Y} \in \mathbb{R}^{c\times n}$ is the label matrix with c categories. The model defined in Eq. (4) employs the label information of training data to guide the model to learn discriminative shared representations $\mathbf{H}$ for multiple modalities. That is, the "good" feature representation learned is expected to boost the classification performance.

Using Eq. (4), we can jointly learn the discriminative shared representation (*i.e.*, $\mathbf{H}$) and the classification/diagnosis model. However, one main issue is that Eq. (4) only defines a shallow (*i.e.*, linear) NMF model, which cannot effectively uncover the complex (*e.g.*, high-level) correlations among multiple modalities. It is well known that deep learning can produce high-quality feature representations and also capture the high-level correlations among features. To this end, a deep NMF (or semi-NMF) model has recently been developed [14,17], with promising results for data representation. Specifically, a multi-layer decomposition process in the deep NMF model is formulated as

$$\begin{aligned}
\mathbf{X}^{(v)} &\approx \mathbf{B}_1^{(v)}\mathbf{H}_1^{(v)} \\
\mathbf{X}^{(v)} &\approx \mathbf{B}_1^{(v)}\mathbf{B}_2^{(v)}\mathbf{H}_2^{(v)} \\
&\vdots \\
\mathbf{X}^{(v)} &\approx \mathbf{B}_1^{(v)}\mathbf{B}_2^{(v)}\cdots\mathbf{B}_l^{(v)}\cdots\mathbf{B}_L^{(v)}\mathbf{H}_L,
\end{aligned} \tag{5}$$

where $\mathbf{B}_l^{(v)}$ $(l = 1,\ldots,L)$ and $\mathbf{H}_l^{(v)}$ $(l = 1,\ldots,L)$ denote the basis matrix and the latent representation matrix of the v-th modality at the l-th layer, respectively. Also, $\mathbf{H}_L$ is the shared latent representation of different modalities at the last layer, and L is the number of decomposition layers. It is worth noting that the latent representation in the last layer is able to identify shared attributes among different modalities. Thus, the deep NMF model can effectively uncover the correlations among multi-modality data by using the high-level feature representations (*i.e.*, $\mathbf{H}_L$).

For an ideal latent representation matrix $\mathbf{H}_L$, it should be able to reconstruct the original data $\mathbf{X}^{(v)}$ via the basis matrices with a small reconstruction error, $\mathbf{X}^{(v)} = \mathbf{B}_1^{(v)} \cdots \mathbf{B}_L^{(v)} \mathbf{H}_L$. On the other hand, it should also be obtained by directly projecting the original data $\mathbf{X}^{(v)}$ into the latent representation space with the aid of the basis matrix [14], *i.e.*, $\mathbf{H}_L = \mathbf{B}_L^{(v)^\top} \cdots \mathbf{B}_1^{(v)^\top} \mathbf{X}^{(v)}$. Accordingly, we have the following formulation for each modality as

$$\min_{\mathbf{B}_l^{(v)}, \mathbf{H}_L} \|\mathbf{X}^{(v)} - \mathbf{B}_1^{(v)} \cdots \mathbf{B}_L^{(v)} \mathbf{H}_L\|_F^2 + \|\mathbf{H}_L - \mathbf{B}_L^{(v)^\top} \cdots \mathbf{B}_1^{(v)^\top} \mathbf{X}^{(v)}\|_F^2, \quad (6)$$

through which the two components (*i.e.*, the non-negative factorization of the original data $\mathbf{X}^{(v)}$ and the task-oriented learning of the latent representation $\mathbf{H}_L$) guide each other during the learning process. In this way, it is able to obtain the ideal latent representation of the original data.

Finally, we integrate the latent representation learning (via deep NMF) and the classification model construction into a unified framework, and our DLMD^2 model is formulated as follows

$$\min_{\substack{\mathbf{B}_1^{(v)} \cdots \mathbf{B}_L^{(v)}, \\ \mathbf{H}_L, \mathbf{W}}} \sum_{v=1}^{V} \left(\|\mathbf{X}^{(v)} - \mathbf{B}_1^{(v)} \cdots \mathbf{B}_L^{(v)} \mathbf{H}_L\|_F^2 + \|\mathbf{H}_L - \mathbf{B}_L^{(v)^\top} \cdots \mathbf{B}_1^{(v)^\top} \mathbf{X}^{(v)}\|_F^2 \right)$$

$$+ \lambda \|(\mathbf{W}\mathbf{H}_L - \mathbf{Y})\mathbf{S}\|_F^2 + \beta \|\mathbf{W}\|_F^2,$$

$$\text{s.t.} \quad \mathbf{H}_L \geq 0, \mathbf{B}_l^{(v)} \geq 0 \ (\forall v = 1, 2, \ldots, V; \forall l = 1, 2, \ldots, L),$$

$$(7)$$

where λ and β are trade-off parameters. Besides, $\mathbf{S}$ is a diagonal matrix used to indicate the labeled samples with $s_{ii} = 1$ if the i-th sample is labeled and 0 otherwise. The label matrix $\mathbf{Y} = [\mathbf{Y}_{\text{labeled}}, \mathbf{Y}_{\text{unlabeled}}]$ includes label information of both labeled and unlabeled subjects, thus ensuring that our model can directly predict labels for unseen test samples.

2.2 Optimization

Initialization. Following [14], we first decompose each modality matrix $\mathbf{X}^{(v)}$ (*i.e.*, minimize $\|\mathbf{X}^{(v)} - \mathbf{B}_1^{(v)} \mathbf{H}_1^{(v)}\|_F^2 + \|\mathbf{H}_1^{(v)} - \mathbf{B}_1^{(v)^\top} \mathbf{X}^{(v)}\|_F^2$), and then decompose the matrix $\mathbf{H}_1^{(v)}$ (*i.e.*, minimize $\|\mathbf{H}_1^{(v)} - \mathbf{B}_2^{(v)} \mathbf{H}_2^{(v)}\|_F^2 + \|\mathbf{H}_2^{(v)} - \mathbf{B}_2^{(v)^\top} \mathbf{H}_1^{(v)}\|_F^2$) until all layers are initialized. Note that we initialize $\mathbf{H}_L$ using $\mathbf{H}_L = \sum_v \mathbf{H}_{L-1}^{(v)}/V$. Then, we utilize an alternative optimization method to optimize the objective function, the detailed steps of which are given as follows.

Step 1: Update $\mathbf{B}_l^{(v)}$. For the v-th modality, we obtain the following equation for $\mathbf{B}_l^{(v)}$ by taking the derivative of Eq. (7) *w.r.t.* $\mathbf{B}_l^{(v)}$:

$$
\begin{aligned}
\mathcal{J}_1(\mathbf{B}_l^{(v)}) = {}& \Theta_{l-1}^{(v)}{}^\top \mathbf{X}^{(v)}\mathbf{X}^{(v)}{}^\top \Theta_{l-1}^{(v)}\mathbf{B}_l^{(v)}\Omega_{l+1}^{(v)}\Omega_{l+1}^{(v)}{}^\top - 2\Theta_{l-1}^{(v)}{}^\top \mathbf{X}^{(v)}\mathbf{H}_L^\top \Omega_{l+1}^{(v)}{}^\top \\
& + \Theta_{l-1}^{(v)}{}^\top \Theta_{l-1}^{(v)}\mathbf{B}_l^{(v)}\Omega_{l+1}^{(v)}\mathbf{H}_L\mathbf{H}_L^\top \Omega_{l+1}^{(v)}{}^\top, \quad s.t. \ \mathbf{B}_l^{(v)} \geq 0,
\end{aligned}
\tag{8}
$$

where $\Theta_{l-1}^{(v)} = \mathbf{B}_1^{(v)}\mathbf{B}_2^{(v)}\cdots\mathbf{B}_{l-1}^{(v)}$, and $\Omega_{l+1}^{(v)} = \mathbf{B}_{l+1}^{(v)}\mathbf{B}_{l+2}^{(v)}\cdots\mathbf{B}_L^{(v)}$.

By using the Karush-Kuhn-Tucker (KKT) condition [1], we can derive the following updating rule:

$$
\mathbf{B}_l^{(v)} \leftarrow
$$

$$
\mathbf{B}_l^{(v)} \odot \frac{2\Theta_{l-1}^{(v)}{}^\top \mathbf{X}^{(v)}\mathbf{H}_L^\top \Omega_{l+1}^{(v)}{}^\top}{\Theta_{l-1}^{(v)}{}^\top \mathbf{X}^{(v)}\mathbf{X}^{(v)}{}^\top \Theta_{l-1}^{(v)}\mathbf{B}_l^{(v)}\Omega_{l+1}^{(v)}\Omega_{l+1}^{(v)}{}^\top + \Theta_{l-1}^{(v)}{}^\top \Theta_{l-1}^{(v)}\mathbf{B}_l^{(v)}\Omega_{l+1}^{(v)}\mathbf{H}_L\mathbf{H}_L^\top \Omega_{l+1}^{(v)}{}^\top}
\tag{9}
$$

Step 2: Update $\mathbf{H}_L$. We obtain the following equation for $\mathbf{H}_L$ by taking the derivative of Eq. (7) *w.r.t.* $\mathbf{H}_L$:

$$
\begin{aligned}
\mathcal{J}_2(\mathbf{H}_L) = {}& \sum_{v=1}^V \left(\Theta_L^{(v)}{}^\top \Theta_L^{(v)}\mathbf{H}_L + \mathbf{H}_L \right) - 2\sum_{v=1}^V \Theta_L^{(v)}{}^\top \mathbf{X}^{(v)} \\
& + \lambda\mathbf{W}^\top\mathbf{W}\mathbf{H}_L\mathbf{S}\mathbf{S}^\top - \lambda\mathbf{W}^\top\mathbf{Y}\mathbf{S}\mathbf{S}^\top, \quad s.t. \ \mathbf{H}_L \geq 0,
\end{aligned}
\tag{10}
$$

where $\Theta_L^{(v)} = \mathbf{B}_1^{(v)}\mathbf{B}_2^{(v)}\cdots\mathbf{B}_L^{(v)}$.

By using the KKT condition, we can obtain the following updating rule:

$$
\mathbf{H}_L \leftarrow \mathbf{H}_L \odot \frac{2\sum_{v=1}^V \Theta_L^{(v)}{}^\top \mathbf{X}^{(v)} + \lambda\mathbf{W}^\top\mathbf{Y}\mathbf{S}\mathbf{S}^\top}{\sum_{v=1}^V \left(\Theta_L^{(v)}{}^\top \Theta_L^{(v)}\mathbf{H}_L + \mathbf{H}_L \right) + \lambda\mathbf{W}^\top\mathbf{W}\mathbf{H}_L\mathbf{S}\mathbf{S}^\top}.
\tag{11}
$$

Step 3: Update $\mathbf{W}$. The associated optimization problem is given as

$$
\min_{\mathbf{W}} \ \lambda\|(\mathbf{W}\mathbf{H}_L - \mathbf{Y})\mathbf{S}\|_F^2 + \beta\|\mathbf{W}\|_F^2.
\tag{12}
$$

Denoting $\mathbf{I}$ as an identity matrix, we have the following updating rule:

$$
\mathbf{W} = \mathbf{Y}\mathbf{S}\mathbf{S}^\top\mathbf{H}_L^\top \left(\mathbf{H}_L\mathbf{S}\mathbf{S}^\top\mathbf{H}_L^\top + \frac{\beta}{\lambda}\mathbf{I} \right)^{-1}.
\tag{13}
$$

We repeat the above updating rules to iteratively optimize $\mathbf{B}_l^{(v)}$ ($l = 1, 2\ldots, L; v = 1, 2, \ldots, V$), $\mathbf{H}_L$, and $\mathbf{W}$, until the model converges. Our model can find at least a locally optimal solution, by seeking an optimal solution for each convex subproblem alternatively. Additionally, several related works have provided the convergence proof associated with the updating rules in Eqs. (9) and (11) using KKT condition [12]. Therefore, the convergence of our model is easily guaranteed.

3   Experiments

3.1   Materials and Neuroimage Preprocessing

The proposed method was evaluated on 379 subjects with complete MRI and PET data at baseline scan from the ADNI dataset, including 101 Normal Control (NC), 185 Mild Cognitive Impairment (MCI), and

Table 1. Demographic information (Mean ± SD). MMSE: mini-mental state examination.

Diagnosis	Gender (M/F)	Education	Age	MMSE
NC	62/39	15.8 ± 3.2	75.8 ± 4.8	28.9 ± 1.1
sMCI	80/34	15.6 ± 3.0	75.5 ± 7.2	27.5 ± 1.6
pMCI	46/25	15.9 ± 2.7	75.4 ± 6.5	26.8 ± 1.7
AD	57/36	14.7 ± 3.2	75.4 ± 7.4	23.5 ± 2.1

93 AD. Within MCI subjects, we defined progressive MCI (pMCI) subjects as MCI subjects that will progress to AD within 24 months, while sMCI subjects remain stable all the time. Subsequently, there were 71 pMCI and 114 sMCI subjects. The MR images were preprocessed via skull stripping, dura and cerebellum removal, intensity correction, tissue segmentation and template registration. Then the processed MR images were divided into 93 pre-defined Regions-Of-Interest (ROIs), and the gray matter volumes were calculated as MRI-based features. We linearly aligned each PET image (*i.e.*, FDG-PET scans) to its corresponding MRI scan, and the mean intensity value of each ROI was calculated as PET-based features. Table 1 summarizes the demographic information of the subjects used in this study.

3.2   Experimental Settings

We evaluated the effectiveness of the proposed model by conducting three binary classification tasks: MCI vs. NC, MCI vs. AD, and sMCI vs. pMCI classification. We used four popular metrics for performance evaluation, including accuracy (ACC), sensitivity (SEN), specificity (SPE), and Fscore. We compared our method with two conventional methods: (1) Baseline method (**Baseline**), which concatenates MRI and PET ROI-based features into a vector for an SVM classifier, and (2) **MKL** method [3]. We further compared our method with four state-of-the-art multi-view/modality learning methods, including (1) shallow **NMF** [4], (2) **MDCR** [16], (3) **MLAN** [8], (4) **DMF** [17], and **Mdl-cw** [9]. We performed 10-fold cross-validation with 10 repetitions for all the methods under comparison, and reported the means and standard deviations of the experimental results. For our method, we determined two parameters (*i.e.*, $\lambda, \beta \in \{10^{-5}, 10^{-4}, \ldots, 10^{2}\}$) and the dimension of each layer (*i.e.*, $h_l \in \{90, 80, \ldots, 20\}$) via an inner cross-validation search on the training data, and we also set $L = 2$ in Eq. (5). For other methods, we used inner cross-validation to determine hyper-parameter values. Note that our method and MLAN can directly perform disease prediction, while the other methods need to resort to SVM for prediction (the parameter C in SVM is selected from $\{10^{-5}, 10^{-4}, \ldots, 10^{2}\}$).

3.3   Results and Discussion

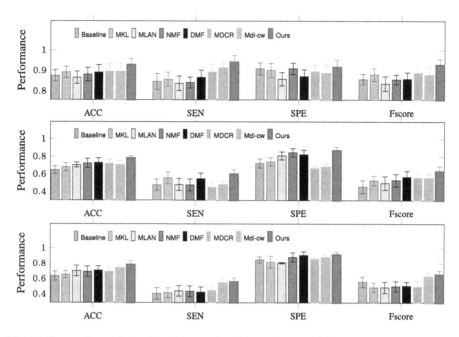

Fig. 2. Comparison of classification results obtained using different methods, on three tasks: (Top) AD vs. NC, (Middle) MCI vs. AD, and (Bottom) pMCI vs. sMCI classification.

Figure 2 shows the comparison results achieved by seven methods on three classification tasks. Note that five competing methods (*i.e.*, Baseline, MKL, NMF, DMF and MDCR) conduct feature learning and model training via two separate steps, while our model, Mdl-cw and MLAN integrate them into a unified framework. From Fig. 2, it can be clearly seen that our proposed method performs better than all the comparison methods in four metrics. This could be partly because our unified framework ensures the classification model to provide feedbacks to the deep NMF step for focusing on learning discriminative features. Although the DMF method also relies on a deep NMF model, its performance

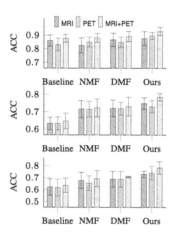

Fig. 3. Influence of using multi-modality data vs. single modality in three classification tasks: (Top) AD vs. NC, (Middle) MCI vs. AD, and (Bottom) pMCI vs. sMCI.

is inferior to ours. One possible reason for this is that DMF only learns the shared representation for multi-modality data, without reconstructing the original features, and it does not use label information to guide the representation learning process (which we do in this work).

Multi-modality Data Fusion. To analyze the benefit of multi-modality fusion, Fig. 3 shows the performance comparison of different methods using multi-modality (*i.e.*, MRI+PET) and single modality (*i.e.*, MRI or PET) data. From Fig. 3, it can be seen that all methods using multi-modality data outperform their counterparts using just a single modality data. However, our method consistently performs better than other comparison methods when using a single modality data (*e.g.*, MRI or PET).

Table 2. Comparison with state-of-the-art methods for pMCI vs. sMCI classification

Algorithm	Methodology	Subject #	Modalities	ACC
Liu *et al.* [6]	Multi-task learning	56 pMCI + 43 sMCI	MRI+PET	0.678
Suk *et al.* [11]	Deep learning	76 pMCI + 128 sMCI	MRI+PET	0.733
Lei *et al.* [5]	Sparse learning	226 pMCI + 167 sMCI	MRI+PET+CSF	0.746
Shi *et al.* [10]	Deep learning	56 pMCI + 43 sMCI	MRI+PET	0.743
DLMD^2 (Ours)	Deep NMF	71 pMCI + 114 sMCI	MRI+PET	0.783

Comparison with State-of-the-Art Methods. We further compare our method with four state-of-the-art methods for pMCI vs. sMCI classification in Table 2. Even though these methods use different numbers of subjects, a rough comparison has demonstrated that our method achieves the best ACC values among the five methods.

4   Conclusion

In this paper, we propose a deep latent multi-modality dementia diagnosis (DLMD^2) framework, by integrating deep latent representation learning and disease prediction into a unified model. The proposed model is able to uncover hierarchical multi-modal correlations and capture the complex data-to-label relationships. Experimental results on three classification tasks, with both MRI and PET data, clearly validate the superiority of our model over several state-of-the-art methods. Besides, we can extend it to problems with incomplete multi-modality data in the future.

References

1. Boyd, S., et al.: Convex Optimization. Cambridge University Press, Cambridge (2004)

2. Chetelat, G., Desgranges, B., De La Sayette, V., Viader, F., Eustache, F., Baron, J.C.: Mild cognitive impairment: can FDG-PET predict who is to rapidly convert to Alzheimer's disease? Neurology **60**(8), 1374–1377 (2003)
3. Hinrichs, C., Singh, V., Xu, G., Johnson, S.: MKL for robust multi-modality AD classification. In: Yang, G.-Z., Hawkes, D., Rueckert, D., Noble, A., Taylor, C. (eds.) MICCAI 2009. LNCS, vol. 5762, pp. 786–794. Springer, Heidelberg (2009). https://doi.org/10.1007/978-3-642-04271-3_95
4. Lee, D.D., Seung, H.S.: Algorithms for non-negative matrix factorization. In: NIPS (2001)
5. Lei, B., Yang, P., Wang, T., Chen, S., Ni, D.: Relational-regularized discriminative sparse learning for Alzheimer's disease diagnosis. IEEE Trans. Cybern. **47**(4), 1102–1113 (2017)
6. Liu, F., Wee, C.Y., et al.: Inter-modality relationship constrained multi-modality multi-task feature selection for Alzheimer's disease and mild cognitive impairment identification. NeuroImage **84**, 466–475 (2014)
7. Liu, S., Liu, S., Cai, W., et al.: Multimodal neuroimaging feature learning for multiclass diagnosis of Alzheimer's disease. IEEE Trans. Biomed. Eng. **62**(4), 1132–1140 (2015)
8. Nie, F., Cai, G., et al.: Auto-weighted multi-view learning for image clustering and semi-supervised classification. IEEE Trans. Image Process. **27**(3), 1501–1511 (2018)
9. Rastegar, S., Soleymani, M., Rabiee, H.R., Mohsen Shojaee, S.: MDL-CW: a multimodal deep learning framework with cross weights. In: CVPR (2016)
10. Shi, J., Zheng, X., Li, Y., Zhang, Q., Ying, S.: Multimodal neuroimaging feature learning with multimodal stacked deep polynomial networks for diagnosis of Alzheimer's disease. IEEE J. Biomed. Health Inf. **22**(1), 173–183 (2018)
11. Suk, H.I., Lee, S.W., Shen, D.: Hierarchical feature representation and multimodal fusion with deep learning for AD/MCI diagnosis. NeuroImage **101**, 569–582 (2014)
12. Wang, J., Tian, F., Yu, H., Liu, C.H., Zhan, K., Wang, X.: Diverse non-negative matrix factorization for multiview data representation. IEEE Trans. Cybern. **48**(9), 2620–2632 (2018)
13. Yang, X., Liu, C., Wang, Z., Yang, J., et al.: Co-trained convolutional neural networks for automated detection of prostate cancer in multi-parametric MRI. Med. Image Anal. **42**, 212–227 (2017)
14. Ye, F., Chen, C., Zheng, Z.: Deep autoencoder-like nonnegative matrix factorization for community detection. In: CIKM, pp. 1393–1402. ACM (2018)
15. Zhang, C., Fu, H., et al.: Generalized latent multi-view subspace clustering. IEEE Trans. Pattern Anal. Mach. Intell. (2018)
16. Zhang, C., Fu, H., Hu, Q., Zhu, P., Cao, X.: Flexible multi-view dimensionality co-reduction. IEEE Trans. Image Process. **26**(2), 648–659 (2017)
17. Zhao, H., et al.: Multi-view clustering via deep matrix factorization. In: AAAI (2017)
18. Zhou, T., et al.: Inter-modality dependence induced data recovery for MCI conversion prediction. In: MICCAI (2019)
19. Zhou, T., Liu, M., Thung, K.H., Shen, D.: Latent representation learning for Alzheimer's disease diagnosis with incomplete multi-modality neuroimaging and genetic data. IEEE Trans. Med. Imaging (2019)
20. Zhou, T., Thung, K.H., Zhu, X., Shen, D.: Effective feature learning and fusion of multimodality data using stage-wise deep neural network for dementia diagnosis. Hum. Brain Mapp. **40**(3), 1001–1016 (2019)

Dynamic Spectral Graph Convolution Networks with Assistant Task Training for Early MCI Diagnosis

Xiaodan Xing[1,2], Qingfeng Li[1,3], Hao Wei[1,4], Minqing Zhang[1,5],
Yiqiang Zhan[1], Xiang Sean Zhou[1], Zhong Xue[1], and Feng Shi[1(✉)]

[1] Shanghai United Imaging Intelligence Co., Ltd., Shanghai, China
feng.shi@united-imaging.com
[2] Medical Imaging Center, Shanghai Advanced Research Institute, Shanghai, China
[3] School of Biomedical Engineering, Southern Medical University, Guangdong, China
[4] School of Computer Science and Engineering, Central South University,
Hunan, China
[5] College of Software Enginerring, Southeast University, Jiangsu, China

Abstract. Functional brain connectome, also known as inter-regional functional connectivity (FC) matrix, is recently considered providing decisive markers for early mild cognitive impairment (eMCI). However, in most existing methods, vectorized static FC matrices and some "off-the-shelf" classifiers were used, which may lead to a deprecation of both spatial and temporal information and thus compromise the diagnosis performance. In this paper, we propose dynamic spectral graph convolution networks (DS-GCNs) for early MCI diagnosis using functional MRI (fMRI). First, a dynamic brain graph is constructed so that the connectivity strengths (edges) are derived by time-varying correlations of fMRI signals, and the node signals are computed from T1 MR images. Then, the spectral graph convolution (GC) based long short term memory (LSTM) network is employed to process long range temporal information from the dynamic graphs. Finally, instead of directly using demographic information as additional inputs as in the conventional methods, we proposed to predict gender and age of each subject as assistant tasks, which in turn captures useful network features and facilitates the main task of eMCI classification; we refer this strategy as assistant task training. Experiments on 294 training and 74 testing subjects show that eMCI classification results achieved 79.7% accuracy (with 86.5% sensitivity and 73.0% specificity) and outperformed the state-of-the-art methods. Notably, the proposed method could be further extended to other Connectomics studies, where the graphs are computed through white matter fiber connections or gray matter characteristics.

1 Introduction

Mild Cognitive Impairment (MCI) is a preclinical stage between expected cognitive decline of normal aging and dementia. It may develop to Alzheimer's disease

© Springer Nature Switzerland AG 2019
D. Shen et al. (Eds.): MICCAI 2019, LNCS 11767, pp. 639–646, 2019.
https://doi.org/10.1007/978-3-030-32251-9_70

(AD) or other types of dementia, remain stable, or sometimes improve. On-time intervention could prevent symptom deterioration and slow down the progression of MCI to AD. However, in early MCI (eMCI), there are no obvious and noticeable abnormalities in structural brain images. Fortunately, studies showed that functional MRI (fMRI), which evaluates the blood oxygen level dependent (BOLD) signals in the brain and reveals activation and inactivation in different brain regions, demonstrates possible functional brain connectivity abnormality between normal controls (NC) and eMCI.

Conventional fMRI diagnosing methods calculated functional connectivity matrix (FC matrix) for the entire time series and generated features by reshaping FC matrix into a vector of features, with which classifiers such as SVM can be employed for diagnosis. However, these methods *neither* considered the dynamics of the blood oxygen level dependent (BOLD) signals across the time-series, thus neglecting the condition-dependent nature of brain activity, *nor* preserved spatial information by reshaping FC matrices into vectors. To preserve both topological and temporal information, researchers have implemented CNN (convolutional neural network) [8] and RNN (recurrent neural networks) [2] for classification. However, their methods are still affected by the noises in fMRI signals, which may overwhelm the desired signals related to neuronal activities.

Brain connectivity network can be described by a graph that describes brain regions and their relationships. Graph convolution networks (GCNs) allow for an implement of neural networks on network/graph structure. Researchers have utilized GCN on disease diagnosis by two means, i.e., node classification and graph classification. Node classification [7] treats subjects as nodes, classifying them on a pre-defined demographic graph. Graph classification [5] assigns a graph for every subject with each brain region as a node. Like aforementioned conventional methods, they only deal with static networks and do not consider the dynamic nature of BOLD signals.

On the other hand, it has been reported a higher incidence of MCI occurring in females than males. Besides, the incidence of MCI increases with the years of age [4]. Thus, gender and age are helpful features for eMCI prediction and are adopted in many studies. However, in many datasets such as ADNI, the guideline of data acquisition is to balance the demographic distribution, i.e., male-female ratio and age distribution, in both patient group and healthy control group, where demographic features weakly correlates with diagnosis and thus has limited influence for diagnosis.

In this study, we propose dynamic spectral graph convolution networks (DS-GCNs), with assistant task training, for early MCI diagnosis using fMRI. To address aforementioned problems, the novelty of the proposed method is summarized in three aspects: (1) a spectral graph convolution operation for graph-like functional connectivity data; (2) an LSTM architecture to further extract temporal information relevant to diagnosis; (3) two assistant networks that use gender and age as extra outputs, respectively, to provide guidance for the main task of eMCI diagnosis.

2 Method

Figure 1 illustrates the framework of the proposed DS-GCNs. The left part (A and B) demonstrates how the dynamic graph is formed. The feature on each node is defined by the volume of the corresponding ROI calculated from T1-weighted MR images. The time-varying edges are calculated based on correlations of BOLD signals within sliding-windows. After defining the graphs, a spectral graph convolution-based LSTM (GC-LSTM) layer with three fully-connected layers is employed to predict status, gender, and age of each patient, respectively. Finally, feature maps from two assistant networks with the same structure but different parameters (C and E) are weighted and combined into the feature maps of the diagnosis network (D), guiding the parameter training and optimization of the diagnosis network.

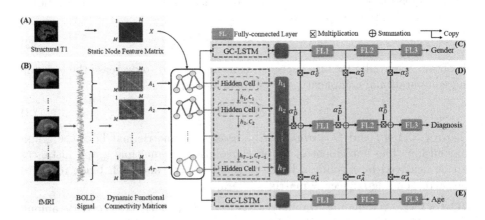

Fig. 1. Overview of the architecture of the proposed DS-GCNs. Graphs are constructed by (A) structural T1 MR image and (B) fMRI, and are fed into (D) the main networks and (C, E) two assistant networks (that share the same structure but different parameters). Here h_t denotes the output of t-th hidden layer, and C_t is the cell state. Alphas are learnable parameters determining the contributions from corresponding networks.

2.1 Graph Convolution LSTM

Graph Construction. A graph $\mathcal{G}(\mathcal{V}, \mathcal{E})$ is formed by nodes and edges. First, a feature description for every node in the graph is summarized in a feature matrix $X^{M \times N}$. Here, M denotes the number of graph nodes. In our case, nodes are defined by anatomical ROIs, and features are their volumes; thus, X is a diagonal matrix, defined by $\{X | x_{ij} = \begin{cases} 0, & i \neq j \\ v_i, & i = j \end{cases}, X \in R^{M \times M}\}$. Here v_i is the volume of the i-th ROI. Second, a structural description of the graph connection is in the form of an adjacency matrix $A^{M \times M}$. That, by applying a sliding window through the entire time-sequences, can be represented by dynamic adjacency matrices $\{A_t | t = 1, 2, ..., T, A_t \in R^{M \times M}\}$.

Spectral Graph Convolution. Since it is difficult to match spatial local neighborhoods for a node and there is no unique mathematical definition of translation on graph from the spatial perspective, we chose the spectral graph convolution in our study for graph classification [1]. Since a convolution in the spatial domain corresponds to a multiplication in the spectral domain, graph convolution can be computed in the Fourier domain. Therefore, the Fourier transforms of a learnable convolutional kernel w and feature map x could be obtained by $\hat{w} = U^T w$ and $\hat{x} = U^T x$. U denotes the eigenvector matrix of the graph Laplacian L:

$$L = D^{-\frac{1}{2}} A D^{-\frac{1}{2}}, \tag{1}$$

Here A is the adjacency matrix of the graph structure, and $D = diag \sum_j a_{i,j}$ is the degree matrix of A. Thus, the graph convolution between convolutional kernel w and feature map x is defined as

$$w * x = U((U^T w) \odot (U^T x)). \tag{2}$$

To obtain a spatially localized spectral convolution and to decrease the learning and computational complexity, we approximate Eq. (2) as:

$$w * x = \tilde{D}^{-\frac{1}{2}} \tilde{A} \tilde{D}^{-\frac{1}{2}} x \Theta, \tag{3}$$

where $\tilde{A} = A + I$ and $\tilde{D} = diag \sum_j \tilde{a}_{i,j}$. Θ is a parametric matrix of the graph convolution. The implement of graph convolution on multiple graph instances can be achieved by forming a block-diagonal matrix, and each block refers to the corresponding adjacency matrix of a graph.

GC-LSTM. A dynamic graph consists of time-varying connectivity among anatomical regions, and to handle temporal information the long short-term memory (LSTM) units are used. LSTM has been widely used for processing recurrent or temporal signals, and it solves the long-term dependencies problem by using hidden layer as states. By replacing matrix multiplication operators in the traditional LSTM with the graph convolution presented above, we come up with a dynamic graph LSTM neural network. Mathematically, according to LSTM, the gates of t-th hidden cell of graph convolution LSTM follows these formula:

$$ForgetGate : f_t = \sigma(\omega_{xf} * x_t + \omega_{hf} * h_{t-1} + \omega_{Cf} \odot C_{t-1} + b_f)$$
$$InputGate : i_t = \sigma(\omega_{xi} * x_t + \omega_{hi} * h_{t-1} + \omega_{Ci} \odot C_{t-1} + b_i)$$
$$MemoryCell : C_t = f_t \odot C_t + i_t \odot tanh(\omega_{xc} * x_t + \omega_{hc} * h_{t-1} + b_c)$$
$$OutputGate : o_t = \sigma(\omega_{xo} * x_t + \omega_{ho} * h_{t-1} + \omega_{Co} \odot C_t + b_o)$$
$$OutputHiddenState : h_t = o \odot tanh(C_t), \tag{4}$$

where $*$ denotes the graph convolution operator, x_t the t-th input of the time series, σ the activate function, w-s graph convolutional kernels and b-s biases. The unfolded LSTM cell is shown in Fig. 2.

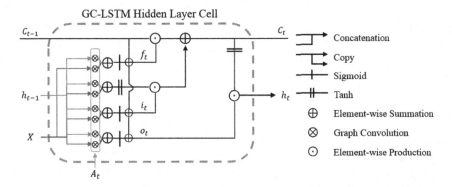

Fig. 2. Details of GC-LSTM hidden cell. Each cell has two sources of input, i.e., the present (A_t and X) and the recent past (h_{t-1} and C_{t-1}). Output sequence $\{h_t|t = 1, 2, \ldots T\}$ were feature maps for following layers.

2.2   Assistant Task Training

Demographic information including gender and age could assist eMCI prediction. Unlike most existing methods, we use them as extra outputs. Such an assistant task training has two advantages. First, brain functional signals contain a lot of noise and thus cause difficulties on appropriate feature extraction. Relevant assistant tasks could help deep learning model focus its attention on relevant features. Second, as mentioned above, gender/age may correlate weakly with diagnosis results in the ADNI dataset. Thus, simply adding gender and age directly as extra inputs will not necessarily improve the classification performance.

However, in conventional multi-task settings different tasks share parameters in convolutional layers, and it is difficult to decide which layers to be shared or split among different tasks. Thus, we allow the networks to learn a linear combination of feature maps from different tasks to determine the shared representations by itself. We adopted this architecture from the cross stitch networks [6], but our networks are task-oriented, i.e., only the main task receives the weighted combination of feature maps. Three networks with the same structure but different parameters were designed for three respective tasks (eMCI classification, gender classification, and age prediction). Consider three activation maps x_D, x_G and x_A generated by layer l from corresponding network, weighted combination of these activation maps was learned and fed into next layer $l+1$ of diagnosis network as inputs,

$$\hat{x}_D^{l+1} = \alpha_D^l x_D + \alpha_G^l x_G + \alpha_A^l x_A. \tag{5}$$

Here, α^l is a learnable parameter in layer l which determines the contributions from assistant tasks. For classification tasks (i.e., diagnosis and gender classification), the cross-entropy loss is used for training. For age prediction, the mean squared loss is used. Our final loss function is a weighted combination of three losses:

$$\mathcal{L} = w_D \mathcal{L}_D + w_G \mathcal{L}_G + w_A \mathcal{L}_A. \tag{6}$$

Considering that gender classification and age prediction are the assistant tasks, we set $w_D = 0.989$, $w_G = 0.01$, $w_A = 0.001$. w_A is smaller than w_G to balance the losses of two assistant tasks.

3   Experiments

3.1   Data

We used T1-weighted and fMRI images from the Alzheimer's Disease Neuroimaging Initiative II (ADNI2) [3] including 177 healthy controls and 191 early MCIs. The 3T T1-weighted MR images were pre-processed under a standard pipeline including image reorientation, resampling into isotropic spatial resolution, bias field correction, skull-stripping, and then parcellated using the anatomical automatic labeling (AAL) template. Functional images include 137 time points with $TR = 2$ s. Image processing included slice time correction, motion correction, spatial and temporal filtering and covariates regression. To calculate the dynamic network, a sliding window of 120 s and stride 2 s was used. We split the subjects into 294 training and 74 testing subjects.

3.2   Results

We computed classification accuracy, specificity and sensitivity with a number of methods, as well as different settings of our proposed algorithm (see Table 1 for more details). There comparison methods are listed as follows:

Algorithms Using Static Connectivity Matrices. In these algorithms, the connectivity matrices are calculated based on the correlations of the entire BOLD signals of each ROI pair. *SVM:* support vector machine was used for classification by reshaping matrices into vectors. *CNN:* convolutional neural network was applied by treating FC matrices and node feature matrices as two-channel images; VGG-16 was used. *GCN:* static graphs were constructed from static FCs and node feature matrices; GCN consisted one graph convolution layer and three fully-connected layers.

Algorithms Using Dynamic Connectivity Matrices. In these algorithms, the dynamic connectivity matrices of each subject was calculated. *LSTM:* the long short term memory network was applied by reshaping dynamic matrices into vectors. *DS-GCN (proposed):* gender and age predicting tasks were not used in the training stage. *DS-GCN + Demographic features (proposed):* gender and age were added as extra inputs into the last fully-connected layer (FL3 in Fig. 1). *DS-GCN + Assistant task training (proposed):* Notice that gender and age were used not as extra input features, but as outputs.

To further evaluate the effectiveness of assistant task training, we plotted α values before each fully-connected layers during training stage in Fig. 3, which

Table 1. Classification results of various methods using static/dynamic connectivity matrices. Note that VGG-16 was used for Static FC, but CNN did not converge in the training stage. These results indicate that dynamic connectivity with graph-based neural networks is a better way for fMRI connectivity analysis. Meanwhile, assistant task training may help improve the performance of classification.

	Method	Accuracy	Sensitivity	Specificity
Static FC	SVM	60.81%	81.08%	40.54%
	CNN	/	/	/
	GCN	70.27%	83.78%	56.76%
Dynamic FC	LSTM	67.56%	70.27%	64.86%
	DS-GCN (Proposed)	71.62%	70.27%	72.97%
	DS-GCN + Demographic features (Proposed)	72.97%	75.67%	64.86%
	DS-GCN + Assistant task training (Proposed)	**79.73%**	**86.49%**	**72.97%**

reflect the amount of each network contributing to the final classification performance. Also, we checked the performance of our assistant tasks. Results show that the average accuracy of gender prediction is 89%, and the mean absolute error of age prediction is 3 years.

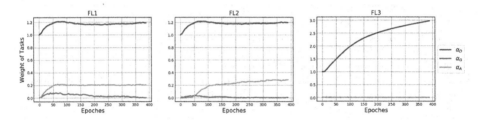

Fig. 3. The curves of task weights for input feature maps of different layers. The weight of the main task α_D was initialized as one, and the weights of assistant tasks, α_G and α_A, were initialized as zeros.

4   Conclusion

A dynamic graph convolution network was proposed for analyzing fMRI connectivity and classifying eMCI from normal controls. In addition, to improve the network stability and classification performance, we proposed a novel assistant task training strategy, i.e., simultaneous prediction of multiple demographic factors, for improving the eMCI classification. Using datasets from ADNI2, we demonstrated that our proposed algorithm can classify eMCI from NC with 79.73% accuracy. It is worth noting that our proposed network can be extended to other connectomics studies.

References

1. Defferrard, M., Bresson, X., Vandergheynst, P.: Convolutional neural networks on graphs with fast localized spectral filtering. In: Advances in Neural Information Processing Systems, pp. 3844–3852 (2016)
2. Dvornek, N.C., Ventola, P., Pelphrey, K.A., Duncan, J.S.: Identifying autism from resting-state fMRI using long short-term memory networks. In: Wang, Q., Shi, Y., Suk, H.-I., Suzuki, K. (eds.) MLMI 2017. LNCS, vol. 10541, pp. 362–370. Springer, Cham (2017). https://doi.org/10.1007/978-3-319-67389-9_42
3. Jack Jr., C.R., et al.: The Alzheimer's disease neuroimaging initiative (ADNI): MRI methods. J. Magn. Reson. Imaging Off. J. Int. Soc. Magn. Reson. Med. **27**(4), 685–691 (2008)
4. Katz, M.J., et al.: Age and sex specific prevalence and incidence of mild cognitive impairment, dementia and Alzheimer's dementia in blacks and whites: a report from the einstein aging study. Alzheimer Dis. Assoc. Disord. **26**(4), 335 (2012)
5. Ktena, S.I., et al.: Distance metric learning using graph convolutional networks: application to functional brain networks. In: Descoteaux, M., Maier-Hein, L., Franz, A., Jannin, P., Collins, D.L., Duchesne, S. (eds.) MICCAI 2017. LNCS, vol. 10433, pp. 469–477. Springer, Cham (2017). https://doi.org/10.1007/978-3-319-66182-7_54
6. Misra, I., Shrivastava, A., Gupta, A., Hebert, M.: Cross-stitch networks for multi-task learning. In: Proceedings of the IEEE Conference on Computer Vision and Pattern Recognition, pp. 3994–4003 (2016)
7. Parisot, S., et al.: Spectral graph convolutions for population-based disease prediction. In: Descoteaux, M., Maier-Hein, L., Franz, A., Jannin, P., Collins, D.L., Duchesne, S. (eds.) MICCAI 2017. LNCS, vol. 10435, pp. 177–185. Springer, Cham (2017). https://doi.org/10.1007/978-3-319-66179-7_21
8. Sarraf, S., Tofighi, G.: Deep learning-based pipeline to recognize Alzheimer's disease using fMRI data. In: 2016 Future Technologies Conference (FTC), pp. 816–820. IEEE (2016)

Bridging Imaging, Genetics, and Diagnosis in a Coupled Low-Dimensional Framework

Sayan Ghosal[1]([⊠]), Qiang Chen[2], Aaron L. Goldman[2], William Ulrich[2],
Karen F. Berman[3], Daniel R. Weinberger[2,4], Venkata S. Mattay[2,4],
and Archana Venkataraman[1]

[1] Department of Electrical and Computer Engineering, Johns Hopkins University,
Baltimore, USA
sghosal3@jhu.edu
[2] Lieber Institute for Brain Development, Baltimore, USA
[3] Clinical and Translational Neuroscience Branch, NIMH, NIH, Bethesda, USA
[4] Department of Neurology and Radiology, Johns Hopkins School of Medicine,
Baltimore, USA

Abstract. We propose a joint dictionary learning framework that couples imaging and genetics data in a low dimensional subspace as guided by clinical diagnosis. We use a graph regularization penalty to simultaneously capture inter-regional brain interactions and identify the representative set anatomical basis vectors that span the low dimensional space. We further employ group sparsity to find the representative set of genetic basis vectors that span the same latent space. Finally, the latent projection is used to classify patients versus controls. We have evaluated our model on two task fMRI paradigms and single nucleotide polymorphism (SNP) data from schizophrenic patients and matched neurotypical controls. We employ a ten fold cross validation technique to show the predictive power of our model. We compare our model with canonical correlation analysis of imaging and genetics data and random forest classification. Our approach shows better prediction accuracy on both task datasets. Moreover, the implicated brain regions and genetic variants underlie the well documented deficits in schizophrenia.

1 Introduction

Neuropsychiatric disorders, such as autism and schizophrenia are hereditary, which suggests a genetic underpinning. These disorders are characterized by behavioral and cognitive deficits linked to atypical neural functioning. Identifying the brain mechanisms through which the genomes confer risk is essential to find targeted biomarkers for these disorders. Functional MRI (fMRI) and Single Neucleotipe Polymorphisms (SNPs) are the most common modalities used to study brain activity and genetic variation, respectively. However, integrating them is hard due to large dimensionality and the complex interactions between them.

© Springer Nature Switzerland AG 2019
D. Shen et al. (Eds.): MICCAI 2019, LNCS 11767, pp. 647–655, 2019.
https://doi.org/10.1007/978-3-030-32251-9_71

Prior work in imaging-genetics can be grouped into three general categories. The first are multivariate regression methods [8] that uses SNPs as feature vectors and the imaging phenotype as the response variables in penalized least square setting. Some of these methods also induce structured sparsity both at the SNP level and gene levels to find unique interactions between the imaging and the genetic components. However, they do not consider inter-regional brain interactions or the impact of diagnosis. The second category uses canonical correlation analysis (CCA) to maximize the correlation between linear projections of the imaging and genetics data [5]. Once again these unsupervised methods do not incorporate the clinical factor, so the implicated features may not be related to the disease. Finally, the recent approach of [1] develops a probabilistic framework that incorporates imaging, genetics and diagnosis. Specifically, they consider the imaging data as an intermediate phenotype between genetics and disease. However, this method cannot identify genetic variants associated with the disease that do not also express themselves in the imaging data.

In contrast to prior work, we propose coupled dictionary learning framework to bridge the three data domains. Our model assumes that the imaging and genetics data share a joint latent space. The shared projection coefficients are used as a low-dimensional feature vector to predict diagnosis. We couple the imaging, genetics and diagnosis terms in a regularized optimization framework. We use alternating minimization to estimate the unknown dictionary atoms, projection coefficients, and regression weights. The coupling between these variables overcomes the drawbacks of previous methods and yields better diagnosis prediction in a nested cross validation setting. We validate our framework on a population study of schizophrenia and compare our model with standard machine learning baselines. Our framework achieves the best classification accuracy while finding the interpretable and clinically relevant biomarkers.

2   Joint Modeling of Imaging, Genetics, and Diagnosis

Figure 1 presents a overview of our joint modelling approach. Let M be the total number of subjects in our study. Our input data for each subject m consists of fMRI activation maps $\mathbf{f_m}$, SNP variants $\mathbf{g_m}$, and binary disease diagnosis y_m. We model the fMRI and SNPs in a parallel dictionary learning framework, where the matrices $\mathbf{A}$ and $\mathbf{B}$ contain the associated dictionary elements. The projection onto these dictionaries is controlled by the latent vector $\mathbf{z}_m$ for both imaging and genetics. Likewise, classification is performed using the projection vector $\mathbf{z}_m$. This joint optimization method allows us to learn the related basis features of both imaging and genetics that are associated with the disease.

Generative Model for Imaging: Mathematically, let N denotes the total number of ROIs in the brain. The imaging data has dimensionality $\mathbf{f}_m \in \mathbb{R}^{N \times 1}$. We assume that this data can be represented by a sparse set of anatomical basis vectors that lie in a lower dimensional latent space:

$$\mathbf{f}_m \approx \mathbf{A}^T \mathbf{z}_m \quad \text{s.t. } \mathbf{A}\mathbf{A}^T = \mathbf{I}$$

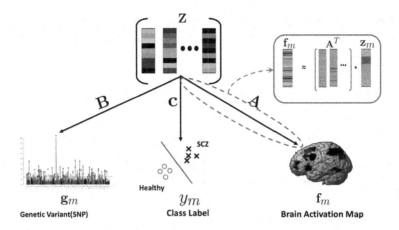

Fig. 1. The generative process linking imaging ($\mathbf{f}_m$), genetics ($\mathbf{g}_m$), and diagnosis (y_m). The imaging model is shown as a linear projection. The genetics model parallels this, whereas the classification is based on a logistic regression.

where rows of $\mathbf{A} \in \mathbb{R}^{d \times N}$ correspond to the basis vectors (common across the group) and $\mathbf{z}_m \in \mathbb{R}^{d \times 1}$ is the subject specific projection to the latent space. The orthogonality constraint ensures that the basis vectors capture different facets of the data. We also introduce a graph based regularizer on $\mathbf{A}$ so that highly correlated brain regions play a similar role in projection:

$$\frac{\lambda_1}{2} Tr(\mathbf{A}\mathbf{L}\mathbf{A}^T) = \frac{\lambda_1}{2} \sum_{(i,j)} \mathbf{W}_{ij} ||\mathbf{a}_i - \mathbf{a}_j||_2^2$$

where $\mathbf{a}_i$ denotes the ith column of $\mathbf{A}$ and $\mathbf{W}_{ij}$ is the Pearson correlation between the activation map of region i and region j across M patients. The standard graph Laplacian, $\mathbf{L}$, is computed from the sample correlation matrix, $\mathbf{W}$.

Generative Model for Genetics: Let G denote the number of genetic variants measured in each subject. This data is captured by the vector $\mathbf{g_m} \in \mathbb{R}^{G \times 1}$. We assume that the genetic data express itself through a sparse set of basis vectors, $\mathbf{g}_m \approx \mathbf{B}^T \mathbf{z}_m$; furthermore, the projection is tied to that of the imaging data. Here $\mathbf{B} \in \mathbb{R}^{d \times G}$ is the genetic basis matrix. We employ a group sparsity penalty over $\mathbf{B}$, in the form of $\ell_{2,1}$ norm. This penalty selects a sparse set of genetic variants through the ℓ_1 penalty across rows. At the same time, the ℓ_2 penalty across columns preserve the genetic representation across basis vectors.

Joint Objective with Diagnosis Prediction: We use the patient-specific projection coefficients $\{\mathbf{z}_m\}_{m=1}^M$ to predict the class labels. Mathematically, $y_m \approx \sigma(\mathbf{z}_m^T \mathbf{c})$ where $\sigma(\cdot)$ is the standard sigmoid function and $\mathbf{c} \in \mathbb{R}^{d \times 1}$ is the regression vector. We combine the dictionary learning and logistic regression terms in a joint objective. For convenience, we concatenate the imaging and genetics data into the matrices $\mathbf{F} = [\mathbf{f}_1, \ldots, \mathbf{f}_M]$ and $\mathbf{G} = [\mathbf{g}_1, \ldots, \mathbf{g}_M]$, respectively. Likewise, we define the latent projection matrix $\mathbf{Z} = [\mathbf{z}_1, \ldots, \mathbf{z}_M]$.

$$\mathcal{J}(\mathbf{A}, \mathbf{B}, \mathbf{Z}, \mathbf{c}) = ||\mathbf{F} - \mathbf{A}^T \mathbf{Z}||_F^2 + ||\mathbf{G} - \mathbf{B}^T \mathbf{Z}||_F^2$$

$$- \sum_{m=1}^{M} (y_m \log(\sigma(\mathbf{z}_m^T \mathbf{c})) + (1 - y_m) \log(1 - \sigma(\mathbf{z}_m^T \mathbf{c})))$$

$$+ \frac{\lambda_1}{2} Tr(\mathbf{A} \mathbf{L} \mathbf{A}^T) + \lambda_2 ||\mathbf{B}||_{2,1} + \frac{\lambda_3}{2} ||\mathbf{Z}||_F^2 + \frac{\lambda_4}{2} ||\mathbf{c}||_2^2 \quad \text{s.t. } \mathbf{A}\mathbf{A}^T = \mathbf{I} \quad (1)$$

where $\{\lambda_1, \lambda_2, \lambda_3, \lambda_4\}$ are the associated regularization parameters. The penalties, $\frac{\lambda_3}{2} ||\mathbf{Z}||_F^2$, and $\frac{\lambda_4}{2} ||\mathbf{c}||_2^2$ are introduced to make the optimization well-posed.

2.1   Optimization Strategy

We use an alternating minimization strategy to optimize the unknown variables $\{\mathbf{A}, \mathbf{B}, \mathbf{Z}, \mathbf{c}\}$ in Eq. (1) from the data $\{\mathbf{f}_m, \mathbf{g}_m, y_m\}$. This procedure iteratively updates each variable while holding the remaining variables constant.

Update for A via Interior Point Solver: The objective $\mathcal{J}(\cdot)$ is a convex function in $\mathbf{A}$ with a nonconvex equality constraint $\mathbf{A}\mathbf{A}^T = \mathbf{I}$. We use an interior point solver to incrementally optimize over $\mathbf{A}$. Specifically, each iteration solves the following modified problem:

$$\mathbf{A}_{t+1} = \min_{\mathbf{A}} \ ||\mathbf{F} - \mathbf{A}^T \mathbf{Z}||_F^2 + \frac{\lambda_1}{2} Tr(\mathbf{A} \mathbf{L} \mathbf{A}^T) \quad \text{subject to: } \mathbf{A}\mathbf{A}^T - \mathbf{I} = 0 \quad (2)$$

The interior point solver uses two methods to solve Eq. (2). It first tries to take a Newton step by solving the augmented Lagrangian problem. If this step fails the algorithm approximates the augmented Lagragian in the least squares sense to solve for the lagrange multipliers and takes a conjugate gradient step to approximately solve Eq. (2) using a trust region method.

Update B, Z, and c Using Trust Region Method: The objective $\mathcal{J}(\cdot)$ is convex in each of the variables $\{\mathbf{B}, \mathbf{Z}, \mathbf{c}\}$ while keeping the other variables constant. So, we solve the minimization problem for each variable in an iterative fashion using an unconstrained trust region solver. At each iteration the trust region method estimates the step size and direction $\mathbf{s}_k$ to optimize the function $f(\mathbf{x})$ through the following quadratic program:

$$\mathbf{s}_k = \text{argmin}_{\mathbf{s}} \ f(\mathbf{x}_k) + \mathbf{g}_k^T \mathbf{s} + \frac{1}{2} \mathbf{s}^T \mathbf{H}_k \mathbf{s} \quad \text{subject to: } ||\mathbf{s}|| < \delta \quad (3)$$

where $\mathbf{g}_k$ and $\mathbf{H}_k$ are the gradient and hessian of $f(\mathbf{x})$ at $\mathbf{x}_k$. The update $\mathbf{x}_k \to \mathbf{x} + \mathbf{s}_k$ is taken such that $f(\mathbf{x}_k + \mathbf{s}_k) < f(\mathbf{x}_k)$. This method is guaranteed to converge to a local minimum in polynomial time.

In our setting $f(\cdot)$ involves the terms of the objective function, $\mathcal{J}(\cdot)$ that involves the variable in consideration. A typical example is minimization of $\mathbf{B}$ where, $f(\mathbf{B}) = ||\mathbf{G} - \mathbf{B}^T \mathbf{Z}||_F^2 + \lambda_2 ||\mathbf{B}||_{2,1}$. $f(\mathbf{Z})$ and $f(\mathbf{c})$ are similarly specified.

Prediction on Unseen Data: We use a tenfold cross validation setup to evaluate the predictive power of our framework. In this case, we optimize the variables $\{\mathbf{A}^*, \mathbf{B}^*, \mathbf{Z}^*, \mathbf{c}^*\}$ based just on the training data. For testing, we use just the imaging and genetics data $\{\mathbf{f}_{test}, \mathbf{g}_{test}\}$ of a new subject to obtain the subject-specific projection $\mathbf{z}_{test}$ while setting the cross-entropy term to zero (since the diagnosis y_{test} in unknown). We then use the same logistic regression $y_{test} = \sigma(\mathbf{z}_{test}^T \mathbf{c}^*)$ to predict the class label. Unlike prior work [1], our setup performs feature selection in a nested fashion, since the bases matrices $\mathbf{A}$ and $\mathbf{B}$, which in turn govern the latent projection, are estimated only from the training data.

Baseline Comparisons: We compare out model with three baseline methods, as described below:

- **Random Forest (RF) Classification:** We construct a RF classifier for diagnosis based on the concatenated imaging and genetics data, $[\mathbf{f}_m^T, \mathbf{g}_m^T]^T$.
- **CCA + RF Classification:** Canonical correlation analysis (CCA) identifies bi-multivariate associations between imaging and genetics data. This approach is similar in spirit to our coupled latent projection, but it does not include the diagnosis to guide the association. The input to the RF classifier is the aligned imaging & genetics data after performing CCA. Once again, we concatenate the modalities into a single feature vector.
- **Imaging Only Variant of Eq. 1:** Finally we consider a variant of our own model with just the imaging terms and ignore the terms that involve genetic information. This baseline will help us to quantify the performance gain for adding genetic data. We again evaluate this model in a nested fashion, where we optimize the variables $\{\mathbf{A}^*, \mathbf{Z}^*, \mathbf{c}^*\}$ over training set and use them to estimate subject specific projection and diagnosis on the testing data.

We use a grid search to fix parameters for each method. Based on this experiment, we fix the genetic regularizer λ_2, the projection regularizer λ_3, and the regression regularizer λ_4 to $\lambda_2 = 7.5$, $\lambda_3 = 0.6$, $\lambda_4 = 0.04$ for both our model variants. The imaging regularizer λ_1 and latent dimension d are sensitive to the complexity of the fMRI paradigm used in the study. We use $\{d = 9, \lambda_1 = 17.5\}$ for the Nback task, and $\{d = 7, \lambda_1 = 12.5\}$ for SDMT task. The baseline RFs produce stable results for 9000 trees, which is what we use in the analysis.

3 Experimental Results

We evaluate our model on two fMRI datasets and a SNP dataset of schizophrenia patients and normal controls. The first fMRI paradigm is a working memory task (NBack), comprised of 2-back working memory trial blocks alternating with 0-back trial blocks. During 0-back trials participants were instructed to press a button corresponding to a number displayed on the screen and during the 2-back working memory trials the participants were instructed to press the button corresponding to the number they saw two stimuli previously. This dataset includes

Table 1. Performance of each of the methods during nested cross validation. We abbreviated Sensitivity to Sens, Specificity to Spec and Accuracy to Acc.

Method	NBack task			SDMT task		
	Sens	Spec	Acc	Sens	Spec	Acc
RF	0.58	0.56	0.57	**0.68**	0.56	0.62
CCA + RF	0.41	0.47	0.44	0.55	0.69	0.62
Our method (Imaging only)	0.66	0.52	0.60	0.63	0.63	0.63
Our method (Imaging+Genetics)	**0.71**	**0.68**	**0.70**	0.60	**0.76**	**0.68**

53 patients and 53 controls, matched on age, IQ and education. The second fMRI paradigm is a simple declarative memory task (SDMT), which involved incidental encoding of complex aversive visual scenes. This dataset includes 46 patients and 47 controls, matched on age, IQ, and education. All fMRI data was acquired on 3-T General Electric Sigma scanner (EPI, TR/TE = 2000/28 ms; flip angle = 90; field of view = 24 cm, res: 3.75 mm in x and y dimensions and 6 mm in the z dimension for NBack and 5 mm for SDMT;). FMRI preprocessing include slice timing correction, realignment, spatial normalization to an MNI template, smoothing and motion regression. SPM12 is used to generate activation and contrast maps for each paradigm. We use the Brainnetome atlas [6] to define 246 cortical and subcortical regions. The input to our model is the contrast map over these 246 ROIs. In parallel, genotyping was done using variate Illumina Bead Chips including 510K/610K/660K/2.5M. Quality control and imputation were performed using PLINK and IMPUTE2 respectively. The resulting 102K linkage disequilibrium independent SNPs are used to calculate the polygenic risk score of schizophrenia via a log-odds ratio of the imputation probability for the reference allele [3]. By selecting $P < 10^{-4}$, we obtain 1252 linkage disequilibrium independent SNPs. We remove the effect of first principal component from the SNP training data and use the same estimated projection matrix to remove the effect of first principal component from the test data.

Table 1 quantifies the classification performance of each method. Notice that both dictionary learning frameworks (with and without genetics) outperform the standard machine learning baselines. Additionally, the genetic information improves the overall performance of our model. This result suggest that our coupled dictionary learning framework is able to identify meaningful features from both the imaging and genetics data that distinctly separates patients and controls.

Figure 2 shows the most significant set of brain region as obtained from the template basis vectors of **A**. We observe that in the Nback dataset the set of regions include the dorsolateral prefrontal cortex that is well known to underlie executive function including working memory. This region has been implicated in the executive functioning deficits of Schizophrenia [2]. The SDMT task implicates hippocampal and parahippocampal regions also thought to be disrupted in

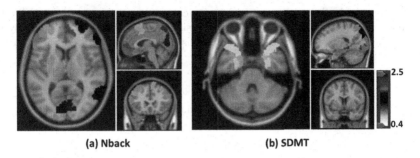

(a) Nback   **(b) SDMT**

Fig. 2. The representative set of regions captured by the matrix, **A**. The color bar shows the level of contribution of each region for classification. (Color figure online)

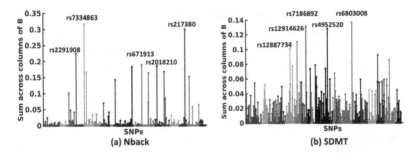

(a) Nback   **(b) SDMT**

Fig. 3. The contribution of each SNP to discriminate the subjects between patients and controls. We have annotated the top five SNPs. The colors indicate the chromosomes on which the SNPs are located. (Color figure online)

schizophrenia [7]. Hence our model is able to find well reported and interpretable aberrations between schizophrenia patients and controls.

Figure 3 illustrates the contribution of individual SNP to the latent vector. It is calculated as the sum of absolute values of the columns in **B**. We have annotated the five most highly implicated SNPs for each dataset as a reference. According to GWAS the overlapping genes of these SNPs are closely related to schizophrenia. Additionally, we ran a gene ontology enrichment analysis based on the genes associated with the top 150 SNPs. The results are shown in Table 2. We found a common biological process for both the datasets implicated in *nervous system development* [4]. These findings verifies the ability of our coupled framework to find clinically relevant biomarkers from both the imaging and genetic data.

Table 2. The table shows the enriched biological processes along with their level of significance obtained via GO enrichment analysis. The processes are arranged by the most specific subclass first, with its parent terms indented directly below it.

Dataset	Biological processes	FDR
Nback	Central nervous system development	0.03
	→ Nervous system development	0.0002
	→ System development	0.001
	Generation of neurons	0.03
	→ Neurogenesis	0.02
	→ Cell differentiation	0.003
SDMT	Forebrain neuron differentiation	0.04
	→ Nervous system development	0.002
	→ Generation of neurons	0.004
	→ Central nervous system neuron differentiation	0.04
	Central nervous system neuron development	0.02
	Regulation of neurogenesis	0.03

4   Conclusion

We have introduced an elegant joint matrix decomposition framework that identifies imaging and genetic biomarkers guided by the clinical diagnosis. Unlike other conventional analysis this framework can robustly and efficiently integrate diverse datatypes while maintaining good prediction accuracy. Moreover, the biomarkers may help us understand the biology underlying cognitive deficits in patients with schizophrenia in relation to genetic variants. This model can easily be adapted to other imaging and genetic modalities. In this work we only explored a linear relationship between imaging, genetics and diagnosis, however in future work we will also explore the non linear relationships across them.

Acknowledgements. This work was supported by NSF CRCNS 1822575, and the National Institute of Mental Health extramural research program.

References

1. Batmanghelich, N.K., et al.: Probabilistic modeling of imaging, genetics and diagnosis. IEEE Trans. Med. Imaging **35**(7), 1765–1779 (2016)
2. Callicott, J.H., et al.: Abnormal fMRI response of the dorsolateral prefrontal cortex in cognitively intact siblings of patients with schizophrenia. Am. J. Psychiatry **160**(4), 709–719 (2003)
3. Chen, Q., et al.: Schizophrenia polygenic risk score predicts mnemonic hippocampal activity. Brain **141**(4), 1218–1228 (2018)
4. Dean, B.: Is schizophrenia the price of human central nervous system complexity? Aust. New Zealand J. Psychiatry **43**(1), 13–24 (2009)

5. Du, L., et al.: Pattern discovery in brain imaging genetics via SCCA modeling with a generic non-convex penalty. Sci. Rep. **7**(1), 14052 (2017)
6. Fan, L., et al.: The human brainnetome atlas: a new brain atlas based on connectional architecture. Cereb. Cortex **26**(8), 3508–3526 (2016)
7. Rasetti, R., et al.: Altered hippocampal-parahippocampal function during stimulus encoding. JAMA Psychiatry **71**(3), 236 (2014)
8. Wang, H., et al.: Identifying quantitative trait loci via group-sparse multitask regression and feature selection: an imaging genetics study of the ADNI cohort. Bioinformatics **28**(2), 229–237 (2012)

Global and Local Interpretability for Cardiac MRI Classification

James R. Clough$^{(\boxtimes)}$, Ilkay Oksuz, Esther Puyol-Antón, Bram Ruijsink,
Andrew P. King, and Julia A. Schnabel

School of Biomedical Engineering and Imaging Sciences,
King's College London, London, UK
james.clough@kcl.ac.uk

Abstract. Deep learning methods for classifying medical images have demonstrated impressive accuracy in a wide range of tasks but often these models are hard to interpret, limiting their applicability in clinical practice. In this work we introduce a convolutional neural network model for identifying disease in temporal sequences of cardiac MR segmentations which is interpretable in terms of clinically familiar measurements. The model is based around a variational autoencoder, reducing the input into a low-dimensional latent space in which classification occurs. We then use the recently developed 'concept activation vector' technique to associate concepts which are diagnostically meaningful (eg. clinical biomarkers such as 'low left-ventricular ejection fraction') to certain vectors in the latent space. These concepts are then qualitatively inspected by observing the change in the image domain resulting from interpolations in the latent space in the direction of these vectors. As a result, when the model classifies images it is also capable of providing naturally interpretable concepts relevant to that classification and demonstrating the meaning of those concepts in the image domain. Our approach is demonstrated on the UK Biobank cardiac MRI dataset where we detect the presence of coronary artery disease.

Keywords: Interpretable ML · Cardiac MRI · Coronary artery disease

This work was supported by an EPSRC programme Grant (EP/P001009/1) and the Wellcome EPSRC Centre for Medical Engineering at the School of Biomedical Engineering and Imaging Sciences, King's College London (WT 203148/Z/16/Z). This research has been conducted using the UK Biobank Resource under Application Numbers 40119 and 17806. The GPU used in this research was generously donated by the NVIDIA Corporation.

Electronic supplementary material The online version of this chapter (https://doi.org/10.1007/978-3-030-32251-9_72) contains supplementary material, which is available to authorized users.

1   Introduction

Heart disease is the leading cause of death globally. Cardiac magnetic resonance (CMR) is the gold-standard imaging tool for assessment and diagnosis of many serious forms of heart disease [11]. As the performance of machine learning (ML) tools for image classification has improved in recent years [3], the interest in the application of ML to the analysis of CMR images and volumes has grown. Such systems have the potential to provide significant benefits to patients such as improved diagnostic quality and decreased time and cost of image analysis. However, ML methods successfully demonstrated in a research setting can face barriers to clinical application due to concerns about reliability and a lack of interpretability. In particular, deep convolutional neural networks (CNN) have proven powerful tools for image analysis but their ability to yield adequate explanations of their decisions to clinicians is still lacking. Interpretable ML models are important in healthcare for the trust of patients and clinicians, to guard against model unreliability in the face of distributional shift [10] (e.g. due to a change in scanner design, imaging protocol and pre-processing, or patient demographics) and for legal reasons such as a patient's 'right to explanation' [5].

In this work we develop a classification framework using variational autoencoders (VAE) [7] which allows for both local and global interpretability of a classification decision. By *local interpretability* we mean the ability to ask 'which features of this particular image led to it being classified in this particular way?'. By *global interpretability* we mean the ability to ask 'which common features were generally associated with images assigned to this particular class?'. Our method first encodes 2D image segmentations into a low-dimensional latent space with a VAE and then classifies using the latent vectors. Using concept activation vectors [6] in the space of activations in the intermediate layers of the classification network provides global interpretability to the model. The VAE contains a decoder which is trained to reconstruct images from the latent vectors and so local interpretability is provided by interpolating in the latent space and visualising the changes in the corresponding decoded images. This approach is demonstrated using cardiac segmentations, obtained from CMR studies in the UK Biobank, and classifying for the presence of coronary artery disease. Our primary contribution in this work is the integration of local and global interpretability methods in the context of a realistic clinical application. Additionally, our proposed classification method utilises temporal information over the full cardiac cycle. This is important as dynamic features, such as regional and global myocardial wall motion, are sensitive markers of disease that are missed when only taking into account images at end-diastolic and/or end-systolic positions.

2   Related Work

The importance of providing interpretability to image classification models is reflected in the growing body of literature around the subject. Some classification models such as simple decision trees or linear models are considered to be inherently interpretable in the sense that a human observer can understand each step in the process by which a model makes a decision. Unfortunately many ML models which have the most impressive classification performance and so are most desirable to use in clinical practice do not have this property.

When a model is too complex for its entire decision process to be understood, interpretability is still possible by supplementing the output decision with information which can help to explain it. Saliency maps [15] are a commonly used approach for interpreting image classification in which the gradient of the loss with respect to the input image is visualised. Although saliency maps can be useful for highlighting relevant regions of images, the level of interpretability that they can provide is often of limited use. Firstly, as explained in [1], *'some widely deployed saliency methods are independent of both the data the model was trained on, and the model parameters'*, which is clearly undesirable. Secondly, as noted in [12], saliency methods only explain 'where the network is looking'. If an image of a dog is misclassified as a cat, and a saliency map highlights the region of the image containing the dog, we still do not know much about why this image was misclassified. Thirdly, the explanation is only relevant for the particular image in question and so an observer must manually assess many images and their saliency maps to draw more general conclusions [6].

Another family of approaches attempts to understand the representations learned by intermediate layers in a deep CNN by visualising the images which strongly activate each neuron [9]. While these methods are helpful for achieving a better understanding of how CNNs work, the images produced do not typically appear realistic and so are often hard to interpret themselves, appearing to capture textures more strongly than wider-scale structure.

Autoencoders are neural networks trained to find efficient representations of a dataset. They do this with an encoder network, which maps images to low-dimensional latent vectors, and a decoder network which approximates the original image from the latent vector. The representations learned by such models can be used to de-noise images or impose prior knowledge about allowed structures [8]. In [4] a classification task (detecting hypertrophic cardiomyopathy from CMR volume segmentations) was performed in the latent space of a variational autoencoder. This allowed the classifier to be understood because one can take the latent vector corresponding to a patient's CMR data, and interpolate it in the direction of the gradient of the classifier's output, and observe the changes to the decoded image. Our method extends this autoencoder approach to use the whole cardiac cycle rather than just two frames, providing local interpretability, and integrates it with concept activation vectors [6], a method for global interpretability.

3   Methods

VAE/Classification Network: Our classification model is described by the diagram in Fig. 1. The model consists firstly of an encoder which finds a latent representation (of dimensionality 128) for each input. In our case, these inputs

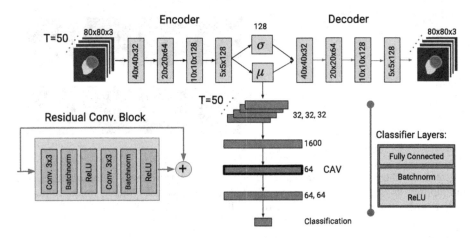

Fig. 1. Diagram showing the architecture of the joint VAE/classification model. The VAE consists of a series of residual convolutional blocks, with the image resolution and number of feature maps denoted in each block. The classification network consists of a series of fully connected layers (number of hidden units in each denoted to the side) which first processes the latent vectors individually, then concatenates them and processes them together.

are 80×80 segmentations of 3 central slices in the stack of short-axis CMR images of the heart, where each slice is treated as a channel in the image. A decoder network is trained to reconstruct the original data from the latent representations. The data for each subject consists of $T = 50$ segmentations per slice, representing one full cardiac cycle. These segmentations are mapped to T latent vectors by the encoder and the classification network then predicts the presence of disease from these T latent vectors using fully connected layers. The vectors are processed individually and are then concatenated into one vector which represents the state of the whole image sequence. More fully connected layers then process this vector to produce the classification.

We denote an input segmentation sequence as $\mathbf{X} = [\mathbf{x}_1, \mathbf{x}_2, ...\mathbf{x}_T]$, and its corresponding latent mean and standard deviation vectors as $\mathbf{M} = [\mu_1, \mu_2, ...\mu_T]$ and $\mathbf{\Sigma} = [\sigma_1, \sigma_2, ...\sigma_T]$ where $(\mu_t, \sigma_t) = \text{Encoder}(\mathbf{x}_t)$. The decoded images are denoted as $\tilde{\mathbf{X}} = [\tilde{\mathbf{x}}_1, \tilde{\mathbf{x}}_2, ...\tilde{\mathbf{x}}_T]$. During training the decoder is provided samples $\tilde{\mathbf{x}}_t = \text{Decoder}(\mu_t + \sigma_t \odot \nu)$ where $\nu \sim \mathcal{N}(0, I)$ is a noise vector and $\odot$ denotes elementwise multiplication. During inference, the only the mean is used and so $\tilde{\mathbf{x}}_t = \text{Decoder}(\mu_t)$. The ground truth label is denoted by y and the predicted label by $\tilde{y} = \text{Classifier}(\mathbf{M})$. The joint loss function for the VAE and classifier can then be written as follows:

$$\mathcal{L}_{\text{total}} = \frac{1}{T} \sum_{t=1}^{t=T} [\mathcal{L}_{\text{recon}}(\mathbf{x}_t, \tilde{\mathbf{x}}_t) + \beta \mathcal{L}_{\text{KL}}(\mu_t, \sigma_t)] + \gamma \mathcal{L}_{\text{class}}(y, \tilde{y}) \tag{1}$$

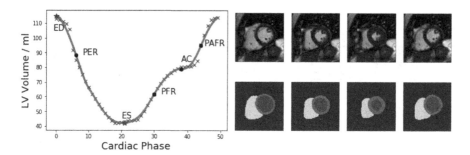

Fig. 2. Left: Curve of LV volume over time, with raw data (crosses), smoothed (curve) and landmarks of the cardiac cycle annotated. Right: Typical cropped image sequence with 4 cardiac phases shown, and corresponding segmentations.

for constants β and γ which weight the components of the loss function. $\mathcal{L}_{\text{recon}}$ was chosen to be the cross-entropy between the input segmentations and the output predictions, and $\mathcal{L}_{\text{class}}$ the binary cross entropy loss for the classification task. $\mathcal{L}_{\text{KL}}$ is the usual Kullback-Leibler divergence between the latent variables and a unit Gaussian, which has the effect of penalising latent vectors far from the origin and so by pulling each input's latent vector towards the origin ensures a smoothness to the latent space. We train the model in two stages, first using only the VAE loss, i.e. $\gamma = 0$, and secondly training both the VAE and classifier together using $\gamma = 1$. We set $\beta = 0.2$ throughout , chosen by manual tuning. The data were augmented during training by randomly applying pixel-wise shifts of up to 5 pixels in the up-down, and left-right directions.

Concept Activation Vectors: CAV [6] aim to provide explanations for a classification network's decision in terms of concepts understandable to a human. The network is trained as usual, and the CAV analysis occurs at test time. Data which do, and do not, contain certain human-understandable concepts are passed through the classifier, and the activations $\mathbf{z}$ at a given intermediate hidden layer are recorded. For our experiments this layer is the fully connected layer with 64 units, labelled 'CAV' in Fig. 1, and the concepts are clinically relevant biomarkers measured from the segmentation. A separate linear classifier is then trained to distinguish between the activations $\mathbf{z}$ produced by these two sets of inputs. The CAV for a concept c is the normal vector, $\mathbf{v}_c$, to this linear classifier. This allows an observer to measure the sensitivity of the classifier to a concept understandable to humans by evaluating the dot product between $\mathbf{v}_c$ and the gradient, at the layer of the classifier in question, of the logit value of that class, $\nabla_{\mathbf{z}}\tilde{y}$. Here we apply this idea to interpret cardiac disease classification in terms of commonly used clinical biomarkers.

4   Materials and Experiments

We demonstrated our approach for interpretable classification of CMR using data from the UK Biobank [11]. The labels for the classification task were derived from

Table 1. The sensitivity of the classifier to clinical biomarkers of poor cardiac health. A biomarker with no relevance would have $\nabla_z \tilde{y} \cdot \mathbf{v}_c = 0$ on average.

CAV	Description	$\nabla \tilde{y} \cdot \mathbf{v}_c > 0$	$\langle \nabla \tilde{y} \cdot \mathbf{v}_c \rangle$
Low EF	Ejection fraction	78.2%	0.0417
Low PER	Peak ejection rate	88.8%	0.0770
Low PFR	Peak filling rate	99.6%	0.1560
Low APFR	Atrial peak filling rate	58.2%	0.0048
High LVT	Variance of LV wall thickening	63.4%	0.0156

the subject's listed medical conditions according to the ICD10 disease classification. Those listed as having any condition under I21, I22 or I25, corresponding to myocardial infarction and coronary artery disease (CAD) were labelled as positive. Subjects who were labelled as negative for CAD but with other serious heart conditions (I00-I52 including hypertensive heart disease, valve disorders, congestive heart failure etc.) or who self-reported having previously had a heart attack were excluded from analysis as they could also have CAD, or very similar symptoms despite not being labelled as such. Using the segmentation method of [2] the left ventricular (LV) myocardium, blood pool, and right ventricle (RV) were each segmented as shown in the examples in Fig. 2. From these segmentations we calculated several established clinical biomarkers of ventricular function which were then used as possible explanatory 'concepts' in the CAV framework. These metrics were calculated from the curve representing blood pool volume over time which was smoothed using a Savitzky-Golay filter [14], as shown in Fig. 2, and described in more detail in [13]. The ejection fraction (EF) is defined as the fractional drop in blood pool volume from end-diastole (ED) to end-systole (ES). The peak ejection rate (PER), peak filling rate (PFR) and peak atrial filling rate (PAFR) were determined by the magnitude of the maximal gradients of the blood pool volume over time in the relevant parts of the cardiac cycle, with the atrial contribution (AC) determined by the inflection point in this curve. LV wall thickening was defined as the variance of LV myocardial thickening during contraction, observed between six predefined segments per image slice. This measure indicates the presence of localised changes in myocardial contraction, and is indicative of poor cardiac health in the hypokinetic region. A rigorous quality control process was used to remove low quality segmentations, which were typically associated with artefacts in the original images. Subjects with short-axis image stacks that did not cover the full LV, or intersect the apex and/or mitral valve plane were discarded. Physiologically unrealistic segmentations were detected from the LV volume curve, determined by their having a difference of >10% in ventricular volume between the first and last segmentation in the cycle.

The final dataset had a total of 10,816 subjects, of which 778 were labelled with CAD. These data were split into a training set of 5,316 subjects (708 positive, 4,608 negative), test set (70 positive, 430 negative) and a held out set of 5,000 CAD-negative subjects used for the CAV analysis. The final trained

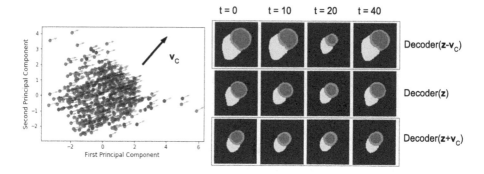

Fig. 3. Left: PCA of the latent space vectors for the 500 test cases, where blue are positive for CAD. Each point's arrow shows the gradient of the classification logit. For the concept 'low peak ejection rate' the CAV $\mathbf{v}_c$ is shown. Right: For a real test case the activations $\mathbf{z}_h$ are calculated. By adding $\pm\mathbf{v}_c$ and decoding the latent vectors the effect of this concept is visible in the image domain, showing noticeable changes in LV contraction. Four of the 50 frames in each sequence are shown here.

binary classifier had an AUC of 0.78, and the reconstructed segmentations had an average Dice Score of 0.93 with reference to the input segmentations, suggesting that the encoder and decoder networks were accurately mapping from segmentations to latent vectors and back. The sets of images describing each human-interpretable concept were determined as follows. In the held-out set of 5000 subjects the 1000 cases with the highest and the lowest recorded quantities of the given concept were used as the positively-labelled and negatively-labelled cases for each concept. To test the CAV concepts the dot product between the gradient of the classification decision with respect to the activations $\nabla_{\mathbf{z}}\tilde{y}$, and the concept activation vector $\mathbf{v}_c$ was measured for each case in the test set. Table 1 shows the proportion of cases in which $\nabla_{\mathbf{z}}\tilde{y} \cdot \mathbf{v}_c > 0$, (meaning the concept had a positive impact on classification for the disease), and its mean value. Figure 3 shows an example of a latent-space interpolation in the direction of the 'low peak ejection rate' concept. A subset of the frames are shown here but the full cardiac cycle is available in the supplementary material.

5   Discussion and Conclusions

Our model not only performs classification, but also allows interpretation of features important during classification. Utilising CAV to interrogate the importance of well established biomarkers we found that biomarkers relating to ventricular ejection and filling rates had a large contribution suggesting that the classifier network identifies these clinically relevant features as significant. Latent space interpolations in the direction of the concept activation vectors, such as that in Fig. 3 illustrate the ability of our method to describe its learned features, providing evidence that these vectors in the latent space correspond to typical clinical interpretations of these biomarkers.

Interpretable models do not just offer clinicians a well-calibrated estimate of the likelihood of disease. Interpretability using known biomarkers allows the model's prediction to be placed in the context of current medical knowledge and clinical decision-making guidelines, which is a key part of translation into clinical practice. It also has the potential to improve care by suggesting explanatory factors in an image that may have been missed or disregarded by a human.

In future work we aim to investigate which kinds of model interpretability are perceived as most informative and trustworthy by clinicians, and study the accuracy/interpretability trade-off. We experimented with using recurrent units such as an LSTM in the classification network to process the time series of latent vectors, but found that simply concatenating them gave a superior classification performance. Nonetheless more sophisticated architectures which more directly make use of the temporal correlations between frames should be investigated. We also trained our model to reconstruct and predict from raw CMR images rather than segmentations. While classification performance was comparable (AUC of 0.81) the quality of reconstructed images and latent space interpolations was not high enough (due to image blurring) to be considered usefully interpretable. We hope to extend our approach to the image domain using adversarial training to ensure high-quality image reconstructions which can then be used to visualise both structural and textural features relevant to the classification.

References

1. Adebayo, J., Gilmer, J., Muelly, M., Goodfellow, I., Hardt, M., Kim, B.: Sanity checks for saliency maps. In: Advances in Neural Information Processing Systems, pp. 9525–9536 (2018)
2. Bai, W., et al.: Automated cardiovascular magnetic resonance image analysis with fully convolutional networks. J. Cardiovasc. Magn. Reson. **20**(1), 65 (2018)
3. Bernard, O., et al.: Deep learning techniques for automatic MRI cardiac multi-structures segmentation and diagnosis: is the problem solved? IEEE Trans. Med. Imaging **37**(11), 2514–2525 (2018)
4. Biffi, C., et al.: Learning interpretable anatomical features through deep generative models: application to cardiac remodeling. In: Frangi, A.F., Schnabel, J.A., Davatzikos, C., Alberola-López, C., Fichtinger, G. (eds.) MICCAI 2018. LNCS, vol. 11071, pp. 464–471. Springer, Cham (2018). https://doi.org/10.1007/978-3-030-00934-2_52
5. Goodman, B., Flaxman, S.: EU regulations on algorithmic decision-making and a "right to explanation". In: ICML Workshop on Human Interpretability in Machine Learning (WHI 2016), New York, NY (2016)
6. Kim, B., et al.: Interpretability beyond feature attribution: quantitative testing with concept activation vectors (TCAV). arXiv:1711.11279 (2017)
7. Kingma, D., Welling, M.: Auto-Encoding Variational Bayes. arXiv preprint arXiv:1312.6114 (2013)
8. Oktay, O., et al.: Anatomically constrained neural networks (ACNNs): application to cardiac image enhancement and segmentation. IEEE Trans. Med. Imaging **37**(2), 384–395 (2018)
9. Olah, C., et al.: The building blocks of interpretability. Distill (2018). https://distill.pub/2018/building-blocks

10. Patel, V., Gopalan, R., Li, R., Chellappa, R.: Visual domain adaptation: a survey of recent advances. IEEE Signal Process. Mag. **32**(3), 53–69 (2015)
11. Petersen, S.E., et al.: UK Biobank's cardiovascular magnetic resonanceprotocol. J. Cardiovasc. Magn. Reson. **18**(1), 8 (2015)
12. Rudin, C.: Please stop explaining black box models for high stakes decisions. arXiv:1811.10154 (2018)
13. Ruijsink, B., et al.: Fully automated, quality-controlled cardiac analysis from CMR: validation and large-scale application to characterize cardiac function. JACC: Cardiovasc. Imaging (2019). https://doi.org/10.1016/j.jcmg.2019.05.030
14. Savitzky, A., Golay, M.J.: Smoothing and differentiation of data by simplified least squares procedures. Anal. Chem. **36**(8), 1627–1639 (1964)
15. Simonyan, K., Vedaldi, A., Zisserman, A.: Deep inside convolutional networks: visualising image classification models and saliency maps. arXiv:1312.6034 (2013)

Let's Agree to Disagree: Learning Highly Debatable Multirater Labelling

Carole H. Sudre[1,2,3(✉)], Beatriz Gomez Anson[4], Silvia Ingala[5], Chris D. Lane[2],
Daniel Jimenez[2], Lukas Haider[6], Thomas Varsavsky[1,3], Ryutaro Tanno[3],
Lorna Smith[7], Sébastien Ourselin[1], Rolf H. Jäger[8], and M. Jorge Cardoso[1,2,3]

[1] School of Biomedical Engineering and Imaging Sciences, KCL, London, UK
carole.sudre@kcl.ac.uk
[2] Dementia Research Centre, UCL Institute of Neurology, London, UK
[3] Department of Medical Physics and Biomedical Engineering, UCL, London, UK
[4] Santa Creu i Sant Pau Hospital, Universitat Autònoma de Barcelona,
Barcelona, Spain
[5] Vrije University Medical Centre Amsterdam, Amsterdam, The Netherlands
[6] Queen Square Multiple Sclerosis Centre, UCL Institute of Neurology, London, UK
[7] Cardiometabolic Phenotyping Group, Institute of Cardiovascular Science,
UCL, London, UK
[8] Brain Repair and Rehabilitation Group, Institute of Neurology, UCL, London, UK

Abstract. Classification and differentiation of small pathological objects may greatly vary among human raters due to differences in training, expertise and their consistency over time. In a radiological setting, objects commonly have high within-class appearance variability whilst sharing certain characteristics across different classes, making their distinction even more difficult. As an example, markers of cerebral small vessel disease, such as enlarged perivascular spaces (EPVS) and lacunes, can be very varied in their appearance while exhibiting high inter-class similarity, making this task highly challenging for human raters. In this work, we investigate joint models of individual rater behaviour and multirater consensus in a deep learning setting, and apply it to a brain lesion object-detection task. Results show that jointly modelling both individual and consensus estimates leads to significant improvements in performance when compared to directly predicting consensus labels, while also allowing the characterization of human-rater consistency.

Keywords: Deep learning · Noisy labels · Classification

1 Introduction

Detection and differentiation between types of pathological objects is a core problem of medical image analysis, generally requiring costly expert labelling. Disagreement between raters can be a result of differences in radiological training schools, rater competence, and sample appearance, among others. This problem is often exacerbated by changes in rater performance caused by retraining or observational bias.

© Springer Nature Switzerland AG 2019
D. Shen et al. (Eds.): MICCAI 2019, LNCS 11767, pp. 665–673, 2019.
https://doi.org/10.1007/978-3-030-32251-9_73

Due to the variability in shape and intensity signatures observed across the full spectrum of lesions, even the most trained raters can present a high inter-rater variability. In such cases, finding a majority voting consensus classification is the most common strategy.

When classifying objects into multiple classes, it is often more complex to separate all object types directly, than it is to first detect all pathological objects followed by their classification, as some class decision boundaries are easier than others. This sequential detection/classification problem is, for instance, present in the context of age-related vascular changes in which macroscopic alterations can be observed on structural MR images. Among these observed changes, small elements such as enlarged perivascular spaces (EPVS) and lacunes are observed on similar image sequences [9]. EPVS, often associated with concomitant neuropathology and deleterious clinical outcome [5], appear as fluid filled structures with a linear shape. However, because of their limited size ($<10\,\mathrm{mm}^3$) and highly variable appearance, EPVS instances are often confused with other concomitant lesions, such as lacunes. Because of this intrinsic uncertainty, the labelling of these small vascular lesions can be seen as a four-class problem, with classes 'EPVS', 'Lacune', 'Undetermined', and 'Nothing'. This classification problem suffers from two concomitant issues: (a) class imbalance with a 100:1 ratio between EPVS and lacunes, and (b) noisy labelling as a result of rater disagreement. Consensus labels are also problematic in this setting, as rater behaviour is non-random and samples are not truly independent.

In this work, we build on a previously described 3-dimensional multirater Regional Convolutional Neural Network (RCNN) model, used here as a lacune and EPVS object detection system. However, rather than only learning the consensus value or a single rater, we propose to jointly learn the consensus majority voting, the associated probability for each class, and each individual rater decision, so as to appropriately model highly debatable label predictions.

2   Related Work and Problem Specificities

Many of the recent publications on classification with noisy labels assume independence between samples and noise, and a constant mislabelling probability [4], which does not hold in the case of difficulty induced variability and rater shift. Strategies for classification in the presence of noise include sample reweighting (importance reweighting) or curriculum-based sample selection [1,3]. Other approaches, normally classed as label/classifier fusion, disentangle rater and label uncertainty either by iteratively favouring raters that agree with the consensus [10], or by reducing sample correlation to construct a balanced classifier [2]. Lastly, the relationships between rater behaviour can also be learned through their confusion matrices [7]. Notably, most of these works focus on the problem of classification, where balanced sampling strategies can be employed, something that is not possible in a joint detection/classification model. In this work, we argue that combining majority voting predictions while learning individual rater behaviour allows for a better model of rater consistency and sample uncertainty.

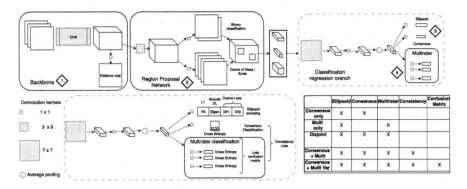

Fig. 1. Detection and multirater classification architecture framework. In this work focus is put on the classification branch (red dashed) further detailed on the second row along with the description of the different training regimes. (Color figure online)

3   Methods

3.1   Network Architecture

The multirater 3D RCNN framework presented in [6] is composed of four stages: (1) a backbone network learning the features using as target a distance map to the objects of interest; (2) a region proposal network (RPN) regressing the location of candidate centres of mass of target objects together with their spatial scale; (3) patches from the RPN representation are fed into a two layer network in order to regress the average object classification and object shape; (4) a multi-branch fully connected layer is used to model the behaviour of each rater (see Fig. 1).

Shape Encoding. Instead of modelling each object by its encompassing cuboid [6], the shape of each candidate object is encoded as a four-parameter simplified encompassing ellipsoid, namely using the largest eigenvalue, the two first components of the associated eigenvector and the value of fractional anisotropy of the associated tensor.

3.2   Multi-rater Classification

The classification of the candidate objects is defined as a four-class problem, i.e. EPVS, Lacune, Undetermined, Nothing. From a human-rater point of view, the classification can be seen in two different ways: a multi-rater consensus, here modeled as the probability of a class to be chosen among the six raters computed as the average rating, and a rater-specific categorical label.

Consensus Average Classification. When modelling the consensus/average rater, the training can be performed using either a hard or a probabilistic classification, or a combination of both. Note, here, the hard classification corresponds simply to the majority voting categorical consensus, while the continuous probability encodes the uncertainty over the final classification. As a consequence, a cross-entropy loss is used to learn the consensus, while a root mean square error loss is used over the resulting class probabilities.

Independent Rater Modelling. In the last stage of classification, a cross-entropy loss is used to learn each rater label independently. Inter-rater behaviour can be enforced through a variability loss (L_{var}) penalizing the difference between the effective and predicted probabilistic confusion matrices. Noting C (resp. $\widehat{C}$) the observed (resp. predicted) confusion matrix, $L_{var} = \sum_{(i,j)} |C_{i,j} - \widehat{C_{i,j}}|$

Ideally, we would also like to have consistency between the predicted group consensus and the consensus of individual prediction. In order to achieve this, the following consistency loss L_{cons} is introduced:

$$L_{cons} = \sqrt{\sum_{k=1}^{K} \widehat{p_k} - \frac{1}{R}\sum_{r=1}^{R} \widehat{p_{kr}}}$$

with $\widehat{p_k}$ denoting the predicted consensus probability, and $\widehat{p_{kr}}$ denoting the predicted probability given by rater r for class k.

Compensating for Inter-rater Variability and Enhancing Individual Rater Characteristics. The EPVS labelling problem is highly variable in terms of rater agreement; sometimes all raters agree with each other, while other times raters converge to completely different decisions. As a consequence, when predicting the group consensus, we have enforced consensus learning from samples of high agreement. To this effect, sample importances were downweighted according to their observed variability, here expressed as $var = 1 - \sum_{k=1}^{K} p_k^2$, where p_k is the observed classification probability for class k. The sample is then weighted by $\exp(-var)$. Conversely, when modelling individual raters, and in order to learn rater-specific behaviours, we promote samples for which the individual rater disagrees with the consensus. This is achieved by weighting each rater-sample combination by the inverse of its contribution to the consensus $(1/p_{kr})$, where p_{kr} is the observed probability for the sample to be classified as k if rater r labels it as k.

4   Data and Experiments

4.1   Data

16 subjects that were part of a large tri-ethnic cohort investigating the relationship between cardiovascular risk factors and brain health [8] were chosen due to their elevated vascular burden. 4147 EPVS and lacunes were manually segmented using jointly $1\,\mathrm{mm}^3$ structural MR sequences (T1, T2, FLAIR) using ITKSnap[1]. Individual segmented lesions, defined using connected components,

---

[1] http://www.itksnap.org/pmwiki/pmwiki.php?n=Main.HomePage.

were then classified by six trained raters using an in house dedicated viewer. Only objects bigger than 5 voxels were used in this study, resulting in a database of 2202 elements. 14 subjects were used for training and two subjects for testing. The test set contained 184 objects that were all classified at least by one rater as EPVS. Inter-rater accuracy ranged from 0.47 to 0.92 with a mean of 0.72.

4.2   Training Modes

In order to investigate the model's ability to handle label noise, different training regimes were adopted (see Fig. 1): (1) Training only the shape + consensus classification (Consensus only); (2) Staged training of the shape encoding followed by the independent rater multihead (Multi Only); (3) Staged training of shape and classification, followed by training the independent rater multihead (Disjoint); (4) Staged training of 'shape and consensus only', followed by 'multihead only' finishing by 'shape, consensus and multihead' with consistency loss (Consensus + Multi); (5) Training as in 4, with an extra loss over the confusion matrix L_{var}. All models were trained for 10000 iterations with a learning rate of 10^{-4} and using the Adam optimiser.

5   Experiments and Results

5.1   Consensus Probability

As a first experiment, we investigate the ability of each training mode to appropriately predict the distribution of EPVS classification probabilities. Figure 2 presents the joint histograms of the target and predicted distributions. The resulting Kullback-Leibler Divergence (KLD) over the distributions are displayed below along with the mean absolute error in prediction. Results show that all methods explicitly learning the average consensus are able to reproduce it well. The ability of the different models to reproduce individual rater behaviour was evaluated by comparing predicted inter-rater agreement with observed inter-rater agreement. Figure 3 presents the pairwise agreement results between observations and between predictions, and measures of correlation and absolute difference between agreement matrices. One can note that, as expected, no inter-rater behaviour is learnt when adopting the 'Consensus only' framework. Furthermore, we observe that the inter-rater agreement learnt with both the 'Multi only' and the 'Disjoint' model is exacerbated compared to the truth. This rater behaviour exacerbation fades away when enforcing consistency between multi-rater consensus predictions and the consensus of individual rater predictions (i.e. 'Consensus + Multi' model).

5.2   Consistency Between Consensus and Multirater Average

This experiment aims to test the efficacy of the loss function introduced in Sect. 3.2 with the aim of promoting the agreement between the multi-rater consensus labelling and the consensus of individual predictions. Figure 4 left presents

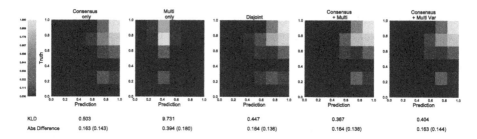

KLD	0.503	9.731	0.447	0.387	0.404
Abs Difference	0.163 (0.143)	0.394 (0.180)	0.164 (0.136)	0.164 (0.138)	0.163 (0.144)

Fig. 2. Comparison of EPVS probability distributions quantitatively evaluated in terms of KLD and absolute error (mean sd).

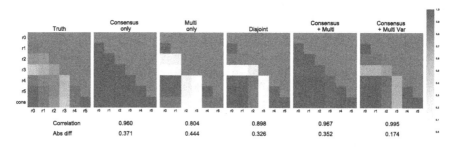

Correlation	0.960	0.804	0.898	0.967	0.995
Abs diff	0.371	0.444	0.326	0.352	0.174

Fig. 3. Pairwise agreement scores between observed rater labels compared to the agreement scores between categorized individual rater predictions for each training mode. The left most element is the target inter-rater behaviour. Pearson correlation coefficient and mean absolute difference against the target inter-rater behaviour are presented below.

the boxplots of the difference between the average of the predicted individual raters and the consensus prediction. Numerical results of median and interquartile range are presented below the graph. Training regimes that promote consistency between the consensus prediction and the average of independent predictions both reach, as expected, a very high level of consistency. Conversely, simpler models only optimising for independent rater predictions do not achieve a good consensus estimation.

5.3   Variability, Disagreements and Individual Rater Quality

In this experiment, we would like to assess if the probabilistic predictions of each individual rater provide a good proxy for sample uncertainty (defined as the variability of individual ratings). To this end, we estimate the Spearman correlation coefficient between each individual prediction and the measured precision defined as $1/var$, displayed on Fig. 4 (right). As already noted from Fig. 3, no rater-specific information can be modeled using only the consensus. Individualized rater predictions were found to be strongly associated with overall variability, primarily when consistency losses were applied.

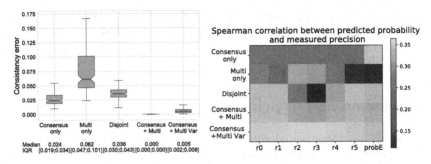

Fig. 4. Left: Boxplot of the consistency error between predicted consensus probability and average of individual raters predictions. Right: Spearman coefficient between predicted probability of classifying the element as an EPVS and measured precision ($1/var$) over multiple models. ProbE refers to the predicted probability of an EPVS for the consensus of raters.

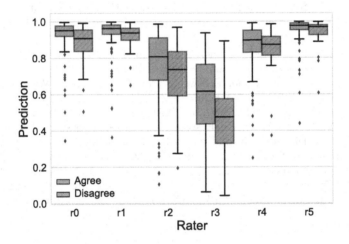

Fig. 5. Boxplot of the predicted probabilities for the agreeing and disagreeing cases for each rater with the best training regime (Consensus + Multi Var).

5.4 Labelling Introspection

We used the best overall model ('Consensus + Multi Var') to study the distribution of probabilistic predictions for objects whose rater classification was in agreement with the consensus versus objects where there was rater disagreement, plotted in Fig. 5. High prediction probabilities for individual raters were found to be a good surrogate marker rater agreement and rater consistency over training samples. Results suggest that rater 3, and to a lesser degree rater 2, displayed inconsistent labelling behaviour. Interestingly, when asked about their rating practice, both raters 2 and 3 indicated having undergone clinical retraining, possibly explaining the observed shift in their labelling. Retraining the model without these two raters resulted in an improvement in the consensus prediction, with a KLD reduced to 0.202 and a mean absolute error over the predicted probability of 0.15. This experiment suggests that one can use the proposed framework to identify not only inter-rater disagreement but also intra-rater inconsistency, and potentially correct for it.

6   Discussion and Conclusion

In this work, we investigated different training regimes in presence of noisy labelling with the aim of predicting both rater consensus and individualized predictions. We found that promoting agreement between predicted multi-rater consensus and the consensus of individualized predictions can provide good model accuracy together with the ability to introspect rater behaviour, thus not only allowing the identification of noisy labels/subjects but also assessing rater skills so as to prevent bias in large scale studies and enforce appropriate radiological training. Future work will explore the use of this information in an active learning setting and develop the accuracy of the multi-rater model estimates.

Acknowledgments. We are extremely grateful to all the participants of the SABRE study, and past and present members of the SABRE team. This work was supported by an Alzheimer's Society Junior Fellowship (AS-JF-17-011), the Wellcome/EPSRC Centre for Medical Engineering [WT 203148/Z/16/Z], IMI2 grant AMYPAD [115952], the MSCA-ITN-Demo [721820], and the Wellcome Flagship Programme in High-Dimensional Neurology. The SABRE study was funded at baseline by the Medical Research Council, Diabetes UK, and the British Heart Foundation. At follow-up, the study was funded by the Wellcome Trust (067100, 37055891 and 086676/7/08/Z), the British Heart Foundation (PG/06/145, PG/08/103/26133, PG/12/29/29497 and CS/13/1/30327) and Diabetes UK (13/0004774). We gratefully acknowledge NVIDIA corporation for the donation of a GPU Tesla K40 that was used in the preparation of this work.

References

1. Bouguelia, M.R., Nowaczyk, S., Santosh, K.C., Verikas, A.: Agreeing to disagree: active learning with noisy labels without crowdsourcing. Int. J. Mach. Learn. Cybern. **9**(8), 1307–1319 (2018)
2. Wang, H., Suh, J.W., Das, S.R., Pluta, J.B., Craige, C., Yushkevich, P.A.: Multi-atlas segmentation with joint label fusion. IEEE TPAMI **35**(3), 611–623 (2013). https://doi.org/10.1109/TPAMI.2012.143
3. Jiang, L., Zhou, Z., Leung, T., Li, L.J., Fei-Fei, L.: MentorNet: Learning Data-Driven Curriculum for Very Deep Neural Networks on Corrupted Labels, December 2017. http://arxiv.org/abs/1712.05055
4. Li, Y., Yang, J., Song, Y., Cao, L., Luo, J., Li, L.J.: Learning From Noisy Labels With Distillation (2017)
5. Ramirez, J., Berezuk, C., McNeely, A.A., Gao, F., McLaurin, J., Black, S.E.: Imaging the perivascular space as a potential biomarker of neurovascular and neurodegenerative diseases. Cell. Mol. Neurobiol. **36**(2), 289–299 (2016)

6. Sudre, C., et al.: 3D multirater RCNN for multimodal multiclass detection and characterization of extremely small objects. In: Proceedings of the 2nd International MIDL Conference on Proceedings of Machine Learning Research, vol. 102, pp. 447–456. PMLR, London, United Kingdom, 08–10 Jul 2019

7. Tanno, R., Saeedi, A., Sankaranarayanan, S., Alexander, D.C., Silberman, N.: Learning from noisy labels by regularized estimation of annotator confusion. In: Conference on Computer Vision and Pattern Recognition (2019)

8. Tillin, T., Forouhi, N.G., McKeigue, P.M., Chaturvedi, N.F.T.S., Chaturvedi, N.: Southall and Brent REvisited: cohort profile of SABRE, a UK population-based comparison of cardiovascular disease and diabetes in people of European, Indian Asian and African Caribbean origins. Int. J. Epidemiol. **41**(1), 33–42 (2012). https://doi.org/10.1093/ije/dyq175

9. Wardlaw, J.M., et al.: Neuroimaging standards for research into small vessel disease and its contribution to ageing and neurodegeneration. Lancet Neurol. **12**, 822–838 (2013)

10. Warfield, S.K., Zou, K.H., Wells, W.M.: Simultaneous truth and performance level estimation (STAPLE): an algorithm for the validation of image segmentation. IEEE TMI **23**(7), 903–921 (2004)

Coidentification of Group-Level Hole Structures in Brain Networks via Hodge Laplacian

Hyekyoung Lee[1](✉), Moo K. Chung[3], Hyejin Kang[2], Hongyoon Choi[1,2],
Seunggyun Ha[4], Youngmin Huh[2], Eunkyung Kim[1], and Dong Soo Lee[1,2]

[1] Seoul National University Hospital, Seoul, Republic of Korea
hklee.brain@gmail.com
[2] Seoul National University, Seoul, Republic of Korea
[3] University of Wisconsin, Madison, USA
[4] The Catholic University of Korea, Seoul ST. Mary's Hospital,
Seoul, Republic of Korea

Abstract. One of outstanding issues in brain network analysis is to extract common topological substructure shared by a group of individuals. Recently, methods to detect group-wise modular structure on graph Laplacians have been introduced. From the perspective of algebraic topology, the modules or clusters are the zeroth topology information of a topological space. Higher order topology information can be found in holes. In this study, we extend the concept of graph Laplacian to higher order Hodge Laplacian of weighted networks, and develop a group-level hole identification method via the Stiefel optimization. In experiments, we applied the proposed method to three synthetic data and Alzheimer's disease neuroimaging initiative (ADNI) database. Experimental results showed that the coidentification of group-level hole structures helped to find the underlying topology information of brain networks that discriminate groups well.

Keywords: Hole structure · Group analysis · Hodge Laplacian · Stiefel optimization · ADNI

1 Introduction

Persistent homology has been widely applied for brain network analysis [4,9]. Especially, the concept of filtration in persistent homology helps to solve the thresholding problem of correlation-based brain networks. During the filtration, a weighted network is decomposed into the sequence of unweighted networks at all possible thresholds, and the change of network shape is observed over thresholds. The persistent homology focuses on the birth and death of topological features, called holes, and the change of their numbers, called Betti numbers, during the filtration. Persistence diagram is a useful tool for analyzing and visualizing the change of holes and Betti numbers during the filtration. The most widely

© Springer Nature Switzerland AG 2019
D. Shen et al. (Eds.): MICCAI 2019, LNCS 11767, pp. 674–682, 2019.
https://doi.org/10.1007/978-3-030-32251-9_74

used algorithm to compute persistent homology was developed by Zomorodian and Carlsson, called the ZC algorithm [11]. It is very efficient in computing a persistence diagram. However, since the ZC algorithm finds only one sparse representation of a hole among many possible representations, it can obscure the identification of holes in practice [6,7].

The k-dimensional holes in a network span in the intersection of the null space of the kth and $(k + 1)$th incidence matrices [5–7,11]. The null space of a matrix is generally estimated by the Gaussian elimination or eigen-decomposition. The ZC algorithm is on the Smith normal form of the incidence matrices, which is the extension of the Gaussian elimination [11]. Another approach to the hole estimation is based on the eigen-decomposition of the kth Hodge Laplacian constructed by the kth and $(k+1)$th incidence matrices [5–7,11]. The Gaussian elimination of sparse incidence matrices gives us the sparse representation of holes. On the other hand, the eigen-decomposition of Hodge Laplacian estimates a dense representation of holes, called a harmonic form. The harmonic form can express all possible paths around a hole with their weights representing the amount of contributions [6]. Another advantage of the harmonic form estimation method is to represent the convex optimization problem on the Stiefel manifold of Hodge Laplacian [8]. If we change the harmonic form estimation method to an optimization problem, we can easily add regularization term such as sparseness constraints as well as extend to group-level analysis [8].

A further consideration when computing holes during the filtration is that the shape of a hole is changed from its birth to death by increasing the number of edges during the filtration. The ZC algorithm chooses the youngest persistent hole at birth for the localization of a hole. However, the best solution in the hole localization is to find the consistent shape of a hole from its birth to death. In this paper, we add the weight to simplexes including edges and higher order counterparts in a network for the consistency of holes during filtration [5]. Since the connections (topology) in a network is not changed by the weight of a simplex, the Betti numbers and the birth and death of holes are not affected by the presence of weights. The harmonic form is affected both by topology and geometry. If we assign large weights to edges at birth and small weights to edges at death, it is possible to reduce the change of the shape of the harmonic form.

The contribution of this paper is (1) to introduce a weighted version of the kth Hodge Laplacian for computing harmonic forms of a brain network during filtration, (2) to propose a harmonic form estimation method based on the Stiefel optimization, and (3) to extend a group analysis of harmonic form estimation by adding the constraint of pairwise similarity between harmonic forms in a group. In experiments, we applied to three synthetic data and the FDG PET dataset in Alzheimer's disease neuroimaging initiative (ADNI) database. The experimental results showed that coidentification of group-level hole structure helped to find the underlying topology information that improves the clustering accuracy between the groups.

2 Methods

2.1 Datasets and Preprocessing

FDG PET images in ADNI data set was used for application[1]. It consists of 4 groups, 181 normal controls (NC), 91 mild cognitive impairment non-converters (MCIn), 77 MCI converters (MCIc), and 135 Alzheimer's disease (AD). The FDG PET images were preprocessed by statistical parametric mapping (SPM8)[2]. The whole brain image was divided into 94 regions of interest (ROIs) based on automated anatomical labeling (AAL2) excluding cerebellum. The distance between two ROIs (nodes) was obtained by diffusion distance on positive correlation between the measurements [2]. We transformed the distance to the similarity (weight) between two nodes by Gaussian kernel with bandwidth 0.005 [1]. The edge weight between nodes i and j are denoted by w_{ij}.

2.2 Hodge Laplacian of Weighted Simplicial Network

Weighted Simplicial Network. Given a non-empty node set V, a k-simplex is an element with nodes, $v_1, ..., v_{k+1} \in V$, denoted by $\sigma_k = [v_1, ..., v_{k+1}]$. An abstract simplicial complex K is a subset of the power set of V, i.e., $K \subseteq 2^V$ such that (1) $\varnothing \in K$, and (2) if $\sigma \in K$ and $\tau \in \sigma$, $\tau \in K$ [11]. The dimension of K, denoted by $\dim K$, is the maximum dimension of $\sigma \in K$. The collection of σ_k's in K is denoted by K_k ($-1 \leqslant k \leqslant \dim K$). The number of simplices in K_k is denoted by $|K_k|$. The $(k-1)$-face of σ_k is obtained by $\sigma_{k,j} = [v_1, \ldots, v_{j-1}, v_{j+1}, \ldots, v_{k+1}] \in K_{k-1}$. We call a simplicial complex a (simplicial) network for convenience [6].

In a weighted simplicial network, each simplex has its own weight function $w : 2^V \to (0, \infty)$. Suppose that a weighted simplicial network has the ordered $\sigma_k^i \in K_k$, $i = 1, \ldots, |K_k|$ for $0 \leqslant k \leqslant \dim K$. The weight matrix of σ_k's are a diagonal matrix such that $\boldsymbol{W}_k = diag\left\{ w(\sigma_k^1), \cdots, w(\sigma_k^{|K_k|}) \right\} \in \mathbb{R}^{|K_k| \times |K_k|}$. In this study, we define the weight of simplexes as follows [10]:

$$\begin{cases} w(\sigma_0 = [v_i]) = 1 (1 \leqslant i \leqslant p), \\ w(\sigma_1 = [v_i, v_j]) = w_{ij} (1 \leqslant i < j \leqslant p), \\ w(\sigma_k) = \min(\sigma_{k,\bar{1}}, \ldots, \sigma_{k,\overline{k+1}}) \text{ for } k > 1. \end{cases}$$

Hodge Laplacian. Given a finite simplicial complex K, a chain complex C_k is defined by $\mathbb{Z}^{|K_k|}$ with $C_{-1} = \mathbb{Z}$. $\mathbb{Z}^k$ is a k-dimensional integer space [11]. The boundary operator ∂_k and coboundary operator $\partial_k^\top$ are functions such that $\partial_k : C_k \to C_{k-1}$ and $\partial_k^\top : C_{k-1} \to C_k$, respectively. For $k = 0$, $\partial_0 : C_0 \to 0$.

---

[1] http://adni.loni.usc.edu.
[2] http://www.fil.ion.ucl.ac.uk/spm.

Given $\sigma_k = [v_1, ..., v_{k+1}] \in C_k$ and its weight $w(\sigma_k)$, the boundary of σ_k is algebraically defined as [5, 10]

$$\partial_k \sigma_k = \sum_{j=1}^{k+1} \frac{w(\sigma_k)}{w(\sigma_{k,\hat{j}})} (-1)^{j-1} \sigma_{k,\hat{j}}. \tag{1}$$

If the sign of σ_{k-1} in $\partial_k \sigma_k$ is positive/negative, it is called positively/negatively oriented with respect to σ_k. It is denoted by $\sigma_{k-1} \in_{+(-)} \sigma_k$.

Given $K_k, K_{k-1} \subset K$, the kth incidence matrix $M_k \in \mathbb{Z}^{|K_{k-1}| \times |K_k|}$ is defined by $[M_k]_{ij} = 1$, if $\sigma_{k-1}^i \in_+ \sigma_k^j$; -1, if $\sigma_{k-1}^i \in_- \sigma_k^j$; 0 otherwise [5]. Then, the boundary operator ∂_k in (1) is written by $\partial_k = W_{k-1}^{-1} M_k W_k$, and The coboundary operator $\partial_k^\top$ is written by $W_k M_k^\top W_{k-1}^{-1}$ [3]. The kth Hodge Laplacian $L_k : C_k \to C_k$ of a weighted simplicial network is defined by [3, 5]

$$\begin{aligned} L_k &= \partial_k^\top \partial_k + \partial_{k+1} \partial_{k+1}^\top \\ &= W_k M_k^\top W_{k-1}^{-2} M_k W_k + W_k^{-1} M_{k+1} W_{k+1}^2 M_{k+1}^\top W_k^{-1}. \end{aligned} \tag{2}$$

Harmonic Form. The kernel of L_k are denoted by $\ker L_k$. The dimension of $\ker L_k$, i.e., the number of zero eigenvalues of L_k is the kth Betti number, denoted by β_k. Eigenvectors with zero eigenvalues in $\ker L_k$ are called a harmonic k-form, denoted by $H_k = [h_{1,k}, \cdots, h_{\beta_k,k}] \in \mathbb{R}^{|K_k| \times \beta_k}$. The eigenvalue of $h_{i,k}$ can be written by $\lambda_{i,k} = h_{i,k}^\top L_k h_{i,k} = 0$ for $i = 1, \cdots, \beta_k$.

2.3 Stiefel Optimization for Group-Level Harmonic Forms

Given a network K, the problem of estimating harmonic k-forms of L_k can be written by an optimization problem on a Stiefel manifold

$$\min_{H_k \in \mathcal{S}(|K_k|, r)} H_k^\top L_k H_k + \beta \| H_k \|_1, \tag{3}$$

where $\mathcal{S}(|K_k|, r)$ is a Stiefel manifold which is the set of all r-tuples of orthonormal vectors in $\mathbb{R}^{|K_k|}$, $\| \cdot \|_1$ is the l_1-norm of $\cdot$, and β is the control parameter for sparseness [8].

Pairwise Similarity Constraint for Group Analysis. Suppose that there are N simplicial networks in a group. Their kth Hodge Laplacians and harmonic forms are denoted by $L_k^{(1)}, \ldots, L_k^{(N)}$ and $H_k^{(1)}, \ldots, H_k^{(N)}$, respectively. To estimate group-level harmonic forms, we extend (3) to

$$\begin{aligned} \min_{H_n \in \mathcal{S}(|K_k|, r)} &\sum_{n=1}^{N} \left((H_k^{(n)})^\top L_k^{(n)} H_k^{(n)} + \beta \| H_k^{(n)} \|_1 \right) \\ &+ \frac{\mu}{2} \sum \sum_{m,n,1 \leqslant m \neq n \leqslant N} \| H_k^{(m)} - H_k^{(n)} \|_2^2, \end{aligned} \tag{4}$$

where μ is a parameter to control pairwise similarity between harmonic forms. When $\mu = 0$, the obtained $\boldsymbol{H}_k^{(n)}$s are an individual-level harmonic form. The larger the μ, the stronger the group-level constraint. The derivative of the optimization problem in (4) is $2\boldsymbol{L}_k^{(n)}\boldsymbol{H}_k^{(n)} + \beta sign(\boldsymbol{H}_k^{(n)}) + \mu\sum_{m=1,m\neq n}^{N}(-\boldsymbol{H}_k^{(m)})$. We used the trust-region algorithm on a Stiefel manifold for the proposed optimization problem (4).

Threshold-Dependency Constraint for Filtration. Suppose that the threshold of weights (similarities between nodes) is given by $\epsilon_1 \geqslant \epsilon_2 \geqslant \cdots \geqslant \epsilon_T$. Here, we mainly consider the 2nd Hodge Laplacians and their harmonic 2-forms ($k = 2$). Therefore, we omit k in $\boldsymbol{L}_k$, $\boldsymbol{h}_{i,k}$ and $\boldsymbol{\lambda}_{i,k}$ in (1–4).

The Hodge Laplacian at ϵ_t in the nth network is now written by $\boldsymbol{L}_{\epsilon_t}^{(n)}$. The group-level harmonic form in (4) is denoted by $\boldsymbol{H}_{\epsilon_t}^{(n)} = [\boldsymbol{h}_{1t}^{(n)} \cdots \boldsymbol{h}_{rt}^{(n)}] \in \mathbb{R}^{q\times r}$, where q is the number of edges in $K^{(n)}$ and r is β_2 at ϵ_t. The eigenvalue of $\boldsymbol{H}_{\epsilon_t}^{(n)}$ is denoted by $\boldsymbol{\lambda}_{\epsilon_t}^{(n)} = [\lambda_{it}^{(n)} = (\boldsymbol{h}_{it}^{(n)})^\top \boldsymbol{L}_{\epsilon_t}^{(n)} \boldsymbol{h}_{it}^{(n)}] \in \mathbb{R}^r$. Then, we have the hole sequence of the nth network at $\epsilon_1, \epsilon_2, \ldots, \epsilon_T$ defined by

$$\mathcal{H}_n : (\boldsymbol{H}_{\epsilon_1}^{(n)}, \boldsymbol{\lambda}_{\epsilon_1}^{(n)}) \to \cdots \to (\boldsymbol{H}_{\epsilon_T}^{(n)}, \boldsymbol{\lambda}_{\epsilon_T}^{(n)}). \tag{5}$$

To impose the dependency between $(\boldsymbol{H}_{\epsilon_{t-1}}^{(n)}, \boldsymbol{\lambda}_{\epsilon_{t-1}}^{(n)})$ and $(\boldsymbol{H}_{\epsilon_t}^{(n)}, \boldsymbol{\lambda}_{\epsilon_t}^{(n)})$, we replace $\boldsymbol{L}_{\epsilon_t}^{(n)}$ in (4) with $\tilde{\boldsymbol{L}}_{\epsilon_t}^{(n)} = (1-\alpha)\boldsymbol{L}_{\epsilon_{t-1}}^{(n)} + \alpha\boldsymbol{L}_{\epsilon_t}^{(n)}$ ($0.5 \ll \alpha \leqslant 1$). Then, a persistent harmonic form lasted from the threshold ϵ_{t-1} will be selected first at ϵ_t.

2.4   Similarity Between Hole Sequences

As eigenvalue $\lambda_{it}^{(n)}$ approaches zero, the corresponding eigenvector $\boldsymbol{h}_{it}^{(n)}$ becomes a harmonic form. Given two hole sequences, $\mathcal{H}_m$ and $\mathcal{H}_n$, we define a similarity between $\mathcal{H}_m$ and $\mathcal{H}_n$ as follows:

$$\Gamma(\mathcal{H}_m, \mathcal{H}_n) = \sum_{i=1}^{r}\sum_{t=1}^{T} w(\lambda_{it}^{(m)}, \lambda_{it}^{(n)}) \left| (\boldsymbol{h}_{it}^{(m)})^\top \boldsymbol{h}_{it}^{(n)} \right|,$$

where $w(\lambda_{it}^{(m)}, \lambda_{it}^{(n)}) = \frac{\exp(-\lambda_{it}^{(m)}/s)\exp(-\lambda_{it}^{(n)}/s)}{\sum_t \exp(-\lambda_{it}^{(m)}/s)\exp(-\lambda_{it}^{(n)}/s)}$. Since $\boldsymbol{h}_{it}^{(m)}$ and $\boldsymbol{h}_{it}^{(n)}$ are an eigenvector, $0 \leqslant \left| (\boldsymbol{h}_{it}^{true})^\top \boldsymbol{h}_{it}^{(n)} \right| \leqslant 1$. When $\mathcal{H}_m = \mathcal{H}_n$, $\Gamma(\mathcal{H}_m, \mathcal{H}_n) = 1$. It compares two hole sequences using the shape of holes in the eigenvectors $\boldsymbol{H}_{\epsilon_t}^{(n)}$ and the existence of the holes in the eigenvalues $\boldsymbol{\lambda}_{\epsilon_t}^{(n)}$.

3   Results

3.1   Experiments on Synthetic Data

The synthetic data used in this experiment were (1) house data with 5 nodes and one hole; (2) snowman data with 11 nodes and two holes; and (3) three

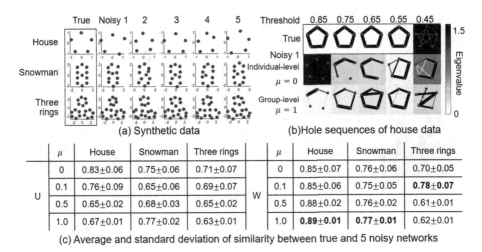

(c) Average and standard deviation of similarity between true and 5 noisy networks

	μ	House	Snowman	Three rings		μ	House	Snowman	Three rings
U	0	0.83±0.06	0.75±0.06	0.71±0.07	W	0	0.85±0.07	0.76±0.06	0.70±0.05
	0.1	0.76±0.09	0.65±0.06	0.69±0.07		0.1	0.85±0.06	0.75±0.05	**0.78±0.07**
	0.5	0.65±0.02	0.68±0.03	0.65±0.02		0.5	0.88±0.02	0.76±0.02	0.61±0.01
	1.0	0.67±0.01	0.77±0.02	0.63±0.01		1.0	**0.89±0.01**	**0.77±0.01**	0.62±0.01

Fig. 1. (a) Synthetic data, house, snowman, and three rings. Each data consists of true network and 5 noisy networks. (b) The first row shows the hole sequence of the true network, and the second and third rows respectively show the individual- and group-level hole sequences of the noisy network 1 in the house data. The similarity between the true and individual-level hole sequences is 0.74, and the similarity between the true and group-level hole sequences is 0.88. (c) Average and standard deviation of the similarities of hole sequences between true and 5 noisy networks. U and W represent when not using and using the weight of simplexes during the harmonic form estimation. (Color figure online)

rings data with 18 nodes and three holes. We generated 5 noisy networks by adding Gaussian noise with mean 0 and standard deviation 0.13 to the position of nodes in the true networks in Fig. 1(a). The measurement of a node is the position of a node in (a), and the edge weight were estimated by Gaussian kernel of the measurements of two nodes. We assumed that the individual-level hole sequences of noisy networks ($\mu = 0$) were different from the true hole sequence, while the group-level hole sequences of 5 noisy networks ($\mu > 0$) were close to true topology. We estimated the group-level hole sequences of 5 noisy networks for $\mu = 0, 0.1, 0.5, 1$, and estimated the similarity between the true and 5 individual- and group-level hole sequences. Figure 1(b) showed the true hole sequence, individual- and group-level hole sequences of house data from top to bottom. The background color of each hole was determined by the eigenvalue of the hole as shown in the right colorbar. In each hole, a thick and dark edge had large weight which is proportional to its contribution to the hole. The average of 5 similarities were shown in Fig. 1(c). The similarity to the true network was maximized when we used the weight of simplexes (W) for $\mu > 0$. It meant that the group-level hole estimation could find the true topology of a network.

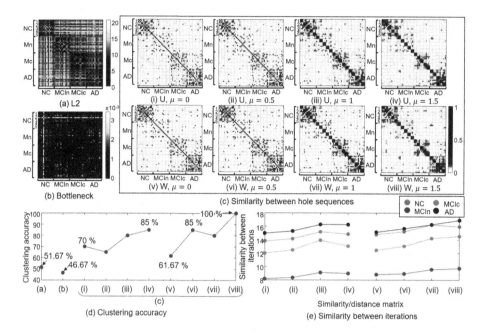

Fig. 2. (a) L2-norm, (b) Bottleneck distance of holes. (c) Similarity matrix between hole sequences for U (top) and W (middle), and $\mu = 0, 0.5, 1.0, 1.5$ from left to right. The similarity matrix of individual-level hole sequences were in (i, v) in (c). When μ increased, the 3 group-level hole sequences in a group resembled each other. Thus, dark 3×3 block matrices with large similarity were found in the diagonal term of the matrices in (iv, viii) in (c). (d) Clustering accuracy. (e) Similarity between hole sequences over CV iterations. The most of maximum accuracy and similarity were found at (viii) W, $\mu = 1.5$ in (c).

3.2   Experiments on ADNI Data

We randomly divided the data of a group into 3 parts, and constructed 3 brain networks for each group, NC, MCIn, MCIc, and AD. We estimated 3 individual- and group-level hole sequences from 3 networks by varying $\mu = 0, 0.5, 1, 1.5$. We repeated this 3-fold cross validation (CV) procedure 5 times, and compared the individual- and group-level hole structures of 5 CV iterations. The number of networks we used was 3 folds/group $\times$ 4 groups $\times$ 5 CV iterations = 60.

Figure 2(c) showed the similarity between 60 hole sequences when μ increased from left to right. If the group-level holes identified the ground truth hole structure of a group, the group-level holes were reproducible over CV iterations. Moreover, the closer the group-level hole structures were to the ground truth, the better the group-level holes discriminated the groups. We clustered 60 hole sequences into 4 groups by Ward's hierarchical clustering method based on the similarity matrix in (c). The clustering accuracy was shown in Fig. 2(d) with the accuracy based on L2-norm and bottleneck distance of holes in (a) and (b). The clustering accuracy when using the weight of simplexes in (v–viii) in (c) was

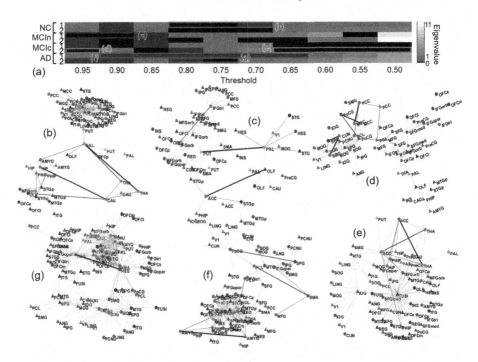

Fig. 3. (a) Sequence of the two smallest eigenvalues of Hodge Laplacian over thresholds. When the eigenvalue was close to zero (dark region), the corresponding eigenvector became a group-level harmonic form. We selected 6 group-level holes from (a). Holes in (b) NC, (c) MCIn, (d, e) MCIc, and (f, g) AD.

better than the clustering accuracy without weights in (i–iv) in Fig. 2(c). The larger the μ, i.e., the stronger the group-level constraint, the better the clustering accuracy. We also estimated the sum of similarity between hole sequences obtained from different CV iterations in Fig. 2(e). The similarity of hole structures increased as μ increased in Fig. 2(e). It meant that the group-level hole structure was reproducible. The similarity was the largest in AD, followed by NC, MCIc, and MCIn. It might be related with the data homogeneity. The sequence of the two smallest eigenvalues over thresholds in each group were shown in Fig. 3(a), and six selected holes were plotted in (b–g). A hole was found in subcortical region in NC in (b), while there were holes in cortico-cortical connections in AD in (f, g).

Acknowledgements. Data used in preparation of this article were obtained from the ADNI database http://adni.loni.usc.edu. This work is supported by NRF Grants funded by the Korean Government (No. 2013R1A1A2064593, No. 2016R1D1A1B03935463, No. 2015M3C7A1028926, No. 2017M3C7A1048079, No. 2016R1D1A1A02937497, No. 2017R1A5A1015626, and No. 2011-0030815), and NIH grant EB022856.

References

1. Bishop, C.M.: Pattern Recognition and Machine Learning. Springer, New York (2006)
2. Coifman, R.R., Lafon, S., Lee, A.B., Maggioni, M., Warner, F., Zucker, S.: Geometric diffusions as a tool for harmonic analysis and structure definition of data: diffusion maps. In: Proceedings of the National Academy of Sciences (2005)
3. Dawson, R.J.M.: Homology of weighted simplicial complexes. Cahiers de Topologie et Géométrie Différentielle Catégoriques **31**(3), 229–243 (1990)
4. Giusti, C., Ghrist, R., Bassett, D.S.: Two's company, three (or more) is a simplex. J. Comput. Neurosci. **41**(1), 1–14 (2016)
5. Horak, D., Jost, J.: Spectra of combinatorial Laplace operators on simplicial complexes. Adv. Math. **244**, 303–336 (2013)
6. Kim, Y.J., Kook, W.: Harmonic cycles for graphs. Linear Multilinear Algebra **67**, 1–11 (2018)
7. Lee, H., Chung, M.K., Kang, H., Lee, D.S.: Hole detection in metabolic connectivity of alzheimer's disease using k-laplacian. In: Golland, P., Hata, N., Barillot, C., Hornegger, J., Howe, R. (eds.) MICCAI 2014. LNCS, vol. 8675, pp. 297–304. Springer, Cham (2014). https://doi.org/10.1007/978-3-319-10443-0_38
8. Lu, C., Yan, S., Lin, Z.: Convex sparse spectral clustering: Single-view to multiview. IEEE Trans. Image Process. **25**(6), 2833–2843 (2016)
9. Wu, P., et al.: Optimal topological cycles and their application in cardiac trabeculae restoration. In: Niethammer, M., et al. (eds.) IPMI 2017. LNCS, vol. 10265, pp. 80–92. Springer, Cham (2017). https://doi.org/10.1007/978-3-319-59050-9_7
10. Zomorodian, A.: Fast construction of the Vietoris-Rips complex. Comput. Graph. **34**, 263–271 (2010)
11. Zomorodian, A., Carlsson, G.: Computing persistent homology. Discrete Comput. Geom. **33**, 249–274 (2005)

Confident Head Circumference Measurement from Ultrasound with Real-Time Feedback for Sonographers

Samuel Budd[1](✉)(iD), Matthew Sinclair[1], Bishesh Khanal[2,3],
Jacqueline Matthew[2], David Lloyd[2], Alberto Gomez[2], Nicolas Toussaint[2],
Emma C. Robinson[2], and Bernhard Kainz[1]

[1] Department of Computing, BioMedIA, Imperial College London, London, UK
`samuel.budd13@imperial.ac.uk`
[2] King's College London, ISBE, London, UK
[3] NAAMII, Kathmandu, Nepal

Abstract. Manual estimation of fetal Head Circumference (HC) from Ultrasound (US) is a key biometric for monitoring the healthy development of fetuses. Unfortunately, such measurements are subject to large inter-observer variability, resulting in low early-detection rates of fetal abnormalities. To address this issue, we propose a novel probabilistic Deep Learning approach for real-time automated estimation of fetal HC. This system feeds back statistics on measurement robustness to inform users how confident a deep neural network is in evaluating suitable views acquired during free-hand ultrasound examination. In real-time scenarios, this approach may be exploited to guide operators to scan planes that are as close as possible to the underlying distribution of training images, for the purpose of improving inter-operator consistency. We train on free-hand ultrasound data from over 2000 subjects (2848 training/540 test) and show that our method is able to predict HC measurements within 1.81 ± 1.65 mm deviation from the ground truth, with 50% of the test images fully contained within the predicted confidence margins, and an average of 1.82 ± 1.78 mm deviation from the margin for the remaining cases that are not fully contained.

1 Introduction

Fetal Ultrasound (US) scanning is a vital part of ensuring good health of mothers and fetuses during and after pregnancy. Accurate anomaly detection and assessment of fetal development from US scans are required to ensure that the best care is given at the earliest identifiable stage. In many countries a mid-trimester US scan is carried out between 18–22 weeks gestation as a part of standard prenatal care. 'Standardized plane' views are used to acquire images in which

Electronic supplementary material The online version of this chapter (https:// doi.org/10.1007/978-3-030-32251-9_75) contains supplementary material, which is available to authorized users.

© Springer Nature Switzerland AG 2019
D. Shen et al. (Eds.): MICCAI 2019, LNCS 11767, pp. 683–691, 2019.
https://doi.org/10.1007/978-3-030-32251-9_75

distinct anatomical features can be extracted [13]. From some of these standard plane views, measurements of the head, abdomen and femur are most commonly used to predict fetal age and weight, and are the key biometrics identified from US. Biometrics acquired longitudinally can be used to predict the fetal development trajectory. Unfortunately, rates for early detection of fetal abnormalities are low, largely due to the high level of skill required by the sonographer to perform such scans and extract the relevant biometrics [12].

Recently, automatic US scanning approaches have been developed using deep learning [2], which mitigate the problems of manual US measurement through automatic detection of diagnostically relevant anatomical planes. Such systems have allowed development of robust automated methods for estimation of anatomical biometrics [14,16] in diverse acquisition conditions with various imaging artefacts, outperforming non-deep learning approaches [3,8,11]. Critically, such methods only provide point estimates of HC without confidence or uncertainty measures, and do not provide any means to assess the quality of individual measurements during real-time scans. This can lead to many, potentially contradicting, measurements without any means to control the trustworthiness of the predictions during examination or retrospectively.

To this end, several approaches have been proposed for estimation of uncertainty in Deep Networks. These include Monte-Carlo Dropout (MC Dropout), the most common dropout method which has been shown to model a posterior mixture of Gaussians well. Weights in a deep neural network are 'dropped' randomly during inference with a given probability p which has been shown to approximate Bayesian inference in deep Gaussian processes [5]. In addition, ensemble approaches produce N prediction samples per input image by training a set of N separate networks for the same task. The results are then combined to produce a final segmentation which seems to offer a good trade-off between robustness and accuracy [6]. Finally, the Probabilistic U-Net represents a generative segmentation model based on a combination of a U-Net with a conditional variational autoencoder. This is capable of producing an unlimited number of plausible hypotheses, reproducing the possible segmentation variants as well as the frequencies with which they occur [7].

Contribution: In this paper, we extend upon a state-of-the-art convolutional Deep Learning approach for automatic fetal HC measurement [14] to develop a new approach for automated probabilistic fetal HC with real-time feedback on measurement robustness. Two probabilistic deep learning methods are evaluated: MC Dropout during inference and Probabilistic U-Net. These are used to return an ensemble of segmentations, from which upper and lower bounds on the measurement are generated. In addition, we propose the derivation of a 'variance score', used to reject acquired images that produce sub-optimal HC measurements. In this way, the system will guide operators towards acquiring optimal US views, resulting in more consistent and accurate measurements.

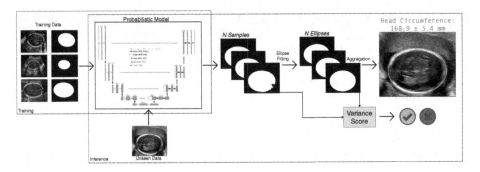

Fig. 1. Overview of our proposed method. We train a probabilistic model using the available training data. During inference we take N samples from our model, fit ellipses to each sample and aggregate these ellipses to extract a HC value and an upper and lower bound on that HC value. Various outputs of the pipeline are used to calculate different variance scores given a set of N samples. As a proof of concept we extract a threshold such that test cases whose variance score is outside the threshold are rejected, and inside are accepted.

2 Method

Biometric Estimation: Our HC estimation builds on the approach developed in [14] which achieves human level performance. First, a U-Net [10] segmentation network masks out the head from an US image. Then, an ellipse is fitted to the segmented contours [4] from which the ellipse parameters can be obtained in mm. We extract ellipse centroid co-ordinates (c_x and c_y), major and minor axis radii (a and b) each in pixels, and the angle of rotation (α) and estimate HC using the Ramanujan approximation II [1] as $HC = \pi(a+b)(1 + \frac{3h}{10+\sqrt{4-3h}})s_{xy}$ where $h = \frac{(a-b)^2}{(a+b)^2}$. The error of this approximation is $O(h^{10})$ which for more circular ellipses is negligible. This ellipse fitting process mimics the sonographer's manual actions when extracting a HC measurement during fetal US screening (Fig. 1).

Probabilistic Segmentation: Given the inherent variability between sonographers' annotations in the training data, we generate a set of N plausible segmentations from a single input using the following methods:

(i) *MC Dropout*: We randomly drop weights of the network with probability p to predict N segmentation samples. Here, single-sample experiments ($N = 1$) were used to optimise the configuration of the network. This led to implementation of a single dropout layer ($p = 0.6$) before the bottleneck layer of the U-Net during inference.

(ii) *Probabilistic U-Net*: We sample a set of N plausible segmentations using this method [7] where we follow the same training scheme as [7].

Variance Estimation: With a probabilistic mapping function $g_P(X) = \hat{X}_i$, in our case a deep probabilistic neural network, we can map a continuous input image to a possible segmentation mask $\hat{X}_i$. We assume a deterministic function $f(\hat{X}_i) = [a, b, \theta, x_c, y_c]^T$, with semi-major axis length a, semi-minor axis length b, angle of orientation θ and center $C(x_c, y_c)$, which provides a least square solution to the ellipse fitting problem to the set of points $\hat{X}$ as proposed by [9]. Based on $f(\hat{X}_i)$ we can evaluate hypotheses for their suitability to act as a metric to measure robustness during inference given N prediction samples from $g_P(X)$. These proposed metrics are

(h1) *Ellipse parameter variance:* $\sum_i^5 (\text{Var}(f(\hat{X}_n)_i))$;

(h2) *Total ring area:* $\sum (f(\bigcup_{i=1}^N \hat{X}_i) - f(\bigcap_{i=1}^N \hat{X}_i)) \cdot s_{xyz}$, where s_{xyz} scales $\hat{X}_i$ to world space in mm;

(h3) *Mask classification entropy:* $\sum_{x,y}^K \underline{\hat{X}}(x, y) \log(\underline{\hat{X}}(x, y))$, where K is the number of pixels in $\underline{\hat{X}} \in \mathbb{Z}_2$ after $argmax(\hat{X}_i)$ class assignment and $\underline{\hat{X}} = \frac{1}{N} \cdot \sum_i^N \hat{X}_i$; and

(h4) *Softmax confidence entropy:* given $\hat{X}_i \in \mathbb{R}$ before class assignment, after conversion of the network's final layer's logits with $Softmax(x_i) = \frac{\exp(x_i)}{\sum^i \exp(x_i)}$, the resulting $\hat{X}_i^*$ can be interpreted as two-element prediction confidence $[p_f, p_b]_i = \hat{X}_i^*(x, y)$ for foreground p_f and background p_b. Thus we can estimate class-agnostic prediction entropy by $\sum_i^K p_i \log(p_i)$ where $p_i = \sum_i^N \max([p_f, p_b]_i)$.

3   Experiments and Results

Data: Our base dataset, named subsequently as Dataset A, consists of 2,724 two-dimensional US examinations from volunteers at 18–22 weeks gestation, acquired and labelled during routine screening by 45 expert sonographers. Several images were taken during each session, including the standard transverse brain view at the posterior horn of the ventricle (TV) plane used for HC measurement. This data was combined with the HC18 Challenge [15] dataset which consists of 1334 two-dimensional US images of the standard plane that is used to measure HC, each image is 800 × 540 pixels with a pixel size ranging from 0.052 mm to 0.326 mm. Each image in the training set has an accompanying manual annotation of the HC (ellipse outline) performed by a single trained sonographer [15]. We resample all images to 320 × 384 pixels, and produce a head mask from the expert ground truth delineation. Training data is randomly flipped both horizontally and vertically, and a random rotation (±5°) is performed.

Single-Sampling Experiments: In the first instance, single-sample experiments, generating a single segmentation and HC measurement ($N = 1$) per subject, were used to verify the performance of the proposed model against the state-of-the-art [14]. Table 1 reports performance measures for all *single-sampling* experiments. These show comparable performance relative to [14] for our U-Net implementation, trained on Dataset A. This result improves further when the same model is trained on Dataset A and HC18 data. MC dropout during training further improves the result. For subsequent analysis, all experiments for MC

Dropout (during inference) use the combined data and are trained using MC dropout.

Table 1. Single sample results of three U-Net's. **Baseline**: Trained on Dataset A data only. **Dataset A + HC18**: Trained on Dataset A data and HC18 Challenge data transformed to same format as Dataset A data. **Dropout**: Trained on Dataset A and HC18 Challenge data with dropout ($p = 0.6$ value found to be best performing in variety of dropout configurations). We compare the Mean absolute difference between the final HC measurement, the DICE overlap of the fitted ellipse with the ground truth ellipse, and the Hausdorff distance between the outline of the fitted ellipse and the outline of the ground truth ellipse. Results calculated on Dataset A test data.

	Mean abs difference ± std (mm)	Mean DICE ± std (%)	Mean Hausdorff distance ± std (mm)
Baseline	2.09 ± 1.97	0.982 ± 0.011	1.289 ± 0.880
Dataset A + HC18	1.90 ± 1.90	0.982 ± 0.010	1.292 ± 0.791
Dropout $p = 0.6$	**1.808 ± 1.65**	**0.982 ± 0.008**	**1.295 ± 0.664**

Multi-sampling Experiments: MC Dropout during inference has been compared against a Probabilistic U-Net. Here, multiple (N) segmentation predictions are made for each US image. From these, the mean and median of the set of fitted ellipse parameters are used to obtain a single HC value for each test case, and the set of N segmentations are used to obtain an upper and lower bound. Table 2 shows the performance measures for our *multi-sampling* experiments. Results show that we lose performance through aggregating multiple results using the mean or median, although this is likely due to dropout not being applied during inference for single sample experiments. However, the *multi-sampling* methods do allow us to produce an upper and lower bound on the HC value, with an average difference of 1.82 ± 1.78 mm between upper-lower bounds and ground truth HC measurement ($N = 10$ samples), for cases where the ground truth is not within the upper-lower bounds (*MC(inf.)*).

Variance Measure Thresholding: Finally, we experiment with each of the variance scores produced over the test set as a means to accept/reject images at test time. We assess their performance by counting the number of accepted/rejected cases for a range of thresholds between zero and one, and how this threshold affects the resulting average performance scores after rejected images are removed from the test set. In this experiment we use only MC dropout during inference ($p = 0.6$) which performs best in our previous experiments. Figure 2 shows graphs depicting how each variance measure can be used to reject test cases, and how rejecting high variance cases can lead to improved performance. In each case we normalise the variance score to lie between 0 and 1, and for each threshold between 0 and 1 we 'reject' cases whose variance score is above the threshold. Plots show the performance for remaining 'accepted' cases, plotted against the number of 'rejected' cases. For most variance scores

Table 2. Multi-sampling results for the two methods. We report the performance measures of a single-sampled point-predictor (*Det. (Deterministic)*), mean/median of $N = 10$ samples from the Probabilistic U-Net (*Prob. U-Net (Probabilistic U-Net)*), and our previous best U-Net with Monte-Carlo dropout during inference (*MC(inf.) (Monte Carlo dropout during inference)*, $p = 0.6$). We report the % ground truth HC values that lie in the calculated upper/lower bound range. This percentage varies significantly with N, for *MC(inf.)*: $N = 2$: 14.8%; $N = 1000$: 50.4%. See Supplementary Material Figures 1–3.

	Mean abs difference ± std (mm)	Mean DICE ± std (%)	Mean Hausdorff distance ± std (mm)	$LB \leq HC_{gt}$ $\leq UB(\%)$
Det.				
MC $p = 0.6$	**1.81 ± 1.65**	**0.982 ± 0.008**	**1.295 ± 0.664**	N/A
Prob. UNet				
Mean	2.22 ± 2.15	0.980 ± 0.011	1.413 ± 0.751	20.4
Median	2.21 ± 2.15	0.980 ± 0.011	1.410 ± 0.748	20.4
MC(inf.)				
Mean	2.15 ± 2.09	0.981 ± 0.010	1.313 ± 0.613	27.8
Median	**2.15 ± 2.07**	**0.981 ± 0.010**	**1.307 ± 0.604**	**27.8**

we obtain an initial performance boost from 'rejecting' the worst cases, but after an initial improvement, the variance scores do not delineate 'good' from 'bad' cases very well. Results suggest that higher measurement variance may indicate sub-optimal imaging plane acquisition.

Qualitative Assessment: Figure 3 shows examples for successful and less model-compliant images using Dropout during inference to produce the samples, where model-compliance captures the proximity of the image to the training data. Note that the best performing examples produce very narrow upper and lower bounds (in this figure where the upper and lower bounds occupy the same pixels the margin is not visible). The worst performing examples show a wider upper and lower bound range but the ground truth ellipse is often not contained within the predicted range. These images often show a lack of clear white presentation of the skull. However, ambiguous segmentation of the regions with missing signal is often reflected in the confidence margin produced, showing greater variation in those image regions, which can be seen clearly in the second example in the bottom row - a wider upper-lower bound area for image regions with low signal from fetal skull. The example on the bottom far right shows missing signal on both sides, which results in a large uncertainty in the ellipses globally due to the compounded effect of missing signal on both sides of the skull.

4   Discussion

While we cannot claim our proposed 'variance scores' represent model uncertainty directly, they show some capability to 'reject' particularly low performing

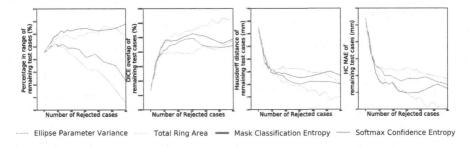

----- Ellipse Parameter Variance   ----- Total Ring Area   ▬▬ Mask Classification Entropy   ——— Softmax Confidence Entropy

Fig. 2. Plots showing performance measures against the number of rejected test cases. Each measure shows improvement after removing a few test cases for each score (these thresholds vary for each score), however after removing an initial low performing set, the scores power to discriminate between 'good' and 'bad' images deteriorate. 'Percentage in range' calculated as the percentage of test cases for which the ground truth HC measurement lies within the predicted upper-lower bounds.

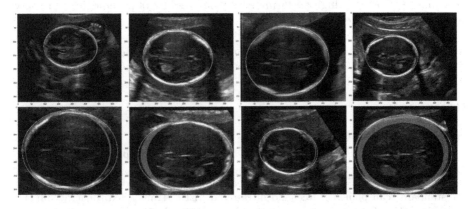

Fig. 3. Results produced by our model. White line: Ground Truth, Orange dashed line: Mean of sampled ellipse parameters, Pink shaded area: Upper/lower bound range. Top row: High performing images. Bottom row: Low performing images. See Supplementary Material Figures 4 and 5 for more examples and a demo video demonstration. (Color figure online)

test cases. In this way, the 'variance scores' can be described as a measurement for the proximity to the variance of the training data of an unseen test sample, which is also desirable, showing the confidence of the network with respect to its capacity and seen training examples. Scenarios in which an operator is present stand to benefit practically using methods introduced in this work, prompting operators to reject sub-optimal measurements by providing real-time feedback during acquisition, thus improving inter-operator consistency. This work lays the foundations for methods by which this can be achieved.

5   Conclusion

We demonstrate the effectiveness of probabilistic CNNs to automatically generate HC measurements from US scans, and produce upper-lower bound confidence intervals in real-time. Using multi-sampling probabilistic networks we derive 'variance scores', which indicate how confident our network is in generating measurements for a given image. This approach could be used to derive a system which rejects images collected from sub-optimal views, forcing sonographers to take measurements from a view for which the network performs optimally. This could lead to techniques for automated fetal HC measurement, which outperform manual approaches in terms of accuracy and consistency.

Future directions of this work include exploring alternative methods for multi-sampling networks, alternative segmentation fusion strategies and alternative 'variance scores'. Analysis of new datasets to investigate network bias towards particular datasets is valuable, as well as analysis of cases with anomalous anatomy to verify high performance in the presence of pathologies, clinically the most important cases to identify.

Acknowledgements. This work is supported by the Wellcome Trust IEH 102431, EPSRC (EP/S022104/1, EP/S013687/1), and Nvidia GPU donations.

References

1. Barnard, R.W., Pearce, K., Schovanec, L.: Inequalities for the perimeter of an ellipse. J. Math. Anal. Appl. **260**(2), 295–306 (2001). https://doi.org/10.1006/JMAA.2000.7128
2. Baumgartner, C.F., et al.: SonoNet: real-time detection and localisation of fetal standard scan planes in freehand ultrasound. IEEE Trans. Med. Imaging **36**(11), 2204–2215 (2017). https://doi.org/10.1109/TMI.2017.2712367
3. Carneiro, G., Georgescu, B., Good, S., Comaniciu, D.: Detection and measurement of fetal anatomies from ultrasound images using a constrained probabilistic boosting tree. IEEE Trans. Med. Imaging **27**(9), 1342–1355 (2008). https://doi.org/10.1109/TMI.2008.928917
4. Fitzgibbon, A., Pilu, M., Fisher, R.: Direct least squares fitting of ellipses. In: 13th ICPR 1996, pp. 253–257. IEEE (1996). https://doi.org/10.1109/ICPR.1996.546029
5. Gal, Y., Ghahramani, Z.: Dropout as a Bayesian approximation: representing model uncertainty in deep learning. In: ICLR 2016, pp. 1050–1059 (2016)
6. Kamnitsas, K., et al.: Ensembles of multiple models and architectures for robust brain tumour segmentation. In: Brainlesion: Glioma, Multiple Sclerosis, Stroke and Traumatic Brain Injuries, pp. 450–462, September 2018. https://doi.org/10.1007/978-3-319-75238-9_38
7. Kohl, S., et al.: A probabilistic U-Net for segmentation of ambiguous images. In: Advances in Neural Information Processing Systems, pp. 6965–6975 (2018)
8. Li, J., et al.: Automatic fetal head circumference measurement in ultrasound using random forest and fast ellipse fitting. IEEE J. Biomed. Health Inform. **22**(1), 215–223 (2018). https://doi.org/10.1109/JBHI.2017.2703890

9. Prasad, D., Leung, M., Quek, C.: ElliFit: an unconstrained, non-iterative, least squares based geometric ellipse fitting method. Pattern Recogn. **46**(5), 1449–1465 (2013). https://doi.org/10.1016/j.patcog.2012.11.007

10. Ronneberger, O., Fischer, P., Brox, T.: U-Net: convolutional networks for biomedical image segmentation. In: Navab, N., Hornegger, J., Wells, W.M., Frangi, A.F. (eds.) MICCAI 2015. LNCS, vol. 9351, pp. 234–241. Springer, Cham (2015). https://doi.org/10.1007/978-3-319-24574-4_28

11. Rueda, S., et al.: Evaluation and comparison of current fetal ultrasound image segmentation methods for biometric measurements: a grand challenge. IEEE Trans. Med. Imaging **33**(4), 797–813 (2014). https://doi.org/10.1109/TMI.2013.2276943

12. Sarris, I., et al.: Intra- and interobserver variability in fetal ultrasound measurements. Ultrasound Obstet. Gynecol. **39**(3), 266–273 (2012). https://doi.org/10.1002/uog.10082

13. UK National Health Service: NHS Fetal Anomaly Screening Programme (FASP) Handbook Valid from August 2018. Technical report (2018)

14. Sinclair, M., et al.: Human-level performance on automatic head biometrics in fetal ultrasound using fully convolutional neural networks. In: 40th EMBC 2018, pp. 714–717. IEEE, July 2018. https://doi.org/10.1109/EMBC.2018.8512278

15. van den Heuvel, T.L.A., de Bruijn, D., de Korte, C.L., Ginneken, B.V.: Automated measurement of fetal head circumference using 2D ultrasound images. PLoS ONE **13**(8), e0200412 (2018). https://doi.org/10.1371/journal.pone.0200412

16. Wu, L., et al.: Cascaded fully convolutional networks for automatic prenatal ultrasound image segmentation. In: IEEE 14th ISBI 2017, pp. 663–666. IEEE, April 2017. https://doi.org/10.1109/ISBI.2017.7950607

Image Reconstruction and Synthesis

Detection and Correction of Cardiac MRI Motion Artefacts During Reconstruction from k-space

Ilkay Oksuz[1]([envelope]), James Clough[1], Bram Ruijsink[1,2], Esther Puyol-Antón[1], Aurelien Bustin[1], Gastao Cruz[1], Claudia Prieto[1], Daniel Rueckert[3], Andrew P. King[1], and Julia A. Schnabel[1]

[1] School of Biomedical Engineering and Imaging Sciences, King's College London, London, UK
ilkay.oksuz@kcl.ac.uk
[2] Guy's and St Thomas' Hospital NHS Foundation Trust, London, UK
[3] Biomedical Image Analysis Group, Imperial College London, London, UK

Abstract. In fully sampled cardiac MR (CMR) acquisitions, motion can lead to corruption of k-space lines, which can result in artefacts in the reconstructed images. In this paper, we propose a method to automatically detect and correct motion-related artefacts in CMR acquisitions during reconstruction from k-space data. Our correction method is inspired by work on undersampled CMR reconstruction, and uses deep learning to optimize a data-consistency term for under-sampled k-space reconstruction. Our main methodological contribution is the addition of a detection network to classify motion-corrupted k-space lines to convert the problem of artefact correction to a problem of reconstruction using the data consistency term. We train our network to automatically correct for motion-related artefacts using synthetically corrupted cine CMR k-space data as well as uncorrupted CMR images. Using a test set of 50 2D+time cine CMR datasets from the UK Biobank, we achieve good image quality in the presence of synthetic motion artefacts. We quantitatively compare our method with a variety of techniques for recovering good image quality and showcase better performance compared to state of the art denoising techniques with a PSNR of 37.1. Moreover, we show that our method preserves the quality of uncorrupted images and therefore can be also utilized as a general image reconstruction algorithm.

Keywords: Cardiac MR · Image reconstruction · Motion artefacts · UK Biobank · Convolutional neural networks

1 Introduction

Ensuring high image quality is essential for image analysis pipelines to extract clinically useful information. Misleading diagnoses can be made when the original data are of low quality, in particular for cardiac magnetic resonance (CMR)

© Springer Nature Switzerland AG 2019
D. Shen et al. (Eds.): MICCAI 2019, LNCS 11767, pp. 695–703, 2019.
https://doi.org/10.1007/978-3-030-32251-9_76

imaging, where cardiac indices are extracted using post-processing techniques including segmentation and registration. CMR images can contain a range of image artefacts [1], which can reduce the accuracy of image analysis. Improving the quality of such images acquired on MR scanners is a challenging task.

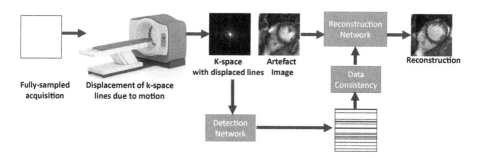

Fig. 1. Detection and correction of MR artefacts using predicted data consistency masks.

One approach for correcting artefacts is image reconstruction using deep neural networks. In deep learning based reconstruction of accelerated (i.e. undersampled) CMR, a pre-determined k-space acquisition trajectory is used and those parts of k-space that have not been sampled are estimated using an inverse problem formulation to reconstruct the image [13]. A different, but related problem exists in fully sampled acquisitions that have been corrupted by motion artefacts, for example due to mis-triggering or arrythmias. In these cases, the data contain correct k-space lines as well as corrupted lines, but it is unknown which are correct and which are corrupted. This problem is our focus in this paper but we draw inspiration from work on accelerated imaging in devising our solution.

We propose a k-space artefact detection network that generates an individual data consistency term for any given acquisition and converts the image artefact correction task to an undersampled image reconstruction problem, which is subsequently addressed by an algorithm developed for reconstruction of undersampled CMR acquisitions (see the illustration in Fig. 1). Our proposed method is evaluated using 300 cine SSFP (2D+time) CMR datasets from the UK Biobank.

The major contributions of this work are as follows: First, we introduce a novel solution for the detection of artefacts in CMR images. Second, we use the output of this k-space artefact detection network to introduce a data consistency term to be used by an image reconstruction network. By training both networks end-to-end we are able to ignore motion corrupted k-space lines during the reconstruction. Finally, our algorithm is trained and tested also on uncorrupted images, which demonstrates its utility as a generic image reconstruction algorithm.

2   Background

Deep learning has recently shown great promise in reconstruction of highly undersampled MR acquisitions with convolutional neural networks (CNNs) [4,12,13]. For example, Schlemper et al. [13] proposed to use a deep cascaded network to generate high quality images, and Hauptmann et al. [3] proposed to use a residual U-net to reduce aliasing artefacts due to undersampling with the purpose of accelerating image acquisition.

For automatic correction of CMR, Lotjonen et al. [7] used reconstructed short-axis and long-axis slices to optimise the locations of the slices using mutual information as a similarity measure. Estimating high quality images from corrupted (or under-sampled) k-space has been a well investigated subject in the literature [2]. The problem can be addressed either in the k-space domain or the image domain. One choice is to correct the k-space before applying the inverse Fourier transform (IFT) as proposed by Han et al. [2]. A more common approach is to use the IFT on k-space and learn a mapping between the corrupted reconstructed images and good quality images. To this end, a variety of image denoising techniques can be utilized such as autoencoders [15], residual learning networks [16] or wide networks [6]. Zhu et al. [17] proposed an end-to-end image reconstruction approach (Automap) for MR and evaluated it on undersampled k-space data.

3   Methods

Our network architecture consists of two sub-networks that are trained jointly as visualized in Fig. 2. The first network is an artefact detection network which is used to identify potentially corrupted k-space lines and hence define a data-consistency term. and the second network is a recurrent convolutional neural network (RCNN) used for reconstruction using this data-consistency term [12]. Details of both networks are provided below.

3.1   Network Architecture

The proposed artefact detection CNN consists of eight layers The architecture of our network follows a similar architecture to [14], which was originally developed for video classification using a spatio-temporal 3D CNN. In our case we use the third dimension as the time component and use 2D+time mid-ventricular sequences as the input to the network. Each image sequence has 50 time frames. The network has 4 convolutional layers and 4 pooling layers, 1 fully-connected layer and a softmax loss layer to predict corrupted k-space lines. After each convolutional layer, a ReLU activation is used. We then apply pooling on each feature map to reduce the filter responses to a lower dimensionality. We apply dropout with a probability of 0.2 at all convolutional layers and after the first fully connected layer for regularization. All of these convolutional layers are applied with appropriate padding of 2 and stride of 1.

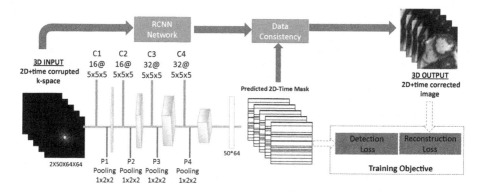

Fig. 2. The CNN architecture for motion artefact correction. The proposed network architecture consists of two building blocks (1) A corrupted k-space line detection network to define the data-consistency term; (2) A recurrent neural network (RCNN) architecture to correct image artefacts.

The reconstruction network features a RCNN architecture [12]. This network reconstructs high quality cardiac MR images from highly undersampled k-space data by jointly exploiting the dependencies of the temporal sequences as well as the iterative nature of traditional optimisation algorithms. In addition, spatio-temporal dependencies are simultaneously learned by exploiting bi-directional recurrent hidden connections across time sequences. Any reconstruction network can replace this network in our architecture. We chose this particular network for its capability to incorporate information from different frames, which is instrumental in correcting the artefacts that occur due to displacement of k-space lines in time.

3.2 Loss Function and Training

Our training objective is a linearly weighted combination of the image reconstruction loss and a cross-entropy loss for the detection of corrupted lines:

$$\mathcal{L}_{\text{total}} = \lambda\mathcal{L}_{\text{detection}} + (1 - \lambda)\mathcal{L}_{\text{reconstruction}}$$

The reconstruction loss is computed using the mean square error, defined as:

$$\mathcal{L}_{\text{reconstruction}} = \frac{1}{N_p}\sum_{p=0}^{N_p}(I_x(p) - I_y(p))^2$$

where p denotes each pixel and N_p denotes the total number of pixels in images I_x and I_y. The detection loss is the cross entropy loss, defined as:

$$\mathcal{L}_{\text{detection}}(pr, y) = \frac{1}{N_l} - (y\log(pr) + (1 - y)\log(1 - pr))$$

where y is a binary indicator (0 or 1) indicating if a k-space line is corrupted or not and pr is predicted probability of the line being uncorrupted. N_p denotes the total number of k-space lines in an image.

We used the Adam optimizer to minimise the binary cross entropy and mean square error loss function. λ, which defines the contribution of each loss was set to 0.3 using the validation set. The cross entropy term represents the dissimilarity of the predicted output distribution to the true distribution of labels after a softmax layer. The detection and reconstruction networks were pre-trained for 50 epochs separately to enable faster convergence. End-to-end training ended when the network did not significantly improve its performance on the validation set for a predefined number of epochs (100). An improvement was considered sufficient if the relative increase in performance was at least 0.5%.

During training, a batch-size of 5 2D+time sequences was used. The momentum of the optimizer was set to 0.90 and the learning rate was 10^{-4}. The parameters of the convolutional and fully-connected layers were initialised randomly from a zero-mean Gaussian distribution. In each trial, training was continued until the network converged. Convergence was defined as a state in which no substantial progress was observed in the training loss. We used Pytorch for implementation of the network and training took around 3 h on a NVIDIA Quadro P6000 GPU. After training, deployment of the network to correct a single image sequence took less than 1 s.

4   Experimental Results

We evaluated our algorithm on a subset of the UK Biobank dataset containing 300 datasets each consisting of 50 2D+time good quality cine CMR acquisitions at a mid-ventricular short axis slice. From each subject, the 50 temporal frames were used to generate synthetic motion artefacts. We used 200 datasets for training, 50 for validation and 50 for testing. The total of 300 subjects were chosen to be free of other types of image quality issues, such as missing axial slices, and were visually verified by an expert cardiologist for sufficient image quality. The details of the acquisition protocol of the UK Biobank dataset can be found in [11].

Data Preprocessing: Given a 2D+time cine CMR sequence of images we first normalise the pixel values between 0 and 1. Since the image dimensions vary from subject to subject, instead of image reshaping we use a motion information based ROI extraction to 64×64 pixels [5]. Briefly, the ROI is determined by performing a Fourier analysis of the sequences of images, followed by a circular Hough transform to highlight the center of periodically moving structures.

K-space Corruption for Synthetic Data: We generated k-space corrupted data in order to simulate motion artefacts. We followed a Cartesian sampling strategy for k-space corruption to generate synthetic but realistic motion artefacts [8,10]. We retrospectively transformed each 2D short axis sequence to the Fourier domain and changed a number (0, 2, 4, 8, 16) of Cartesian sampling k-space lines to the corresponding lines from other cardiac phases to mimic motion artefacts. These lines were selected randomly in order to mimic the randomness of real motion artefacts. The newly introduced k-space lines were also selected randomly from all other frames in the image sequence. In this way CMR images with artefacts were generated from the original 'good quality' images in the training set. This is a realistic approach as the motion artefacts that occur from mis-triggering arise from similar displacement (in time) of an arbitrary set of k-space lines.

Methods of Comparison: We compared our algorithm to a variety of classes of artefact correction strategy as outlined in Sect. 2. For image-to-image to artefact removal (i.e. post-reconstruction), we used a deep network based on residual learning (DNCNN) as well as a wide network with larger receptive fields and more channels in each layer as proposed in [6] (WIN5). We also compared our method to a reconstruction algorithm that uses an end-to-end correction methodology [9] (Automap-GAN) based on Automap [17]. Additionally, we compared our approach to its variants: (1) training detection and reconstruction networks separately (Proposed-separate); and (2) considering the corruption mask as a pre-determined mask to illustrate the top performance achievable in this setup (Proposed-known mask).

Table 1. Mean image quality results of image quality correction for motion artefacts for corrupted and uncorrupted inputs. Uncorrupted results use the correct k-space as input and indicates the potential of our method to be used as a global image reconstruction framework.

Methods	Corrupted			Uncorrupted		
	PSNR	RMSE	SSIM	PSNR	RMSE	SSIM
Baseline	26.3	0.068	0.821	–	–	–
DNCNN [16]	30.8	0.049	0.845	36.7	0.005	0.905
Win5 [6]	32.2	0.041	0.853	37.2	0.004	0.913
Automap-GAN [9]	34.8	0.028	0.878	38.7	0.003	0.927
Proposed-separate	34.7	0.026	0.879	39.3	0.003	0.947
Proposed-end to end	**37.1**	**0.023**	**0.890**	**40.8**	**0.002**	**0.972**
Proposed-known Mask	38.9	0.019	0.901	–	–	–

Quantitative Results: Table 1 shows the image quality metrics for the corrected images produced by each image artefact correction algorithm for corrupted and original images. For these experiments the ground truth was the uncorrupted original 2D+time image sequence and we use peak signal to noise ratio (PSNR), root mean square error (RMSE) and structural similarity index metric (SSIM) for evaluation. The proposed end-to-end k-space detection and correction algorithm outperforms the other methods. As can be appreciated, the joint end-to-end network performs better compared to separate training of both architectures. Compared to the image-to-image denoising techniques (Win5, DNCNN), k-space based correction (Automap-GAN) results in improved reconstructions of the images. We have also shown results on using original images as input to illustrate the capability of our method as a general image reconstruction algorithm. Our method outperforms the other state of the art techniques and does not diminish the image quality of the original k-space thanks to the detection network. Baseline and proposed-known mask methods provide perfect image quality in case of uncorrupted images and therefore omitted.

Original   **Win5**   **Automap-GAN**   **Proposed**

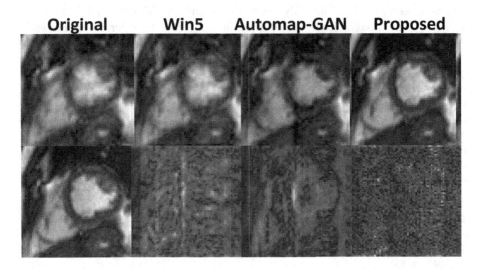

Fig. 3. The results produced by Win5 (second column), Automap-GAN (third column) and proposed algorithm (final column). In the first column, the top row shows the corrupted image and the bottom row shows the corresponding uncorrupted image. It is evident from the difference images in the bottom row that image quality is recovered at the septum using proposed method.

Qualitative Results: In Fig. 3 we illustrate the performance of our technique on artefact correction in comparison to the top state-of-the-art techniques [6,9]. The difference image shows improved image quality with the proposed technique, especially in the left ventricular and right ventricular regions and with regard to the sharpness of the myocardial boundaries. These results demonstrate that the network reduced the impact of k-space corruption on reconstruction quality, as the (beating) ventricles and their myocardial borders are mostly affected by such corruption.

5   Discussion and Conclusion

In this paper, we have proposed a CNN-based technique for correcting motion-related artefacts in a large 2D+time CINE CMR dataset. We have addressed the issue of incorrect k-space lines using a combined architecture to detect, correct and reconstruct images. The proposed network clearly outperforms competing algorithms. Moreover, the current architecture can also be used as a global image reconstructor, as we have shown that it does not diminish the quality of uncorrupted images, compared to the original reconstruction performed on the scanner.

We have shown for the first time that a 3D CNN based neural network architecture is capable of classifying k-space lines that cause motion artefacts. Our work brings fully automated assessment of ventricular function from CMR imaging a step closer to clinically acceptable standards, enabling reconstruction of high quality images from data containing artefacts in order to enable their analysis in large imaging datasets such as the UK Biobank. In future work, we plan to validate our method on the entire UK Biobank cohort, which is eventually expected to be 100,000 CMR images.

Acknowledgments. This work was supported by an EPSRC programme Grant (EP/P001009/1) and the Wellcome EPSRC Centre for Medical Engineering at the School of Biomedical Engineering and Imaging Sciences, King's College London (WT 203148/Z/16/Z). This research has been conducted using the UK Biobank Resource under Application Number 17806. The GPU used in this research was generously donated by the NVIDIA Corporation.

References

1. Ferreira, P.F., et al.: Cardiovascular magnetic resonance artefacts. JCMR **15**(1), 1–41 (2013)
2. Han, Y., et al.: k-Space Deep Learning for Accelerated MRI. arXiv:1805.03779 (2018)
3. Hauptmann, A., et al.: Real-time cardiovascular MR with spatio-temporal artifact suppression using deep learning-proof of concept in congenital heart disease. Magn. Reson. Med. **81**, 1143–1156 (2019)
4. Hyun, C.M., et al.: Deep learning for under sampled MRI reconstruction. Phys. Med. Biol. **63**(13), 135007 (2018)
5. Korshunova, I., et al.: Diagnosing heart diseases with deep neural networks (2016). http://irakorshunova.github.io/2016/03/15/heart.html
6. Liu, P., Fang, R.: Wide inference network for image denoising. arXiv preprint arXiv:1707.05414 (2017)
7. Lotjonen, J., et al.: Correction of motion artifacts from cardiac cine magnetic resonance images. Acad. Radiol. **12**(10), 1273–1284 (2005)
8. Oksuz, I., et al., Deep learning using k-space based data augmentation for automated cardiac MR motion artefact detection. In: MICCAI, pp. 250–258 (2018)
9. Oksuz, I., et al.: Cardiac MR motion artefact correction from k-space using deep learning-based reconstruction. In: MICCAI-MLMIR (2018)
10. Oksuz, I., et al.: Automatic CNN-based detection of cardiac MR motion artefacts using k-space data augmentation and curriculum learning. MedIA **55**, 250–258 (2018)
11. Petersen, S.E., et al.: UK Biobank's cardiovascular magnetic resonance protocol. JCMR **18**(1), 1–8 (2016)

12. Qin, C., et al.: Convolutional recurrent neural networks for dynamic MR image reconstruction. IEEE TMI **38**(1), 280–290 (2019)
13. Schlemper, J., et al.: A deep cascade of convolutional neural networks for dynamic MR image reconstruction. IEEE TMI **37**(2), 491–503 (2018)
14. Tran, D., et al.: Learning spatiotemporal features with 3D convolutional networks. In: ICCV, pp. 4489–4497 (2015)
15. Xie, J., et al.: Image denoising and inpainting with deep neural networks. In: Advances in Neural Information Processing Systems, pp. 341–349 (2012)
16. Zhang, K., et al.: Beyond a Gaussian denoiser: residual learning of deep CNN for image denoising. IEEE TIP **26**(7), 3142–3155 (2017)
17. Zhu, B., et al.: Image reconstruction by domain-transform manifold learning. Nature **555**(7697), 487 (2018)

Exploiting Motion for Deep Learning Reconstruction of Extremely-Undersampled Dynamic MRI

Gavin Seegoolam[1]([⊠]), Jo Schlemper[1], Chen Qin[1], Anthony Price[2], Jo Hajnal[2], and Daniel Rueckert[1]

[1] BioMedIA, Department of Computing, Imperial College London,
London SW7 2AZ, UK
{kgs13,js3611,dr}@ic.ac.uk
[2] Biomedical Engineering Department, Kings College London,
London WC2R 2LS, UK
{jo.hajnal,anthony.price}@kcl.ac.uk

Abstract. The problem of accelerated acquisition for dynamic MRI has been recently tackled with deep learning techniques. However, current state-of-the-art approaches do not incorporate a strategy to exploit the full temporal information of the k-space acquisition which would aid in producing higher quality reconstructions. In this paper, we propose a novel method for exploiting the full temporal dynamics for dynamic MRI reconstructions. Specifically, motion estimates are derived from undersampled MRI sequences. These are used to fuse data along the entire temporal axis to produce a novel *data-consistent motion-augmented cine* (DC-MAC). This is generated and utilised within an end-to-end trainable deep learning framework for MRI reconstruction. In particular, we find that for aggressive acceleration rates of ×51.2 on our cardiac dataset, our method with 3-fold cross-validation, ME-CNN, outperforms the current widely-accepted state-of-the-art, DC-CNN, with an improvement of 12% and 16% in PSNR and SSIM respectively. We report an average PSNR of 27.3 ± 2.5 and SSIM of 0.776 ± 0.054. We also explore the robustness of using ME-CNN for unseen, out-of-domain examples.

1 Introduction

The problem of image reconstruction for accelerated MRI has been a well-explored problem with approaches ranging from sensitivity encoding to Bayesian dictionary learning [3,5]. The process of MR image reconstruction typically involves the reconstruction of an image, vectorised as $\mathbf{y}$, from a set of data collected in the Fourier space (or 'k-space') of the scanner, $\hat{\mathbf{x}}$. The physics of

Electronic supplementary material The online version of this chapter (https://doi.org/10.1007/978-3-030-32251-9_77) contains supplementary material, which is available to authorized users.

D. Shen et al. (Eds.): MICCAI 2019, LNCS 11767, pp. 704–712, 2019.
https://doi.org/10.1007/978-3-030-32251-9_77

MR imaging relates $\hat{\mathbf{x}}$ and $\mathbf{y}$ through an encoding matrix $\mathbf{E}$ which applies coil-sensitivity maps, k-space undersampling and a Fourier transform to the image domain. This can be summarised as:

$$\hat{\mathbf{x}} = \mathbf{E}\mathbf{y} + \epsilon, \tag{1}$$

where ϵ represents the noise in the data acquisition. Since MRI data acquisition takes place in k-space, accelerated acquisition typically involves acquiring fewer samples in k-space whilst trying to reconstruct with the same resolution in image space. This is known as undersampling. Given the acquired undersampled k-space data, $\hat{\mathbf{x}}$, the process of finding the true image, $\mathbf{y}$, violates the Nyquist criterion and is thus ill-posed and typically ill-conditioned.

In this paper, we propose a novel deep learning approach for extremely-accelerated dynamic MR image reconstruction by exploiting motion present in MRI cines. The proposed method consists of three components: a motion estimation network; a *data-consistent motion-augmented cine* (DC-MAC) formed by intelligently propagating k-space information along the temporal axis; and a 3D CNN for MR image reconstruction. The use of the DC-MAC incorporates the full temporal k-space information into the reconstruction algorithm, where data across the whole sequence can be utilised for dealiasing each frame. The network is trained end-to-end by minimising a composite loss function which comprises of a motion estimation loss and an image reconstruction loss.

2 Related Work

More recently, there has been a shift towards deep learning for the reconstruction of MRI via compressed sensing approaches. However, a direct zero-filled reconstruction of the k-space data, $\hat{\mathbf{x}}$, leaves behind aliasing artefacts which drastically reduces perceptual quality. Instead, deep learning has been used to recover useful information from aliasing artefacts and subsequently improve image quality [4,7,9]. For dynamic MRI, the current widely accepted state-of-the-art is the DC-CNN studied by [9] which uses cascades of convolutional neural networks, with a residual connection from the input of each cascade to its reconstruction output. In addition to this, a *data consistency* (DC) step is applied to ensure the output of each cascade is consistent with the original k-space information.

In order to exploit the entire temporal domain, motion field estimation is required as will be explained in Sect. 3. Whilst motion estimation in the context of dynamic MRI reconstruction has been studied previously [2,10], we focus on a method for harvesting the *original* k-space acquisition within a *fast, deep learning framework* with performance highlighted for *extreme* undersampling. [6] studied the use of unsupervised learning for motion estimation in order to perform joint cardiac MRI segmentation and motion estimation [1,6]. This study used fully sampled MRI cines within a U-Net architecture trained to produce an optical flow estimate between a given frame and a target. The motion estimation technique used was based on [1]. In this study, we propose a novel pipeline to combine the methodology by [1,9]. The result is a unique, end-to-end-trainable *motion-estimating convolutional neural network*, or ME-CNN, which can reconstruct extremely undersampled dynamic MRIs. By explicitly exploiting motion, we contribute towards building MRI reconstruction models that can harness the full temporal domain of the original k-space sequence.

3   Methods

In brief, DC-CNN consists of N dealiasing units or 'cascades'. Each cascade takes a complex-valued estimate of the reconstruction as input (with additional 'data sharing' channels for neighbouring frames). It subsequently produces another, higher-quality cine as an output. This output cine is then subject to data consistency [9]. With our ME-CNN, we additionally provide each cascade with a novel *data-consistent motion-augmented cine*, also called x-DC-MAC, which exploits the full temporal information present in the original k-space data (with no data sharing required). As an additional set of channels, we also provide a method to motion-augmented the individual frame predictions from the previous cascade so that they can also be used for dealiasing. This is called y-DC-MAC. These DC-MACs are produced by learning a motion field, $\mathbf{u}_c$, for each cascade, c. The resulting process is illustrated in Fig. 1 and forms the ME-CNN architecture.

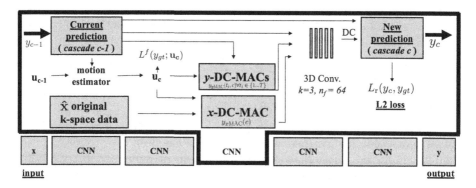

Fig. 1. The proposed ME-CNN architecture with one example cascade illustrated. The motion estimator is based on the U-net architecture [8] as shown in Supplementary Fig. 1. The motion field, $\mathbf{u}_c$, is used to produce the DC-MACs which are then concatenating with the prediction from the previous cascade i.e. y_{c-1}.

In terms of training, each cascade, c, outputs two values - an optical flow representation and a predicted MRI reconstruction. These are used in the total loss function described in Sect. 5 which consists of an optical flow loss and a reconstruction loss. In general, the predicted reconstruction, y_c, should improve in quality as you look at the output of deeper cascades. The prediction from the final cascade is used to produce the reconstruction loss. The optical flow, $\mathbf{u}_c^t$, of the MRI cine for each frame $t \in \{1...T\}$ is used to produce the optical flow loss. In our study $c \in \{1...N\}$ where $N = 5$ and $T = 30$ as thirty different cardiac phases were used in the construction of the dataset.

3.1   Motion Estimation

Within each cascade, a prediction of the motion field is made using an optical flow approach performed on the output of the previous cascade. In the case of the first cascade of the network, the original zero-filled reconstruction is used.

[1,6] showed that by training on the MSE loss between a motion-warped frame and its associated ground-truth, it is possible to learn the optical flow between frames in an unsupervised fashion. The important part of the loss for the motion field produced by a single cascade, c, is given by:

$$L_w^f(y_{\text{gt}}; \mathbf{u}_c) = \sum_{\mathbf{r},t} ||W(y_{\text{gt}}^t, \mathbf{u}_c^t) - y_{\text{gt}}^{t+1}||^2, \tag{2}$$

where y_{gt}^t is frame t of the ground truth, $\mathbf{u}_c^t$ is the motion field prediction from cascade c at time frame t and $W(y_{gt}^t, \mathbf{u}_c^t)$ warps frame y_{gt}^t using $\mathbf{u}_c^t$ and bilinear interpolation. There are two additional terms L_s^f and L_t^f which regularise the motion field, $\mathbf{u}_c$, with respect to its first order spatial and temporal gradients respectively. The total loss for the motion field output for a given cascade output in the network becomes Eq. (3) with hyperparameters α and β.

$$L^f(y_{gt}; \mathbf{u}_c) = L_w^f(y_{gt}; \mathbf{u}_c) + \alpha L_s^f(\mathbf{u}_c) + \beta L_t^f(\mathbf{u}_c). \tag{3}$$

3.2   Data-Consistent Motion-Augmented Cine (DC-MAC)

In order to better incorporate temporal information into the reconstruction of each frame, the full temporal-axis of the original k-space information is used to produce an intermediate cine reconstruction. The motion field, $\mathbf{u}_c$, from Sect. 3.1 is used to propagate the acquired k-space information from one frame, t, to the next frame, $t + 1$, whilst also acquiring the k-space information at frame $t + 1$. This can be repeated iteratively for all subsequent frames until a k-space is achieved that has collected data from the entire temporal-axis of the original data. Given the aquisition data, $\mathbf{x}$ and a motion field, $\mathbf{u}$, the DC-MAC generation process is summarised by Algorithm 1 in the supplementary material and Supplementary Figure 2. In particular, Eq. (4) shows the intermediate steps in the DC-MAC production process and Eq. (5) shows how the original k-space information, $\hat{x}$, is used in the generation of f_c^t, noting that x^t represents the zero-filled reconstruction for frame t.

$$f_c^{t+1}(t') = DC^{t+1} \circ W(f_c^t(t'), \mathbf{u}_c^t), \tag{4}$$

where DC^{t+1} is data consistency with the original k-space data, $\hat{x}$, at frame $t+1$ and t' is the frame number of the original k-space data to use as the first frame in the iterative warping process.

$$f_c^t(t) = x^t \tag{5}$$

When using the initial condition set by Eq. (5), the desired DC-MAC, which is referred to as x-DC-MAC, using the motion field from cascade c is given by Eq. (6).

$$y_{x\text{MAC}}^t(c) = f_c^{t+T}(t) \tag{6}$$

Using y_{c-1} to Generate a Set of DC-MACs for the Reconstruction of y_c. In addition to the x-DC-MAC, we can use the output prediction of the previous cascade, y_{c-1}, with the motion estimation of the current cascade, $\mathbf{u_c}$, to make further warped projections of the output cine. This is achieved by using a different initial condition from Eq. (5) within Eq. (4). Instead $f_c^t(t) = y_{c-1}^t$ is used. The result is the generation of T additional predictive cines (since there are T frames to create different initial conditions from). This is summarised by $y_{y\text{MAC}}^t(t_i, c) = f_c^t(t_i)$, where t_i is the frame number of the output from the previous cascade to use as the first frame in the iterative warping process.

4   Experiments

Architecture and Comparison to DC-CNN. The ME-CNN architecture is depicted in Fig. 1. DC-CNN is trained with a data-sharing width $n_d = 5$ and feature map size of $n_f = 96$, giving a total of 3.9M parameters in the full network. Our proposed model uses $n_f = 64$ and introduces an additional motion estimation branch bringing the total network to 3.8M parameters. Like DC-CNN, ME-CNN uses residual connections between cascades.

The total loss function combining all cascades $c = \{1...N\}$ becomes:

$$L(x, \{y_1...y_N\}, \{\mathbf{u_1}...\mathbf{u_N}\}, y_{gt}) = \sum_c^N w_c(L_r(y_c, y_{gt}) + \gamma L^f(y_{gt}; \mathbf{u_c})), \tag{7}$$

where $w_i = 2^{-(N-i)}$ is the cascade-weight parameter. It is important to note that the motion estimation network produces predictions based on undersampled and intermediate network reconstructions y_c but is trained on warping ground-truth frames, y_{gt}^t.

Dataset and Data Augmentation. In this study, the same dataset from the study in Schlemper et al. is used [9]. This consists of ten 256×256 short-axis cardiac MRI cines acquired with an SSFP sequence and $T = 30$ frames. Seven scans are used for training, one for validation and two for testing. In order to help prevent overfitting and generalise the de-aliasing process, the dataset was split into patches with a width of 32 pixels and retaining the original height of 256 pixels (which ensures that data-consistency can be applied). It was also augmented with on-the-fly random translations (± 50 pixels), random rotations ($\pm 45^o$) and randomly generated Gaussian-centered variable density undersampling masks. For testing, we generated 1000 undersampling masks per test example resulting in a large augmented test set of 2000 cines.

Hyper-parameters and Configuration. As advised in the study by Qin et al. (2018), we use $\alpha = 1 \times 10^{-3}$, $\beta = 1 \times 10^{-4}$ [6] and $\gamma = 50.0$. We sampled 2 central lines in the k-space.

Training. Each model was trained with a learning rate of 1×10^{-5} for 4×10^4 backpropagations, and then 1×10^{-6} for 2×10^4 backpropagations. This took 5 days on a NVIDIA Tesla P40 GPU but there are further advancements that will increase training speed in the near future. He initialisation was used with an Adam optimiser and parameters $\beta_1 = 0.9$, $\beta_2 = 0.999$ and $\epsilon = 1 \times 10^{-8}$. The model was developed using the TensorFlow v1.8 Python API.

5   Results

Our model was evaluated using three-fold cross validation. On an initialised model, each cine took an average of 55 s to reconstruct on an NVIDIA Tesla P40 GPU with 24 GB of memory. Table 1 shows the PSNR and SSIM statistics when computed across all three folds of the dataset. Across all three folds, ME-CNN performed better than DC-CNN with respect to SSIM for 100% of the test cases, and 89% of the time for PSNR. Figure 2 and Supplementary Figures 3 and 4 shows examples where ME-CNN have produced a perceptually better quality reconstruction. There are cases where the PSNR for DC-CNN are greater than that of ME-CNN. However, upon inspection, the ME-CNN still visually outperforms DC-CNN as is made clear by possessing a greater SSIM index (see Supplementary Figure 5).

(a)   **(b)**   **(c)**   **(d)**

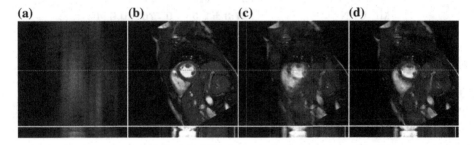

Fig. 2. (a) x51.2 undersampled frame (b) Ground truth mid-motion frame (c) Baseline model. PSNR: 25.9, SSIM: 0.74 (d) Proposed model. PSNR: 27.7, SSIM: 0.80. The images on the bottom row shown the temporal variation (vertical axis) of the slice given by the blue dotted line. The cines for the full ground-truth, DC-CNN, ME-CNN and DC-MAC (from the final cascade of ME-CNN) are found in Supplementary Figures. 6a, 6b, 6c and 6d respectively. (Color figure online)

5.1   Using the Motion Field for Reconstruction

The x-DC-MAC produced in this study was also examined. Using the model trained to reconstruct x51.2 undersampled cines, we evaluate our test set on much less aggressive undersampling rates of x9. Whilst the reconstruction outputs from DC-CNN were poor, ME-CNN produced more robust reconstructions.

Furthermore, the x-DC-MAC produced from the final cascade of ME-CNN produced a quality greater than that of both DC-CNN and ME-CNN. This is shown in Fig. 3. The motion field was used to warp each frame to the next frame in the ground-truth cine sequence, thus generating a new cine upon which motion field quality can be partially determined. For the x51.2 experiment, the cine produced an average PSNR of 39.5 ± 1.9 which is comparable to that of the x9 experiment of 39.6 ± 1.8 which indicates that whilst the dealiasing part of the network has not generalised well to other undersampling rates, the motion estimation network has. The generalisability of the motion estimation arguably helps provide more robustness to the neural network to unseen examples. Indeed, the perceptual quality of the reconstructions from ME-CNN outperform that of DC-CNN as shown in Table 2. Further experiments are required to see if there exists domain shifts where ME-CNN doesn't outperform DC-CNN.

Table 1. A comparison of the reconstructions produced by 3 different models, DC-CNN, DC-MAC and ME-CNN. The DC-MAC is from the final cascade of ME-CNN, $y_{x\mathrm{MAC}}^{t}(N)$. The difference in performance of each method on the same test sample is also recorded with the mean difference given by the entries starting with a 'Δ'.

Model	PSNR	SSIM
DC-CNN	24.4 ± 2.4	0.670 ± 0.081
DC-MAC	23.0 ± 1.8	0.628 ± 0.041
ME-CNN	$\mathbf{27.3 \pm 2.5}$	$\mathbf{0.776 \pm 0.054}$
Δ(ME-CNN − DC-CNN)	$\mathbf{2.82 \pm 2.34}$	$\mathbf{0.106 \pm 0.079}$
Δ(DC-MAC − DC-CNN)	-1.42 ± 1.77	-0.042 ± 0.062

Table 2. Video quality metrics when testing the generalisability of the trained x51.2-acceleration reconstruction models on x9-accelerated test data.

Model	PSNR	SSIM
DC-CNN	21.9 ± 5.3	0.570 ± 0.190
DC-MAC	$\mathbf{34.3 \pm 1.9}$	$\mathbf{0.930 \pm 0.023}$
ME-CNN	31.5 ± 1.5	0.874 ± 0.019
Δ(ME-CNN − DC-CNN)	9.57 ± 5.44	0.305 ± 0.182
Δ(DC-MAC − DC-CNN)	$\mathbf{12.44 \pm 5.45}$	$\mathbf{0.361 \pm 0.188}$

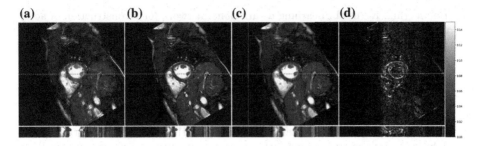

Fig. 3. (a) Baseline. PSNR: 28.29, SSIM: 0.75 (b) ME-CNN. PSNR: 32.2, SSIM: 0.89 (c) x-DC-MAC. PSNR: 35.2, SSIM: 0.94 (d) Absolute difference between x-DC-MAC and ground truth with colorbar (cine dynamic range is 1.0). The ground truth image is found in Fig. 2. The full ground-truth, x-DC-MAC for the final cascade and the absolute error cines are found in Supplementary Figures 10a, 10b and 10c respectively.

6   Conclusion

In conclusion, we observe that for aggressive undersampling rates where the DC-CNN approach is not able to effectively exploit the full temporal domain, the proposed ME-CNN is able to outperform the state-of-the-art approach. The proposed end-to-end trainable model was able to generate motion field estimations which were used to produce the DC-MACs. The increased performance of the network is largely due to the DC-MACs which allow the entire temporal axis to be exploited. We have demonstrated that ME-CNN is a more robust approach to dealiasing unseen examples of different acceleration rates. For future work, we will explore the use of ME-CNN for 3D reconstructions. We will also modify the ME-CNN to explore potential real-time imaging applications.

Acknowledgements. GS is funded by the KCL & ICL EPSRC CDT in Medical Imaging (EP/L015226/1). Additionally, this work was supported by EPSRC programme Grant (EP/P001009/1).

References

1. Ahmadi, A., Patras, I.: Unsupervised convolutional neural networks for motion estimation. In: 2016 IEEE International Conference on Image Processing (ICIP), pp. 1629–1633. IEEE (2016)
2. Aviles-Rivero, A.I., Williams, G., Graves, M.J., Schonlieb, C.B.: Compressed Sensing Plus Motion (CS+M): A New Perspective for Improving Undersampled MR Image Reconstruction. arXiv e-prints arXiv:1810.10828 (2018)
3. Caballero, J., Rueckert, D., Hajnal, J.V.: Dictionary learning and time sparsity in dynamic MRI. In: Ayache, N., Delingette, H., Golland, P., Mori, K. (eds.) MICCAI 2012. LNCS, vol. 7510, pp. 256–263. Springer, Heidelberg (2012). https://doi.org/10.1007/978-3-642-33415-3_32

4. Hammernik, K., et al.: Learning a variational network for reconstruction of accelerated MRI data. Magn. Reson. Med. **79**(6), 3055–3071 (2018)

5. Pruessmann, K.P., Weiger, M., Scheidegger, M.B., Boesiger, P.: Sense: sensitivity encoding for fast MRI. Magn. Reson. Med. **42**(5), 952–962 (1999)

6. Qin, C., et al.: Joint learning of motion estimation and segmentation for cardiac MR image sequences. In: Frangi, A.F., Schnabel, J.A., Davatzikos, C., Alberola-López, C., Fichtinger, G. (eds.) MICCAI 2018. LNCS, vol. 11071, pp. 472–480. Springer, Cham (2018). https://doi.org/10.1007/978-3-030-00934-2_53

7. Qin, C., Schlemper, J., Caballero, J., Price, A.N., Hajnal, J.V., Rueckert, D.: Convolutional recurrent neural networks for dynamic MR image reconstruction. IEEE Trans. Med. Imaging **38**(1), 280–290 (2019)

8. Ronneberger, O., Fischer, P., Brox, T.: U-Net: convolutional networks for biomedical image segmentation. In: Navab, N., Hornegger, J., Wells, W.M., Frangi, A.F. (eds.) MICCAI 2015. LNCS, vol. 9351, pp. 234–241. Springer, Cham (2015). https://doi.org/10.1007/978-3-319-24574-4_28

9. Schlemper, J., Caballero, J., Hajnal, J.V., Price, A.N., Rueckert, D.: A deep cascade of convolutional neural networks for dynamic MR image reconstruction. IEEE Trans. Med. Imaging **37**(2), 491–503 (2018)

10. Zhao, N., O'Connor, D., Basarab, A., Ruan, D., Sheng, K.: Motion compensated dynamic MRI reconstruction with local affine optical flow estimation. IEEE Trans. Biomed. Eng. 1 (2019). https://doi.org/10.1109/TBME.2019.2900037

VS-Net: Variable Splitting Network for Accelerated Parallel MRI Reconstruction

Jinming Duan[1,2(✉)], Jo Schlemper[2], Chen Qin[2], Cheng Ouyang[2], Wenjia Bai[2], Carlo Biffi[2], Ghalib Bello[3], Ben Statton[3], Declan P. O'Regan[3], and Daniel Rueckert[2]

[1] School of Computer Science, University of Birmingham, Birmingham, UK
j.duan@cs.bham.ac.uk
[2] Biomedical Image Analysis Group, Imperial College London, London, UK
[3] MRC London Institute of Medical Sciences, Imperial College London, London, UK

Abstract. In this work, we propose a deep learning approach for parallel magnetic resonance imaging (MRI) reconstruction, termed a variable splitting network (VS-Net), for an efficient, high-quality reconstruction of undersampled multi-coil MR data. We formulate the generalized parallel compressed sensing reconstruction as an energy minimization problem, for which a variable splitting optimization method is derived. Based on this formulation we propose a novel, end-to-end trainable deep neural network architecture by unrolling the resulting iterative process of such variable splitting scheme. VS-Net is evaluated on complex valued multi-coil knee images for 4-fold and 6-fold acceleration factors. We show that VS-Net outperforms state-of-the-art deep learning reconstruction algorithms, in terms of reconstruction accuracy and perceptual quality. Our code is publicly available at https://github.com/j-duan/VS-Net.

1 Introduction

Magnetic resonance imaging (MRI) is an important diagnostic and research tool in many clinical scenarios. However, its inherently slow data acquisition process is often problematic. To accelerate the scanning process, parallel MRI (p-MRI) and compressed sensing MRI (CS-MRI) are often employed. These methods are designed to facilitate fast reconstruction of high-quality, artifact-free images from minimal k-space data. Recently, deep learning approaches for MRI reconstruction [1–10] have demonstrated great promises for further acceleration of MRI acquisition. However, not all of these techniques [1,2,5,7,8] are able to exploit parallel image acquisitions which are common in clinical practice.

In this paper, we investigate accelerated p-MRI reconstruction using deep learning. We propose a novel, end-to-end trainable approach for this task which

---

J. Duan and J. Schlemper—Contributed equally.

Electronic supplementary material The online version of this chapter (https://doi.org/10.1007/978-3-030-32251-9_78) contains supplementary material, which is available to authorized users.

© Springer Nature Switzerland AG 2019
D. Shen et al. (Eds.): MICCAI 2019, LNCS 11767, pp. 713–722, 2019.
https://doi.org/10.1007/978-3-030-32251-9_78

we refer to as a variable splitting network (VS-Net). VS-Net builds on a general parallel CS-MRI concept, which is formulated as a multi-variable energy minimization process in a deep learning framework. It has three computational blocks: a denoiser block, a data consistency block and a weighted average block. The first one is a denoising convolutional neural network (CNN), while the latter two have point-wise closed-form solutions. As such, VS-Net is computationally efficient yet simple to implement. VS-Net accepts complex-valued multi-channel MRI data and learns all parameters automatically during offline training. In a series of experiments, we monitor reconstruction accuracies obtained from varying the number of stages in VS-Net. We studied different parameterizations for weight parameters in VS-Net and analyzed their numerical behaviour. We also evaluated VS-Net performance on a multi-coil knee image dataset for different acceleration factors using the Cartesian undersampling patterns, and showed improved image quality and preservation of tissue textures.

To this end, we point out the differences between our method and related works in [1–4,8], as well as highlight our novel contributions to this area. First, data consistency (DC) layer introduced in [1] was designed for single-coil images. MoDL [4] extended the cascade idea of [1] to a multi-coil setting. However, its DC layer implementation was through iteratively solving a linear system using the conjugate gradient in their network, which can be very complicated. In contrast, DC layer in VS-Net naturally applies to multi-coil images, and is also a point-wise, analytical solution, making VS-Net both computationally efficient and numerically accurate. Variational network (VN) [3] and [8] were applicable to multi-coil images. However, they were based gradient-descent optimization and proximal methods respectively, which does not impose the exact DC. Compared ADMM-net [2] to VS-Net, the former was also only applied to single-coil images. Moreover, ADMM-Net was derived from the augmented Lagrangian method (ALM), while VS-Net uses a penalty function method, which results in a simpler network architecture. ALM introduces Lagrange multipliers to weaken the dependence on penalty weight selection. While these weights can be learned automatically in network training, the need for a network with a more complicated ALM is not clear. In ADMM-Net and VN, the regularization term was defined via a set of explicit learnable linear filter kernels. In contrast, VS-Net treats regularization implicitly in a CNN-denoising process. Consequently, VS-Net has the flexibility of using varying advanced denoising CNN architectures while avoiding expensive dense matrix inversion - a encountered problem in ADMM-Net. A final distinction is that the effect of different weight parameterizations is studied in VS-Net, while this was not investigated previously.

2   VS-Net for Accelerated p-MRI Reconstruction

General CS p-MRI Model: Let $m \in \mathbb{C}^N$ be a complex-valued MR image stacked as a column vector and $y_i \in \mathbb{C}^M$ ($M < N$) be the under-sampled k-space data measured from the ith MR receiver coil. Recovering m from y_i is an ill-posed inverse problem. According to compressed sensing (CS) theory, one can estimate the reconstructed image m by minimizing:

$$\min_{m} \left\{ \frac{\lambda}{2} \sum_{i=1}^{n_c} \|\mathcal{DFS}_i m - y_i\|_2^2 + \mathcal{R}(m) \right\}, \tag{1}$$

In the data fidelity term (first term), n_c denotes the number of receiver coils, $\mathcal{D} \in \mathbb{R}^{M \times N}$ is the sampling matrix that zeros out entries that have not been acquired, $\mathcal{F} \in \mathbb{C}^{N \times N}$ is the Fourier transform matrix, $S_i \in \mathbb{C}^{N \times N}$ is the ith coil sensitivity, and λ is a model weight that balances the two terms. Note that the coil sensitivity S_i is a diagonal matrix, which can be pre-computed from the fully sampled k-space center using the E-SPIRiT algorithm [11]. The second term is a general sparse regularization term, e.g. (nonlocal) total variation [12,13], total generalized variation [12,14] or the $\ell 1$ penalty on the discrete wavelet transform of m [15].

Variable Splitting: In order to optimize (1) efficiently, we develop a variable splitting method. Specifically, we introduce the auxiliary splitting variables $u \in \mathbb{C}^N$ and $\{x_i \in \mathbb{C}^N\}_{i=1}^{n_c}$, converting (1) into the following equivalent form

$$\min_{m,u,x_i} \frac{\lambda}{2} \sum_{i=1}^{n_c} \|\mathcal{DF}x_i - y_i\|_2^2 + \mathcal{R}(u) \ s.t. \ m = u, \ S_i m = x_i, \ \forall i \in \{1,2,...,n_c\}.$$

The introduction of the first constraint $m = u$ decouples m in the regularization from that in the data fidelity term so that a denoising problem can be explicitly formulated (see Eq. (3) top). The introduction of the second constraint $S_i m = x_i$ is also crucial as it allows decomposition of $S_i m$ from $\mathcal{DF}S_i m$ in the data fidelity term such that no dense matrix inversion is involved in subsequent calculations (see Eq. (4) middle and bottom). Using the penalty function method, we then add these constraints back into the model and minimize the single problem

$$\min_{m,u,x_i} \frac{\lambda}{2} \sum_{i=1}^{n_c} \|\mathcal{DF}x_i - y_i\|_2^2 + \mathcal{R}(u) + \frac{\alpha}{2} \sum_{i=1}^{n_c} \|x_i - S_i m\|_2^2 + \frac{\beta}{2} \|u - m\|_2^2, \tag{2}$$

where α and β are introduced penalty weights. To minimize (2), which is a multi-variable optimization problem, one needs to alternatively optimize m, u and x_i by solving the following three subproblems:

$$\begin{cases} u^{k+1} = \arg\min_{u} \frac{\beta}{2} \|u - m^k\|_2^2 + \mathcal{R}(u) \\ x_i^{k+1} = \arg\min_{x_i} \lambda \sum_{i=1}^{n_c} \|\mathcal{DF}x_i - y_i\|_2^2 + \frac{\alpha}{2} \sum_{i=1}^{n_c} \|x_i - S_i m^k\|_2^2, \\ m^{k+1} = \arg\min_{m} \frac{\alpha}{2} \sum_{i=1}^{n_c} \|x_i^{k+1} - S_i m\|_2^2 + \frac{\beta}{2} \|u^{k+1} - m\|_2^2 \end{cases} \tag{3}$$

Here $k \in \{1,2,...,n_{it}\}$ denotes the kth iteration. An optimal solution (m^*) may be found by iterating over u^{k+1}, x_i^{k+1} and m^{k+1} until convergence is achieved or the number of iterations reaches n_{it}. An initial solution to these subproblems can be derived as follows

$$\begin{cases} u^{k+1} = denoiser(m^k) \\ x_i^{k+1} = \mathcal{F}^{-1}((\lambda \mathcal{D}^T \mathcal{D} + \alpha I)^{-1}(\alpha \mathcal{F} S_i m^k + \lambda \mathcal{D}^T y_i)) \quad \forall i \in \{1, 2, ..., n_c\} \\ m^{k+1} = (\beta I + \alpha \sum_{i=1}^{n_c} S_i^H S_i)^{-1}(\beta u^{k+1} + \alpha \sum_{i=1}^{n_c} S_i^H x_i^{k+1}) \end{cases} \quad (4)$$

Above S_i^H is the conjugate transpose of S_i and I is the identity matrix of size N by N. $\mathcal{D}^T \mathcal{D}$ is a diagonal matrix of size N by N, whose diagonal entries are either zero or one corresponding to a binary sampling mask. $\mathcal{D}^T y_i$ is an N-length vector, representing the k-space measurements (ith coil) with the unsampled positions filled with zeros. In this step we have turned the original problem (1) into a denoising problem (denoted by *denoiser*) and two other equations, both of which have closed-form solutions that can be computed point-wise due to the nature of diagonal matrix inversion. We also note that the middle equation efficiently imposes the consistency between k-space data and image space data coil-wisely, and the bottom equation simply computes a weighted average of the results obtained from the first two equations. Next, we will show an appropriate network architecture can be derived by unfolding the iterations of (4).

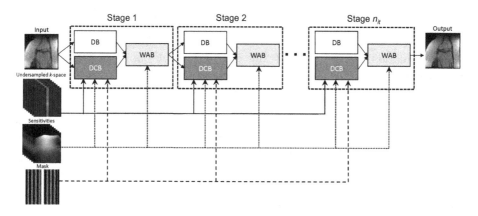

Fig. 1. Overall architecture of the proposed variable splitting network (VS-Net).

Network Architecture: We propose a deep cascade network that naturally integrates the iterative procedures in Eq. (4). Figure 1 depicts the network architecture. Specifically, one iteration of an iterative reconstruction is related to one stage in the network. In each stage, there are three blocks: denoiser block (DB), data consistency block (DCB) and weighted average block (WAB), which respectively correspond to the three equations in (4). The network takes four inputs: (1) the single sensitivity-weighted undersampled image which is computed using $\sum_i^{n_c} S_i^H \mathcal{F}^{-1} \mathcal{D}^T y_i$; (2) the pre-computed coil sensitivity maps $\{S_i\}_{i=1}^{n_c}$; (3) the binary sampling mask $\mathcal{D}^T \mathcal{D}$; (4) the undersampled k-space data $\{\mathcal{D}^T y_i\}_{i=1}^{n_c}$. Note

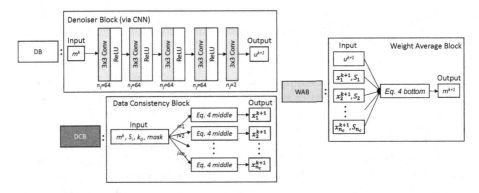

Fig. 2. Detailed structure of each block in VS-net. DB, DCB and WAB stand for Denoiser Block, Data Consistency Block and Weighted Average Block, respectively.

that the sensitivity-weighted undersampled image is only used once for DB and DCB in Stage 1. In contrast, $\{\mathcal{D}^T y_i\}_{i=1}^{n_c}$, $\{S_i\}_{i=1}^{n_c}$ and the mask are required for WAB and DCB at each stage (see Figs. 1 and 2). As the network is guided by the iterative process resulting from the variable splitting method, we refer to it as a Variable Splitting Network (VS-Net).

In Fig. 2, we illustrate the detailed structures of key building blocks of the network (DB, DCB and WAB) at Stage k in VS-Net. In DB, we intend to denoise a complex-valued image with a convolutional neural network (CNN). To handle complex values, we stack real and imaginary parts of the undersampled input into a real-valued two-channel image. ReLU's are used to add nonlinearities to the *denoiser* to increase its denoising capability. Note that while we use a simple CNN here, our setup allows for incorporation of more advanced denoising CNN architectures. In DCB, m^k from the upstream block, $\{S_i\}_{i=1}^{n_c}$, $\{k_i\}_{i=1}^{n_c}$ (i.e. the undersampled k-space data of all coils) and the mask are taken as inputs, passing through the middle equation of (4) and outputting $\{x_i^{k+1}\}_{i=1}^{n_c}$. The outputs u^{k+1} and $\{x_i^{k+1}\}_{i=1}^{n_c}$ from DCB and WAB, concurrently with the coil sensitivity maps, are fed to WAB producing m^{k+1}, which is then used as the input to DB and DCB in the next stage in VS-Net. Due to the existence of analytical solutions, no iteration is required in WAB and DCB. Further, all the computational operations in WAB and DCB are point-wise. These features make the calculations in the two blocks simple and efficient. The process proceeds in the same manner until Stage n_{it} is reached.

Network Loss and Parameterizations: Training the proposed VS-Net is another optimization process, for which a loss function must be explicitly formulated. In MR reconstruction, the loss function often defines the similarity between the reconstructed image and a clean, artifact-free reference image. For example, a common choice for the loss function used in this work is the mean squared error (MSE), given by

$$\mathcal{L}(\boldsymbol{\Theta}) = \min_{\boldsymbol{\Theta}} \frac{1}{2n_i} \sum_{i=1}^{n_i} \|m_i^{n_{it}}(\boldsymbol{\Theta}) - g_i\|_2^2, \tag{5}$$

where n_i is the number of training images, and g is the reference image, which is a sensitivity-weighted fully sampled image computed by $\sum_j^{n_c} S_j^H \mathcal{F}^{-1} f_j$. Here f_j represents the fully sampled raw data of the jth coil. $\boldsymbol{\Theta}$ above are the network parameters $\boldsymbol{\Theta}$ to be learned. In this work we study two parameterizations for $\boldsymbol{\Theta}$, i.e., $\boldsymbol{\Theta^1} = \{\{\mathbf{W}^l\}_{l=1}^{n_{it}}, \lambda, \alpha, \beta\}$ and $\boldsymbol{\Theta^2} = \{\{\mathbf{W}^l, \lambda^l, \alpha^l, \beta^l\}_{l=1}^{n_{it}}\}$. Here $\{\mathbf{W}^l\}_{l=1}^{n_{it}}$ are learnable parameters for all (n_{it}) CNN denoising blocks in VS-Net. Moreover, in both cases we also make the data fidelity weight λ and the penalty weights α and β learnable parameters. In contrast, for $\boldsymbol{\Theta^1}$ we let the weights λ, α and β be shared by the WABs and DCBs across VS-Net, while for $\boldsymbol{\Theta^2}$ each WAB and DCB have their own learnable weights. Since all the blocks are differentiable, backpropagation (BP) can be effectively employed to minimize the loss with respect to the network parameters $\boldsymbol{\Theta}$ in an end-to-end fashion.

3   Experiments Results

Datasets and Training Details: We used a publicly available clinical knee dataset[1] in [3], which has the following 5 image acquisition protocols: coronal proton-density (PD), coronal fat-saturated PD, axial fat-saturated T_2, sagittal fat-saturated T_2 and sagittal PD. For each acquisition protocol, the same 20 subjects were scanned using an off-the-shelf 15-element knee coil. The scan of each subject cover approximately 40 slices and each slice has 15 channels ($n_c = 15$). Coil sensitivity maps provided in the dataset were precomputed from a data block of size 24×24 at the center of fully sampled k-space using BART [16]. For training, we retrospectively undersampled the original k-space data for 4-fold and 6-fold acceleration factors (AF) with Cartesian undersampling, sampling 24 lines at the central region. For each acquisition protocol, we split the subjects into training and testing subsets (each with sample size of 10), and trained VS-Net to reconstruct each slice in a 2D fashion. The network parameters was optimized for 200 epochs, using Adam with learning rate 10^{-3} and batch size 1. We used PSNR and SSIM as quantitative performance metrics.

Parameter Behaviour: To show the impact of the stage number n_{it} (see Fig. 1), we first experiment on the subjects under the coronal PD protocol with 4-fold AF. We set $n_{it} = \{1, 3, 5, 7, 10, 15, 20\}$ and plotted the training and testing quantitative curves versus the number of epochs in the upper portion of Fig. 3. As the plots show, increasing the stage number improves network performance. This is obvious for two reasons: (1) as number of parameters increases, so does the network's learning capability; (2) the embedded variable splitting minimization is an iterative process, for which sufficient iterations (stages) are required to converge to an ideal solution. We also found that: (i) the performance difference between $n_{it} = 15$ and $n_{it} = 20$ is negligible as the network gradually converges

---

[1]   https://github.com/VLOGroup/mri-variationalnetwork.

after $n_{it} = 15$; (ii) there is no overfitting during network training despite the use of a relatively small training set. Second, we examine the network performance when using two different parameterizations: $\Theta^1 = \{\{\mathbf{W}^l\}_{l=1}^{n_{it}}, \lambda, \alpha, \beta\}$ and $\Theta^2 = \{\{\mathbf{W}^l, \lambda^l, \alpha^l, \beta^l\}_{l=1}^{n_{it}}\}$. For a fair comparison, we used the same initialization for both parameterizations and experimented with two cases $n_{it} = \{5, 10\}$. As shown in the bottom portion of Fig. 3, in both cases the network with Θ^1 performs slightly worse than the one with Θ^2. In penalty function methods, a penalty weight is usually shared (fixed) across iterations. However, our experiments indicated improved performance if the model weights (λ, α and β) are non-shared or adaptive at each stage in the network.

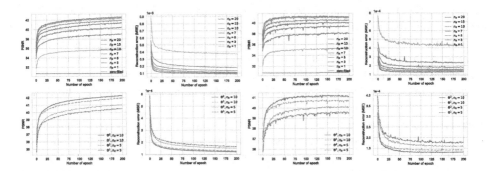

Fig. 3. Quantitative measures versus number of epochs at training (first two columns) and testing (last two columns). 1st row shows the network performance using different stage numbers. 2nd column shows the network performance using different parameterizations of Θ in the loss (5).

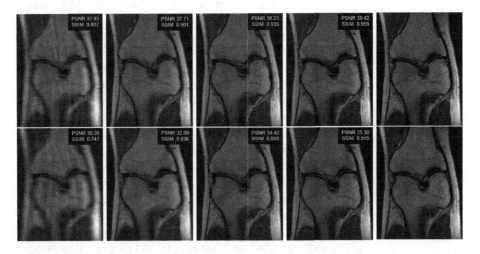

Fig. 4. Visual comparison of results obtained by different methods for Cartesian undersampling with AF 4 (top) and 6 (bottom). From left to right: zero-filling results, $\ell 1$-SPIRiT results, VN results, VS-Net results, and ground truth. See the supplementary for more visual comparison.

Numerical Comparison: We compared our VS-Net with the iterative $\ell1$-SPIRiT [17] and the variational network (VN) [3], with the zero-filling reconstruction as a reference. For VS-Net, we used n_{it} (10) and Θ^2, although the network's performance can be further boosted with a larger n_{it}. For VN, we carried out training using mostly default hyper-parameters from [3], except for the batch size, which (using original image size) was set to 1 to better fit GPU memory. For both VS-Net and VN, we trained a separate model for each protocol, resulting in a total of 20 models for the 4-fold and 6-fold AFs. In Table 1, we summarize the quantitative results obtained by these methods. As is evident, learning-based methods VS-Net and VN outperformed the iterative $\ell1$-SPIRiT. VN produced comparable SSIMs to VS-Net in some scenarios. The resulting PNSRs were however lower than that of VS-Net for all acquisition protocols and AFs, indicating the superior numerical performance of VS-Net. In Fig. 4, we present a visual comparison on a coronal PD image reconstruction for both AFs. Apart from zero-filling, all methods removed aliasing artifacts successfully. Among $\ell1$-SPIRiT, VN and VS-Net, VS-Net recovered more small, textural details and thus achieved the best visual results, relative to the ground truth. The quantitative metrics in Fig. 4 further show that VS-Net is the best.

Table 1. Quantitative results obtained by different methods on the test set including ~2000 image slices across 5 acquisition protocols. Each metric was calculated on ~400 image slices, and mean ± standard deviation are reported.

Protocol	Method	4-fold AF		6-fold AF	
		PSNR	SSIM	PSNR	SSIM
Coronal fat-sat. PD	Zero-filling	32.34 ± 2.83	0.80 ± 0.11	30.47 ± 2.71	0.74 ± 0.14
	$\ell1$-SPIRiT	34.57 ± 3.32	0.81 ± 0.11	31.51 ± 2.21	$\mathbf{0.78 \pm 0.08}$
	VN	35.83 ± 4.43	$\mathbf{0.84 \pm 0.13}$	32.90 ± 4.66	$\mathbf{0.78 \pm 0.15}$
	VS-Net	$\mathbf{36.00 \pm 3.83}$	$\mathbf{0.84 \pm 0.13}$	$\mathbf{33.24 \pm 3.44}$	$\mathbf{0.78 \pm 0.15}$
Coronal PD	Zero-filling	31.35 ± 3.84	0.87 ± 0.11	29.39 ± 3.81	0.84 ± 0.13
	$\ell1$-SPIRiT	39.38 ± 2.16	0.93 ± 0.03	34.06 ± 2.41	0.88 ± 0.04
	VN	40.14 ± 4.97	0.94 ± 0.12	36.01 ± 4.63	0.90 ± 0.13
	VS-Net	$\mathbf{41.27 \pm 5.25}$	$\mathbf{0.95 \pm 0.12}$	$\mathbf{36.77 \pm 4.84}$	$\mathbf{0.92 \pm 0.14}$
Axial fat-sat. T_2	Zero-filling	36.47 ± 2.34	0.94 ± 0.02	34.90 ± 2.39	0.92 ± 0.02
	$\ell1$-SPIRiT	39.38 ± 2.70	0.94 ± 0.03	35.44 ± 2.87	0.91 ± 0.03
	VN	42.10 ± 1.97	$\mathbf{0.97 \pm 0.01}$	37.94 ± 2.29	$\mathbf{0.94 \pm 0.02}$
	VS-Net	$\mathbf{42.34 \pm 2.06}$	0.96 ± 0.01	$\mathbf{39.40 \pm 2.10}$	$\mathbf{0.94 \pm 0.02}$
Sagittal fat-sat. T_2	Zero-filling	37.35 ± 2.69	0.93 ± 0.07	35.25 ± 2.68	0.90 ± 0.09
	$\ell1$-SPIRiT	41.27 ± 2.95	0.94 ± 0.06	36.00 ± 2.67	0.92 ± 0.05
	VN	42.84 ± 3.47	$\mathbf{0.95 \pm 0.07}$	38.92 ± 3.23	$\mathbf{0.93 \pm 0.09}$
	VS-Net	$\mathbf{43.10 \pm 3.44}$	$\mathbf{0.95 \pm 0.07}$	$\mathbf{39.07 \pm 3.33}$	0.92 ± 0.09
Sagittal PD	Zero-filling	37.12 ± 2.58	0.96 ± 0.04	35.96 ± 2.57	0.94 ± 0.05
	$\ell1$-SPIRiT	44.52 ± 1.94	0.97 ± 0.02	39.14 ± 2.12	0.96 ± 0.02
	VN	46.34 ± 2.75	$\mathbf{0.98 \pm 0.05}$	39.71 ± 2.58	$\mathbf{0.96 \pm 0.05}$
	VS-Net	$\mathbf{47.22 \pm 2.89}$	0.98 ± 0.04	$\mathbf{40.11 \pm 2.46}$	$\mathbf{0.96 \pm 0.05}$

4   Conclusion

In this paper, we proposed the variable spitting network (VS-Net) for accelerated reconstruction of parallel MR images. We have detailed how to formulate VS-Net as an iterative energy minimization process embedded in a deep learning framework, where each stage essentially corresponds to one iteration of an iterative reconstruction. In experiments, we have shown that the performance of VS-Net gradually plateaued as the network stage number increased, and that setting parameters in each stage as learnable improved the quantitative results. Further, we have evaluated VS-Net on a multi-coil knee image dataset for 4-fold and 6-fold acceleration factors under Cartesian undersampling and showed its superiority over two state-of-the-art methods.

Acknowledgements. This work was supported by the EPSRC Programme Grant (EP/P001009/1) and the British Heart Foundation (NH/17/1/32725). The TITAN Xp GPU used for this research was kindly donated by the NVIDIA Corporation.

References

1. Schlemper, J., et al.: A deep cascade of convolutional neural networks for dynamic MR image reconstruction. IEEE Trans. Med. Imag. **37**(2), 491–503 (2018)
2. Yan, Y., et al.: Deep ADMM-Net for compressive sensing MRI. In: NIPS, pp. 10–18 (2016)
3. Hammernik, K., et al.: Learning a variational network for reconstruction of accelerated MRI data. Magn. Reson. Med. **79**(6), 3055–3071 (2018)
4. Aggarwal, H.K., et al.: MoDL: model-based deep learning architecture for inverse problems. IEEE Trans. Med. Imag. **38**(2), 394–405 (2019)
5. Han, Y., et al.: k-space deep learning for accelerated MRI. arXiv:1805.03779 (2018)
6. Akcakaya, M., et al.: Scan-specific robust artificial-neural-networks for k-space interpolation (RAKI) reconstruction: database-free deep learning for fast imaging. Magn. Reson. Med. **81**(1), 439–453 (2018)
7. Jin, K., et al.: Self-supervised deep active accelerated MRI. arXiv:1901.04547 (2019)
8. Mardani, M., et al.: Deep generative adversarial neural networks for compressive sensing MRI. IEEE Trans. Med. Imag. **38**(1), 167–179 (2019)
9. Tezcan, K., et al.: MR image reconstruction using deep density priors. IEEE Trans. Med. Imag. (2018)
10. Zhang, P., Wang, F., Xu, W., Li, Y.: Multi-channel generative adversarial network for parallel magnetic resonance image reconstruction in K-space. In: Frangi, A.F., Schnabel, J.A., Davatzikos, C., Alberola-López, C., Fichtinger, G. (eds.) MICCAI 2018. LNCS, vol. 11070, pp. 180–188. Springer, Cham (2018). https://doi.org/10.1007/978-3-030-00928-1_21
11. Uecker, M., et al.: ESPIRiT an eigenvalue approach to autocalibrating parallel MRI: where sense meets grappa. Magn. Reson. Med. **71**(3), 990–1001 (2014)
12. Lu, W., et al.: Implementation of high-order variational models made easy for image processing. Math. Method Appl. Sci. **39**(14), 4208–4233 (2016)
13. Lu, W., et al.: Graph-and finite element-based total variation models for the inverse problem in diffuse optical tomography. Biomed. Opt. Express **10**(6), 2684–2707 (2019)

14. Duan, J., et al.: Denoising optical coherence tomography using second order total generalized variation decomposition. Biomed. Signal Process. Control **24**, 120–127 (2016)
15. Liu, R.W., et al.: Undersampled CS image reconstruction using nonconvex nonsmooth mixed constraints. Multimed. Tools Appl. **78**(10), 12749–12782 (2019)
16. Uecker, M., et al.: Software toolbox and programming library for compressed sensing and parallel imaging, Citeseer
17. Murphy, M., et al.: Fast l1-spirit compressed sensing parallel imaging MRI: Scalable parallel implementation and clinically feasible runtime. IEEE Trans. Med. Imag. **31**(6), 1250–1262 (2012)

A Novel Loss Function Incorporating Imaging Acquisition Physics for PET Attenuation Map Generation Using Deep Learning

Luyao Shi[1], John A. Onofrey[1], Enette Mae Revilla[1],
Takuya Toyonaga[1], David Menard[2], Joseph Ankrah[2],
Richard E. Carson[1], Chi Liu[1], and Yihuan Lu[1(✉)]

[1] Yale University, New Haven, CT 06520, USA
Yihuan.lu@yale.edu
[2] Yale New Haven Hospital, New Haven, CT 06520, USA

Abstract. In PET/CT imaging, CT is used for PET attenuation correction (AC). Mismatch between CT and PET due to patient body motion results in AC artifacts. In addition, artifact caused by metal, beam-hardening and count-starving in CT itself also introduces inaccurate AC for PET. Maximum likelihood reconstruction of activity and attenuation (MLAA) was proposed to solve those issues by simultaneously reconstructing tracer activity (λ-MLAA) and attenuation map (μ-MLAA) based on the PET raw data only. However, μ-MLAA suffers from high noise and λ-MLAA suffers from large bias as compared to the reconstruction using the CT-based attenuation map (μ-CT). Recently, a convolutional neural network (CNN) was applied to predict the CT attenuation map (μ-CNN) from λ-MLAA and μ-MLAA, in which an image-domain loss (IM-loss) function between the μ-CNN and the ground truth μ-CT was used. However, IM-loss does not directly measure the AC errors according to the PET attenuation physics, where the line-integral projection of the attenuation map (μ) along the path of the two annihilation events, instead of the μ itself, is used for AC. Therefore, a network trained with the IM-loss may yield suboptimal performance in the μ generation. Here, we propose a novel line-integral projection loss (LIP-loss) function that incorporates the PET attenuation physics for μ generation. Eighty training and twenty testing datasets of whole-body ^{18}F-FDG PET and paired ground truth μ-CT were used. Quantitative evaluations showed that the model trained with the additional LIP-loss was able to significantly outperform the model trained solely based on the IM-loss function.

Keywords: Synthetic attenuation map · Deep learning · PET

1 Introduction

Positron Emission Tomography (PET) is used to assess physiological or pathological processes, e.g., cancer staging, via the use of specific tracers. Those assessments rely on *in vivo* radiotracer quantification based on PET images, which require accurate attenuation correction (AC). CT-based AC is commonly used for PET/CT studies. However, mismatch between CT and PET due to patient body motion [1] results in AC artifacts

© Springer Nature Switzerland AG 2019
D. Shen et al. (Eds.): MICCAI 2019, LNCS 11767, pp. 723–731, 2019.
https://doi.org/10.1007/978-3-030-32251-9_79

and thus inaccurate PET quantification. In addition, artifact caused by metal, beam-hardening and count-starving in CT itself also introduces inaccurate AC for PET. Therefore, a method that can generate an accurate attenuation map (μ) is critical for accurate radiotracer quantification in PET.

The maximum likelihood reconstruction of activity and attenuation (MLAA) algorithm [2] was proposed to simultaneously reconstruct tracer activity (λ-MLAA) and artifact-free attenuation map (μ-MLAA) based on the time-of-flight (TOF) PET raw data only. However, mainly due to the limited TOF timing resolution, μ-MLAA suffers from high noise and λ-MLAA suffers from large bias [3] as compared to the standard maximum likelihood expectation maximization reconstruction using the CT-based attenuation map (μ-CT). Recently, Hwang et al. [4] proposed to use a convolutional neural network (CNN) to predict the CT attenuation map (μ-CNN) from λ-MLAA and μ-MLAA. Similar to other image-to-image translation work [5, 6], Hwang et al. [4] used the L1-norm between the μ-CNN and the ground truth μ-CT in the image domain as a loss function (IM-loss). However, this loss choice does not directly measure the AC errors according to the PET attenuation physics, where the line-integral of the μ along the path of the two annihilation events, instead of μ itself, is used for AC. Therefore, a CNN trained using the IM-loss function may yield suboptimal performance in the μ generation task. In this study, we propose a novel loss function that uses the line-integral projection (LIP-loss) of μ as the loss, in addition to the IM-loss, for μ generation. Our hypothesis is that the additional LIP-loss will provide a stronger constraint than the IM-loss alone for μ generation, and therefore a more accurate μ can be generated.

We evaluated our method on real whole-body PET/CT datasets. Experimental results demonstrate that incorporating the proposed LIP-loss in the network training significantly improved the accuracy of the predicted μ and yielded more accurate quantification in the final attenuation corrected PET images compared with the conventional training strategy using only the IM-loss.

2 Datasets

For this study, 220 whole-body, i.e., skull to feet, ^{18}F-FDG PET/CT scan data of patients were acquired using a Siemens Biograph mCT 40 scanner. Based on careful human-observer examination, i.e., visual comparison between λ-MLAA/μ-MLAA and CT, 100 scans with minimal mismatch, i.e., body motion free, between the ground truth μ-CT and PET, were selected for training (N = 80) and testing (N = 20). The CTs for the 100 selected scans were also without artifacts. All scans were performed ~ 60 min after intravenous injection of ~ 10 mCi ^{18}F-FDG. The entire body of each patient with arm-down position was scanned using the continuous bed motion protocol for ~ 20 min. For MLAA, we used the same implementation as in [3] with 3 iterations by 21 subsets. Both λ-MLAA and μ-MLAA were originally reconstructed using 2 mm voxel size followed by 5 mm Gaussian post-smoothing, and were further down-sampled to 4 mm. CT attenuation maps were generated using the Siemens e7 toolkit and down-sampled to 4 mm voxel in width to save GPU memory in the later network training.

3   Methods

3.1   Line-Integral Projection Loss (LIP-Loss) Function

The LIP-loss measures the line-integral difference between the image patch X of the predicted μ and the ground-truth patch Y of μ-CT in the projection domain:

$$L_{LIP}(X, Y) = \frac{1}{N_{\mathbb{K}}} \sum_{k \in \mathbb{K}} \frac{\sum_{i=1}^{N_k} \left([P_k X]_i - [P_k Y]_i\right)^2}{N_k} \qquad (1)$$

where $\mathbb{K}$ is the set of line-integral projection (LIP) angles, k is the index for the projection angles, $N_{\mathbb{K}}$ is the total number of angles in $\mathbb{K}$, P_k is the LIP operator on the image X and Y at the k-th angle, i is the pixel index in the projection domain and N_k is the total number of pixels in the LIP $P_k X$ and $P_k Y$. Set $\mathbb{K}$ was designed such that $N_{\mathbb{K}}$ angles were uniformly sampled over $180°$, i.e., $\mathbb{K} = \{0°, 45°, 90°, 135°\}$ in the case of $N_{\mathbb{K}} = 4$. In our implementation, we rotated the images (using bilinear interpolation) and perform LIP at a single angle, instead of performing LIP at different angles. Note that the LIP-loss can be easily back-propagated to update the weights in the network, since the LIP operator P_k is a linear operation so that the loss function is differentiable.

In terms of loss function, the conventional IM-loss is constructed as

$$L_{IM}(X, Y) = L_{L1}(X, Y) + \lambda_1 L_{GDL}(X, Y), \qquad (2)$$

where L_{L1} is an L1-norm loss, which was reported [5, 6] to better preserve anatomical structures than an L2-norm loss. L_{GDL} is an image gradient difference loss defined as:

$$L_{GDL}(X, Y) = ||\nabla X_x| - |\nabla Y_x||^2 + ||\nabla X_y| - |\nabla Y_y||^2 + ||\nabla X_z| - |\nabla Z_z||^2, \qquad (3)$$

where ∇ is the gradient operator. L_{GDL} is used to further discourage image blurring [7].

To enforce the additional similarity in the projection domain between the predicted and ground-truth μ-CT, the proposed LIP-loss (L_{LIP}) was added to the IM-loss as:

$$L_{TOTAL}(X, Y) = L_{L1}(X, Y) + \lambda_1 L_{GDL}(X, Y) + \lambda_2 L_{LIP}(X, Y), \qquad (4)$$

where λ_1 and λ_2 are the weights for the L_{GDL} and L_{LIP} terms, respectively. The proposed framework for the training phase is illustrated in Fig. 1. In this paper, we refer the proposed method, i.e., training using L_{TOTAL}, as line-integral projection enforced deep learning method (LIPDL), and the conventional method, i.e., training using L_{IM}, as deep learning method (DL).

3.2   Network Architectures

In this work, we used a modified version of the fully-convolutional U-net architecture [8] for predicting the attenuation map from λ-MLAA and μ-MLAA. The network operates on 3D patches and uses $3 \times 3 \times 3$ convolution kernels. Different from the original U-net, where $2 \times 2 \times 2$ max pooling operations are used at the end of each stage, we reduced the resolution by using convolution operations with $2 \times 2 \times 2$ kernels and stride 2 [9]. In addition, symmetric padding was applied to the input image (and the feature maps in later layers) prior to the convolution operations to avoid reducing the image (or feature map) sizes due to the convolution. This allows the network's output layer to have the same size as the input layer. Batch normalization was applied after each convolutional layer and before the ReLU. Dropout with a rate of 0.15 was applied to the bottleneck layer of the U-net in the training phase to prevent overfitting, however, was removed in the testing phase.

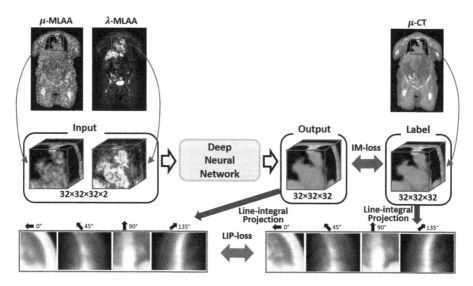

Fig. 1. Proposed framework (training phase). Both image domain loss (IM-loss) and line-integral projection loss (LIP-loss) are used to update the deep neural network.

3.3 Image Preprocessing

Image normalization is a key pre-processing step for deep learning algorithms [10]. Unlike CT images, in which the image intensity (Hounsfield Unit, HU) represents attenuation as relative to water and the intensity range is consistent across all the patients, the PET image intensity represents the tracer uptake level. The use of standardized uptake value (SUV) in PET helps to normalize the tracer injection dose and patient weight, however, the biological uptake range is intrinsically broad for FDG PET, e.g., the contrast between brain and muscle can be 10:1, and even 100:1 between bladder and muscle tissue. Additional image normalization is needed in order to obtain more stable results. In this study, the λ-MLAA images were normalized using $\lambda_{norm} = \tanh(\lambda/\sigma)$ before training and testing, where λ and λ_{norm} are the λ-MLAA images (in SUV) before and after normalization; σ is a parameter controlling the range of the active gradient zone of the hyperbolic tangent (tanh) function, which was empirically set to 5 to ensure that the organs of interests, i.e., except bladder, are in the active gradient zone. The μ-CT and μ-MLAA images were normalized by 0.15 cm^{-1}, which corresponds to skull bone attenuation coefficient at 511 keV, to match the value range of λ_{norm}. The normalized λ-MLAA and μ-MLAA were concatenated as a multi-channel image and used as the input to the deep neural networks for training and testing.

3.4   Evaluation

In this study, 80 subjects were included in training, and 20 subjects were used for evaluation. The predicted attenuation maps from the proposed LIPDL method (μ-LIPDL) were compared with those trained using only the image domain loss L_{IM} (μ-DL) and μ-MLAA, using the μ-CT as the reference.

The quality of the predicted attenuation maps was evaluated regarding the normalized mean absolute error (NMAE), the mean squared error (MSE), peak signal-to-noise ratio (PSNR), structural similarity index (SSIM), line-integral normalized mean absolute error (LINMAE) and line-integral mean squared error (LIMSE). The NMAE was defined as $NMAE = \left(\sum_{x,y,z} |X(x,y,z) - Y(x,y,z)|\right)/(N(\max(Y) - \min(Y)))$, where X and Y present the predicted attenuation map and the reference CT-attenuation map, *max* and *min* operators calculate the maximum and minimum intensities of the reference image. N is the total number of voxels. The LINMAE and LIMSE measure the error in line-integral projection domain. LINMAE was defined as: $LINMAE = \left[\sum_{k \in \mathbb{K}} \sum_{i=1}^{N_k} |[P_k X]_i - [P_k Y]_i|/(N_k(\max(P_k Y) - \min(P_k Y)))\right]/N_{\mathbb{K}}$. The definition of LIMSE can be found in Eq. 1.

For each patient, 4 PET reconstructions, using the ordered subset expectation maximization (3 iterations by 21 subsets, 5 mm Gaussian smoothing) algorithm, were performed using μ-LIPDL, μ-DL, μ-MLAA, and the ground-truth μ-CT as the attenuation map, respectively. All the attenuation maps were resliced to 2 mm voxel in width prior to the PET reconstructions. 2 mm voxel in width was used in PET reconstruction. Using the PET reconstructed with μ-CT as the reference, NMAE and MSE were computed for μ-LIPDL, μ-DL and μ-MLAA, respectively, on the entire body as well as 5 anatomical regions: head, neck to chest, abdomen, pelvis and legs, which correspond to the 0%–10%, 10%–30%, 30%–40%, 40%–50% and 50%-100% segments of each patient.

4   Experimental Results

For both LIPDL and DL methods, we trained the networks for 80 epochs, respectively. In each epoch, 40,000 32 × 32 × 32 patches were randomly sampled from the training data and batch size of 16 was used for updating the network. The networks were trained with the Adam optimizer. An initial learning rate of 10^{-3} was used, which was decayed by a factor of 0.99 after each epoch. λ_1 and λ_2 were set to 1 and 0.02, respectively. In the testing phase, to reduce the stitching artifacts caused by overlapping small image patches, we used relatively a large patch size of 200 × 200 × 32 and stride size of 200 × 200 × 16 (i.e., no striding in the first 2 dimensions). We implemented our framework using Tensorflow. The training takes about 40 h on an NVIDIA GTX 1080 Ti GPU.

4.1   Attenuation Map Evaluation

Figure 2 shows one example of different attenuations maps. Qualitatively, both μ-DL and the proposed μ-LIPDL yielded much less noisy attenuation maps as compared to the μ-MLAA, and visually, both μ-DL and μ-LIPDL are very similar to the μ-CT. However, μ-LIPDL showed more consistent intestine cavity area (yellow arrow) than the μ-DL as compared to the μ-CT. Note that the CT reconstruction artifacts in μ-CT (red arrow) were also removed in both μ-DL and μ-LIPDL.

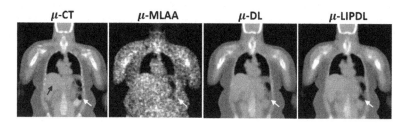

Fig. 2. Visual comparison for the original μ-CT, the μ-MLAA, the predicted μ-DL and μ-LIPDL. Improved intestine cavity area (yellow arrow) prediction can be seen in the proposed μ-LIPDL, as compared to the standard μ-DL. Red arrow in the μ-CT points at the CT reconstruction artifacts (mild). The same gray-scale window is used for all images. (Color figure online)

Table 1. Evaluation of the attenuation maps generated by three methods over 20 subjects using the image domain quality metrics and the line integral projection (LIP) domain quality metrics.

	Metric	μ-MLAA	μ-DL	μ-LIPDL
Image domain quality metrics	NMAE	6.29% ± 1.16%	1.66% ± 0.25%	**1.61% ± 0.24%***
	MSE	3.26E-4 ± 6.22E-5	3.20E-5 ± 9.24E-6	3.23E-5 ± 9.66E-6
	PSNR	28.1 ± 1.06	38.2 ± 1.02	38.2 ± 1.06
	SSIM	93.1% ± 0.007%	99.8% ± 0.0009%	99.8% ± 0.0008%
LIP domain quality metrics	LINMAE	7.95% ± 1.10%	1.29% ± 0.24%	**1.08% ± 0.19%****
	LIMSE	0.769 ± 0.144	0.024 ± 0.010	**0.018 ± 0.008****

mean ± STD, *indicates μ-LIPDL and μ-DL's difference is significant (*: $p < 10^{-5}$, **: $p < 10^{-8}$)

Table 1 quantitatively shows that both μ-DL and μ-LIPDL yielded statistically significant superior performance than the μ-MLAAover all evaluation metrics (maximum $p < 10^{-13}$). A paired t-test was used to evaluate statistical significance cross subjects (N = 20). Interestingly, no significant difference was found between μ-DL and μ-LIPDL when the conventional image domain quality metrics, i.e., MSE, PSNR and SSIM, were used. Only 3% reduced error from μ-DL to μ-LIPDL was observed for NMAE although it was statistically significant. In contrast, when the line-integral domain quality metrics were used, large improvements in μ-LIPDL were found as compared to μ-DL. Specifically, μ-LIPDL yielded a 16.3% reduction in LIMAE and 33.3% reduction in LIMSE as compared to the μ-DL. We note that for the PET attenuation correction (AC) task, the line integral of μ is used, therefore, an attenuation map yielding lower line-integral error will provide superior performance in the AC task than one with larger line-integral error. These results suggest that training with only the conventional image domain loss might produce suboptimal results, since the image domain loss cannot distinguish a better attenuation map, i.e., μ-LIPDL, than a sub-optimal attenuation map, i.e., μ-DL, for the AC task.

4.2   Attenuation Correction Performance in PET Reconstruction

PET images corrected by μ-LIPDL and μ-DL yielded significantly lower NMAE and MSE than those corrected by μ-MLAA, respectively (maximum $p < 10^{-3}$). Reconstructed PET images corrected by the μ-LIPDL yielded statistically significant lower NMAE and MSE than those corrected by μ-DL. As shown in Table 2, under both metrics, the LIPDL-obtained results with substantially and significantly smaller errors than DL on all the 5 body regions as well as on the whole body.

Table 2. Using PET images corrected by the μ-CT as the reference, the NMAE and MSE of the PET images corrected by μ-MLAA, μ-LIPDL and μ-DL, respectively, were shown. Evaluations were performed on 5 different anatomical regions as well as on the whole body.

AC method		Head	Neck/Chest	Abdomen	Pelvis	Legs	Whole-body
NMAE	μ-MLAA	21.4%	7.8%	9.4%	9.2%	8.5%	11.26%
	μ-DL	3.5%	4.2%	4.8%	4.4%	3.6%	4.1%
	μ-LIPDL	**3.2%***	**3.7%****	**4.1%***	**3.6%*****	**3.2%****	**3.6%*****
MSE	μ-MLAA	1.3E-01	7.4E-03	1.2E-02	1.4E-02	3.3E-03	3.4E-02
	μ-DL	2.7E-02	3.5E-03	4.1E-03	7.7E-03	9.2E-04	8.7E-03
	μ-LIPDL	**1.9E-02***	**2.7E-03***	**3.1E-03***	**4.8E-03***	**7.4E-04***	**6.0E-03****

* indicates μ-LIPDL and μ-DL's difference is significant (*: $p < 10^{-2}$, **: $p < 10^{-4}$, ***: $p < 10^{-6}$)

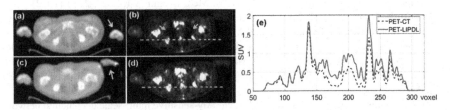

Fig. 3. (a) Coronal μ-CT, (b) PET corrected by μ-CT, (c) μ-LIPDL, (d) PET corrected by μ-LIPDL and (e) line profile measured on PET images corrected by μ-CT and μ-LIPDL.

4.3   Clinical Impact

Clinically, patient motion introduced mismatch between PET and CT that not only can generate AC inaccuracy in the PET reconstruction, but also can result in scatter correction (SC) inaccuracy. Figure 3 shows a case that patient right arm moved substantially between CT (a) and PET (b). Such mismatch caused erroneous SC, which is compounded with the AC artifact in the PET (dark area, arrows in (b)). μ-LIPDL(c) removed such mismatch and yielded stable SC in the PET reconstruction (d). Figure 3 (e) shows the line profile (dashed line in (b) and (d)) comparison between the PET corrected by μ-CT and μ-LIPDL. High uptakes in the PET indicate bone metastasis.

5   Summary

We have proposed a novel line integral loss function which incorporates imaging acquisition physics for PET attenuation map generation using deep learning. We showed that by enforcing the image projection domain consistency while training the deep neural networks, the generated attenuation maps perform significantly better for the task of PET attenuation correction, compared with conventional training that focuses solely on image domain consistency. In this study we used a modified version of U-net to demonstrate the effectiveness of the proposed training strategy, although the proposed method can be applied with any other neural networks. At the point of writing this paper, we empirically set the weight of the proposed line integral loss to 0.02 and obtained substantial improvement, we anticipate that fine tuning this parameter in the future could further improve the results. Furthermore, the proposed method is not only applicable to PET-CT image synthesis, but also to MRI-CT synthesis (for PET/MRI systems) for the purpose of generating attenuation maps.

References

1. Hunter, C.R., Klein, R., Beanlands, R.S., et al.: Patient motion effects on the quantification of regional myocardial blood flow with dynamic PET imaging. Med. Phys. **43**, 1829 (2016)
2. Rezaei, A., Defrise, M., Bal, G., et al.: Simultaneous reconstruction of activity and attenuation in time-of-flight PET. IEEE Trans. Med. Imaging **31**, 2224–2233 (2012)
3. Hamill, J., Panin, V.: TOF-MLAA for attenuation correction in thoracic PET/CT. In: 2012 IEEE Nuclear Science Symposium and Medical Imaging Conference (2012)
4. Hwang, D., Kang, S.K., Kim, K.Y., et al.: Generation of PET attenuation map for whole-body time-of-flight (18)F-FDG PET/MRI using a deep neural network trained with simultaneously reconstructed activity and attenuation maps. J. Nucl. Med. **60**(8), 1183–1189 (2019)
5. You, C., Yang, Q., Gjesteby, L., et al.: Structurally-sensitive multi-scale deep neural network for low-dose CT denoising. IEEE Access **6**, 41839–41855 (2018)
6. Isola, P., Zhu, J.-Y., Zhou, T., et al.: Image-to-image translation with conditional adversarial networks. In: Proceedings of the IEEE Conference on Computer Vision and Pattern Recognition, pp. 1125–1134 (2017)
7. Nie, D., Trullo, R., Lian, J., et al.: Medical image synthesis with deep convolutional adversarial networks. IEEE Trans. Biomed. Eng. **65**, 2720–2730 (2018)

8. Ronneberger, O., Fischer, P., Brox, T.: U-Net: convolutional networks for biomedical image segmentation. In: Navab, N., Hornegger, J., Wells, W.M., Frangi, A.F. (eds.) MICCAI 2015. LNCS, vol. 9351, pp. 234–241. Springer, Cham (2015). https://doi.org/10.1007/978-3-319-24574-4_28

9. Milletari, F., Navab, N., Ahmadi, S.-A.: V-net: fully convolutional neural networks for volumetric medical image segmentation. In: 2016 Fourth International Conference on 3D Vision (3DV), pp. 565–571. IEEE (2016)

10. Onofrey, J.A., Casetti-Dinescu, D.I., Lauritzen, A.D., et al.: Generalizable multi-site training and testing of deep neural networks using image normalization. In: 2019 IEEE 16th International Symposium on Biomedical Imaging (ISBI), pp. 1–4 (2019)

A Prior Learning Network for Joint Image and Sensitivity Estimation in Parallel MR Imaging

Nan Meng, Yan Yang, Zongben Xu, and Jian Sun$^{(\boxtimes)}$

Xi'an Jiaotong University, Xi'an 710049, China
{mnnedna168,yangyan92}@stu.xjtu.edu.cn, {zbxu,jiansun}@xjtu.edu.cn

Abstract. Parallel imaging is a fast magnetic resonance imaging technique through spatial sensitivity coding using multi-coils. To reconstruct a high quality MR image from under-sampled k-space data, we propose a novel deep network, dubbed as Blind-PMRI-Net, to simultaneously reconstruct the MR image and sensitivity maps in a blind setting for parallel imaging. The Blind-PMRI-Net is a novel deep architecture inspired by the iterative algorithm optimizing a novel energy model for joint image and sensitivity estimation based on image and sensitivity priors. The network is designed to be able to automatically learn these two priors by learning their corresponding proximal operators using convolutional neural networks. Blind-PMRI-Net naturally combines the physical constraint of parallel imaging and prior learning in a single deep architecture. Experiments on a knee MRI dataset show that our network can effectively reconstruct MR image with improved accuracy than previous methods, with fast computational speed. For example, Blind-PMRI-Net takes 0.72 s on GPU to reconstruct 15-channel sensitivity maps and a complex-valued MR image in size of 320×320.

Keywords: Parallel imaging · Prior learning · Deep learning

1 Introduction

Parallel imaging (PI) has been a routine method for accelerating Magnetic Resonance (MR) imaging. It relies on spatial sensitivity differences of multi-coils to reduce the data acquisition in k-space of multi-channels [3,8]. Combining with compressed sensing, parallel imaging can be further accelerated by under-sampling in k-space, followed by image reconstruction methods using better image priors [6]. In this paper, we aim to tackle the challenging task for

---

N. Meng and Y. Yang—Both authors contributed equally to this work.

Electronic supplementary material The online version of this chapter (https://doi.org/10.1007/978-3-030-32251-9_80) contains supplementary material, which is available to authorized users.

© Springer Nature Switzerland AG 2019
D. Shen et al. (Eds.): MICCAI 2019, LNCS 11767, pp. 732–740, 2019.
https://doi.org/10.1007/978-3-030-32251-9_80

reconstructing high quality MR image from limited samples in k-space of multi-channels.

Sensitivity profiles of multi-coils are important for parallel imaging. The calibration methods require pre-scans or auto-calibration signals (ACS) for calibration to estimate sensitivity maps in image domain [8,11] or interpolation kernels in k-space [3,7]. The inaccuracy of estimated sensitivity may deteriorate the quality of reconstructed MR image by introducing artifacts. The calibration-less methods do not require an external calibration process. They may treat PI as a blind image reconstruction task that simultaneously estimates the MR image and sensitivity, or directly reconstructs multi-channel images using an iterative algorithm optimizing a model regularized by the MR image sparse prior [13], sensitivity prior [10], or the correlation of multi-channel images [2,12]. Although these methods can improve the performance of PI reconstruction, they suffer from high computational complexity. It is also challenging to choose optimal priors of MR image and sensitivity, or determine the optimal hyper-parameters in models and algorithms.

Deep learning has been successfully applied to parallel imaging. A multi-layer perceptron [5] and a multi-channel generative adversarial network [14] were proposed to learn a mapping from k-space data to aliasing-free multi-channel images. Schlemper et al. [9] further introduced the data consistency into the design of deep network. These methods are computationally fast and achieved promising results for PI. However, since they can not estimate sensitivity maps, they often synthesize a real-valued MR image by SOS (square root of the sum of squares) on the reconstructed multi-channel images, which may not be consistent with the physical mechanism of parallel imaging and lose phase information. Methods in [1,4] learn a de-aliasing network or a Fields of Experts (FOE) model by unrolling a (conjugate) gradient descent procedure for a variational reconstruction model. The sensitivity maps embedded in the networks are estimated by a calibration step, e.g., SENSE, ESPIRiT [8,11].

In this work, we propose a novel deep architecture that can simultaneously reconstruct a complex-valued MR image and sensitivity maps from undersampled multi-channel k-space data. It naturally integrates the parallel imaging model and learning of priors of MR image and sensitivity maps into a single deep network. Specifically, we first formulate the blind reconstruction problem as an energy model with imaging model as data term, regularized by image and sensitivity priors. Then we design an iterative algorithm based on half-quadratic splitting to alternately estimate multi-channel images, sensitivity maps and the reconstructed MR image. Instead of setting these two priors by hand, we use deep CNNs to learn their corresponding proximal operators. In this way, by unfolding the iterative algorithm, we derive a deep architecture, dubbed as **Blind-PMRI-Net** shown in Fig. 1, to jointly estimate sensitivity maps and the MR image.

Compared with other deep learning-based PI methods, our approach incorporates prior learning of sensitivity into the network architecture, which allows the network to not only reconstruct a high-quality complex-valued MR image, but also estimate sensitivity maps optimized to be consistent with reconstructed MR image according to the parallel imaging model.

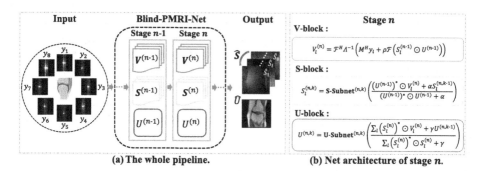

Fig. 1. (a) The architecture of Blind-PMRI-Net. Inputting a set of multi-channel measurements in k-space, it outputs optimal sensitivity maps and MR image. (b) Each stage of the net consists of V-block, S-block and U-block.

2 Method

Assume that we are given sampled k-space data $\{y_l \in \mathbb{C}^s\}_{l=1}^L$ of L channels captured by multi-coils, we aim to estimate both L sensitivity maps $\mathbf{S} = \{S_l \in \mathbb{C}^d\}_{l=1}^L$ and reconstructed MR image $U \in \mathbb{C}^d$, where d, s denote the number of image pixels and sampled k-space data. Based on the parallel imaging model, we design the following energy model:

$$E(\mathbf{V}, \mathbf{S}, U) = \frac{1}{2}\sum_l \|M\mathcal{F}V_l - y_l\|_2^2 + \frac{\rho}{2}\sum_l \|S_l \odot U - V_l\|_2^2 + \beta\sum_l R(S_l) + \lambda P(U),$$

$$(1)$$

where $M \in \mathbb{C}^{s \times d}$ is sampling matrix in k-space and $\mathcal{F} \in \mathbb{C}^{d \times d}$ is Fourier transform. $\mathbf{V} = \{V_l \in \mathbb{C}^d\}_{l=1}^L$ and U denote the images of L channels and the final MR image to be reconstructed. The first term enforces that the per-channel image V_l should be consistent with sampled data y_l in k-space, and the second term enforces that V_l is related to MR image U by $S_l \odot U = V_l$. We regularize sensitivity maps and MR image by $R(\cdot)$ and $P(\cdot)$ respectively.

2.1 Model Optimization

To estimate the unknown variables, the energy model of Eq. (1) can be minimized by iteratively updating $\mathbf{V}, \mathbf{S}, U$ based on half-quadratic splitting (HQS). The updating formulas at iteration n $(n = 1, 2, \cdots, N)$ are discussed as follows.

Coil Image Updating: Given $\mathbf{S}$ and U at iteration $n-1$, coil image V_l of l-th channel $(l \in \{1, 2, \cdots, L\})$ in n-th iteration can be updated as:

$$V_l^{(n)} = \arg\min_{V_l} \frac{1}{2}\|M\mathcal{F}V_l - y_l\|_2^2 + \frac{\rho}{2}\|S_l^{(n-1)} \odot U^{(n-1)} - V_l\|_2^2.$$

It has a closed-form solution:

$$V_l^{(n)} = \mathcal{F}^H \Lambda^{-1}(M^H y_l + \rho \mathcal{F}(S_l^{(n-1)} \odot U^{(n-1)})), \tag{2}$$

where $\Lambda = M^H M + \mathrm{diag}(\boldsymbol{\rho})$, $\boldsymbol{\rho} \in \mathbb{C}^d$ is a vector with elements of ρ. The initialized $S_l^{(0)}$ is estimated by SENSE from $\mathcal{F}^H M^H y_l$, and $U^{(0)} = \sum_l (S_l^{(0)})^* \odot (\mathcal{F}^H M^H y_l)$.

Sensitivity Updating: Given $\boldsymbol{V}^{(n)}$ and $U^{(n-1)}$, the sensitivity map S_l of l-th channel ($l \in \{1, 2, \cdots, L\}$) in n-th iteration can be updated as:

$$S_l^{(n)} = \arg\min_{S_l} \frac{\rho}{2}||S_l \odot U^{(n-1)} - V_l^{(n)}||_2^2 + \beta R(S_l).$$

By HQS and introducing auxiliary variable $\tilde{S}_l$, it is equivalent to optimizing:

$$\min_{\tilde{S}_l, S_l} \frac{1}{2}||\tilde{S}_l \odot U^{(n-1)} - V_l^{(n)}||_2^2 + \frac{\alpha}{2}||S_l - \tilde{S}_l||_2^2 + \frac{\beta}{\rho} R(S_l),$$

where $\alpha \to \infty$ during optimization. We alternately solve two sub-problems of $\tilde{S}_l$ and S_l. Substituting closed-form solution of $\tilde{S}_l$ to sub-problem of S_l, we derive the iterative updating formula for S_l:

$$S_l^{(n,k)} = \mathrm{Prox}_{\frac{\beta}{\alpha\rho}R} \left(\frac{(U^{(n-1)})^* \odot V_l^{(n)} + \alpha S_l^{(n,k-1)}}{(U^{(n-1)})^* \odot U^{(n-1)} + \alpha} \right), k = 1, \cdots, K, \tag{3}$$

where the division is a pixel-wise operation, $\mathrm{Prox}(\cdot)$ is the proximal operator defined as: $\mathrm{Prox}_{\eta R}(O) = \arg\min_X \frac{1}{2}||X - O||_2^2 + \eta R(X)$. $S_l^{(n,0)}$ is initialized as $S_l^{(n-1)}$. The updated sensitivity map of l-th channel is $S_l^{(n)} = S_l^{(n,K)}$.

MR Image Updating: Given updated multi-channel images $\boldsymbol{V}^{(n)}$ and sensitivity maps $\boldsymbol{S}^{(n)}$, the MR image U in n-th iteration can be updated as:

$$U^{(n)} = \arg\min_U \frac{\rho}{2} \sum_l ||S_l^{(n)} \odot U - V_l^{(n)}||_2^2 + \lambda P(U).$$

Similar to sensitivity updating, by HQS, U can be iteratively optimized by:

$$U^{(n,k)} = \mathrm{Prox}_{\frac{\lambda}{\rho\gamma}P} \left(\frac{\sum_l (S_l^{(n)})^* \odot V_l^{(n)} + \gamma U^{(n,k-1)}}{\sum_l (S_l^{(n)})^* \odot S_l^{(n)} + \gamma} \right), k = 1, \cdots, K. \tag{4}$$

$U^{(n,0)} = U^{(n-1)}$ and γ is a introduced parameter in HQS. Thus $U^{(n)} = U^{(n,K)}$.

2.2 Unfolded Network for Image and Sensitivity Priors Learning

Instead of setting regularization terms of sensitivity maps (i.e., $R(\cdot)$) and the MR image (i.e., $P(\cdot)$) by hand, we learn these terms implicitly by learning deep

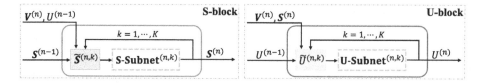

Fig. 2. The structure of S-block and U-block.

CNNs, through unfolding the above iterative optimization algorithm to be a novel deep architecture, dubbed as Blind-PMRI-Net.

As illustrated in Fig. 1(a), n-th stage of the network corresponds to n-th iteration of the algorithm. As shown in Fig. 1(b), each stage of the net consists of **V-block**, **S-block** and **U-block**, which implement Eqs. (2), (3), (4) for updating the multi-channel images, sensitivity maps and the reconstructed MR image respectively. Since regularization terms $R(\cdot)$ and $P(\cdot)$ correspond to proximal operators $\text{Prox}_{\frac{\beta}{\alpha\rho}R}(\cdot)$ and $\text{Prox}_{\frac{\lambda}{\rho\gamma}P}(\cdot)$ in the iterative algorithm, we substitute the proximal operators by CNNs to model the complex non-linear mappings:

$$S_l^{(n,k)} = \text{Prox}_{\frac{\beta}{\alpha\rho}R}(\tilde{S}_l^{(n,k)}) \triangleq \textbf{S-Subnet}^{(n,k)}(\tilde{S}_l^{(n,k)}),$$

$$U^{(n,k)} = \text{Prox}_{\frac{\lambda}{\rho\gamma}P}(\tilde{U}^{(n,k)}) \triangleq \textbf{U-Subnet}^{(n,k)}(\tilde{U}^{(n,k)}),$$

where $\tilde{S}_l^{(n,k)}$ and $\tilde{U}_l^{(n,k)}$ represent the terms in brackets of Eqs. (3) and (4) respectively. **S-Subnet**$(\cdot)$ is implemented as 6 cascaded convolutional (conv) blocks and an extra conv layer with residual connection. Each block consists of a conv layer, a batch normalization layer and a LeakyReLU activation layer. The conv layers in the first and the following five blocks have 32 filters in size of 5×5 and 7×7 respectively. The final conv layer has 2 filters in size of 9×9. **U-Subnet**$(\cdot)$ has a similar structure with 9 convolutional blocks and an extra convolutional layer. Each convolutional layer in the blocks has 64 filters in size of 3×3. The final layer has 2 filters in size of 3×3. Figure 2 shows the network structures of S-block and U-block in Blind-PMRI-Net.

Network Training. The training loss is defined as:

$$\mathcal{L}(\hat{\textbf{S}}, \hat{U}) = \sum_l \|\hat{S}_l - S_l^{gt}\|_1 + \sum_l \| |\hat{S}_l| - |S_l^{gt}| \|_1 + \sum_l \text{TV}(|\hat{S}_l|) + \xi\|\hat{U} - U^{gt}\|_2^2,$$

where $\hat{\textbf{S}} = \{\hat{S}_l\}_{l=1}^L$ and $\hat{U}$ are outputs of our network, $|\cdot|$ is for the magnitude of complex value and ξ is a hyper-parameter. TV is the regularization of total variation. $\{S_l^{gt}\}_{l=1}^L$ and U^{gt} are targeting sensitivity maps and MR image generated from fully-sampled k-space data. Therefore given multi-channel sampled k-space data, our net learns to output sensitivity and MR image approximating the corresponding targets using fully-sampled k- space data. The gradients of loss w.r.t. the parameters of **S-Subnet**, **U-Subnet**, ρ, α, γ can be computed by

Table 1. Comparison of average performance on the testing knee dataset.

Rate	Measure	Zero-filling	GRAPPA	Fast-JTV	MoDL	DC-CNN	Our net
15%	PSNR	23.64	26.47	26.10	28.93	30.58	**31.15**
	nRMSE	0.068	0.049	0.051	0.038	0.031	**0.029**
20%	PSNR	24.71	28.83	27.10	29.42	31.06	**32.03**
	nRMSE	0.060	0.038	0.046	0.036	0.030	**0.027**
30%	PSNR	26.38	30.49	31.42	31.39	32.96	**33.52**
	nRMSE	0.050	0.032	0.028	0.029	0.023	**0.022**

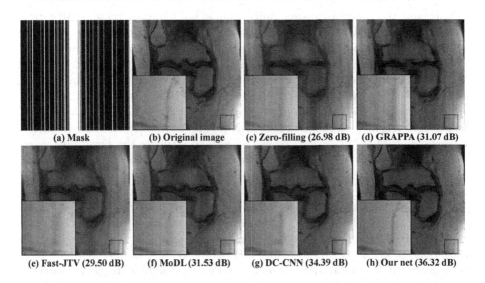

(a) Mask   (b) Original image   (c) Zero-filling (26.98 dB)   (d) GRAPPA (31.07 dB)

(e) Fast-JTV (29.50 dB)   (f) MoDL (31.53 dB)   (g) DC-CNN (34.39 dB)   (h) Our net (36.32 dB)

Fig. 3. Results for a knee MR image using 20% 1D Cartesian sampling.

auto-differentiation. Note that these parameters are not shared across different stages, and parameters of two subnets are initialized using Xavier random initialization. We learn these parameters using Adam with learning rate of 1e-4 by PyTorch, implemented on a ubuntu 16.04 system with GTX 1080 Ti GPU.

3   Experiments

We train and test Blind-PMRI-Net on a knee MR dataset from NYU dataset[1]. The raw data consists of 15-channel k-space data with resolution of 320×320. Because we aim to train our Blind-PMRI-Net to map the multi-coil undersampled k-space data to both sensitivity maps and MR image by approximating the targets generated from k-space data without sampling. Based on fully-sampled k-space data, we generate targeting multi-channel sensitivities by

---

[1] http://mridata.org.

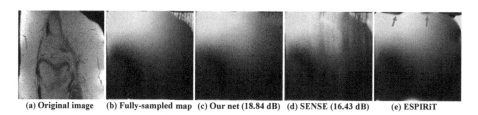

(a) Original image   (b) Fully-sampled map   (c) Our net (18.84 dB)   (d) SENSE (16.43 dB)   (e) ESPIRiT

Fig. 4. Estimated sensitivity maps.

SENSE, and MR image by fusing multi-channel images using these sensitivities. We take 354 and 100 multi-channel data for training and testing respectively, and 1D Cartesian sampling masks with sampling rates of 15%, 20% and 30%.

We compare our Blind-PMRI-Net ($K = 1, N = 3$)[2] with three traditional methods including Zero-filling (Zf), GRAPPA [3] estimating interpolation kernels for sensitivity by ACS, and calibration-less method Fast-JTV [2] solving a model with joint total variation prior on images. We also compare with state-of-the-art deep learning methods of DC-CNN [9] and MoDL [1]. In order to obtain the complex-valued MR image, we use SENSE to estimate the sensitivity maps from under-sampled data for MoDL method. Since only multi-channel images are reconstructed by Fast-JTV and DC-CNN, for fair comparison, we synthesize the complex-valued MR image for them by combining multi-channel images using weights computed based on the synthesized MR image by SOS. Table 1 shows the quantitative results with 15%, 20% and 30% sampling rates. Compared with Zero-filling, GRAPPA and Fast-JTV, our method produces significantly higher recovery accuracy. For example, using 15% sampling rate, Blind-PMRI-Net outperforms GRAPPA by 4.68 dB. In average, our method achieves better reconstruction accuracy in nRMSE using 5% less sampled data compared with two deep learning methods DC-CNN and MoDL. The visual comparisons of reconstructed images with 20% sampling rate are shown in Fig. 3. Our method produces the higher-quality image with clearer details and without obvious artifacts.

Sensitivity Maps. Our Blind-PMRI-Net can also output the sensitivity maps. Figure 4 compares our estimated sensitivity map with SENSE and ESPIRiT methods in 20% sampling rate. Compared with SENSE, our net and ESPIRiT achieve smoother maps which are closer to the sensitivity map estimated based on fully-sampled k-space data. The sensitivity map from ESPIRiT has some missing information (e.g., the region near the boundary as indicated by the arrows). Our Blind-PMRI-Net takes 0.72 s on GPU to reconstruct both sensitivity maps and complex-valued MR image in average, while ESPIRiT takes 46.64 s to estimate the sensitivity using the public code[3].

---

[2] We empirically found that increasing N is more important than increasing K for network performance, therefore we mainly increase N and set $K = 1$ for simplicity.

[3] https://www.eecs.berkeley.edu/%7Emlustig/Software.html.

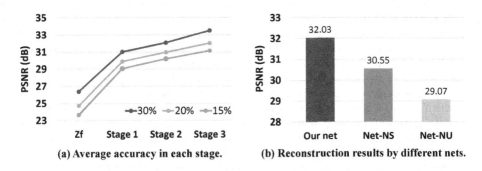

Fig. 5. Performance comparison for different network settings.

Ablation Study. To explore the effect of the number of stages (i.e., N) on the reconstruction performance, we greedily train our Blind-PMRI-Net from stage 1 to 3. The average PSNR values of the testing results with different sampling rates and different stages are shown in Fig. 5(a). The accuracy of reconstruction gradually increases with the increase of stages. To test the effectiveness of networks **S-Subnet(·)** and **U-Subnet(·)** for learning sensitivity and image priors, we respectively set **S-Subnet(·)** and **U-Subnet(·)** as an identity mapping without learning, and the corresponding nets are denoted as Net-NS and Net-NU. The results of trained Net-NS and Net-NU with $N = 3$ using 20% sampled data are shown in Fig. 5(b). Both subnets are beneficial for improving the reconstruction quality, e.g., the results are improved by 5.84 dB and 4.36 dB compared with baseline Zero-filling.

4   Conclusion

In this work, we proposed a novel Blind-PMRI-Net to simultaneously estimate the MR image and sensitivity maps for parallel imaging from sampled k-space data. After building an energy model using priors of MR image and sensitivity maps, we unfold its optimization algorithm to be a deep architecture, in which the two priors are learned by substituting corresponding proximal operators using deep CNNs. To the best of our knowledge, this is the first deep architecture that uses CNNs to learn both sensitivity maps and MR image priors for parallel imaging. In the future, we are interested in incorporating more advanced deep learning techniques, e.g., attention or GAN, into our learning framework.

Acknowledgement. This work was supported by National Natural Science Foundation of China under Grants 11622106, 11690011, 61721002, U1811461.

References

1. Aggarwal, H.K., Mani, M.P., Jacob, M.: MoDL: model-based deep learning architecture for inverse problems. IEEE Trans. Med. Imaging **38**(2), 394–405 (2019)
2. Chen, C., Li, Y., Huang, J.: Calibrationless parallel MRI with joint total variation regularization. In: Mori, K., Sakuma, I., Sato, Y., Barillot, C., Navab, N. (eds.) MICCAI 2013. LNCS, vol. 8151, pp. 106–114. Springer, Heidelberg (2013). https://doi.org/10.1007/978-3-642-40760-4_14
3. Griswold, M.A., et al.: Generalized autocalibrating partially parallel acquisitions (GRAPPA). Magn. Reson. Med. **47**(6), 1202–1210 (2002)
4. Hammernik, K., et al.: Learning a variational network for reconstruction of accelerated MRI data. Magn. Reson. Med. **79**(6), 3055–3071 (2018)
5. Kwon, K., Kim, D., Park, H.: A parallel MR imaging method using multilayer perceptron. Med. Phys. **44**(12), 6209–6224 (2017)
6. Liang, D., Liu, B., Wang, J., Ying, L.: Accelerating SENSE using compressed sensing. Magn. Reson. Med. **62**(6), 1574–1584 (2009)
7. Lustig, M., Pauly, J.M.: SPIRiT: iterative self-consistent parallel imaging reconstruction from arbitrary k-space. Magn. Reson. Med. **64**(2), 457–471 (2010)
8. Pruessmann, K.P., Weiger, M., Scheidegger, M.B., Boesiger, P.: SENSE: sensitivity encoding for fast MRI. Magn. Reson. Med. **42**(5), 952–962 (1999)
9. Schlemper, J., et al.: A deep cascade of convolutional neural networks for dynamic MR image reconstruction. IEEE Trans. Med. Imaging **37**(2), 491–503 (2018)
10. She, H., et al.: Sparse BLIP: BLind iterative parallel imaging reconstruction using compressed sensing. Magn. Reson. Med. **71**(2), 645–660 (2014)
11. Uecker, M., et al.: ESPIRiT-an eigenvalue approach to autocalibrating parallel MRI: where SENSE meets GRAPPA. Magn. Reson. Med. **71**(3), 990–1001 (2014)
12. Wang, S., et al.: Learning joint-sparse codes for calibration-free parallel MR imaging. IEEE Trans. Med. Imaging **37**(1), 251–261 (2018)
13. Ying, L., Sheng, J.: Joint image reconstruction and sensitivity estimation in SENSE (JSENSE). Magn. Reson. Med. **57**(6), 1196–1202 (2007)
14. Zhang, P., Wang, F., Xu, W., Li, Y.: Multi-channel generative adversarial network for parallel magnetic resonance image reconstruction in K-space. In: Frangi, A.F., Schnabel, J.A., Davatzikos, C., Alberola-López, C., Fichtinger, G. (eds.) MICCAI 2018. LNCS, vol. 11070, pp. 180–188. Springer, Cham (2018). https://doi.org/10.1007/978-3-030-00928-1_21

Consensus Neural Network for Medical Imaging Denoising with Only Noisy Training Samples

Dufan Wu[1,2], Kuang Gong[1,2], Kyungsang Kim[1,2], Xiang Li[1,2],
and Quanzheng Li[1,2(✉)]

[1] Center for Advanced Medical Computing and Analysis, Massachusetts General
Hospital and Harvard Medical School, Boston, MA 02114, USA
{dwu6,kgong,kkim24,xli60,li.quanzheng}@mgh.harvard.edu
[2] Gordon Center for Medical Imaging, Massachusetts General Hospital and Harvard
Medical School, Boston, MA 02114, USA

Abstract. Deep neural networks have been proved efficient for medical image denoising. Current training methods require both noisy and clean images. However, clean images cannot be acquired for many practical medical applications due to naturally noisy signal, such as dynamic imaging, spectral computed tomography, arterial spin labeling magnetic resonance imaging, etc. In this paper we proposed a training method which learned denoising neural networks from noisy training samples only. Training data in the acquisition domain was split to two subsets and the network was trained to map one noisy set to the other. A consensus loss function was further proposed to efficiently combine the outputs from both subsets. A mathematical proof was provided that the proposed training scheme was equivalent to training with noisy and clean samples when the noise in the two subsets was uncorrelated and zero-mean. The method was validated on Low-dose CT Challenge dataset and NYU MRI dataset and achieved improved performance compared to existing unsupervised methods.

Keywords: Image denoising · Neural network · Unsupervised learning

1 Introduction

Deep neural network has been proved efficient for noise and artifacts reduction in medical imaging reconstruction [1,2]. Despite of the superior image quality achieved by neural networks compared to handcrafted prior functions [3], almost all the neural network based methods require both noisy and clean images during the training. However, such clean images are not always accessible due to naturally noisy signals acquired in many medical applications. Dynamic imaging,

Supported by National Institute of Health under grant 5P41EB022544 and 1RF1AG052653.

D. Shen et al. (Eds.): MICCAI 2019, LNCS 11767, pp. 741–749, 2019.
https://doi.org/10.1007/978-3-030-32251-9_81

including dynamic positron emission tomography (PET), dynamic magnetic resonance (MR), and computed tomography (CT) perfusion, acquires signals with rapid temporal change, and the signal quality is limited due to short acquisition time. Spectral CT has very noisy material images due to the ill-posed decomposition procedure [4]. Arterial spin labeling (ASL) MR also has noisy images due to the low efficiency in labeling arterial blood with magnetic field, which results in noisy signals emitted by the labeled blood [5].

A recent work proposed in 2018, Noise2noise [6], demonstrated that denoising networks can be learned by mapping a noisy image to another noisy realization of the same image, and the performance was similar to that using noisy-clean pairs. However, it requires at least two noise realizations for each training sample, which is not readily available for most medical images. Even if two noise realizations are given, Noise2noise framework can only effectively use one of them, which degraded the achievable image quality. Last but not least, [6] did not clarify the conditions for Noise2noise to work, which can be problematic for medical imaging due to the complicated noise characteristics.

In this work we proposed a consensus network for medical imaging which required only noisy data for training. Our consensus network was inspired by Noise2noise but with major improvements for medical imaging. The Noise2noise framework was first analyzed with a newly proposed mathematical theorem, which further clarified its applicable condition. Based on conditions derived from the theorem, the acquired signals were split to two sets to reconstruct images with different noise realizations. The denoising network was then trained to map one noise realization to the other, with a novel loss function which efficiently aggregated both noise realizations during testing time. The proposed method was evaluated on Low-dose CT (LDCT) Challenge dataset [7] for quarter-dose CT image denoising, and New York University (NYU) MR dataset [8] for 4× undersampling parallel imaging. Results from both datasets demonstrated improved performance compared to the original Noise2noise framework and iterative reconstruction methods.

2   Methodology

We will first provide proof for Noise2Noise training, then derive loss function for the proposed consensus network based on our theorem.

2.1   Noise2noise Training

Given paired clean and noisy images $\mathbf{x}_i, \mathbf{x}_i + \mathbf{n}_i \in \mathbb{R}^n$, conventional method to train denoising network under L2-loss is:

$$\mathbf{\Theta}_c = \underset{\mathbf{\Theta}}{\operatorname{argmin}} \frac{1}{N} \sum_{i=1}^{N} \|f(\mathbf{x}_i + \mathbf{n}_i; \mathbf{\Theta}) - \mathbf{x}_i\|_2^2, \tag{1}$$

where $f(\mathbf{x}; \mathbf{\Theta}) : \mathbb{R}^n \to \mathbb{R}^n$ is the denoising neural network and $\mathbf{\Theta} \in \mathbb{R}^m$ is the parameters to be trained. Equation (1) is referred as Noise2clean training.

Noise2noise training uses two independent noise realizations of each sample for the training:

$$\boldsymbol{\Theta}_n = \underset{\boldsymbol{\Theta}}{\operatorname{argmin}} \frac{1}{N} \sum_{i=1}^{N} \|f(\mathbf{x}_i + \mathbf{n}_{i1}; \boldsymbol{\Theta}) - (\mathbf{x}_i + \mathbf{n}_{i2})\|_2^2, \tag{2}$$

where $\mathbf{n}_{i1}, \mathbf{n}_{i2} \in \mathbb{R}^n$ are two independent noise samples.

The equivalence between Noise2noise (2) and Noise2clean (1) is guaranteed by Theorem 1, which is one of our main contributions:

Theorem 1. *If conditional expectation $E\{\mathbf{n}_{i2}|\mathbf{x}_i + \mathbf{n}_{i1}\} = \mathbf{0} \ \forall \ \boldsymbol{\Theta} \in \mathbb{R}^m$ and i, then $\lim_{N \to \infty} \boldsymbol{\Theta}_n = \boldsymbol{\Theta}_c$.*

Proof. Let $\mathbf{y}_i := f(\mathbf{x}_i + \mathbf{n}_{i1}; \boldsymbol{\Theta})$ and expand the loss function in (2):

$$\frac{1}{N} \sum_{i=1}^{N} \|\mathbf{y}_i - (\mathbf{x}_i + \mathbf{n}_{i2})\|_2^2$$

$$= \frac{1}{N} \sum_{i=1}^{N} \|\mathbf{y}_i - \mathbf{x}_i\|_2^2 - \frac{1}{N} \sum_{i=1}^{N} 2\mathbf{n}_{i2}^T \mathbf{y}_i + \frac{1}{N} \sum_{i=1}^{N} (\mathbf{n}_{i2}^T \mathbf{n}_{i2} + 2\mathbf{n}_{i2}^T \mathbf{x}_i) \tag{3}$$

The first term is Noise2clean loss (1) and the last term is irrelevant to $\boldsymbol{\Theta}$.

For the second term, according to Lindeberg-Levy central limit theorem:

$$\sqrt{N}\left(\frac{1}{N} \sum 2\mathbf{n}_{i2}^T \mathbf{y}_i - E\{2\mathbf{n}_{i2}^T \mathbf{y}_i\}\right) \xrightarrow{d} N(0, Var\{2\mathbf{n}_{i2}^T \mathbf{y}_i\}), \tag{4}$$

where $Var\{x\}$ is the variance of x, and $N(0, \sigma^2)$ is a normal distribution with variance σ^2. As $Var\{2\mathbf{n}_{i2}^T \mathbf{y}_i\}$ is finite, the second term in (3) will converge to $E\{2\mathbf{n}_{i2}^T \mathbf{y}_i\}$ as $N \to \infty$.

The expectation can be written as conditional expectation:

$$E\{2\mathbf{n}_{i2}^T \mathbf{y}_i\} = 2E\{E^T\{\mathbf{n}_{i2}|\mathbf{y}_i\}\mathbf{y}_i\} = 2E\{E^T\{\mathbf{n}_{i2}|\mathbf{x}_i + \mathbf{n}_{i1}\}f(\mathbf{x}_i + \mathbf{n}_{i1}; \boldsymbol{\Theta})\}, \tag{5}$$

the last equivalence was due to that $\mathbf{y}_i = f(\mathbf{x}_i + \mathbf{n}_{i1}; \boldsymbol{\Theta})$ was deterministic.

Equation (5) equals to 0 given the theorem's assumption, which lead to diminishing second term in (3) as $N \to \infty$. As the third term was irrelevant to $\boldsymbol{\Theta}$, we have:

$$\underset{\boldsymbol{\Theta}}{\operatorname{argmin}} \frac{1}{N} \sum_{i=1}^{N} \|\mathbf{y}_i - \mathbf{x}_i\|_2^2 = \underset{\boldsymbol{\Theta}}{\operatorname{argmin}} \frac{1}{N} \sum_{i=1}^{N} \|\mathbf{y}_i - (\mathbf{x}_i + \mathbf{n}_{i2})\|_2^2, \tag{6}$$

as $N \to \infty$, which implies $\boldsymbol{\Theta}_n = \boldsymbol{\Theta}_c$. $\qquad\square$

2.2   Consensus Loss Function

The key to Noise2noise training is finding independent and zero-mean noise realizations $\mathbf{n}_{i1}$ and $\mathbf{n}_{i2}$. For medical imaging, it can be achieved by splitting the measurement to independent sets which are reconstructed separately. For example, in low-dose CT, $\mathbf{x}_i + \mathbf{n}_{i1}$ and $\mathbf{x}_i + \mathbf{n}_{i2}$ can be images reconstructed from odd and even projections respectively.

The major drawback of this "data splitting" method was that both $\mathbf{x}_i + \mathbf{n}_{i1}$ and $\mathbf{x}_i + \mathbf{n}_{i2}$ were noisier than the original noisy image, which restricted the quality of denoised images. To efficiently aggregate both noise realizations, they should be taken into consideration in the same loss function. According to Theorem 1, such loss function can be designed under the Noise2clean framework first, then substituting clean images $\mathbf{x}_i$ with its noisy version when appropriate. The following Noise2clean model was considered to derive our consensus loss:

$$
\begin{aligned}
L_c &= \frac{1}{N} \sum_{i=1}^{N} \left\| \frac{\mathbf{y}_{i1} + \mathbf{y}_{i2}}{2} - \mathbf{x}_i \right\|_2^2 \\
&= \frac{1}{N} \sum_{i=1}^{N} \left\{ \frac{1}{2} \|\mathbf{y}_{i1} - \mathbf{x}_i\|_2^2 + \frac{1}{2} \|\mathbf{y}_{i2} - \mathbf{x}_i\|_2^2 - \frac{1}{4} \|\mathbf{y}_{i1} - \mathbf{y}_{i2}\|_2^2 \right\},
\end{aligned}
\tag{7}
$$

where $\mathbf{y}_{i1} := f(\mathbf{x}_i + \mathbf{n}_{i1}; \mathbf{\Theta}_1)$ and $\mathbf{y}_{i2} := f(\mathbf{x}_i + \mathbf{n}_{i2}; \mathbf{\Theta}_2)$. $\mathbf{\Theta}_1, \mathbf{\Theta}_2 \in \mathbb{R}^m$ were the trainable variables. The second equivalence was just simple factorization. This model effectively aggregated $\mathbf{x}_i + \mathbf{n}_{i1}$ and $\mathbf{x}_i + \mathbf{n}_{i2}$ by taking both of them into consideration in the same loss function.

Similar to Theorem 1, $\mathbf{x}_i$ can be substituted with $\mathbf{x}_i + \mathbf{n}_{i1}$ or $\mathbf{x}_i + \mathbf{n}_{i2}$ during training, and our Noise2noise consensus loss is given as:

$$
\begin{aligned}
L_n = \frac{1}{N} \sum_{i=1}^{N} \Big\{ &\frac{1}{2} \|f(\mathbf{x}_i + \mathbf{n}_{i1}; \mathbf{\Theta}_1) - (\mathbf{x}_i + \mathbf{n}_{i2})\|_2^2 + \\
&\frac{1}{2} \|f(\mathbf{x}_i + \mathbf{n}_{i2}; \mathbf{\Theta}_2) - (\mathbf{x}_i + \mathbf{n}_{i1})\|_2^2 - \\
&\frac{1}{4} \|f(\mathbf{x}_i + \mathbf{n}_{i1}; \mathbf{\Theta}_1) - f(\mathbf{x}_i + \mathbf{n}_{i2}; \mathbf{\Theta}_2)\|_2^2 \Big\}
\end{aligned}
\tag{8}
$$

and the denoised image is given by:

$$
\mathbf{z}_i = \frac{f(\mathbf{x}_i + \mathbf{n}_{i1}; \mathbf{\Theta}_1) + f(\mathbf{x}_i + \mathbf{n}_{i2}; \mathbf{\Theta}_2)}{2}
\tag{9}
$$

2.3   Regularization

In practice, $\mathbf{n}_{i1}$ and $\mathbf{n}_{i2}$ could be correlated due to aliasing related to structures, and N may not be large enough in mini-batch training. Two regularization terms were added beside L_n for artifacts reduction and detail preservation.

The first term was weight decay defined as:

$$
L_w = \|\mathbf{\Theta}_1\|_2^2 + \|\mathbf{\Theta}_2\|_2^2,
\tag{10}
$$

which was effective at eliminating artifacts due to noise correlation.

The second term was image consistency:

$$L_r = \frac{1}{N} \sum_{i=1}^{N} \left\| \mathbf{z}_i - \mathbf{x}_i^{est} \right\|_2^2, \tag{11}$$

where $\mathbf{z}_i$ is given by (9) and $\mathbf{x}_i^{est}$ is an estimation of $\mathbf{x}_i$. It could be the original noisy images, or reconstructed with artifacts-suppressing algorithms.

The final loss function for training was

$$L = L_n + \beta_w L_w + \beta_r L_r, \tag{12}$$

where β_w could be tuned first with $\beta_r = 0$ to remove artifacts, then β_r could be tuned for image details with fixed β_w. The denoised image was given by (9).

3 Experiments

3.1 Data Preparation

We validated the proposed methods on two datasets: LDCT Grand Challenge [7] and NYU MR images [8]. Both datasets have high quality images which provided reference for evaluation.

The LDCT dataset consisted of abdomen CT scans from 10 patients. Quarter-dose raw data was synthesized from the acquisitions by realistic noise insertion. The raw data was rebinned to multi-slice fanbeam sinogram for image reconstruction. We randomly chose 50 slices from each patients for our study, and used 8 patients for training with the other 2 patients for testing. For each slice, we split the 2304 quarter-dose projections to odd and even set and used filtered backprojection (FBP) with Hann filter to reconstruct the $\mathbf{x}_i + \mathbf{n}_{i1}$ and $\mathbf{x}_i + \mathbf{n}_{i2}$ required for the training of consensus network.

The NYU MR dataset used in this study consisted of sagittal knee MR scans with Turbo Spin Echo sequence from 20 patients. $4\times$ cartesian downsampling was synthesized by downsampling the original kspace data with different random masks for each slice. The central 48 lines were kept for aliasing reduction and sensitivity map estimation. Each patients had 31 to 35 slices and we randomly chose 16 patients for training with 4 patients for testing. For each patient, the sampled lines were further randomly split to two sets with $8\times$ downsampling each. The central 48 lines were kept for both sets.

Zero-filling was used to reconstruct $\mathbf{x}_i + \mathbf{n}_{i1}$ and $\mathbf{x}_i + \mathbf{n}_{i2}$ due to its linear property so that the artifacts was zero-mean. The random sampling part of the kspace data was also amplified by a factor of 8 to enforce the zero-mean property.

3.2 Parameters

We used UNet [1,9] as $f(\mathbf{x}; \boldsymbol{\Theta})$ in all the studies. 32 and 64 basic featuremaps were used for LDCT and NYU MR datasets respectively. For MR study, the real and imaginary part of the images were fed to the network as two channels.

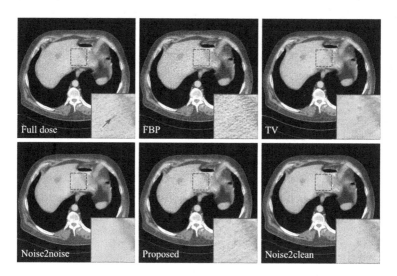

Fig. 1. A testing CT slice processed with different methods. A small lesion is marked with blue arrow on the full-dose image. The display window is $[-160, 240]$ HU. (Color figure online)

The $\mathbf{x}_i^{est}$ in CT and MR studies were quarter-dose FBP results and SENSE [10] results respectively. The hyperparameters, β_w and β_r, were tuned according to Sect. 2.3. LDCT study used $\beta_w = 5 \times 10^{-6}$ and $\beta_r = 0.5$. MR study used $\beta_w = 1 \times 10^{-6}$ and $\beta_r = 5$.

The networks were trained on 96×96 local patches with mini-batch size of 40. At each epoch, 40 patches were randomly extracted from each training slice. The networks were trained by Adam algorithm with learning rate of 10^{-4} for 100 epochs. CT images were normalized to HU/1000 and MR images were normalized to $[-1, 1]$ before being fed to the networks.

4   Results

The root mean squares error (RMSE), and structural similarity index (SSIM) on the testing quarter-dose CT dataset are given in Table 1, and one of the testing slices with two lesions is given in Fig. 1. Beside the proposed method, we also gave the results from quarter-dose FBP, iterative reconstruction with total variation (TV) minimization [3], original Noise2noise (2) and Noise2clean (1). All the methods did not require clean images for training or testing except for the Noise2clean, which was supervised learning.

The proposed method achieved the best SSIM among all the unsupervised methods. Although Noise2noise had lower RMSE compared to the proposed method, its images were significantly oversmoothed as shown in Fig. 1. The higher RMSE of the proposed methods were mainly due to mismatch in noise patterns in the reference images and the proposed results. The proposed method

Table 1. RMSEs and SSIMs of the testing CT images. SSIMs were calculated within the liver window [−160, 240] HU. Noise2clean required clean images for training.

Index	FBP	TV	Noise2noise	Proposed	Noise2clean
RMSE(HU)	27.6 ± 5.3	36.9 ± 4.4	17.4 ± 3.2	18.4 ± 2.9	14.7 ± 2.8
SSIM	81.5 ± 4.7	81.8 ± 3.5	84.2 ± 4.6	87.1 ± 3.4	87.7 ± 3.3

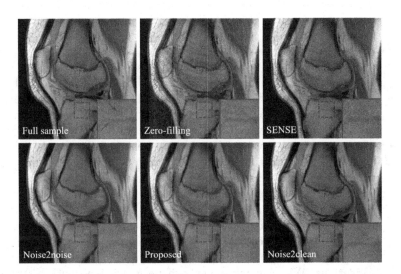

Fig. 2. Amplitude images of a testing MR slice processed with different methods. Structures are marked with blue arrows on the fully sampled image. (Color figure online)

preserved both the small lesion structure and textures compared to TV and Noise2noise. The structural details recovered by the proposed method were very similar to that by the Noise2clean training, and they achieved close SSIMs.

The 4× downsampling MR testing results are given in Table 2 and Fig. 2. Results from Zero-filling, SENSE, Noise2noise and Noise2clean are given beside the proposed method.

In the MR study, the proposed method achieved the best RMSE and SSIM among all the unsupervised methods. Noise2noise results were still over-smoothed. The proposed method preserved detailed structures of the knee compared to Noise2noise, and had significantly reduced artifacts and noise compared to zero-filling and SENSE. Compared to Noise2clean result, the proposed method recovered almost the same amount of structures despite of some slight loss in contrast. The artifacts and noise level were also similar for the two results.

Table 2. RMSEs and SSIMs of the testing MR images. SSIMs were calculated for the amplitude images. Noise2clean required clean images for training.

Index	Zero-filling	SENSE	Noise2noise	Proposed	Noise2clean
RMSE(10^{-3})	36.3 ± 7.6	38.4 ± 4.6	27.7 ± 6.3	23.4 ± 4.2	21.0 ± 4.5
SSIM	90.1 ± 1.9	86.5 ± 1.1	94.6 ± 1.3	95.2 ± 0.6	96.4 ± 0.8

5   Conclusion and Discussion

In this paper we proposed an unsupervised learning method for medical image denoising which only required noisy samples during training. A novel theorem was proposed for the Noise2noise framework. Our consensus network was proposed based on the theorem with novel framework and loss functions designed for medical imaging. The proposed loss function efficiently utilized both noise realizations of the same object and achieved improved performance compared to Noise2noise under the same framework. The proposed method achieved better performance than other unsupervised methods. Its image quality was close to that of supervised denoising networks.

The proposed method had weak assumption on the property of noise and images. It worked for both local noise in CT and non-local undersampling artifacts in MR. The noise was only required to be zero-mean and independent in the two realizations. Whereas zero-mean can be guaranteed with appropriate reconstruction algorithms, the independence property could be breached due to various factors. The artifacts caused by correlations were successfully compensated with the proposed regularizations.

Although the proposed method need to split the raw data to create the training dataset, its deployment can work in image domain only. After the consensus network was trained, another network could be trained to map noisy images to the output of consensus network in a conventional supervised manner. Hence, the networks' deployment does not need to interfere existing workflow of scanners.

We achieved promising results on existing public datasets where high-quality reference images were available, which provided reliable evaluation of the method's performance. The method can be applied to more challenging applications where only noisy images are available, such as dynamic PET, ASL MR, and spectral CT. Furthermore, the method itself could also be improved, such as replacing the image consistency (11) with data consistency; or replacing UNet with reconstruction networks.

References

1. Jin, K.H., McCann, M.T., Froustey, E., Unser, M.: Deep convolutional neural network for inverse problems in imaging. IEEE Trans. Image Process. **26**(9), 4509–4522 (2017)

2. Kang, E., Min, J., Ye, J.C.: A deep convolutional neural network using directional wavelets for low-dose X-ray CT reconstruction. Med. Phys. **44**(10), e360–e375 (2017)
3. Sidky, E.Y., Pan, X.: Image reconstruction in circular cone-beam computed tomography by constrained, total-variation minimization. Phys. Med. Biol. **53**(17), 4777–4807 (2008)
4. Niu, T., Dong, X., Petrongolo, M., Zhu, L.: Iterative image-domain decomposition for dual-energy CT. Med. Phys. **41**, 041901 (2014)
5. Bibic, A., Knutsson, L., Ståhlberg, F., Wirestam, R.: Denoising of arterial spin labeling data: wavelet-domain filtering compared with Gaussian smoothing. Magn. Reson. Mater. Phys. Biol. Med. **23**(3), 125–137 (2010)
6. Lehtinen, J., Munkberg, J., Hasselgren, J., Laine, S., Karras, T., Aittala, M., et al.: Noise2Noise: learning image restoration without clean data. Proc. Mach. Learn. Res. **80**, 2965–2974 (2018)
7. McCollough, C.H., Bartley, A.C., Carter, R.E., Chen, B., Drees, T.A., Edwards, P., et al.: Low-dose CT for the detection and classification of metastatic liver lesions: results of the 2016 low dose CT grand challenge. Med. Phys. **44**(10), e339–e352 (2017)
8. Hammernik, K., Klatzer, T., Kobler, E., Recht, M.P., Sodickson, D.K., Pock, T., et al.: Learning a variational network for reconstruction of accelerated MRI data. Magn. Reson. Med. **79**(6), 3055–3071 (2018)
9. Ronneberger, O., Fischer, P., Brox, T.: U-Net: convolutional networks for biomedical image segmentation. In: Navab, N., Hornegger, J., Wells, W.M., Frangi, A.F. (eds.) MICCAI 2015. LNCS, vol. 9351, pp. 234–241. Springer, Cham (2015). https://doi.org/10.1007/978-3-319-24574-4_28
10. Pruessmann, K.P., Weiger, M., Scheidegger, M.B., Boesiger, P.: Sense: sensitivity encoding for fast MRI. Magn. Reson. Med. **42**(5), 952–962 (1999)

Consistent Brain Ageing Synthesis

Tian Xia[1]([✉]), Agisilaos Chartsias[1], Sotirios A. Tsaftaris[1,2],
and for the Alzheimer's Disease Neuroimaging Initiative

[1] School of Engineering, University of Edinburgh, Edinburgh, UK
tian.xia@ed.ac.uk
[2] The Alan Turing Institute, London, UK

Abstract. Brain ageing is associated with morphological changes and cognitive degeneration, and can be affected by neurodegenerative diseases which can accelerate the ageing process. The ability to separate accelerated from healthy ageing is useful from a diagnostic perspective and towards developing subject-specific models of progression. In this paper we start with the 'simpler' problem of synthesising age-progressed 2D slices. We adopt adversarial training to learn the joint distribution of brain images and ages, and simulate aged images by a network conditioned on age (a continuous variable) encoded as an ordinal embedding vector. We introduce a loss to help preserve subject identity despite that we train with cross-sectional (unpaired) data. To evaluate the quality of aged images, a pre-trained age predictor is used to estimate an apparent age. We show qualitatively and quantitatively that our method can progressively synthesise realistic brain images of different target ages.

Keywords: Brain ageing · GAN · Conditioning

1 Introduction

Brain ageing is a complex process characterised by morphological and cognitive changes over a subject's lifespan. This process is influenced by age [18], neurodegenerative disease(s) [8], gender [9], education [4], and other factors. The separation of these factors is of great value for research and clinical applications to detect early stages of degenerative diseases [6,13]. One approach to achieve this separation task is to simulate the ageing process w.r.t. different factors, i.e. synthesise brain images given different factors as input [2,13]. In this paper, we focus on synthesising brain images conditioned on age.

One challenge with brain ageing synthesis is inter-subject variation, i.e. different individuals have different brain ageing trajectories. Previous studies used regression [7,13] to learn population models, which only represented the average brain images of different ages. However, this approach may not traverse a

Electronic supplementary material The online version of this chapter (https://doi.org/10.1007/978-3-030-32251-9_82) contains supplementary material, which is available to authorized users.

© Springer Nature Switzerland AG 2019
D. Shen et al. (Eds.): MICCAI 2019, LNCS 11767, pp. 750–758, 2019.
https://doi.org/10.1007/978-3-030-32251-9_82

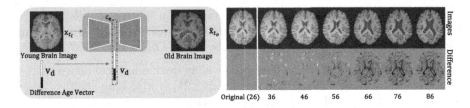

Fig. 1. Left: The network synthesises an image x_{t_o} of age t_o from input x_{t_i}, conditioned on vector v_d, derived by ordinal encoding of age difference $d = t_o - t_i$. **Right:** Top row shows the *synthetic output* at different age. Observe the progressive change between input and output (highlighted in bottom row).

subject-specific ageing trajectory [4]. Another challenge is lack of diverse longitudinal data, since it is difficult to acquire brain images of the same subject at different ages hindering the use of supervised learning.

In this paper, we overcome these challenges by proposing an adversarial deep neural network that learns the joint distribution of age and brain images. We introduce, and motivate, a loss function that helps preserve the identity of the subject –a classical problem in synthesis with cross-sectional (unpaired) data [23]– and induces progressively modulated changes on the brain. A simplified illustration of the proposed network and some example results are presented in Fig. 1. Given a brain image and a vector representing the target age difference, our method can synthesise it at an older age. For quantitative evaluation, we train a VGG-like network [17] as an age estimator to predict apparent age given an image. The estimated age is used as a proxy metric to evaluate the quality of output images in terms of *age accuracy*. We compare our method with conditional GAN [14] and CycleGAN [22]. The results show that we outperform these baselines in terms of *age accuracy*, and we consistently synthesize visually realistic images. **Contributions:**

1. We model ageing progression as a conditional network that is trained adversarially from cross-sectional (unpaired) data.
2. An age embedding mechanism that is used for synthesis and to teach an adversary to learn the joint distribution of age and brain appearance.
3. A regularisation loss to preserve age-modulated subject identity.

2   Related Work

Brain Ageing: Previous studies can be classified as: *prediction* (where ages are predicted from brain images) and *simulation* (where brain images are synthesised given age as input) [23]. For *prediction*, convolutional neural networks [5] and Gaussian Process Regression [6] have been used to estimate ages from MRI images as a marker for detecting neurodegenerative diseases. For *simulation*, [13] used partial regression to learn a model which represents the mean morphological change with age, while [7] proposed a regression method to learn a longitudinal growth model to synthesise population-average brain images of different ages. However, these regression-based methods did not consider subject-specific simulation and their performance was limited by the use of hand-crafted features.

Adversarial Networks: GANs have been widely used in medical image synthesis, with [3] converting MR to CT images and [1,21] synthesising healthy images from pathological ones. However, these approaches focused on translating images between different discrete states, and did not model a continuous time progression. The progression of Alzheimer's Disease (AD), was approached by [2] with image arithmetic. They synthesised images from random latent vectors and simulated AD progression using linear interpolation in latent space. However, they assumed a linear progression of the disease and did not address the problem of identity preservation. Instead, we directly model age progression, as a non-linear process [18], and focus on preserving subject identity.

3   Methods

3.1   Problem Overview and Notation

We denote a brain image as x_t of age t, and the distribution of brain images of age t as $\mathcal{X}_t$, such that $x_t \sim \mathcal{X}_t$. Our goal is to synthesise a brain image $\hat{x}_{t_o}$ of desired age t_o given an input image x_{t_i} of age t_i conditioned on the age difference d between input and output $d = t_o - t_i$, $t_o \geq t_i$. The objective is to generate $\hat{x}_{t_o}$ that is realistic (i.e. the distribution $\hat{\mathcal{X}}_{t_o}$ of output images $\hat{x}_{t_o}$ matches the data distribution $\mathcal{X}_{t_o}$) and retains the 'identity' of the subject throughout the ageing process. The contribution of our approach, shown in Fig. 2, is the design of the conditioning mechanism, a loss to preserve age-modulated identity and an adversary that learns the joint distribution of age and brain appearance.

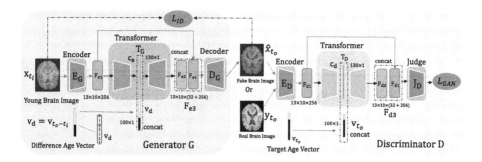

Fig. 2. Proposed method (training). x_{t_i} is the input image of age t_i; $\hat{x}_{t_o}$ is the output (aged) image (supposedly of the same subject as x_{t_i}) at the age t_o; v_{t_o} is the target age vector representing age t_o and v_d is the difference age vector corresponding to $d = t_o - t_i$. The *Generator* takes as input x_{t_i} and v_d, and outputs $\hat{x}_{t_o}$; the *Discriminator* takes as input an image and a target age vector, and outputs a Wasserstein score.

3.2   Model

Ordinal Encoding of Age: we use ordinal vectors to encode age (a continuous variable), to ensure that the *mean absolute error* between two age vectors positively correlates with age difference [11]. Assuming a max age of 100, we use a 100-d vector v_t to encode age t, where the first t elements are 1 and the rest are 0. (Fig. S3, in the *supplemental*, shows the benefit of ordinal vs. one-hot encoding.)

Model: Our model consists of a *Generator* and a *Discriminator*, shown in Fig. 2. These are detailed below. Note images x_{t_i}, $\hat{x}_{t_o}$ and y_{t_o} represent the input, the aged output and a real older brain image from another subject, respectively.

Generator: 'G' takes as input a 2D brain image x_{t_i} and an ordinal age vector v_d ($d = t_o - t_i$), and outputs a 2D older image $\hat{x}_{t_o}$. We condition on v_d such that when input and output ages are equal ($d = 0$) the network is drawn to recreate its input. This works in synergy with our identity-preserving loss described below.

The *Generator* consists of three subnetworks: '*Encoder*' E_G, '*Transformer*' T_G, and '*Decoder*' D_G. E_G extracts latent features F_{e1} from input x_{t_i}: $F_{e1} = E_G(x_{t_i})$. T_G outputs a feature map $F_{e2} = T_G(F_{e1}, v_d)$ by first transforming F_{e1} to a bottleneck vector c_{e1}, and by concatenating c_{e1} with v_d. To keep networks parameters low we empirically set the size of c_{e1} to *130*. Afterwards, to preserve information of x_i, and achieve accurate synthetic results, we introduce a skip connection between F_{e1} and F_{e2}: $F_{e3} = cat(F_{e1}, F_{e2})$, where cat($\cdot$) concatenates the elements of the given tensors along the channel dimension. Finally, the *Decoder* D_G synthesises the aged output $\hat{x}_t$ from F_{e3}. $\hat{x}_{t_o}$ should manifest the characteristics of brains at age t_o whilst preserving the identity of input x_{t_i}, i.e. $\hat{x}_{t_o}$ should be the brain image of the same subject as x_{t_i} at age t_o.

Discriminator: D contains an *Encoder* E_D and a *Transformer* T_D to condition on target age and a *Judge* J_D to output a discriminator score. Note here we condition on v_{t_o}, instead of v_d, to learn the joint distribution of brain appearance and age, such that it can discriminate real vs. synthetic images of correct age.

To summarise, the forward pass for the *Generator* is $\hat{x}_t = G(x_{t_i}, v_d)$, and for the *Discriminator* is $w_{fake} = D(\hat{x}_{t_o}, v_{t_o})$ and $w_{real} = D(y_{t_o}, v_{t_o})$.

3.3   Adversarial and Identity-Preserving Training Losses

The overall training loss is defined as:

$$\mathcal{L} = \max_{G}\min_{D}\mathcal{L}_{GAN} + \min_{G}\lambda_{ID}\mathcal{L}_{ID},$$

where $\mathcal{L}_{GAN}$ is the *GAN loss*, $\mathcal{L}_{ID}$ is an *age-modulated identity-preserving loss* and $\lambda_{ID} = 100$ the weight of $\mathcal{L}_{ID}$. $\mathcal{L}_{GAN}$ pushes the solution towards realistic images of correct age, whereas $\mathcal{L}_{ID}$ pushes towards subject-specific synthesis. $\mathcal{L}_{GAN}$ is a Wasserstein loss with gradient penalty for stable training [10]:

$$\mathcal{L}_{GAN} = \mathbb{E}_{y_{t_o} \sim \mathcal{X}_{t_o}, \hat{x}_{t_o} \sim \hat{\mathcal{X}}_{t_o}}[D(y_{t_o}, v_{t_o}) - D(\hat{x}_{t_o}, v_{t_o}) + \lambda_{GP}(\|\nabla_{\tilde{z}_{t_o}} D(\tilde{z}_{t_o})\|_2 - 1)^2],$$

where $\tilde{z}_t$ is the average sample defined as $\tilde{z}_t = \epsilon \hat{x}_t + (1 - \epsilon) y_t$, $\epsilon \sim U[0, 1]$. First two terms measure the Wasserstein distance between real and fake samples; last term is the gradient penalty. As in [10] we set $\lambda_{GP} = 10$.

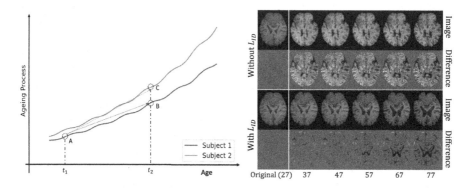

Fig. 3. Left: Illustration of ageing trajectories for two subjects showing that for an input image of age t_1 (A), the network may learn a mapping from A to C, which can still fool the *Discriminator* but lose the identity of Subject 1. **Right:** When $\mathcal{L}_{ID}$ is not used (top two rows) image differences are large (2nd row) and identity is lost, implying that we have an A to C potential mapping (left panel). In contrast, when $\mathcal{L}_{ID}$ is used (bottom two rows) changes are smooth and *consistent* (observe the gradually enlarging ventricles, 3rd row) and differences appear progressive (4th row).

$\mathcal{L}_{ID}$ defends against loss of identity, due to lack of longitudinal data and use of $\mathcal{L}_{GAN}$. We offer an illustration in Fig. 3 as motivation, where we show ageing trajectories for two subjects and 3 points A,B and C. We want to 'age' subject 1 of initial age t_1 (point A) to age t_2 (point B), but we do not have ground truth to ensure we stay on the trajectory (of subject 1). Instead, as training data we have images of subject 2 (and of many others) of age t_2 (point C). Without any restrictions, the *Generator* may learn a mapping from A to C to fool the *Discriminator*. This will break the identity of subject 1. To alleviate this and encourage mappings from A to B (ie. along the trajectory), we adopt:

$$\mathcal{L}_{ID} = \mathbb{E}_{x_{t_i} \sim \mathcal{X}_{t_i}, \hat{x}_{t_o} \sim \hat{\mathcal{X}}_{t_o}} \|x_{t_i} - \hat{x}_{t_o}\|^2 \cdot e^{-\frac{|t_o - t_i|}{|t_{max} - t_{min}|}},$$

where t_{max} and t_{min} are the maximal and minimal age in the training dataset, respectively. The regularisation $e^{-\frac{|t_o - t_i|}{|t_{max} - t_{min}|}} = e^{-\frac{|d|}{|t_{max} - t_{min}|}}$ captures that if age difference is small, then the change between x_{t_i} and $\hat{x}_{t_o}$ should also be small. In the special case of $d = 0$ it pushes the solution to reconstruct (auto-encode) the input (ie. $x_{t_i} \approx \hat{x}_{t_o}$). Right panel of Fig. 3, demonstrates the importance of this loss, via an ablation on training the network without and with $\mathcal{L}_{ID}$.

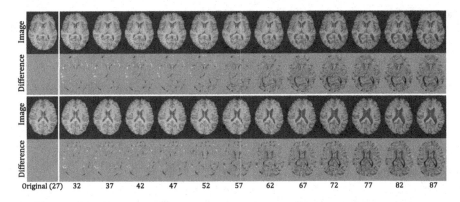

Fig. 4. Example results of synthetically aged brain images. Two slices of subjects with age 27, and synthetically aged outputs at different target ages (rows 1 and 3) are shown. The difference (rows 2 and 4) between input and output demonstrates progression.

4   Experiments

4.1   Experimental Setup

Dataset and Preprocessing: We apply our 2D method on two datasets. We use the Cam-CAN [19] and ADNI datasets [15]. For each dataset, we use FSL [20] to perform brain extraction and volumetric registration to MNI 152 space. We normalise the resulting intensities to $[-1,1]$. For every 5-year span, we select 38 volumes with 30 used for training and 8 for testing. Thus, there are 360 training and 96 testing volumes for CAM-CAN, and 240 training and 64 testing volumes for ADNI. We select the middle 60 axial slices from each volume and use these 2D slices to perform experiments.

Baselines: We set up 2 baselines with conditional GAN [14] and CycleGAN [22]. Since both frameworks only translate images between two discrete styles, for each dataset, we train different models for transforming the youngest group to different target age groups (where each group covers 10 years).

Implementation Details: The method is implemented in Python using Keras (https://keras.io). The *Generator* is a U-net [16] with the bottleneck layer modified to be a *Transformer*. The *Discriminator* is a ResNet [12] with a latent layer modified as *Transformer*. The detailed structures are shown in *Supplemental*.

Evaluation Metric: Due to lack of sufficient longitudinal data, it is hard to evaluate the synthetic output. As a proxy, we train an *age predictor*, f_{pred}, to estimate apparent age of outputs, and use the estimated age to evaluate *age accuracy*, i.e. how close the output is to the desired target age. The *age predictor* is a VGG-like network [17] with *mean absolute error* of 3.2 years on training dataset and 5.3 years on testing (detailed structure in *supplemental*). Formally, we use *predicted age difference (PAD)*: $PAD = \mathbb{E}_{x_{t_i} \sim \mathcal{X}_{t_i}} |f_{pred}(G(x_{t_i}, v_{t_o-t_i})) - t_o|$.

Table 1. Testing test ($N = 480$ images) PAD results (defined in Sect. 4.2) on Cam-CAN and ADNI of proposed and baseline methods. Best values shown in **bold**. Paired t-tests (5% level) between our method and the best baseline are significant.

	Cam-CAN					ADNI		
Target Age	(30,40)	(40, 50)	(50, 60)	(60, 70)	(70, 80)	(60, 70)	(70,80)	(80,90)
Conditional GAN	$13.5_{\pm 6.2}$	$11.3_{\pm 5.4}$	$9.3_{\pm 5.1}$	$10.4_{\pm 4.7}$	$9.5_{\pm 5.2}$	$10.3_{\pm 4.7}$	$9.3_{\pm 4.5}$	$8.9_{\pm 4.9}$
CycleGAN	$12.7_{\pm 7.2}$	$11.5_{\pm 6.3}$	$9.5_{\pm 5.4}$	$9.4_{\pm 6.4}$	$9.7_{\pm 5.8}$	$9.6_{\pm 5.4}$	$9.8_{\pm 4.7}$	$9.6_{\pm 5.2}$
Proposed method	$\mathbf{7.2}_{\pm 3.4}$	$\mathbf{6.1}_{\pm 3.6}$	$\mathbf{4.6}_{\pm 3.2}$	$\mathbf{4.3}_{\pm 3.1}$	$\mathbf{4.1}_{\pm 3.5}$	$\mathbf{4.6}_{\pm 3.1}$	$\mathbf{5.4}_{\pm 3.6}$	$\mathbf{4.9}_{\pm 3.8}$

4.2 Experiments and Results

Ageing Progression: We visualise differences between input and output images in Fig. 4 for two subjects (more results in the *supplemental*, including higher zoom to show sharpness). Observe that the output gradually changes as age increases. At an early stage, the brains do not change much. After around age 52, *ageing* is accelerated. This observation is consistent with [18], implying that our method captures known age-modulated changes in the brain.

Comparison with Baselines: We apply the pre-trained age predictor to quantitatively evaluate the proposed method and compare it with baselines. The results for each age group are shown in Table 1. *Conditional GAN* and *Cycle-GAN* are trained as described in Sect. 4.1, to synthesise images of a particular group. Instead, our method can generate images of any age. Therefore, in order to make it comparable with the baselines, we use the middle age of each group as the target age. The quantitative results show that our method, can achieve more *age-consistent* output compared to the baselines. The higher *PAD* in the early stage (before age 50) could be caused by the slow rate of brain ageing, i.e. when ageing process is slow, prediction becomes more difficult.

Longitudinal Evaluation: We also evaluated our method using a small number (15) of follow-up studies from ADNI which start from an age between 55–60 years and end at an age larger than 60. The MAE between the ground-truth images and predicted aged images are 0.08, 0.21 and 0.20 for proposed model, conditional GAN and CycleGAN, respectively. These results show that our method synthesizes realistic aged images and preserves subject identity well.

5 Conclusion

We proposed a deep adversarial neural network to model brain ageing. The method learns the joint distribution of age and brain morphology. We also proposed a loss to encourage the preservation of subject identity. Due to lack of longitudinal data, quantitative evaluation of synthetic images remains challenging. Here, we used an age predictor to predict apparent age of output images as a proxy to evaluate quality. Both qualitative and quantitative results show that our method can smoothly and consistently simulate subject-specific ageing.

We evaluated on 2D healthy brain images. As future work, we envision involving 3D data and other factors (e.g. gender). A longitudinal and diverse dataset with large age span will be ideal for evaluation, however, this is currently lacking as a community resource.

Acknowledgements. This work was supported by the University of Edinburgh by a PhD studentship. This work was partially supported by EPSRC (EP/P022928/1) and by The Alan Turing Institute under the EPSRC grant EP/N510129/1. This work was supported in part by the US National Institutes of Health (R01HL136578). We also thank Nvidia for donating a Titan-X GPU. S.A. Tsaftaris acknowledges the support of the Royal Academy of Engineering and the Research Chairs and Senior Research Fellowships scheme.

References

1. Baumgartner, C.F., Koch, L.M., Can Tezcan, K., Xi Ang, J., Konukoglu, E.: Visual feature attribution using wasserstein GANs. In: CVPR, pp. 8309–8319 (2018)
2. Bowles, C., Gunn, R., Hammers, A., Rueckert, D.: Modelling the progression of Alzheimer's disease in MRI using generative adversarial networks. In: Medical Imaging 2018: Image Processing. International Society for Optics and Photonics (2018)
3. Chartsias, A., Joyce, T., Dharmakumar, R., Tsaftaris, S.A.: Adversarial image synthesis for unpaired multi-modal cardiac data. In: Tsaftaris, S.A., Gooya, A., Frangi, A.F., Prince, J.L. (eds.) SASHIMI 2017. LNCS, vol. 10557, pp. 3–13. Springer, Cham (2017). https://doi.org/10.1007/978-3-319-68127-6_1
4. Cole, J.H., Franke, K.: Predicting age using neuroimaging: innovative brain ageing biomarkers. Trends Neurosci. **40**(12), 681–690 (2017)
5. Cole, J.H., et al.: Predicting brain age with deep learning from raw imaging data results in a reliable and heritable biomarker. NeuroImage **163**, 115–124 (2017)
6. Cole, J.H., et al.: Brain age predicts mortality. Mol. Psychiatry (2017)
7. Davis, B.C., Fletcher, P.T., Bullitt, E., Joshi, S.: Population shape regression from random design data. Int. J. Comput. Vis. **90**(2), 255–266 (2010)
8. Franke, K., Gaser, C.: Longitudinal changes in individual BrainAGE in healthy aging, mild cognitive impairment, and Alzheimer's disease. GeroPsych J. Gerontopsychology Geriatr. Psychiatry **25**(4), 235 (2012)
9. Goyal, M.S., et al.: Persistent metabolic youth in the aging female brain. PNAS **116**(8), 3251–3255 (2019)
10. Gulrajani, I., Ahmed, F., Arjovsky, M., Dumoulin, V., Courville, A.C.: Improved training of Wasserstein GANs. In: NIPS, pp. 5767–5777 (2017)
11. Gutiérrez, P.A., Perez-Ortiz, M., Sanchez-Monedero, J., Fernandez-Navarro, F., Hervas-Martinez, C.: Ordinal regression methods: survey and experimental study. IEEE Trans. Knowl. Data Eng. **28**(1), 127–146 (2016)
12. He, K., Zhang, X., Ren, S., Sun, J.: Deep residual learning for image recognition. In: CVPR (2016)
13. Huizinga, W., et al.: A spatio-temporal reference model of the aging brain. NeuroImage **169**, 11–22 (2018)
14. Mirza, M., Osindero, S.: Conditional generative adversarial nets. arXiv preprint arXiv:1411.1784 (2014)

15. Petersen, R.C., et al.: Alzheimer's Disease Neuroimaging Initiative (ADNI): clinical characterization. Neurology **74**(3), 201–209 (2010)

16. Ronneberger, O., Fischer, P., Brox, T.: U-net: convolutional networks for biomedical image segmentation. In: Navab, N., Hornegger, J., Wells, W.M., Frangi, A.F. (eds.) MICCAI 2015. LNCS, vol. 9351, pp. 234–241. Springer, Cham (2015). https://doi.org/10.1007/978-3-319-24574-4_28

17. Simonyan, K., Zisserman, A.: Very deep convolutional networks for large-scale image recognition. In: ICLR (2015)

18. Singh-Manoux, A., et al.: Timing of onset of cognitive decline: results from Whitehall II prospective cohort study. BMJ **344**, d7622 (2012)

19. Taylor, J.R., et al.: The Cambridge centre for ageing and neuroscience (Cam-CAN) data repository: structural and functional MRI, MEG, and cognitive data from a cross-sectional adult lifespan sample. NeuroImage **144**, 262–269 (2017)

20. Woolrich, M.W., et al.: Bayesian analysis of neuroimaging data in FSL. Neuroimage **45**(1), S173–S186 (2009)

21. Xia, T., Chartsias, A., Tsaftaris, S.A.: Adversarial pseudo healthy synthesis needs pathology factorization. In: International Conference on Medical Imaging with Deep Learning (2019)

22. Zhu, J.Y., Park, T., Isola, P., Efros, A.A.: Unpaired image-to-image translation using cycle-consistent adversarial networks. In: CVPR (2017)

23. Ziegler, G., Dahnke, R., Gaser, C.: Models of the aging brain structure and individual decline. Front. Neuroinf. **6**, 3 (2012)

Hybrid Generative Adversarial Networks for Deep MR to CT Synthesis Using Unpaired Data

Guodong Zeng[1,2,3] and Guoyan Zheng[1,2(✉)]

[1] School of Biomedical Engineering, Shanghai Jiao Tong University, Shanghai, China
guoyan.zheng@sjtu.edu.cn
[2] Institute of Medical Robotics, Shanghai Jiao Tong University, Shanghai, China
[3] ARTORG Center for Biomedical Engineering, University of Bern,
Bern, Switzerland

Abstract. Many different methods have been proposed for generation of synthetic CT from MR images. Most of these methods depend on pairwise aligned MR and CT training images of the same patient, which are difficult to obtain. 2D cycle-consistent Generative Adversarial Networks (2D-cGAN) have been explored before for generating synthetic CTs from MR images but the results are not satisfied due to spatial inconsistency. There exists attempt to develop 3D cycle GAN (3D-cGAN) for image translation but its training requires large number of data which may not be always available. In this paper, we introduce two novel mechanisms to address above mentioned problems. First, we introduce a hybrid GAN (hGAN) consisting of a 3D generator network and a 2D discriminator network for deep MR to CT synthesis using unpaired data. We use 3D fully convolutional networks to form the generator, which can better model the 3D spatial information and thus could solve the discontinuity problem across slices. Second, we take the results generated from the 2D-cGAN as weak labels, which will be used together with an adversarial training strategy to encourage the generator's 3D output to look like a stack of real CT slices as much as possible. Experimental results demonstrated that our approach achieved better results than the state-of-the-art when limited number of unpaired data are available.

Keywords: Deep learning · CT synthesis · MRI · Generative Adversarial Networks

1 Introduction

Despite the fact that Computed Tomography (CT) images have limited soft tissue contrast and result in extra radiation to the patients, CT imaging is critical for various applications, e.g., radiotherapy treatment planning and Positron Emission Tomography (PET) attenuation correction. This is because CT images offer accurate presentation of patient geometry and more importantly, CT values

© Springer Nature Switzerland AG 2019
D. Shen et al. (Eds.): MICCAI 2019, LNCS 11767, pp. 759–767, 2019.
https://doi.org/10.1007/978-3-030-32251-9_83

in Hounsfield units (HU), which measure tissue attenuation coefficients, can be directly converted to electron density for radiation dose calculation. Recently, interests in replacing CT with magnetic resonance imaging (MRI) have grown rapidly due to MRI's free of ionizing radiation, excellent soft tissue contrast, and ability of multiparametric imaging through various MRI sequences. The main challenges in replacing CT with MRI, however, are (a) the MRI intensity values, unlike CT values, are not directly related to electron densities; and (b) conventional MRI sequences pose dramatic limitations for distinguishing cortical bone from air. It is therefore desirable to have a method to derive CT-equivalent information from MR images. Such MR-based CT-equivalent data are often referred to as synthetic CT (sCT) in the literature.

Many different methods have been proposed for generation of synthetic CT from MR images [1–13]. Most of these methods depend on pairwise aligned MR and CT training images of the same patient, which are difficult to obtain. Any error in aligning MR and CT images could lead to errors in generating sCT. Inspired by the work of [14], Wolterink et al. [5] introduced a 2D method for automated MR-to-CT synthesis using cycle-consistent Generative Adversarial Networks (2D-cGAN), which could be trained without the need for paired training data. The results generated by 2D-cGAN look good along the view used for training but spatial inconsistency is observed when the images generated by 2D-cGAN are used to construct a 3D volume. There exist attempts to develop 3D cycle GAN (3D-cGAN) for image translation [10,15] but its training requires large number of data which may not be always available. For example, Zhang et al. [16] used a dataset with 4,496 cardiovascular 3D images in MRI and CT modalities, while Pan et al. [15] takes 1457 MR images and 649 PET images. In contrast, Wolterink et al. [5] only used brain MR and CT images of 24 patients to train their 2D-cGAN.

In this paper, we introduced two novel mechanisms to address above mentioned problems. First, we introduce a hybrid GAN (hGAN) consisting of a 3D generator network and a 2D discriminator network for deep MR to CT synthesis using unpaired data. We use 3D fully convolutional networks to form the generator, which can better model the 3D spatial information and thus could solve the discontinuity problem across slices. Second, we take the results generated from the 2D-cGAN as weak labels, which will be used together with an adversarial training strategy to encourage the generator's 3D output to look like a stack of real CT slices as much as possible. The reason why we choose to use a 2D discriminator network instead of a 3D one are based on following observations. Due to GPU memory restrictions caused by moving to 3D, a 3D discriminator network depends on patch processing where sampled patches only contain a local view of the data, lack of global context. Additionally, a 3D discriminator network has much more parameters to be learned than a 2D discriminator network. Thus, its training requires large number of data as shown in [10,15]. In contrast, a 2D discriminator network takes complete slices as the input which have a global view of the data. Its training requires much smaller number of data as shown in [5].

The paper is organized as follows. In the next section we present our method. We then describe experimental results in Sect. 3, followed by discussions in Sect. 4.

2   Methods

In this section, we first present an overview of the present method, followed by presentation of the loss functions, the network architectures, and the implementation details.

Overview of the Proposed hGAN. Assume we have a set of unpaired data containing $\{X^i\}_{i=1}^N$ MR images and $\{Y^j\}_{j=1}^M$ CT images, we first extract slices along the axial view to train a 2D-cGAN. After that, for each MR image X^i, there will be a sCT image which can be used as a weak label $\tilde{Y}^i$. As shown in Fig. 1, our hGAN consists of a 3D generator network G and a 2D discriminator network D. The 3D generator network G has a 3D Fully Convolutional Networks (FCN) architecture and can directly map an input MR volume to a sCT volume in arbitrary size. During training, the 3D generator is trained in a weakly supervised way. Specifically, we randomly sample a number of K continuous slices along the axial view from a MR volume X^i and from the corresponding weak label volume $\tilde{Y}^i$ that was constructed from the results obtained from the trained 2D-cGAN, which are taken as 3D patch inputs P_x^i and $\tilde{P}_y^i$ respectively to the 3D generator network (i.e., when training the 3D generator network, we chose the batch size to be 1). The 3D generator is optimized by a reconstruction L1 loss between the prediction $G(P_x^i)$ and the weak labels $\tilde{P}_y^i$. The output from the 3D generator will be converted into a batch of 2D K slices $\{\hat{s}_y^k\}_{k=1}^K$ (3D to 2D conversion), which will then be used together with K slices $\{s_y^k\}_{k=1}^K$ sampled from an unpaired real CT data Y^j as the input to train the 2D discriminator network D (i.e., when training the 2D discriminator network, the batch size is chosen to be K) in order to discriminate whether the input are real or fake. The adversarial loss will encourage the generator's 3D output to look like a stack of real CT slices as much as possible.

Discriminator Loss. The 2D discriminator network D is trained to discriminate between sCT slices $\{\hat{s}_y^k\}_{k=1}^K$ and the unpaired real CT slices $\{s_y^k\}_{k=1}^K$. Specifically, the discriminator D is trying to tell whether the input CT slice is real or fake, where real is 1 and fake is 0. The loss function for D is defined as:

$$L_D = \sum_k \left(1 - D(s_y^k)\right)^2 + \sum_k (D(\hat{s}_y^k))^2 \tag{1}$$

Generator Loss. For the generator network G, it aims to generate a sCT image patch $\hat{P}_y^i$ from an input MR patch P_x^i and its corresponding weak label patch $\tilde{P}_y^i$ obtained from the trained 2D-cGAN. Additionally, the generator network also

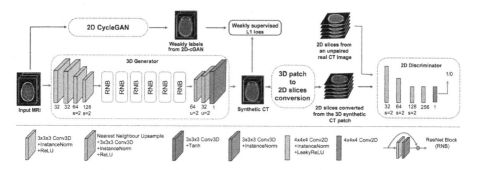

Fig. 1. A schematic view of the proposed hGAN for MR-to-CT synthesis using unpaired data. hGAN consists of a 3D generator network and a 2D discriminator network. The 3D generator is trained in a weakly supervised way by using paired sCT images generated from a 2D-cGAN as weak labels. The 2D discriminator constrains the generator's 3D output to look like a stack of real CT slices as much as possible. The number below each block in generator and discriminator is the channel number. 's = 2' means stride is 2 in convolutional layers, and 'u = 2' means 2 times upscaling.

aims to generate a sCT image patch, which after 3D to 2D conversion, cannot be discriminated from a stack of real CT slices by the discriminator network D. Thus, the loss of G includes a reconstruction error and an adversarial term. It is defined as:

$$L_G = \left\| G(P_x^i) - \tilde{P}_y^i \right\|_1 + \lambda \sum_k \left(1 - D(\hat{s}_y^k)\right)^2 \qquad (2)$$

Network Architecture. As shown in Fig. 1, the 3D generator network follows an encoding and decoding structure. The encoding path consists of four convolutional layers (with 32, 32, 64 and 128 channels, respectively). Each of them is immediately followed by an instance normalization (IN) and ReLU layer. Then the encoder path is connected with 6 residual blocks. Each residual block consists of 2 convolutional layers while the first one is followed by an IN and a ReLU layer, and the second one is only followed by an IN layer. Finally, the decoding path consists of 2 upscaling blocks (with 64 and 32 channels, respectively), a Conv layer and a Tanh output layer. Each upscaling block consists of a nearest-neighbor interpolation layer, an IN and a ReLU layer. The 2D discriminator network D contains 5 convolution layers(with 32, 64, 128, 256 and 1 channels, respectively). All convolutional layers in D are followed by an IN and a LeakyReLU (leak = 0.2) layer except for the last output layer. All kernel size of the convolutions in the 3D Generator network is $3 \times 3 \times 3$ and all kernel size of the convolutions in the 2D Discriminator network is 4×4.

Implementation Details. The proposed hGAN was implemented in python using TensorFlow framework on a desktop with a 3.6 GHz Intel(R) i7 CPU and a GTX 1080 Ti graphics card with 11 GB GPU memory. We first trained a 2D-cGAN with slices of axial plane to get the weak image labels. All experiment

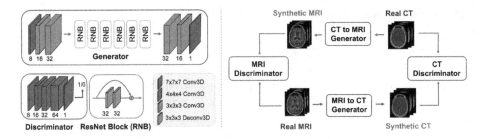

Fig. 2. The architecture of the 3D-cGAN.

settings are the same as used in [14]. We then start to train the hGAN. During the training, we randomly cropped patches containing $K = 32$ slices of the associated data. We trained the hGAN from scratch. All parameters were initialized from a Truncated normal distribution ($\mu = 0, \sigma = 0.02$) and then updated by the Adam algorithm. We trained the network for 200 epoches in total. The initial learning rate was 5×10^{-4} and kept the same for the first 100 epoches. In the next 100 epoches, it was linearly decayed to 0. λ in Eq. 2 was set as 0 and 5 for the first and second 100 epoches, respectively. It means the network was only optimized by the L1 loss for the first 100 epoches. During testing phase, we fed the whole MR image to the neural network. Following Wolterink et al. [5], we use Mean Absolute Error (MAE) and Peak Signal-to-Noise Ratio (PSNR) as evaluation metrics. Please note that it is difficult to compare MAE and PSNR results reported in different papers as different CT HU ranges are used. For example, the HU range of CT images in [5] was $[-600, 1400]$ while in our paper, the HU range of our CT images was $[-1024, 2253]$. Thus, we also adopted relative MAE as a new evaluation metric, which was defined as the MAE value divided by the range of HU values of ground truth CT.

3   Experiments and Results

3.1   Dataset Description

We evaluated our data on MR and CT images of 50 subjects [13]. The MR images were acquired with a 3T Siemens Magnetom Skyra scanner (Siemens Healthcare, Erlangen, Germany) using 3D T1-weighted magnetization-prepared rapid gradient-echo (MP-RAGE). For each patient, the MR imaging was followed by a CT scan on the Biograph mCT scanner (Siemens Healthcare, Erlangen, Germany). The two modalities were aligned with a rigid registration. The CT voxel values were in the range of $[-1024, 2253]$ Hounsfield Unit (HU). All the images are resampled to have the size of $256 \times 288 \times 112$.

3.2   Experimental Results

Validation Study. With a standard 2-fold cross-validation study setup, we compared the proposed approach with the state-of-the-art methods when unpaired data were used: 2D-cGAN [14] and 3D-cGAN [10]. For 2D-cGAN, we obtained the results by running the official code from the original authors and kept the same parameters as reported in their paper. For 3D-cGAN, we implemented it by ourselves and the network architecture is shown in Fig. 2, which is an extension of 2D-cGAN. Due to the size of the 3D-cGAN, we used a fixed patch size of $256 \times 288 \times 16$ to train the 3D-cGAN. The results are shown in Table 1, which demonstrated the efficacy of the proposed method. Our proposed hGAN outperforms the 2D-cGAN and the 3D-cGAN in all metrics, and reported a MAE of 75.04 HU, an average PSNR of 25.69, and a relative MAE of 2.29%. Although the method introduced in [5] reported a MAE of 73.7 HU and an average PSNR of 32.3, their relative MAE was 3.69%, which was larger than our method, indicating a lower performance than ours.

Table 1. Quantitative evaluation results

MAE	Mean	Relative MAE	Mean	PSNR	Mean
2D-cGAN	111.35	2D-cGAN	3.40%	2D-cGAN	23.43
3D-cGAN	118.34	3D-cGAN	3.61%	3D-cGAN	22.41
hGAN	**75.04**	hGAN	**2.29%**	hGAN	**25.69**

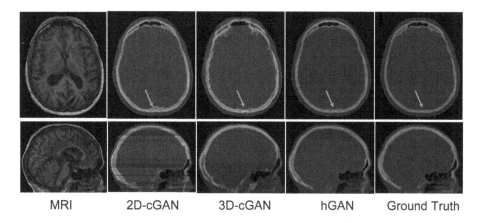

| MRI | 2D-cGAN | 3D-cGAN | hGAN | Ground Truth |

Fig. 3. Visual comparison of sCTs generated with different methods.

Figure 3 visually compares the sCTs generated with different methods. We can observe that the proposed hGAN shows better results in terms of spatial consistency and smoothness. Further, the results from the proposed hGAN look much closer to the ground truth in details than 2D-cGAN and the 3D-cGAN. For the 2D-cGAN, the is caused by the spatial inconsistency while for the 3D-cGAN, it probably needs more data to generalize.

Ablation Study. To investigate the influence of different discriminators in hGAN, we conducted a comparison study to compare the performance of three variants of our method: (a) without using any discriminator network; (b) using the 2D discriminator network as we proposed; and (c) using a 3D discriminator network. In this study, we randomly chosen data of 25 subjects as the training data and the data of remaining 25 subjects as the testing data. The results are shown in Fig. 4. Without using any discriminator, the 3D generator network was trained with purely weak labels generated from the 2D-cGAN. A MAE of 81.66 was obtained. With the 2D discriminator network, it was improved to 74.82. However, when a 3D discriminator was used, the MAE increased when compared with the case when no discriminator was used. Such a finding indicates that when only limited unpaired data are available, it is difficult to train a 3D discriminator and it is better to use a 2D discriminator for an improved performance.

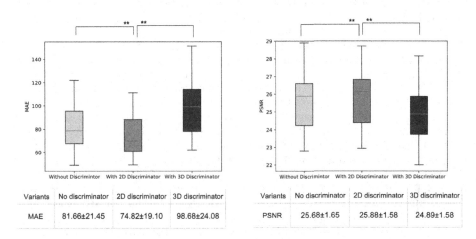

Fig. 4. MAE and PSNR boxplots of three different variants of our method. The box shows the interquartile range (IQR) and extends from first quartile (Q1) to third quartile (Q3) values of the data, with a line at the median data. The whiskers extend up to 1.5 times of the IQR. ** indicates significant improvement with significance level of 0.01

4 Discussion

In summary, we presented hybrid generative adversarial networks consisting of a 3D generator network and a 2D discriminator network to address the problem of generating synthetic CT images from MR images when only limited number of unpaired data were available. 3D fully convolutional networks formed the generator to better model the 3D spatial information and to solve the discontinuity problem across slices. Due to the GPU memory constrain and due to the fact that 3D discriminator network had much more parameters to be learned than a 2D one, we chose to use 2D discriminator network in our hGAN. We took the results generated from a 2D-cGAN as weak labels together with an adversarial training strategy to train the hGAN. Our results demonstrated that the present method achieved better results than the state-of-the-art when only limited number of unpaired data were available.

Acknowledgment. This study was partially supported by a start-up funding from Shanghai Jiao Tong University, China with the Grant No. WF220882002. We are grateful to the data provided by Dr. H Arabi and Prof. H Zaidi in Geneva University Hospital, Dept. of Medical Imaging & Information Sciences, Geneva, Switzerland, which were used in our previous study [13].

References

1. Nie, D., Cao, X., Gao, Y., Wang, L., Shen, D.: Estimating CT image from MRI data using 3D fully convolutional networks. In: Carneiro, G., et al. (eds.) LABELS/DLMIA-2016. LNCS, vol. 10008, pp. 170–178. Springer, Cham (2016). https://doi.org/10.1007/978-3-319-46976-8_18
2. Han, X.: MR-based synthetic CT generation using a deep convolutional neural network. Med. Phys. **44**(4), 1408–1419 (2017)
3. Burgos, N., et al.: Iterative framework for the joint segmentation and CT synthesis of MR images: application to MRI-only radiotherapy treatment planning. Phys. Med. Biol. **62**, 4237–4253 (2017)
4. Nie, D., et al.: Medical image synthesis with context-aware generative adversarial networks. In: Descoteaux, M., Maier-Hein, L., Franz, A., Jannin, P., Collins, D.L., Duchesne, S. (eds.) MICCAI 2017. LNCS, vol. 10435, pp. 417–425. Springer, Cham (2017). https://doi.org/10.1007/978-3-319-66179-7_48
5. Wolterink, J.M., Dinkla, A.M., Savenije, M.H.F., Seevinck, P.R., van den Berg, C.A.T., Išgum, I.: Deep MR to CT synthesis using unpaired data. In: Tsaftaris, S.A., Gooya, A., Frangi, A.F., Prince, J.L. (eds.) SASHIMI 2017. LNCS, vol. 10557, pp. 14–23. Springer, Cham (2017). https://doi.org/10.1007/978-3-319-68127-6_2
6. Liu, F., Jang, H., Kijowski, R., Bradshaw, T., McMillan, A.B.: Deep learning MR imaging-based attenuation correction for PET/MR imaging. Radiology **286**(2), 676–684 (2017)
7. Chartsias, A., Joyce, T., Dharmakumar, R., Tsaftaris, S.A.: Adversarial image synthesis for unpaired multi-modal cardiac data. In: Tsaftaris, S.A., Gooya, A., Frangi, A.F., Prince, J.L. (eds.) SASHIMI 2017. LNCS, vol. 10557, pp. 3–13. Springer, Cham (2017). https://doi.org/10.1007/978-3-319-68127-6_1
8. Huo, Y., Xu, Z., Bao, S., Assad, A., Abramson, R.G., Landman, B.A.: Adversarial synthesis learning enables segmentation without target modality ground truth. arXiv preprint arXiv:1712.07695 (2017)
9. Ladefoged, C.N., et al.: A multi-centre evaluation of eleven clinically feasible brain PET/MRI attenuation correction techniques using a large cohort of patients. NeuroImage **147**, 346–359 (2017)
10. Zhang, Z., Yang, L., Zheng, Y.: Translating and segmenting multimodal medical volumes with cycle-and shape-consistency generative adversarial network. In: Proceedings CVPR, pp. 9242–9251 (2018)
11. Hiasa, Y., et al.: Cross-modality image synthesis from unpaired data using Cycle-GAN. In: Gooya, A., Goksel, O., Oguz, I., Burgos, N. (eds.) SASHIMI 2018. LNCS, vol. 11037, pp. 31–41. Springer, Cham (2018). https://doi.org/10.1007/978-3-030-00536-8_4

12. Yang, H., et al.: Unpaired brain MR-to-CT synthesis using a structure-constrained CycleGAN. In: Stoyanov, D., et al. (eds.) DLMIA/ML-CDS-2018. LNCS, vol. 11045, pp. 174–182. Springer, Cham (2018). https://doi.org/10.1007/978-3-030-00889-5_20

13. Arabi, H., Zeng, G., Zheng, G., Zaidi, H.: Novel adversarial semantic structure deep learning for MRI-guided attenuation correction in brain PET/MRI. Eur. J. Nucl. Med. Mol. Imaging, 1–14 (2019)

14. Zhu, J.Y., Park, T., Isola, P., Efros, A.: Unpaired image-to-image translation using cycle-consistent adversarial networks. In: Proceedings ICCV, pp. 2242–2251. IEEE (2017)

15. Pan, Y., Liu, M., Lian, C., Zhou, T., Xia, Y., Shen, D.: Synthesizing missing PET from MRI with cycle-consistent generative adversarial networks for Alzheimer's disease diagnosis. In: Frangi, A.F., Schnabel, J.A., Davatzikos, C., Alberola-López, C., Fichtinger, G. (eds.) MICCAI 2018. LNCS, vol. 11072, pp. 455–463. Springer, Cham (2018). https://doi.org/10.1007/978-3-030-00931-1_52

16. Zhang, S., Yang, J., Schiele, B.: Occluded pedestrian detection through guided attention in CNNs. In: Proceedings CVPR (2018)

Arterial Spin Labeling Images Synthesis via Locally-Constrained WGAN-GP Ensemble

Wei Huang[1] , Mingyuan Luo[1], Xi Liu[1], Peng Zhang[2], Huijun Ding[3], and Dong Ni[3(✉)]

[1] School of Information Engineering, Nanchang University, Nanchang, China
[2] School of Computer Science, Northwestern Polytechnical University, Xi'an, China
[3] Guangdong Provincial Key Laboratory of Biomedical Measurements and Ultrasound Imaging, School of Biomedical Engineering, Health Science Center, Shenzhen University, Shenzhen, China
nidong@szu.edu.cn

Abstract. Arterial spin labeling (ASL) images begin to receive much popularity in dementia diseases diagnosis recently, yet it is still not commonly seen in well-established image datasets for investigating dementia diseases. Hence, synthesizing ASL images from available data is worthy of investigations. In this study, a novel locally-constrained WGAN-GP model ensemble is proposed to realize ASL images synthesis from structural MRI for the first time. Technically, this new WGAN-GP model ensemble is unique in its constrained optimization task, in which diverse local constraints are incorporated. In this way, more details of synthesized ASL images can be obtained after incorporating local constraints in this new ensemble. The effectiveness of the new WGAN-GP model ensemble for synthesizing ASL images has been substantiated both qualitatively and quantitatively through rigorous experiments in this study. Comprehensive analyses reveal that, this new WGAN-GP model ensemble is superior to several state-of-the-art GAN-based models in synthesizing ASL images from structural MRI in this study.

Keywords: Medical images synthesis · GAN · Dementia diagnosis

1 Introduction

Adequate medical images are often indispensable in contemporary deep learning-based medical imaging studies, although the acquisition of certain image modalities may become limited due to several factors including high acquisition cost, patients' concern, etc. However, thanks to recent advances in deep learning techniques, the above challenging problem can be substantially alleviated by medical images synthesis, by which various modalities including T1/T2/DTI MRI images [1,2], PET images [3], cardiac ultrasound images [4], retinal images [5], etc., have already been successfully synthesized from other available data. Among various deep learning techniques incorporated in those above-mentioned medical

© Springer Nature Switzerland AG 2019
D. Shen et al. (Eds.): MICCAI 2019, LNCS 11767, pp. 768–776, 2019.
https://doi.org/10.1007/978-3-030-32251-9_84

images synthesis studies, the generative adversarial network (GAN) [6] receives much popularity in recent years.

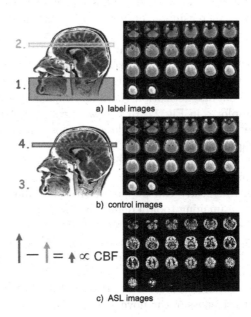

a) label images

b) control images

c) ASL images

Fig. 1. An illustration of ASL images acquisition with example images (i.e., from the transverse view) obtained from one patient in this study.

Although the original GAN has noticeable merits in synthesizing images because of its unique model structure composed of a generator and a discriminator that are co-trained together with a competing strategy, its shortcomings should not be neglected. *First*, the metric to be optimized in the original GAN (i.e., either the Kullback-Leibler divergence or the Jensen-Shannon divergence) cannot reasonably reflect the true difference between distributions of real data and synthesized data. *Second*, the problem of vanishing gradients is often inevitable in the original GAN, so that the model itself is often quite challenging to be well-trained. In order to tackle the above dilemmas, GAN-based alternatives, including WGAN [7], WGAN-GP [8], etc., have been proposed in recent years. Technically, WGAN mainly replaces the Kullback-Leibler divergence in the original GAN with the Wasserstein distance, which is more convenient to derive gradients for training the model [7] (i.e., for tackling the above-mentioned problem (1). However, the weight clipping utilized in WGAN for enforcing the well-known Lipschitz constraint is not beneficial to tackle the problem of vanishing gradients (i.e., for tackling the above-mentioned problem (2). In order to solve both the two problems simultaneously, WGAN-GP is proposed and the gradient penalty is introduced as an alternative towards the weight clipping [8].

In this study, a novel WGAN-GP model ensemble with new local constraints is proposed to realize medical images synthesis for the first time, and arterial spin labeling (ASL) images are successfully synthesized from structural MRI. Generally speaking, ASL is widely acknowledged as a non-invasive fMRI technique, which utilizes arterial water as an endogenous tracer to measure the perfusion signal. Also, it receives increasing attention in dementia diseases diagnosis only beginning from recent years [9–11]. Technically, an ASL image is produced via a label image and a control image. When a certain scanned region within the brain of a patient is determined (i.e., illustrated as Area 2 of subplot a in Fig. 1), arterial blood supplying into the interested region is magnetically labeled by inverting its longitudinal magnetization via radio-frequency pulses (i.e., occurred within Area 1 of subplot a in Fig. 1). In this way, water molecules within arterial blood will serve as tracers, and ASL label images can be acquired, therein. For ASL control images, the arterial blood is not magnetically labeled, and ASL images can be finally produced as the direct difference via subtracting ASL label images from ASL control images.

Contributions of this study can be summarized as follows. *First*, although ASL is a relatively new imaging tool in dementia diseases diagnosis, ASL images do lack in many well-established image-based datasets for studying dementia diseases, unfortunately. Synthesizing ASL images from other commonly seen data (e.g., structural MRI in this study) is undoubtedly a beneficial supplement. *Second*, a novel WGAN-GP model ensemble composed of several sub-WGAN-GP models with special emphasis on local attributes of synthesized images is proposed. *Third*, the effectiveness of the novel WGAN-GP model ensemble for ASL images synthesis has been quantitatively verified based on rigorous experiments and comprehensive analyses in this study.

2 Methodology

Technical details of the novel locally-constrained WGAN-GP model ensemble is introduced in this section. This new model ensemble is unique in two aspects, i.e., its locally-constrained optimization task and its model's structure, whose details are elaborated in Sect. 2.1 and Sect. 2.2, respectively.

2.1 The Locally-Constrained Optimization of WGAN-GP Ensemble

The explicit form of the locally-constrained optimization task in the new WGAN-GP model ensemble is represented in Eq. 1.

$$E = \frac{1}{\sum_R \alpha_R} \sum_R \alpha_R E_R + \lambda_1 C_F + \lambda_2 C_S + \lambda_3 C_L \tag{1}$$

where, α_R describes the weight of regional objective function E_R (i.e., of region R), and α_R is to be automatically determined within the end-to-end training process of the whole ensemble. C_F, C_S, and C_L are diverse local constraints, whose Lagrange multipliers are denoted as λ_1, λ_2, and λ_3, respectively. In the following, key components of the locally-constrained optimization problem in Eq. 1 are described in detail.

The objective function E_R in each individual generator/discriminator of the new WGAN-GP model ensemble can be explicitly represented in Eq. 2.

$$E_R = \mathbb{E}_{x_s \sim \mathbb{P}_s}[D(G(x_s))] - \mathbb{E}_{x_t \sim \mathbb{P}_t}[D(x_t)] + \gamma \mathbb{E}_{x_{\hat{t}} \sim \mathbb{P}_{\hat{t}}}[(\left\|\nabla_{x_{\hat{t}}} D(x_{\hat{t}})\right\|_2 - 1)^2] \quad (2)$$

in which, the 1st, 2nd and 3rd term of RHS (i.e., the right hand side) of Eq. 2 denote the discriminator's loss, the generator's loss, and the gradient penalty, respectively; D and G represent the discriminator and the generator, separately; x_s denotes the source data (i.e., structural MRI in this study), which follows the data distribution $\mathbb{P}_s$; x_t represents the target data (i.e., ASL in this study), which also follows the data distribution $\mathbb{P}_t$; $x_{\hat{t}} = \epsilon x_t + (1 - \epsilon)G(x_s)$, in which ϵ is randomly chosen between $[0, 1]$; γ is the weight of the gradient penalty. Moreover, E_R in Eq. 2 needs to work together with three local constraints (i.e., C_F, C_S, and C_L) in Eq. 1. Details of them are explained as follows.

The first regional constraint C_F in Eq. 1 can be represented via Eq. 3, in which m_R indicates the number of local regions and w_R suggests regional weights. Hence, different local regions will be distinctively emphasized in the synthesis task according to their diverse notions of importance suggested from Eq. 3.

$$C_F = \frac{1}{m_R} \sum_R std(w_R) \quad (3)$$

Furthermore, more locally spatial constraints of C_S and C_L in Eq. 1 can be represented using Eqs. 4 and 5, in which the $3D$ 1st operator f (e.g., the conventional Sobel operator is utilized in this study) and the $3D$ 2nd operator l (e.g., the popular Laplacian of Gaussian operator is incorporated in this study) are employed, respectively.

$$C_S = -\frac{1}{m_t} \sum_{t \in T} \left| \sqrt{(T(t) * f_x(t))^2 + (T(t) * f_y(t))^2 + (T(t) * f_z(t))^2} \right| \quad (4)$$

$$C_L = -\frac{1}{m_t} \sum_{t \in T} \left| \sqrt{(T(t) * l_x(t))^2 + (T(t) * l_y(t))^2 + (T(t) * l_z(t))^2} \right| \quad (5)$$

It is also valuable to point out that, the locally-constrained optimization task in Eq. 1 is significantly different from the original one in WGAN-GP, provided the fact that local constraints in Eqs. 3, 4 and 5 are incorporated in the novel WGAN-GP model ensemble for the first time. These constraints emphasize local attributes of images from different perspectives (i.e., regions in Eq. 3 as well as edges in Eqs. 4 and 5) during the whole images synthesis procedure. They are beneficial to improve the quality of synthesized images in this study.

2.2   The Model Structure of WGAN-GP Ensemble

An illustration depicting the structure of the novel WGAN-GP model ensemble with local constraints to realize ASL images synthesis from structural MRI is demonstrated in Fig. 2. It can be noticed that, the model ensemble is composed

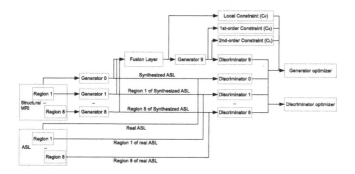

Fig. 2. The structure of the novel WGAN-GP model ensemble with local constraints to realize ASL images synthesis from structural MRI in this study.

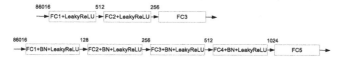

Fig. 3. Model structures of each individual discriminator (top) and each individual generator (bottom) in the newly proposed WGAN-GP model ensemble.

of 10 generators and 10 discriminators. To be specific, Generator 0 and Discriminator 0 focus on the whole image, while Generators 1–8 and Discriminators 1–8 emphasize different local regions. Moreover, Generator 9 and Discriminator 9 are associated with three local constraints (i.e., C_F, C_S, and C_L) in the WGAN-GP model ensemble. It is necessary to point out that, each individual discriminator (i.e., or generator) in the WGAN-GP model ensemble actually share the same topological structure, which is illustrated in Fig. 3. It can be noticed that, the number of neurons in each FC layer is annotated separately in Fig. 3. It is also clear that, essential sub-structures of "FC+leakyReLu" are mainly adopted in those discriminators and generators. The reason to incorporate the leaky ReLu function (i.e., $f(x) = \max(\alpha x, x)$, $\alpha \in [0, 1]$), rather than other conventional activation functions is that, it is more effective in dealing with the "dying ReLu" problem that always outputs the same value for any input. For each individual generator in Fig. 3, BN (i.e., batch normalization) is adopted in each sub-structure of "FC+BN+leakyReLu", in order to avoid potential problems of vanishing/exploding gradients as well as speed up the ensemble's training that is realized by the popular Adam optimization algorithm. In Sect. 3, the effectiveness of the novel WGAN-GP model ensemble in synthesizing ASL images from structural MRI will be substantiated based on rigorous experiments. Their comprehensive analyses are also conducted from the statistical perspective.

3   Experimental Analyses

The dataset of this study was constructed from an on-going demented population-based study. There are totally 355 real patients in this dataset, including 38 AD (i.e., Alzheimer's disease) patients, 185 MCI (i.e., mild cognitive impairments) patients, and 132 NCI (i.e., non-cognitive impairments) patients as normal controls. The average age of these patients is 70.56 ± 7.20 years old, and informed consents were obtained from all patients for conducting this study. High-resolution MPRAGE (i.e., magnetization prepared rapid acquisition gradient echo) T1-weighted MRI images were acquired as structural MRI using a SIEMENS 3T TIM Trio MR scanner. Meanwhile, the pseudo-continuous ASL scanning was applied for acquiring ASL images from each individual patient as well. Acquisition parameters mainly include: labeling duration = 1500 ms, post-labeling delay = 1500 ms, TR/TE = 4000/9.1 ms, ASL voxel size = $3 \times 3 \times 5$ mm^3, etc. Spatial resolutions of all MRI images in this study are $64 \times 64 \times 21$. After obtaining raw MRI data, a series of processes are applied via the well-known SPM toolbox, including motion correction, brain extraction (i.e., skull removal), intra-modality registration (i.e., using the first slice as the reference) separately within ASL and structural MRI images, inter-registration between ASL and structural MRI, etc.

In order to demonstrate the effectiveness of the newly proposed WGAN-GP model ensemble in synthesizing ASL images from structural MRI, both qualitative and quantitative analyses are applied. For qualitative evaluation, the novel WGAN-GP ensemble has been compared with several state-of-the-art GAN models, including WGAN-GP [8], LSGAN [12], and CycleGAN [13]. All implemented GANs in this study are trained using the Adam optimization algorithm (i.e., hyper-parameters β_1 and β_2 controlling two exponentially weighted averages are 0.5 and 0.999, respectively). The batch size, the epoch and the learning rate are 4, 200, and 0.0002, respectively for all GANs. All parameters are determined through trail-and-error for optimal synthesis performance. Also, the ensemble learning is adopted for mitigating the imbalance data problem [14].

Figure 4 illustrates examples of synthesized ASL images and their corresponding difference images towards golden standards (i.e., real images acquired via actual scanning) obtained by all compared models. It is necessary to mention that, images in Column 2 of Fig. 4 are produced as the direct absolute difference between synthesized images (i.e., Column 1) and their corresponding golden standards. It can be observed that, the ideal case of difference images certainly belongs to Row 1, in which no difference exists after subtracting the golden standard from itself. For Rows 2–5, it is clear that difference images produced by WGAN-GP model ensemble are the least (i.e., the voxel-to-voxel variation between synthesized ASL images and golden standards is also calculated and WGAN-GP ensemble provides the lowest variance, i.e., 1.7544, among all compared models). Hence, the synthesis performance of WGAN-GP ensemble is promising.

Another more detailed quantitative experiment is also carried out based on the accuracy performance of incorporating synthesized ASL images in

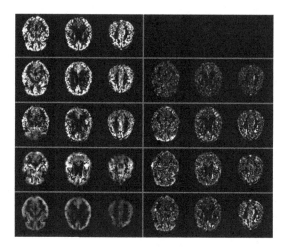

Fig. 4. Synthesized ASL images and corresponding difference images obtained by compared models based on an example patient in this study. Rows 1: Golden standard (real ASL images), 2: locally-constrained WGAN-GP model ensemble, 3: WGAN-GP, 4: LSGAN, 5: CycleGAN; Columns 1: Real/Synthesized ASL images, 2: Difference images (i.e., the absolute difference between images of Columns I and their golden standards).

Table 1. Statistics of dementia diseases diagnosis accuracies based on real/synthesized ASL images.

	WGAN-GP	LSGAN	CycleGAN	WGAN-GP ensemble	Real ASL
Regression	93.20% ± 3.58%	92.29% ± 2.73%	91.71% ± 2.84%	93.34% ± 2.77%	93.71% ± 2.16%
Ranking	89.71% ± 5.17%	89.71% ± 5.17%	89.71% ± 5.17%	90.00% ± 5.08%	90.00% ± 4.92%
CNN-2	46.20% ± 6.80%	46.20% ± 5.63%	49.20% ± 6.55%	49.80% ± 6.67%	55.60% ± 3.72%
CNN-20	46.80% ± 7.24%	48.20% ± 5.30%	46.00% ± 3.94%	48.60% ± 4.87%	49.80% ± 5.03%
Average	68.97% ± 5.69%	69.10% ± 4.70%	69.15% ± 4.62%	70.43% ± 4.84%	72.27% ± 3.95%

differentiating diverse progressions of dementia diseases (i.e., AD, MCI, and NCI) in this study. There are four diagnosis tools applied on all real/synthesized ASL images for dementia diseases diagnosis, including non-linear SVM-based regression (i.e., "Regression" in Table 1), non-linear SVM-based ranking (i.e., "Ranking"), and classic CNN models with different numbers of layers (i.e., "CNN-2" and "CNN-20"). Each element in Table 1 represents the average accuracy of 5-fold cross validation and its corresponding standard deviation. It can be observed that, synthesized ASL images obtained by the novel WGAN-GP model ensemble can provide the highest diagnosis accuracy (i.e., 70.43% ± 4.84%) among all compared GAN-based synthesis models in Table 1. It is also necessary to highlight that, the mean accuracy using real sMRI alone is 69.61% based on the four diagnosis tools. Thus, only the new WGAN-GP ensemble provides an improvement (i.e., 70.43%), compared with other GAN models (i.e., mean averages from WGAN-GP, LSGAN, and CycleGAN are 68.97%, 69.10%, and 69.15%, respectively). It can be concluded that, the superiority of the new WGAN-GP model ensemble for synthesizing ASL images from structural MRI in this study is significant.

4   Conclusions

In this study, a novel WGAN-GP model ensemble is proposed for the first time to realize ASL images synthesis from structural MRI. Novelties of this study can be summarized as follows. *First*, ASL images synthesis studies are not commonly seen, although ASL receives more and more popularity in dementia diseases diagnosis nowadays. This study is the first attempt to synthesize ASL images based on popular GAN-based models from the deep learning perspective. *Second*, the WGAN-GP model ensemble is technically novel, since its locally-constrained optimization task as well as the model's structure are completely new. The high notion of similarity in synthesized ASL images obtained by the WGAN-GP model ensemble towards real ASL images obtained by actual scanning has been demonstrated and substantiated both qualitatively and quantitatively in this study. Future efforts will be focused on investigating more sophisticated deep learning-based diagnosis tools to improve the diagnosis accuracy based on synthesized ASL images obtained from the WGAN-GP model ensemble.

Acknowledgements. This work was supported by the grant 61862043 approved by National Natural Science Foundation of China, and the key grant 20181ACB20006 approved by Natural Science Foundation of Jiangxi Province.

References

1. Huang, Y., et al.: Cross-modality image synthesis via weakly coupled and geometry co-regularized joint dictionary learning. IEEE TMI **37**(3), 815–827 (2018)
2. Duchateau, N., Sermesant, M., Delingette, H., Ayache, N.: Model-based generation of large databases of cardiac images: synthesis of pathological cine MR sequences from real healthy cases. IEEE TMI **37**(3), 755–766 (2018)
3. Wang, Y., Zhou, L., Yu, B., et al.: 3D auto-context-based locality adaptive multi-modality GANs for PET synthesis. IEEE TMI **38**(6), 1328–1339 (2018)
4. Zhou, Y., Giffard-Roisin, S., De Craene, M., et al.: A framework for the generation of realistic synthetic cardiac ultrasound and magnetic resonance imaging sequences from the same virtual patients. IEEE TMI **37**(3), 741–754 (2018)
5. Costa, P., Galdran, A., Meyer, M., et al.: End-to-end adversarial retinal image synthesis. IEEE TMI **37**(3), 781–791 (2018)
6. Goodfellow, I., et al.: Generative adversarial networks. arXiv:1406.2661 (2014)
7. Arjovsky, M., Chintala, S., Bottou, L.: Wasserstein GAN. arXiv:1701.07875 (2017)
8. Gulrajani, I., Ahmed, F., Arjovsky, M., et al.: Improved training of wasserstein GANs, arXiv:1704.00028 (2017)
9. Huang, W.: A novel disease severity prediction scheme via big pair-wise ranking and learning techniques using image-based personal clinical data. Sign. Process. **124**, 233–245 (2016)

10. Huang, W., et al.: Arterial Spin labeling images synthesis from sMRI using unbalanced deep discriminant learning. IEEE TMI (2019). https://doi.org/10.1109/TMI.2019.2906677
11. Huang, W., Zeng, S., Wan, M., Chen, G.: Medical media analytics via ranking and big learning: a multi-modality image-based disease severity prediction study. Neurocomputing **204**, 125–134 (2016)
12. Mao, X., Li, Q., Xie, H., et al.: Least squares generative adversarial networks. arXiv:1611.04076 (2016)
13. Zhu, J., Park, T., Isola, P., Efros, A.: Unpaired image-to-image translation using cycle-consistent adversarial networks. arXiv:1703.10593 (2017)
14. Rezaei, M., et al.: Conditional generative refinement adversarial networks for unbalanced medical image semantic segmentation. arXiv:1810.03871 (2018)

SkrGAN: Sketching-Rendering Unconditional Generative Adversarial Networks for Medical Image Synthesis

Tianyang Zhang[1,2], Huazhu Fu[3(✉)], Yitian Zhao[2(✉)], Jun Cheng[2,4],
Mengjie Guo[5], Zaiwang Gu[6], Bing Yang[2], Yuting Xiao[5], Shenghua Gao[5],
and Jiang Liu[6]

[1] University of Chinese Academy of Sciences, Beijing, China
[2] Cixi Institute of Biomedical Engineering, Chinese Academy of Sciences,
Ningbo, China
yitian.zhao@nimte.ac.cn
[3] Inception Institute of Artificial Intelligence, Abu Dhabi, United Arab Emirates
hzfu@ieee.org
[4] UBTech Research, Shenzhen, China
[5] ShanghaiTech University, Shanghai, China
[6] Southern University of Science and Technology, Shenzhen, China

Abstract. Generative Adversarial Networks (GANs) have the capability of synthesizing images, which have been successfully applied to medical image synthesis tasks. However, most of existing methods merely consider the global contextual information and ignore the fine foreground structures, e.g., vessel, skeleton, which may contain diagnostic indicators for medical image analysis. Inspired by human painting procedure, which is composed of stroking and color rendering steps, we propose a Sketching-rendering Unconditional Generative Adversarial Network (SkrGAN) to introduce a sketch prior constraint to guide the medical image generation. In our SkrGAN, a sketch guidance module is utilized to generate a high quality structural sketch from random noise, then a color render mapping is used to embed the sketch-based representations and resemble the background appearances. Experimental results show that the proposed SkrGAN achieves the state-of-the-art results in synthesizing images for various image modalities, including retinal color fundus, X-Ray, Computed Tomography (CT) and Magnetic Resonance Imaging (MRI). In addition, we also show that the performances of medical image segmentation method has been improved by using our synthesized images as data augmentation.

Keywords: Deep learning · Generative Adversarial Networks · Medical image synthesis

1 Introduction

In the last decade, deep learning techniques have shown to be very promising in many visual recognition tasks [3,5], including object detection, image

D. Shen et al. (Eds.): MICCAI 2019, LNCS 11767, pp. 777–785, 2019.
https://doi.org/10.1007/978-3-030-32251-9_85

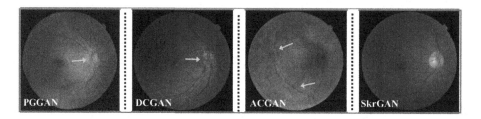

Fig. 1. Synthesized retinal images by PGGAN [7], DCGAN [14], ACGAN [11] and our SkrGAN. Compared with these methods, our method performs better in retaining structural details, e.g., blood vessels, disc and cup regions, as indicated by green arrows. (Color figure online)

classification, face recognition, and medical image analysis. The large scale training data is extremely important for training accurate and deep models. Although it is easy to collect data in conventional computer vision tasks, it is often difficult to obtain sufficient high quality data in medical imaging area. Recently, Generative Adversarial Networks (GANs) are proposed to generate a distribution that matches the real data distribution via an adversarial process [4]. Due to the powerful capability of image generation, GANs have been successfully applied to many medical image synthesis tasks, including retinal fundus [2,19], X-Ray [9], CT and MRI images [18] synthesizing.

The GANs algorithms can be divided into the conditional and unconditional manners. The conditional GANs direct the data generation process by conditioning the model on additional information [10], which have been widely used in cross-modality synthesis and conditioned segmentation. For example, the pix2pix method is proposed to translate images from one type to another [6]. An auxiliary classifier GAN (ACGAN) is provided to produce higher quality sample by adding more structures to the GAN latent space [11]. In [18], a CT and MRI translation network is provided to segment multimodal medical volumes. By contrast, the unconditional GANs synthesize images from random noise without any conditional constraint, which are mainly used to generate images. For example, Deep Convolutional GAN (DCGAN) [14] uses deep convolution structure to generate images. S^2-GAN [17] materializes a two-stage network and depth maps to generate images with realistic surface normal map (i.e., generate RGBD images). However, the S^2-GAN requires depth maps of the training dataset, while we usually do not have medical image datasets with paired depth maps. Wasserstein GAN (WGAN) [1] improves the loss and training stability of previous GANs to obtain a better performance. Progressive Growing GAN (PGGAN) [7] grows the depth of convolution layers to produce the high resolution natural images.

In this paper, we aim to generate high quality medical images with correct anatomical objects and realistic foreground structures (Fig. 1). Inspired by realistic drawing procedures of human painting [12], which is composed of stroking and color rendering, we propose a novel unconditional GAN named Sketching-rendering Unconditional Generative Adversarial Network (SkrGAN) for medical

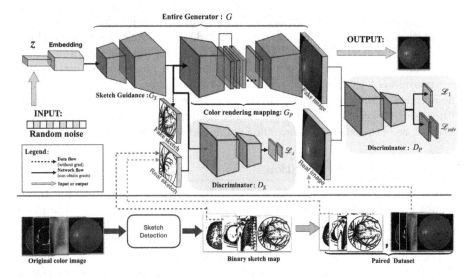

Fig. 2. Illustration of our SkrGAN structure, which can generate medical images from the input noises. The sketch guidance module G_S (blue block) obtains the representations based on sketch structure discriminator D_S. The color render mapping G_P (green block) embeds the sketch representations to generate the final color image with a discriminator D_P. Moreover, We also extract a sketch draft dataset (bottom) for training the model. (best viewed in color) (Color figure online)

image synthesis. Our SkrGAN decomposes into two tractable sub-modules: one sketch guidance module generating the structural sketch from random noise; and one color render mapping module producing the structure-preserved medical images. The main contributions of this paper are summarized as follows:

(1) An unconditional GAN, named SkrGAN, is proposed for medical image synthesis. By decomposing the whole image generation into sketch guidance and color rendering stages, our SkrGAN could embed the sketch structural representations to guide the high quality medical image generation.
(2) The experiments in four medical imaging modalities synthesizing tasks show that our SkrGAN is more accurate and robust to variations in the size, intensity inhomogeneity and modality of the data than other state-of-the-art GAN methods.
(3) The medical image segmentation experiments demonstrate that our SkrGAN could be applied as a data augmentation method to improve the segmentation performance effectively.

2   Proposed Method

Inspired by realistic drawing skills of the human painting [12], which suggests that the painting is usually accomplished from simple to difficult procedures, i.e., from sketching to color rendering, we propose a novel Sketching-rendering Unconditional Generative Adversarial Networks (SkrGAN), to generate high quality medical images with realistic anatomical structures. As shown in Fig. 2, we decompose the entire image generator G into two phases, as a sketch guidance module G_S (in Sect. 2.2) and a color render mapping G_P (in Sect. 2.3). The sketch guidance module G_S generates the sketch structural representations with a sketch discriminator D_S, while the color render mapping G_P embeds the sketch representations to generate the final image with a color discriminator D_P.

2.1 Sketch Draft Preparation

In order to train our SkrGAN, the sketch draft corresponding to the input training image is required by sketch discriminator D_S. We aim to retain the main structural information of the given images, such as the blood vessels of retinal fundus, and bones of X-ray images. In our method, firstly the Sobel edge detection method is used to extract the initial structural boundaries, and then a Gaussian lowpass filtering is applied to remove the isolated noise and pixels. Finally, a morphological operation consisting of an opening process followed by a closing process is employed to remove noise further and fill the vessel-like structures. This procedure will greatly reduce the complexity of sketch images, which makes the sketch synthetic process easier than just using traditional edge detection methods. An example of sketch draft detection method could be found at the bottom of Fig. 2, where the main sketch structures (e.g., vessels and bones) are extracted.

2.2 Sketch Guidance Module

With the given dataset X and corresponding sketch draft set Y by the sketch draft extraction, the sketch guidance module G_S is trained by using loss $\mathcal{L}_s$ in sketch discriminator D_S:

$$\begin{cases} \mathcal{L}_s = \mathbb{E}_{z \sim p_{noise}}[\log(D_S(G_S(z \odot l)))] + \mathbb{E}_{x \sim p_x}[\log(1 - D_S(y))] \\ D_S = D_S^{(n)} \cdots D_S^{(1)} D_S^{(0)} \\ G_S = G_S^{(n)} \cdots G_S^{(1)} G_S^{(0)} \end{cases} \qquad (1)$$

where $z \sim p_{noise}$ and l represent the noise pattern and latent code respectively; p_x represents the distribution of x and $\odot$ is the element-wise multiplication. $D_S^{(i)}, i = 0, 1, ..., n$ denote discriminating layers of the discriminator in different levels, whose inputs are determined to different resolutions. $G_S^{(i)}, i = 0, 1, ..., n$ are the generating layers of different resolutions, respectively. More concretely, our method iteratively adds convolutional layers of the generator and the discriminator during the training period, which guarantees to synthesize images at $\{2^{k+1} \times 2^{k+1} | k = 1, 2, ..., 8\}$ resolutions. Additionally, the training process fades in the high resolution layer smoothly by using skip connections and the smooth coefficients. For simplicity, we utilize the network structure in PGGAN [7] as the backbone of G_S.

2.3   Color Render Mapping

The color render mapping G_P translates the generated sketch representations to color images, which contains the U-net [15] structure as backbone, and a color discriminator D_P for adversarial training. Two losses $\mathcal{L}_{adv}$ and $\mathcal{L}_1$ for training G_P are described as:

$$\begin{cases} \mathcal{L}_{adv} = \mathbb{E}_{y \sim Y}[\log(D_P(G_P(y), y))] + \mathbb{E}_{(x,y) \sim (X,Y)}[\log(1 - D_P(x, y))] \\ \mathcal{L}_1 = \lambda \mathbb{E}_{(x,y) \sim (X,Y)} \|G_P(y) - x\|_1 \end{cases} \quad (2)$$

where $(x, y) \sim (X, Y)$ represent the training pair of real image and sketch. The $\mathcal{L}_{adv}$ is utilized to provide adversarial loss for training G_P, while $\mathcal{L}_1$ is utilized to calculate the $L1$ norm for accelerating training. Finally, the full objective of our SkrGAN is given by the combination of the loss functions in Eqs. (1) and (2):

$$G_S^*, G_P^*, D_S^*, D_P^* = \arg[\underbrace{\min_{G_S} \max_{D_S} \mathcal{L}_s}_{sketch\ guidance} + \underbrace{\min_{G_P} \max_{D_P} (\mathcal{L}_{adv} + \mathcal{L}_1)}_{color\ rendering}]. \quad (3)$$

3   Experiments

Datasets: Three public datasets and one in-house dataset are utilized in our experiments: Chest X-Ray dataset [8][1] with 5,863 images categorized into Pneumonia and normal; Kaggle Lung dataset[2] with 267 CT images; Brain MRI dataset[3] with 147 selected images and a local retinal color fundus dataset (RCF) with 6,432 retinal images collected from local hospitals. In our unconditional experiment, we do not need labeling information.

Evaluation Metrics: In this work, we employ the following three metrics to evaluate the performance in the synthetic medical images, including multi-scale structural similarity (**MS-SSIM**), Sliced Wasserstein Distance (**SWD**) [13], and Freshet Inception Distance (**FID**) [7]. MS-SSIM is a widely used metric to measure the similarity of paired images, where the higher MS-SSIM the better performance. SWD is an efficient metric to compute random approximation to earth mover's distance, which has also been used for measuring GAN performance, where the lower SWD the better performance. FID calculates the distance between real and fake images at feature level, where the lower FID the better performance.

---

[1] https://www.kaggle.com/paultimothymooney/chest-xray-pneumonia.
[2] https://www.kaggle.com/kmader/finding-lungs-in-ct-data/data/.
[3] http://neuromorphometrics.com.

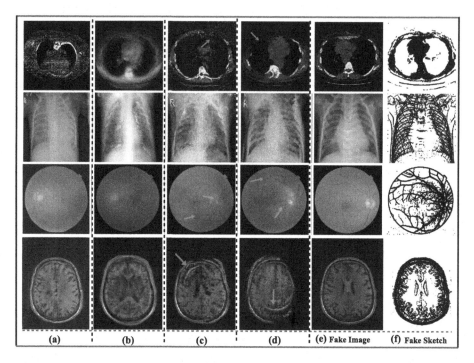

Fig. 3. These images are generated by different GANs: from left to right are results by: (a) PGGAN [7], (b) WGAN [1], (c) DCGAN [14], (d) ACGAN [11] and (e) Our SkrGAN. The synthetic sketches generated from random noise are shown in the figure (f). From top to bottom, we show results from: CT, X-ray, Retina color fundus and MRI. The green arrows illustrate the structural distortions in the generated images. (Color figure online)

Experimental Results: The images from all datasets are firstly resized to $512 \times 512 \times 3$. In G_S, D_S, G_P and D_P, we use Adam optimizers, where the learning rate of G_S and D_S are set to 0.001, and the learning rate of our G_P and D_P are set to 0.0002. Based on experience, we set the value of λ in Eq. (2) to 100 and a small change of λ does not affect much the performance. The batch size of our model is set to 16. The proposed SkrGAN is implemented on PyTorch library with two NVIDIA GPUs (GeForce TITAN XP).

To justify the performance of the proposed method, we compare our Skr-GAN with four state-of-the-art GANs: DCGAN [14], ACGAN [11], WGAN [1] and PGGAN [7]. These different methods are used to generate 100 images, and the aforementioned metrics are used for quantitative comparisons by using these generated images. Table 1 summarizes the results. It can be seen that our Skr-GAN achieves SWD of 0.025, 0.026, 0.020 and 0.028, MS-SSIM of 0.614, 0.506, 0.359 and 0.436 and FID of 27.59, 114.6, 79.97 and 27.51 on the generated retinal color fundus, Chest X-ray, lung CT and brain MRI images, better than other GANs. On one hand, as DCGAN, ACGAN, WGAN and PGGAN are

Table 1. Performances (mean) of different GANs on Retinal color fundus, chest X-Ray, lung CT and Brain MRI.

Evaluation		Method				
Dataset	Metric	SkrGAN	DCGAN [14]	ACGAN [11]	WGAN [1]	PGGAN [7]
Color Fundus	SWD ↓	**0.025**	0.160	0.149	0.078	0.036
	MS-SSIM ↑	**0.614**	0.418	0.490	0.584	0.537
	FID ↓	**27.59**	64.83	96.72	240.7	110.8
Chest X-ray	SWD ↓	**0.026**	0.118	0.139	0.196	0.031
	MS-SSIM ↑	**0.506**	0.269	0.301	0.401	0.493
	FID ↓	**114.6**	260.3	235.2	300.7	124.2
Lung CT	SWD ↓	**0.020**	0.333	0.317	0.236	0.057
	MS-SSIM ↑	**0.359**	0.199	0.235	0.277	0.328
	FID ↓	**79.97**	285.0	222.5	349.1	91.89
Brain MRI	SWD ↓	**0.028**	0.163	0.122	0.036	0.042
	MS-SSIM ↑	**0.436**	0.277	0.235	0.314	0.411
	FID ↓	**27.51**	285.0	222.5	176.1	33.76

not designed for generating high resolution images from a small dataset. Therefore, these methods produce relatively poor results on generating medical images from small training datasets. On the other hand, these methods only consider the global contextual information and ignore the foreground structures, which lead to the discontinued and distorted sketch structures, such as the discontinued vessel and distorted disc cup in retinal color fundus, the discontinued bones and the distorted lung in chest X-ray, the discontinued ribs in CT and the distorted textures in MRI. By contrast, our method uses sketch to guide the intermediate training step, which guarantees the network to generate high quality medical images with realistic anatomical structures.

Figure 3 illustrates examples of the synthetic images by DCGAN, ACGAN, WGAN, PGGAN, and our method in the four different medical image modalities: CT, X-Ray, retinal color fundus and MRI. It can be observed that SkrGAN presents visually appealing results, where most of the structural features such as the vessel in color fundus, bones in X-ray, ribs and backbone in CT, texture distribution in MRI are close to those in real images. On the contrary, there are some structural distortions in images, which are generated by other GANs, as illustrated by green arrows in Fig. 3.

Application to Vessel Segmentation: Besides the above quantitative and qualitative comparisons, we further apply the proposed SkrGAN as a data augmentation method on a vessel segmentation task in DRIVE[4] [16] (including 20 training images and 20 testing images). The DRIVE dataset provides two expert manual annotations, and the first one is chosen as the ground truth for performance evaluation in the literature. We generated 2000 synthetic images

---

[4] https://www.isi.uu.nl/Research/Databases/DRIVE/.

and utilized the generated sketches as the label to pretrain a vessel detection network. In this paper, we use the U-net [15], which is widely used in many biomedical segmentation tasks. The pretrained model is then further finetuned for vessel detection using 20 training images and tested in 20 testing images.

To justify the benefits of the synthetic images for training the segmentation network, we compared the trained model using synthetic images with the model without pretraining. The following metrics were calculated to

Table 2. Segmentation performance of U-net

Pretrain	SEN	ACC	AUC
With	**0.8464**	**0.9513**	**0.9762**
Whithout	0.7781	0.9477	0.9705

provide an objective evaluation: $sensitivity(SEN) = TP/(TP + FN)$, $accuracy(ACC) = (TP+TN)/(TP+FP+TN+FN)$, and the Area Under the ROC Curve (AUC). The results summarized in Table 2 shows that: pretraining with synthetic images improves SEN of the vessel detection by 8.78%, while ACC and AUC are improved by pretraining with the synthetic pairs too.

4   Conclusion

In this paper, we have proposed an unconditional GAN named Sketching-rendering Unconditional Generative Adversarial Network (SkrGAN) that is capable of generating high quality medical images. Our SkrGAN embedded the sketch representation to guide the unconditional medical image synthesis and generate images with realistic foreground structures. The experiments on four types of medical images, including retinal color fundus, chest X-ray, lung CT and brain MRI, showed that our SkrGAN obtained state-of-the-art performances in medical image synthesis. It demonstrated that the sketch information can benefit the structure generation. Besides, the application of retina vessel segmentation showed that the SkrGAN could be used as a data augmentation method to improve deep network training.

References

1. Arjovsky, M., Chintala, S., Bottou, L.: Wasserstein GAN. arXiv:1701.07875 (2017)
2. Costa, P., Galdran, A., et al.: End-to-end adversarial retinal image synthesis. IEEE TMI **37**(99), 781–791 (2017)
3. Fu, H., Cheng, J., Xu, Y., Wong, D.W.K., Liu, J., Cao, X.: Joint optic disc and cup segmentation based on multi-label deep network and polar transformation. IEEE Trans. Med. Imaging **37**(7), 1597–1605 (2018)
4. Goodfellow, I.J., Pouget-Abadie, J., et al.: Generative adversarial networks. In: NIPS (2014)
5. Gu, Z., et al.: CE-Net: context encoder network for 2D medical image segmentation. IEEE Trans. Med. Imaging (2019)
6. Isola, P., Zhu, J.Y., et al.: Image-to-image translation with conditional adversarial networks. In: CVPR, pp. 1125–1134 (2017)

7. Karras, T., Aila, T., et al.: Progressive growing of GANs for improved quality, stability, and variation. arXiv:1710.10196 (2017)
8. Kermany, D.S., Goldbaum, M., et al.: Identifying medical diagnoses and treatable diseases by image-based deep learning. Cell **172**(5), 1122–1131 (2018)
9. Madani, A., Moradi, M., et al.: Semi-supervised learning with generative adversarial networks for chest X-ray classification with ability of data domain adaptation. In: ISBI, pp. 1038–1042 (2018)
10. Mirza, M., Osindero, S.: Conditional generative adversarial nets. arXiv:1411.1784 (2014)
11. Odena, A., Olah, C., Shlens, J.: Conditional image synthesis with auxiliary classifier GANs. In: ICML, pp. 2642–2651 (2017)
12. Ostrofsky, J., Kozbelt, A., Seidel, A.: Perceptual constancies and visual selection as predictors of realistic drawing skill. Psychol. Aesthetics Creativity Arts **6**(2), 124–136 (2012)
13. Peyré, G., Cuturi, M., et al.: Computational optimal transport. Found. Trends® Mach. Learn. **11**(5–6), 355–607 (2019)
14. Radford, A., Metz, L., Chintala, S.: Unsupervised representation learning with deep convolutional generative adversarial networks. In: International Conference on Learning Representations (2016)
15. Ronneberger, O., Fischer, P., Brox, T.: U-net: convolutional networks for biomedical image segmentation. In: Navab, N., Hornegger, J., Wells, W.M., Frangi, A.F. (eds.) MICCAI 2015. LNCS, vol. 9351, pp. 234–241. Springer, Cham (2015). https://doi.org/10.1007/978-3-319-24574-4_28
16. Staal, J., Abramoff, M.D., et al.: Ridge-based vessel segmentation in color images of the retina. IEEE TMI **23**(4), 501–509 (2004)
17. Wang, X., Gupta, A.: Generative image modeling using style and structure adversarial networks. In: Leibe, B., Matas, J., Sebe, N., Welling, M. (eds.) ECCV 2016. LNCS, vol. 9908, pp. 318–335. Springer, Cham (2016). https://doi.org/10.1007/978-3-319-46493-0_20
18. Zhang, Z., Yang, L., Zheng, Y.: Translating and segmenting multimodal medical volumes with cycle-and shape-consistency generative adversarial network. In: CVPR, pp. 9242–9251 (2018)
19. Zhao, H., Li, H., et al.: Synthesizing retinal and neuronal images with generative adversarial nets. Med. Image Anal. **49**, 14–26 (2018)

Wavelet-based Semi-supervised Adversarial Learning for Synthesizing Realistic 7T from 3T MRI

Liangqiong Qu, Shuai Wang, Pew-Thian Yap$^{(\boxtimes)}$, and Dinggang Shen$^{(\boxtimes)}$

Department of Radiology and BRIC, University of North Carolina at Chapel Hill, Chapel Hill, NC 27599, USA
{ptyap,dgshen}@med.unc.edu

Abstract. Ultra-high field 7T magnetic resonance imaging (MRI) scanners produce images with exceptional anatomical details, which can facilitate diagnosis and prognosis. However, 7T MRI scanners are often cost prohibitive and hence inaccessible. In this paper, we propose a novel wavelet-based semi-supervised adversarial learning framework to synthesize 7T MR images from their 3T counterparts. Unlike most learning methods that rely on supervision requiring a significant amount of 3T-7T paired data, our method applies a semi-supervised learning mechanism to leverage unpaired 3T and 7T MR images to learn the 3T-to-7T mapping when 3T-7T paired data are scarce. This is achieved via a cycle generative adversarial network that operates in the joint spatial-wavelet domain for the synthesis of multi-frequency details. Extensive experimental results show that our method achieves better performance than state-of-the-art methods trained using fully paired data.

1 Introduction

The first 7T magnetic resonance (MR) scanner was approved for clinical use by the United States Food and Drug Administration in 2017. Compared to routine 3T MRI, 7T MRI typically affords greater anatomical details and higher signal-to-noise ratio, potentially facilitating diagnosis and prognosis [8]. However, 7T MR scanners are cost-prohibitive and hence less accessible at the clinics. For example, to date, there are less than 100 7T MR scanners compared with more than 20,000 3T MR scanners worldwide. Synthesizing 7T MR images from their 3T counterparts is thus valuable for both clinical and research applications.

In the past decades, a large number of learning based methods have been proposed for 7T MR image synthesis, including sparse learning, random forest, and deep learning. For example, Bahrami *et al.* [4] proposed a convolutional neural network taking into account appearance and anatomical features to learn the nonlinear 3T-to-7T mapping. Zhang *et al.* [9] utilized two multi-stage linear regression streams in both spatial and frequency domains for 7T MR image synthesis. While effective, these methods often share the following limitations. (i) Existing methods usually require a large amount of paired data (i.e., 3T and

© Springer Nature Switzerland AG 2019
D. Shen et al. (Eds.): MICCAI 2019, LNCS 11767, pp. 786–794, 2019.
https://doi.org/10.1007/978-3-030-32251-9_86

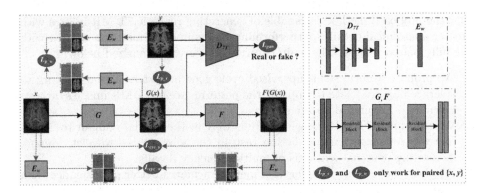

Fig. 1. Architecture of SemiWave. We show only $x \rightarrow G(x) \rightarrow F(G(x))$ for simplicity. SemiWave consists of two mapping functions ($G : x \rightarrow y$ and $F : y \rightarrow x$), an adversarial discriminator D_{7T}, and a wavelet coefficient extractor E_w. Four kinds of losses are used to regularize these two mapping functions: Adversarial loss $\mathcal{L}_{gan}$, pair-wise reconstruction loss $\mathcal{L}_{p\_s}$, cycle consistency loss $\mathcal{L}_{cyc\_s}$, and wavelet losses $\mathcal{L}_{p\_w}$ and $\mathcal{L}_{cyc\_w}$. $\mathcal{L}_{p\_s}$ and $\mathcal{L}_{p\_w}$ are for paired data and $\mathcal{L}_{gan}$, $\mathcal{L}_{cyc\_s}$ and $\mathcal{L}_{cyc\_w}$ are for both paired and unpaired data.

7T MR images of the same subject) for training. However, acquiring paired data can be challenging and they are hence not always available in large quantities. (ii) Existing methods often fail to capture sufficient anatomical details and produce blurred results.

In this paper, we propose a wavelet-based semi-supervised adversarial network to synthesize 7T T1-weighted MR images from their 3T counterparts. Our method, called SemiWave, learns a two-way mapping by a small number of paired data together with a large amount of unpaired data. To learn from unpaired data, we couple the primal 3T-to-7T mapping task with a dual 7T-to-3T mapping task and impose a cycle-consistent loss [10] to regularize these two tasks, i.e., a synthetic 7T MR image generated by 3T-to-7T mapping should be mapped back to the original 3T MR image via a 7T-to-3T mapping. Specifically, we further transform these two mapping tasks from the spatial domain to a flexible wavelet coefficient predication task in a joint spatial-wavelet domain. Emphasis on the prediction of low-frequency wavelet coefficients enforces consistency in global information, whereas emphasis on high-frequency wavelet coefficients promotes reconstruction with better anatomical details. A flexible wavelet loss with adaptive weights on wavelet coefficients of different bands is introduced to help generate realistic 7T MR images.

As shown in Fig. 1, SemiWave consists of four main modules: (i) a standard adversarial loss module, (ii) a standard pair-wise reconstruction loss module, (iii) a cycle consistency loss module, and (iv) a wavelet loss module. Specifically, the cycle consistency loss is introduced to alleviate the need of large amounts of paired data and the wavelet loss is utilized to facilitate effective reconstruction with multi-frequency details. Extensive experimental results demonstrate that the proposed method is capable of generating realistic 7T MR images with greater anatomical details, outperforming the competing methods trained with the fully paired images. The main contributions are summarized below:

1. We propose a novel semi-supervised cycle generative adversarial network to leverage unpaired data to improve the performance of 7T MR image synthesis when 3T-7T paired data are scarce.
2. We transform 7T MR image synthesis task in the spatial domain to a flexible wavelet coefficient prediction task in the joint spatial-wavelet domain, facilitating effective synthesis of multi-frequency details.
3. We show that our semi-supervised method achieves better performance than competing state-of-the-art methods trained with fully paired data.

2 Method

Our goal is to learn the mapping from 3T MR images in domain X to 7T MR images in domain Y, given a set of training samples $\{x_i\}_{i=1}^{N} \subset X$ and $\{y_i\}_{i=1}^{M} \subset Y$, where $X = X' \bigcup X''$ and $Y = Y' \bigcup Y''$. The training samples in X' and Y' are paired 3T-7T MR images, whereas the samples in X'' and Y'' are unpaired. To learn from unpaired data, we couple the primal 3T-to-7T mapping task with a dual 7T-to-3T mapping task. As shown in Fig. 1, SemiWave consists of two mapping functions: a primal 3T-to-7T mapping $(G : x \rightarrow y)$ and a dual 7T-to-3T mapping $(F : y \rightarrow x)$, two associated adversarial discriminators $(D_{3T}$ and $D_{7T})$, and one wavelet coefficient extractor (E_w). Discriminator D_{7T} tries to distinguish between the real 7T MR image y and the synthesized 7T MR image $G(x)$. Similarly, D_{3T} tries to distinguish between x and $F(y)$. The wavelet coefficient extractor E_w computes the wavelet coefficients of four frequency bands. Four losses are involved to regularize these two mappings: adversarial loss, pair-wise reconstruction loss, cycle consistency loss, and wavelet loss.

2.1 Adversarial Loss

Adversarial loss is applied to both mapping functions, aiming to match the distribution of the synthetic images to the distribution of the target images. For generator G and its corresponding discriminator D_{7T}, the adversarial loss is defined as

$$\mathcal{L}_{\text{gan}}(G, D_{7T}) = \mathbb{E}_{y \in Y} \left[\log D_{7T}(y) \right] + \mathbb{E}_{x \in X} \left[1 - \log D_{7T}(G(x)) \right], \quad (1)$$

where G tries to generate a synthetic 7T MR image $G(x)$ that resembles real 7T MR image y in Y, whereas D_{7T} aims to distinguish between a synthetic 7T MR image $G(x)$ and a real image y. G tries to minimize this objective function, whereas D_{7T} aims to maximize it, i.e., arg $\min_G \max_{D_{7T}} \mathcal{L}_{\text{gan}}(G, D_{7T})$. Similarly, adversarial loss is also applied to generator F and its discriminator D_{3T} as

$$\mathcal{L}_{\text{gan}}(F, D_{3T}) = \mathbb{E}_{x \in X} \left[\log D_{3T}(x) \right] + \mathbb{E}_{y \in Y} \left[1 - \log D_{3T}(F(y)) \right]. \quad (2)$$

2.2   Pair-Wise Reconstruction Loss

Networks with adversarial loss are often affected by model collapse and training instability. We incorporate a pair-wise reconstruction loss to impose additional constraints on the generators with a small number of paired images. Specifically, the generator is tasked not only to fool the discriminator but also to minimize the pixel-wise intensity difference between synthetic and real images.

Given a set of paired 3T and 7T MR images $\{X', Y'\}$, the pair-wise reconstruction loss is defined as

$$\mathcal{L}_{\text{p\_s}}(G, F) = \mathbb{E}_{x \in X', y \in Y'} \left[\|y - G(x)\|_1 + \|x - F(y)\|_1 \right]. \tag{3}$$

We choose L1 distance rather than L2 to encourage image sharpness.

2.3   Cycle Consistency Loss

Training an effective 7T MR image synthesis model with adversarial loss and pair-wise reconstruction loss often requires a significant amount of 3T-7T paired data. However, acquiring paired data is often challenging due to factors such as prolonged scanning time, patient discomfort, and costs. Acquisition of unpaired data is relatively straightforward. In light of this, we design a semi-supervised learning mechanism to leverage both the paired and unpaired data to learn the 3T-to-7T mapping. Specifically, to learn from extra unpaired data, a cycle consistency constraint is enforced on G and F. Following [10], the cycle consistency constraint encourages similarity between each synthetic 7T MR image $G(x)$ generated by the 3T-to-7T mapping G with the original 3T image x when mapped back via the 7T-to-3T mapping F, i.e., $F(G(x)) \approx x$. Similarly, $G(F(y)) \approx y$. The cycle consistency loss is defined as

$$\mathcal{L}_{\text{cyc\_s}}(G, F) = \mathbb{E}_{x \in X} \left[\|x - F(G(x))\|_1 \right] + \mathbb{E}_{y \in Y} \left[\|y - G(\text{F}(\text{y}))\|_1 \right]. \tag{4}$$

2.4   Wavelet Loss

The pair-wise reconstruction loss and cycle consistency loss aim at keeping the pixel/voxel-wise intensity consistency between synthetic and real images. These L1/L2 driven pixel-wise losses tend to produce over-smoothed outputs and fail to capture anatomical details [5].

We thus introduce a wavelet loss to encourage the network to generate images with realistic details. Specifically, a wavelet coefficient extractor E_w is first utilized to decompose the image into its wavelet coefficients in four bands. Given a 7T MR image y, we denote its wavelet coefficients in four bands as $\{y_w^A, y_w^H, y_w^V, y_w^D\}$. The approximation coefficients y_w^A capture the global topology information, and the detail coefficients $\{y_w^H, y_w^V, y_w^D\}$ store the high-frequency details. The wavelet loss $\mathcal{L}_{p\_w}(G)$ between the generated image $G(x)$ and real image y is defined as

$$\begin{aligned}
\mathcal{L}_{\text{p\_w}}(G) = \mathbb{E}_{x \in X', y \in Y'} \Big[&\lambda_1 \big\| y_w^A - (G(x))_w^A \big\|_1 \\
&+ \lambda_2 \big(\big\| y_w^H - (G(x))_w^H \big\|_1 + \big\| y_w^V - (G(x))_w^V \big\|_1 \big) \\
&+ \lambda_3 \big\| y_w^D - (G(x))_w^D \big\|_1 \Big],
\end{aligned} \tag{5}$$

where λ_1, λ_2, and λ_3 are the weights for balancing the contributions of wavelet coefficients of different bands. Emphasis on the reconstruction of high-frequency wavelet coefficients helps recover better anatomical details, whereas emphasis on the prediction of low-frequency wavelet coefficients enforces consistency in global information. During training, we gradually increase the weights λ_2 and λ_3 in order to generate more realistic 7T MR images with greater anatomical details.

Similarly, we also apply wavelet loss $\mathcal{L}_{\text{p\_w}}(F)$ between the synthetic image $F(y)$ and real image x, and the wavelet loss $\mathcal{L}_{\text{cyc\_w}}(G, F)$ between real images $\{x, y\}$ and reconstructed images $\{F(G(x)), G(F(y))\}$.

2.5   Overall Objective Function

The overall objective function is defined as

$$\mathcal{L}(G, F, D_{3T}, D_{7T}) = \mathcal{L}_{\text{gan}} + \alpha\mathcal{L}_{\text{p\_s}} + \beta\mathcal{L}_{\text{cyc\_s}} + \gamma\mathcal{L}_{\text{p\_w}} + \delta\mathcal{L}_{\text{cyc\_w}}, \qquad (6)$$

where $\mathcal{L}_{\text{p\_s}}$ and $\mathcal{L}_{\text{p\_w}}$ are only valid for paired data $\{X', Y'\}$, and the others are valid for all the training data $\{X, Y\}$. Parameters $\alpha, \beta, \gamma, \delta$ balance the contributions of the different losses.

2.6   Network Architecture

The detailed network architecture of SemiWave is shown in Fig. 1. Similar to [10], our generators G and F contain two stride-2 convolutions, six residual blocks, and two fractionally-strided convolutions with a stride of $1/2$. Instance normalization is applied after each convolutional layers. For discriminators D_{7T} and D_{3T}, a 70×70 PatchGans scheme [6,10] is applied to classify whether 70×70 overlapping patches are real or fake. The wavelet coefficient extractor E_{w} is based on one-level Haar wavelet packet decomposition [1]. It is composed of a stride-2 convolution with its filter weights determined by Haar-based filters.

3   Experiments

3.1   Dataset

We utilized 15 pairs of 3T and 7T T1 weighted MR brain images in our study. The 3T MR images were acquired using a Siemens Magnetom Trio 3T scanner with voxel size $1 \times 1 \times 1\,\text{mm}^3$, TR $= 1990\,\text{ms}$, and TE $= 2.16\,\text{ms}$. The 7T MR images were acquired using a Siemens Magnetom 7T whole-body MR scanner, with voxel size $0.65 \times 0.65 \times 0.65\,\text{mm}^3$, TR $= 6000\,\text{ms}$, and TE $= 2.95\,\text{ms}$. These images were linearly aligned and skull-stripped to remove non-brain voxels. After skull stripping, the intensity values of each image were linearly scaled to $[-1,1]$.

We adopt leave-one-out cross validation for performance evaluation. One pair of 3T and 7T MR images were used for testing, and the remaining 14 pairs were used for training. Specifically, we divided the training set into two subsets: four pairs for paired training and the remaining ten pairs were randomly shuffled for unpaired training.

3T MRI   7T MRI   MCCA [4]   RF [2]   CAAF [3]   DDCR [9]   SemiWave

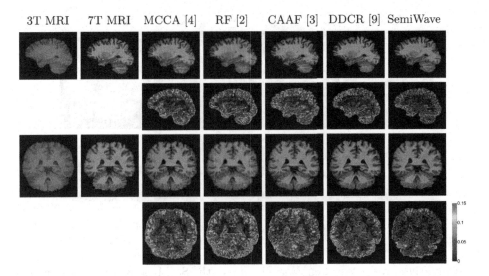

Fig. 2. 7T MR images synthesized using SemiWave and four other methods shown in sagittal and coronal views, along with the prediction error maps.

3.2 Implementation Details

SemiWave was implemented with Pytorch and optimized with Adam [7]. In our implementation, the negative log likelihood objectives in (1) and (2) were replaced by a more stable least-square loss [10]. In order to stabilize the training, we set the batch size to 2 with one batch from paired data and another from unpaired data. The learning rate was set to 0.0002 for the first 100 epochs and linearly decayed to zero in subsequent 100 epochs. Parameters α, γ were set to 30, and parameters β, δ were set to 10. Parameters λ_2 and λ_3 were initially set to be small and were gradually increased for greater contribution from high-frequency wavelet coefficients. Specifically, we linearly increased parameters $\lambda_1, \lambda_2, \lambda_3$ from $1, 1, 1$ to $1, 3, 5$ for the first 50 epochs and then fixed them for the following epochs. In the training phase, we extracted several consecutive axial slices from the 3D images as the training images. Horizontal flipping, randomly scaling, and random rotation were applied to augment the training data.

3.3 Prediction Performance

To validate the effectiveness of the proposed method, we compared our method with four state-of-the-art fully-supervised 7T MR image synthesis methods: MCCA [4], RF [2], CAAF [3] and DDCR [9]. We evaluated the performance of these methods with two commonly accepted metrics: peak signal-noise ratio (PSNR), and structural similarity (SSIM). Table 1 shows the quantitative comparison results of the different 7T MR image synthesis methods. Even with only 28.5% paired data, SemiWave still achieves superior performance compared with the competing fully-supervised methods. Specifically, with the cycle consistency

| 3T MRI | 7T MRI | No $\mathcal{L}_{p\_w}, \mathcal{L}_{cyc\_w}$ | SemiWave |

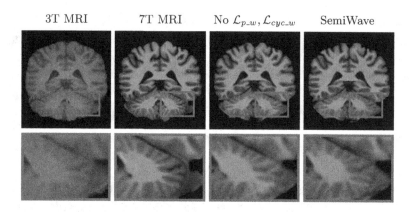

Fig. 3. Ablation study: Effectiveness of wavelet loss.

loss and the wavelet loss, SemiWave improves the SSIM value from 0.8580 given by [9] to 0.8740. The visual comparison results in Fig. 2 also demonstrate the ability of SemiWave in generating realistic 7T MR images with greater anatomical details.

Table 1. Mean PSNR and SSIM for different 7T MR image synthesis methods. All the competing methods were trained with the fully paired data. SemiWave was trained with around 28.5% paired data and 71.5% unpaired data.

	MCCA [4]	RF [2]	CFFA [3]	DDCR [9]	SemiWave
PSNR	25.52	26.55	27.05	27.51	**27.85**
SSIM	0.4840	0.5728	0.8406	0.8580	**0.8740**

3.4   Ablation Study

We investigated the contributions of the three main loses of SemiWave, i.e., pair-wise reconstruction loss ($\mathcal{L}_{p\_s}$ and $\mathcal{L}_{p\_w}$), cycle consistency loss ($\mathcal{L}_{cyc\_s}$ and $\mathcal{L}_{cyc\_w}$), and wavelet loss ($\mathcal{L}_{p\_w}$ and $\mathcal{L}_{cyc\_w}$). We removed each of these losses from SemiWave and train variant models using a strategy similar to SemiWave. Figure 3 and Table 2 compare SemiWave and its variants.

Without pair-wise reconstruction loss, the performance drops dramatically, i.e., the PSNR value drops from 27.85 to 26.72. With the cycle consistency loss, SSIM is improved from 0.8697 to 0.8740. With wavelet loss, realistic images with greater anatomical details can be generated, as depicted in Fig. 3 and Table 2.

Table 2. Ablation study: Effectiveness of different loses in SemiWave.

	Without $\mathcal{L}_{p\_s}, \mathcal{L}_{p\_w}$	Without $\mathcal{L}_{cyc\_s}, \mathcal{L}_{cyc\_w}$	Without $\mathcal{L}_{p\_w}, \mathcal{L}_{cyc\_w}$	SemiWave
PSNR	26.72	27.42	27.60	**27.85**
SSIM	0.8417	0.8697	0.8702	**0.8740**

4   Conclusion

In this paper, we propose a novel semi-supervised cycle generative adversarial network called SemiWave for 7T MR image synthesis, considering information in both spatial and wavelet domains. Adversarial loss, pair-wise loss, cycle consistency loss, and wavelet loss are incorporated to capture both global and local information. Comprehensive qualitative and quantitative experiments show that our method generates realistic 7T MR images with greater anatomical details than competing fully-supervised methods. Future work will focus on boosting the performance of SemiWave with large-scale unpaired images and extending SemiWave to tackle general cross-modality image synthesis problems.

Acknowledgement. This work was supported in part by NIH grant EB006733.

References

1. Akansu, A.N., Haddad, P.A., Haddad, R.A.: Multiresolution Signal Decomposition: Transforms, Subbands, and Wavelets. Academic Press, Orlando (2001)
2. Bahrami, K., Shi, F., Rekik, I., Gao, Y., Shen, D.: 7T-guided super-resolution of 3T MRI. Med. Phys. **44**(5), 1661–1677 (2017)
3. Bahrami, K., Shi, F., Rekik, I., Shen, D.: Convolutional neural network for reconstruction of 7T-like images from 3T MRI using appearance and anatomical features. In: Carneiro, G., et al. (eds.) LABELS/DLMIA-2016. LNCS, vol. 10008, pp. 39–47. Springer, Cham (2016). https://doi.org/10.1007/978-3-319-46976-8_5
4. Bahrami, K., Shi, F., Zong, X., Shin, H.W., An, H., Shen, D.: Hierarchical reconstruction of 7T-like images from 3T MRI using multi-level CCA and group sparsity. In: Navab, N., Hornegger, J., Wells, W.M., Frangi, A.F. (eds.) MICCAI 2015. LNCS, vol. 9350, pp. 659–666. Springer, Cham (2015). https://doi.org/10.1007/978-3-319-24571-3_79
5. Huang, H., He, R., Sun, Z., Tan, T.: Wavelet-SRNet: a wavelet-based CNN for multi-scale face super resolution. In: Proceedings IEEE ICCV, pp. 1689–1697 (2017)
6. Isola, P., Zhu, J.Y., Zhou, T., Efros, A.A.: Image-to-image translation with conditional adversarial networks. In: Proceedings IEEE CVPR, pp. 1125–1134 (2017)
7. Kingma, D.P., Ba, J.: Adam: a method for stochastic optimization. arXiv preprint arXiv:1412.6980 (2014)
8. Van der Kolk, A.G., Hendrikse, J., Zwanenburg, J.J., Visser, F., Luijten, P.R.: Clinical applications of 7T MRI in the brain. Eur. J. Radiol. **82**(5), 708–718 (2013)

9. Zhang, Y., Cheng, J.-Z., Xiang, L., Yap, P.-T., Shen, D.: Dual-domain cascaded regression for synthesizing 7T from 3T MRI. In: Frangi, A.F., Schnabel, J.A., Davatzikos, C., Alberola-López, C., Fichtinger, G. (eds.) MICCAI 2018. LNCS, vol. 11070, pp. 410–417. Springer, Cham (2018). https://doi.org/10.1007/978-3-030-00928-1_47

10. Zhu, J.Y., Park, T., Isola, P., Efros, A.A.: Unpaired image-to-image translation using cycle-consistent adversarial networks. In: Proceedings IEEE CVPR, pp. 2223–2232 (2017)

DiamondGAN: Unified Multi-modal Generative Adversarial Networks for MRI Sequences Synthesis

Hongwei Li[1], Johannes C. Paetzold[1], Anjany Sekuboyina[1,2], Florian Kofler[1], Jianguo Zhang[3,4(✉)], Jan S. Kirschke[2], Benedikt Wiestler[2], and Bjoern Menze[1,5]

[1] Department of Informatics, Technical University of Munich, Munich, Germany
{hongwei.li,bjoern.menze}@tum.de
[2] Department of Neuroradiology, Klinikum rechts der Isar, Munich, Germany
[3] Department of Computer Science and Engineering,
Southern University of Science and Technology, Shenzhen, China
jgzhang@ieee.org
[4] Shenzhen Institute of Artificial Intelligence and Robotics for Society,
Shenzhen, China
[5] Institute for Advanced Study, Technical University of Munich, Munich, Germany

Abstract. Synthesizing MR imaging sequences is highly relevant in clinical practice, as single sequences are often missing or are of poor quality (e.g. due to motion). Naturally, the idea arises that a target modality would benefit from multi-modal input, as proprietary information of individual modalities can be synergistic. However, existing methods fail to scale up to multiple non-aligned imaging modalities, facing common drawbacks of complex imaging sequences. We propose a novel, scalable and multi-modal approach called *DiamondGAN*. Our model is capable of performing flexible non-aligned cross-modality synthesis and data infill, when given multiple modalities or any of their arbitrary subsets, learning structured information in an end-to-end fashion. We synthesize two MRI sequences with clinical relevance (i.e., double inversion recovery (DIR) and contrast-enhanced T1 (T1-c)), reconstructed from three common sequences. In addition, we perform a multi-rater visual evaluation experiment and find that trained radiologists are unable to distinguish synthetic DIR images from real ones.

1 Introduction

In clinical practice, magnetic resonance imaging (MRI) datasets often consists of high-dimensional image volumes with multiple imaging protocols and repeated scans acquired at multiple time points. Given the multiplicity of possible sequence parameters, protocols largely vary depends on the imaging centers,

---

H. Li and J. C. Paetzold—Equal contribution.

© Springer Nature Switzerland AG 2019
D. Shen et al. (Eds.): MICCAI 2019, LNCS 11767, pp. 795–803, 2019.
https://doi.org/10.1007/978-3-030-32251-9_87

hindering their comparability. This often leads to repeated exams or severely limits the clinical information that can be drawn from those MRI studies. Particularly, in the case of multiple sclerosis, longitudinal comparisons of MRI studies are the main reason for treatment decisions and existing lesion quantification tools require complete identical modalities at multiple time points. Potentially, cross-modality image synthesis technique can resolve those obstacles through efficient data infilling and re-synthesis.

Recently, generative adversarial networks (GANs) have been applied in translating MRI sequences, positron emission tomography (PET) and computed tomography (CT) images. Most of them are one-to-one cross-modality synthesis approaches, for example, PET [12] synthesis and MRI sequences translation [3]. A recent multi-modal synthesis method [10] has limited scalability because the input and output modalities are required to be spatially aligned. Although there are several multi-domain translation algorithms [2] in the computer vision community, these approaches design one-to-multiple domain translation but do not model the multiple-to-one domain mapping. Especially in medical images synthesis, *multiple-to-one* cross-modality mapping is highly relevant as proprietary information of individual and non-aligned modalities can be synergistic.

There are three main challenges in the scenario of multi-modal cross-modality medical image synthesis: (1) the input and target modalities are assumed to be *not* spatially-aligned because registration methods for aligning multiple modalities may fail, restricting the applicability of conventional regression approaches. (2) input modalities may be missing due to different clinical settings between centers, thus a traditional regression-based data infill would be restricted to the smallest uniform subset or rely on iterative data infill methods. (3) existing approaches have limited scalability, e.g. in a *Cycle-GAN* [14] setting, one would therefore have to train individual models for possible combinations of the input modalities.

Contributions (1) We propose *DiamondGAN*, which is a unified, scalable multi-modal generative adversarial network. It learns the multiple-to-one cross-modality mapping among non-aligned modalities using only a pair of generators and discriminators, optimized with a multi-modal cycle-consistency loss function. (2) We provide both qualitative and quantitative results on two clinically-relevant MRI sequences synthesis tasks, showing *DiamondGAN's* superiority over baseline models. (3) We present the results of extensive visual evaluation, performed by fourteen experienced radiologists to confirm the quality of synthetic images.

2   Methodology

2.1   Multi-modal Cross-Modality Synthesis

Given an input set of n modalities: $X = \{x_i | i = 1, ..., n\}$ and a target modality T. Our goal is to learn a generator G that learns mappings from multiple input modalities to one target modality. We assume that (1) all the modalities,

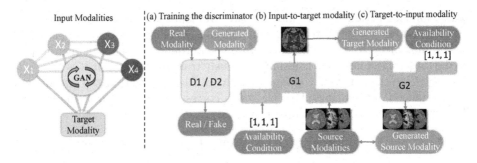

Fig. 1. Left: The high-level idea behind *DiamondGAN*, which is capable of learning mappings between any subset of multiple input modalities (X) to a target modality in a single model. This mapping represents a diamond-shape topology. Right: Overview of *DiamondGAN*. It consists of two modules, a pair of discriminators D and a pair of generators G. (a) *D1* and *D2* learn to distinguish between the real and synthetic images from multi-modal input and the target output respectively. (b) *G1* takes both multi-modal input and the condition as input and generates a target modality. The condition c is a binary vector: $c = \{c_1, c_2, ..., c_n\}$, where c_i indicates the corresponding input modality as available (1) or not (0). It is spatially replicated and concatenated with the input modalities in the feature level. (c) *G2* tries to generate the original modalities from the synthetic target modality given the original availability condition.

i.e., X and T, are *not* spatially-aligned because it is rather difficult to obtain *strictly* spatially-aligned images as mentioned in Sect. 1; (2) the input modalities can be any subset of X, denoted as X' during the training and inference stages as some modalities of a subject may be missing in clinical practice.

We enforce G to be capable of translating any subset X' into a target modality T using a condition c which indicates the presence of the input modalities, i.e., $G(X', c) \to T$. This condition handles the missing modality issue and makes it a scalable model in both the training and the inference stages. We further introduce a multi-modal cycle-consistency loss to handle the "non-aligned modalities" issue among the input and output. Figure 1 illustrates the main idea of our proposed approach. We regularly generate the condition c and the corresponding multi-modal data X_c of all possible combinations, so that G learns to flexibly translate the arbitrary multi-modal input. As mentioned in the caption of Fig. 1, we use an *availability* condition to serve as an indicator of the input modalities. It is spatially replicated to the image size ($1 \times H \times W$) and is a part of the two-stream network input. In the case of 3 modalities as the input, the condition $c = [1, 1, 1]$ would indicate that every input modality is given.

Multi-modal Reconstruction Loss. We aim to train G to guarantee that a generated target modality preserves the content of its input modalities. The input modalities are assumed to be not spatially aligned or not from the same subject as mentioned above. In this situation, the traditional cycle loss [14] as well as the regression loss [5] would fail to tackle the multi-modal and non-alignment issues. To alleviate the two problems, we extend the traditional cycle-consistency loss [14] to a multi-modal one. Specifically, we concatenate the source modalities into a multi-channel input and define a multi-channel output as the target modality. We then simultaneously train two generators $G_1 : X \rightarrow T$ and $G_2 : T \rightarrow X$ in a cycle-consistency fashion. Please note that the output target modality is in multiple channels which correspond to the input modalities. The loss function of the generator is defined as:

$$\mathcal{L}_{rec} = \mathbb{E}_{X,T,c}[||X - G_2(G_1(X,c),c)||_1 + ||T - G_1(G_2(T,c),c)||_1] \qquad (1)$$

Adversarial Loss. To make the generated images indistinguishable from real images, we adopt an adversarial loss:

$$\begin{aligned} \mathcal{L}_{adv} = &\, \mathbb{E}_{X,T}\{log\;[D_1(X) \cdot D_2(T)]\} \\ &+ \mathbb{E}_{X,T,c}\{log\;[(1 - D_2(G_1(X,c))) \cdot (1 - D_1(G_2(T,c)))]\} \end{aligned} \qquad (2)$$

where G_1 generates a target modality $G_1(X, c)$ conditioned on the presence of input modalities X, while D_1 tries to distinguish between real input modalities and generated ones. Similarly, G_2 generates the original input modalities $G_2(T, c)$ conditioned on the presence of original input modalities X and D_2 tries to distinguish between the real target modality and the generated one. The generators try to minimize this objective, while the discriminators to maximize it.

Full Objective. The objective functions to optimize D and G respectively are

$$\mathcal{L}_D = -\mathcal{L}_{adv}; \quad \mathcal{L}_G = \mathcal{L}_{adv} + \lambda_{rec}\mathcal{L}_{rec} \qquad (3)$$

where λ_{rec} is the hyper-parameter that balances the reconstruction loss and adversarial loss.

2.2   Implementation

Two-Stream Network Architecture. To leverage the information from both input modalities and corresponding availability conditions, we build a two-stream network architecture based on the popular encoder-decoder network [6]. It takes the multi-modal images and condition as two inputs and merges them in the feature level. This network contains stride-2 convolutions, residual blocks [4] and fractionally-strided convolutions (1/2 stride). We use 6 blocks for the input size of $N \times H \times W$, where N, H and W are the number of modalities, height and width of the images respectively. The input and availability conditions pass through two encoders and are merged in the last feature layer before the decoder. *PatchGANs* [6] is used for the discriminator network, which classifies the patch feature maps to real or fake, instead of using a fully-connected layer.

Training Details. We apply two recent techniques to stabilize the training of the model. First, for $\mathcal{L}_{adv}$ (Eq. 2), we replace the negative log likelihood objective by a least-squares loss [9]. Second, to reduce the model oscillation, we update the discriminators using a history of generated images rather than the ones produced by the latest generators, as proposed in [11]. Thus we put the 25 previously generated images in an image buffer. We set $\lambda_{rec} = 10$ in Eq. 3 for all the experiments. We use the Adam solver [7] with a batch size of 5. All networks were trained from scratch with a learning rate of 0.0002 and for 20 epochs. When given n input modalities, for each epoch the parameters in both generator and discriminator are updated for $2^n - 1$ times given $2^n - 1$ training subsets of input modalities excluding empty set. The implementations of our model are available in https://github.com/hongweilibran/DiamondGAN.

2.3   Visual Rating and Evaluation Protocol

Quantitative evaluation of generated images in terms of standard scores for errors and correlation remains a debatable task [1]. Additionally, the evaluation with common metrics such as PSNR and MAE [13] would not tell us to whether the algorithm captures clinically relevant small substructures. Therefore, we strive to get experts' estimates of the image quality. We design a multi-rater quality evaluation experiment. Neuro-radiologists rated the images in a browser-application. In each trial, they were provided with two images. On the left side, one real source image of a T1 or Flair images is presented. On the other side, a paired image of the target modality is shown which is either a real image or a generated one. The displayed paired images were randomly chosen in the pool of generated images and real ones. This particular setup enables the experts to identify very small inconsistency or implausibility between the two images immediately. For evaluation, the experts were asked to rate the plausibility of the image on the right based on the real image on the left, to assign a 6-star rating, where 6 stars denoted a perfectly plausible image and 1 star a completely implausible image. The images were presented in 280 trials.

3   Experiments

Datasets. *Dataset 1* consists of 65 scans of patients with MS lesions from a local hospital, acquired with a multi-parametric protocol, which includes co-registered Flair, T1, T2, double inversion recovery (DIR) and contrast-enhanced T1 (T1-c) after skull-stripping. The first three modalities are common modalities in most MS lesion exams. DIR is a MRI pulse sequence, which suppresses signal from the cerebrospinal fluid and the white matter, enhancing the inflammatory lesion. T1-c is a MRI sequence which requires a paramagnetic contrast agent (usually gadolinium) that reduces the T1 relaxation time and thereby increases the signal intensity. Synthesizing DIR and T1-c is of clinical relevance because it can substantially reduce medical costs. We mainly report our result on *Dataset 1*. Additional *Dataset 2* is used to demonstrate that our approach can work on multiple datasets with incomplete and non-aligned modalities. It is a part of the public MICCAI-WMH dataset

[8], and includes 40 subjects with two modalities (Flair and T1). 2D axial slices are used for training the network. All the slices are cropped or padded to a uniform size of 240×240 and intensity values are rescaled to $[-1, 1]$.

Reconstructing DIR and T1-c from Common Modalities. We perform two image synthesis tasks on two clinically-relevant MRI sequences (DIR and T1-c), using three common modalities (i.e., Flair, T1 and T2). We separate the *Dataset 1* into a training set, a validation set and a test set, resulting in 30 scans (2015 slices for each modality) for training and 35 scans for testing (2100 slices for each modality). To obtain the optimal hyper-parameters of the model, we use 5 out of the 30 training scans as a validation set. A common approach for quantitative evaluation of medical GAN images is to calculate relative errors and signal to noise ratio between the synthetic image and the real image [13]. Table 1 shows the results of peak signal-to-noise ratio (PSNR) and mean absolute error (MAE) by comparing the synthetic images and real T1-c and DIR images. For the synthetic DIR and T1-c images, we report the highest PSNR and the lowest MAE for a combined T1+T2+Flair input to our model. In the DIR synthesis experiment, the listed scores of using multiple inputs to our GAN are comparable (MAE 0.058-0.065). Whereas, the scores for single inputs are substantially worse (MAE 0.073-0.084). For the T1-c synthesis task, we find that any combination of multi-modal inputs involving the T1 modality (MAE 0.045-0.048) results in better scores compared to other inputs. This indicates that our model successfully extracts the relevant information, as T1-c is a T1 scan with a contrast enhancing agent. For comparison, we implement *CycleGAN* [14] to perform one-to-one cross-modality synthesis, the best results of *CycleGAN* are listed in Table 1. For DIR synthesis, using Flair images as the input of *CycleGAN* achieves the highest PSNR and lowest MAE while for T1-c, using T1 as the input gets the best performance. The proposed model outperforms *CycleGAN* in both

Table 1. Quantitative evaluation of our generated images compared to the real DIR and T1-c image using PSNR and MAE as evaluation metrics. Results show that the generated images benefit from a multi-modal input. ↑ indicates that higher values corresponds to better image qualities.

	DIR $_{PSNR}$↑	DIR $_{MAE}$↓	T1-c $_{PSNR}$↑	T1-c $_{MAE}$↓
CycleGAN [14]	17.34	0.068	20.36	0.045
DiamonGAN$_{T1}$	15.46	0.084	20.21	0.048
DiamonGAN$_{T2}$	15.99	0.073	19.34	0.054
DiamonGAN$_{Flair}$	16.16	0.078	17.15	0.068
DiamonGAN$_{T1+T2}$	17.41	0.065	20.75	0.046
DiamonGAN$_{T2+Flair}$	18.58	0.059	19.78	0.051
DiamonGAN$_{T1+Flair}$	18.02	0.062	20.40	0.047
DiamonGAN$_{T1+T2+Flair}$	**18.63**	**0.058**	**20.86**	**0.045**

tasks. We further replace a part of the training Flair and T1 images in *Dataset 1* with images from *Dataset 2* (totally 794 images for each modality) and we find the result on same testing set is comparable to using the original *Dataset 1*.

Wilconxon signed-rank tests are conducted on the PSNR and MAE pairs generated by *DiamondGAN* (with 3 modalities) and *CycleGAN* respectively. Although the improvements of PSNR and MAE look small in whole image level, they are statistically significant (p-value < 0.0001) in the case of DIR in Table 1. This improvement is highly relevant for biomaker synthesis and for pathological evaluation especially in the case of MS lesions with small volumes. The samples of synthetic T1-c and DIR images are shown in Fig. 2.

Visual Evaluations by Neuroradiologists. Fourteen neuro-radiologists with median 5+ years of professional experience participated. Each evaluated 210 synthetic images and 70 original images. The 210 synthetic images are generated enforcing 6 different input conditions in which each condition includes 35 samples. The rating results of the 14 raters are averaged and the box plots of the results are shown in Fig. 3. For the synthesis of T1-c images, we found that three multi-modal combinations (i.e., *T1*, *T1+Flair* and *T1+T2+Flair*) gave comparable results, while the ones based solely on a Flair were consistently rated as implausible. The plausibility of DIR images synthesized with *T1+T2+Flair* input was rated on average 0.83 stars higher than that with solely T1 input. This is plausible as the DIR is a complex sequence containing proprietary information, its synthesis thus benefits from multiple input sources. For the synthetic

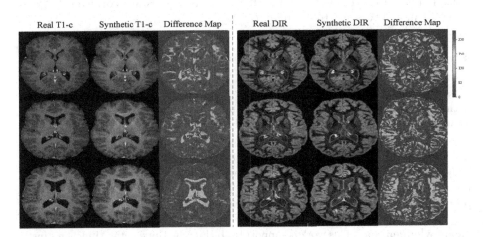

Fig. 2. Samples of synthetic T1-c and DIR images given the combination of T1, T2 and Flair modalities. Difference images are generated and visualized in heat maps. The synthetic images preserve the tissue contrast and the anatomy information. However, we find more differences in synthetic DIR images than in synthetic T1-c ones, especially around the brain boundary. This could be due to the alignment error by registration methods.

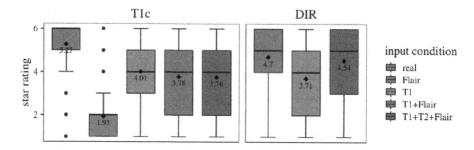

Fig. 3. Box plots showing the rating scores of synthetic images and real ones for T1-c modality on the left and DIR modality on the right. The means are shown as black numbers. *DiamondGAN* achieves comparable plausibility levels for the DIR modality.

images with $T1+T2+Flair$ input, the experts assigned an identical rating to the synthetic and original images (4.54 stars *vs* 4.7 stars).

We conduct Wilcoxon rank-sum tests on the paired rating scores of synthetic and real images from 14 raters on 6 conditions which results in 6 pairs of 14 observations. Results show that the pair of rating scores on synthetic DIR images by $T1+T2+Flair$ input and real DIR images are not significantly different (p-value = 0.1432) while all other pairs are significantly different (p-values < 0.0001). This demonstrates that trained radiologists are unable to distinguish our synthetic DIR images from real ones. Furthermore, the experts ratings for the individual conditions of synthetic images are in agreement with the metrical evaluation in Table 1. For T1-c synthesis, the PSNR and MAE scores are consistently good when T1 modality is fed to *DiamondGAN*.

4   Conclusion and Discussion

This work introduces a novel approach for multi-modal medical image synthesis, with extensive multi-rater experiments and statistical tests. This multi-modal approach allows us to mine the structured information inside the existing extensive MRI sequences. Pathological evaluation is the ultimate goal of this work. Our approach is evaluated by clinical partners who contributed the datasets. We compared synthetic DIR sequence with conventional FLAIR sequence in a MS lesions detection task in a cohort study. The proposed *DiamondGAN* has the potential to reduce medical costs in clinical practice.

Acknowledgement. This work is support by Technische Universität München - Institute for Advanced Study, funded by the German Excellence Initiative and European Union 7th Framework Programme under grant agreement No. 291763. HL and BW are supported by the funding from Zentrum Digitalisierung Bayern.

References

1. Borji, A.: Pros and cons of gan evaluation measures. Comput. Vis. Image Underst. **179**, 41–65 (2019)
2. Choi, Y., et al.: StarGAN: unified generative adversarial networks for multi-domain image-to-image translation. In: CVPR, pp. 8789–8797 (2018)
3. Dar, S.U., et al.: Image synthesis in multi-contrast MRI with conditional generative adversarial networks. IEEE Trans. Med. Imaging (2019)
4. He, K., et al.: Deep residual learning for image recognition. In: CVPR, pp. 770–778 (2016)
5. Isola, P., et al.: Image-to-image translation with conditional adversarial networks. In: CVPR, pp. 1125–1134 (2017)
6. Johnson, J., Alahi, A., Fei-Fei, L.: Perceptual losses for real-time style transfer and super-resolution. In: Leibe, B., Matas, J., Sebe, N., Welling, M. (eds.) ECCV 2016. LNCS, vol. 9906, pp. 694–711. Springer, Cham (2016). https://doi.org/10.1007/978-3-319-46475-6_43
7. Kingma, D.P., Ba, J.: Adam: a method for stochastic optimization. arXiv preprint arXiv:1412.6980 (2014)
8. Kuijf, H.J., et al.: Standardized assessment of automatic segmentation of white matter hyperintensities; results of the WMH segmentation challenge. IEEE Trans. Med. Imaging (2019)
9. Mao, X., et al.: Least squares generative adversarial networks. In: CVPR, pp. 2794–2802 (2017)
10. Sharma, A., Hamarneh, G.: Missing MRI pulse sequence synthesis using multi-modal generative adversarial network. arXiv preprint arXiv:1904.12200 (2019)
11. Shrivastava, A., et al.: Learning from simulated and unsupervised images through adversarial training. In: CVPR, pp. 2107–2116 (2017)
12. Wang, Y., et al.: 3D conditional generative adversarial networks for high-quality PET image estimation at low dose. Neuroimage **174**, 550–562 (2018)
13. Welander, P., et al.: Generative adversarial networks for image-to-image translation on multi-contrast MR images-a comparison of cyclegan and unit. arXiv preprint arXiv:1806.07777 (2018)
14. Zhu, J.Y., et al.: Unpaired image-to-image translation using cycle-consistent adversarial networks. In: CVPR, pp. 2223–2232 (2017)

Author Index

Printed in the United States
By Bookmasters